'e show"

PRINCIPLES of EXERCISE TESTING and INTERPRETATION

INCLUDING PATHOPHYSIOLOGY AND CLINICAL APPLICATIONS   Fourth Edition

PRINCIPLES of EXERCISE TESTING and INTERPRETATION

INCLUDING PATHOPHYSIOLOGY AND CLINICAL APPLICATIONS

Fourth Edition

KARLMAN WASSERMAN, M.D., Ph. D.
Professor of Medicine, UCLA School of Medicine
Division of Respiratory and Critical Care Physiology and Medicine
Department of Medicine
Harbor–UCLA Medical Center
Torrance, California

JAMES E. HANSEN, M.D.
Professor of Medicine, UCLA School of Medicine
Division of Respiratory and Critical Care Physiology and Medicine
Department of Medicine
Harbor–UCLA Medical Center
Torrance, California

DARRYL Y. SUE, M.D.
Professor of Medicine, UCLA School of Medicine
Division of Respiratory and Critical Care Physiology and Medicine
Department of Medicine
Harbor–UCLA Medical Center
Torrance, California

WILLIAM W. STRINGER, M.D.
Associate Professor of Medicine, UCLA School of Medicine
Chair, Department of Medicine
Harbor–UCLA Medical Center
Torrance, California

BRIAN J. WHIPP, Ph.D., D.Sc.
Principle Research Fellow
School of Sport and Exercise Science
University of Leeds
Leeds, United Kingdom

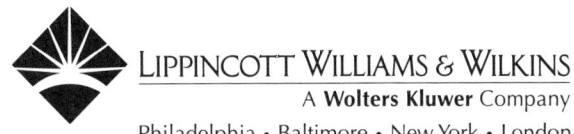

LIPPINCOTT WILLIAMS & WILKINS
A **Wolters Kluwer** Company

Philadelphia • Baltimore • New York • London
Buenos Aires • Hong Kong • Sydney • Tokyo

Acquisitions Editor: Ruth W. Weinberg
Developmental Editors: Lisa Consoli and LuzSelenia Loeb
Project Manager: Fran Gunning
Production Editor: Print Matters, Inc.
Manufacturing Manager: Ben Rivera
Marketing Manager: Sara Bodison
Production Services: Print Matters Inc.
Compositor: Compset, Inc.
Printer: Edwards Brothers

© 2005 by LIPPINCOTT WILLIAMS & WILKINS
530 Walnut Street
Philadelphia, PA 19106 USA
LWW.com

Printed in the USA

Library of Congress Cataloging-in-Publication Data

Principles of exercise testing and interpretation : including pathophysiology and clinical applications / Karlman Wasserman ... [et al.]. — 4th ed.
    p. ; cm.
   Rev/ ed/ of: Principles of exercise testing & interpretation. 3rd ed. ©1999.
   Includes bibliographical references and index.
   ISBN 13: 978-0-7817-4876-6
   ISBN 10: 0-7817-4876-3
     1. Exercise tests. 2. Heart function tests. 3. Pulmonary function tests. I. Wasserman, Karlman. II. Principles of exercise testing & interpretation.
   [DNLM: 1. Exercise Test. 2. Exertion—physiology. WG 141.5.F9 P957 2004]
   RC683.5.E94P75 2004
   616.1'20754—dc22

                                                200457602

---

10 9 8 7 6 5

To Our Families

Preface

In this fourth edition of *Principles of Exercise Testing and Interpretation,* it was our purpose to incorporate new conceptual advances in the physiology and pathophysiology of exercise, particularly as related to the practice of medicine. The underlying theme of the book continues to be the recognition that the most important requirement for exercise performance is transport of oxygen to support the bioenergetic processes in the muscle cells (including, of course, the heart) and elimination of the carbon dioxide formed as a by-product of exercise metabolism. Thus, appropriate cardiovascular and ventilatory responses are required to match those of muscle respiration in meeting the energy requirement of exercise. Appropriate treatment of exercise intolerance requires that patients' symptoms be thought of in terms of a gas exchange defect between the cell and the environment. The defect may be in the lungs, heart, peripheral or pulmonary circulations, or the muscles themselves, or there may be a combination of defects. This book describes the pathophysiology in gas exchange resulting from diseases affecting each site in the cardiorespiratory coupling mechanism, and illustrates how the functional competency of each component can be evaluated by cardiopulmonary exercise testing. To achieve this, 85 actual clinical cases are used to illustrate the wide spectrum of pathophysiology capable of causing exercise intolerance.

The primary symptoms causing exercise intolerance, typically dyspnea or fatigue, are shown to have a rational pathophysiological basis. Without cardiopulmonary exercise testing, the treatment of patients with exercise intolerance is often improperly focused because the pathophysiology *causing* the exercise intolerance is not well understood. Exertional dyspnea or fatigue at unusually low levels of exercise can usually be traced to abnormal coupling of the cardiopulmonary mechanisms required for normal gas exchange. And so by measuring gas exchange during cardiopulmonary exercise tests, not only can the exercise limitation be quantified, but also the functional adequacy of the heart, circulatory systems, and lungs can be established. Fortunately, this can usually be done noninvasively.

A new chapter has been added to this edition describing the changes in arterial, mixed venous, and femoral vein blood gases during lower extremity exercise. In it, mechanisms are described that enable favorable shifts in the oxyhemoglobin and CO_2 dissociation curves to optimize arterial-venous differences while minimizing changes in muscle capillary P_{O_2} and P_{CO_2}. In addition, we have considerably updated the chapter on applications of cardiopulmonary exercise testing, which was added to the third edition, in light of the major advances that have occurred in this area over the past 5 years.

The gas exchange responses to exercise can indicate to the investigator which organs are functioning poorly and which are functioning well. Because the pattern of the gas exchange response is characteristic of the disease process, it can enable a clinical diagnosis. For instance, cardiopulmonary exercise testing might not only detect cardiovascular limitation, but could be used to distinguish *which* cardiovascular disease restricts the patient's exercise performance when several might coexist (e.g., coronary artery disease, chronic heart failure, and peripheral vascular disease). Chapter 8 describes a flow chart approach to assist in making a clinical diagnosis, using the physiological data obtained during cardiopulmonary exercise testing. It is likely that no test in medicine can be used to diagnose the broad spectrum of diseases, while also quantifying severity of organ dysfunction or improvement in the pathophysiology of exercise intolerance, better than cardiopulmonary exercise testing. As a referral center for problematic cases, we are often impressed with the revelations of pathophysiology provided by cardiopulmonary exercise testing.

This book describes how to evaluate the patient with exercise intolerance using the physiology and pathophysiology of exercise gas exchange as frames of reference. The absence of detailed electrocardiographic (ECG) displays in this book should not be interpreted to mean that the authors do not regard the ECG to be an essential component of exercise testing. On the contrary, we routinely record and analyze a 12-lead ECG throughout the exercise test. But it is not the purpose of this monograph to teach how to interpret the exercise ECG; this is thoroughly covered elsewhere. We therefore only provide the interpretation of the ECG records in the case discussions in Chapter 10, rather than occupying pages of print with the records themselves.

As important background chapters to the interpretation of exercise tests, we devote the first three chapters to bioenergetic and physiological principles underpinning exercise performance. In the fourth chapter, we apply this knowledge to define specific variables that can be used to detect abnormalities in function during exercise. The fifth chapter describes the pathophysiology of exercise limitation caused by diseases of the cardiovascular, respiratory, musculoskeletal, and other systems. The sixth chapter describes how to prepare the patient for, and how to perform, a cardiopulmonary exercise test. Chapter 7 provides an analysis of normal values. Chapter 8 presents an interpretive approach for making specific diagnoses, using flow charts and physiologic data derived from the cardiopulmonary exercise test. Chapter 9 describes the many applications in which the expanding uses of cardiopulmonary exercise testing have been applied. Importantly it describes certain clinical diagnoses that can *only* be made by cardiopulmonary exercise testing. The final chapter consists of 85 cases in which cardiopulmonary exercise tests are used to illustrate causes of exercise intolerance or show the effect of therapy. Each case was selected to make a teaching point with respect to the pathophysiology of specific diseases. This chapter might therefore serve as an atlas of disorders that result in exercise limitation.

Detailed practical information is provided in the Appendix to assist in the technical support of a new

laboratory, testing the subject, and making necessary calculations. Although this is of special importance to anyone wishing to establish a laboratory, this information is also very helpful to the interpreter's understanding of the technical aspects of the measurements and calculations used in cardiopulmonary exercise testing.

We designed the content of this book to help cardiologists, pulmonologists, and exercise physiologists maximize the knowledge gained from computerized measurements of gas exchange during exercise. Thus, it serves as a guide for those who wish to use cardiopulmonary exercise testing to (a) diagnose the pathophysiology of exercise limitation; (b) evaluate the severity of a patient's pathophysiology; (c) evaluate the effect of medical or surgical therapy; and (d) provide a physiological basis for assessing training strategies for patients undergoing exercise rehabilitation or athletes in training. This book spans the field of exercise, from teaching basic concepts in exercise physiology to providing a meaningful report for the medical record. In summary, our goal was to write a comprehensive, and yet practical book that could be used for multiple purposes by physiologists, cardiologists, pulmonologists, and other physicians, and exercise technicians.

KARLMAN WASSERMAN
JAMES E. HANSEN
DARRYL Y. SUE
WILLIAM W. STRINGER
BRIAN J. WHIPP
Torrance, California

Acknowledgments

We are very much indebted to Leah Kram for her highly intelligent editing of the chapters of this book as they became available from the authors. Her dedication to this book made its completion possible in a timely fashion. We are also indebted to William L Beaver, Ph.D., for the analysis of oscillatory gas exchange of Case 26 of Chapter 10, Xing-Guo Sun, M.D., for his preparation of the figures in Chapter 3, and to Samuel E. Cohen for his preparation of Fig. 9.9. We are also very thankful to the talented Deanna and Don Hockett for most of the high quality art work in this book.

We are grateful to our colleagues, our former fellows and students, and the many physicians and scientists who have participated in our semi-annual postgraduate course (practicum) in Exercise Testing and Interpretation over the past 21 years, for which the three prior editions served as a syllabus. This fourth edition benefits from the many useful discussions we have had with former course participants, as well as the knowledge gained from new research. These have served as a milieu for improving our understanding of exercise physiology and pathophysiology and have helped to close the gap between physiologic knowledge and the application of cardiopulmonary exercise testing to clinical problems.

K.W. is especially indebted to his wife, Gail, for tolerating his diversions during innumerable evenings and weekends in his effort to see this edition completed in a timely fashion.

K.W.
J.E.H.
D.Y.S.
W.W.S.
B.J.W.

Contents

4   Measurements During Integrative Cardiopulmonary Exercise Testing 76

5   Pathophysiology of Disorders Limiting Exercise 111

6   Clinical Exercise Testing 133

10   Case Presentations 242

CHAPTER 1

Exercise Testing and Interpretation: An Overview

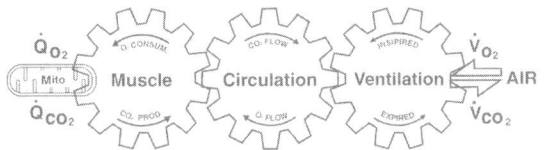

T HE ENERGY TO SUPPORT LIFE and its changing levels of physical activity is obtained from the oxidation of metabolic substrate. Oxygen (O_2) is the key that unlocks the energy from metabolic substrate by serving as the proton acceptor in the oxidative processes that yield high-energy compounds. The energy is in the bond of a phosphate anion in high-energy compounds, mainly as adenosine triphosphate (ATP). Splitting of these high-energy phosphate bonds ($\sim P$) is controlled by enzymatic reactions at the myofibril such that the energy released is transduced into mechanical energy of muscular contraction.

Because the reserve of $\sim P$ in the cell is quite small relative to the need, $\sim P$ production, and therefore O_2 consumption, must increase to sustain exercise. Because there is a relatively precise relation between the O_2 consumption and $\sim P$ production, measurement of O_2 consumption reveals the rate of $\sim P$ expended for physical work.

CELL RESPIRATION AND BIOENERGETICS

The most immediate requirement of exercise is the release of the energy of the terminal phosphate bond of adenosine triphosphate to fuel the energy demands of muscular exercise. The bioenergetic process for the regeneration of ATP in the muscle is achieved by three mechanisms (Fig. 1.1): the aerobic (O_2-requiring) oxidation of substrates (primarily glycogen and fatty acids), the anaerobic hydrolysis of creatine phosphate (phosphocreatine, PCr), and the anaerobic (non-O_2-requiring) oxidation of glycogen or glucose via pyruvate to yield lactic acid—or, more precisely, the lactate ion and its associated proton. Each of these processes is critically important for the normal exercise response, and

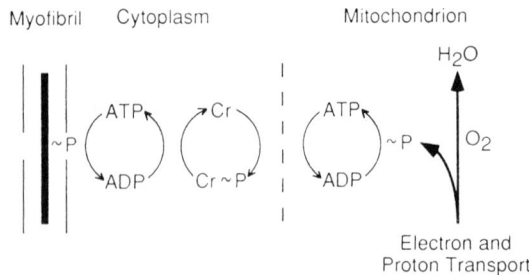

FIGURE 1.2. Scheme by which phosphocreatine (creatine phosphate, PCr or $Cr\sim P$) supplies high-energy phosphate ($\sim P$) to adenosine diphosphate (ADP) at the myofibril. Because of its quantity in muscle, PCr serves as a reservoir of readily available $\sim P$ as well as a shuttle mechanism to translocate $\sim P$ from mitochondria to the myofibril contractile sites.

each plays a different role in the total bioenergetic response.

The aerobic oxidation of carbohydrate and fatty acids provides the major source of ATP regeneration, and becomes the unique source during sustained exercise of moderate intensity. In a normally nourished individual, about five-sixths of the energy comes from aerobic oxidation of carbohydrate, and one-sixth from fatty acids (1–3). To sustain a given level of exercise, the cardiorespiratory response must be adequate to supply the O_2 needed to regenerate, aerobically, all the ATP needed for the activity. Local stores of PCr are a source of high-energy phosphate in the early phase of exercise. PCr is quickly hydrolyzed by creatine kinase to creatine and inorganic phosphate (Pi). The energy released in this reaction is used to regenerate ATP at the myofibril during early exercise (Fig. 1.2). A person with less fitness for aerobic exercise has a greater decrease in PCr at a given work rate, or O_2 consumption, than a more fit person. PCr, like adenosine diphosphate (ADP), is intimately linked to the control of O_2 consumption. Thus, the profile of change of PCr is often considered to be a proxy variable of muscle O_2 consumption during the early period of exercise when its intracellular concentration is changing (4–7).

During the process of glycolysis, the coenzyme nicotinamide adenine dinucleotide (NAD^+) is reduced to $NADH + H^+$. If it is not reoxidized aerobically at the mitochondrial site of O_2 utilization, $NADH + H^+$ can be reoxidized anaerobically by pyruvate ($NADH + H^+ + $ pyruvate $\rightarrow NAD^+ + $ lactate). Thus, pyruvate can serve as the oxidant to regenerate NAD^+ when the cell becomes critically O_2 poor. The reoxidation of $NADH + H^+$ to NAD^+ is required for glycolysis to proceed.

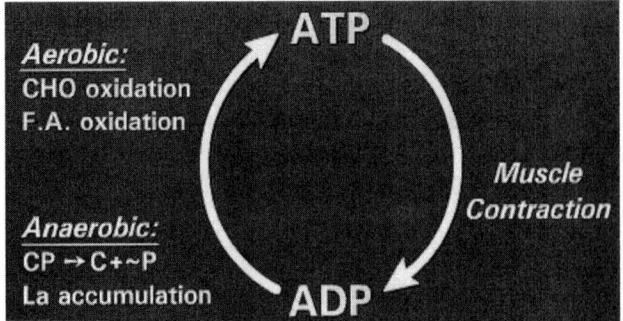

FIGURE 1.1. Sources of energy for adenosine triphosphate (ATP) regeneration from adenosine diphosphate (ADP).

The energy produced by anaerobic glycolysis is relatively small per unit glycogen and glucose consumed. Two molecules of lactate are produced with the consumption of each six-carbon moiety of glycogen or glucose molecule. Because a H^+ is produced with each lactate that accumulates, anaerobic glycolysis has important implications with respect to acid–base balance during exercise, and therefore with respect to gas exchange.

Gas exchange [O_2 uptake ($\dot{V}O_2$) and CO_2 output ($\dot{V}CO_2$)] is affected in a different way by each of the three sources of *ATP* regeneration. For instance, when the regeneration of *ATP* is aerobic, O_2 is consumed and CO_2 is produced in proportion to the ratio of carbohydrate to fatty acid in the substrate being oxidized in the muscle cells. On the other hand, when *PCr* is split, it is converted to creatine (*Cr*) and inorganic phosphate. Because *Cr* is neutral in water whereas *PCr* reacts like a relatively strong acid, the splitting of *PCr* decreases cell acidity. This reaction therefore consumes CO_2 produced from cellular metabolism by its conversion to HCO_3^- in the tissues (8,9) This reduces CO_2 output at the airway relative to O_2 uptake, creating a disparity between the early kinetics in $\dot{V}CO_2$ relative to $\dot{V}O_2$ (to be discussed more thoroughly in the next chapter) (10,11). Finally, when high-energy phosphate is generated from anaerobic glycolysis, the H^+ produced with lactate is buffered primarily by HCO_3^-, thereby adding CO_2 to that produced by aerobic metabolism. This is usually sufficient to increase $\dot{V}CO_2$ above $\dot{V}O_2$.

Because these different mechanisms in *ATP* regeneration have different effects on gas exchange, study of the gas exchange responses to exercise can reveal information regarding the kinetics of the relative contributions of aerobic respiration, *PCr* hydrolysis, and anaerobic glycolysis to the total bioenergetic response.

WHAT IS CARDIOPULMONARY EXERCISE TESTING?

Cardiopulmonary exercise testing (CPET) allows the simultaneous study of the responses of the cardiovascular and ventilatory systems to a known exercise stress through the measurement of gas exchange at the airway. The gas exchange measurements are accompanied by the electrocardiogram (ECG), heart rate, and blood pressure measurements. Importantly, the cardiovascular measurements are interrelated with the gas exchange measurements. The interrelation adds meaning to the non–gas exchange measurements because it relates them to the actual energy expended during exercise rather than relying on indirect estimates of energy expenditure. It also provides information regarding the stroke volume response to exercise by the measure of the O_2 extracted from each heartbeat at specified work intensities.

WHY MEASURE GAS EXCHANGE TO EVALUATE CARDIOVASCULAR FUNCTION AND CELLULAR RESPIRATION?

Physical exercise requires the interaction of physiological control mechanisms to enable the cardiovascular and ventilatory systems to couple their behaviors to support their common function, that of meeting the increased respiratory demands [O_2 consumption ($\dot{Q}O_2$) and CO_2 production ($\dot{Q}CO_2$)] of the contracting muscles (Fig. 1.3). Thus, both systems are stressed during exercise to meet the increased need for O_2 by the exercising muscles and the removal of metabolic CO_2. Therefore, by studying external respiration in response to exercise, it is possible to address the functional competence or "health" of the organ systems coupling external to cellular respiration.

CPET offers the investigator the unique opportunity to study the cellular, cardiovascular, and ventilatory systems' responses, simultaneously, under precise conditions of metabolic stress. Exercise tests in which gas exchange is not determined, cannot realistically evaluate the ability of the cardiovascular and ventilatory systems to subserve their common major function, support of cellular respiration. CPET allows the investigator to distinguish between a normal and a diseased state, grade the adequacy of the coupling mechanisms, and assess the effect of therapy on a diseased organ system. CPET is one of the most inexpensive ways of diagnosing the pathophysiology of the cardiovascular and ventilatory systems because, in contrast to other diagnostic tests that evaluate one organ system, CPET evaluates each and every organ system essential for exercise, simultaneously. An exercise test that restricts its measurements to the electrocardiogram can only support a diagnosis of myocardial ischemia. However, an individual patient may have mixed defects (e.g., cardiac and pulmonary). CPET

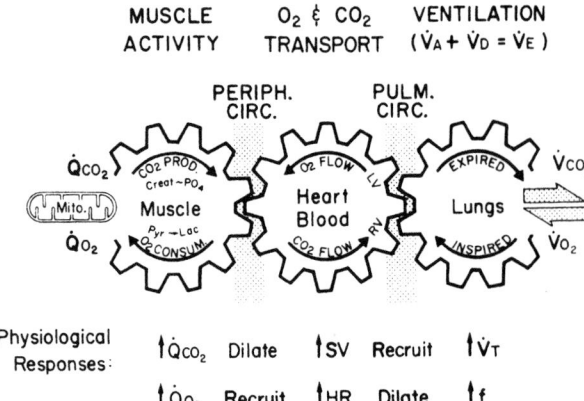

FIGURE 1.3.   Gas transport mechanisms for coupling cellular (internal) to pulmonary (external) respiration. The gears represent the functional interdependence of the physiological components of the system. The large increase in O_2 utilization by the muscles ($\dot{Q}O_2$) is achieved by increased extraction of O_2 from the blood perfusing the muscles, the dilatation of selected peripheral vascular beds, an increase in cardiac output (stroke volume and heart rate), an increase in pulmonary blood flow by recruitment and vasodilatation of pulmonary blood vessels, and finally, an increase in ventilation. Oxygen is taken up ($\dot{V}O_2$) from the alveoli in proportion to the pulmonary blood flow and degree of O_2 desaturation of hemoglobin in the pulmonary capillary blood. In the steady state, $\dot{V}O_2 = \dot{Q}O_2$. Ventilation [tidal volume (V_T) × breathing frequency (f)] increases in relation to the newly produced CO_2 ($\dot{Q}CO_2$) arriving at the lungs and the drive to achieve arterial CO_2 and hydrogen ion homeostasis. These variables are related in the following way: $\dot{V}CO_2 = \dot{V}A \times PaCO_2/PB$, where $\dot{V}CO_2$ is minute CO_2 output, $\dot{V}A$ is minute alveolar ventilation, $PaCO_2$ is arterial or ideal alveolar CO_2 tension, and PB is barometric pressure. $\dot{V}O_2$, $\dot{V}CO_2$, $\dot{Q}O_2$, and $\dot{Q}CO_2$ are expressed as STPD.

The representation of uniformly sized gears is not intended to imply equal changes in each of the components of the coupling. For instance, the increase in cardiac output is relatively small for the increase in metabolic rate. This implies an increased extraction of O_2 from and CO_2 loading into the blood by the muscles. In contrast, at moderate work intensities, minute ventilation increases in approximate proportion to the new CO_2 brought to the lungs by the venous return. The development of metabolic acidosis at heavy and very heavy work intensities accelerates the increase in ventilation to provide respiratory compensation for the metabolic acidosis.

can be used to determine which of these defects is responsible for the patient's symptoms before embarking on major therapeutic procedures directed at either one (12).

CARDIAC STRESS TEST AND PULMONARY STRESS TEST: NOMENCLATURE FALLACIES

The authors would like to dispel a concept that has been, and remains, prevalent in clinical exercise testing, namely, that there is *cardiac stress testing* and *pulmonary stress testing*. It is impossible to stress only the heart or only the lungs. Exercise requires the coordinated function of the heart, the lungs, and the peripheral and pulmonary circulations to meet the increased cellular respiratory demands of work. Diseases of the heart cause both abnormal breathing and gas exchange responses to exercise, as do many disorders of the lungs.

Abnormalities of the heart might cause abnormalities in lung gas exchange during exercise, with "pulmonary symptoms" (13–16). Similarly, pulmonary disorders might result primarily in abnormalities in cardiovascular responses to exercise (17,18). Although the cardiovascular and pulmonary gas exchange responses to exercise tend to be relatively uniform and, to a large extent, predictable in normal subjects, specific diseases affect the gas exchange responses in specific ways, depending on the particular pathophysiology. Thus, the knowledgeable examiner can not only detect abnormality, but can often define the contributory disease process. Because CPET is quantitative, it also allows the severity of dysfunction to be graded.

NORMAL COUPLING OF EXTERNAL TO CELLULAR RESPIRATION

Figure 1.3 schematizes the coupling of pulmonary ($\dot{V}O_2$ and $\dot{V}CO_2$) to cellular ($\dot{Q}O_2$ and $\dot{Q}CO_2$) respiration by the circulation. Obviously, the circulation must increase at a rate that is adequate to meet the O_2 requirement ($\dot{Q}O_2$) of the cells. Cardiac output increases in proportion to the $\dot{Q}O_2$. In normal subjects, in the steady state, muscle blood flow must increase by approximately 5 to 6 liters per liter of O_2 consumption (19,20). Since 5 liters of arterial blood contain approximately 1 liter of O_2 when the hemoglobin concentration is 15 g/dL, the normal steady-state circulatory response must exceed this flow to meet the energy requirement. O_2 cannot be completely extracted from the muscle blood flow since a gradient for O_2 diffusion must be maintained between the end-capillary blood and myocyte (20). If $\dot{V}O_2$ fails to increase at a rate appropriate to $\dot{Q}O_2$, such as seen in diseases of the cardiovascular system (21,22), lactic acidosis will result, usually at a low work rate.

Because the total H^+ in the body is only on the order of 3.4 micromoles, and the total H^+ equivalent produced per minute from metabolism in the form of CO_2, even for a moderate walking speed, is about 40,000 micromoles per minute (approximately 10,000 times), elimination of the increased CO_2 must be accomplished quickly and precisely. Therefore, to regulate arterial pH at physiological levels, the ventilatory control mechanism(s) must increase ventilation at a rate closely linked to the CO_2 delivered to the lungs. Even a very small error in the linkage of the ventilatory control system to these CO_2 demands will cause a respiratory acidosis or respiratory alkalosis. A very slight respiratory acidosis, but not an alkalosis, can be encountered in normal subjects during moderate exercise (23), and a metabolic acidosis is characteristic at heavier work intensities. Ventilation must increase more steeply, relative to work rate, when a lactic acidosis is superimposed on the respiratory acid (CO_2) load to meet the demands of clearing the additional CO_2 produced in the HCO_3^- buffering reactions. To constrain the fall of pH, it must increase even further (24) to lower arterial P_{CO_2}. However, the hyperventilatory response is typically inadequate to avoid development of arterial acidemia when lactate increases during exercise (25).

PATTERNS OF CHANGE IN EXTERNAL RESPIRATION (OXYGEN UPTAKE AND CARBON DIOXIDE OUTPUT) AS RELATED TO FUNCTION, FITNESS, AND DISEASE

This book is devoted largely to describing patterns of gas exchange that relate to function, fitness, and disease states. As described earlier, increases in external respiration ($\dot{V}_{O_2}$ and $\dot{V}_{CO_2}$) need to be intimately coupled to the increases in cellular respiration ($\dot{Q}_{O_2}$ and $\dot{Q}_{CO_2}$). Because of the increased need for O_2 to regenerate *ATP* and the proportional increase in the production of acid equivalents during exercise, the circulatory and ventilatory systems must be tightly coupled to cellular bioenergetics.

The proportional contributions of aerobic and anaerobic regeneration of *ATP* during exercise can often be inferred from measurements of external respiration. For example, gas exchange kinetics differ in response to exercise depending on whether work is performed above or below the anaerobic threshold (*AT*) (Fig. 1.4). For work performed below the *AT* (without a lactic acidosis), O_2 flow through the muscles is adequate to supply all of the O_2 needed for the aerobic regeneration of *ATP*, and the patterns of $\dot{V}_{O_2}$ and $\dot{V}_{CO_2}$ increase as shown in the right side of the "without a lactic acidosis" panel of Figure 1.4. In contrast, if the O_2 supply is inadequate to meet the total O_2 need, lactic acidosis develops and the patterns of increase in $\dot{V}_{O_2}$ and $\dot{V}_{CO_2}$

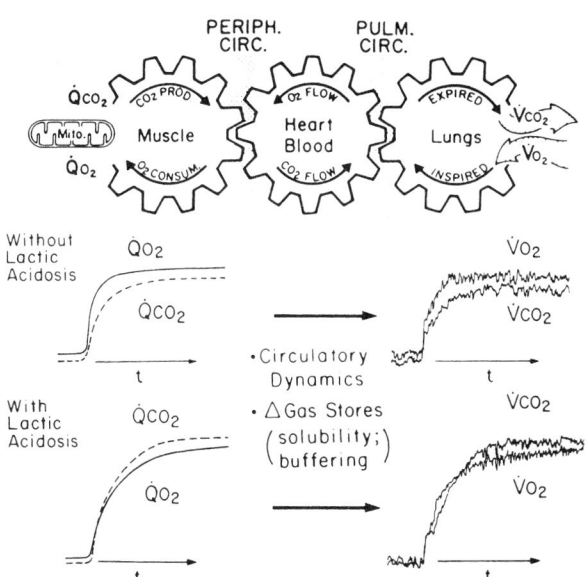

FIGURE 1.4. Scheme of coupling of external to cellular respiration for constant-load exercise. The right side of the figure shows breath-by-breath data for 6 minutes of constant work rate exercise for work with and without lactic acidosis. Each study is an overlay of four repetitions to reduce random noise in the data and enhance the physiological features. Measurements of external respiration (right) can be used as a basis for reconstructing the changes in muscle cellular respiration. The left side of the figure shows, schematically, the changes in muscle cellular respiration that would account for the observed changes in external respiration. The factors that modulate the relationship between cellular respiration and external respiration are shown in the center. At the start of exercise, there is normally a step increase in both $\dot{V}_{O_2}$ and $\dot{V}_{CO_2}$ consequent to the abrupt increase in pulmonary blood flow due to an immediate increase in heart rate and stroke volume. After an approximate 15-second "delay," $\dot{V}_{O_2}$ and $\dot{V}_{CO_2}$ increase further, when venous blood, formed after exercise started, arrives at the lungs, albeit with $\dot{V}_{CO_2}$ increasing more slowly than $\dot{V}_{O_2}$. The slower rise in $\dot{V}_{CO_2}$ than $\dot{V}_{O_2}$, for exercise capable of being performed without a lactic acidosis, is accounted for by chemical reactions in the tissues that store some of the metabolic CO_2. For work rates without a lactic acidosis, $\dot{V}_{O_2}$ reaches a steady state by approximately 3 minutes and $\dot{V}_{CO_2}$ by 4 minutes. For work rates with a lactic acidosis, $\dot{V}_{O_2}$ does not reach a steady state by 3 minutes and may not reach a steady state before the subject fatigues. In contrast, $\dot{V}_{CO_2}$ kinetics remain relatively unchanged, with the level of $\dot{V}_{CO_2}$ exceeding $\dot{V}_{O_2}$ after the first several minutes of heavy-intensity exercise (see text for discussion of mechanisms).

change as shown in the right side of the "with lactic acidosis" panel of Figure 1.4. In the former state, work is done in a true steady state, where $\dot{V}_{O_2}$ is equal to $\dot{Q}_{O_2}$. In the latter state, if the cardiopulmonary system fails to transport enough O_2 to meet the cellular O_2 requirement, $\dot{V}_{O_2}$ does not reach a steady state and work is performed with a lactic acidosis. Consequently, $\dot{V}_{CO_2}$ increases in excess of $\dot{V}_{O_2}$ due to the CO_2 release from bicarbonate as it buffers lactic acid.

Individuals who are fit for endurance work do not develop a lactic acidosis until work rates are high relative to less fit subjects. Their $\dot{V}O_2$ kinetics are relatively rapid compared with less fit subjects (26). Patients with circulatory disorders usually have slow $\dot{V}O_2$ kinetics, even at relatively low work rates (27). Thus, the difference between the steady-state $\dot{V}O_2$ requirement and the actual $\dot{V}O_2$ during the transition from rest to exercise (i.e., the O_2 deficit) varies depending on the subject's fitness for aerobic work.

FACTORS LIMITING EXERCISE

Symptoms that stop people from performing exercise are fatigue, dyspnea, and pain (angina or claudication). By observing external respiration during a quantitative exercise test in which large muscle groups are stressed (walking, running, or cycling), it can be determined if exercise tolerance is reduced and, if so, whether abnormal cardiovascular, ventilatory, or metabolic responses to exercise account for the reduction.

Fatigue

A muscle is considered to fatigue when its force output decreases for a given stimulus. However, the exact mechanisms of muscle fatigue remain a topic of debate. Because lactic acidosis accompanies an increased rate of anaerobic *ATP* production, and the inorganic phosphate concentration increases in proportion to the time constant of the $\dot{V}O_2$ change, it is tempting to attribute the fatigue to the intracellular consequences of these mediators, and possibly decreased levels of *ATP*. Low cellular pH and increased inorganic phosphate have been shown to reduce force production via reduction of myofibrillar calcium sensitivity and impaired calcium release from the sarcoplasmic reticulum. However, regardless of the precise mechanisms (13), the consistent physiological signal for impending fatigue during exercise is the failure of $\dot{V}O_2$ to reach a steady state and to meet the cellular O_2 requirement.

A number of investigators have measured $\dot{V}O_2$ during increasing work rate exercise in both patients with heart failure and normal subjects (21, 22,28) and observed that $\dot{V}O_2$ increases more slowly, relative to the increase in work rate, before the onset of fatigue. This places further demands on anaerobic mechanisms of *ATP* regeneration. Although this phenomenon is seen as work rate is in-

creased toward peak $\dot{V}O_2$ in normal subjects, it is particularly notable in heart failure patients as they approach their symptom-limited maximum work rate.

Dyspnea

Dyspnea is a common exercise-induced symptom of disease states. It occurs in patients with pathophysiology that results in inefficient gas exchange due to ventilation–perfusion mismatching (high physiological dead space), low work rate lactic acidosis (e.g., low cardiac output response to exercise), exercise-induced hypoxemia, and disorders associated with impaired ventilatory mechanics. These pathophysiological changes can occur singly, but more commonly they occur in combination. For example, patients with chronic obstructive pulmonary disease have a combination of impaired ventilatory mechanics that limits their maximal ability to ventilate their lungs and of ventilation–perfusion mismatching that causes ventilation to be inefficient. In addition, they may have exercise-induced hypoxemia that further stimulates ventilatory drive.

Another example is patients with left ventricular failure. They have a low work rate lactic acidosis as well as inefficient lung gas exchange due to ventilation–perfusion mismatching (high physiological dead space). Both of these mechanisms stimulate ventilatory drive. Any pathophysiology that increases ventilatory drive can cause dyspnea.

Arterial hypoxemia is a common disorder in lung and pulmonary vascular diseases. If the oxygen tension decreases during exercise, it stimulates the carotid body chemoreceptors to increase ventilatory drive. This stimulus to ventilation can cause the symptom of dyspnea. The carotid bodies are the chemoreceptors that drive ventilation in response to both hypoxemia and acute exercise lactic acidosis (24). Mechanisms of dyspnea in health and disease are discussed further in later chapters.

Pain

Pain in the chest, arm, or neck is the most common symptom of acute myocardial ischemia brought on by exercise (angina pectoris) in patients with coronary artery disease. This is a reflection of an inadequate O_2 supply to the myocardium relative to the myocardial O_2 demand. Reducing the O_2 demand by decreasing myocardial work or increasing myocardial O_2 supply can eliminate anginal pain. These are established cardiologic therapeutic practices for treating anginal pain. The successful treatment of myocardial ischemia might be documented with cardiopulmonary exercise testing.

Claudication occurs because of an O_2 supply/demand imbalance in the muscles of the lower exercising extremities. Walking at a normal pace requires an increase in $\dot{Q}O_2$ of the muscles of locomotion of approximately 20-fold compared to rest. Therefore, the ability of muscle blood flow to increase appropriately is critically important to enable walking without ischemic pain. If stenotic, atherosclerotic changes in the conducting vessels to the lower extremity limit the increase in leg blood flow in response to exercise, an O_2 supply/demand imbalance will occur. This will result in critically low levels of O_2 in the muscles (29), causing local lactate and H^+ accumulation secondary to the ischemia. These accumulated metabolites might account for the exercise-induced leg pain. The impaired blood supply will be reflected in slow O_2 uptake kinetics (30).

EVIDENCE OF SYSTEMIC DYSFUNCTION UNIQUELY REVEALED BY INTEGRATIVE CARDIOPULMONARY EXERCISE TESTING

Chapter 9 describes pathophysiological diagnoses uniquely made by cardiopulmonary exercise testing. Obligatory changes in the normal exercise gas exchange responses occur when diseases of the cardiovascular or ventilatory systems or both decrease their effective function. Thus, the gas exchange responses to exercise could indicate which organ or organs are functioning poorly and which are functioning well. CPET might not only distinguish between lung and cardiovascular disease, but also distinguish one cardiovascular disease from another as the cause of exercise limitation. For instance, coronary artery disease, chronic heart failure, and peripheral vascular disease have abnormal patterns of exercise gas exchange unique to each and therefore can be distinguished one from the other (31). The gas exchange measurements can confirm ischemia-induced left ventricular dysfunction during exercise and the precise metabolic rate at which the ischemia and dysfunction take place.

The unique ability of CPET to detect pulmonary vasculopathy leading to pulmonary hypertension early in the course of disease, and to detect an exercise-induced right-to-left shunting, is addressed in Chapter 9.

The cardiopulmonary exercise test, in which gas exchange is measured with the ECG, should be among the most sensitive tests to evaluate causes of exercise intolerance because exercise amplifies the abnormalities of all organs that couple external to cellular respiration (Fig. 1.3). Also, no test is likely to be capable of quantifying improvement or worsening of function of these organs better than CPET. Thus, CPET with gas exchange, ECG, blood pressure, and spirometry measurements early in the evaluation of the patient with exercise limitation would greatly reduce unneeded diagnostic tests, thereby decreasing medical costs. However, maximal benefit cannot be obtained from a cardiopulmonary exercise test unless the diagnosing physician is trained to recognize both the normal responses to exercise and the pathophysiological changes brought about by disease states.

To facilitate recognition of the pattern of disease, we believe that the data collected during a cardiopulmonary exercise study should be displayed graphically so that the relations between the functional variables can be seen. We illustrate this approach in Chapter 10, which shows the cardiopulmonary exercise test data from patients with a large variety of diseases. A nine-panel graphical display was developed to view critical variables simultaneously. This nine-panel graphical array is shown on a single page to provide a picture of all of the critical data needed to determine the physiological state of each of the links in the coupling of external to cellular respiration. It was developed over time from an extensive practice experience.

Because CPET makes important contributions to the diagnosis and treatment course of patients, is relatively inexpensive and has a low morbidity, it is surprising that it is not used more frequently by specialists who treat patients with heart and lung diseases. Nevertheless, we do recognize that it is becoming used with a greater frequency now than in preceding years. It is likely that its greater use in the future will result from the recognition that it shortens time to diagnosis and reduces medical costs.

SUMMARY

Organ dysfunction that limits exercise can usually be detected by an abnormality in the coupling of external (pulmonary) respiration to cellular respiration. Integrative cardiopulmonary exercise tests, in which gas exchange is measured dynamically at the airway rather than as a single steady-state measurement, can usually identify the pathophysiology of reduced exercise tolerance. Knowing the pathophysiology of exercise performance might be sufficient information to make an anatomical diagnosis. If not, it might suggest other tests that could narrow the diagnostic choices. When the cause of the patient's exercise intolerance is not clinically obvious, we believe that it is cost-effective to do a cardiopulmonary exercise test before proceeding with more invasive and expensive testing.

References

1. Beaver WL, Wasserman K. Muscle RQ and lactate accumulation from analysis of the $\dot{V}CO_2$-$\dot{V}O_2$ relationship during exercise. *Clin J Sport Med* 1991;1:27–34.
2. Cooper CB, Whipp BJ, Cooper DM, Wasserman K. Factors affecting the components of the alveolar CO_2 output-O_2 uptake relationship during incremental exercise in man. *Exp Physiol* 1992;77:51–64.
3. Sue DY, Chung MM, Grosvenor M, Wasserman K. Effect of altering the proportion of dietary fat and carbohydrate on exercise gas exchange on normal subjects. *Am Rev Respir Dis* 1989;139:1430–1434.
4. Balaban R. Regulation of oxidative phosphorylation in mammalian cell. *Am J Physiol* 1990;258:C377–C389.
5. Chance B, Leigh J, Clark B, Maris J, Kent J, Nioka S, Smith D. Control of oxidative metabolism and oxygen delivery in human skeletal muscle: a steady-state analysis of the work/energy cost transfer function. *Proc Natl Acad Sci USA* 1985;82:8384–8388.
6. Mahler M. First-order kinetics of muscle oxygen consumption, and an equivalent proportionality between $\dot{Q}O_2$ and phosphorylcreatine level: implications for the control of respiration. *J Gen Physiol* 1985;86:135–165.
7. Rossiter HB, Ward SA, Doyle VL, Howe FA, Griffiths JR, Whipp BJ. Inferences from pulmonary O_2 uptake with respect to intramuscular [phosphocreatine] kinetics during moderate exercise in humans. *J Physiol* 1999;518:921–932.
8. Piiper J. Production of lactic acid in heavy exercise and acid-base balance. In: Moret PR, Weber J, Haissly J, Denolin H, eds. *Lactate: physiologic, methodologic and pathologic approach*. New York: Springer-Verlag, 1980: 35–45.
9. Wasserman K, Stringer W, Casaburi R, Zhang YY. Mechanism of the exercise hyperkalemia: an alternate hypothesis. *J Appl Physiol* 1997;83:631–643.
10. Wasserman K, Stringer W, Sun X-G, Koike A. Circulatory coupling of external to muscle respiration during exercise. In: Wasserman K, ed. *Cardiopulmonary exercise testing and cardiovascular health*. Armonk, NY: Futura Publishing, 2002:3–26.
11. Chuang ML, Ting H, Otsuka T, Sun XG, Chiu FY, Beaver WL, Hansen JE, Lewis DA, Wasserman K. Aerobically generated CO_2 stored during early exercise. *J Appl Physiol* 1999;87:1048–1058.
12. Weber KT. What can we learn from exercise testing beyond the detection of myocardial ischemia? *Clin Cardiol* 1997;20:684–696.
13. Kleber F, Reindl I, Wernecke K, Baumann G. Dyspnea in heart failure. In: Wasserman K, ed. *Exercise gas exchange in heart disease*. Armonk, NY: Futura Publishing, 1996:95–108.
14. Metra M, Raccagni D, Carini G, Orzan F, Papa A, Nodari S, Cody RJ, Dejours P. Ventilatory and arterial blood gas changes during exercise in heart failure. In: Wasserman K, ed. *Exercise gas exchange in heart disease*. Armonk, NY: Futura Publishing, 1996:125–143.
15. Sullivan MJ, Higginbotham MB, Cobb FR. Increased exercise ventilation in patients with chronic heart failure: intact ventilatory control despite hemodynamic and pulmonary abnormalities. *Circulation* 1988;77:552–559.
16. Wasserman K, Zhang YY, Gitt A, Belardinelli R, Koike A, Lubarsky L, Agostoni PG. Lung function and exercise gas exchange in chronic heart failure. *Circulation* 1997;96:2221–2227.
17. Butler J, Schrijen F, Polu JM, Albert RK. Cause of the raised wedge pressure on exercise in chronic obstructive pulmonary disease. *Am Rev Respir Dis* 1988;138: 350–354.
18. Hansen JE, Wasserman K. Pathophysiology of activity limitation in patients with interstitial lung disease. *Chest* 1996;109:1566–1576.
19. Weber KT, Janicki JS. *Cardiopulmonary exercise testing: physiological principles and clinical applications*. Philadelphia: W.B. Saunders, 1986:200, 238–243.
20. Wasserman K. Coupling of external to cellular respiration during exercise: the wisdom of the body revisited. *Am J Physiol* 1994;266:E519–E539.
21. Kitzman DW, Higginbotham MB, Cobb FR, Sheikh KH, Sullivan MJ. Exercise intolerance in patients with heart failure and preserved left ventricular systolic function: failure of the Frank-Starling mechanism. *J Am Coll Cardiol* 1991;17:1065–1072.
22. Wilson JR, Ferraro N, Weber KT. Respiratory gas analysis during exercise as a noninvasive measure of lactate concentration in chronic congestive heart failure. *Am J Cardiol* 1983;51:1639–1643.
23. Stringer W, Casaburi R, Wasserman K. Acid-base regulation during exercise and recovery in man. *J Appl Physiol* 1992;72:954–961.
24. Wasserman K, Whipp BJ, Koyal SN, Cleary MG. Effect of carotid body resection on ventilatory and acid-base control during exercise. *J Appl Physiol* 1975;39:354–358.

25. Wasserman K, VanKessel A, Burton GB. Interaction of physiological mechanisms during exercise. *J Appl Physiol* 1967;22:71–85.
26. Sietsema KE, Daly JA, Wasserman K. Early dynamics of O_2 uptake and heart rate as affected by exercise work rate. *J Appl Physiol* 1989;67:2535–2541.
27. Koike A, Hiroe M, Itoh H. Time constant for $\dot{V}O_2$ and other parameters of cardiac function in heart failure. In: Wasserman K, ed. *Cardiopulmonary exercise testing and cardiovascular health*. Armonk, NY: Futura Publishing, 2002:89–102.
28. Sullivan MJ, Cobb FR. Relation between central and peripheral hemodynamics during exercise in patients with chronic heart failure. *Circulation* 1989;80:769–781.
29. Bylund-Fellenius AC, Walker PM, Elander A, Holm S, Holm J, Schersten T. Energy metabolism in relation to oxygen, partial pressure in human skeletal muscle during exercise. *Biochem J* 1981;200:247–255.
30. Auchincloss JH, Ashutosh K, Rana S, Peppi D, Johnson LW, Gilbert R. Effect of cardiac, pulmonary, and vascular disease on one-minute oxygen uptake. *Chest* 1976;70:486–493.
31. Wasserman K. Diagnosing cardiovascular and lung pathophysiology from exercise gas exchange. *Chest* 1997;112:1091–1101.

Physiology of Exercise

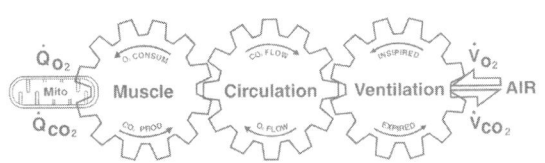

THE PERFORMANCE OF muscular work requires the physiological responses of the cardiovascular and ventilatory systems to be coupled to the increase in metabolic rate. Efficient coupling minimizes the stress to the component mechanisms supporting the energy transformations. In other words, cellular respiratory requirements (internal respiration) can only be met by the interaction of physiological mechanisms that link gas exchange between the muscle cells and the atmosphere (external respiration) (see Fig. 1.3). Inefficient coupling increases the stress to these systems and, when sufficiently severe, can impair or limit work performance. Efficient gas exchange between the cells and the environment requires the following:

- Appropriate intracellular structure, energy substrate, and enzyme concentrations
- A heart capable of pumping the quantity of oxygenated blood needed to sustain energy production
- An effective system of blood vessels that can selectively distribute blood flow to match local tissue gas exchange requirements
- Blood with normal hemoglobin of adequate concentration
- An effective pulmonary circulation through which the regional blood flow is matched to the appropriate ventilation
- Normal lung mechanics and chest bellows
- Ventilatory control mechanisms capable of regulating arterial blood gas tensions and pH

The response of each of the coupling links in the gas exchange process is usually quite predictable and can be used as a frame of reference for considerations of impaired responses.

This chapter reviews the essentials of skeletal muscle physiology, including the relation of structure and function, cellular respiration, substrate metabolism, and the effect of an inadequate O_2 supply. After considering internal respiration, it examines the circulatory and ventilatory links between internal and external respiration. These include the factors that determine the magnitude and time course of the cardiovascular and ventilatory responses and how they are coupled with the metabolic stress of exercise.

SKELETAL MUSCLE

Mechanical Properties and Fiber Types

Human skeletal muscles consist of two basic fiber types: types I and II (Table 2.1). These fiber types are classified on the basis of both their contractile and biochemical properties (1). Type I (or "slow-twitch") fibers take a relatively long time to develop peak tension following their activation, that is, some 80 msec, compared with the 30-msec average for type II (or "fast-twitch") fibers. The slow contractile properties of type I fibers appear to result largely from the relatively low activity of the myosin *ATPase* at the myofibril that catalyzes the splitting of the terminal high-energy phosphate of *ATP*, the lower Ca^{++} activity of the regulatory protein, troponin, and the slower rate of Ca^{++} uptake by sarcoplasmic reticulum. These same properties appear to confer a relatively high resistance to fatigue on the type I fibers.

Biochemical differences between the two basic fiber types focus chiefly on their capacity for oxidative and glycolytic activities. Type I fibers, being especially rich in myoglobin, are classified as red fibers, whereas type II fibers, which contain considerably less myoglobin, are classified as white fibers. The type I slow-twitch fibers tend to have significantly higher levels of oxidative enzymes than the type II fast-twitch fibers, which typically have a high glycolytic activity and enzyme profile. The type II fibers are further classified into type IIa and type IIx (formally classified as Type IIb)(2), based on the greater oxidative and lesser glycolytic potential of the type IIa fibers compared with the type IIx fibers (Table 2.1). With respect to substrate stores, muscle glycogen concentration is, in fact, similar in type I and type II fibers, but the triglyceride content is two to three times greater in the type I slow-twitch fibers. Evidence suggests that the type I slow-twitch fibers are more efficient than the type II fast-twitch

TABLE 2.1.   Characteristics of Muscle Fiber Types

	Slow Oxidative (Type 1)	Fast Oxidative (Type IIa)	Fast Glycolytic (Type IIx)
Contraction	Slow twitch	Fast twitch	Fast twitch
Fiber size	Small	Intermediate	Large
Color	Red	Red	White
Myoglobin concentration	High	High	Low
Mitochondrial content	High	High	Low

fibers, performing more work or developing more tension per unit of substrate energy utilized (3).

Considerable potential for change by specific training exists in the enzyme concentrations of a particular fiber. For example, a fast-twitch fiber in an endurance-trained athlete could have higher concentrations of oxidative enzymes than slow-twitch fibers in a chronically sedentary subject (4).

These structural and functional differences between fiber types depend to a large extent on the neural innervation of the fibers. A single motor neuron supplies numerous individual muscle fibers; this functional assembly is termed a *motor unit*. These fibers are distributed throughout the muscle, rather than being spatially contiguous. Fibers comprising a motor unit are characteristically of the same "fiber type," and substrate depletion occurs rather uniformly within each fiber of the contracting unit.

Fiber type distribution within human skeletal muscle varies from muscle to muscle. For example, the soleus muscle typically has a much higher density of slow-twitch fibers (greater than 80%) than the gastrocnemius muscle (about 50%) or the triceps brachii (about 20% to 50%). The vastus lateralis muscle (on average, approximately 50% slow-twitch fibers) has been used widely for analysis of fiber type characteristics in humans. The basic fiber type pattern of this muscle varies in different subjects. Elite endurance-trained athletes typically have a high percentage of slow-twitch fibers in this muscle (greater than 90% not being uncommon) compared with untrained, control subjects (about 50%) or elite sprinters (20% to 30%).

Whereas basic fiber type pattern is genetically determined, it is greatly influenced by the neural characteristics of the efferent motor neuron. When the motor nerves innervating the fast flexor digitorum longus and the slow soleus muscles of the cat are cut and cross-spliced, the contractile and biochemical characteristics of the muscle begin to resemble the features of the muscle originally innervated by the nerve (5). Thus, an important trophic influence on muscle function is conferred by its nerve supply. Although phenotypic changes within a muscle fiber can be induced by activity, with mechanical factors such as stretch considered to be contributory to the fast-to-slow shift, a typical program of exercise training does not cause appreciable interchanges between type I and type II fibers, but can cause changes within type II fibers (e.g., from type IIx to type IIa) (6). Evidence is accumulating, however, that long-term inactivity and/or

chronic disease can result in a shift toward a greater percentage of type II fibers.

The pattern of activation of fiber types depends on the form of exercise. For low-intensity exercise, the type I slow-twitch fibers tend to be recruited predominantly, whereas the type II fast-twitch fibers (which produce greater force) are recruited at higher work rates, especially at or above 70% to 80% of the maximal aerobic power (7).

Energetics

Skeletal muscle may be considered to be a machine that is fueled by the chemical energy of substrates derived from ingested food and stored as carbohydrates and lipids in the body. Although protein is a perfectly viable energy source, it is not used to fuel the energy needs of the body to any appreciable extent, except under conditions of starvation.

The free energy of the substrate (i.e., that fraction of the total chemical energy that is capable of doing work) is not used directly for muscle contraction. It must first be stored in the terminal phosphate bond of adenosine triphosphate (*ATP*). The terminal phosphate bond of this compound has a high free energy of hydrolysis (ΔG) and is designated as a *high-energy* phosphate bond ($\sim P$). Current estimates of ΔG per $\sim P$ for physiological conditions such as those occurring in contracting muscle are as high as 12 to 14 Kcal/mole. Muscle is ultimately, therefore, a digital device operating in discrete multiple units of $\sim P$ energy, with one $\sim P$ thought to be utilized per myosin cross-bridge linkage to and subsequent release from actin. The muscle uses this energy for the conformational changes externally manifested by shortening or increasing tension. Thus, muscular exercise depends on the intrinsic structural characteristics of muscle and on the body's systems, which maintain an appropriate physico-chemical milieu for adequate ATP regeneration.

Sources of High-Energy Phosphate and Cell Respiration

Energy for muscular contraction is obtained predominantly by the oxidation in the mitochondria of three-carbon (pyruvate) and two-carbon (acetate) metabolic intermediaries from carbohydrate and fatty acid catabolism (Fig. 2.1). A small additional amount of energy comes from biochemical mechanisms in the cell cytoplasm that metabolize glucose and glycosyl units (from glycogen) to pyruvate (Fig. 2.1). Both the mitochondrial and cytosolic sources of energy are transformed into high-energy phos-

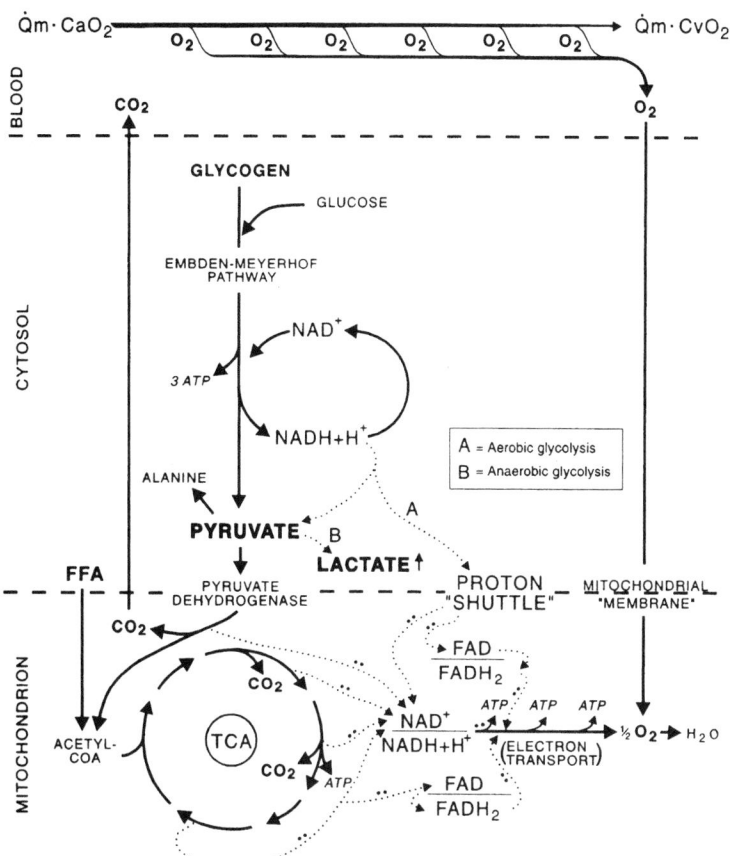

FIGURE 2.1. Scheme of the major biochemical pathways for production of adenosine triphosphate (*ATP*). The transfer of H^+ and electrons to O_2 by the electron transport chain in the mitochondrion and the "shuttle" of protons from the cytosol to the mitochondrion (Pathway A) are the essential components of aerobic glycolysis. This allows the efficient use of carbohydrate substrate in regenerating *ATP* to replace that consumed by muscle contraction. Also illustrated is the important O_2 flow from the blood to the mitochondrion, without which the aerobic energy generating mechanisms within the mitochondrion would come to a halt. At the sites of inadequate O_2 flow to mitochondria, Pathway B serves to reoxidize $NADH + H^+$ to NAD^+ with a net increase in lactic acid production (lactate accumulation). Lactate will increase relative to pyruvate as $NADH + H^+/NAD^+$ increases in the cytosol.

phate compounds, predominantly as creatine phosphate and *ATP*. During the splitting of ~*P* from these compounds, energy is released for cellular reactions such as biosynthesis, active transport, and muscle contraction. Exercise entails an acceleration of these energy-yielding reactions in the muscles to regenerate ~*P* at the increased rate needed for the increased energy expenditure of physical work. Thus, the cellular consumption of O_2 is increased; this must be matched by an increased delivery of O_2 from the atmosphere to the mitochondria. Simultaneously, CO_2, the major catabolic end product of exercise, is removed from the cell by muscle blood flow and excreted by the lungs.

Acetate, produced from the catabolism of carbohydrates, fatty acids, or (in nutritionally deficient states) amino acids, reacts with oxaloacetate in the mitochondrion, after esterification with coenzyme-A (also known as acetyl-CoA), to form citrate in the Krebs or tricarboxylic acid (TCA) cycle (Fig. 2.1). Here, catabolic reactions result in CO_2 release and the transfer of hydrogen ions (protons) and their associated electrons to the mitochondrial electron transport chain. These then flow down the energy gradient of the electron transport chain, transfer-

ring energy to resynthesize *ATP* from adenosine diphosphate (*ADP*) and inorganic phosphate (*Pi*) (i.e., oxidative phosphorylation). At the end of the electron transport chain, cytochrome oxidase catalyzes the reaction of each pair of protons and electrons with an atom of oxygen to form a molecule of water. For each transfer of a pair of protons and electrons, sufficient energy is released to form either two or three *ATP* molecules: three if the electron transport process begins at nicotinamide adenine dinucleotide (NAD^+), but only two if it begins at flavin adenine dinucleotide (FAD) (Fig. 2.1).

Six *ATP* molecules are gained during the catabolism of glucose to pyruvate if the reduced nicotinamide adenine dinucleotide ($NADH + H^+$) in the cytosol, formed during glycolysis, is reoxidized by the proton shuttle and FAD (Pathway A of Fig. 2.1) (8). Of the six *ATP* molecules regenerated from glucose (seven from glycogen) by this mechanism, two are formed in the cytosol by the Embden-Meyerhof (glycolytic) pathway and four in the mitochondrion during the coupled reoxidation of cytosolic $NADH + H^+$ by the mitochondrion, via the mitochondrial membrane proton shuttle and the cytochrome electron transport chain (8). The shuttle accepts hydrogen ions from the cytosolic NADH + H$^+$ and transfers them to mitochondrial coenzymes, NAD$^+$ or FAD, as illustrated in Figure 2.1. This method of regenerating oxidized NAD$^+$ in the cytosol maintains the cytosolic redox state and enables glycolysis to continue. Because O$_2$ is the ultimate recipient of the protons that are generated by glycolysis and transported into the mitochondria, this glycolysis is aerobic (Pathway A, Fig. 2.1).

The formation of acetyl-CoA from pyruvate and its subsequent entry into the TCA cycle yields a total of 5 reduced mitochondrial NAD molecules (i.e., NADH + H$^+$). Since the reoxidation of each NADH + H$^+$ by the electron transport chain yields 3 *ATP* molecules, there is a net gain of 15 ATP. However, 2 molecules of acetyl-CoA are formed from each glucose molecule, so the total gain is 30 *ATP* from these reactions. When added to the 2 *ATP* gained from glycolysis and the 4 others obtained from reoxidation of cytosolic NADH + H$^+$ by the proton shuttle with the subsequent transfer of its protons and electrons to oxygen (Fig. 2.1), the total gain in *ATP* from the complete oxidation of glucose is 36. However, because glycogen is the major carbohydrate source in the normally nourished person, an additional ~P is obtained because when a glycosyl unit combines with inorganic phosphate it becomes ~P. Thus, there is a net yield of 37 *ATP* molecules from the aerobic oxidation of each glycosyl unit. Because 6 molecules of O$_2$ are used for glucose (glycosyl) oxidation and 36 high-energy phosphate bonds are formed, the ratio of ~P to O$_2$ is 6 for glucose (6.18 for glycogen). Six molecules of CO$_2$ and H$_2$O are catabolic end products of these reactions.

Under conditions in which the mitochondrial proton shuttles fail to reoxidize the NADH + H$^+$ generated by glycolysis at a rate sufficient to keep cytosolic NADH + H$^+$/NAD$^+$ normal (Fig. 2.1), the redox state of the cytosol is lowered. As NADH + H$^+$ accumulates in the cytosol at the expense of NAD$^+$, glycolysis would slow if it were not for an alternate pathway capable of reoxidizing cytosolic NADH + H$^+$. When NADH + H$^+$ accumulates, pyruvate can reoxidize the NADH + H$^+$ to NAD$^+$. However, pyruvate is reduced to lactate in this process (Pathway B, Fig. 2.1). This pyruvate oxidation of NADH + H$^+$ results in lactate accumulation. Because the breakdown of glucose or glycosyl to lactate occurs without use of oxygen, it is termed *anaerobic glycolysis*. The substrate price for the production of energy from this reaction is expensive compared with the complete oxidation of glycogen to CO$_2$ and H$_2$O. The net gain in *ATP* is only 3 from

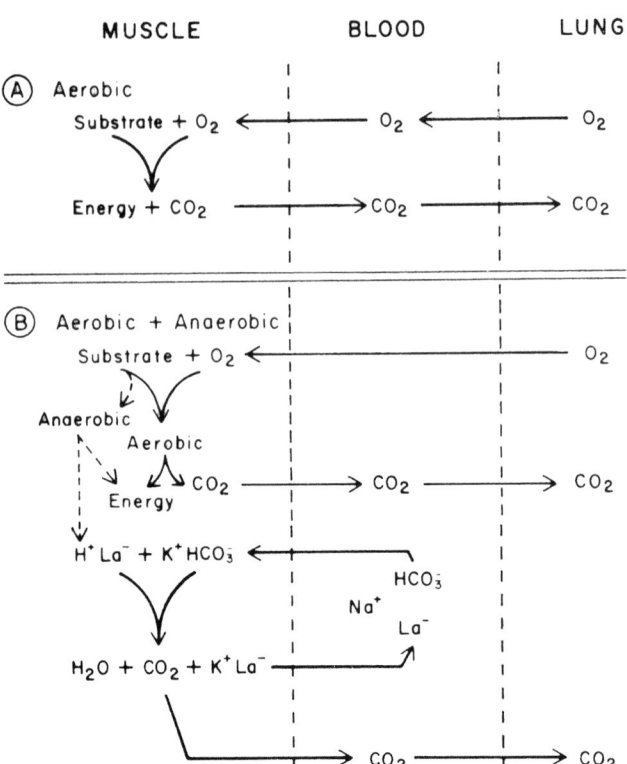

FIGURE 2.2. Gas exchange during aerobic **(A)** and aerobic plus anaerobic **(B)** exercise. The acid–base consequence of the latter is a net increase in cell lactic acid production. The buffering of the accumulating lactic acid takes place in the cell at the site of formation, predominantly by bicarbonate. The latter mechanism will increase the CO$_2$ production of the cell by approximately 22 ml per mEq of bicarbonate buffering of lactic acid. The increase in cell lactate and decrease in cell bicarbonate will result in chemical concentration gradients, causing lactate to be transported out of and bicarbonate to be transported into the cell.

each glycosyl unit instead of 37. For the same work rate, therefore, this pathway causes glycogen (and glucose) to be used at a considerably faster rate than when the production of ~P is totally aerobic (9,10). Moreover, the two lactic acid molecules that accumulate when each glucose molecule or glycosyl unit undergoes anaerobic metabolism cause a disturbance in acid–base balance in the cell and blood (Fig. 2.2). That the turn-on of anaerobic *ATP* production does not signal the turn-off of aerobic *ATP* production deserves emphasis. Both aerobic and anaerobic mechanisms share in energy generation at high work rates, with the anaerobic mechanism providing an increasing proportion of energy as the work rate is increased.

Phosphocreatine Kinetics

Oxygen uptake ($\dot{V}O_2$) during exercise is inextricably linked to increased rates of high-energy phosphate utilization. It is the major source of resynthesis of

ATP, which is used to fuel muscular contraction, through the process of oxidative phosphorylation. Phosphocreatine (*PCr*), with an intracellular concentration some five times greater than that of *ATP*, also serves as a mediator of *ATP* resynthesis through the creatine kinase reaction; that is,

$$PCr + ADP + H^+ \leftrightarrow Cr + ATP$$

(Note that the breakdown of *PCr* produces an alkalinizing reaction.)

Kushmerick and Conley (11) have termed *PCr* a "chemical capacitor" for *ATP*. Consequently, the decrease in *PCr* concentration as work rate increases contributes to the O_2 deficit by an amount that is greater the slower the time course of the $\dot{V}O_2$ increase. In fact, for moderate-intensity exercise, it appears that the sum of the utilization of *PCr* and O_2 stores is sufficient to account for the O_2 deficit. At higher work rates, however, these stored resources are supplemented by anaerobic energy transfer from lactate production.

In addition to serving as what has been termed an energy buffer, *PCr* is also considered to play an important role in the control of oxidative phosphorylation, likely in its link to local *ADP*. For example,

$$[ADP] = ([ATP][Cr])/([PCr]\,[H^+]\,Keq)$$

where Keq is the equilibrium constant of the creatine kinase reaction. *ADP* consequently increases as *PCr* decreases; thus, the *ADP* increase and/or *PCr* decrease might be the signal that triggers mitochondrial O_2 uptake (12). In fact, the time course of the change in [*PCr*], measured by nuclear magnetic resonance spectroscopy, has been shown to be indistinguishable from that of $\dot{V}O_2$ (and, by extension, $\dot{Q}O_2$) in exercising humans (13).

Substrate Utilization and Regulation

At this point, several terms need to be clarified for precision and to avoid possible confusion (see Fig. 1.3). The symbol $\dot{V}O_2$ indicates O_2 uptake by the lungs. It is distinguished from O_2 consumption by the cells, which is symbolized by $\dot{Q}O_2$. The symbol $\dot{V}CO_2$ indicates CO_2 output by the lungs, to distinguish it from CO_2 production by the cells, symbolized by $\dot{Q}CO_2$. Thus, the substrate mixture undergoing oxidation is characterized by the net rates of CO_2 yield or production ($\dot{Q}CO_2$) and oxygen utilization or consumption ($\dot{Q}O_2$). The ratio $\dot{V}CO_2/\dot{V}O_2$ as measured at the mouth (i.e., the gas exchange ratio, R) reflects $\dot{Q}CO_2/\dot{Q}O_2$, the metabolic respiratory

quotient (RQ), only when there is a steady state, that is, when CO_2 is not being added to or being removed from the body CO_2 stores and the O_2 stores are constant (i.e., when $\dot{Q}CO_2 = \dot{V}CO_2$ and $\dot{Q}O_2 = \dot{V}O_2$).

During acute hyperventilation (resulting, for example, from acute hypoxia, pain, or anxiety, or of volitional origin), considerably more CO_2 is unloaded from the body CO_2 stores than O_2 is loaded into the O_2 stores. This is because hemoglobin is almost completely saturated with O_2 at the end of the pulmonary capillaries at sea level and the physical solubility of O_2 in blood is low; on the other hand, appreciable amounts of CO_2 can be unloaded from blood and tissue stores as alveolar ventilation is increased and $PaCO_2$ is reduced. Thus, the gas exchange ratio, R, will exceed the metabolic RQ until a steady state (CO_2 output equals CO_2 production) is again attained at the new level of ventilation. Similarly, during the acute metabolic acidosis of exercise, "extra" CO_2 is evolved when HCO_3^- buffers lactic acid (Fig. 2.2). This, too, will result in R exceeding RQ until a new steady state in CO_2 stores is attained (i.e., the CO_2 pool size is again constant, although depleted, and CO_2 output equals production), at which time R again equals RQ. Differences between R and RQ will also occur during acute hypoventilation and recovery from metabolic acidosis, but in the opposite direction.

As seen in the following equations, carbohydrate (e.g., glycogen or glucose) is oxidized with RQ = 1.0 (i.e., six CO_2 molecules produced and six O_2 molecules consumed) and has a ~P:O_2 = 6.0 or 6.18 depending on whether glucose or glycogen is the substrate:

$$C_6H_{12}O_6 + 6\,O_2 \rightarrow 6\,CO_2 + 6\,H_2O + 36 \text{ or } 37\,ATP \tag{1}$$

Lipid (e.g., palmitate) is oxidized with RQ = 0.71 (i.e., 16 CO_2 produced to 23 O_2 consumed) and has a ~P:O_2 = 5.65 (i.e., 130 *ATP*/23 O_2):

$$C_{16}H_{32}O_2 + 23\,O_2 \rightarrow 16\,CO_2 + 16\,H_2O + 130\,ATP \tag{2}$$

Intermediate steady-state RQ values reflect different proportions of carbohydrate and fat being utilized in the metabolic process (Fig. 2.3). For storage economy, fat is the more efficient energy; however, for economy of O_2 utilization, carbohydrate is the more efficient substrate.

When a steady state of gas exchange exists, R provides an accurate reflection of RQ. During exer-

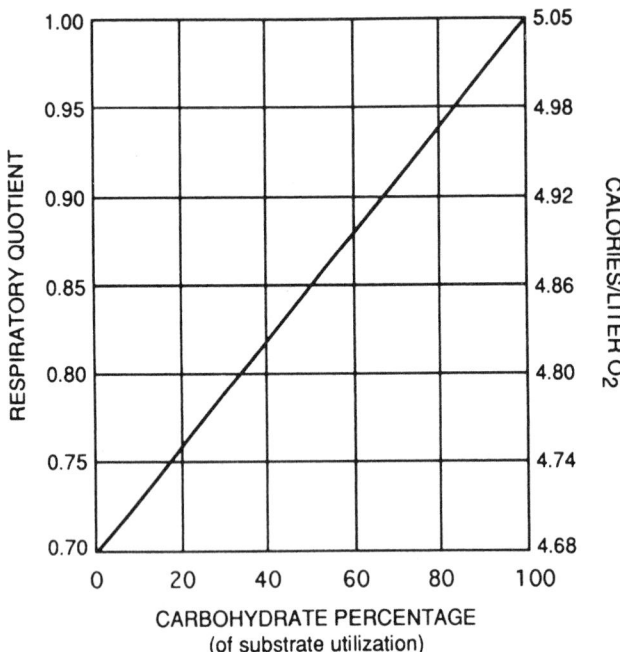

FIGURE 2.3.   The percentage of carbohydrate substrate in the diet estimated from the respiratory quotient measurement. The calories of energy obtained per liter of oxygen consumed for each combination is given on the right ordinate. (Plot of data from Lusk G. *Science of nutrition.* New York: Johnson Reprint, 1976:65, with permission.)

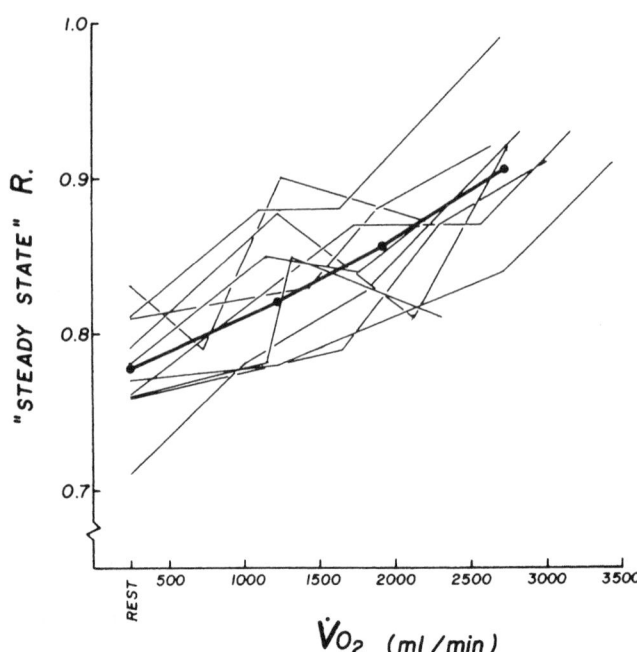

FIGURE 2.4.   The steady state R (RQ) at various levels of exercise for the whole body determined as the ratio of steady state $\dot{V}CO_2$ to $\dot{V}O_2$ for the levels of exercise indicated on the *x*-axis for ten subjects. The heavy line is the average response.

cise, the muscle RQ can be estimated from the increase in $\dot{V}CO_2$ relative to the increase in $\dot{V}O_2$ over the range of moderate work rates. These gas exchange measurements (14–16) suggest that the muscle substrate RQ during exercise is approximately 0.95. This is in close agreement with the muscle substrate RQ in normal humans found by Bergstrom and associates (17) based on the rate of muscle glycogen consumption during exercise determined from repeated muscle biopsies. Thus, a greater proportion of carbohydrate than of fatty acids is used for energy during muscular work as compared with the resting state.

Because muscle RQ is high relative to that of most other organs (the nervous system excluded), the total body RQ increases from a resting value of approximately 0.8 (on an average "Western diet") toward approximately 0.95 during moderate exercise, depending on the exercise metabolic rate (Fig. 2.4). An RQ of 0.95 indicates that about 84% of the substrate during exercise is derived from carbohydrate (Fig. 2.3). Although the fuel mixture for the total body derives proportionally more from carbohydrate than from lipid stores during exercise as work rate increases (Fig. 2.4), RQ decreases slowly over time during prolonged constant-load exercise (Fig. 2.5), reflecting a decrease in the proportional utilization of carbohydrate associated with a reduc-

tion in muscle glycogen stores. When muscle glycogen becomes depleted, the exercising subject senses exhaustion (18). Acute ingestion of glucose allows the work to continue (19).

The rate of decrease in muscle glycogen during exercise can be slowed by raising blood glucose levels with a continued infusion of glucose (20). The importance of muscle glycogen in work tolerance is well described by the experiments of Bergstrom et al. (17), who demonstrated a high positive correlation between the tolerable duration of high-intensity work and the muscle glycogen content before exercise.

Physical fitness affects the substrate utilization pattern. A fitter subject uses a greater proportion of fatty acids for energy than an unfit one for submaximal work (21). This mechanism conserves glycogen, allowing more work to be performed before glycogen depletion and consequent exhaustion. The specific regulation of different substrates is considered in the following sections.

Carbohydrates. Skeletal muscle in humans contains, on average, 80 to 100 mmol (15 to 18 g) glucose per kilogram of wet weight stored as glycogen. For the "standard" 70-kg man, this amounts to approximately 400 g of muscle glycogen. Note that this represents an estimate of the total skeletal muscle carbohydrate pool, whereas a contracting

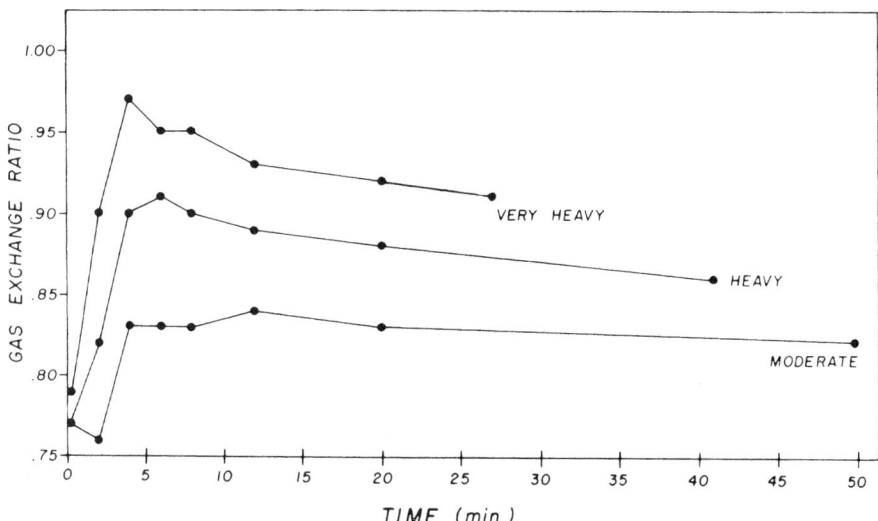

muscle can draw only on its own glycogen reserves and not on the pools in noncontracting muscles.

Normally, there are 5 to 6 g of glucose available in the blood (100 mg/100 ml). Although muscle uptake of blood glucose increases considerably during exercise, the blood concentration does not fall, due to an increased rate of glucose release from the liver, except during prolonged work. The liver represents a highly labile glycogen reserve of some 50 to 90 g. This glycogen is broken down into glucose by glycogenolysis and released into the blood. Glucose can also be produced in the liver (gluconeogenesis) from lactate, pyruvate, glycerol, and alanine precursors. The rate of glucose release from the liver into the circulation depends on both the blood glucose concentration and a complex interaction of hormones such as insulin, glucagon, and the catecholamines epinephrine and norepinephrine (22,23). As exercise intensity and duration increase, the circulating levels of catecholamines and glucagon increase, thereby maintaining the level of blood glucose despite its increased utilization by the exercising muscles. These regulatory processes maintain physiologically adequate concentrations of glucose except when muscle and liver glycogen stores become greatly depleted.

Lipids. Skeletal muscles have access to their own intramuscular store of lipids, averaging 20 g of triglycerides per kilogram wet weight. This source accounts for a considerable proportion of the total energy required by the muscles, depending on the duration of exercise and the rate of depletion of muscle glycogen.

Extramuscular lipid sources are also utilized during exercise. These derive from adipose tissue where triglycerides undergo hydrolysis to glycerol and free fatty acids (mainly palmitic, stearic, oleic, and linoleic acids). The fatty acids are transported in the blood, bound predominantly to albumin. The store of extramuscular lipid is large. In the "standard" 70-kg man, fat accounts for approximately 15 kg of triglycerides, equivalent to about 135,000 Kcal of energy.

The sympathetic nervous system, along with catecholamines from the adrenal medulla, regulates adipose tissue lipolysis. Epinephrine and norepinephrine increase the local concentration of cyclic 3',5'-AMP through activation of adenyl cyclase. This leads to increased rates of hydrolysis of the stored adipose tissue triglycerides. Other factors reduce the rate of adipose tissue lipolysis during exercise, including increased blood lactate and exogenous glucose loads.

The free fatty acids account for only a small proportion (usually less than 5%) of the total plasma fatty acid pool; the remainder are triglycerides. Resting plasma free fatty acid concentrations are approximately 0.5 mmol/L, rising during exercise to approximately 2 mmol/L. The turnover rate of the plasma free fatty acid pool is high, with a half-time of 2 to 3 minutes at rest and less during exercise. As a consequence, the flux of free fatty acids to the exercising muscle (i.e., plasma flow × plasma free fatty acid concentration) is an important determinant of skeletal muscle uptake.

The plasma concentration of free fatty acids does not increase, and may even decrease slightly, with physical training. Therefore, the increased proportional contribution of free fatty acid oxidation to exercise energetics, when measured at a specific work rate after training, may reflect increased utilization from intramuscular sources. Adipose tissue lipolysis does not appear to be enhanced by training and may even be depressed.

Amino Acids. During exercise, the rate of release of intramuscular alanine increases appreciably, but with little or no change in other amino acids (24). The arterial alanine concentration increases as much as twofold during severe exercise (25). The source of the alanine released from muscle is predominantly from the transamination of pyruvate (derived from increased rates of carbohydrate metabolism). The amino groups are derived from the deamination of inosine monophosphate during purine nucleotide metabolism and the branch-chain amino acids (valine, leucine, and isoleucine).

A highly linear relation exists between the plasma concentrations of alanine and pyruvate at rest and during exercise. A decreased muscle release of alanine is observed in phosphorylase-deficient muscle (McArdle's syndrome), associated with the decreased output of pyruvate (26). The alanine formed by transamination in muscle is transported in the blood to the liver, where it serves as a precursor for gluconeogenesis. Thus, an alanine–glucose cycle is established between muscle and liver, with the carbon skeleton of alanine supporting hepatic glucose synthesis.

OXYGEN COST OF WORK

The oxygen cost of performing work depends on the work rate. Figure 2.6 shows the time course of oxygen uptake ($\dot{V}_{O_2}$) from unloaded cycling for various levels of cycle ergometer exercise in a normal individual. Note that, in this individual, a steady state is reached by 3 minutes up to a work rate of 150 watts. At higher work rates, $\dot{V}_{O_2}$ continues to increase above the 3-minute value. In this range of work rate, the rate at which $\dot{V}_{O_2}$ increases is greater the higher the work rate (27,28). The maximum $\dot{V}_{O_2}$ for each of the work rates above 200 watts is the same, thereby identifying the subject's $\dot{V}_{O_2}$max. Note that the $\dot{V}_{O_2}$max is reached earlier the higher the work rate, causing the subject to fatigue earlier. The subject cannot sustain exercise at $\dot{V}_{O_2}$max. The $\dot{V}_{O_2}$ kinetics shown in Figure 2.6 are typical of all subjects, but the work rate at which the non-steady-state pattern of $\dot{V}_{O_2}$ increases is seen differs depending on the subject's fitness for aerobic work.

When plotting the steady-state $\dot{V}_{O_2}$ values for those cycle ergometer work rates in which a steady state is achieved, such as shown for 50, 100, and 150 watts in Figure 2.6, a linear relation between

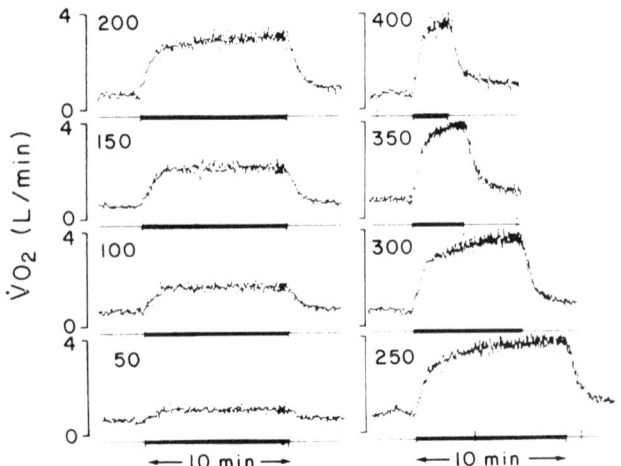

FIGURE 2.6. Breath-by-breath time course of oxygen uptake for eight levels of constant work rate cycle ergometer exercise, starting from unloaded cycling. The work rate (watts) for each study is shown in the respective panel. The bar on the x-axis indicates the period of the imposed work rate. The $\dot{V}_{O_2}$ asymptote (steady state) is significantly delayed for work above the anaerobic threshold. (From Whipp BJ, Mahler M. Dynamics of pulmonary gas exchange during exercise. In: West JB, ed. *Pulmonary gas exchange.* New York: Academic Press, 1980:2:33–96, with permission.)

$\dot{V}_{O_2}$ and work rate is obtained (Fig. 2.7). The slope of this relationship is approximately the same for all normal people (approximately 10 ml/min/watt). This means that work efficiency in humans is relatively fixed for a given work task. However, while the slope of the $\dot{V}_{O_2}$–work rate relationship is not affected by training, age, or gender, the position of the relation depends on body weight.

On the cycle ergometer, obese subjects exhibit an upward displacement of approximately 5.8 ml/min/kg body weight (29). This reflects the added work rate generated as a result of moving the heavier lower extremities. The effect of body weight on $\dot{V}_{O_2}$ is more pronounced on the treadmill since an even greater work rate must be done to support the movement of the entire body through space.

Work Efficiency

Cycle ergometer work rate and the steady-state $\dot{V}_{O_2}$ measurement are commonly used interchangeably when describing the level of exercise being performed, because work efficiency or the increase in work rate (ΔWR) as related to the increase in $\dot{V}_{O_2}$ required to perform the work ($\Delta\dot{V}_{O_2}$) varies only slightly from one individual to another (30). Trained and untrained individuals, whether old or young, male or female, all have similar work efficiencies. This similarity reflects the basic biochemical en-

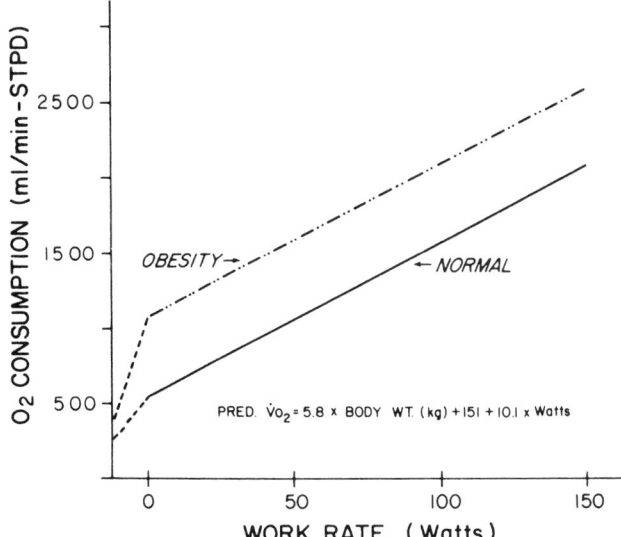

FIGURE 2.7. The effect of work rate on steady-state oxygen consumption during cycle ergometer exercise. The oxygen consumption response in normal subjects is quite predictable for cycle ergometer work regardless of age, gender, or training. The predicting equation is given in the figure. In obese subjects, the oxygen requirement to perform work is displaced upward, with the displacement dependent on body weight. (From Wasserman K, Whipp BJ. Exercise physiology in health and disease. *Am Rev Respir Dis* 1975;112:219–249, with permission.)

ergy-yielding reactions needed for muscle contraction. However, it is important to recognize that the $\dot{V}O_2$ of the "unloaded" ergometer can vary considerably from one subject to another because of differences in subject size and actual work rate of the "unloaded" cycle. Thus, $\Delta \dot{V}O_2/\Delta WR$ is much more uniform among subjects than $\dot{V}O_2/WR$.

Care must be taken not to confuse changes in skill or motor efficiency due to practice with the assessment of work efficiency. To measure work efficiency, relatively simple tasks must be employed that do not depend on technique and for which the work output can be measured (e.g., cycling). To calculate muscle work efficiency, the caloric equivalent of the steady-state $\dot{V}O_2$ (4.98 Cal/L $\dot{V}O_2$ at RQ = 0.95, see Fig. 2.3) and the external power (0.014 Cal/min/watt) for at least two measured work rates must be known. For lower extremity cycle ergometer work, normal subjects have an efficiency of approximately 28% (29,31).

$\dot{V}O_2$ Non–Steady State

The continued slow increase in $\dot{V}O_2$ observed after 3 minutes during constant work rate exercise is only seen for work rates that are accompanied by a lactic acidosis (27,28,32). The rate of increase in $\dot{V}O_2$ in

response to constant work rate exercise correlates well with the increase in blood lactate (27,32–34), as discussed in the section "Gas Exchange Kinetics" later in this chapter. At least six mechanisms may contribute to the slow increase in $\dot{V}O_2$ after 3 minutes of exercise:

1. Reduced muscular efficiency during heavy work by recruiting more low-efficiency fast-twitch muscle fibers.
2. Increase in $\dot{V}O_2$ needed to satisfy the increased work of the muscles of respiration and the heart at high ventilatory and cardiac output responses.
3. Calling into play additional groups of muscles (such as more forceful pulling on the handlebars).
4. Acidemia facilitating O_2 unloading from hemoglobin by shifting the oxyhemoglobin dissociation curve downward for a given PO_2.
5. Progressive vasodilation to the local muscle units by metabolic vasodilators (e.g., $\uparrow[H^+]$, $\uparrow PCO_2$, $\downarrow PO_2$), thereby increasing O_2 flow and O_2 consumption at the O_2-deficient sites.
6. While the O_2 cost of conversion of lactate to glycogen in the liver as the lactate concentration rises is also contributory, its magnitude is quite small compared with the rate of $\dot{V}O_2$ increase during the slow phase (35).

LACTATE INCREASE

Lactate Increase as Related to Work Rate

Figure 2.8 shows the arterial blood lactate concentration as related to $\dot{V}O_2$ in three groups of subjects performing progressively increasing cycle ergometer work: normal subjects who are relatively active, sedentary normal subjects, and patients with heart disease. All show similar resting and low-level exercise lactate concentrations. The pattern of lactate increase is the same for each group, but the $\dot{V}O_2$ at which the lactate starts to increase differs. Lactate does not start to increase in subjects who are relatively physically active until $\dot{V}O_2$ is increased to as much as 10 times the resting metabolic rate. In contrast, the $\dot{V}O_2$ at which lactate starts to increase in sedentary subjects is about 4 times the resting level (equivalent to the $\dot{V}O_2$ required for adults to walk at a normal pace). In cardiac patients with a low, symptom-limited maximum $\dot{V}O_2$, arterial lactate increases at exceedingly low exercise levels. Activity that only doubles the resting metabolic rate can result in a marked increase in lactate.

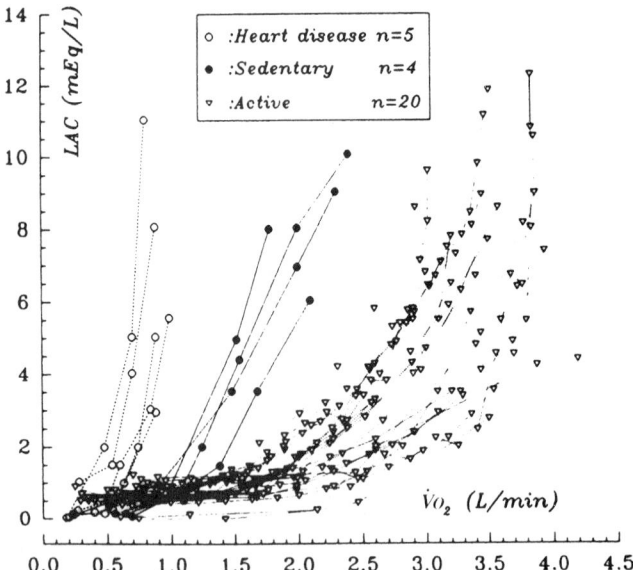

FIGURE 2.8. Pattern of increase in arterial lactate in active and sedentary healthy subjects and patients with heart disease as related to increasing exercise oxygen uptake ($\dot{V}o_2$). Lactate (LAC) concentration rises from approximately the same resting value to approximately the same concentration at maximal exercise in each of the three groups. The fitter the subject for aerobic work, the higher the $\dot{V}o_2$ before lactate starts to increase significantly above resting levels. (Modified from Wasserman K. Coupling of external to cellular respiration during exercise: the wisdom of the body revisited. *Am J Physiol* 1994;266:E519–E539.)

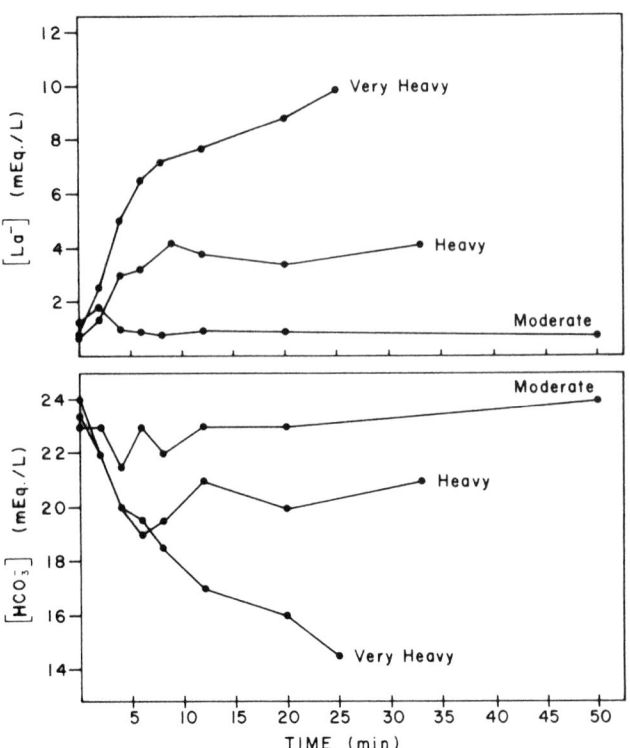

FIGURE 2.9. Arterial lactate increase and bicarbonate decrease with time for moderate, heavy, and very heavy exercise intensities for a normal subject. Bicarbonate changes in an opposite direction to lactate and in a quantitatively similar manner. Although the target exercise duration was 50 minutes for each work rate, the endurance time was reduced for the heavy and very heavy work rates.

The $\dot{V}o_2$ at which lactate starts to increase in normal subjects is, on average, about 50% to 60% of their $\dot{V}o_2$max, but with a range extending from 40% to more than 80%. However, it can be considerably higher in aerobically fit subjects. Because both the lactate threshold and $\dot{V}o_2$max increase by approximately the same amount with endurance training, the threshold fraction of the $\dot{V}o_2$max is increased. As we age, the $\dot{V}o_2$ at which lactate starts to increase, as a percentage of $\dot{V}o_2$max, increases on average because $\dot{V}o_2$max decreases at a proportionately faster rate than the lactate threshold in older than in younger people; this ratio is also slightly higher for females than males.

Lactate Increase as Related to Time

Work rate or power output is an absolute quantity of work performed per unit of time. However, a given work rate may be stressful for one individual, limiting the duration that the work can be sustained, whereas not a significant physical stress for a more fit individual. Therefore, we use adjectives to describe the degree of physical stress (e.g., moderate, heavy, very heavy) based on the pattern of arte-

rial lactate change, as suggested by Wells et al. (36), since the magnitude of arterial lactate increase for a given work rate closely reflects the fitness of an individual for endurance (aerobic) exercise (37).

For constant-load cycle ergometer exercise, three patterns of arterial blood lactate concentration are observed (Fig. 2.9) (38). The first pattern is one in which either no increase in lactate is observed or lactate transiently rises and then returns to its resting value as $\dot{V}o_2$ reaches a steady state. This is defined as *moderate work intensity* and implies that the work is not uncomfortable and hence can be sustained in a true steady state. *Heavy-intensity exercise* is defined as a sustained but constant increase in arterial lactate resulting from a balance between increased rate of production and increased rate of utilization. This work can only be sustained for a limited duration (Figs. 2.9 and 2.10), and a true metabolic steady state does not exist. The latter is evident from a continuously increasing minute ventilation and development of a metabolic acidosis (39).

When arterial lactate continues to increase throughout the exercise to the point of fatigue (Fig.

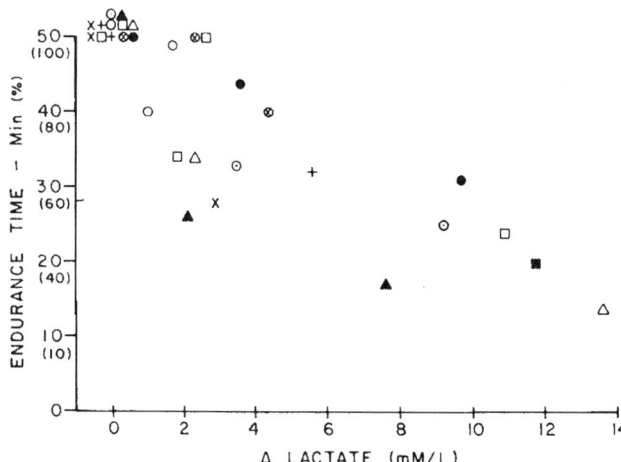

FIGURE 2.10. The endurance time as related to the increase in arterial lactate (above the pre-exercise resting value) during the last minute of constant work rate cycle ergometer exercise. Data are from 30 experiments on ten male subjects studied at three work rates, each for a target time of 50 minutes. Endurance time is reduced when lactate is increased. (From Wasserman K. The anaerobic threshold measurement to evaluate exercise performance. *Am Rev Respir Dis* 1984;129(Suppl):535–540, with permission.)

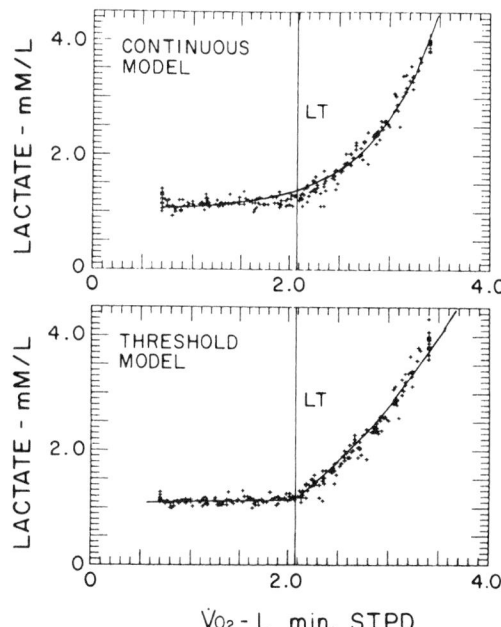

$\dot{V}_{O_2}$ - L min, STPD

FIGURE 2.11. The threshold behavior of arterial lactate increase as related to $\dot{V}_{O_2}$ in response to exercise. Data are arterial lactate measurements from 17 active healthy subjects (shown in Figure 2.8). Points are plotted only up to a lactate level of 4.5 mmol/L (the region of interest in evaluating threshold versus a continuous exponential model). The vertical solid line shows the average threshold for the 17 subjects. The points for the individual subjects are plotted in the same relation to the threshold $\dot{V}_{O_2}$ as existed in their individual plots. In the upper panel, the solid curve describes the continuous exponential model. Lactate values fall above the exponential model curve at the lowest $\dot{V}_{O_2}$, whereas the lactate values are below the model curve in the region of the threshold. In contrast, the threshold model (solid lines, lower panel) is a better fit to the actual lactate measurements. Details of the mathematical analysis for a smaller number of subjects are presented in Wasserman et al. Gas exchange theory and the lactic acidosis (anaerobic) threshold. *Circulation* 1990;81(Suppl II):II13–II30.

2.9), this is termed *very heavy work*. At these work rates, arterial lactate typically continues to increase to levels greater than 5 mmol/L. The higher the lactate, the earlier the fatigue, whether arterial lactate is in the heavy or very heavy work intensity range (Fig. 2.10).

Lactate Increase in Response to Increasing Work Rate

As illustrated in Figure 2.8, arterial lactate does not appreciably increase above resting values until a $\dot{V}_{O_2}$ is reached above which lactate increases at a progressively steeper rate. To determine the best-fit mathematical model describing the $\dot{V}_{O_2}$ at which lactate starts to increase, we tested both continuous-exponential and threshold models (40–42). The purpose of this model testing was to better understand the physiological events that accompany the development of the highly reproducible lactic acidosis engendered by heavy exercise. To obtain a better picture of the systematic pattern of the change in arterial lactate with increasing $\dot{V}_{O_2}$, we plotted the arterial blood lactate against the simultaneously measured $\dot{V}_{O_2}$, after the $\dot{V}_{O_2}$ scale was normalized to that demonstrating a significant increase in arterial lactate for the 17 physically active, healthy young male subjects shown in Figure 2.11. In this plot, the data points are distributed with the same deviation relative to the average curve as they were distributed in the individual curves for each

subject. Because lactate increases steeply with little increase in $\dot{V}_{O_2}$ as $\dot{V}_{O_2}$max is approached, the data examined to address the question of model behavior for lactate increase are restricted to the region of interest, from resting lactate to that below an arterial lactate of 4.5 mmol/L.

As illustrated in Figure 2.11 (upper panel), a mono-exponential model of lactate increase from rest as a function of $\dot{V}_{O_2}$ does not describe the lactate data well. Lactate points fall above the model curve at the low $\dot{V}_{O_2}$ values, whereas in the region of $\dot{V}_{O_2}$ just below that at which lactate starts to rise (identified as the threshold in the threshold model), the points fall below the model curve. In contrast, the points distribute evenly around the two components of the threshold model (Fig. 2.11, lower panel). This threshold is denoted the *lactate threshold* (*LT*).

Neither the threshold nor the mono-exponential models is a perfect fit for the lactate–$\dot{V}_{O_2}$ relationship at all work levels. But the data in the region of interest (i.e., below 4.5 mmol/L) clearly fit the threshold model better than the exponential model. Supporting the threshold model are numerous muscle biopsy studies that show that muscle lactate does not increase at work rates within the moderate-intensity domain (43–47). The $\dot{V}O_2$ at which lactate begins to increase in arterial blood coincides with that of the muscle (43).

Mechanisms of Lactate Increase

Several mechanisms have the potential to yield increases in lactate production as $\dot{V}O_2$ increases during exercise.

Overload of the Tricarboxylic Acid Cycle

Lactate can accumulate in the muscle and blood during exercise if glycolysis proceeds at a rate faster than pyruvate can be utilized by the mitochondrial tricarboxylic acid cycle (Fig. 2.1). This mechanism should cause lactate to increase *as a result of* and *in proportion to* pyruvate increase—that is, a mass action effect.

Sequential Recruitment of Fiber Types

Another mechanism proposed for the increase in lactate during exercise is the increased recruitment of type IIx muscle fibers above the lactate threshold (48). These fibers contain high levels of glycogen. However, it has never been demonstrated that these fibers are activated at the lactate threshold. Furthermore, it would be necessary to demonstrate that type IIx fibers have a redox state with a higher NADH + H⁺ to NAD⁺ ratio and, therefore, higher lactate-to-pyruvate (L/P) ratio than types I or IIa fibers. Additionally, there is no evidence that activation of type IIx fiber types is influenced by changes in oxygenation, as is the case for arterial lactate concentration.

Change in Cytosolic Redox State

When cytosolic nicotinamide adenine dinucleotide (NADH + H⁺), reduced in the process of glycolysis, cannot be reoxidized rapidly enough by Pathway A of Fig. 2.1 (the mitochondrial membrane proton shuttle–electron transport chain–cytochrome oxidase–O_2 pathway), reoxidation of cytosolic NADH + H⁺ can take place by Pathway B of Fig. 2.1 (Pyruvate + NADH + H⁺ → Lactate + NAD⁺). This mechanism is operative when the oxygen required by the exercising muscles cannot be

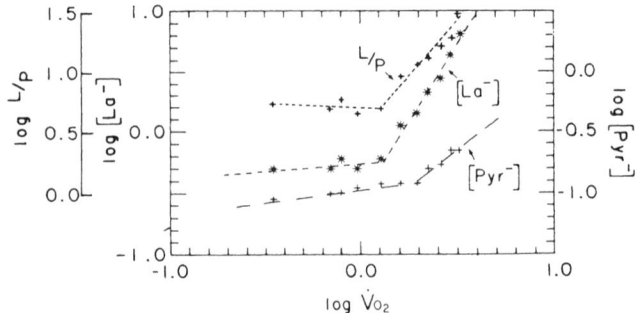

FIGURE 2.12.   Log lactate (La⁻), log pyruvate (Pyr⁻), and log lactate-to-pyruvate (L/P) ratio plotted against log $\dot{V}O_2$. The loglog transform of the lactate–$\dot{V}O_2$ and pyruvate–$\dot{V}O_2$ relationships allows easy detection of the lactate and pyruvate inflection points. The pyruvate inflection point is at a higher $\dot{V}O_2$ than the lactate inflection point. Because the prethreshold pyruvate slope is the same as the lactate slope, the L/P ratio does not increase until the lactate inflection point. (From Wasserman K, Beaver WL, Davis JA, et al. Lactate, pyruvate, and lactate to pyruvate ratio during exercise and recovery. *J Appl Physiol* 1985;59:935–940, with permission.)

supplied at a sufficiently rapid rate to reoxidize NADH + H⁺ by Pathway A. Thus, the cell redox state is lowered, forcing lactate to be increased *relative* to pyruvate.

Figure 2.12 shows a plot of the log-log transformation of arterial lactate, pyruvate, and L/P ratio as a function of $\dot{V}O_2$ in one normal subject who was representative of the average response of ten healthy subjects (49). Below the lactate threshold, lactate increased by a few tenths of a mmol/L as pyruvate increased, but the L/P ratio did not increase until the *LT* was reached. Pyruvate also increased steeply, but not until a $\dot{V}O_2$ was reached that was well above that of the *LT*. Also, the rate of increase in pyruvate was always slower than lactate. Consequently, the L/P ratio increased at the *LT* and continued to increase until $\dot{V}O_2$max. A similar phenomenon has been observed in the muscle cells of humans (50). The increase in muscle L/P was accompanied by a reduction in the muscle energy charge, indicated by an increase in the *ADP/ATP* ratio (50).

The increase in lactate with an increase in L/P ratio indicates that the increase in lactate during exercise is not simply a mass action phenomenon resulting from increased glycolysis. Rather, the lactate increase results from a shift in equilibrium between lactate and pyruvate *as a result of* change in the NADH + H⁺/NAD⁺ ratio (cytosolic redox state) (Fig. 2.1). The conversion of pyruvate to lactate results in the reoxidation of cytosolic NADH + H⁺, providing NAD⁺ for continued glycolysis even under anaerobic conditions. Because no O_2 is used in the reoxidation of Pathway B (Fig. 2.1), this gly-

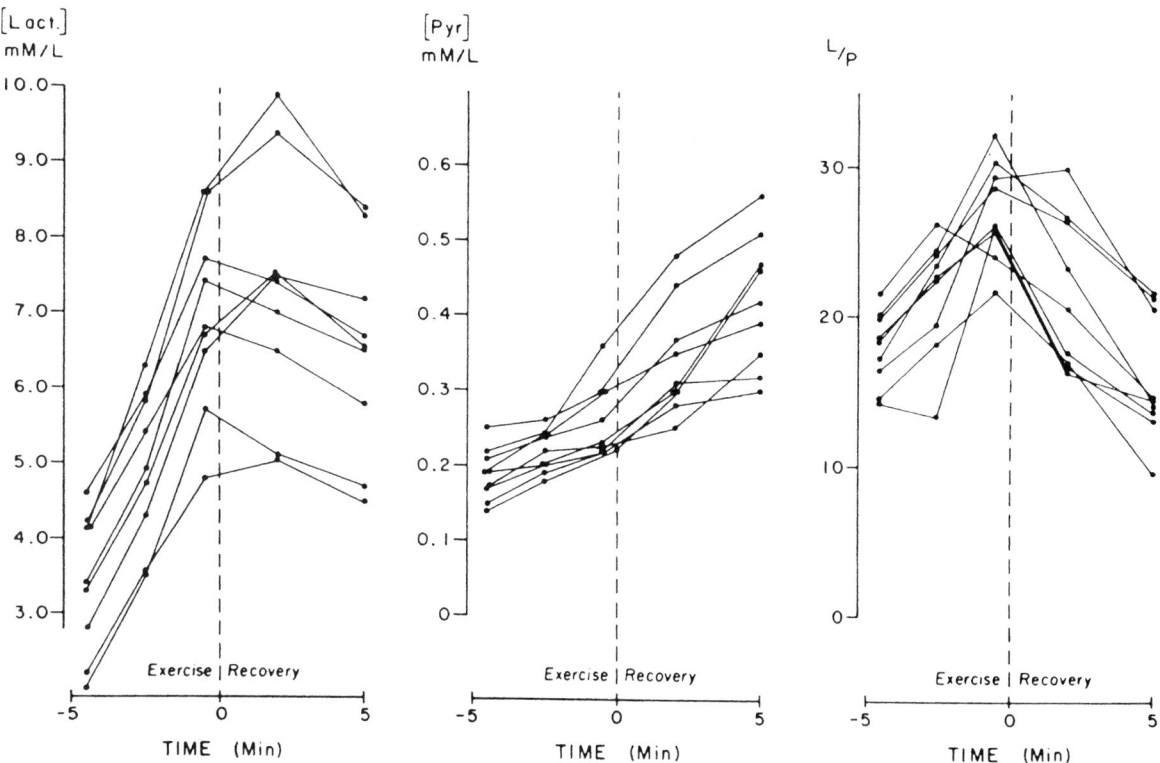

FIGURE 2.13.   Lactate (*Lact*), pyruvate (*Pyr*), and lactate-to-pyruvate (L/P) ratio during last 5 minutes (highest three work rates) of exercise and first 5 minutes of recovery. Studies show that lactate either increases or decreases slightly by 2 minutes of recovery. All subjects show a decrease by 5 minutes of recovery. In contrast, pyruvate continues to rise through the first 5 minutes of recovery. As a consequence, L/P ratio decreases by 2 minutes and continues to decrease by 5 minutes of recovery toward control value. (From Wasserman K, Beaver WL, Davis JA, et al. Lactate, pyruvate, and lactate-to-pyruvate ratio during exercise and recovery. *J Appl Physiol* 1985;59:935–940, with permission.)

colysis is *an*aerobic. Simultaneously, reoxidation of cytosolic NADH + H[+] can take place aerobically in better-oxygenated contracting muscle cells by Pathway A, that is, aerobic glycolysis (Fig. 2.1). A reversal of the exercise-induced increase in arterial L/P is seen at the start of recovery (Fig. 2.13). This provides an important clue to the mechanism(s) of the lactic acidosis during the exercise. The exercise-induced rise in arterial lactate continues into the recovery phase, but at a slowed rate before it starts to decrease. Pyruvate concentration, on the other hand, actually increases more rapidly at the start of recovery (Fig. 2.13, middle panel). Thus, as soon as exercise stops (and the O_2 requirement decreases), the L/P ratio reverses, supporting the evidence obtained during exercise that the exercise-induced lactate increase is not simply a mass action effect consequent to pyruvate increase. A similar reversal in L/P ratio, with lactate decreasing and pyruvate increasing, takes place in the muscle cell at the start of recovery (51).

In summary, it is difficult to attribute the increase in lactate with an increase in L/P ratio, as seen with heavy exercise, to accelerated glycolysis, inadequate tricarboxylic acid cycle enzymes, or changes in contracting muscle fiber type. Rather, the experimental studies support the concept that the major mechanism accounting for the lactate increase at the lactate threshold is the lowering of cytosolic redox state induced by a net increase in anaerobic glycolysis.

Oxygen Supply, Critical Capillary PO_2, and Lactate Increase

O_2 is extracted from the capillary blood as it flows through the actively contracting muscles because O_2 is required for the aerobic production of *ATP* (Fig. 2.1). Although isolated mitochondria can respire and rephosphorylate *ADP* to *ATP* at a PO_2 of 1 mm Hg or less (52), the capillary PO_2 must be appreciably greater than 1 mm Hg to provide the pressure for O_2 to diffuse from the red cell to the sarcoplasm to sustain muscle mitochondrial respiration during exercise. Wittenberg and Wittenberg estimated this pressure to be 15 to 20 mm Hg (53). It was termed the *critical* capillary PO_2 because it represents the lowest capillary PO_2 that allows the muscle mitochondria to receive the O_2 required to perform exercise aerobically. The major factors determining the P_{O_2} difference between red cell and sarcoplasm are the resistances to O_2 diffusion by the red cell membrane, plasma, capillary endothelium, interstitial space, and sarcolemma (53). By measuring oxymyoglobin saturation in the dog gracilis muscle during a moderate level of exercise, Gayeski and Honig (54) estimated the P_{O_2} in the sarcoplasm to be about 5 mm Hg. The P_{50} for oxymyoglobin in humans is 3 to 6 mm Hg (55). Because it would be less than one-half saturated, oxymyoglobin can serve as an O_2 store to support only very short bursts of heavy exercise. However, it may play a role in facilitating O_2 diffusion in muscle fibers containing myoglobin.

To obtain a P_{O_2} of 15 mm Hg at the end capillary, a muscle blood flow of at least 6 liters would be needed for a muscle O_2 consumption of 1 L/min, assuming a hemoglobin concentration of 15 g/dl and an alveolar P_{O_2} adequate to saturate the arterial oxyhemoglobin to at least 95%. Thus, less than one-sixth of the O_2 inflow into the capillary bed would remain at the venous end of the capillary.

Figure 2.14 illustrates the change in P_{O_2} along a muscle capillary for various blood flow–metabolic rate ratios ($\dot{Q}m/\dot{V}_{O_2}m$) thought to be physiologic. This model allows for the Bohr effect resulting from aerobic metabolism (decreasing pH in the capillary from aerobic CO_2 production) but not for anaerobic metabolism (lactic acidosis). A blood flow–O_2 consumption ratio of 5:1 would cause obligatory anaerobiosis and lactic acidosis since P_{O_2} would fall below the critical level well before the blood has reached the venous end of the capillary bed.

A lactic acidosis secondary to cellular hypoxia would be expected only if the critical capillary P_{O_2} was reached in the muscle capillary blood before reaching the vein. When reaching the critical capillary P_{O_2}, capillary blood P_{O_2} could no longer decrease despite increasing work and metabolic rate. As work rate increased further, lactate would increase because the critical capillary P_{O_2} would be reached earlier in the course of the blood flow through the capillary. In contrast to the metabolic rate increase of the exercising muscles (including respiratory muscles and heart), the metabolic rates of other tissues do not change appreciably as work rate increases. It may therefore be assumed that the increase in $\dot{V}_{O_2}$ during leg cycling exercise is due primarily to the increase in lower extremity muscle metabolism. Consequently, because the vast major-

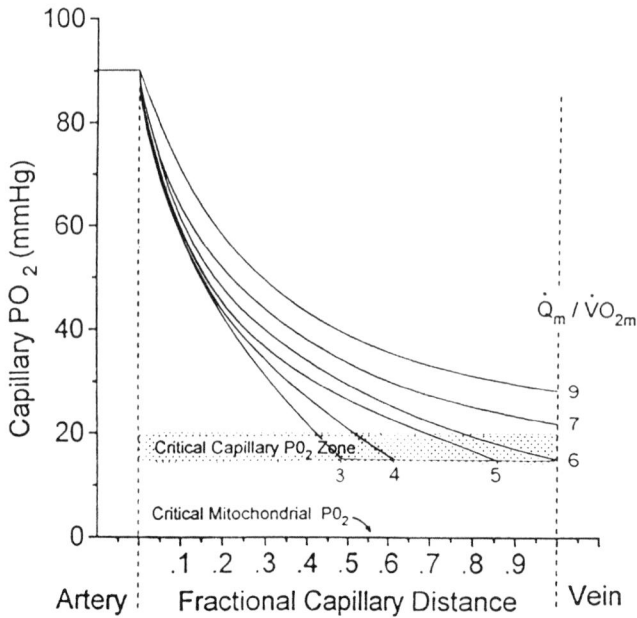

FIGURE 2.14. Model of muscle capillary bed O_2 partial pressure (P_{O_2}) as blood travels from artery to vein. The model assumes hemoglobin concentration of 15 g/dl, arterial P_{O_2} of 90 mmHg, and a linear O_2 consumption along the capillary. The rate of fall of capillary P_{O_2} depends on the muscle blood flow ($\dot{Q}m$)/muscle $\dot{V}_{O_2}$ ($\dot{V}_{O_2}m$) ratio. The curves include a Bohr effect due to a respiratory CO_2 production. The capillary P_{O_2} is heterogeneous along the capillary bed even with a homogenous $\dot{Q}m/\dot{V}_{O_2}m$. The end capillary P_{O_2} cannot decrease below the critical capillary P_{O_2}. Any muscle unit with a theoretical $\dot{Q}m/\dot{V}_{O_2}m$ less than 6 will have increased anaerobic metabolism and lactate production. See text for application of model. (From Wasserman K. Coupling of external to cellular respiration during exercise: the wisdom of the body revisited. *Am J Physiol* 1994;266: E519–E539, with permission.)

ity of the blood flowing past the sampling site is from the contracting units, it may further be assumed that femoral vein P_{O_2} and lactate closely approximate the average end-capillary values.

Because the blood enters the muscle with a P_{O_2} of 90 mm Hg (in a normal subject at sea level) and leaves the capillary bed at a P_{O_2} that is approximately equal to that of the femoral vein P_{O_2}, the P_{O_2} in the muscle fiber depends on the anatomical relation between the arterial and the venous end of the muscle capillary bed, and the blood flow–metabolic rate ratio of the muscle unit (Fig. 2.14). The "critical" capillary P_{O_2} would be the lowest P_{O_2} to which the end-capillary P_{O_2} could fall. The capillary P_{O_2} cannot decrease below the critical capillary P_{O_2} because the mitochondrial P_{O_2} would be too low to consume O_2. That the critical capillary P_{O_2} was reached would be evidenced by the failure of end-capillary or femoral vein P_{O_2} to decrease further despite increasing work rate.

CHAPTER 2 Physiology of Exercise   **25**

Critical Capillary P_{O_2}

The model shown in Figure 2.14 is instructive in several respects: It illustrates that the capillary P_{O_2} is heterogeneous, ranging from high values at the arterial end to low values at the venous end of the capillary bed, even when the muscle blood flow–metabolic rate ratios ($\dot{Q}m/\dot{V}_{O_2}m$) for individual capillary beds in the muscle are homogeneous; and it shows that estimates of "mean" muscle P_{O_2}, calculated from femoral vein P_{O_2}, are erroneous unless it is certain that there is no heterogeneity in $\dot{Q}m/\dot{V}_{O_2}m$ ratios and that the $\dot{Q}m/\dot{V}_{O_2}m$ ratio is at least 6 (i.e., lactate is not increased). Rather than the "mean" capillary P_{O_2}, the question must be asked whether the muscle blood flow and therefore capillary P_{O_2} are sufficiently high to prevent a muscle lactic acidosis. When exercise is performed above the *LT*, aerobic and anaerobic metabolism take place simultaneously, because O_2 is consumed from the blood by the muscle at the arterial end while lactate is released by muscle on the venous end. If the increase in *ATP* required exceeds the capability of the circulation to supply O_2 at the rate needed to regenerate the *ATP* aerobically, the critical capillary P_{O_2} will be reached in the muscle capillary, and lactate will be produced by the muscle toward the venous end.

Experimental support for the critical capillary P_{O_2} concept has been provided by the studies of Stringer et al. (56) and Koike et al. (57), in which femoral vein P_{O_2} and lactate were measured during leg cycling exercise in normal subjects and patients with chronic heart failure, respectively. During progressively increasing work rate studies, femoral vein

blood P_{O_2} reached a "floor" or lowest value in the middle of the subjects' work capacities and before lactate concentration started to increase (Fig. 2.15). To determine the critical capillary P_{O_2} in normal subjects, ten healthy adults were studied with femoral vein and arterial catheters, five during progressively increasing work rate cycling exercise and five during two levels of constant work rate leg cycling exercise, one below and one above the *LT*. As would be predicted from the critical capillary P_{O_2} concept, femoral vein and therefore end-capillary P_{O_2} decreased to its lowest value before lactate started to increase (Fig. 2.16). This was true of all subjects, whether performing incremental or heavy constant work rate exercise, consistent with the model shown in Figure 2.14. When end-capillary blood reached a "floor" or "critical" value of 15 to 20 mm Hg, anaerobic metabolism developed and lactate concentration increased. It is important to note that femoral vein lactate increased before arterial lactate increased, and lactate remained higher in the femoral venous than the arterial blood (Fig. 2.17). This is in agreement with prior studies on lactate balance across the exercising extremity (58–60).

To further investigate the hypothesis that femoral vein P_{O_2} reached a floor value by the time the *LT* was reached, normal subjects performed two constant work rate exercise tests for 6 minutes, one at a moderate work rate and one at a heavy work rate. The moderate work rate was calculated to be at 80% of the *LT* (avg = 113 W, $\dot{V}_{O_2}$ = 1.76 L/min). The heavy work rate studied was calculated to be at the *LT* plus 75% of the difference between the *LT* and $\dot{V}_{O_2}$max (avg = 265 W, $\dot{V}_{O_2}$ = 3.36 L/min). These tests were done with a high sampling density of femoral vein

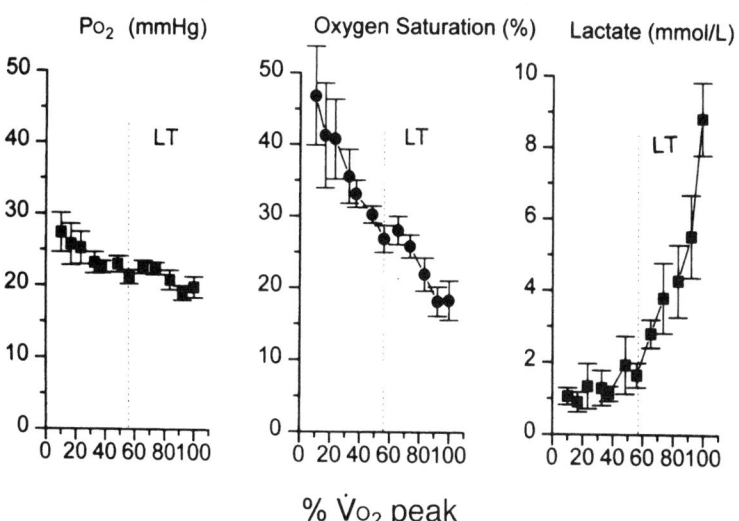

% $\dot{V}_{O_2}$ peak

FIGURE 2.15. Average (five normal subjects) femoral vein oxygen tension (P_{O_2}) **(left panel)**, oxyhemoglobin saturation **(middle panel)**, and lactate concentration **(right panel)** during increasing work rate exercise in ramp pattern to the maximal $\dot{V}_{O_2}$. Vertical dashed line indicates the average lactate threshold (*LT*) determined by gas exchange using the V-slope method (80). Vertical bars indicate standard error of mean. There is no significant difference between the P_{O_2} values from the *LT* to $\dot{V}_{O_2}$max, but the oxyhemoglobin saturation decreased significantly above the *LT*. (Modified from data reported in Stringer WW, Wasserman K, Casaburi R, et al. Lactic acidosis as a facilitator of oxyhemoglobin dissociation during exercise. *J Appl Physiol* 1994;76:1462–1467.)

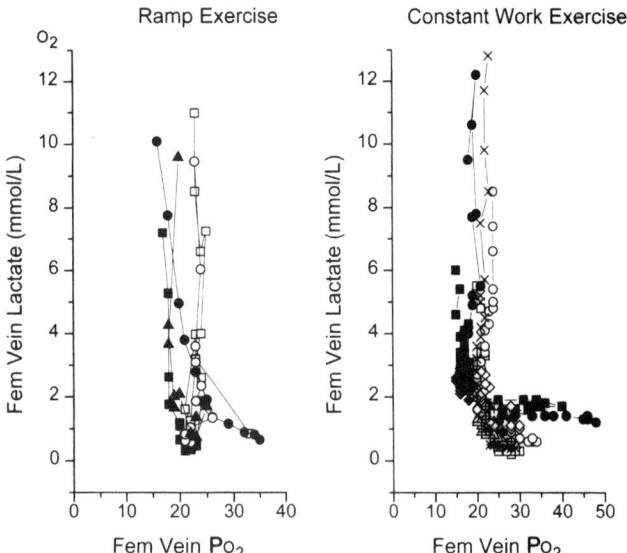

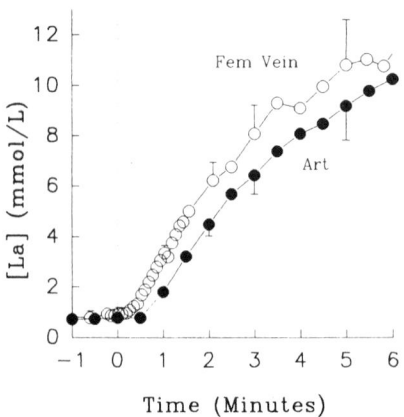

FIGURE 2.17. Average (five normal adult subjects) femoral vein and arterial lactate concentrations during heavy constant work rate leg cycling exercise. By rapid blood sampling, it is clear that the increase in arterial lactate lags the increase in femoral vein lactate concentration. Vertical bars on points are standard errors of the mean.

FIGURE 2.16. Femoral vein lactate as function of femoral vein P_{O_2} for incremental (ramp) exercise in five normal subjects **(left panel)** and ten constant work rate exercise tests (five below and five above the *LT*) in five normal subjects **(right panel)**. The highest P_{O_2} values are where exercise starts. Different symbols represent different subjects. (Modified from Stringer WW, Wasserman K, Casaburi R, et al. Lactic acidosis as a facilitator of oxyhemoglobin dissociation during exercise. *J Appl Physiol* 1994;76:1462–1467.)

blood (every 5 seconds during the first 2 minutes and then every 30 seconds for 4 minutes) to accurately describe the changes. The results of these studies are shown in Figure 2.18. The femoral vein P_{O_2} decreased to the same floor value at 30 to 60 seconds after the start of exercise for both the moderate and heavy work intensities (Fig. 2.18, left panel). The femoral vein P_{O_2} values remained unchanged thereafter as the exercise continued in time, and were not different despite the large difference in work rate and $\dot{V}_{O_2}$. In

contrast to P_{O_2}, oxyhemoglobin saturation continued to decrease past the time when the end-capillary P_{O_2} (as evidenced from the femoral vein measurements) became constant (middle panel of Fig. 2.18).

Oxyhemoglobin Dissociation Above the Lactic Acidosis Threshold

As shown in Figure 2.18, for the work rates selected to be below the *LT*, oxyhemoglobin desaturation proceeded rapidly for the first minute and then more slowly for the next 1 to 2 minutes before reaching a constant value. The change after 1 minute followed the decrease in pH. For the work rate above the *LT*, the oxyhemoglobin desaturation was much more marked and continued for the entire 6 minutes of exercise. The femoral vein oxyhe-

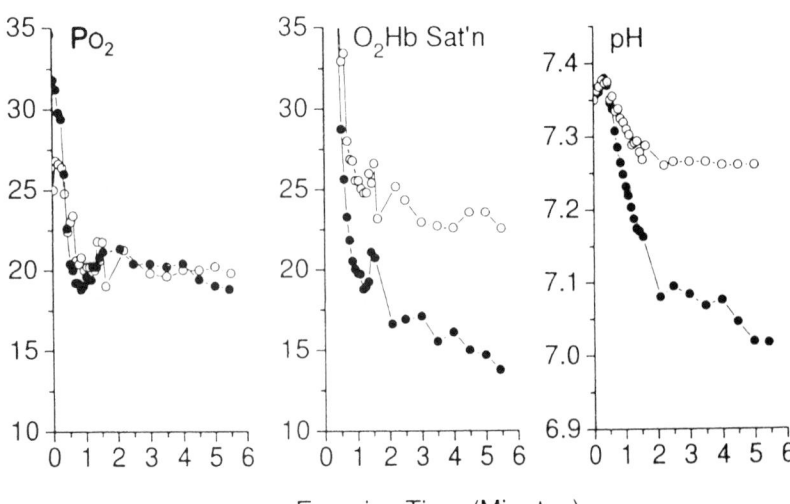

Exercise Time (Minutes)

FIGURE 2.18. Femoral venous P_{O_2}, oxyhemoglobin saturation (*O₂Hb Sat'n*) and pH as related to time of exercise for two constant work rate tests, one below (*open circles*) and one above (*solid circles*) the lactate threshold (*LT*). The data are the average of five subjects. The below- and above-*LT* work rates averaged 113 and 265 watts, respectively. Note that O₂Hb saturation is lower during the higher-intensity exercise despite identical P_{O_2} values. This is related to the Bohr effect resulting from the decreasing pH in the high-intensity test. (Modified from Stringer WW, Wasserman K, Casaburi R, et al. Lactic acidosis as a facilitator of oxyhemoglobin dissociation during exercise. *J Appl Physiol* 1994;76:1462–1467.)

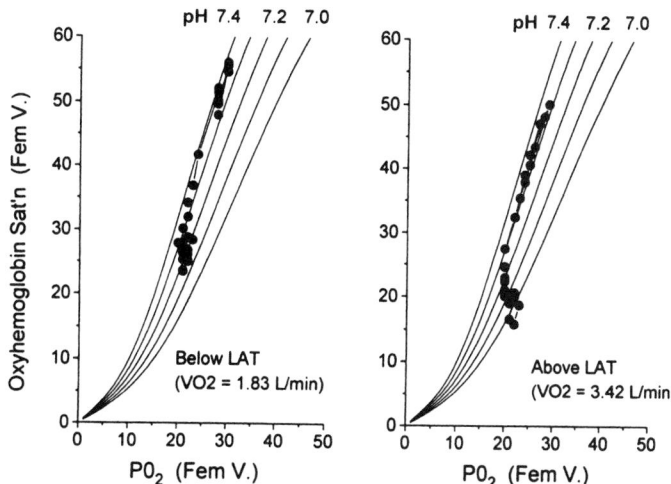

FIGURE 2.19.   Changing femoral vein oxyhemoglobin saturation ($O_2Hb\ Sat'n$; see Fig. 2.18, middle panel) as a function of femoral vein P_{O_2} (Fig. 2.18, left panel) for the 6-minute constant work rate exercise tests shown in Figure 2.18. Superimposed are the lower part of oxyhemoglobin dissociation curves with superimposed pH isopleths ranging from 7.0 to 7.4, calculated from equations reported by Severinghaus. (Severinghaus JW. Simple accurate equations for human blood $\dot{Q}o_2$ dissociation computations. *J Appl Physiol* 1979;46:599–602.) **Left panel:** Data for below LT. **Right panel:** Data for above-LT exercise. Start of exercise is where O_2Hb saturation is highest. Femoral vein oxyhemoglobin saturation progressively decreased as exercise continued, as shown in Figure 2.18. Oxyhemoglobin saturations fell on pH isopleths in agreement with measured pH (Fig. 2.18, right panel). Thus the entire decrease in O_2Hb saturation that took place after P_{O_2} reached its lowest value could be accounted for by Bohr effect. (From Stringer WW, Wasserman K, Casaburi R, et al. Lactic acidosis as a facilitator of oxyhemoglobin dissociation during exercise. *J Appl Physiol* 1994;76:1462–1467, with permission.)

moglobin desaturation, which was not accounted for by the P_{O_2} decrease, could be completely accounted for by the pH decrease (Fig. 2.18, right panel). To illustrate this, the data shown in Figure 2.18 were replotted, with femoral vein oxyhemoglobin saturation values plotted against the independently measured femoral vein P_{O_2} values (Fig. 2.19); pH isopleths are overlaid on these data. This plot, when compared with the pH changes shown in the right panel of Figure 2.18, shows that the decrease in oxyhemoglobin saturation that could not be accounted for by a decrease in P_{O_2} could be completely accounted for by the decrease in measured pH. Also, Figure 2.19 shows that the decrease in oxyhemoglobin saturation below 25% was completely accounted by the Bohr effect (acidification of the capillary blood). Thus, blood acidification appears to account for oxyhemoglobin dissociation for work above the *LT*. Although to a much lesser degree, acidification from increasing P_{CO_2} should also contribute to oxyhemoglobin dissociation

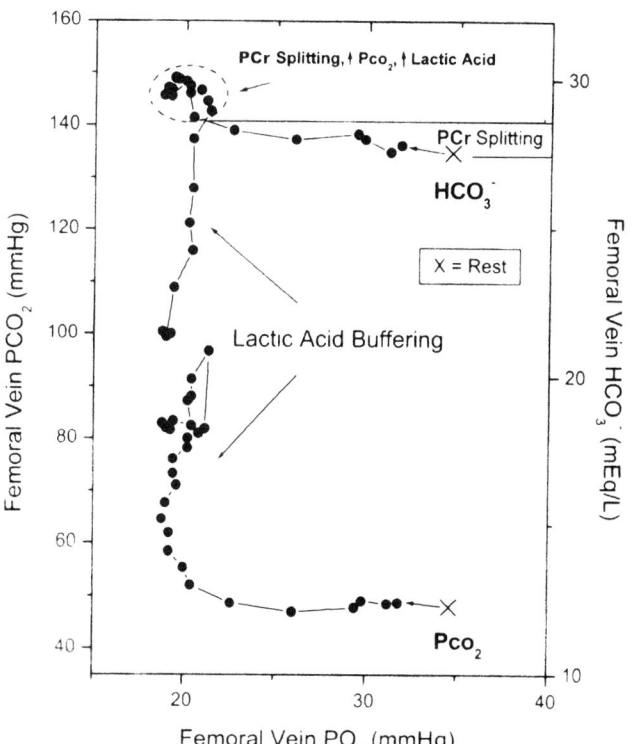

FIGURE 2.20.   Change in femoral vein P_{CO_2} and HCO_3^- as P_{O_2} decreases after the start of heavy (85% of $\dot{V}o_2$max) exercise. The direction of change is from the resting value (X), leftward. Each subsequent point leftward is recorded from femoral vein blood sampled at 5-second intervals. The increase in femoral vein HCO_3^- during the first 30 seconds occurs without an increase in P_{CO_2}. Thus this is a true metabolic alkalosis, likely resulting from the splitting of phosphocreatine (see text). Lactic acid production starts after the minimal (critical) capillary P_{O_2} is reached (about 18 mm Hg in this figure). Thus, femoral vein HCO_3^- decreases and P_{CO_2} increases due to the HCO_3^- buffering of lactic acid in the exercising muscle, without a further fall in femoral vein P_{O_2}. The data are the average of five normal subjects, taken from Stringer W, Wasserman K, Casaburi R, et al. Lactic acidosis as a facilitator of oxyhemoglobin dissociation during exercise. *J Appl Physiol* 1994;76:1462–1467.

below the *LT*, along with the much more important decrease in P_{O_2}.

Because the net increase in lactic acid production during exercise is buffered by intracellular HCO_3^-, additional CO_2 is produced in the muscle over that expected from aerobic metabolism as HCO_3^- dissociates. This results in an increase in end-capillary P_{CO_2} without a further fall in P_{O_2} (Fig. 2.20). Simultaneously, the decrease in intracellular HCO_3^- results in a decrease in extracellular and therefore femoral vein HCO_3^-. Both the decrease in femoral vein HCO_3^- and the increase in P_{CO_2} reflect acidification of the capillary blood of the muscle cells producing lactate (61). The lactic acidosis of exercise thereby facilitates oxyhemoglobin dissociation. Consequently, it is an essential mechanism for achieving maximal O_2 extraction while simultaneously maintaining the partial pressure gradient needed to allow O_2 to diffuse into the myocyte at an adequate rate to perform heavy exercise. Thus, for work rates demanding more O_2 than that at the *LT*, the further extraction of O_2 from oxyhemoglobin is H^+ concentration dependent.

BUFFERING THE EXERCISE-INDUCED LACTIC ACIDOSIS

Lactic acid (as lactate ions and associated protons) is the predominant fixed acid produced during exercise. It has a pK of approximately 3.9 and therefore is essentially totally disassociated at the pH of the muscle cell (approximately 7.0). The H^+ produced in the cell as lactate accumulates must be buffered immediately on its formation. Because HCO_3^- is a volatile buffer, the resulting H_2CO_3 does not remain in the cell but leaves on its formation as CO_2, thereby removing H^+ from the intracellular environment. Thus, CO_2 production by the cell increases at a rate commensurate with the *rate* of HCO_3^- buffering of lactic acid. Approximately 22.3 mL CO_2 will be produced over that generated from aerobic metabolism for each mmol of lactic acid buffered by HCO_3^- (Fig. 2.2). The increase in cell lactate and decrease in cell HCO_3^- concentrations stimulate transmembrane exchange of these ions, with $[HCO_3^-]$ decreasing in the blood almost mmol for mmol with the increase in lactate concentration (Fig. 2.21) (38,62–66).

The mechanism for lactate movement out of the cell is primarily carrier mediated. The studies of Trosper and Philipson, working with cardiac sarcolemmal vesicles, suggest that transport is accelerated by the pH gradient across the sarcolemmal mem-

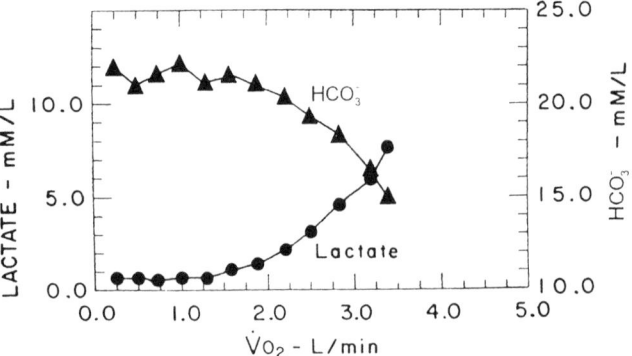

FIGURE 2.21.   The increase in arterial lactate and decrease in standard HCO_3^- as related to the increase in O_2 uptake ($\dot{V}_{O_2}$) during a progressively increasing work rate test on a cycle ergometer in a normal subject. (Modified from Wasserman K, Beaver WL, Davis JA, et al. Lactate, pyruvate, and lactate-to-pyruvate ratio during exercise and recovery. *J Appl Physiol* 1985;59:935–940.)

brane (67). At the cellular level, this will be established primarily by the $[HCO_3^-]$ gradient since the intra- and extracellular fluid will have similar partial pressures of CO_2. Mainwood et al. (68) and Hirsche et al. (69) found that lactate efflux from muscle was highly influenced by the HCO_3^- concentration of the muscle perfusate. The reciprocal changes of lactate and HCO_3^- in the extracellular fluid during heavy exercise suggest that permeation of lactate across the sarcolemmal membrane is a coupled HCO_3^-–lactate antiport carrier mechanism. This is supported by the study of Korotzer et al. (70), which shows that intravenous injection of the carbonic anhydrase inhibitor acetazolamide prior to performing heavy exercise significantly attenuates the increase in arterial lactate and decrease in bicarbonate. Replacing the intracellular HCO_3^-, which is consumed when it buffers newly produced lactic acid, with HCO_3^- from the bloodstream, minimizes the decrease in intracellular pH.

To better appreciate the dynamics of lactate and HCO_3^- movement between the cell and perfusing blood, arterial lactate and standard (Std) HCO_3^- were measured every 7.5 seconds during the first 3 minutes and then every 30 seconds during the remaining 3 minutes of a 6-minute constant-load exercise at three different intensities: moderate, heavy, and very heavy (Fig. 2.22). For the latter two work intensities, lactate started to increase at about 40 seconds and Std HCO_3^- started to decrease at about 50 seconds, on average. Thereafter, lactate and Std HCO_3^- changed reciprocally. The simultaneous decrease in Std HCO_3^- and lactate increase for all arterial samples for heavy and very heavy exercise intensities for the eight subjects whose data contribute to the concentration–time plots shown

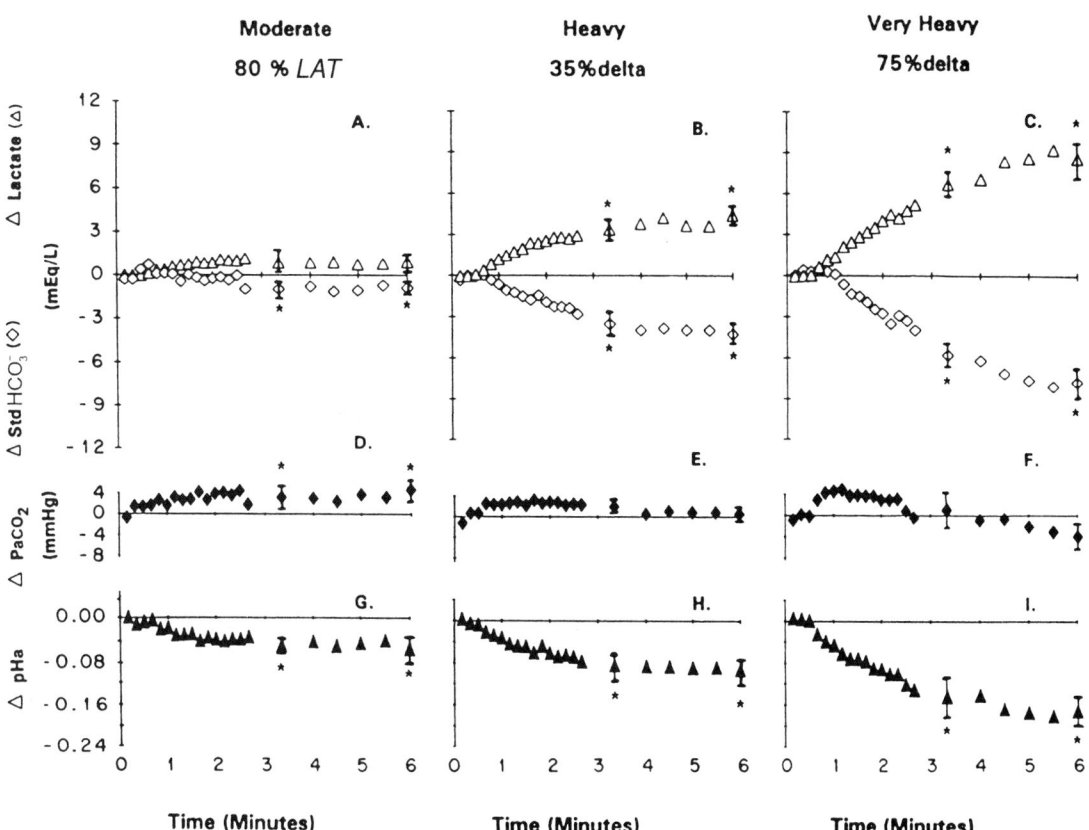

FIGURE 2.22.   Average responses to three exercise intensities displayed as change from resting measurements for arterial lactate, standard bicarbonate (Std HCO_3^-), P_{CO_2}, and pH (n = 8 subjects). Resting values for arterial pH, P_{CO_2}, Std HCO_3^-, lactate, and hemoglobin are 7.40 ± 0.03 (standard deviation), 39.8 ± 3.1 torr, 24.5 ± 1.3 mEq/L, 0.89 ± 0.47 mEq/L, and 14.2 g/dl, respectively. Significant differences from baseline (zero time) are shown at 3 and 6 minutes (*$P < 0.05$ from rest). (From Stringer W, Casaburi R, Wasserman K. Acid-base regulation during exercise and recovery in man. *J Appl Physiol* 1992;72:954–961, with permission.)

in Figure 2.22 are shown in Figure 2.23. Std HCO_3^- and lactate changes were highly correlated after lactate increased by about 0.5 mmol/L and 1.0 mmol/L for heavy and very heavy intensity exercise, respectively (63). This suggests that the earliest H^+ produced with lactate is buffered by a mechanism other than HCO_3^- buffer, or that new HCO_3^- buffer is produced at the start of exercise.

Supporting the latter mechanism is the study of Wasserman et al. (71) showing the development of a femoral vein alkalemia during the first 30 seconds of exercise before the development of the expected acidemia. This alkalemia was due to the early release of K^+ from the muscle cell, accompanied by a stoichiometric increase in HCO_3^- (Fig. 2.24). This development of a metabolic alkalosis during the first 30 seconds of exercise accounts for the failure of arterial HCO_3^- to decrease until lactate increased by approximately 0.5 to 1.0 mmol/L. The release of muscle K^+, and the development of muscle and femoral vein metabolic alkalosis, is thought to be due to the increase in intracellular pH caused by the hydrolysis of phosphocreatine (71) (Fig

2.25). This early exercise-induced metabolic alkalosis masks the initial metabolic acidosis caused by the increase in lactate. Thus, the lactate threshold (i.e., the $\dot{V}_{O_2}$ above which there is a sustained lactate increase) slightly precedes the decrease in arterial Std HCO_3^-, that is, the $\dot{V}_{O_2}$ above which metabolic acidosis develops, as previously shown by Beaver et al. (62) and Stringer et al. (63). Consequently, the lactic acidosis develops at a slightly higher $\dot{V}_{O_2}$ as compared to that of the *LT*.

The lactic acidosis threshold (*LAT*) contrasts with the *LT* in methodology only. The latter is determined from actual measurements of arterial lactate increase, whereas the former is determined by the decrease in arterial standard HCO_3^- concentration due to buffering lactic acid or the gas exchange consequence of the buffering, that is, CO_2 produced over that from aerobic metabolism. This excess CO_2 derives from the dissociation of HCO_3^- as it buffers lactic acid. The *LT* and *LAT* are systematically related and conceptually interchangeable, but they are not quantitatively identical, although the difference is small.

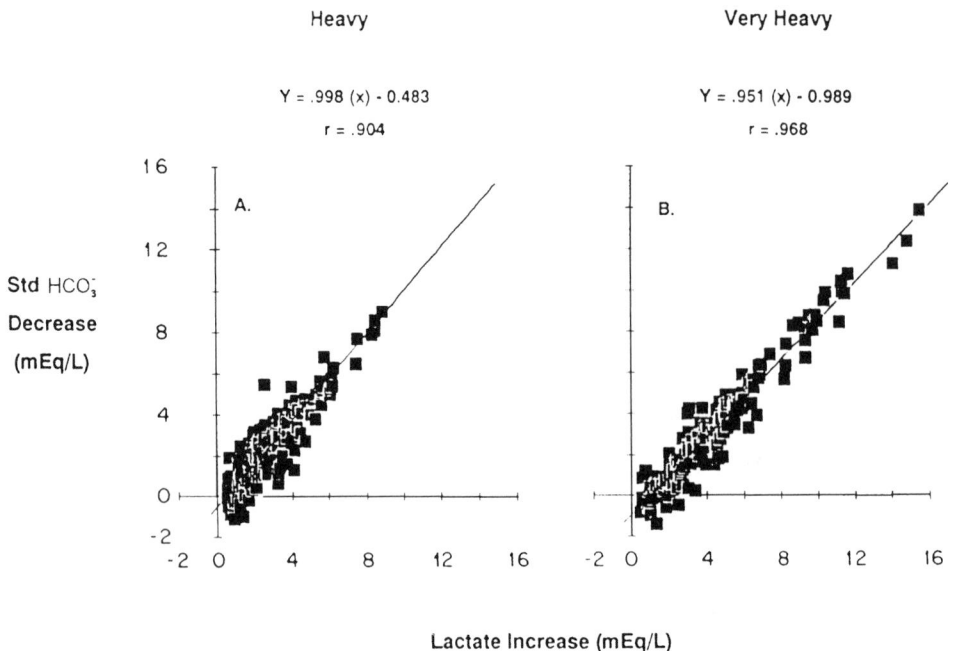

FIGURE 2.23.   Standard (Std) HCO_3^- decrease as a function of lactate increase from resting values for the heavy and very heavy work intensities shown in Figure 2.22. Fall in Std HCO_3^- is delayed until after lactate starts to increase (see regression equations). Thereafter, changes are approximately equal and opposite [heavy, n = 181: slope = 0.998 (CI 0.92 to 1.06), intercept = −0.48 (CI −0.71 to −0.26); very heavy, n = 141: slope = 0.951 (CI 0.92 to 0.98), intercept = −0.99 (CI −1.12 to −0.78)]. (From Stringer W, Casaburi R, Wasserman K. Acid-base regulation during exercise and recovery in man. *J Appl Physiol* 1992;72:954–961, with permission.)

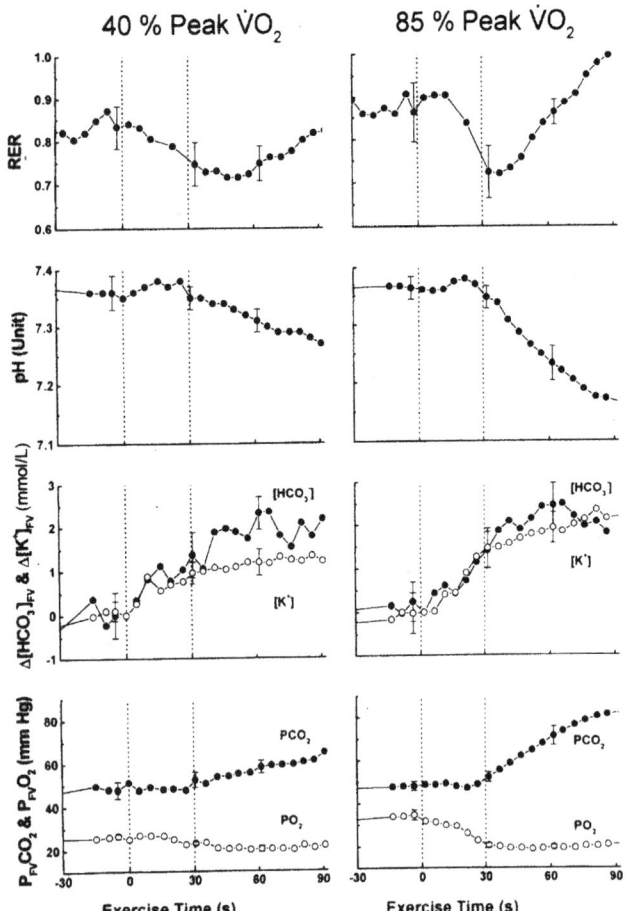

THE ANAEROBIC THRESHOLD CONCEPT

The finding that the lactic acidosis of exercise does not take place until after the critical capillary P_{O_2} is reached supports the concept that lactate accumulation in the active muscle takes place when the muscle O_2 supply becomes critical. Thus, the anaerobic threshold, measured by arterial lactate increase, arterial HCO_3^- decrease, or the CO_2 generated from the HCO_3^- buffering of lactic acid (61), describes the $\dot{V}_{O_2}$ at which the critical capillary P_{O_2} has been reached for a given work task. The decrease in P_{O_2} to its lowest or critical value before lactate concentration starts to increase in femoral vein blood during an incremental test lends sup-

FIGURE 2.24.   Respiratory exchange ratio (RER, **upper panels**), femoral vein pH (**panels second from top**), change (Δ) in femoral vein HCO_3^- and K^+ concentration (**panels third from the top**) and femoral vein P_{CO_2} and P_{O_2} (**bottom panels**) in response to the start of exercise (zero time) for the first 90 seconds of upright leg cycling exercise at 40% (**left panels**) and 85% (**right panels**) of $\dot{V}_{O_{2peak}}$. Each point is the average of five subjects. Vertical bars on select points are standard error values. (Modified from Wasserman K, Stringer W, Casaburi R, et al. Mechanism of the exercise hyperkalemia: an alternate hypothesis. *J Appl Physiol* 1997; 83:631–643.)

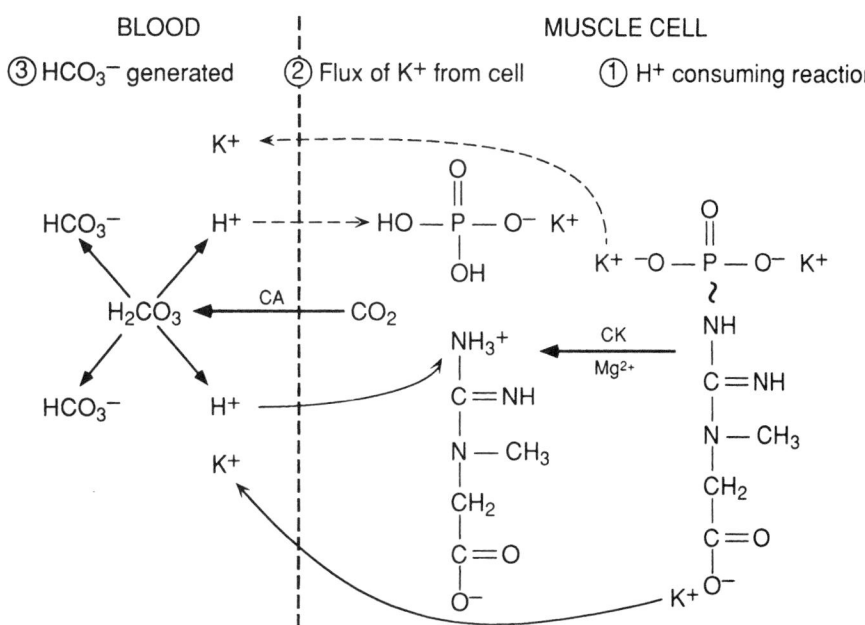

FIGURE 2.25. Hypothesis describing the mechanism for early changes in femoral vein pH, HCO_3^- and K^+ in response to exercise. *Step 1* shows that when phosphocreatine (*PCr*) is hydrolyzed into creatine and inorganic phosphate, H^+ is consumed, resulting in a reduction of negative charges in the cell and an alkalinizing reaction. *Step 2* illustrates that the excess in intracellular cation and a shortage of H^+ causes K^+ to leave the cell and H^+ to enter the cell. *Step 3* shows that the resulting efflux of K^+ from the cell is balanced by newly formed HCO_3^- in the interstitial fluid and therefore the effluent blood of the muscle. Thus, metabolic CO_2, when hydrated, becomes H_2CO_3, which dissociates into H^+ (which is taken up by the alkaline myocyte) and HCO_3^- anion (which serves to balance the positive charge of K^+). (From Wasserman K, Stringer W, Casaburi R, et al. Mechanism of the exercise hyperkalemia: an alternate hypothesis. *J Appl Physiol* 1997;83:631–643, with permission.)

port to the concept that the lactate increase during exercise is dependent on tissue O_2 supply.

That the lactic acidosis of exercise results from tissue hypoxia is further supported by the observation that the muscle L/P ratio, a measure of the cell redox state, increases when the lactate threshold is reached (50,72,73). Arterial blood lactate and pyruvate measurements in humans also show that the arterial L/P ratio increases at the lactate threshold (42). Because the cytosolic $[NADH + H^+]/NAD^+$ ratio is regulated by the mitochondrial redox state through the mitochondrial membrane shuttle (Fig. 2.1), failure to reoxidize mitochondrial coenzymes with molecular O_2 would also limit the reoxidation of cytosolic $NADH + H^+$ to NAD^+, thereby causing the cytosolic L/P ratio to increase.

Experimental observations demonstrate that blood lactate concentration can be reduced or increased as a result of increases or decreases, respectively, in blood oxygenation (9,33,74–76). For example, increasing blood O_2 content during exercise above the *LT* reduces arterial blood lactate, whereas reducing it increases blood lactate (37,76). The diversion of pyruvate from the tricarboxylic acid cycle to the production of lactate results in accelerated use of carbohydrate stores (9,10). Thus, the rate of anaerobic glycolysis is affected by blood oxygenation.

The Oxygen Flow-Independent and Oxygen Flow-Dependent Work Rate Zones and the Anaerobic Threshold

The anaerobic threshold (*AT*) concept implies that there is an exercise $\dot{V}O_2$ below which exercise $\dot{V}O_2$ is determined by the work rate performed and not the O_2 transport to the muscles and above which $\dot{V}O_2$ is determined by O_2 transport as well as the work rate. In other words, below the *AT*, $\dot{V}O_2$ is O_2 flow independent, and above the *AT*, $\dot{V}O_2$ is O_2 flow dependent. To test this hypothesis, Hansen et al. (77) increased work rate at slow, medium, and fast rates and found that below the *AT*, $\dot{V}O_2$ increased at a rate that did not vary as the rate of increase in work rate varied, in contrast to changing work rate above the *AT* (Fig. 2.26); however, peak $\dot{V}O_2$ was unchanged.

The failure of $\dot{V}O_2$ to fully track work rate change above the *AT* was also shown by Haouzi et al. (78), who changed work rate in sine wave pattern below and above the *AT* (Fig. 2.27). Below the *AT*, the am-

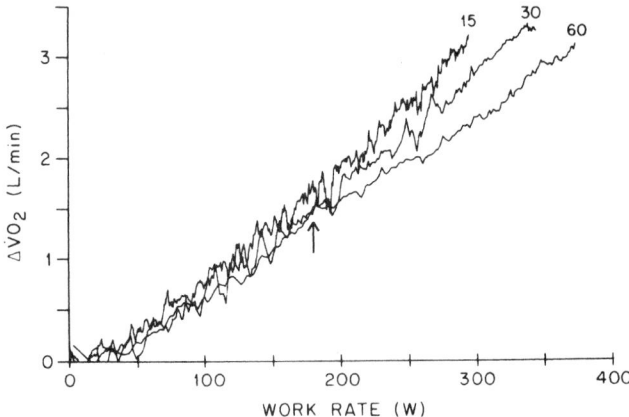

FIGURE 2.26.   Effect of rate of increase in work rate from unloaded cycling on rate of increase in $\dot{V}O_2$ in a normal subject. Below the anaerobic threshold (approximately 180 W, *arrow*), the rate of increase in $\dot{V}O_2$ is independent of the rate of increase in work rate. Above the anaerobic threshold, the increase in $\dot{V}O_2$ is slower the faster the rate of increase in work rate, although the peak $\dot{V}O_2$ is unchanged. (From Hansen JE, Sue DY, Oren A, et al. Relation of oxygen uptake in work rate in normal men and men with circulatory disorders. *Am J Cardiol* 1987;59:669–674.)

plitude in $\dot{V}O_2$ for a work rate period of 4 minutes varied with the amplitude of work rate in an approximate ratio of 10 ml/min/W. In contrast, the amplitude of change in $\dot{V}O_2$ for the same period and work rate change above the *AT* was only about two-thirds as much. This reduction in the $\dot{V}O_2$–work rate relation supports the hypothesis that $\dot{V}O_2$ does not reach the O_2 requirement above the *AT*; that is, the work rate is in the O_2 flow-dependent zone.

Koike et al. demonstrated that the AT demarcates the O_2 flow-independent from the O_2 flow-dependent work rate zones (33,79). In this study, blood O_2 content was decreased in a controlled

fashion in normal subjects by taking up O_2 binding sites on hemoglobin with carbon monoxide (Fig. 2.28). The blood O_2 content was reduced by approximately 10% and 20% before performing exercise. The *AT* and peak $\dot{V}O_2$ were reduced by a percentage consistent with the percent reduction in blood O_2 content. While $\dot{V}O_2$ increased at an unchanged rate for different levels of carboxyhemoglobin (COHb) at the work rates below the *AT*, the rate of increase in $\dot{V}O_2$ was reduced for the work rates above the *AT*.

Identifying the Anaerobic Threshold by Gas Exchange

Figure 2.29 shows the effect of an increasing work rate on ventilation and gas exchange for a cycle ergometer exercise test in which the work rate was increased at 1-minute intervals after a 4-minute warm-up period of pedaling without load. As the work rate is increased, $\dot{V}O_2$, $\dot{V}CO_2$, and $\dot{V}E$ increase linearly with work rate, after a time delay of less than 1 minute, until the exercise lactic acidosis develops. At work rates above the *LAT*, CO_2 output increases more rapidly than O_2 uptake because CO_2 generated by the bicarbonate buffering of lactic acid is added to the metabolic CO_2 production. This is the basis of the V-slope plot for measuring the anaerobic threshold (80) (described later in the chapter).

Isocapnic Buffering Period Above the Anaerobic Threshold

Initially, $\dot{V}E$ increases in proportion to the increased CO_2 output when the lactic acidosis first develops, resulting in no increase in $\dot{V}E/\dot{V}CO_2$ or decrease in

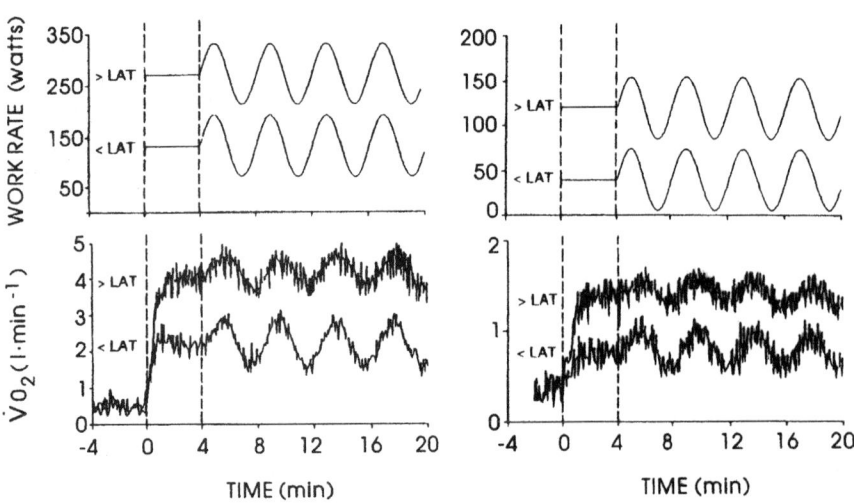

FIGURE 2.27.   Effect of continuously changing work rate in sinusoidal pattern **(upper panel)** on $\dot{V}O_2$ kinetics **(lower panel)** for a range of changing work rates below (<*LAT*) and above (>*LAT*) the lactic acidosis (anaerobic) threshold (*LAT*). (From Haouzi P, Fukuba Y, Casaburi R, et al. O_2 uptake kinetics above and below the lactic acidosis threshold during sinusoidal exercise. *J Appl Physiol* 1993;75:1644–1650, with permission.)

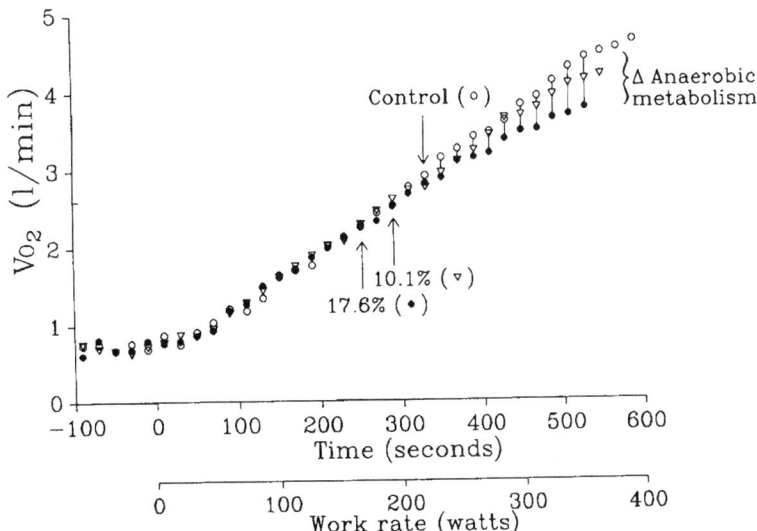

FIGURE 2.28. $\dot{V}O_2$ response to three ramp tests (work rate increased at 40 watt/min) during air breathing (control test) and two tests of air plus carbon monoxide breathing that resulted in COHb levels of 10.1% and 17.6%, respectively, in one subject. Points to the left of 0 are measured during unloaded cycling. Each point is an average of 20 seconds of data. The order of tests was randomized. There was no effect on $\dot{V}O_2$ as work rate was increased until the anaerobic threshold (*AT, arrow*) of the respective study was surpassed. Then the increase in $\dot{V}O_2$ was slower the higher the COHb. The difference between the $\dot{V}O_2$ of the control and the reduced blood O_2 content studies represents the reduced $\dot{V}O_2$ caused by the reduced blood O_2 content. The *AT* and peak $\dot{V}O_2$ systematically decreased as the blood O_2 content was decreased. The difference enclosed by brackets on the right is the metabolic equivalent of increased anaerobic metabolism caused when COHb was increased to 17.6%. (From Koike A, Weiler-Ravell D, McKenzie DK, et al. Evidence that the metabolic acidosis threshold is the anaerobic threshold. *J Appl Physiol* 199;8:2521–2526, with permission.)

$PETCO_2$ (isocapnic buffering, Fig. 2.29). Thus, $\dot{V}E$ retains a linear relation with $\dot{V}CO_2$ ($\dot{V}E/\dot{V}CO_2$ is constant or decreases slightly) while it increases relative to $\dot{V}O_2$ ($\dot{V}E/\dot{V}O_2$ increases) above the *LAT* (Fig. 2.29). As described in Chapter 4, the increase in $\dot{V}E/\dot{V}O_2$ without an increase in $\dot{V}E/\dot{V}CO_2$ is another gas exchange method for detecting the *AT* (81).

Further increasing work rate results in $\dot{V}E$ increasing more rapidly than $\dot{V}CO_2$ (increase in $\dot{V}E/\dot{V}CO_2$), causing $PaCO_2$ and $PETCO_2$ to decrease (Fig. 2.29). This additional ventilatory response reflects the ventilatory compensation for the exercise-induced lactic acidosis. The increased H^+ concentration stimulates the carotid bodies to increase ventilatory drive (39). By increasing the ventilatory drive, arterial PCO_2 is reduced, providing a ventilatory constraint to the lactic acid–induced fall in pH (82). Table 2.2 describes the exercise gas exchange responses for constant work rate exercise performed above the *AT*.

Buffering Lactic Acid and the V-Slope Method for Identifying the Anaerobic Threshold

Figure 2.2 shows the effect of buffering the cellular lactic acidosis with HCO_3^- on $\dot{V}CO_2$ relative to $\dot{V}O_2$. The increases in $\dot{V}O_2$ and $\dot{V}CO_2$, as a function of progressively increasing work rate, are shown in Figure 2.30. Plotting $\dot{V}CO_2$ as a function of $\dot{V}O_2$ for a progressively increasing work rate test (V-slope plot), after the first minute or so of increasing work rate, yields a progression of points that are linear with a slope of 1.0 or slightly less. The curve then breaks, with $\dot{V}CO_2$ increasing faster than $\dot{V}O_2$ so that the slope is now clearly above 1.0. The break point where the slopes coincide is the anaerobic or lactic acidosis threshold (Fig. 2.31). This slope transition coincides with the *LAT*, as confirmed with arterial standard HCO_3^- measurements. It is slightly higher than the *LT* for the reasons described earlier in this section (80). The slope of the increase in $\dot{V}CO_2$ relative to $\dot{V}O_2$ below the threshold (S_1 in Fig. 2.31) has an average value of 0.95, with a small variation (14,16). The transition to a slope greater than 1.0 (S_2 in Fig. 2.31) occurs, on average, in the midrange of healthy subjects' aerobic capacities.

The $\dot{V}CO_2$ Versus $\dot{V}O_2$ Slopes. The intercept of S_1 and S_2 of the $\dot{V}CO_2$ versus $\dot{V}O_2$ relationship is the *LAT*, measured by gas exchange, and estimates the *AT*. The term *lactic acidosis threshold* describes the biochemical event that causes the $\dot{V}CO_2$ vs. $\dot{V}O_2$ slope to exceed 1, although the underlying mechanism is the lactic acidosis resulting from exercise above the *AT*. Hyperventilation (reduction in ideal alveolar

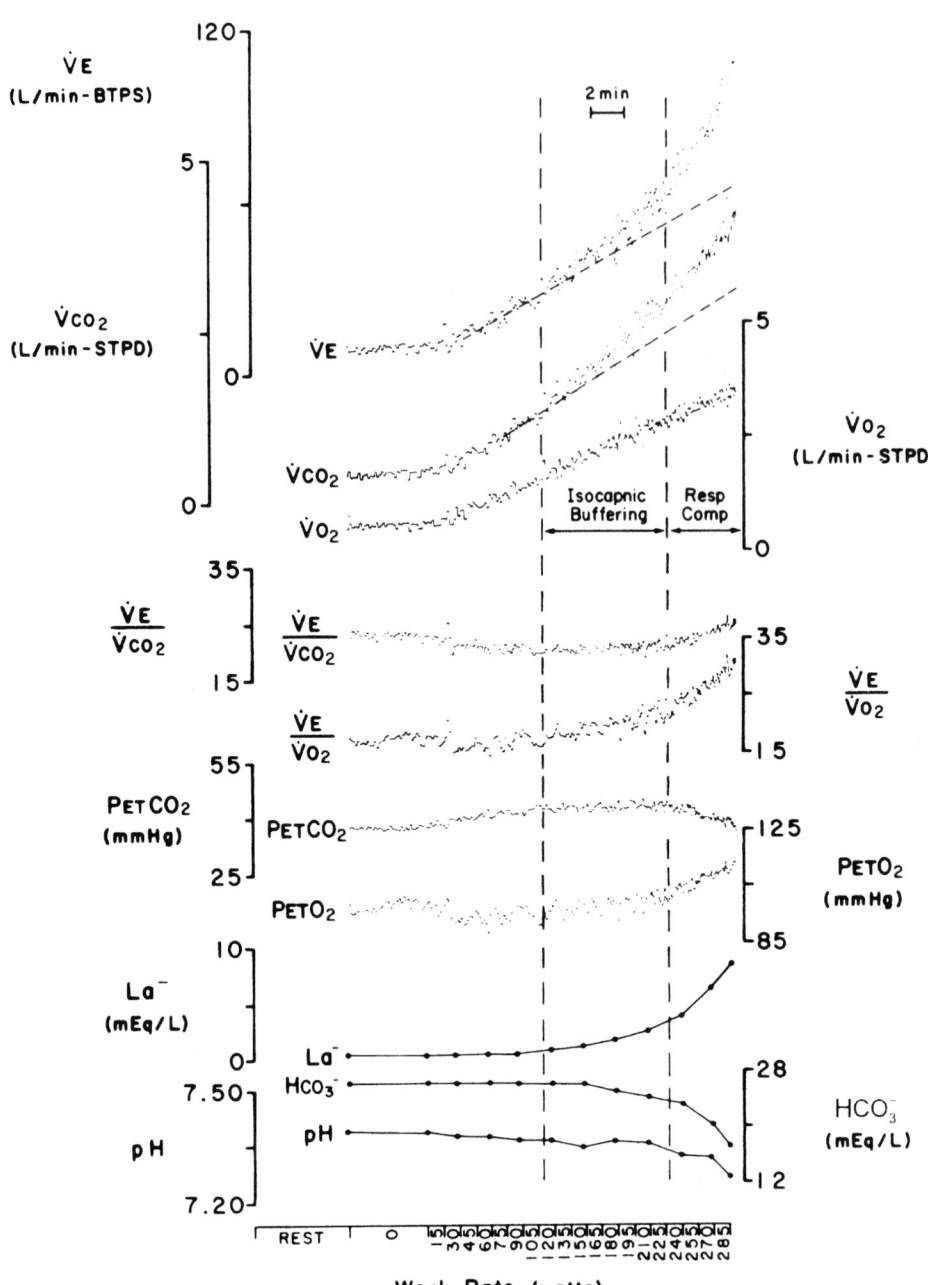

FIGURE 2.29.   Breath-by-breath measurements of minute ventilation ($\dot{V}E$), CO_2 output ($\dot{V}CO_2$), O_2 uptake ($\dot{V}O_2$), $\dot{V}E/\dot{V}CO_2$, $\dot{V}E/\dot{V}O_2$, $PETCO_2$, $PETO_2$, arterial lactate and bicarbonate, and pH for a 1-minute incremental exercise test on a cycle ergometer. The lactic threshold (*LT*) occurs when lactate increases (*left vertical dashed line*). This is accompanied by a fall in HCO_3^- (*LAT*) and generally an increase in $\dot{V}E/\dot{V}O_2$. "Isocapnic buffering" refers to the period when $\dot{V}E$ and $\dot{V}CO_2$ increase curvilinearly at the same rate without an increase in $\dot{V}E/\dot{V}CO_2$, thus retaining a constant $PETCO_2$. After the period of isocapnic buffering, $PETCO_2$ decreases and $\dot{V}E/\dot{V}CO_2$ increases, reflecting ventilatory compensation for the metabolic acidosis of exercise.

PCO_2 or $PaCO_2$ and increase in $\dot{V}E/\dot{V}CO_2$) almost never occurs at the *LAT* and for several minutes thereafter. When hyperventilation does occur during a progressively increasing work rate test, it does so at a higher $\dot{V}O_2$ (at the upper downward-directed arrow in Fig. 2.31) and represents the ventilatory compensation for the lactic acidosis. S_2 being steeper than a slope of 1.0 during the progressively increas-

ing work rate test signifies that CO_2 is being released from cell HCO_3^- as it dissociates during the buffering of lactic acid (Fig. 2.2).

It has been consistently demonstrated in the literature that S_2 becomes steeper the faster the work rate increases (16,83,84), presumably because of the faster rate of lactate formation relative to $\dot{V}O_2$ increase. However, with glycogen depletion, S_1 be-

TABLE 2.2. Altered Physiological Responses to Exercise above the Anaerobic Threshold

1. Accelerated muscle glycogen utilization and anaerobic regeneration of *ATP*
2. Reduced exercise endurance
3. Metabolic acidosis
4. Delay in $\dot{V}O_2$ steady state
5. Increased $\dot{V}CO_2$ over that predicted from aerobic metabolism
6. Increased ventilatory drive
7. Decreasing $PaCO_2$ and $PETCO_2$ with time
8. Bohr effect rather than decreasing capillary PO_2 increases O_2 extraction from blood
9. Increased plasma electrolyte concentration
10. Hemoconcentration
11. Increased production of metabolic intermediaries (e.g., glycerol phosphate and alanine)
12. Increased catecholamine levels
13. Increased double product

comes shallower, consistent with the lower respiratory quotient of the metabolic substrate (16).

Altered Physiological Responses to Exercise Above the Anaerobic Threshold

The *AT* appears to be an excellent discriminator of the highest work rate that can be endured for a prolonged period of exercise, such as a marathon (85,

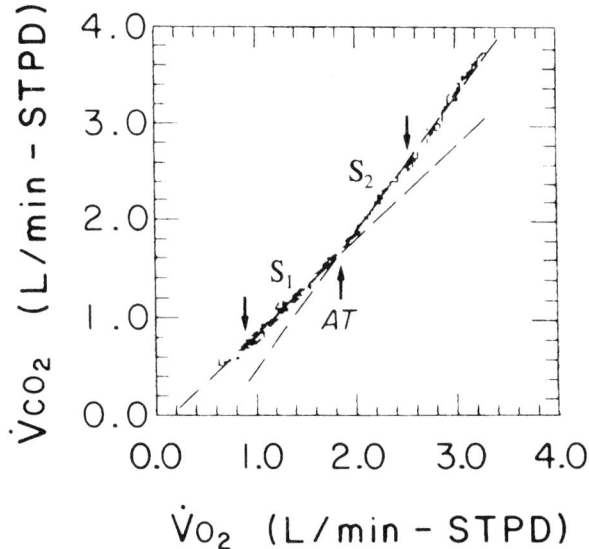

FIGURE 2.31. CO_2 output ($\dot{V}CO_2$) as a function of oxygen uptake ($\dot{V}O_2$) during a progressively increasing work rate test (V-slope plot). The transition from aerobic metabolism, in which $\dot{V}CO_2$ increases linearly with $\dot{V}O_2$ with a slope (S_1) slightly less than 1, to anaerobic plus aerobic metabolism, where the slope increases to a value greater than 1 (S_2), defines the lactic acidosis threshold (*LAT*) or anaerobic threshold (*AT*) by gas exchange. The steeper S_2 reflects the production of additional CO_2 from HCO_3^- buffering of lactic acid over that produced by aerobic metabolism. Hyperventilation does not occur at the AT during a progressively increasing work rate test and, therefore, does not contribute to the steepening of S_2. The lower downward-directed arrow indicates where CO_2 stores are no longer increasing and calculation of S_1 starts. The upper downward-directed arrow indicates the $\dot{V}O_2$ above which hyperventilation in response to metabolic acidosis starts. S_1 and S_2 are calculated from the data between these two arrows. (Modified from Beaver WL, Wasserman K, Whipp BJ. A new method for detecting the anaerobic threshold by gas exchange. *J Appl Physiol* 1986;60:2020–2027.)

86). $\dot{V}O_2$ and $\dot{V}E$ reach a steady state early for exercise at or below the *AT*. However, a steady state in $\dot{V}O_2$ and $\dot{V}E$ is delayed or not achieved for exercise above the *AT*. Acid–base balance is essentially unchanged from rest for work rates below the *AT* (acid–base homeostasis). In contrast, there is a metabolic acidosis above the *AT*, with $PaCO_2$ decreasing several minutes after lactic acidosis develops.

Table 2.2 lists the physiological changes that take place when performing exercise above the *AT*. These include important functional adaptations that affect *ATP* production and mitochondrial O_2 supply, such as further vasodilatation in the vascular bed with high H^+ production (87); a shift in the oxyhemoglobin dissociation curve to the right, allowing O_2 to unload more readily from hemoglobin (88); and increase in hemoglobin concentration (89). A description of the physiological responses to exercise that are altered above the *AT* follows.

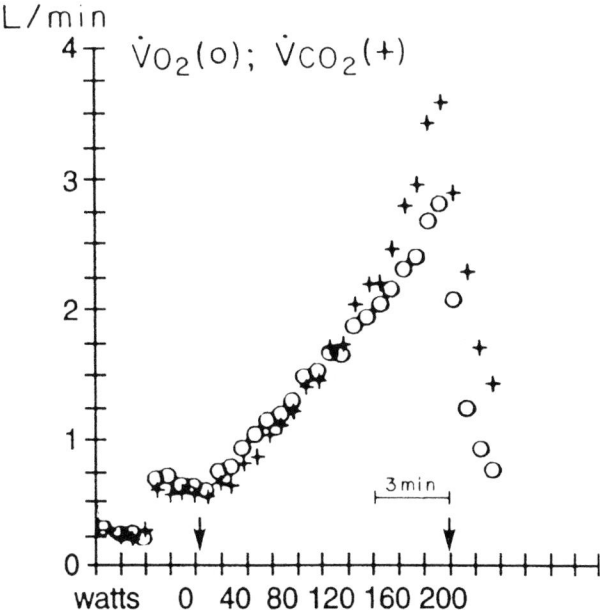

FIGURE 2.30. $\dot{V}CO_2$ and $\dot{V}O_2$ as related to work rate for 1-minute incremental (20 W/min) cycle ergometer exercise test. $\dot{V}CO_2$ starts to increase more steeply than $\dot{V}O_2$ in the middle work rate range, reflecting buffering of lactic acid above the lactic acidosis threshold.

Accelerated Glycolysis

Hill and associates (90) showed a correlation between blood lactate increase and the O_2 debt (the amount of O_2 consumed, over resting levels, during the recovery from exercise). When the mechanism for glycolysis was better understood, it was appreciated that three *ATP* molecules are generated during the anaerobic metabolism of one glycosyl unit of glycogen to two lactate molecules (91). By this mechanism, anaerobic glycolysis provides energy without use of molecular oxygen (Fig. 2.1). Although this mechanism provides *ATP* without use of O_2, the *ATP* yield from each glycosol molecule anaerobically metabolized to lactate is only one-twelfth of that from each glycosol aerobically metabolized to CO_2 and H_2O. Thus, the rate of glycolysis in muscle is markedly accelerated above the *AT*, thereby accelerating the depletion of muscle glycogen stores.

Exercise Endurance

Exercise endurance is reduced for work rates above the *AT*, the reduction being greater the higher the blood lactate that the exercise engenders (Fig. 2.10). Reduced endurance may not be due to the increased lactate concentration or the associated increase in H^+ per se, but rather due to the inadequate rate of aerobic production of *ATP*, reflected by the rising lactate concentration (and decreasing rate of rise in $\dot{V}O_2$, particularly evident in patients with cardiovascular diseases) as work rate approaches the subject's peak $\dot{V}O_2$ and the glycolytic flux is inadequate to increase glycolytic *ATP* production to make up for the reduced $\dot{V}O_2$ component.

Oxyhemoglobin Dissociation

Perhaps the most important beneficial effect of net lactate accumulation during exercise is to cause H^+ to increase in the capillary bed where lactate is produced. This mechanism serves to facilitate the dissociation of oxyhemoglobin (Bohr effect). As described, the rightward shift in the oxyhemoglobin dissociation curve caused by H^+ defends the capillary PO_2 and allows arterial–venous O_2 difference to increase maximally when performing heavy-intensity exercise (61). Dissociation of oxyhemoglobin at work rates above the *AT* occurs because of the Bohr effect created by the increase in lactic acid. Thus, in McArdle's syndrome (92) or other disorders of glycolysis in which lactate cannot increase, it is not possible to extract O_2 to the extent seen in normal subjects during maximal exercise. This has been ex-

perimentally demonstrated by the finding that the maximum $C(a - \bar{v})O_2$ is relatively small at the exercise work rate at which the patient with McArdle's syndrome is forced to stop exercise due to muscle fatigue (92). In healthy subjects, above the *AT*, end-capillary oxyhemoglobin saturation continues to decrease in accordance with the pH decrease, while PO_2 remains constant at its critical value. Thus, for normal extraction of O_2 by the muscles, two factors—decreasing PO_2 and increasing H^+—are required. The former appears to play a more important role in oxyhemoglobin dissociation below the *AT*, whereas the latter has a major role above it (Fig. 2.19).

The biochemical interactions between capillary blood and muscle cell for optimizing the O_2 supply to mitochondria during heavy exercise are summarized in Figure 2.32. At the arterial end of the capillary, as the muscle consumes O_2, capillary PO_2 decreases and oxyhemoglobin dissociates. As capillary PO_2 falls to its "critical" value for diffusion, lactic acid starts to increase in the cell. Capillary blood H^+ quickly increases because the lactic acid–producing cells generate additional CO_2 from HCO_3^- as it dissociates when buffering lactic acid. Simultaneously, capillary blood HCO_3^- is consumed by the cell as cellular lactate exchanges with interstitial HCO_3^-. Although the intracellular buffering of lactic acid by HCO_3^- minimizes the change in cell pH, it acidifies blood more quickly than if a non-HCO_3^- buffer neutralized the cellular lactic acidosis. This is a most remarkable physiological mechanism, since the Bohr effect would not be as great with any other buffer than as with HCO_3^-. Thus, the lactic acidosis–facilitated oxyhemoglobin dissociation ensures a higher blood O_2 extraction and thereby a higher maximal $\dot{V}O_2$ than would otherwise be possible.

Plasma Electrolyte Concentrations

During an incremental exercise test, arterial plasma sodium and chloride concentrations and total cation and anion concentrations increase (Fig 2.33) above the *LT* (93). This suggests that extracellular water volume has decreased. Because the total exercise duration was only about 15 minutes, with only a few minutes of heavy exercise, it is unlikely that the extracellular fluid loss is due to sweating. Rather, the most likely cause is the increase in intracellular osmolality due to increase in intracellular lactate and other by-products of metabolism that accompany lactate increase. This increase in intracellular osmotic force must occur and thereby

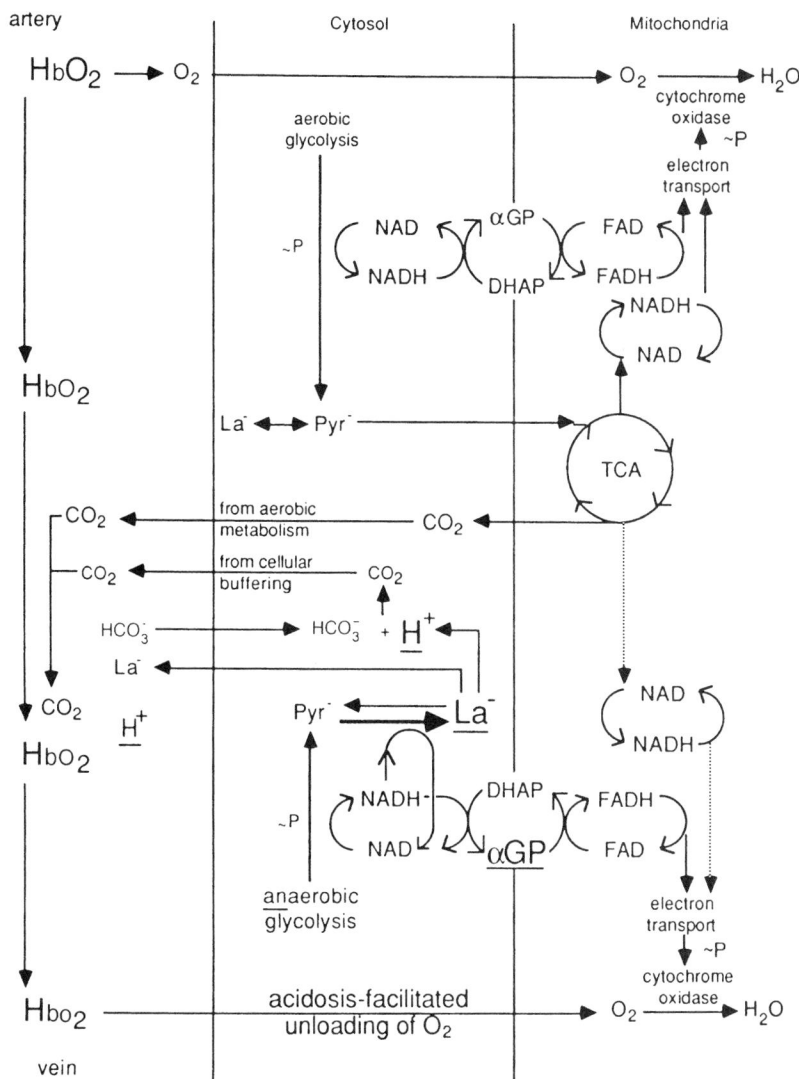

FIGURE 2.32.   Scheme of changing capillary oxyhemoglobin (HbO_2) saturation during blood transit from artery to vein during heavy-intensity exercise. At the arterial end of the capillary, HbO_2 dissociates primarily due to decrease in Po_2. Glycolysis proceeds aerobically, without an increase in lactate (La^-), because mitochondrial membrane redox shuttles (e.g., dihydroxyacetone acetone phosphate, DHAP) regulate cytosolic redox state $(NADH+H^+)/NAD^+$, abbreviated NADH/NAD. The primary substrate for the tricarboxylic acid (TCA) cycle is pyruvate (Pyr). As pyruvate is metabolized in the mitochondria, protons and electrons flow through the electron transport chain to O_2, generating high-energy phosphate ($\sim P$) with H_2O and CO_2 as by-products.

As blood reaches the venous end of the capillary, where Po_2 becomes critically low, mitochondrial membrane redox shuttle fails to reoxidize NADH to NAD^+ at an adequate rate. Thus, the $NADH/NAD^+$ ratio increases. Accordingly, pyruvate is converted to La^-, and DHAP is converted to glycerol 3-phosphate (G3P) in proportion to the change in cell redox state (97). The effect is an increase in cell La^- with a stoichiometric increase in H^+. The latter is immediately buffered by HCO_3^- in the cell. Decreasing cellular HCO_3^- and increasing cellular La^- results in intracellular–extracellular La^- and HCO_3^- exchange (Fig. 2.2). Simultaneously, CO_2, formed during intracellular buffering, leaves the cell. The sum of aerobically and anaerobically produced CO_2 (from buffering), along with decreasing blood HCO_3^- (see Fig. 2.20) further acidifies the capillary blood toward the venous end of the capillary, enhancing dissociation of HbO_2 (Bohr effect). This acidosis-facilitated dissociation of HbO_2 allows aerobic metabolism to proceed at a rate proportional to the rate of acidification of blood, without a further reduction in capillary Po_2. (Modified from Wasserman K. Coupling of external to cellular respiration during exercise: the wisdom of the body revisited. *Am J Physiol* 1994;266:E519–E539.)

obligate water flux into the cell to balance the osmotic forces on both sides of the cell membrane.

Change in plasma K^+ differs from Na^+ and Cl^- ions in that its concentration starts to increase below the *AT*, although its rate of increase is faster above the *AT*. Wasserman et al. (71) suggested that

K^+ release from cells is linked to the hydrolysis of phosphocreatine. When the latter is hydrolyzed, it creates an alkaline reaction in the cell. Thus, strong cations are in relative excess compared with the extracellular fluid. Since K^+ is the primary intracellular cation, it would be this cation that would

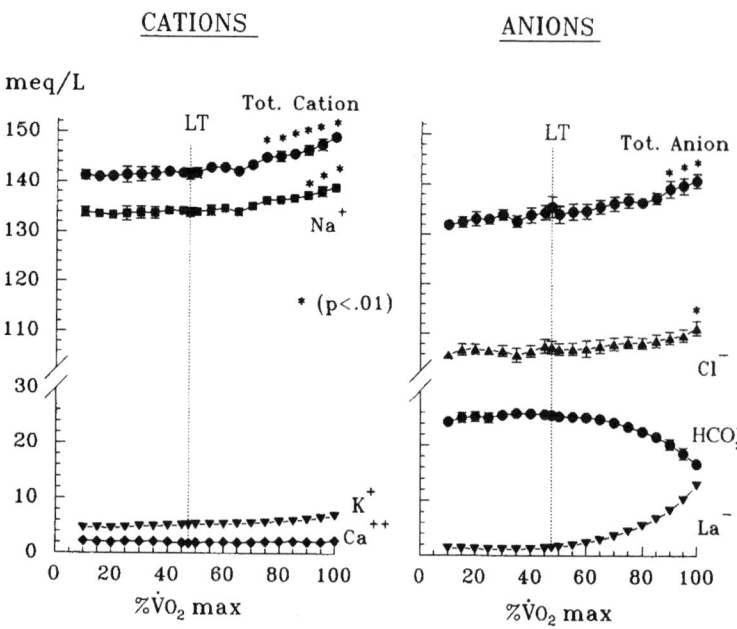

FIGURE 2.33. Change in arterial plasma Na⁺, K⁺, Ca⁺⁺, and total measured cations **(left panel)** and Cl⁻, HCO₃⁻, La⁻, and total measured anions **(right panel)** during a progressively increasing exercise test to maximum level tolerated. Data are the average for ten normal adult subjects. The vertical bars on points are the standard errors of means. The vertical line passing through all the curves is the average lactate threshold.

leave the cell to balance the charge across the cell membrane. It has been shown that the anion balancing the K^+ released during early exercise is HCO_3^- (71).

Hemoconcentration

That hemoconcentration occurs when humans perform exercise has been described in a number of studies (94–96). Whereas, in certain animals, this is due to splenic contraction, this does not appear to be the mechanism in humans. Jung et al. (89) found that the hemoconcentration occurs primarily during exercise above the *LT*, as illustrated in Figure 2.34. The clue for the mechanism of hemoconcentration resides in the observation that the concentration of the total extracellular cations and anions increases above the *LT* (Fig. 2.33). Since the cell osmolality must increase above the *LT*, extracellular fluid would move into cells rich in lactate. The shrinkage of the extracellular fluid would increase the red cell and therefore the arterial O_2 concentration, providing more O_2 per ml of blood flow at exercise levels that cause lactate to increase. This could benefit the subject during exercise in which the O_2 supply limits exercise performance.

Metabolic Intermediaries

Katz and Sahlin (97) found, in muscle biopsy studies performed immediately at the cessation of exercise in humans, that cellular alpha-glycerol phosphate increased in proportion to the increase in lactate. Muscle cell pyruvate and alanine also increased above the *LT*. These changes are most likely secondary to the change in cytosol redox state and the accelerated rate of muscle glycolysis, which takes place above the *LT*.

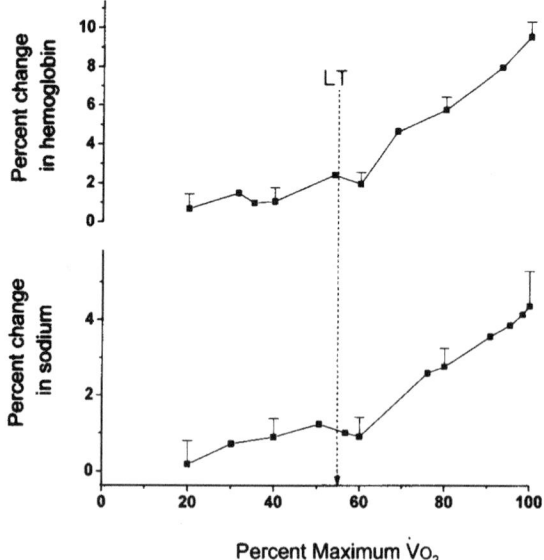

FIGURE 2.34. Change in arterial hemoglobin, and plasma sodium concentration during progressively increasing work rate exercise. Data are the average for ten normal adult subjects. The vertical bars on points are the standard errors of means. The vertical line passing through the curves is the average lactate threshold for the group. The standard deviation of the lactate threshold is ±4.8%.

$\dot{V}O_2$ and $\dot{V}CO_2$ Kinetics: Constant Work Rate Exercise. Figure 1.4 shows the typical onset responses of $\dot{V}O_2$ and $\dot{V}CO_2$ for moderate-intensity exercise (i.e., exercise that does not engender a lactic acidosis) and heavy-intensity exercise (i.e., exercise that results in a sustained lactic acidosis). The patterns of gas exchange differ between exercise performed at work rates with and without lactic acidosis, making it possible to discern if the work rate is above or below the *LAT* from gas exchange measurements at the airway (61,98). In the absence of lactic acidosis, $\dot{V}O_2$ reaches a steady state by 3 minutes, whereas $\dot{V}CO_2$ increases more slowly, reaching a steady state by 4 minutes.

In the steady state of moderate-intensity exercise, $\dot{V}CO_2$ is slightly lower than $\dot{V}O_2$ (Fig. 2.35A) because the metabolic substrate respiratory quotient is less than 1.0. For constant-load exercise above the *LAT* (Fig. 2.35B and C), $\dot{V}CO_2$ generally exceeds

$\dot{V}O_2$, the excess CO_2 being generated when HCO_3^- buffers lactic acid (Fig. 2.35G, H, and I).

Panels D, E, and F of Figure 2.35 illustrate that $\dot{V}CO_2$ kinetics are slow relative to $\dot{V}O_2$ within the first minute of exercise. This slow CO_2 output relative to O_2 uptake during this early exercise period is accounted for in part by the early increase in blood HCO_3^- and K^+, described earlier (71).

For exercise performed above the *AT*, the overall $\dot{V}O_2$ dynamics are slow compared with exercise performed below the *AT*, and a steady state in $\dot{V}O_2$ is often not reached before the subject fatigues (Fig. 2.6). In contrast to $\dot{V}O_2$ dynamics, $\dot{V}CO_2$ dynamics do not change appreciably during above-*AT* exercise (Fig. 2.36), and, usually after 1 minute of such exercise, $\dot{V}CO_2$ exceeds $\dot{V}O_2$ (Figs. 2.35 and 2.36), the magnitude depending on the rate of lactate increase (98,99). The extra CO_2 generated by heavy-intensity exercise can be accounted for by the CO_2

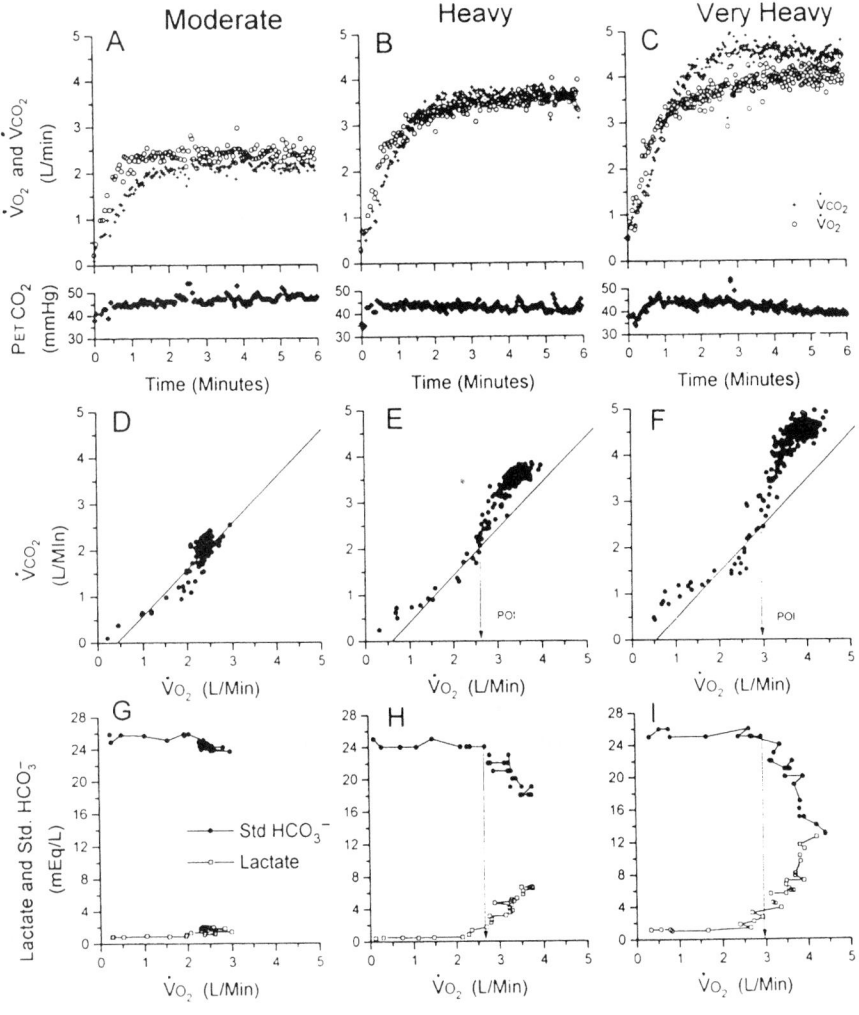

FIGURE 2.35. O_2 uptake ($\dot{V}O_2$), CO_2 output ($\dot{V}CO_2$), and $P_{ET}CO_2$ plotted as a function of time **(A, B and C)** and $\dot{V}CO_2$, arterial lactate HCO_3^-, and standard (Std) HCO_3^- plotted as a function of $\dot{V}O_2$ **(D–I)** for constant work rate tests of moderate, heavy, and very heavy work intensity. Steepening of $\dot{V}CO_2$ relative to $\dot{V}O_2$ (*arrow* in **E** and **F**) occurs simultaneously with the increase in lactate and decrease in HCO_3^- (*arrow* in **H** and **I**), reflecting the buffering of the lactic acid by HCO_3^-. (Modified from Stringer WW, Wasserman K, Casaburi R. The $\dot{V}CO_2/\dot{V}O_2$ relationship during heavy, constant work rate exercise reflects the rate of lactate accumulation. *Eur J Appl Physiol* 1995;72: 25–31.)

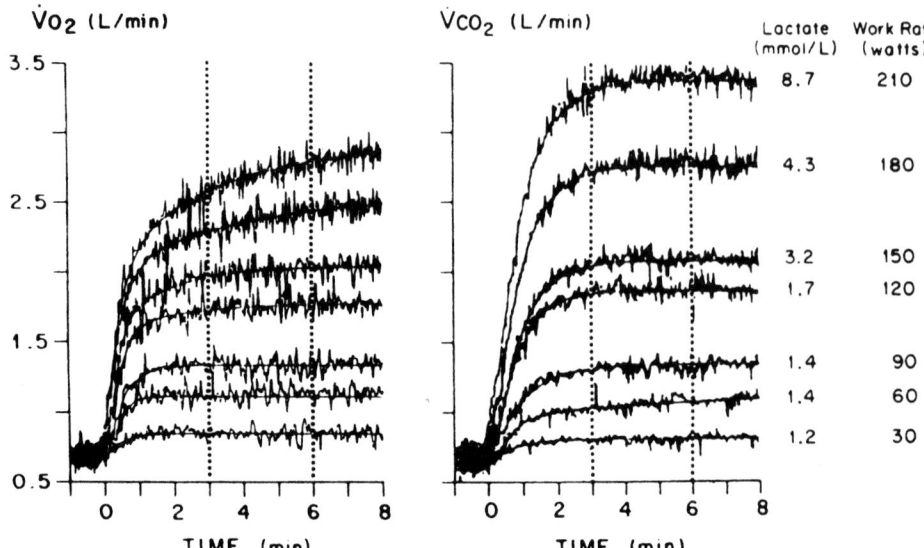

FIGURE 2.36. O_2 uptake ($\dot{V}O_2$) and CO_2 output ($\dot{V}CO_2$) as related to time at seven different levels of work for a healthy subject. The three lowest work rates are below the subject's lactic acidosis threshold (*LAT*), whereas the four highest work rates are above it. The $\dot{V}O_2$ continues to rise for the four work rates above the *LAT*, the rate of rise being more marked the higher the work rate. In contrast, the $\dot{V}CO_2$ kinetics are relatively unchanging, reaching a constant level by 3 to 4 minutes in all seven tests. (Modified from Casaburi R, Barstow TJ, Robinson T, et al. Influence of work rate on ventilatory and gas exchange kinetics. *J Appl Physiol* 1989;67:547–555.)

produced as HCO_3^- buffers the H^+ from lactic acid, and to a lesser degree, by CO_2 unloading from body stores due to hyperventilation, if Pa_{CO_2} is decreased (Figs. 2.2 and 2.29).

Ventilatory Drive

Ventilation tracks the acidity added to the blood as a result of metabolism. Thus, the addition of CO_2 from the HCO_3^- buffering of lactic acid, as well as the reduction in plasma HCO_3^- concentration, adds acid equivalents to the blood. The ventilatory control mechanisms are stimulated to provide levels of ventilation that continue to increase during exercise as long as the arterial pH remains reduced. The proposed control mechanisms are discussed in greater detail later in this chapter. The magnitude of the added ventilatory drive is illustrated in Figure 2.37 and Table 2.3.

Although net lactic acid production, through its H^+, stimulates breathing, causing hyperventilation, it might induce dyspnea in the ventilatory-limited subject. However, the lactic acidosis might provide more benefit than hindrance to the normal subject during the performance of high-intensity exercise because of the following:

1. The facilitation of oxyhemoglobin dissociation through the Bohr effect, thereby allowing increased O_2 extraction from blood

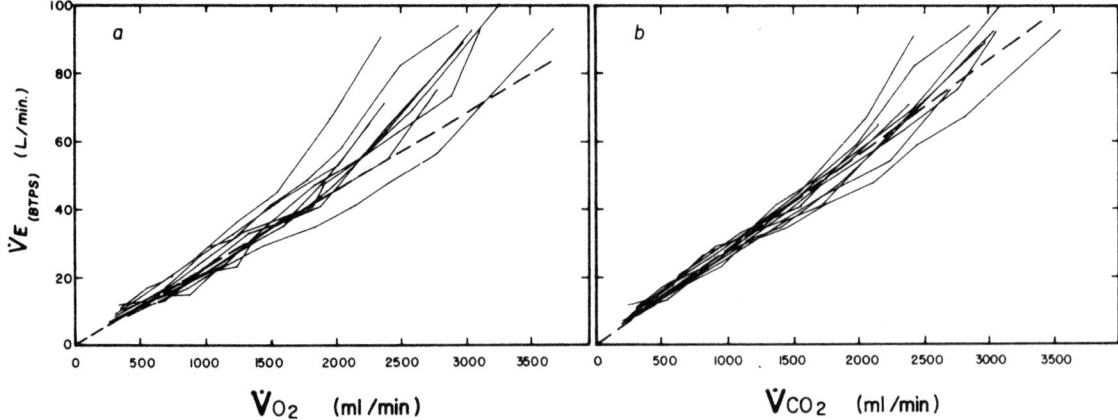

FIGURE 2.37.   Relationship between steady-state minute ventilation ($\dot{V}E$) and oxygen consumption ($\dot{V}O_2$), and CO_2 production ($\dot{V}CO_2$) in ten normal subjects. The curvilinear increase in ventilation at high metabolic rates reflects respiratory compensation for the metabolic acidosis. The reduced dispersion noted in the correlation between $\dot{V}E$ and $\dot{V}CO_2$, as compared with $\dot{V}E$ and $\dot{V}O_2$, reflects the functional dependence of ventilation on CO_2 flow to the lungs and the effect of differences in RQ among the subjects. (From Wasserman K, VanKessel AL, Burton GG. Interaction of physiological mechanisms during exercise. *J Appl Physiol* 1967;22:71–85, with permission.)

TABLE 2.3. Increase in Blood Lactate (Δ Lactate), V̇E, and Heart Rate at 6 Minutes of Work Rate of 200 W

Subject	Δ Lactate (Mmol/L)	V̇E (L/min)	Heart Rate (beats/min)
1	1.9	60	156
2	2.7	81	163
3	5.0	79	151
4	5.1	85	153
5	9.7	151	186

2. The increased arterial O_2 content resulting from the hemoconcentration that takes place above the *AT*
3. The local vasodilatation caused by the tissue acidosis
4. The hyperventilation-induced increase in Pa_{O_2}, which can maintain or even increase Pa_{O_2}, particularly important to the subject performing exercise at high altitude

Catecholamines

The plasma catecholamines increase at work rates above the *LT* (100). Therefore, increases in epinephrine and norepinephrine concentrations cannot account for the *LT*. The increases might represent a cardiovascular compensatory mechanism for the anaerobic stress. Similar changes are reported to take place, but at lower work rates, in patients with chronic heart failure (101,102).

Rate–Pressure Product

The product of heart rate and systolic pressure increases during exercise, becoming more steep above the *AT* (103). The increase in slope suggests that myocardial work is increasing. The increasing catecholamine levels possibly contribute to the steepening in the rate–pressure product. The increasing rate–pressure product above the *AT* might be a mechanism that serves to enhance O_2 delivery to muscle when there is an imbalance between O_2 demand and O_2 supply.

Anaerobic, Lactate, and Lactic Acidosis Thresholds

When increasing work rate, an energetic demand is reached at which aerobic regeneration of *ATP* is partially limited by the O_2 supply. Thus, at this V̇o₂,

anaerobic glycolysis supplements the aerobic *ATP*-regenerating mechanism, resulting in increases in lactate and lactate/pyruvate (L/P) ratio. This V̇o₂ has been termed the *anaerobic threshold* (*AT*) (104). The mechanistic basis for the anaerobic threshold, and the changes in gas exchange that accompany it, are as follows.

1. During exercise, the increased O_2 required by the metabolically active muscles can create an O_2 supply/demand imbalance so that capillary P_{O_2} falls to its lowest value compatible with diffusion (critical capillary P_{O_2}); this is reflected in a minimal end-capillary P_{O_2} and a net increase in lactate production as work rate or exercise time increases further (Fig. 2.16).
2. The imbalance between the O_2 supply and O_2 requirement causes the proton-scavenging mitochondrial membrane proton shuttle (Fig. 2.1) to lose pace with the rate of $NADH + H^+$ production in the cytosol, resulting in a reduction in cytosolic redox state, reflected in an increase in L/P ratio.
3. The accumulating lactic acid is immediately buffered intracellularly, predominantly by HCO_3^-, generating additional CO_2 (Fig. 2.2).
4. HCO_3^- exchanges for lactate across the muscle cell membrane (Fig. 2.2), causing arterial blood HCO_3^- to decrease as lactate increases (Figs. 2.21, 2.22, 2.35, and 2.38).
5. The buffering and acid–base disturbances produce predictable changes in gas exchange (Figs. 2.25, 2.27, and 2.38).

The *AT*, *LT*, and *LAT* are all part of the same physiological phenomenon, an O_2 supply/demand imbalance in the muscle. The distinction in terminology describes the method of measurement and does not dispute their common underlying mechanism, anaerobic metabolism (105). Although these terms are often used interchangeably, we regard the technically correct definitions to be as follows:

- *Anaerobic threshold (AT):* The exercise V̇o₂ above which anaerobically produced high-energy phosphate (~*P*) supplements the aerobically produced ~*P*, with consequent lowering of the cytosolic redox state, increasing L/P ratio, and lactate production at the site of cellular anaerobiosis.
- *Lactate threshold (LT):* The exercise V̇o₂ above which a net increase in lactate production is observed to result in a sustained increase in lactate concentration in the circulating blood, accompanied by an increase in L/P ratio.

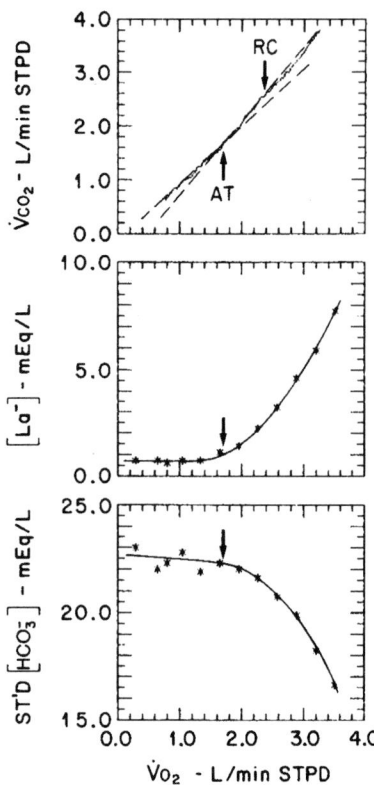

FIGURE 2.38.   Plots of arterial lactate and standard HCO_3^- concentrations and $\dot{V}CO_2$ as a function of $\dot{V}O_2$ for a single subject. Arrows indicate estimates of the anaerobic threshold (AT) from the $\dot{V}CO_2$ vs. $\dot{V}O_2$ plot, which are seen to also represent reasonable estimates of lactate increase and HCO_3^- decrease versus $\dot{V}O_2$. RC is the respiratory compensation point.

• *Lactic acidosis threshold (LAT):* The exercise $\dot{V}O_2$ above which arterial standard HCO_3^- (the principal buffer of lactic acid) is observed to decrease because of a net increase in lactic acid production. During an increasing work rate exercise test, this can be detected by an increase in CO_2 output above that which would be predicted from aerobic metabolism (because of dissociation of HCO_3^- as it buffers lactic acid). The threshold measured by gas exchange is the *LAT*.

METABOLIC-CARDIOVASCULAR-VENTILATORY COUPLING

Cellular Respiration and High-Energy Phosphate Regeneration

Chemical energy, in the form of high-energy phosphate (~P), is utilized at an increased rate when muscles contract. This is regenerated during exercise when mitochondrial respiration (O_2 consumption and CO_2 production) increases. The rate of regeneration of ~P is proportional to cellular O_2 consumption. Creatine ~P concentration rapidly decreases in proportion to the work rate performed (106), and its concentration remains reduced as the work is sustained, returning to the preexercise resting level within the first few minutes of recovery (107).

A scheme describing the gas transport mechanisms for coupling cellular (internal) to pulmonary (external) respiration is shown in Figure 1.3. When exercise is initiated, high-energy phosphate bonds of preexisting *ATP* are split to support the immediate energy requirements of contracting muscle. The resulting *ADP* is rapidly rephosphorylated to *ATP* from creatine phosphate and the conversion of substrate energy to chemical energy (~P), primarily in muscle mitochondria. Experimental evidence suggests that the increases in concentration of creatine, inorganic phosphate, and *ADP* in the muscle stimulate oxidative phosphorylation, thereby replenishing *ATP* (52,108). This keeps the *ATP* relatively constant during exercise as the metabolic requirement approaches the subject's maximal exercise capacity. Only as maximal work rates are approached does muscle *ATP* concentration start to decrease and the less phosphorylated adenosine compounds increase (50).

Sources of ATP Regeneration Reflected in $\dot{V}O_2$ and $\dot{V}CO_2$ Kinetics

Although the mitochondria are the major site of *ATP* regeneration, two anaerobic sources of *ATP* are used during exercise, the magnitude depending on the work level and the subject's fitness. These are the factors that determine the $\dot{V}O_2$ kinetics and hence the O_2 deficit. The kinetics of $\dot{V}O_2$ are naturally dependent on how adequately the circulation couples external respiration to muscle respiration (see Fig. 1.3). The contributions of the two anaerobic sources for regenerating *ATP*—splitting of phosphocreatine (*PCr*) and anaerobic glycolysis—also depend on how effectively the circulation couples external to cellular respiration. The two anaerobic mechanisms of *ATP* regeneration operate only transiently during moderate and heavy-intensity exercise and need to be restored by aerobic (O_2-requiring) mechanisms in recovery. These mechanisms account for a major part of the O_2 debt.

Of the two anaerobic sources of ~P that contribute to exercise bioenergetics (see Fig. 1.3), the first in time sequence is that derived from the hydrolysis of intramuscular *PCr* (109). Because the circulation cannot respond as quickly as muscle contraction can be initiated, muscle *PCr* serves as a source of ~*P* to regenerate muscle *ATP* at the myofibril during early exercise. This source of ~*P* is immediately available at the start of exercise to supplement the *ATP* in the muscle. Its contribution is complete by the time $\dot{V}_{O_2}$ reaches a steady state (110,111).

When *PCr* is split, the cell pH turns alkaline because *PCr*, an acid molecule at cell pH, produces neutral creatine and a mix of dibasic and monobasic phosphate with a pK (6.8) close to the pH of the cell (112). The resulting alkalinization of the cell causes cation (K^+) excess in the cell and a deficit of H^+ (71). Thus, CO_2, hydrated to H_2CO_3, dissociates into HCO_3^- and H^+. The alkaline cell takes up the H^+, while the HCO_3^- serves to balance the positive charge of K^+ liberated by the decrease in negative charges in the myocyte when PCr undergoes hydrolysis (Fig. 2.25). The net effect of this reaction is the fixation of metabolic CO_2 as HCO_3^- during this early period of exercise. The increase in HCO_3^- balancing the K^+, as it leaves the myocyte, is reflected in the venous blood draining the exercising muscle (71). Thus, femoral vein pH, HCO_3^-, and K^+ increase concurrently (Fig. 2.24).

Femoral vein P_{CO_2} does not increase during this early period of exercise, despite an increase in $\dot{V}_{O_2}$ and decrease in femoral vein P_{O_2}, because metabolic CO_2 is being fixed as HCO_3^- (Fig. 2.24). Because O_2 is being consumed by the body, producing CO_2 that is being fixed as HCO_3^- rather than coming out in the expired gas, the respiratory exchange ratio (RER) decreases during the first minute of exercise (Figs. 2.24 and 2.39). Chuang et al. (113) point out that about two-thirds of the metabolic CO_2 retained in the body during this early period of exercise accounts for the slow increase in $\dot{V}_{CO_2}$ relative to $\dot{V}_{O_2}$ and the decrease in RER during the first minute of exercise (Fig. 2.39). The remainder is attributable to the increase in CO_2 dissolved in tissues as tissue P_{CO_2} increases and to the increase in CO_2 in venous blood due to the Haldane effect (increased binding of CO_2 due to decreasing venous oxyhemoglobin saturation). The increase in CO_2 content in venous blood, other than that due to the Haldane effect, is not part of this component because it is closely offset by the unmeasured O_2 consumed from the venous blood during the same period of exercise.

The second anaerobic mechanism, the anaerobic degradation of glycogen or glucose to lactate, starts after 30 seconds of exercise if the circulatory delivery of O_2 is inadequate (71). This source of *ATP* is particularly important when the energy requirement ex-

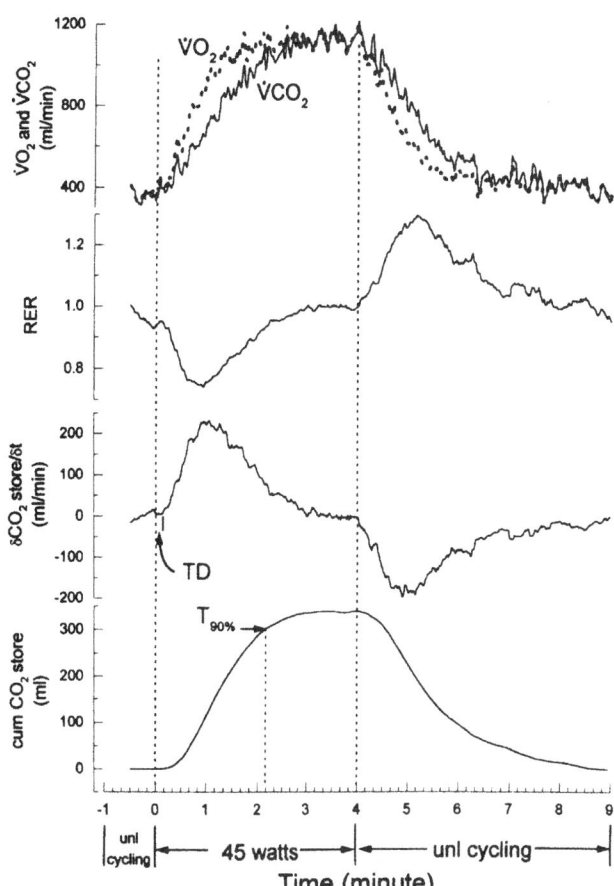

FIGURE 2.39. $\dot{V}_{O_2}$ and $\dot{V}_{CO_2}$ **(top)**, respiratory exchange ratio (RER) **(second from top)**, rate of change in CO_2 **(third from top)**, and the cumulative change in CO_2 store **(bottom)** in response to a 4-minute 60-W constant work rate upright leg cycling exercise, starting at zero time from unloaded cycling, followed by 5-minute unloaded cycling recovery period. The data are second-by-second averages of four replicate tests. TD, time delay for increase in CO_2 stores to be reflected in lung gas exchange; T90%, time for completion of 90% of CO_2 stores. (From Chuang M-L, Ting H, Otsuka T, et al. Aerobically generated CO_2 stored during early exercise. *J Appl Physiol* 1999;87: 1048–1058, with permission.)

ceeds the sum of *PCr* splitting and the aerobic regeneration of ~*P*, for example, when cytoplasmic redox state decreases. This is an exercise intensity defined as being above the subject's anaerobic threshold (Pathway B of Fig. 2.1) (80,81). The *AT* should therefore be a particularly important index of the work rate that can be sustained aerobically (49).

Cardiovascular Coupling to Metabolism: Muscle Oxygen Supply

Cardiac output increases at the start of exercise in the upright position by increasing stroke volume and heart rate. Heart rate increases as vagal tone decreases. Stroke volume increases due to increased venous return resulting from pressure gradients caused by the compression of veins by contracting muscles and decreased intrathoracic pressure accompanying increased depth of breathing (114) and also to increased cardiac inotropy. As exercise continues, further increases in cardiac output are achieved predominantly by increasing heart rate, with stroke volume remaining relatively constant, especially at work rates above approximately 50% of peak $\dot{V}o_2$.

The pulmonary vascular bed dilates at the start of exercise in concert with the increase in right ventricular output and pulmonary artery pressure. This dilatation results in the perfusion of previously unperfused and underperfused lung units in the normal pulmonary vascular bed, accounting for the fact that there is only a small increase in pulmonary artery pressure as pulmonary blood flow increases in the normal lung. A low pulmonary vascular resistance is essential for the normal exercise response of the left ventricle. Without it, the weakly muscled right ventricle could not readily pump the venous blood through the pulmonary circulation to the left side of the heart at a rate fast enough to achieve the increase in cardiac output needed to support cellular respiration.

Because the proportional increase in cardiac output is less than that of $\dot{V}o_2$, the extraction of O_2 from and addition of CO_2 to the muscle capillary blood must increase. Muscle blood flow increases according to its metabolic activity (115). Because of the falling capillary Po_2 and the Bohr effect, it is possible to extract 75% to 85% of the O_2 going through the capillary bed of maximally working muscle.

The oxygen supply to the muscle cells is dependent on five factors:

1. Cardiac output
2. Distribution of perfusion to the tissues in need of O_2
3. Partial pressure profile of O_2 in the capillary blood
4. Hemoglobin concentration
5. Hemoglobin's affinity for O_2

As previously stated, the transport of O_2 from blood to mitochondria is dependent on maintaining an adequate diffusion gradient for O_2 as the blood travels through the contracting muscle. The Po_2 gradient between blood and cell is high at the arterial end of the capillary but decreases as the blood approaches the venous end of the capillary, depending on the O_2 flow–metabolic rate ratio (Fig. 2.14). The critical capillary Po_2 limiting diffusion during exercise appears to be about 20 mm Hg (56,57, 116–119).

Cardiac Output

The cardiac output obviously must play a key role in the O_2 supply to the cells. At the start of exercise in the upright posture, stroke volume increases virtually immediately (120), the magnitude being dependent on the relative degree of the individual's fitness, age, and size (114). In the exceptionally fit young person, the stroke volume can increase by as much as 100%; the increase is much smaller in less fit and elderly people. After the initial increase in stroke volume that takes place at low levels of exercise, cardiac output increase comes about predominantly by increasing heart rate; that is, heart rate usually increases linearly with $\dot{V}o_2$ (see the case studies of normal subjects in Chapter 10). A method for estimating the stroke volume noninvasively from the $\dot{V}o_2$–heart rate relation during progressively increasing exercise is presented in Chapter 9.

Distribution of Peripheral Blood Flow

If the increase in cardiac output is not distributed appropriately to the sites of $\dot{V}o_2$ requirement, their O_2 supply will be compromised. During exercise, the fraction of the cardiac output diverted to the skeletal muscles increases, while the fraction perfusing organs such as the kidney, liver, and gastrointestinal tract decreases (114). The increase in blood flow through the working muscles, and a small fraction through the skin to eliminate some of the heat generated during exercise, accounts for almost all of the increase in cardiac output that takes place during exercise. The mechanism by which blood flow is distributed during exercise depends on the response of the autonomic nervous system and local humoral control. The blood flow–metabolic rate relation affects the level of local humoral factors, such as increased $[H^+]$, Pco_2, $[K^+]$, osmolarity, adenosine, temperature, nitric oxide, and Po_2. These can act locally to regulate blood flow (87).

Arterial Po_2

In the normal subject, arterial Po_2 (Pao_2) is a function of mean alveolar Po_2 (Pao_2). For an idealized lung (all lung units having the same ventilation–perfusion ratio and no diffusion impairment) where the gas exchange ratio is 0.8 and $Paco_2$ is equal to 40 mm Hg, Pao_2 would equal approximately 102 mm Hg at sea level. Reductions in Pao_2 relative to the ideal Pao_2 are due to one or more of the following mechanisms: a right-to-left shunt; O_2 diffusion disequilibrium at the alveolar–capillary interface; or

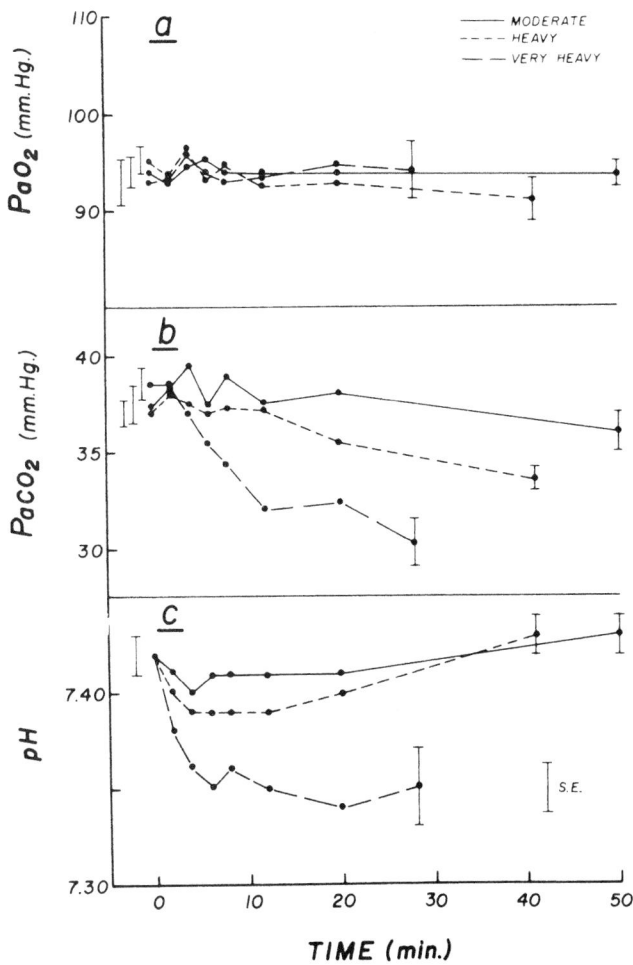

FIGURE 2.40. Effect of prolonged constant work rate exercise of moderate, heavy, and very heavy work intensity on arterial blood gases and pH. Each point is the average of ten subjects. (From Wasserman K, VanKessel AL, Burton GG. Interaction of physiological mechanisms during exercise. *J Appl Physiol* 1967;22:71–85, with permission.)

maldistribution of alveolar ventilation ($\dot{V}A$) with respect to lung perfusion ($\dot{Q}$). Normal young adults have a PaO_2 of about 92 mm Hg (Fig. 2.40) with a $P(A - a)O_2$ of approximately 10 mm Hg during exercise (38). This difference between the alveolar and arterial PO_2 can be attributed to a small right-to-left shunt (possibly the thebesian blood vessels in the heart and the bronchial circulation) and the lack of total uniformity of $\dot{V}A/\dot{Q}$ within the lungs. In highly fit subjects, diffusion impairments have also been described at very high work rates with $P(A - a)O_2$ exceeding 30 mm Hg (121).

Oxyhemoglobin Dissociation in Tissue

Oxyhemoglobin dissociation and the essential role played by the Bohr effect on oxygen extraction were discussed previously (Figs. 2.19 and 2.32). Altered

hemoglobin affinity for O_2, as seen with either congenital or acquired abnormal hemoglobin, may impair muscle O_2 supply. This might be due to either the effect on the arterial O_2 content or on the P_{50} of the hemoglobin (the partial pressure of O_2 in the blood when active hemoglobin is 50% saturated with O_2). Genetic defects causing a shift in the oxyhemoglobin dissociation curve to the left (low P_{50}) can impair O_2 extraction by the exercising muscle, since a "floor" PO_2 for diffusion is reached at a reduced $\dot{V}O_2$. This may induce polycythemia (122).

Hemoglobinopathies that shift oxyhemoglobin dissociation curve to the right (high P_{50}) allow O_2 to unload from hemoglobin more readily and are generally associated with anemia (122). Shifts in P_{50} are common even in normal subjects. A rightward shift resulting from acidosis, increased temperature, or high levels of 2,3-diphosphoglycerate (2,3-DPG) favors diffusion of O_2 from the capillaries into the mitochondria. This contrasts with the leftward shift resulting from alkalosis, carbon monoxide toxicity, or low 2,3-DPG concentration, where the O_2 diffusion gradient is reduced.

Hemoglobin and Arterial Oxygen Content

The arterial O_2 content depends on the arterial PO_2 and hemoglobin concentration that is free to take up O_2. Thus, anemia, resulting in a decreased blood O_2 content, can compromise the supply of O_2 to the tissues during exercise. Hemoglobin that is inactive (methemoglobin) or has carbon monoxide on the O_2 binding sites (as in cigarette smokers) will also result in a reduced O_2 content. All of these conditions will result in a more rapid decrease in capillary PO_2 than normal, and the minimal capillary PO_2 needed for diffusion will be reached at a lower metabolic rate than if all of the hemoglobin were available for O_2 transport. In the presence of anemia or increased concentration of inactive hemoglobin, the blood flow–metabolic rate ratio of the muscle ($\dot{Q}m/\dot{V}O_2m$) must increase to enable a given level of cellular respiration.

Ventilatory Coupling to Metabolism

To remove the CO_2 produced during muscle respiration, the muscles must be perfused by arterialized blood, that is, blood with a PCO_2 low enough to allow CO_2 produced in the cells to diffuse into the muscle blood supply at a rate sufficient to match production. To achieve this, the blood passing through the lungs must be arterialized by eliminating the CO_2 added by the cells while replenishing the O_2 consumed and, simultaneously, achieving

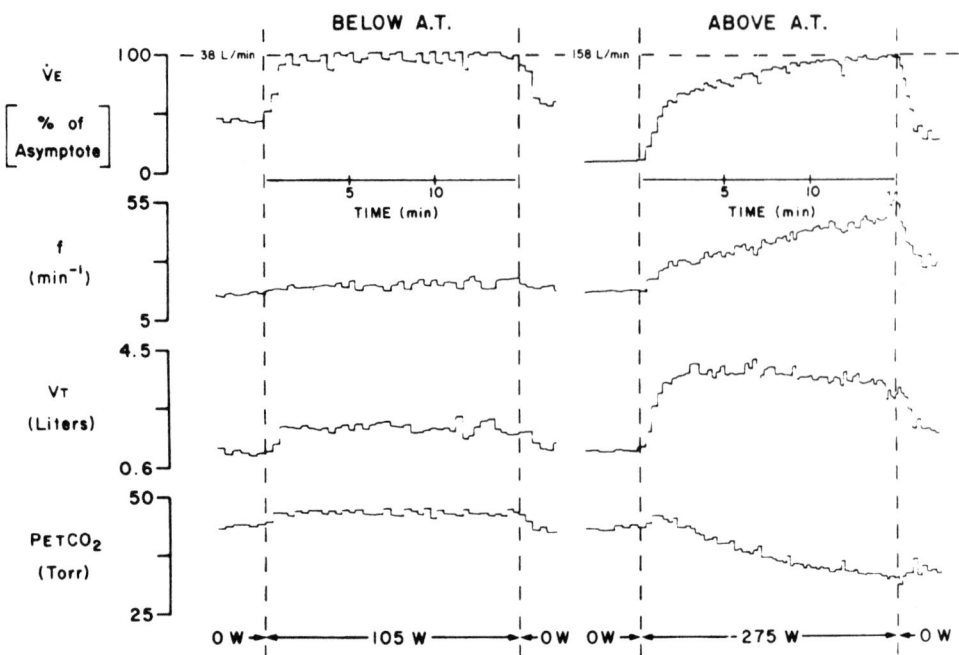

<figure>FIGURE 2.41. Minute ventilation ($\dot{V}E$) plotted as percentage of its asymptotic value, tidal volume (V_T) breathing rate (f), and end-tidal P_{CO_2} (PET_{CO_2}) for exercise below and above the anaerobic threshold in the same subject. The absolute values of minute ventilation are shown to the left of the vertical dashed line at the transition from unloaded cycling (0 W) to the indicated work rate. For the work rate below the anaerobic threshold, $\dot{V}E$, f, V_T, and PET_{CO_2} reach a constant value after several minutes. For the work rate above the anaerobic threshold, $\dot{V}E$ and f continue to increase, and PET_{CO_2} continues to decrease (without a significant change or slight decrease in V_T), signifying the lack of ventilatory steady state.</figure>

pH homeostasis. Minute ventilation ($\dot{V}E$) normally increases at a rate required to remove the CO_2 added to the capillary blood by metabolism and minimize the increase in H^+ concentration when lactic acidosis develops. Below the *AT*, $\dot{V}E$ generally increases so precisely that arterial P_{CO_2} and pH are regulated at approximately resting values (39). Above the *AT*, the metabolic acidosis stimulates ventilation, thereby reducing Pa_{CO_2} and consequently constraining the fall in pH. The ventilatory increase is usually achieved at low and moderate work rates primarily by an increase in tidal volume and, to a lesser degree, breathing frequency (Fig. 2.41). The latter increases to a greater extent at work rates above the *AT*.

Carbon Dioxide Elimination

CO_2 production increases during exercise because of the increase in metabolic activity of the exercising muscles. The amount of CO_2 generated by this process is related to O_2 consumption by the RQ of the muscle substrate. As described earlier and illustrated in Figures 2.35 and 2.36, a substantial amount of additional CO_2 is derived from CO_2 stores when bicarbonate buffers lactic acid at work rates above the *AT*. CO_2 from stores is also added to the expired gas when the ventilatory control mechanism compensates by hyperventilation for the lactic acidosis. In contrast to tissue oxygen supply, the actual cardiac output needed for CO_2 elimination is not critical because CO_2 output is regulated by alveolar ven-

tilation and the resulting arterial P_{CO_2} (Fig. 2.42). However, the cardiac output does determine the venous–arterial CO_2 content difference [$C(a − \bar{v})_{O_2}$] for a given metabolic (exercise) activity.

The venous CO_2 content for a given venous P_{CO_2} is dependent on changes in buffer base and O_2 content (Christiansen-Douglas-Haldane effect) (123). The latter changes most over the lower work rate range (below the *AT*). The former changes

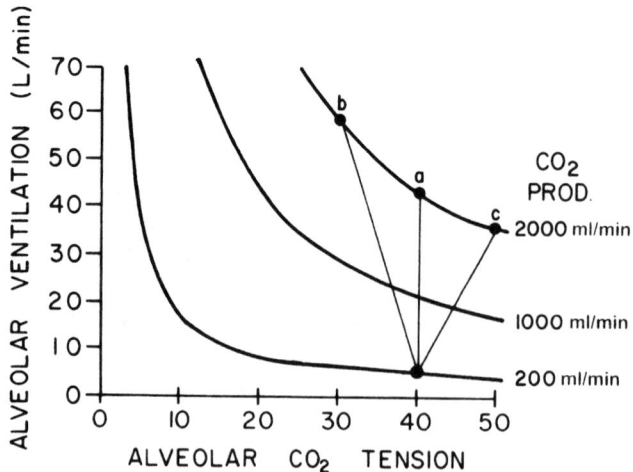

FIGURE 2.42. Effect of changing ideal alveolar (which is equated to arterial) P_{CO_2} during exercise on alveolar ventilation. The point on the CO_2 output isopleth of 200 ml/min represents the normal resting value. Points *a*, *b* and *c* illustrate the alveolar ventilation for isocapnia, hypocapnia (−10 mm Hg), and hypercapnia (+10 mm Hg) for an exercise CO_2 output of 2,000 ml/min. (From Wasserman K. Breathing during exercise. *N Engl J Med* 1978;298:780–785, with permission.)

most over the heavy-intensity range (above the *AT*) due to HCO_3^- buffering of lactic acid. Since these factors affect the position of the CO_2 dissociation curve, estimates of CO_2 content from mixed venous P_{CO_2} alone must be suspect for work rates above the *AT*.

Alveolar Ventilation

The quantity of ventilation required to clear a given amount of CO_2 from the blood ($\dot{V}_{CO_2}$) depends on the CO_2 concentration (F_{ACO_2}) in the alveolar gas ($F_{ACO_2} = P_{ACO_2}/P_B$), where P_B is the barometric pressure and P_{ACO_2} is the ideal alveolar P_{CO_2}. Mass balance considerations dictate that, in an idealized lung, the ventilation–perfusion ratios of all lung units are the same, thereby making the CO_2 concentration the same in all alveolar spaces:

$$\dot{V}_{CO_2} = \dot{V}_A \times (P_{ACO_2}/P_B)$$

or

$$\dot{V}_A = \dot{V}_{CO_2} \times (P_B/P_{ACO_2})$$

This equation derives the theoretical alveolar ventilation ($\dot{V}_A$) required for maximally efficient lungs to regulate P_{ACO_2} for a given $\dot{V}_{CO_2}$. This important relation is plotted in Figure 2.42.

Dead Space Ventilation

Not all respired air ventilates the lungs effectively, because some must ventilate the conducting airways, uninvolved in gas exchange, and some ventilates nonperfused or underperfused alveoli. The difference between the ideal alveolar ventilation and the total ventilation is the physiological dead space ventilation (V_D/V_T). Uneven ventilation relative to perfusion will result in a calculated increase in V_D/V_T and an increase in $\dot{V}_E$ to clear a given volume of CO_2 from the lungs. The reason for this can be seen by referring to Figure 2.42. Given a P_{ACO_2} of 40 mm Hg, composed of equal blood flow from compartments with P_{CO_2} of 50 and 30 mm Hg, the increase in true alveolar ventilation would be dominated by the lung unit with the low alveolar P_{CO_2} (i.e., high-$\dot{V}_A/\dot{Q}$ lung unit). Thus, the mixed expired CO_2 would be relatively low with mismatching of $\dot{V}_A/\dot{Q}$ as compared with that for an ideal lung in which $\dot{V}_A/\dot{Q}$ was perfectly matched.

See Figures 2.43 and 2.44 for illustration of the effect of increase in V_D/V_T on $\dot{V}_E$, and the section "Physical Factors" under "Control of Breathing" later in this chapter for a quantification of the effect

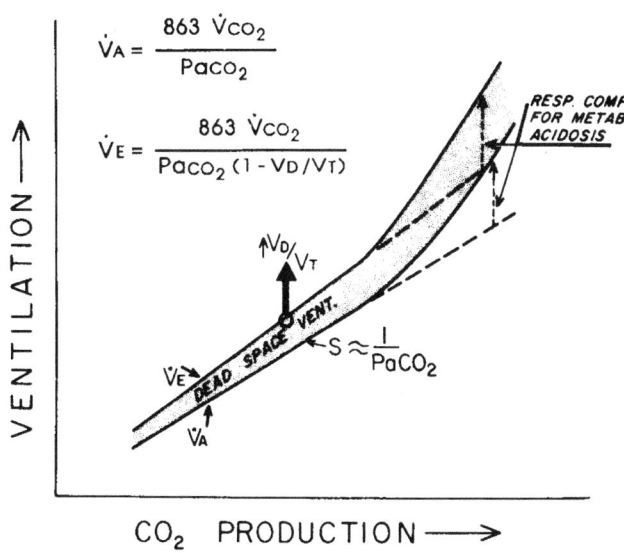

FIGURE 2.43. Factors that determine alveolar and minute ventilation ($\dot{V}_A$ and $\dot{V}_E$, respectively) during exercise are shown in the equations on top of the figure, and the relationships are shown as a graph. V_D/V_T is the ratio of the physiological dead space to the tidal volume, and *S* is the slope of the relationship, shown to be proportional to the reciprocal of the P_{ACO_2}. Respiratory compensation for the metabolic acidosis reduces the P_{ACO_2} value. As P_{ACO_2} decreases, the ventilatory curves become more steep. (Modified from Wasserman K. Breathing during exercise. *N Engl J Med* 1978;298:780–785.)

of increased dead space on the ventilatory response to exercise.

Acid–Base Balance

Because there are acidic end products of the bioenergetic pathways for generating $\sim\!P$ (i.e., the volatile carbonic and the nonvolatile lactic acid), ventilation must keep pace with the acid load if pH homeostasis of body fluids is to be preserved. Figures 2.22 and 2.45 show the acid–base changes in response to constant work rates of moderate, heavy, and very heavy intensity exercise. The ventilatory response does not overshoot the ventilation needed to regulate arterial pH. Characteristically, below the *AT*, the arterial pH is regulated at the resting level or slightly below because of a small increase in P_{ACO_2} (82). For exercise above the *AT*, the acidosis becomes more marked because of the decrease in HCO_3^- caused by net increase in lactic acid production.

Because the change in pH is minimal during moderate-intensity exercise, recovery of pH following exercise is rapid, involving only maintaining P_{ACO_2} at the resting set-point value (Fig. 2.46). At this exercise intensity, only the ventilatory excretion of the exercise-induced increase in CO_2 stores is required. If the exercise is of heavy or very heavy intensity, recovery of pH is slow because it is linked to the rate of regen-

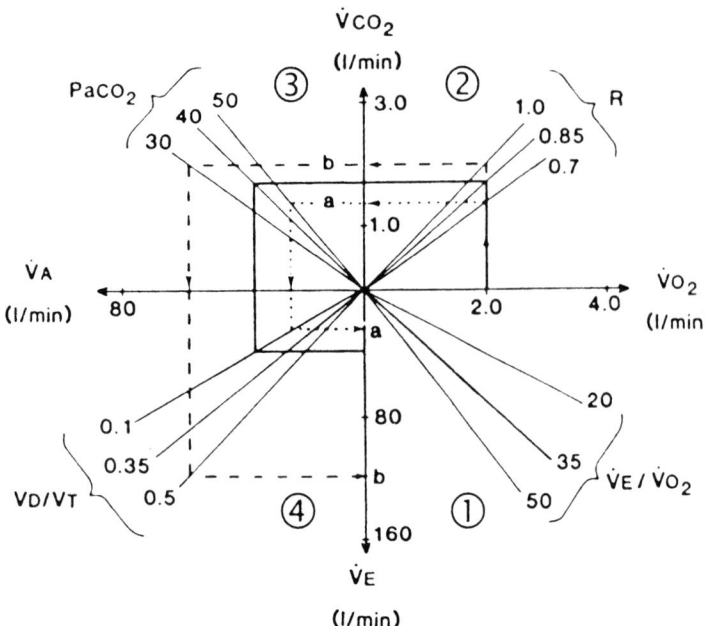

FIGURE 2.44.   Graphic display of influence of respiratory exchange ratio (R), arterial partial pressure of CO_2 ($PaCO_2$), and dead-space fraction of the breath (V_D/V_T) on ventilatory requirement ($\dot{V}_E$) for exercise with an O_2 consumption ($\dot{V}_{O_2}$) of 2 L/min (STPD). The ventilatory requirement can be significantly altered from normal response (*solid line*), with a particular combination of determining variables leading to reduced (*arrow a*) or markedly increased (*arrow b*) $\dot{V}_E$. $\dot{V}_A$, alveolar ventilation. See text for equations showing how the parameter affects the variables in each quadrant. (Modified from Whipp BJ, Pardy RL. Breathing during exercise. In: American Physiological Society, *Handbook of Physiology*, Sect. 3, Vol. III. Bethesda, MD: American Physiological Society, 1985:605.)

eration of HCO_3^-, which, in turn, is dependent on the rate of lactate catabolism (Fig. 2.46) (39).

Effect of Dietary Substrate

Oxygen Consumption

Table 2.4 shows the theoretical high-energy phosphate–gas exchange equivalents for pure carbohydrate and pure fatty acid substrate. Slightly more *ATP* is generated per molecule of O_2 utilized when carbohydrate is the substrate compared with fatty acids ($\sim P{:}O_2 = 6.0$ vs. 5.65, respectively). Consequently, steady-state $\dot{V}_{O_2}$ should be slightly increased for a given work rate when fatty acids are the predominant substrate. This is demonstrated by the experiment shown in Fig. 2.47 (left panel). $\dot{V}_{O_2}$ was measured during constant work rate cycle ergometry

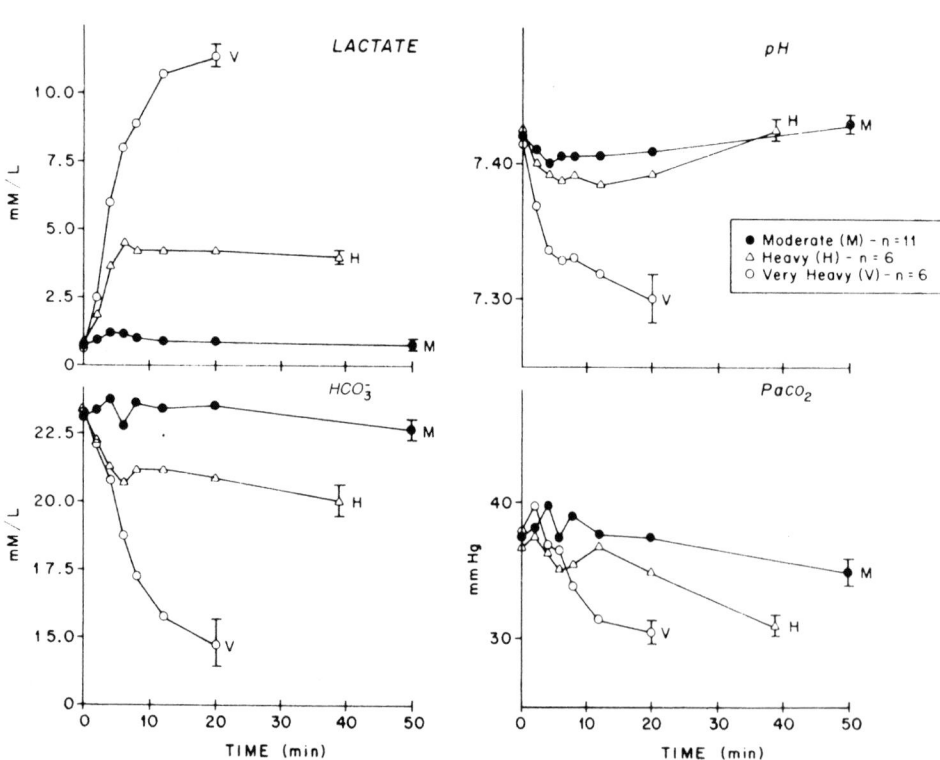

FIGURE 2.45. Time course of change in arterial lactate, bicarbonate, pH, and $PaCO_2$ for moderate, heavy, and very heavy exercise following the onset of constant-load cycle ergometer exercise. Moderate exercise intensity (N = 11) refers to an increase in arterial lactate level of less than 0.8 mmol/L above rest. Heavy exercise intensity (N = 6) refers to an arterial lactate increase at the end of exercise of 2.5 to 4.9 mmol/L above rest. Very heavy intensity exercise (N = 6) refers to a lactate increase of 7 mmol/L or greater above rest at the end of exercise. (Data computed from subjects previously reported in Wasserman K, VanKessel AL, Burton GG. Interaction of physiological mechanisms during exercise. *J Appl Physiol* 1967;22:71–85.)

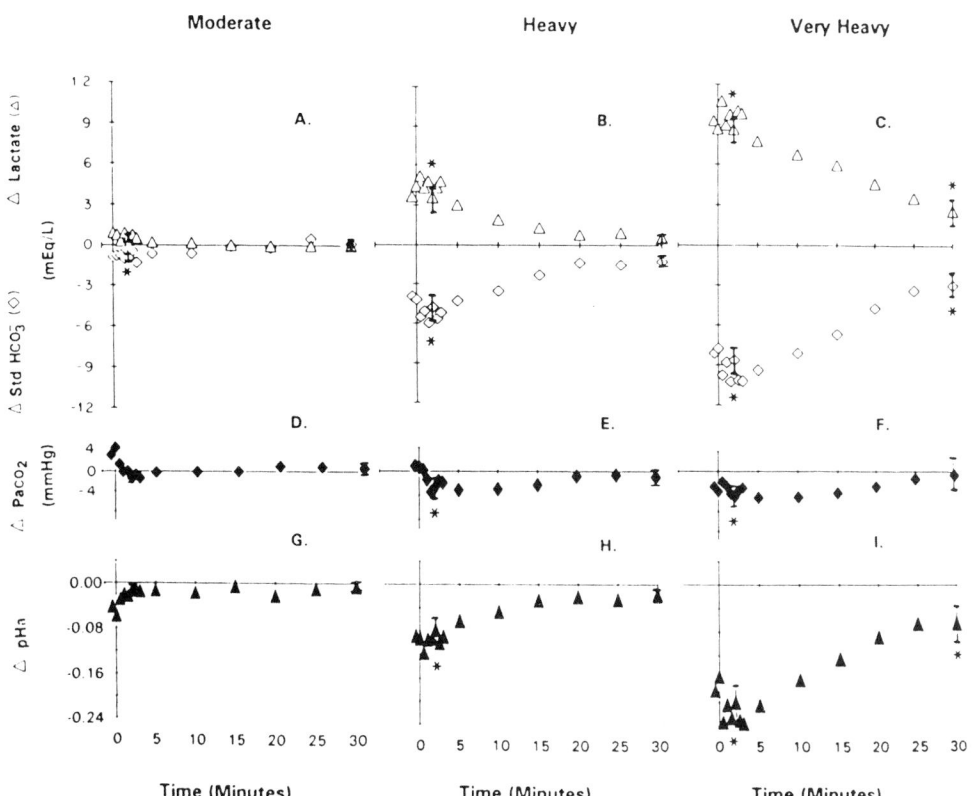

FIGURE 2.46. Changes in lactate, Std HCO_3^-, pHa, and $PaCO_2$ relative to resting values during 30 minutes of recovery from 6 minutes of moderate, heavy, and very heavy constant work rate exercise. Points are the average of eight subjects. At selected times during recovery (2 and 30 minutes), standard errors and significant differences (*$P < 0.05$ from resting value) are provided. (From Stringer W, Casaburi R, Wasserman K. Acid-base regulation during exercise and recovery in man. *J Appl Physiol* 1992; 72:954–961, with permission.)

after the subject consumed a high-carbohydrate diet for three days and a high-fat diet for a similar duration. The $\dot{V}O_2$ is slightly increased, as predicted, when the work task is performed with fatty acids as the dominant substrate than with carbohydrate.

Heart Rate

Because cardiac output increases linearly with $\dot{V}O_2$, the higher $\dot{V}O_2$ required for a given level of exercise when fatty acids are oxidized should predictably demand a higher cardiac output. This is reflected in a slightly higher heart rate when fatty acids are the dominant substrate than when carbohydrate is the predominant fuel (Fig. 2.47, right panel).

Carbon Dioxide Production

While $\dot{V}O_2$ and heart rate are less at a given work rate when carbohydrate is the major substrate, $\dot{V}CO_2$ decreases when fat is the major source of energy (124,125). This is predicted on the basis of the lower RQ for fat than for carbohydrate (Table 2.4). However, the effect is more striking at rest than during exercise. Sue et al. (124) found that a low-carbohydrate diet affected resting much more than exercise $\dot{V}CO_2$, RQ, and $\dot{V}E$. Apparently, the muscles are able to extract carbohydrate from even a low-carbohydrate diet, making the muscle substrate RQ higher than most other organs in the body except for the brain. Thus, the muscles select the most oxygen-efficient fuel possible for aerobic work (Fig. 2.3).

Ventilation

Ventilation is less for a given work rate with a predominant fat substrate, consistent with the hypothesis that the ventilatory control mechanisms are linked to CO_2 exchange (125). When $\dot{V}E$ is plotted as

TABLE 2.4. **Theoretical Gas Exchange and High-Energy Phosphate Yield from Carbohydrate and Free Fatty Acid Oxidation for a Standardized Exercise Bout Requiring an O_2 Uptake of 1 L/min**

	RQ	$\dot{V}O_2$ (L/min)	$\dot{V}CO_2$ (L/min)	~P:O_2	~P:CO_2	O_2:~P	CO_2:~P
Carbohydrate (glucose)	1.0	1.0	1.0	6.00	6.00	0.17	0.17
Free fatty acid (palmitate)	0.7	1.0	0.7	5.65	8.13	0.18	0.12

a function of $\dot{V}CO_2$, the relation is the same whether the RQ is high or low. Thus, a consistent relation is observed among normal subjects when $\dot{V}E$ is plotted against $\dot{V}CO_2$ (Fig. 2.37). However, when $\dot{V}E$ is plotted against $\dot{V}O_2$, there is considerably more variability among subjects. The greater intersubject variability in $\dot{V}E$ with $\dot{V}O_2$ as the independent variable is due to RQ differences among subjects. When a high-RQ substrate is consumed, subjects have a steeper $\dot{V}A$–$\dot{V}O_2$ slope than when a low-RQ substrate is consumed (Fig. 2.44). The mechanism for the curvilinear steepening of $\dot{V}E$ at the higher metabolic rates is accounted for by the ventilatory compensation for metabolic acidosis of heavy exercise shown in Figure 2.43.

CONTROL OF BREATHING

Despite a manifold increase in CO_2 production and O_2 utilization during exercise, the ventilatory control mechanisms normally keep arterial PCO_2 and $[H^+]$ remarkably constant over a wide range of metabolic rates (39,126). Therefore, before getting into specifics on reflex mechanisms controlling ventilation, it is appropriate to review precisely how the ventilatory control mechanisms regulate acid–base balance during exercise.

Acid–Base Regulation

Ventilation appears to be coupled by physiological control mechanisms to CO_2 exchange during exercise. If $\dot{V}E$ did not increase adequately for the increased rate of CO_2 output, a respiratory acidosis would result, with associated disturbances in cellular function. Likewise, if ventilation increased proportionally more than the rate of CO_2 exchange, respiratory alkalosis would result, which would impair cellular function and O_2 unloading from hemoglobin in the muscles. However, exercise usually is an almost isocapnic, isohydric, hypermetabolic state during moderate-intensity exercise (Figs. 2.22 and 2.45). A metabolic acidosis is normally present only for heavy or higher exercise intensities, due to increased blood lactate accumulation. Respiratory acidosis is usually only present transiently in normal subjects because ventilation increase lags the increase in CO_2 output (127). Patients with abnormal respiratory mechanics or impaired chemoreceptor function, or normal subjects breathing through an apparatus that imparts a high resistive load, can develop a significant respiratory acidosis. However, respiratory alkalosis does not typically develop during exercise in normal subjects and is rarely seen in pathophysiological states. Therefore, the physiological mechanism or mechanisms controlling breathing appear to operate with a small transient pH error to the acid side. The ventilatory control mechanism corrects this by increasing ventilation and regulating $PaCO_2$. The precision with which this occurs can best be appreciated by comparing the total H^+ in body water relative to the rate of production. There are only 30 to 40 micromoles of H^+ in the total body water, whereby about 40 millimoles of H^+ equivalents ($\sim 1,000\times$) are produced each minute when walking at about 3 mph.

Figures 2.22 and 2.45 show the acid–base changes in response to constant work rates of moderate, heavy, and very heavy intensity. The ventilatory response does not overshoot that needed to regulate pH. Characteristically, below the AT, the arterial pH is regulated at resting levels or slightly less because of a small increase in $PaCO_2$ (82). For exercise above the AT, the acidosis becomes more marked due to a net increase in lactic acid production. This has a great effect on the ventilatory response to exercise because it increases the CO_2 produced (22.3 mL of CO_2 for each mmol of HCO_3^- decrease in the buffering of lactic acid). To constrain the fall in arterial pH caused by the elevation in lactate, a large ventilatory increase takes place (Fig. 2.29 and Table 2.3). In recovery, as during exercise, pH homeostasis, rather than the level of $PaCO_2$, seems to be the important metabolic determinant of ventilatory control (Fig. 2.46).

Physical Factors

The physical factors that determine the alveolar ventilation were discussed earlier, in the section "Ventilatory Coupling to Metabolism." The current section is concerned with the physical factors that determine the actual ventilation ($\dot{V}E$), that is, the sum of the alveolar ventilation and the respired air that does not participate in normal gas exchange with the pulmonary circulation. $\dot{V}E$ includes ventilation going to the anatomical dead space (conducting, non-alveoli-containing airways) and nonperfused or underperfused alveoli. This is the physiological dead space and is calculated as follows:

$$VD = VT (PaCO_2 - PECO_2)/PaCO_2$$

where $PECO_2$ is the CO_2 concentration in the mixed expired gas, VT is the tidal volume, and VD is the physiological dead space volume. Thus, the differ-

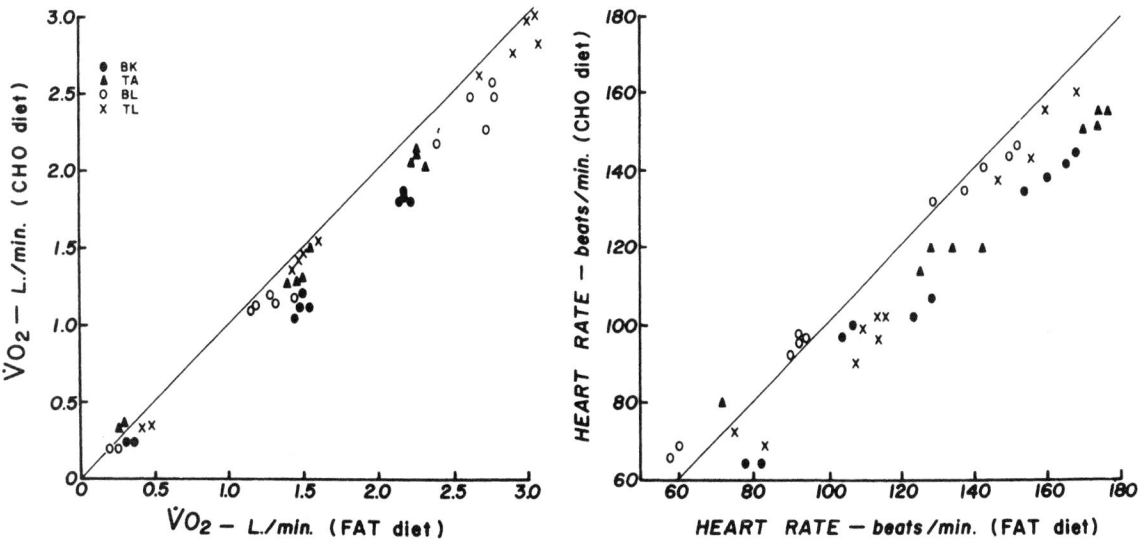

FIGURE 2.47.   Effect of dietary substrate on oxygen consumption and heart rate during exercise. Studies were done on four subjects at rest and during two levels of exercise after three days on a high-carbohydrate diet (RQ at rest = 0.97) and three days on a high-fat diet (RQ at rest = 0.75). The oxygen consumption is higher on the high-fat diet than on the high-carbohydrate diet during the performance of a given work rate. This is consistent with the biochemical evidence that the high-energy phosphate yield from fat is less than that from carbohydrate for a given O_2 cost. Heart rate during exercise is higher on the high-fat diet than on the high-carbohydrate diet, reflecting the link between oxygen consumption and cardiac output.

ence between the actual volume of air respired during breathing ($\dot{V}E$) and the theoretical alveolar ventilation ($\dot{V}A$) is dictated by VD/VT as follows:

$$\dot{V}A = \dot{V}E \,(1 - VD/VT)$$

To determine the $\dot{V}E$ needed to eliminate a given quantity of CO_2, substitute $\dot{V}E\,(1 - VD/VT)$ for $\dot{V}A$ in the alveolar ventilation equation, shown in Figure 2.43, and solve for $\dot{V}E$. The resulting equation is

$$\dot{V}E\ (BTPS) = 863\,\dot{V}CO_2\ (STPD)/PaCO_2\ (1 - VD/VT)$$

where 863 is the product of the barometric pressure, temperature, and water vapor correction factors needed to express $\dot{V}E$ as BTPS, $\dot{V}CO_2$ as STPD, and CO_2 as a partial pressure. From this equation, the quantity of breathing required for exercise is defined by three factors: the $\dot{V}CO_2$; the level or set point at which $PaCO_2$ is regulated by the ventilatory control mechanisms; and the physiological dead space–tidal volume ratio. The influences of these three factors on $\dot{V}E$ are graphically illustrated in Figure 2.43. (By substituting values in the equations shown in the figure, the axes in the figure can be scaled.) At work rates above the AT, $\dot{V}E$ and $\dot{V}A$ increase nonlinearly and steeply as $\dot{V}CO_2$ increases because of the reduction in $PaCO_2$ as part of the ventilatory compensation for the exercise lactic acidosis.

Quadrant 1 of Figure 2.44 shows that the exercise $\dot{V}E$ for a given O_2 cost of exercise (right-going horizontal axis) can be quite variable. The cause for this variability can be described by the physiological factors that contribute to $\dot{V}E$. The first factor is the CO_2 produced as a result of the O_2 cost of work. This is defined by the equation $\dot{V}CO_2 = R \times \dot{V}O_2$ and plotted in quadrant 2. The R isopleths describe the ratio of CO_2 output resulting from aerobic metabolism and HCO_3^- buffering of lactic acid, relative to $\dot{V}O_2$. Quadrant 3 is derived from the alveolar ventilation equation, $\dot{V}CO_2 = \dot{V}A \times PaCO_2$, and takes into account variability in $PaCO_2$. Finally, $\dot{V}E$ is determined by adding the dead space ventilation to $\dot{V}A$ as described in the equation for $\dot{V}E$ given earlier (quadrant 4).

Reflexes Regulating Breathing During Exercise

Despite extensive research, there is no general agreement on the reflexes controlling ventilation during exercise. The observation that arterial pH, PCO_2, and PO_2 are essentially unchanged during moderate-intensity exercise has been difficult to explain mechanistically within the framework of the currently recognized stimuli and the manner by which they are thought to produce their reflex effects. Repeated efforts to discover chemoreceptors in locations where potential stimuli are available (e.g., pulmonary circulation or exercising limbs) in order to explain the exercise hyperpnea, have been largely unsuccessful. The only chemoreceptors that have been clearly demonstrated to play an important role in the hyperpnea of exercise are the carotid bodies; they exert a greater influence above the *AT*, since these are the organs that account for the acute ventilatory compensation for the exercise metabolic acidosis. The carotid bodies also contribute to the speed at which ventilation increases in response to exercise (82,128–130). The following is a brief review of the reflex mechanisms proposed to have a role in exercise hyperpnea. See the reviews by Whipp (126,131) and Wasserman, Whipp, and Casaburi (39) for a more detailed discussion of this subject.

Corticogenic or Conditioned Reflexes

The magnitude of the abrupt increase in $\dot{V}E$ at the start of exercise (Fig. 2.48) varies appreciably from individual to individual. However, high work rates generally result in only a slightly further increase at the start of exercise over that observed for the lightest loads. Consequently, for a mild work rate, the initial increase in $\dot{V}E$ is a larger fraction of the total ventilatory response than that for a heavy work rate (Fig. 2.49). The magnitude of the initial increase in $\dot{V}E$ is also not appreciably affected by different degrees of arterial oxygenation or functionality of the carotid bodies (82). The ventilatory pattern that follows the initial increase is greatly influenced by the work rate in relation to the *AT* (Fig. 2.41) and by carotid body chemosensitivity.

Anxiety might account for part of the immediate ventilatory increase at the start of exercise (phase I) in some subjects. Krogh and Lindhard (132) suggested that the immediate $\dot{V}E$ increase at the start of exercise might originate from the cerebral cortex as a conditioned reflex. Fink and associates (133) suggest that the cerebral cortex may play a role in the exercise hyperpnea beyond the initial ventilatory response. Martin and Mitchell (134) proposed that there may be a strong learning component to the ventilatory response—although this appears to be less prominent, if at all, in humans (135). The studies of Eldridge et al. (136) and DiMarco et al. (137), in cats, suggest that the initial ventilatory stimulus for the exercise hyperpnea might be mediated by the hypothalamus. Despite these important observations describing a neurogenic link to the initial

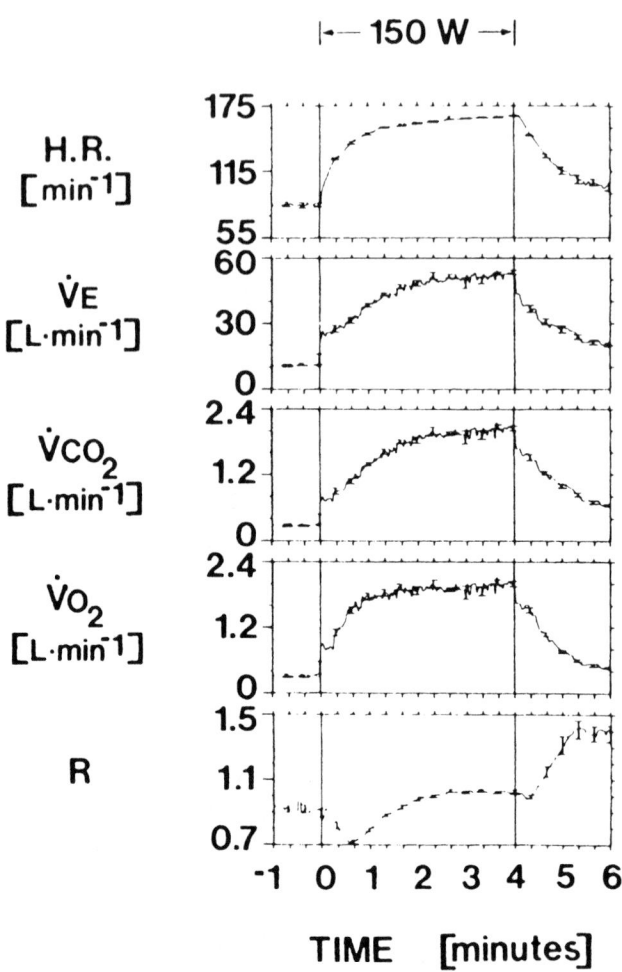

|— 150 W —|

FIGURE 2.48.   Changes in ventilation and gas exchange during cycle ergometer constant work rate exercise starting from rest (zero time) and ending at 4 minutes in a normal subject. This study is the average of six similar repetitions in which gas exchange was measured breath by breath. The vertical bars are the standard errors of the data. The abrupt increase in $\dot{V}E$, $\dot{V}CO_2$, and $\dot{V}O_2$ at the start of exercise (zero time) is termed phase I and thought to be related, mechanistically, to the abrupt increase in cardiac output at the start of exercise. R is usually unchanged from rest for about 15 seconds. The start of phase II is signaled by a decrease in R and is the period of exponential-like increase in $\dot{V}E$, $\dot{V}CO_2$, and $\dot{V}O_2$ to their asymptotes (phase III). This is the period when increasing cellular respiration is reflected in lung gas exchange. R decreases transiently during phase II because $\dot{V}O_2$ increases faster than $\dot{V}CO_2$ due to gas solubility differences in tissues. It usually then increases to a value higher than rest because the RQ of the muscle substrate, being primarily glycogen, is higher than the average RQ of the body, which depends on the RQ of the diet.

and sustained ventilatory response to exercise, the patterns of ventilatory and gas exchange responses in humans suggest that the sustained ventilatory response is predominantly metabolically coupled and that the initial ventilatory (phase I) response might also be linked to the circulatory response to exercise (34,129–131,135–138).

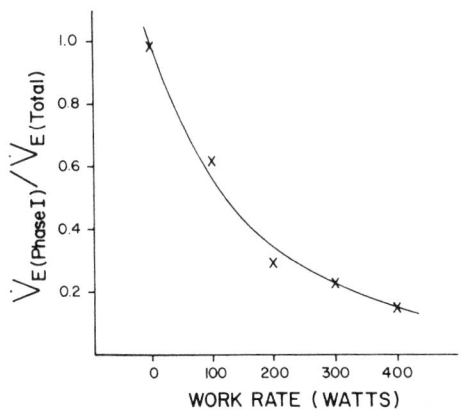

FIGURE 2.49. The magnitude of the phase I ventilatory response to exercise (from rest) as related to steady-state ventilation for various work rates. The higher the work rate, the smaller the fraction of the total ventilatory response attributable to phase I.

Respiratory Center and Central Chemoreceptors

The respiratory center includes collections of neurons in the brainstem that yield a rhythmic discharge to stimulate motor neurons to the respiratory muscles. Medullary lesions associated with tumors, primary hypoventilation syndromes, or central respiratory depression associated with hypoxia-inducing pulmonary diseases can cause the respiratory pacemaker mechanisms to depend on peripheral chemoreceptor input for providing a controlled rhythmic output. The apnea produced by O_2 administration in some patients with arterial hypoxemia is evidence that these pacemaker mechanisms may lose the required rhythmic discharge properties.

The role of the medullary chemoreceptors in ventilatory control during exercise hyperpnea is unclear. Although these chemoreceptors respond to local changes in pH, cerebrospinal fluid acidosis does not occur during exercise. In fact, a respiratory alkalosis is evident in the cerebrospinal fluid at high work rates as a consequence of arterial hypocapnia (132). The central chemoreceptors do not appear to respond to the acute exercise-induced metabolic acidosis (82,133). In adult patients with primary alveolar hypoventilation syndrome (patients with normal pulmonary function but with hypercapnia and markedly diminished or absent ventilatory response to CO_2 breathing), the ventilatory response to exercise is diminished not only because they have rest and exercise hypercapnia (high CO_2 set point) but also because their arterial P_{CO_2}

increases further with exercise (139). However, it is difficult to know if this occurs secondary to central insensitivity to CO_2 or if it is due to a failure of the respiratory center to effectively integrate the afferent stimuli to give an appropriate ventilatory output. Furthermore, children with this syndrome have been reported to have normal ventilatory response to exercise despite absence of response to inhaled CO_2 (140).

Carotid Bodies

Much has been learned about the role of carotid bodies during muscular exercise from studies on selected asthmatic patients who had both carotid bodies resected, but whose baroreceptors were left intact (128,130). The ventilatory response to exercise was studied in these subjects when they (a) were asymptomatic; (b) had normal, or near normal, respiratory function; and (c) had normal exercise tolerance. Their ventilatory responses to exercise were different from those of normal subjects in three ways:

1. The subjects without carotid bodies did not increase their ventilatory drive in response to hypoxia (129), nor did they decrease their ventilatory drive, even transiently, in response to hyperoxia (128).
2. They failed to develop ventilatory compensation for the exercise-induced metabolic acidosis (82) and consequently evidenced a greater arterial acidemia during high-intensity exercise.
3. The rate of increase in ventilation in response to constant-load exercise was slow compared with that of normal subjects, causing a transient arterial hypercapnia (82).

In normal subjects, the ventilatory response to the transition from low work rate to high work rate exercise is slowed and the amplitude is reduced by O_2 breathing (141). Also, O_2 breathing in normal subjects slowed the ventilatory response to a constant work rate challenge in the presence of a lactic acidosis (142). The greater the baseline acidosis, the greater was the attenuation of the ventilatory response. Studies on the acute effect of hyperoxia on $\dot{V}_E$ support the concept that the carotid bodies have an important role in the normal ventilatory response to exercise (143). Although the exact mechanisms mediating this response remain to be elucidated, several potential stimuli of the carotid bodies include increases in P_{CO_2}, K^+, osmolarity, catecholamines, and H^+ and reduction in P_{O_2}. Whatever the precise role of these potential stimuli in the control of breathing during exercise, studies in which exercise ventilation is continuously measured during a switch of the inspired gas from air to 100% O_2 show that ventilation is reduced transiently by only approximately 15% to 20% in normal subjects. However, in patients who develop arterial hypoxemia during exercise, the carotid bodies may account for a much greater proportion of the exercise hyperpnea (see Fig. 4.29).

Aortic Bodies

The aortic bodies seem to be unimportant as ventilatory chemoreceptors in humans, in contrast with their role in some other animal species (e.g., cats and dogs). Removal of the carotid bodies alone has been shown to eliminate the ventilatory response to hypoxia and the acute metabolic acidosis of exercise (82,129).

Vagal Reflexes

The lungs are richly innervated by branches of the vagus nerve. Although investigators have postulated that the vagus nerve might contribute importantly to the exercise hyperpnea, studies on the ventilatory response to exercise in awake dogs by Phillipson et al. (144) showed that vagal blockade, induced by bilateral cooling of the cervical vagus nerves, did not change the overall ventilatory response to exercise, although the breathing pattern was altered. The authors concluded that the vagus nerves were not important in the overall ventilatory response to exercise in dogs at the exercise levels studied (up to 4 times resting $\dot{V}_{O_2}$).

Mechanoreceptors in the Extremities

To explain the exercise hyperpnea, it had been widely postulated that stimulation of position receptors or muscle spindles in the exercising muscle plays a major role in the genesis of exercise hyperpnea (145). The principal argument in favor of an appreciable role for the neural afferents or ergo- or metaboreceptors from exercising muscles stems from the observation of an immediate increase in $\dot{V}_E$ at the start of exercise (phase I) (Fig. 2.48), in advance of the predicted arrival of the products of exercise metabolism to known chemoreceptors.

Neurophysiological studies have helped clarify the possible role of afferents from the exercising limb in mediating the exercise hyperpnea (146). Studies in which the transmission of stimuli in large, myelinated fibers (e.g., transmitting proprioception) was interrupted (147) demonstrate that these receptors play only a small role, if any. Hornbein et al. (148), Hodgson and Mathews (149), and Waldrop et al. (150), using different approaches to stimulate the muscle spindles, demonstrated no significant role for these organs in the exercise hyperpnea. Stimulation of the type III and IV muscle afferents (i.e., unmyelinated or small myelinated neurons) has been demonstrated to induce hyperpnea (151). However, blocking their afferent transmission does not appreciably impair the exercise hyperpnea (152). This is consistent with work that demonstrates that the coupling of $\dot{V}_E$ to metabolic rate ($\dot{V}_{CO_2}$) is not abnormal in human subjects with complete spinal cord transection who are caused to "exercise" by means of electrical stimulation of the leg muscles (153,154). Ponikowski and colleagues (155) have postulated that stimulation of muscle ergoreceptors accounts for the increased ventilatory response found in patients with heart failure. But even if ventilatory stimuli originating in the exercising muscles are active during exercise, respiration is not stimulated with enough intensity by these signals to override the mechanisms that regulate arterial pH in normal subjects or patients with heart failure (156).

Cardiodynamic Hyperpnea

Cardiovascular reflexes linked to the ventilatory control mechanism have been put forth as an alternative explanation to that of ergo- or mechanoreceptors in the extremities to account for the immediate increase in $\dot{V}_E$ at the start of exercise (39,138, 157,158). The abrupt increase in venous return at the start of exercise could deliver increased quantities of blood to receptor sites downstream from the pulmonary capillaries (i.e., arterial chemoreceptors). If $\dot{V}_A$ did not keep pace with the increase in pulmonary blood flow, P_{CO_2} and $[H^+]$ would increase and P_{O_2} would decrease at these sites. These changes could provide feedback stimuli to the respiratory control mechanism in less than the circulation time from muscles to arterial chemoreceptors. That this mechanism plays a role in the rapid, immediate (phase I) $\dot{V}_E$ response to upright exercise is evidenced by the observation that the phase I increase in ventilation is attenuated if the same exercise is performed in the supine position so that static, desaturated, CO_2-rich blood is not stored in dependent parts of the body and the resting stroke volume is already at the level found during exercise (159,160).

Linking the phase I increase in $\dot{V}E$ to the abrupt increase in cardiac output (cardiovascular reflex) rather than involving nonmetabolic, neurogenic mechanisms is notionally attractive in that two unlinked neurogenic mechanisms, one for blood flow and one for ventilation, would be unlikely to produce the near-isocapnic hyperpnea so consistently observed from the start through the steady state of moderate-intensity exercise. These control mechanisms, in some way, regulate pH in a predictable fashion. How this is achieved is by no means clear.

GAS EXCHANGE KINETICS

The $\dot{V}E$, $\dot{V}O_2$, and $\dot{V}CO_2$ responses following the onset of constant work rate exercise from rest can be characterized by three time-related phases, as shown by the experimental data in Figure 2.48. The mechanisms of the gas exchange dynamics in response to exercise, as seen in Figure 2.48, are schematized in Figure 2.50.

Phase I is usually characterized by an immediate increase in gas exchange at the start of exercise. It lasts for about 15 seconds and is accounted for by the abrupt increase in pulmonary blood flow consequent to the increase in heart rate and stroke volume at the start of exercise. This is the period before blood from the exercising muscles, modified by cellular metabolism, has appeared in the lungs. Because the composition of this blood was determined under conditions of rest, R characteristically is the same as that at rest (Fig. 2.48).

Phase II for $\dot{V}O_2$ lasts from about 15 seconds after exercise onset to the third minute or so of exercise. It reflects the period of major increase in cellular respiration. If the exercise is below the AT, a steady state in $\dot{V}O_2$ is achieved by 3 minutes for healthy

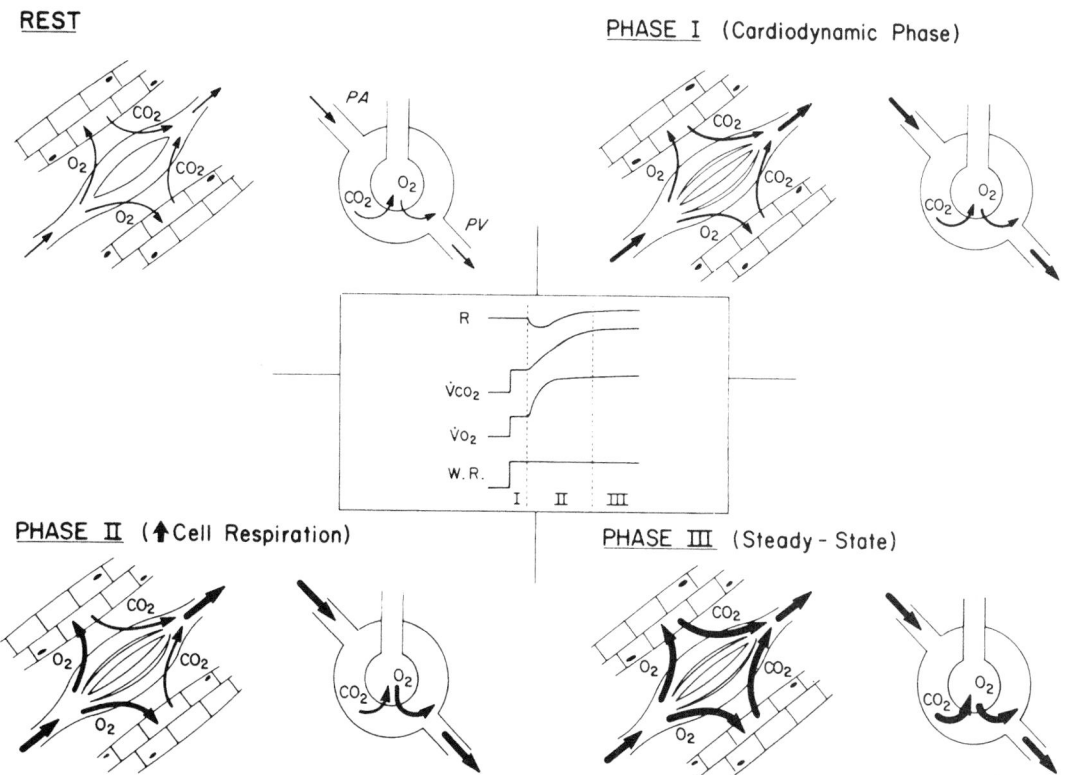

FIGURE 2.50. Gas exchange at the lungs in response to constant work rate exercise **(center diagram)**. Gas exchange at the cell **(left side of each quadrant)** couples to cardiorespiratory gas exchange **(right side of each quadrant)** through cardiovascular adjustments in the lungs and tissues. Phase I gas exchange is postulated to be caused by the immediate increase in cardiac output (pulmonary blood flow) at the start of exercise (cardiodynamic gas exchange). Phase II gas exchange reflects the decreased O_2 content and increased CO_2 content of the venous blood secondary to increased cell respiration as well as a further increase in cardiac output. (See the text section "Sources of *ATP* Regeneration Reflected in $\dot{V}O_2$ and $\dot{V}CO_2$ Kinetics" for an explanation of the decrease in R during phase II). Eventually, a steady state is reached between internal and external respiration (phase III). PA, pulmonary artery; PV, pulmonary vein; W.R., work rate. (From Wasserman K. Coupling of external to internal respiration. *Am Rev Respir Dis* 1984;129(Suppl):S21–S24, with permission.)

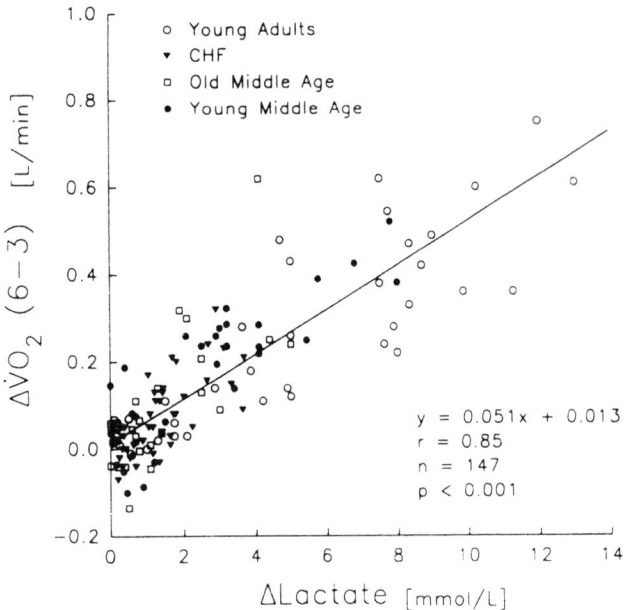

FIGURE 2.51. Increase in blood lactate (above resting value) as related to the difference in oxygen consumption between 3 and 6 minutes of constant work rate exercise in normal, young middle-aged, and late middle-aged adults and in patients with heart failure. Normally, $\dot{V}_{O_2}$ does not increase after 3 minutes when the work is performed below the anaerobic threshold [$\dot{V}_{O_2}$ (6 − 3) = 0]. (Data from Roston WL, Whipp BJ, Davis JA, et al. Oxygen uptake kinetics and lactate concentration during exercise in humans. *Am Rev Respir Dis* 1987;135:1080–1084, and Zhang YY, Wasserman K, Sietsema KE, et al. O_2 uptake kinetics in response to exercise: a measure of tissue anaerobiosis in heart failure. *Chest* 1993;103:735–741, with the data on late middle-aged adults added.)

young subjects (see Fig. 1.4). If the exercise is above the *AT*, the steady state in $\dot{V}_{O_2}$ is delayed or not achieved before the subject fatigues (see Figs. 1.4 and 2.6). Phase III reflects the start of the $\dot{V}_{O_2}$ steady-state period if the work rate is below the *AT*. If the work rate is above the subject's *AT*, the rate of increase in $\dot{V}_{O_2}$ correlates with the magnitude of the lactate increase (Fig. 2.51) (27,32,34).

Oxygen Uptake Kinetics

During the steady state, oxygen uptake from the lungs ($\dot{V}_{O_2}$) reflects the oxygen consumed by the cells (Fig. 2.6). During phase II of exercise, $\dot{V}_{O_2}$ is equal to the O_2 consumed by the cells minus the creditors of the O_2 debt (decrease in oxyhemoglobin of the venous blood, physically dissolved O_2, oxymyoglobin in muscles, *PCr* splitting, and anaerobic glycolysis) (Fig. 2.48). Change in gas stores in the lungs have little effect on $\dot{V}_{O_2}$ kinetics for two reasons: (a) the concentrations of alveolar gases change very little, and (b) in normal subjects, the functional residual capacity (FRC) may decrease, but by no more

than 0.5 liter. Since 0.5 liter of alveolar gas contains about 75 mL of O_2, a change in FRC during phase I or II would have little impact on gas exchange kinetics.

Despite these being relatively small changes, an approach has been described to correct $\dot{V}_{O_2}$ and $\dot{V}_{CO_2}$ kinetics for both change in alveolar concentration and change in lung volume (161). The increase in $\dot{V}_{O_2}$ is determined by the hemodynamic response to exercise [cardiac output and C(a − $\bar{v}$)O_2]. At the onset of moderate exercise, oxygen uptake from the lungs approximately doubles the resting $\dot{V}_{O_2}$ and then remains relatively unchanged during phase I. If C(a − $\bar{v}$)O_2 did not increase during phase I, cardiac output could be inferred to have increased twofold. During upright exercise starting from the motionless sitting position, Casaburi et al. (162) have shown that about one-third of the phase I $\dot{V}_{O_2}$ may be accounted for by the increase in C(a − $\bar{v}$)O_2. This is apparently due to blood stasis during rest in the upright resting condition. If stasis is prevented with elastic wraps on the legs, the abrupt increase in C(a − $\bar{v}$)O_2 at the start of exercise disappears (160). The phase I increase is greatly reduced when exercise is performed in the supine position (159) or following prior mild exercise (163).

During phase II, $\dot{V}_{O_2}$ increases as a single-exponential function with a time constant of approximately 30 to 45 seconds for a work rate below the *AT* (98,164). If the exercise intensity is heavy or very heavy for a normal subject, or if the subject is so impaired that the cardiovascular response is inadequate to supply the total oxygen need, the overall increase in $\dot{V}_{O_2}$ can be significantly slowed, and a steady state is not achieved by 3 minutes (see Figs. 1.4 and 2.36). In this metabolic condition, lactate continues to increase until the $\dot{V}_{O_2}$ reaches an asymptote (165). A steady state in $\dot{V}_{O_2}$ is achieved and can be sustained only when all of the cellular energy requirements are derived from reactions using oxygen transferred from the atmosphere.

Oxygen Deficit

The O_2 deficit is traditionally computed as the difference between the total oxygen uptake during an exercise bout and the product of the steady-state $\dot{V}_{O_2}$ and the exercise duration (Fig. 2.52). A correct estimate of O_2 deficit can be obtained for exercise below the *AT* because the steady state is approached mono-exponentially (166). Above the lactate threshold, however, the complexity of judg-

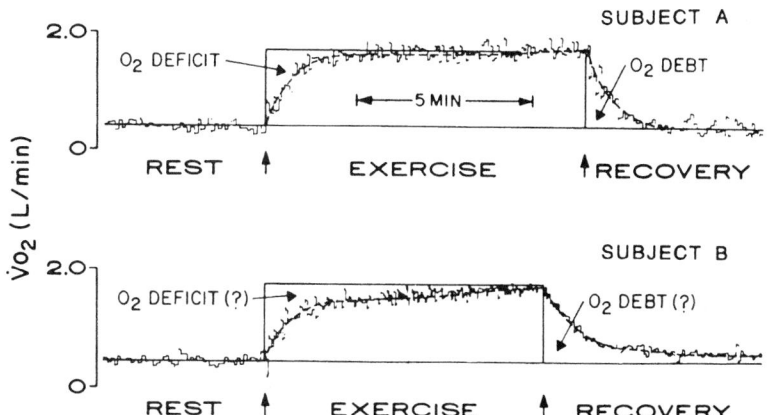

FIGURE 2.52. O_2 uptake kinetics in response to constant work rate exercise of 100 watts in two subjects at different levels of fitness. This figure illustrates the effect of fitness on O_2 deficit and O_2 debt. See the text for precise definitions of O_2 deficit and O_2 debt.

ing the asymptote of the slow phase, and even of assuming that there is a single asymptote, makes a justifiable computation of the deficit tenuous.

Oxygen Debt

The oxygen debt is the difference between the total oxygen uptake in excess of the resting oxygen uptake, or other appropriate control level, during the recovery period (Fig. 2.52) (90). Once $\dot{V}O_2$ reaches a steady state during exercise, the oxygen debt no longer increases, regardless of the exercise duration (167). In this instance, the O_2 debt will be repaid within about 5 minutes of recovery. If the work is above the *AT*, the O_2 debt can be quite high and may not be repaid for an hour or more. The size of the O_2 debt is linked to the increase in blood lactate concentration (168). As long as the oxygen uptake does not reach a steady state and lactate continues to rise during constant work rate exercise, the O_2 deficit and debt will continue to increase. For work levels at which a true steady state in $\dot{V}O_2$ can be achieved (i.e., below the *AT*), the size of the O_2 debt approximates that of the O_2 deficit (166).

Mean Response Time

The averages of replicate, second-by-second measurements of $\dot{V}O_2$, $\dot{V}CO_2$, and R for four different levels of constant work rate exercise are shown in Figure 2.53 for a normal subject. The data are the second-by-second average of four replicate studies. For the 25-watt exercise level, it is evident that about 80% of the $\dot{V}O_2$ required to perform the work (steady-state $\dot{V}O_2$) was achieved during phase I (within 15 seconds of the start of exercise), the cardiodynamic phase of gas exchange. The fraction of the phase I contribution to the steady-state $\dot{V}O_2$ decreases at higher work

rates, so that phase II kinetics become more important in achieving the O_2 requirement.

The subject in this example seems to be at his *AT* at about 100 watts, with $\dot{V}CO_2$ being in steady state by 3 minutes. However, the subject is clearly above his *AT* at 150 watts since $\dot{V}O_2$ continues to increase and $\dot{V}CO_2$ increases above $\dot{V}O_2$. Because the $\dot{V}O_2$ kinetics are informative with respect to determining fitness and the presence of disease in the gas transfer function, there has been considerable interest in quantifying them. Because the actual data do not conform to a single-exponential relation, the *mean response time* (MRT) has been used for quantification of the kinetics of response. The MRT characterizes the combination of the phase I and II $\dot{V}O_2$ dynamics and is obtained by performing a single-exponential fit through the overall response, treated as if it were mono-exponential from exercise onset. The time constant of the exponential (63% of the asymptotic response) is defined as the MRT (Fig. 2.54).

The $\dot{V}O_2$ MRTs of ten different subjects at five different work rates as related to their fitness (maximum $\dot{V}O_2$/kg) are shown in Figure 2.55. This figure shows that MRT is similar among subjects of differing fitness at very low work rates (e.g., unloaded cycling) because even unfit individuals can virtually achieve their steady-state response during phase I of very light work. However, as work rate is increased, the discrimination becomes more obvious; that is, the subjects with the highest $\dot{V}O_2$max have the lowest MRT.

In summary, if phase I is a large fraction of the steady-state response for a given work rate, the O_2 deficit (Fig. 2.52) and debt will be small. In contrast, if phase I is small, the O_2 deficit and debt will be relatively large. The O_2 deficit and debt will also be large if the phase II $\dot{V}O_2$ kinetics for a given work rate

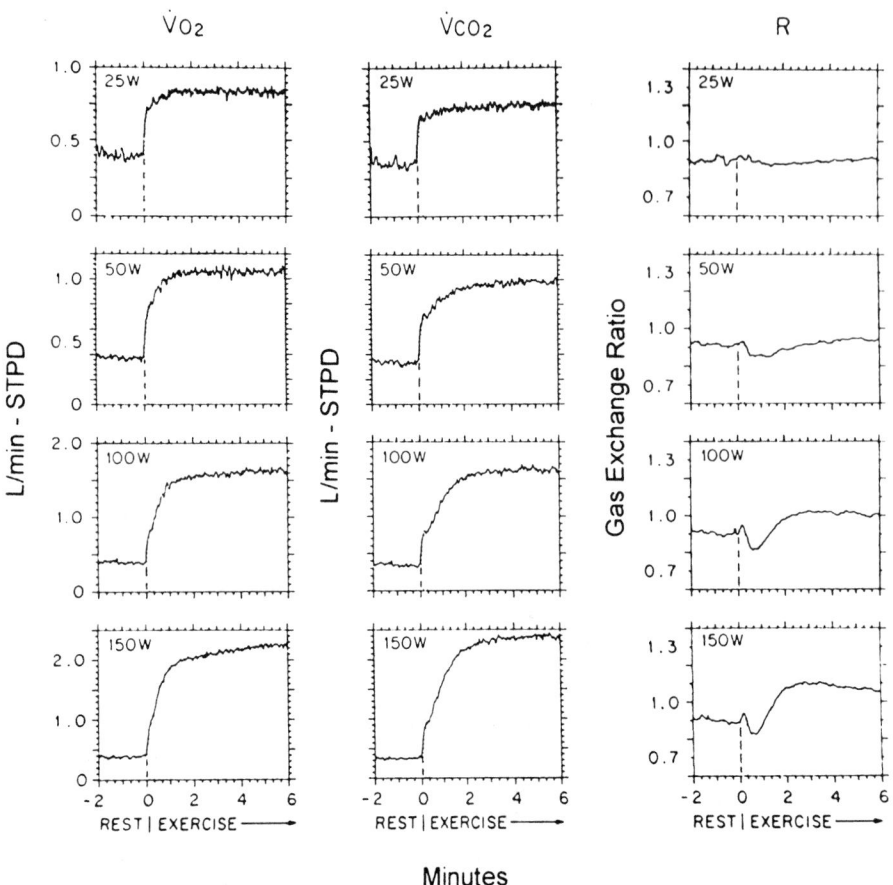

FIGURE 2.53. $\dot{V}O_2$, $\dot{V}CO_2$, and the respiratory gas exchange ratio (R) at four cycle ergometer work rates, starting from rest and cycling for 6 minutes at the work rates indicated. The vertical dashed line indicates the time of start of exercise. The shaded area (15 sec) identifies the period of phase I. Each work rate was repeated four times on different days, and the breath-by-breath data were interpolated second by second. These values were then time-aligned to zero and time-averaged each second to reduce random noise and enhance the reproducible responses. (Data taken from study reported in Sietsema K, Daly JA, Wasserman K. Early dynamics of O_2 uptake and heart rate as affected by exercise work rate. *J Appl Physiol* 1989;67: 2535–2541.)

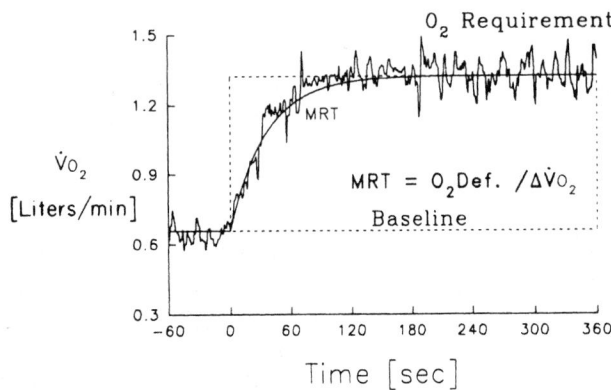

FIGURE 2.54.   Illustration of method for calculating $\dot{V}O_2$ mean response time (MRT) for constant work rate exercise from breath-by-breath data. A single exponential best-fit curve is put through the data, and the time constant (63% of the asymptotic response) for the increase in $\dot{V}O_2$ above baseline is calculated. If there were no O_2 deficit, the $\dot{V}O_2$ would reach a steady state during the first breath, and the MRT would be 0. As shown in the equation, the O_2 deficit can be calculated from the MRT and the increase in $\dot{V}O_2$ above baseline at steady state.

are slow (e.g., the 150-watt work rate in Figure 2.53). Because $\dot{V}O_2$ kinetics are faster for the more fit subject (Fig. 2.55), he or she will have a smaller O_2 deficit and debt for a given work rate.

Carbon Dioxide Output Kinetics

For below-*AT* exercise, $\dot{V}CO_2$ has slower kinetics than $\dot{V}O_2$ (steady state may not occur until approximately 4 minutes). The time of maximum reduction in R is usually at about 30 to 45 seconds (Figs. 2.48 and 2.53). The period of the decrease in R identifies when CO_2 produced aerobically is not being entirely eliminated by the lungs, but is being stored in the tissues (113). The relatively slow kinetics for $\dot{V}CO_2$ might be explained by the following reactions:

1. The hydrolysis of phosphocreatine fixes CO_2 as HCO_3^-.
2. As venous oxyhemoglobin saturation decreases, the reduced hemoglobin is capable of holding more CO_2 at the same PCO_2 (Haldane effect).

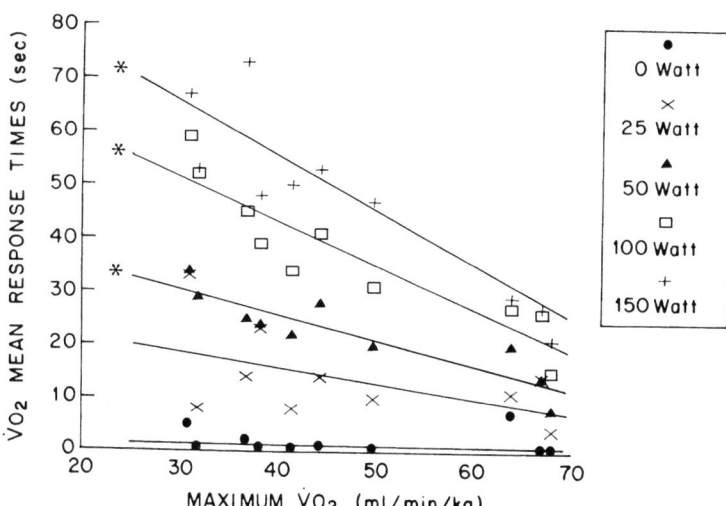

FIGURE 2.55.   Mean response times (MRT) in ten normal subjects, at the work rates indicated, as related to the subject's maximum $\dot{V}O_2$ (peak $\dot{V}O_2$). At work rates of 50 watts and higher, the MRT is greater, the less fit the subject. (From Sietsema K, Daly JA, Wasserman K. Early dynamics of O_2 uptake and heart rate as affected by exercise work rate. *J Appl Physiol* 1989;67:2535–2541, with permission.)

3. The increase in muscle P_{CO_2} puts more CO_2 in physical solution at the same pH.

Because hydrolysis of phosphocreatine contributes to the ~P consumption at the beginning of exercise, and this reaction produces an alkalinizing reaction (169,170), CO_2 produced in the muscle from aerobic metabolism is fixed as HCO_3^-. Thus, $\dot{V}CO_2$ increases more slowly than $\dot{V}O_2$, and R decreases (from approximately 15 to 45 seconds after the onset of constant work rate exercise) before it increases (Figs. 2.48 and 2.53) (113). The increase in R to a constant value (after the decrease) reflects the effect of the substrate RQ in the muscle. If a lactic acidosis occurs during the exercise, $\dot{V}CO_2$ increases faster than $\dot{V}O_2$ due to the additional CO_2 formed as HCO_3^- dissociates during the buffering reaction (Fig. 2.42). This generally starts after about 40 seconds of constant work rate exercise (Fig. 2.35). Thus, R will overshoot the steady-state R, as seen at 150 watts for the subject illustrated in Figure 2.53, until lactate stops increasing.

If the work rate being studied is below the *AT*, true homeostasis occurs in phase III, and $\dot{V}O_2$ and $\dot{V}CO_2$ achieve true steady-state values (Fig. 1.4, upper panel, and three lowest work rates in Figs. 2.36 and 2.53). For exercise above the *AT*, $\dot{V}O_2$ will not achieve a steady state by 3 minutes but will continue to increase (Fig. 1.4, lower panel; four highest work rates of Fig. 2.36; and 150 watts of Fig. 2.53). In contrast, the slow increase observed for $\dot{V}O_2$ is not observed for $\dot{V}CO_2$. The additional CO_2 produced when HCO_3^- buffers the lactate causes $\dot{V}CO_2$ to increase to a higher value than $\dot{V}O_2$ (Figs. 2.35 and 2.36).

SUMMARY

The major physiological responses to exercise are summarized in Figure 1.3. Approximately 28% of the calories generated during work are transformed into useful external work, while the remaining 72% are lost primarily as heat. The oxidative energy obtained from oxygen creditors (hemoglobin, myoglobin, creatine ~P, and pyruvate conversion to lactate) during the O_2 deficit period, which must be repaid during the recovery period of exercise as the O_2 debt, varies with the work rate. If the subject is very fit for the work rate, the O_2 deficit and debt are relatively small. At moderate work rates, the pyruvate-to-lactate mechanism provides none or a very small fraction of the creditors of the O_2 deficit; in contrast, for very heavy work rates the pyruvate-to-lactate mechanism may account for upward of 80% of the total deficit (38).

Gas exchange during exercise should be considered from the standpoint of cellular respiration and how cardiovascular and ventilatory mechanisms are coupled to it. Not only does the magnitude of cellular respiration affect external respiration, but, importantly, the degree to which the work rate is above the subject's *AT* has a major influence on the ventilatory response to exercise. Exercise above the *AT* causes increased CO_2 and H^+ production, both having powerful effects as ventilatory stimuli. The gas exchange kinetics are also altered and exercise endurance is reduced above the *AT*.

The peripheral blood flow distribution appears to depend on the work rate and local humoral factors that optimize the O_2 (blood) flow–metabolic rate relationship. Normally, cardiac output is linearly correlated with oxygen consumption. Because of local control mechanisms, uniformity in the ratio of muscle blood flow to O_2 consumption keeps the slope relatively low (approximately 6 liters flow per liter O_2 consumption). The uniformity enables the muscle end-capillary PO_2 to be sufficiently high to allow as much as 85% of the O_2 to be extracted from the capillary blood during maximal exercise.

During exercise, minute ventilation responds to the changing rate of CO_2 delivered to the lungs, including that generated by aerobic oxidation of energy substrate and that generated by the buffering of lactic acid by HCO_3^-. In addition, the carotid bodies are stimulated by H^+, providing further ventilatory drive. Exercise ventilation is also determined by the size of the physiological dead space ventilation and the level at which arterial PCO_2 is regulated. Arterial PO_2 remains relatively constant during exercise, despite increasing $\dot{V}O_2$.

Incremental exercise tests that dynamically measure $\dot{V}O_2$ and $\dot{V}CO_2$ allow detection of the *AT* by gas exchange. Also, breath-by-breath measurements of $\dot{V}O_2$ and $\dot{V}CO_2$ during constant work rate exercise can be used to determine if the exercise is being performed with or without a lactic acidosis and to estimate the magnitude of the lactate increase at the work rate performed.

$\dot{V}O_2$, $\dot{V}CO_2$, and $\dot{V}E$ abruptly increase at the start of exercise (phase I), particularly when the exercise is performed in the upright position. After the first 15 seconds of constant-load exercise, $\dot{V}O_2$, $\dot{V}CO_2$, and $\dot{V}E$ rise exponentially (phase II) to a steady state or an asymptote (phase III). Their kinetics are influenced by cellular metabolism and the O_2 and CO_2 storage capacities in tissues. During phases II and III, $\dot{V}E$ closely follows the changing rate of CO_2 delivery to the lungs rather than the actual CO_2 produced or the O_2 consumed, if the exercise is performed without a lactic acidosis. $\dot{V}E$ increases disproportionately to $\dot{V}CO_2$ when the exercise induces a lactic acidosis. Breath-by-breath gas exchange measurements provide insight into mechanisms of respiratory control and the state of cellular respiration.

References

1. Saltin B, Gollnick PD. Skeletal muscle adaptability: significance for metabolism and performance. In: Peachey LD, Adrian RH, Greiger SR, eds. *Handbook of physiology*. Bethesda, MD: American Physiological Society, 1983:555–631.

2. Goldspink G. Gene expression in skeletal muscle. *Biochem Soc Trans* 2002;30:285–290.

3. Gibbs CL, Gibson WR. Energy production of rat soleus muscle. *Am J Physiol* 1972;223:874–881.

4. Henrickson I, Reitman IS. Quantitative measures of enzyme activities in type I and type II muscle fibres of man after training. *Acta Physiol Scand* 1976;97:392–397.

5. Buller A, Eccles I, Eccles R. Differentiation of fast and slow muscles in the cat hind limb. *J Physiol* 1960;97:399–416.

6. Karlsson J. Introduction: basics in human skeletal muscle metabolism. *Int J Sports Med* 1982;2:1–5.

7. Essen B. Intramuscular substrate utilization. *Ann N Y Acad Sci* 1977;301:30–44.

8. Lehninger AL. *Biochemistry*. New York: Worth Publishers, 1971:407.

9. Cooper DM, Wasserman DH, Vranic M, Wasserman K. Glucose turnover in response to exercise during high- and low-FIO_2 breathing in man. *Am J Physiol* 1986;251:E209–E214.

10. Idstrom J-P, Subramanian VH, Chance B, Schersten T, Bylund-Fellenius AC. Oxygen dependence of energy metabolism in contracting and recovering rat skeletal muscle. *Am J Physiol* 1985;248:H40–H48.

11. Kushmerick MJ, Conley KE. Energetics of muscle contraction: the whole is less than the sum of its parts. *Biochem Soc Trans* 2002;30:227–231.

12. Wilson DF. Factors affecting the rate and energetics of mitochondrial oxidative phosphorylation. *Med Sci Sports Exerc* 1993;26:37–43.

13. Rossiter HB, Ward SA, Kowalchuk JM, Howe FA, Griffiths JR, Whipp BJ. Dynamic asymmetry of phosphocreatine concentration and O_2 uptake between the on- and off-transients of moderate- and high-intensity exercise in humans. *J Physiol (Lond)* 2002;541: 991–1002.

14. Beaver WL, Wasserman K. Muscle RQ and lactate accumulation from analysis of the $\dot{V}CO_2$-$\dot{V}O_2$ relationship during exercise. *Clin J Sport Med* 1991;1:27–34.

15. Clode M, Campbell EJM. The relationship between gas exchange and changes in blood lactate concentrations during exercise. *Clin Sci* 1969;37:263–272.

16. Cooper CB, Whipp BJ, Cooper DM, Wasserman K. Factors affecting the components of the alveolar CO_2 output-O_2 uptake relationship during incremental exercise in man. *Exp Physiol* 1992;77:51–64.

17. Bergstrom J, Hermansen L, Hultman E, Saltin B. Diet, muscle glycogen and physical performance. *Acta Physiol Scand* 1967;71:140–150.

18. Rosell S, Saltin B. Energy need, delivery, and utilization in muscular exercise. In: Bourne GH, ed. *The structure and function of muscle*. New York: Academic Press, 1973.

19. Simonsen E. Depletion of energy yielding substances. In: Simonsen E, ed. *Physiology of work capacity and fatigue*. Springfield: Charles C. Thomas, 1971.

20. Ahlborg B, Bergstrom J, Ekelund LG, Hultman E. Muscle glycogen and muscle electrolytes during prolonged physical exercise. *Acta Physiol Scand* 1967;70: 129–142.

21. Jones NL. Exercise testing in pulmonary evaluation: rationale, methods, and the normal respiratory response to exercise. *N Engl J Med* 1975;293:541–544.

22. Wasserman DH, Lickley LA, Vranic M. Interactions between glucagon and other counter-regulatory hormones during normoglycemic and hypoglycemic exercise in dogs. *J Clin Invest* 1984;74:1404–1413.

23. Wasserman DH, Cherrington AD. Hepatic fuel metabolism during muscular work: role and regulation. *Am J Physiol* 1991;260:E811–E824.

24. Pozefsky T, Felig P, Tobin ID. Amino acid balance across tissues of the forearm in postabsorptive man. Effects of insulin at two dose levels. *J Clin Invest* 1969;48:2273–2282.

25. Wahren J. Substrate utilization by exercising muscle in man. In: Yin PN, Goodwin IF, eds. *Progress in cardiology*. Philadelphia: Lea & Febiger, 1973:255–280.

26. Wahren J, Felig P, Havel RJ, Jorfeldt L, Pernow B, Saltin B. Amino acid metabolism in McArdle's syndrome. *N Engl J Med* 1973;288:774–777.

27. Whipp BJ, Wasserman K. Oxygen uptake kinetics for various intensities of constant load work. *J Appl Physiol* 1972;33:351–356.

28. Whipp BJ, Mahler M. Dynamics of pulmonary gas exchange during exercise. In: West JB, ed. *Pulmonary gas exchange*. New York: Academic Press, 1980:33–96.

29. Wasserman K, Whipp BJ. Exercise physiology in health and disease (state of the art). *Am Rev Respir Dis* 1975; 112:219–249.

30. Astrand PO, Rodahl K. *Textbook of work physiology*. 2nd ed. New York: McGraw-Hill, 1977.

31. Whipp BJ, Wasserman K. Efficiency of muscular work. *J Appl Physiol* 1969;26:644–648.

32. Roston WL, Whipp BJ, Davis JA, Effros RM, Wasserman K. Oxygen uptake kinetics and lactate concentration during exercise in man. *Am Rev Respir Dis* 1987;135:1080–1084.

33. Koike A, Wasserman K, McKenzie DK, Zanconato S, Weiler-Ravell D. Evidence that diffusion limitation determines oxygen uptake kinetics during exercise in humans. *J Clin Invest* 1990;86:1698–1706.

34. Zhang YY, Wasserman K, Sietsema KE, Barstow TJ, Mizumoto G, Sullivan CS, Ben-Dov I. O_2 uptake kinetics in response to exercise: a measure of tissue anaerobiosis in heart failure. *Chest* 1993;103:735–741.

35. Whipp BJ, Wasserman K. Exercise. In: Murray JF, Nadel JA, eds. *Textbook of respiratory medicine*. Philadelphia: W.B. Saunders, 2000:197–229.

36. Wells JG, Blake B, VanFossan DD. Lactic acid accumulation during work. A suggested standardization of work classification. *J Appl Physiol* 1957;10:51–55.

37. Wasserman K. The anaerobic threshold measurement to evaluate exercise performance. *Am Rev Respir Dis* 1984;129(Suppl):535–540.

38. Wasserman K, VanKessel A, Burton GG. Interaction of physiological mechanisms during exercise. *J Appl Physiol* 1967;22:71–85.

39. Wasserman K, Whipp BJ, Casaburi R. Respiratory control during exercise. In: Cherniack NS, Widdicombe G, eds. *Handbook of physiology*. Bethesda, MD: American Physiological Society, 1986:595–619.

40. Hughson RH, Weisiger KW, Swanson GD. Blood lactate concentration increases as a continuous function in progressive exercise. *J Appl Physiol* 1987; 62:1975–1981.

41. Beaver WL, Wasserman K, Whipp BJ. Improved detection of the lactate threshold during exercise using a log-log transformation. *J Appl Physiol* 1985;59: 1936–1940.

42. Wasserman K, Beaver WL, Whipp BJ. Gas exchange theory and the lactic acidosis (anaerobic) threshold. *Circulation* 1990;81(Suppl II):II-14–II-30.

43. Knuttgen HG, Saltin B. Muscle metabolites and oxygen uptake in short-term submaximal exercise in man. *J Appl Physiol* 1972;32:690–694.

44. Jorfeldt L, Juhlin-Dannfelt A, Karlsson J. Lactate release in relation to tissue lactate in human skeletal muscle during exercise. *J Appl Physiol* 1978;44:350–352.

45. Lindholm A, Saltin B. The physiological and biochemical response of standard-lined horses to exercise of varying speed and duration. *Acta Vet Scand* 1974;15:310–324.

46. Katz A, Sahlin K. Regulation of lactic acid production during exercise. *J Appl Physiol* 1988;65:509–518.

47. Chwalbinska-Moneta J, Rogbergs RA, Costillo DL, Fink WJ. Threshold for muscle lactate accumulation during progressive exercise. *J Appl Physiol* 1983;55: 1178–1186.

48. Ivy JL, Withers RT, Van Handel PJ, Elger DH, Costillo DL. Muscle respiratory capacity and fiber type as determinants of the lactate threshold. *J Appl Physiol* 1980;48:523–527.

49. Wasserman K, Beaver WL, Davis JA, Pu J-Z, Heber D, Whipp BJ. Lactate, pyruvate, and lactate-to-pyruvate ratio during exercise and recovery. *J Appl Physiol* 1985;59:935–940.

50. Bylund-Fellenius AC, Walker PM, Elander A, Holm S, Holm J, Schersten T. Energy metabolism in relation to oxygen, partial pressure in human skeletal muscle during exercise. *Biochem J* 1981;200:247–255.

51. Sahlin K, Harris RD, Nylind B, Hultman E. Lactate content and pH in muscle samples obtained after dynamic exercise. *Pflugers Arch* 1976;367:143–149.

52. Chance B, Mauriello G, Aubert XM. ADP arrival at muscle mitochondria following a twitch. In: Rodahl K, Horvath SM, eds. *Muscle as a tissue*. New York: McGraw-Hill, 1962:128–145.

53. Wittenberg BA, Wittenberg JB. Transport of oxygen in muscle. *Ann Rev Physiol* 1989;51:857–878.

54. Gayeski TEJ, Honig CR. Intracellular P_{O_2} in long axis of individual fibers in working dog gracilis muscle. *Am J Physiol* 1988;254:H1179–H1186.

55. Roughton FJW. Transport of oxygen and carbon dioxide. *Handbook of Physiology*. Bethesda, MD: American Physiological Society, 1964:767–825.

56. Stringer W, Wasserman K, Casaburi R, Porszasz J, Maehara K, French W. Lactic acidosis as a facilitator of oxyhemoglobin dissociation during exercise. *J Appl Physiol* 1994;76:1462–1467.

57. Koike A, Wasserman K, Taniguichi K, Ohtomo N, Hiroe M, Marumo F. The critical capillary P_{O_2} and the anaerobic threshold during exercise in patients with cardiovascular diseases. *J Am Coll Cardiol* 1994;23: 1644–1650.

58. Anderson P, Saltin B. Maximal perfusion of skeletal muscle in man. *J Appl Physiol* 1985;366:233–249.

59. Donald KW, Gloster J, Harris AE, Reeves J, Harris P. The production of lactate acid during exercise in normal subjects and in patients with rheumatic heart disease. *Am Heart J* 1961;62:273–293.

60. Sullivan MJ, Cobb FR. Relation between central and peripheral hemodynamics during exercise in patients with chronic heart failure. *Circulation* 1989;80: 769–781.

61. Wasserman K. Coupling of external to cellular respiration during exercise: the wisdom of the body revisited. *Am J Physiol* 1994;266:E519–E539.

62. Beaver WL, Wasserman K, Whipp BJ. Bicarbonate buffering of lactic acid generated during exercise. *J Appl Physiol* 1986;60:472–478.

63. Stringer W, Casaburi R, Wasserman K. Acid-base regulation during exercise and recovery in man. *J Appl Physiol* 1992;72:954–961.

64. Owles WH. Alterations in the lactic acid content of the blood as a result of light exercise, and associated changes in the CO_2-combining power of the blood and in the alveolar CO_2 pressure. *J Physiol* 1930;69: 214–237.

65. Bouhuys A, Pool J, Binkhorst RA, VanLeeuwen P. Metabolic acidosis of exercise in healthy males. *J Appl Physiol* 1966;21:1040–1046.

66. Yoshida T, Udo M, Chida M, Makiguchi K, Ichioka M, Muraoka I. Arterial blood gases, acid-base balance, and lactate and gas exchange variables during hypoxic exercise. *Int J Sports Med* 1989;10:279–285.

67. Trosper TL, Philipson KD. Lactate transport by cardiac sarcolemmal vesicles. *Am J Physiol* 1987;252: C483–C489.

68. Mainwood GW, Worsley-Brown P, Paterson RA. The metabolic changes in frog satorius muscles during recovery from fatigue at different external bicarbonate concentrations. *Can J Physiol Pharmacol* 1971;50:143–155.

69. Hirsche H, Hombach V, Langhor VD, Wacker U, Busse J. Lactic acid permeation rate in working gastrocnemii of dogs during metabolic alkalosis and acidosis. *Pflugers Arch* 1975;56:209–222.

70. Korotzer B, Jung T, Stringer W, Nguyen P, Jones A, Wasserman K. Effect of acetazolamide on lactate, lactate threshold and acid-base balance during exercise. *Am J Respir Crit Care Med* 1997;83:631–643.

71. Wasserman K, Stringer W, Casaburi R, Zhang YY. Mechanism of the exercise hyperkalemia: an alternate hypothesis. *J Appl Physiol* 1997;83:631–643.

72. Karlsson J. Pyruvate and lactate ratios in muscle tissue and blood during exercise in man. *Acta Physiol Scand* 1971;81:455–458.

73. Sahlin K, Katz A, Henriksson J. Redox state and lactate accumulation in human skeletal muscle during dynamic exercise. *Biochem J* 1987;245:551–556.

74. Vogel JA, Gleser MA. Effect of carbon monoxide on oxygen transport during exercise. *J Appl Physiol* 1972; 32:234–239.

75. Yoshida T, Udo M, Chida M, Ichioka M, Makiguchi K. Effect of hypoxia on arterial and venous blood levels of oxygen, carbon dioxide, hydrogen ions and lactate during incremental forearm exercise. *Eur J Appl Physiol* 1989;58:772–777.

76. Lundin G, Strom G. The concentration of blood lactic acid in man during muscular work in relation to the partial pressure of oxygen of the inspired air. *Acta Physiol Scand* 1947;13:253–266.

77. Hansen JE, Sue DY, Oren A, Wasserman K. Relation of oxygen uptake in work rate in normal men and men with circulatory disorders. *Am J Cardiol* 1987;59: 669–674.

78. Haouzi P, Fukuba Y, Casaburi R, Stringer W, Wasserman K. O_2 uptake kinetics above and below the lactic acidosis threshold during sinusoidal exercise. *J Appl Physiol* 1993;75:1644–1650.

79. Koike A, Weiler-Ravell D, McKenzie DK, Zanconato S, Wasserman K. Evidence that the metabolic acidosis threshold is the anaerobic threshold. *J Appl Physiol* 1990;68:2521–2526.

80. Beaver WL, Wasserman K, Whipp BJ. A new method for detecting the anaerobic threshold by gas exchange. *J Appl Physiol* 1986;60:2020–2027.

81. Wasserman K, Whipp BJ, Koyal S, Beaver WL. Anaerobic threshold and respiratory gas exchange during exercise. *J Appl Physiol* 1973;35:236–243.

82. Wasserman K, Whipp BJ, Koyal SN, Cleary MG. Effect of carotid body resection on ventilatory and acid-base control during exercise. *J Appl Physiol* 1975;39:354–358.

83. Scheuermann BW, Kowalchuk JM. Attenuated respiratory compensation during rapidly incremented ramp exercise. *Respir Physiol* 1998;114:227–238.

84. Ward SA, Whipp BJ. Influence of body CO_2 stores on ventilatory metabolic coupling during exercise. In: Honda Y, Miyamoto Y, Konno K, Widdicombe JG, eds. *Control of breathing and its modeling perspective.* New York: Plenum Press, 1992:425–431.

85. Tanaka K, Matsuura Y, Matsuzaka A, Hirakoba K, Kumagai, Sun SO, Asano K. A longitudinal assessment of anaerobic threshold and distance-running performance. *Med Sci Sports Exerc* 1984;16:278–282.

86. Zoladz JA, Sargeant AJ, Emmerich J, Stoklosa J, Zychowski A. Changes in acid-base status of marathon runners during incremental field test. *Eur J Appl Physiol* 1993;67:71–76.

87. Duling BR. Control of striated muscle blood flow. In: Crystal RG, West JB, eds. *The lung: scientific foundations.* New York: Raven Press, 1991:1497.

88. Kilmartin JV, Rossi-Bernardi L. Interaction of hemoglobin with hydrogen ions, carbon dioxide, and organic phosphates. *Physiol Rev* 1973;53:836–890.

89. Jung T, Korotzer B, Stringer W, Jones A, Wasserman K. Lactate concentration increase and transcellular fluid flux during exercise. *Am J Respir Crit Care Med* 1996; 154(4):A647.

90. Hill AV, Long CNH, Lupton H. Muscular exercise, lactic acid, and the supply and utilization of oxygen. VI. *Proc R Soc Lond* 1924;97:127–137.

91. McGilvery RW. Quantitative significance of lactate production. In: *Biochemistry: a functional approach.* Philadelphia: W.B. Saunders, 1970:268–270.

92. Lewis SF, Vora S, Haller RG. Abnormal oxidative metabolism and O_2 transport in muscle phosphofructokinase deficiency. *J Appl Physiol* 1991;70:391–398.

93. Wasserman K, Nguyen P, Korotzer B, Jung T, Fu P, Stringer W. Arterial plasma electrolyte changes above the lactate threshold. *FASEB J* 1997;11:A214.

94. Kaltreider N, Menely G. The effect of exercise on the volume of the blood. *J Clin Invest* 1940;19:634–637.

95. Beaumont W. Red cell volume with changes in plasma osmolarity during maximal exercise. *J Appl Physiol* 1973;35:47–50.

96. Senay LC, Rogers G, Jooste P. Changes in blood plasma during progressive treadmill and cycle exercise. *J Appl Physiol* 1980;49:59–65.

97. Katz A, Sahlin K. Effect of decreased oxygen availability on NADH and lactate contents in human skeletal muscle during exercise. *Acta Physiol Scand* 1987;131:119–127.

98. Casaburi R, Barstow TJ, Robinson T, Wasserman K. Influence of work rate on ventilatory and gas exchange kinetics. *J Appl Physiol* 1989;67:547–555.

99. Zhang YY, Sietsema KE, Sullivan S, Wasserman K. A method for estimating bicarbonate buffering of lactic acid during constant work rate exercise. *Eur J Appl Physiol* 1994;69:309–315.

100. Weltman A, Wood CM, Womack CJ, Davis SE, Blumer JL, Alvarez J, Sauer K, Gaesser GA. Catecholamine and blood lactate responses to incremental rowing and running exercise. *J Appl Physiol* 1994;76:1144–1149.

101. Richards AM, Nicholls MG, Espiner EA, Lainchbury JG, Troughton RW, Elliott J, Frampton C, Turner J, Crozier IG, Yandle TG. B-Type natriuretic peptides and ejection fraction for prognosis after myocardial infarction. *Circulation* 2003;107:2786–2792.

102. Cohn JN, Levine TB, Olivari MT, Garberg V, Lura D, Francis GS, Simon AB, Rector T. Plasma norepinephrine as a guide to prognosis in patients with chronic congestive heart failure. *N Engl J Med* 1984;311:819–823.

103. Riley M, Maehara K, Porszasz J, Engelen M, Barstow T, Tanaka H, Wasserman K. Association between the anaerobic threshold and the break-point in the double-product-work rate relationship. *Eur J Appl Physiol* 1997;75:14–21.

104. Wasserman K, McIlroy MB. Detecting the threshold of anaerobic metabolism in cardiac patients during exercise. *Am J Cardiol* 1964;14:844–852.

105. Patessio A, Casaburi R, Carone M, Appendini L, Donner CF, Wasserman K. Comparison of gas exchange, lactate and lactic acidosis thresholds in COPD patients. *Am Rev Respir Dis* 1993;148:622–626.

106. Mahler M. First-order kinetics of muscle oxygen consumption, and an equivalent proportionality between QO_2 and phosphorylcreatine level: implications for the control of respiration. *J Gen Physiol* 1985;86:135–165.

107. Yoshida T, Watari H. ^{31}P-Nuclear magnetic resonance spectroscopy study of the time course of energy metabolism during exercise and recovery. *Eur J Appl Physiol* 1993;66:494–499.

108. Chance B, Leigh J, Clark B, Maris J, Kent J, Nioka S, Smith D. Control of oxidative metabolism and oxygen delivery in human skeletal muscle: a steady-state analysis of the work/energy cost transfer function. *Proc Natl Acad Sci USA* 1985;82:8384–8388.

109. Bessman SP, Geiger PJ. Transport of energy in muscle: the phosphorylcreatine shuttle. *Science* 1981;211:448–452.

110. Barstow TJ, Buchthal S, Zanconato S, Cooper DM. Muscle energetics and pulmonary oxygen uptake kinetics during moderate exercise. *J Appl Physiol* 1994;74:1742–1749.

111. Rossiter HB, Ward SA, Doyle VL, Howe FA, Griffiths JR, Whipp BJ. Inferences from pulmonary O_2 uptake with respect to intramuscular [phosphocreatine] kinetics during moderate exercise in humans. *J Physiol* 1999;518:921–932.

112. Yoshida T, Watari H. Changes in intracellular pH during repeated exercise. *Eur J Appl Physiol* 1993;67: 274–278.

113. Chuang ML, Ting H, Otsuka T, Sun XG, Chiu FY, Beaver WL, Hansen JE, Lewis DA, Wasserman K. Aerobically generated CO_2 stored during early exercise. *J Appl Physiol* 1999;87:1048–1058.

114. Rowell LB. *Human circulation regulation during physical stress.* New York: Oxford University Press, 1986: 215.

115. Guyton AC, Jones CE, Coleman TG. Cardiac output in muscular exercise. In: *Cardiac output and its regulation.* Philadelphia: W.B. Saunders, 1973.

116. Agostoni P, Wasserman K, Perego GB, Marenzi GC, Guazzi M, Assanelli E, Lauri G, Guazzi MD. Oxygen transport to muscle during exercise in chronic congestive heart failure secondary to idiopathic dilated cardiomyopathy. *Am J Cardiol* 1997;79:1120–1124.

117. Grassi B, Poole DC, Richardson RS, Knight DR, Erickson BK, Wagner PD. Muscle O_2 uptake kinetics in humans: implications for metabolic control. *J Appl Physiol* 1996;80:988–998.

118. Wagner PD. Diffusive resistance to O_2 transport in muscle. *Acta Physiol Scand* 2000;168:609–614.

119. Maltais F, Jobin J, Sullivan MJ, Bernard S, Whittom F, Killian KJ, Desmeules M, Belanger M, LeBlanc P. Metabolic and hemodynamic responses of lower limb during exercise in patients with COPD. *J Appl Physiol* 1998;84:1573–1580.

120. Loeppky JA, Greene ER, Hoekenga DE, Caprihan A, Luft UC. Beat-by-beat stroke volume assessment by pulsed Doppler in upright and supine exercise. *J Appl Physiol* 1981;50:1173–1182.

121. Dempsey JA, Hanson P, Henderson K. Exercise-induced arterial hypoxemia in healthy humans at sea-level. *J Physiol (Lond)* 1984;355:161–175.

122. Bunn HF, Forget BG. *Hemoglobin: molecular, genetic and clinical aspects.* Philadelphia: W.B. Saunders, 1986:595–616.

123. Christiansen J, Douglas CG, Haldane JS. The absorption and dissociation of carbon dioxide by human blood. *J Physiol* 1914;48:244–271.

124. Sue DY, Chung MM, Grosvenor M, Wasserman K. Effect of altering the proportion of dietary fat and carbohydrate on exercise gas exchange on normal subjects. *Am Rev Respir Dis* 1989;139:1430–1434.

125. Brown SE, Wiener S, Brown RA, Marcarelli PA, Light RW. Exercise performance following a carbohydrate load in chronic airflow obstruction. *J Appl Physiol* 1985;58:1340–1346.

126. Whipp BJ. The control of exercise hyperpnea. In: Hornbein TF, ed. *Regulation of breathing.* New York: Marcel Dekker, 1981:1069–1139.

127. Casaburi R, Whipp BJ, Wasserman K, Beaver WL, Koyal SN. Ventilatory and gas exchange dynamics in response to sinusoidal work. *J Appl Physiol* 1977;42: 300–311.

128. Whipp BJ, Wasserman K. Carotid bodies and ventilatory control dynamics in man. Symposium on recent advances in carotid body physiology. *Fed Proc* 1980; 39:2668–2673.

129. Lugliani R, Whipp BJ, Seard C, Wasserman K. Effect of bilateral carotid-body resection on ventilatory control at rest and during exercise in man. *N Engl J Med* 1971;285:1105–1111.

130. Wasserman K, Whipp BJ. The carotid bodies and respiratory control in man. In: Paintal AS, ed. *Morphology and mechanisms of chemoreceptors.* Delhi: Vallabhbhai Patel Chest Institute, 1976:156–175.

131. Whipp BJ. Breathing during exercise. In: Fishman AP, ed. *Fishman's pulmonary diseases and disorders.* New York: McGraw Hill, 1998:229–241.

132. Krogh A, Lindhard J. The regulation of respiration and circulation during the initial stages of muscular work. *J Physiol* 1913;47:112–136.

133. Fink GR, Adams L, Watson JD, et al. Hyperpnea during and immediately after exercise in man. Evidence of motor cortical involvement. *J Physiol (Lond)* 1995; 489:663–675.

134. Martin PA, Mitchell GS. Long-term modulation of the exercise ventilatory response in goats. *J Physiol (Lond)* 1993;470:601–617.

135. Moosavi SH, Guz A, Adams L. Repeated exercise paired with "imperceptible" dead space loading does not alter VE of subsequent exercise in humans. *J Appl Physiol* 2002;92:1159–1168.

136. Eldridge FL, Millhorn DE, Waldrop TG. Exercise hyperpnea and locomotion: parallel activation from the hypothalamus. *Science* 1981;211:844–846.

137. DiMarco AF, Romaniuk JR, Euler CV, Yamamoto Y. Immediate changes in ventilation and respiratory pattern associated with onset and cessation of locomotion in the cat. *J Physiol (Lond)* 1983;343:1–16.

138. Jones PW, Huszczuk A, Wasserman K. Cardiac output as a controller of ventilation through changes in right ventricular load. *J Appl Physiol* 1982;53:218–224.

139. Lugliani R, Whipp BJ, Brinkman J, Wasserman K. Doxapram hydrochloride: a respiratory stimulant for patients with primary alveolar hypoventilation. *Chest* 1992;76:414–419.

140. Shea SA, Andrews LP, Shannon DC, Banzett RB. Ventilatory responses to exercise in humans lacking ventilatory chemosensitivity. *J Physiol (Lond)* 1993; 469:623–640.

141. Casaburi R, Stremel RW, Whipp BJ, Beaver WL, Wasserman K. Alteration by hyperoxia of ventilatory dynamics during sinusoidal work. *J Appl Physiol* 1980; 48:1083–1091.

142. Oren A, Whipp BJ, Wasserman K. Effect of acid-base status on the kinetics of the ventilatory response to moderate exercise. *J Appl Physiol* 1982;52:1013–1017.

143. Griffiths TL, Henson LC, Whipp BJ. Influence of inspired oxygen concentration on the dynamics of the

exercise hyperpnea in man. *J Physiol* 1986;380:387–403.

144. Phillipson EA, Hickey RF, Bainton CR, Nadel JA. Effect of vagal blockade on regulation of breathing in conscious dogs. *J Appl Physiol* 1970;29:475–479.

145. Dejours P. Control of respiration in muscular exercise. In: Fenn WO, Rahn H, eds. *Handbook of physiology.* Washington, DC: American Physiological Society, 1964:631–638.

146. McCloskey DI, Mitchell JH. Reflex cardiovascular and respiratory responses originating in exercising muscle. *J Physiol (Lond)* 1972;224:173–186.

147. Kao FF. An experimental study of the pathways involved in exercise hyperpnea employing cross-circulation techniques. In: Cunningham DJC, Lloyd BB, eds. *The regulation of human respiration.* Oxford, UK: Blackwell, 1963:461–502.

148. Hornbein TF, Sorensen SC, Parks CR. Role of muscle spindles in lower extremities in breathing during bicycle exercise. *J Appl Physiol* 1969;27:476–479.

149. Hodgson HJF, Mathews PBC. The ineffectiveness of excitation of the primary ending of the muscle spindle by vibration as a respiratory stimulant in the decerebrate cat. *J Physiol (Lond)* 1968;194:555–563.

150. Waldrop TG, Rybicki K, Kaufman MP. Chemical activation of group I and group II muscle afferents has no cardiorespiratory effects. *J Appl Physiol* 1984;56:1223–1228.

151. Kaufman MP, Waldrop TG, Rybicki K, Ordway GA, Mitchell JH. Effects of static and rhythmic contractions on the discharge of group III and IV muscle afferents. *Cardiovasc Res* 1984;18:663–668.

152. Fernandes A, Galbo H, Kjer M, Mitchell JH, Secker NH, Thomas S. Cardiovascular and ventilatory responses to dynamic exercise during epidural anaesthesia in man. *J Physiol (Lond)* 1990;420:281–293.

153. Brice AG, Forster HV, Pan LG, Funahashi A, Hoffman MD, Murphy CL, Lowry TF. Is the hyperpnea of muscular contractions critically dependent on spinal afferents? *J Appl Physiol* 1988;64:226–233.

154. Adams L, Frankel H, Garlic J, Guz A, Murphy K, Semple SJG. The role of spinal cord transmission in the ventilatory response to exercise in man. *J Physiol* 1984;355:85–97.

155. Ponikowski PP, Chua TP, Francis DP, Capucci A, Coats AJS, Piepoli MF. Muscle ergoreceptor overactivity reflects deterioration in clinical status and cardiorespiratory reflex control in chronic heart failure. *Circulation* 2001;104:2324–2330.

156. Wasserman K, Zhang YY, Gitt A, Belardinelli R, Koike A, Lubarsky L, Agostoni PG. Lung function and exercise gas exchange in chronic heart failure. *Circulation* 1997;96:2221–2227.

157. Wasserman K, Whipp BJ, Castagna J. Cardiodynamic hyperpnea: hyperpnea secondary to cardiac output increase. *J Appl Physiol* 1974;36:457–464.

158. Innes JA, Solarte I, Huszczuk A, Yeh E, Whipp BJ, Wasserman K. Respiration during recovery from exercise: effects of trapping and release of femoral blood flow. *J Appl Physiol* 1989;67:2608–2613.

159. Weiler-Ravell D, Whipp BJ, Cooper DM, Wasserman K. The control of breathing at the start of exercise as influenced by posture. *J Appl Physiol* 1983;55:1460–1466.

160. Casaburi R, Cooper CB, Effros RM, Wasserman K. Time course of mixed venous oxygen saturation following various modes of exercise transition. *FASEB J* 1989;3:A849.

161. Beaver WL, Lamarra N, Wasserman K. Breath-by-breath measurement of true alveolar gas exchange. *J Appl Physiol* 1981;51:1662–1675.

162. Casaburi R, Daly J, Hansen JE, Effros RM. Abrupt changes in mixed venous blood gas composition after the onset of exercise. *J Appl Physiol* 1989;67:1106–1112.

163. Whipp BJ, Ward SA, Lamarra N, Davis JA, Wasserman K. Parameters of ventilatory and gas exchange dynamics during exercise. *J Appl Physiol* 1982;52:1506–1513.

164. Brittain CJ, Rossiter HB, Kowalchuk JM, Whipp BJ. Effect of prior metabolic rate on the kinetics of oxygen uptake during moderate-intensity exercise. *Eur J Appl Physiol* 2001;86:125–134.

165. Wasserman K, Casaburi R, Beaver WL, Roston WL, Whipp BJ. Assessing the adequacy of tissue oxygenation during exercise. In: Bryan-Brown CW, Ayres SM, eds. *Oxygen transport and utilization.* Fullerton, CA: Society of Critical Care Medicine, 1987:109–144.

166. Whipp BJ, Seard C, Wasserman K. Oxygen deficit-oxygen debt relationships and efficiency of anaerobic work. *J Appl Physiol* 1970;28:452–456.

167. Schneider EG, Robinson S, Newton JL. Oxygen debt in aerobic work. *J Appl Physiol* 1968;25:58–62.

168. Margaria R, Edwards HT, Dill DB. The possible mechanisms of contracting and paying the oxygen debt and the role of lactic acid in muscular contraction. *Am J Physiol* 1933;106:689–715.

169. Piiper J. Production of lactic acid in heavy exercise and acid-base balance. In: Moret PR, Weber J, Haissly J, Denolin H, eds. *Lactate: physiologic, methodologic and pathologic approach.* New York: Springer-Verlag, 1980: 35–45.

170. Roussel M, Mattei JP, Le Fur Y, Ghattas B, Cozzone PJ, Bendahan D. Metabolic determinants of the onset of acidosis in exercising human muscle: a ^{31}P-MRS study. *J Appl Physiol* 2003;94:1145–1152.

Changes in Blood Gases and pH During Exercise

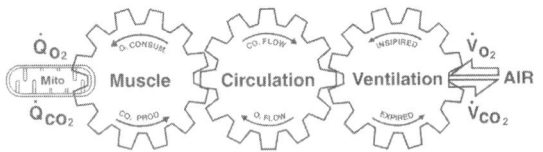

THE ENERGY REQUIREMENT of exercise is supported by the blood transport of oxygen, carbon dioxide, and H$^+$ ion, and the amount of aerobically and anaerobically produced energy dramatically affects the values of these variables in blood. The changes in arterial, venous, and muscle capillary blood gas composition reflect the efficiency of lung gas exchange, cardiovascular function, peripheral blood flow distribution, and muscle metabolism. This chapter describes the changes in oxygen and carbon dioxide content in arterial, mixed venous, and muscle venous blood, the effects of H$^+$ ion concentration on these values, the likely mechanisms responsible for these changes, and the relation of cardiac output to oxygen uptake during exercise in normal subjects.

OXYGEN, CARBON DIOXIDE, AND H$^+$ ION TRANSPORT

Po$_2$

During progressively increasing work (ramp-pattern) cycle ergometer exercise, arterial Po$_2$ at sea level remains high (>80 mm Hg) and relatively constant throughout the exercise bout (Fig. 3.1A), while mixed venous and femoral vein blood Po$_2$ values fall very rapidly to approximately 20 mm Hg, reflecting the increased extraction of O$_2$ in support of muscle metabolism. The mixed venous and femoral vein Po$_2$ values are virtually superimposed from the anaerobic threshold (~54% $\dot{V}o_2$max) to end exercise.

Oxygen Content

Blood oxygen content (Fig. 3.1B) is calculated from hemoglobin concentration [Hb], oxygen saturation (So$_2$), and arterial Po$_2$ (1):

O$_2$ content (ml O$_2$/100 ml)
$$= [Hb] \ (g/dl) \times So_2 \times 1.39 \ ml \ O_2/g \ Hb$$
$$+ \ (0.003 \times Po_2)$$

The oxygen content of blood as a function of Po$_2$ (mm Hg) has a sigmoid relationship (Fig. 3.2), with a plateau value in arterial blood of approximately 20 ml/100 ml in normal adults (using a value of 15 g/dL of hemoglobin). The P$_{50}$, or the partial pressure of oxygen at which the hemoglobin is 50% saturated, is approximately 28 mm Hg at pH = 7.4, Pco$_2$ = 40, and temperature = 37°C. The remarkable characteristic of blood is the increase in oxygen content above that physically dissolved, which is

only 0.3 ml/100 ml at a Po$_2$ of 100 mm Hg. This is related to the strong oxygen-binding properties of the hemoglobin molecule. Arterial oxygen content increases slightly as a function of exercise intensity above the lactic acidosis threshold (*LAT*)(Fig. 3.1B). The values and mechanisms are discussed in Chapter 2.

Mixed venous and femoral vein oxygen contents decrease progressively during exercise. However, the decrease in mixed venous oxygen content above the *LAT* is primarily due to increasing blood acidification (Fig. 3.1E, F) since the Po$_2$ values are virtually unchanged above the *LAT* (Fig. 3.1A). Arteriovenous oxygen content differences [C($\bar{v}$ − a)o$_2$] are maximally increased during peak exercise due to a progressive fall in the mixed venous values and an increase in the arterial oxygen content (Fig. 3.1B).

Several mechanisms assist oxygen content loading in the pulmonary circulation and unloading in the peripheral circulation (1), including hemoglobin.

- *Hemoglobin:* In the lung, hemoglobin exhibits increased O$_2$ affinity as more oxygen molecules are bound to each successive subunit, and hemoglobin has a decreased affinity for oxygen as oxygen molecules are unbound in the muscle capillary bed (steep part of the oxyhemoglobin dissociation curve).
- *Bohr effect:* O$_2$ affinity for hemoglobin increases in the pulmonary capillary blood as H$^+$ and Pco$_2$ are decreased, as in the lung, and O$_2$ affinity decreases in the peripheral capillary blood as H$^+$ and Pco$_2$ increase, as in the muscle.
- *Temperature:* Decreasing temperature shifts the oxyhemoglobin dissociation curve to the left, increasing affinity of hemoglobin for O$_2$, whereas increasing temperature, such as in an active muscle generating heat, shifts the curve to the right, thereby facilitating O$_2$ dissociation from hemoglobin.
- *2,3-diphosphoglycerate (2,3-DPG):* Increasing 2,3-DPG concentrations shift the curve to the right, whereas decreasing concentrations shift the curve to the left (this effect is small compared with H$^+$ ion effect).

A leftward shift of the oxyhemoglobin dissociation curve in the pulmonary capillary bed, where Pco$_2$ decreases and pH increases, assists oxygen loading, whereas a rightward shift enhances oxygen unloading in the muscle, where increased Pco$_2$, reduced pH, and increased temperature are present, particularly during exercise. Therefore, the characteristics of the oxygen content curve with re-

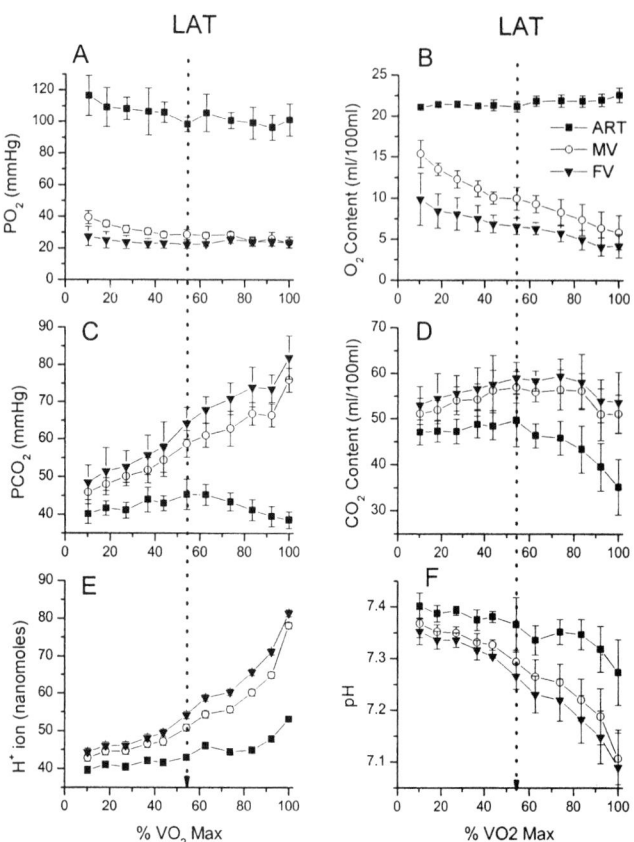

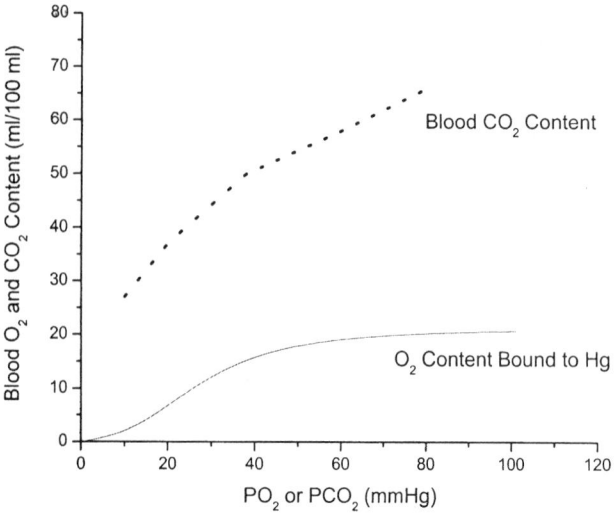

FIGURE 3.2.   Blood carbon dioxide content, oxygen content, and dissolved oxygen in ml/100 ml as a function of partial pressure of O_2 and CO_2. (pH = 7.4, T = 37°C, P_{50} = 28 mm Hg, hemoglobin =15 g/100 ml.) Dissolved oxygen content is 0.3 ml/100 ml at 100 mm Hg P_{O_2}. The increase in arterial oxygen content as a function of P_{O_2} is primarily related to oxygen bound to hemoglobin. Blood CO_2 content as a function of increase in P_{CO_2} is quite steep in the physiologic range. (CO_2 content data are from Christiansen J, Douglas CG, Haldane JS. The dissociation of CO_2 by human blood. *J Appl Physiol* 1913;47:ii).

FIGURE 3.1. P_{O_2} **(A)**, O_2 content **(B)**, P_{CO_2} **(C)**, CO_2 content **(D)**, H^+ ion concentration **(E)**, and pH **(F)** as a function of exercise intensity (%$\dot{V}_{O_2}$max) (mean ± standard deviation) in arterial (■, ART), mixed venous (○, MV), and femoral vein (▼, FV) blood during ramp pattern increasing work rate exercise (N = 5). Lactic acidosis threshold (*LAT*) (54% of $\dot{V}_{O_2}$max) is shown by the vertical dashed line. The results are the average of five normal male subjects. (From Stringer W, Hansen J, Wasserman K. Cardiac output estimated non-invasively from oxygen uptake ($\dot{V}_{O_2}$) during exercise. *J Appl Physiol* 1997;82: 908–912, with permission.)

spect to P_{O_2} are not static, but are subject to change depending on the local environmental and metabolic factors (2).

P_{CO_2}

Arterial P_{CO_2} increases slightly on average during moderate exercise up to the *LAT*, and then decreases below the resting value by the end of exercise (Fig. 3.1C). Mixed venous and femoral vein P_{CO_2} values increase progressively during exercise, with the highest values in the femoral vein. CO_2 content is high relative to arterial oxygen content, approximately 48 ml/100 ml at an arterial P_{CO_2} of 40 mm Hg, compared with an arterial O_2 content of 20 ml/100 ml at a P_{O_2} of 100 mm Hg (Fig. 3.2). Arterial CO_2 content (Fig. 3.1D) remains essentially

constant around 46 ml/100 ml up to the *LAT* metabolic rate. Above that, it decreases dramatically (to 35 ml/100 ml) due to the marked fall in arterial pH and arterial P_{CO_2}. Mixed venous and femoral vein CO_2 content are markedly elevated relative to arterial values and progressively increase until the *LAT*, where progressive acidosis decreases the CO_2 contents. The maximal increase in venous–arterial CO_2 content difference [$C(\bar{v} - a)_{CO_2}$] is due to a more rapid fall in arterial CO_2 content rather than to an increase in mixed venous CO_2 content for exercise above the *LAT*.

H^+ Ion

Arterial H^+ concentration as a function of exercise intensity (Fig. 3.1E) is only slightly increased up to the *LAT*. Above the *LAT* work rate, it begins to increase much more rapidly. Mixed venous and femoral vein H^+ are higher than arterial H^+ during all phases of exercise, increasing more rapidly above the *LAT* to the highest levels at end of exercise. In addition, the values for the mixed venous and femoral vein H^+ were similar throughout exercise, with the femoral vein H^+ being slightly higher. Arterial pH (Fig. 3.1F) decreases slightly up to the

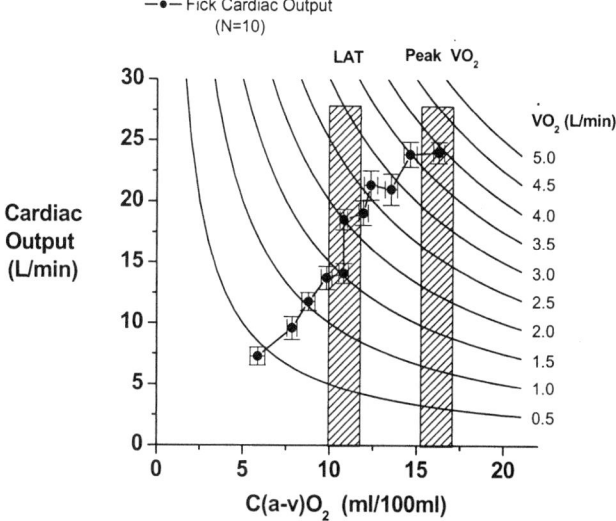

FIGURE 3.3.   Fick cardiac output (C.O.) as a function of arterial–mixed venous oxygen content difference [C(a − v̄)o₂] (mean ± standard error of mean) during exercise for ten studies in five young normal men with mean resting hemoglobin of 15 g/100 ml. V̇o₂ isopleths, as well as the average lactic acidosis threshold (*LAT*) and peak V̇o₂ values (*hashed bars*), are shown. Cardiac output increases on average from 7.5 L/min (unloaded cycling) to approximately 25 L/min at end of exercise, with a value of approximately 15 to 17 L/min at the *LAT*. C(a − v̄)o₂ increases on average from 5 ml/100 ml at rest to 16 ml/100 ml at peak exercise. V̇o₂ increases from below 0.5 L/min for unloaded cycling to 2 L/min at the *LAT*, to nearly 4 L/min at peak exercise. Peak V̇o₂ is dependent upon maximal increases in Fick cardiac output and C(a − v̄)o₂ content difference. (From Stringer W, Hansen J, Wasserman K. Cardiac output estimated non-invasively from oxygen uptake (V̇o₂) during exercise. *J Appl Physiol* 1997;82:908–912, with permission.)

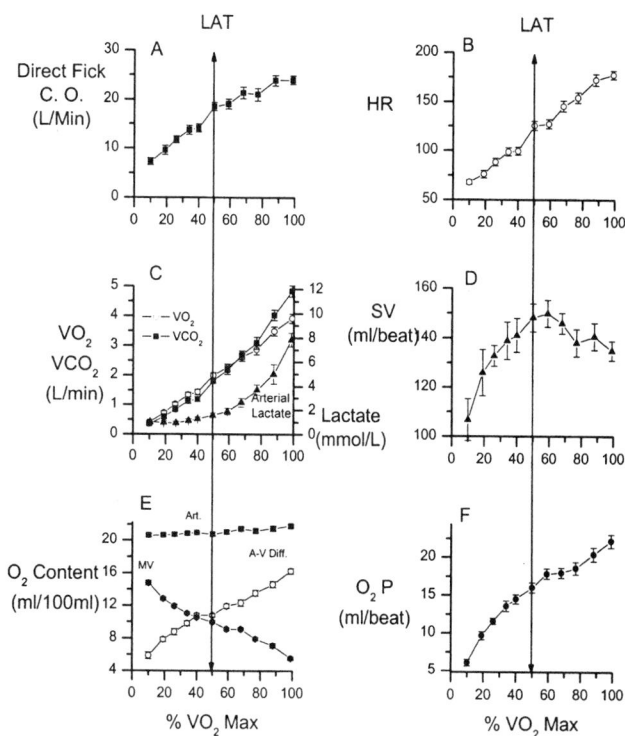

FIGURE 3.4.   Measurement (mean ± standard error of mean of ten studies in five subjects) during a ramp protocol cycle ergometer exercise test for the same subjects shown in Figure 3.3. Cardiac output (C.O., L/min, **A**); heart rate (HR, beats/min, **B**); oxygen uptake (V̇o₂, L/min), carbon dioxide output (V̇co₂, L/min), and arterial lactate (mmol/L) **(C)**; stroke volume (ml/beat, **D**); arterial and mixed venous oxygen contents and a–v oxygen content differences (ml/100 ml, **E**); and O₂ pulse (ml O₂/beat, **F**) (mean ± standard error of mean) in the same subjects as Figure 3.3, as a function of percent V̇o₂max during ramp pattern progressive work rate exercise. Vertical arrows at 50% V̇o₂max mark the mean lactic acidosis threshold (*LAT*). (From Stringer W, Hansen J, Wasserman K. Cardiac output estimated non-invasively from oxygen uptake (V̇o₂) during exercise. *J Appl Physiol* 1997;82:908–912, with permission.)

LAT, and then more rapidly above the *LAT*. Mixed venous and femoral vein pH progressively decrease throughout exercise.

THE RELATION BETWEEN CARDIAC OUTPUT AND OXYGEN UPTAKE DURING EXERCISE

Oxygen uptake (V̇o₂) during exercise (Fig. 3.3) is related to the product of cardiac output and arterial–mixed venous oxygen content difference [C(a − v̄)o₂]:

$$\dot{V}o_2 = Cardiac\ output \times C(a - \bar{v})o_2$$

The highest V̇o₂ isopleth, or highest aerobic production of *ATP*, is obtained by simultaneously, and maximally, increasing the cardiac output and the arterial–mixed venous oxygen content difference (Fig. 3.3).

Cardiac output has been well studied during exercise (3–11) and is a function of heart rate (HR) and stroke volume (SV) (cardiac output = HR × SV). Figure 3.4 typifies the changes in cardiac output that are found in healthy young adult male subjects. Cardiac output progressively increases during exercise (Fig. 3.4A). The heart rate response is essentially linear as a function of percent V̇o₂ max from 70 to 180 beats per minute (Fig. 3.4B). V̇o₂, V̇co₂, and lactate as a function of work intensity all increase dramatically during a ramp-pattern work rate forcing, with V̇co₂ exceeding V̇o₂ when the anaerobic threshold is exceeded due to bicarbonate buffering of lactic acid (Fig. 3.4C). Stroke volume increased from 100 ml per beat at rest to 150 ml per beat at the *LAT*. Above the *LAT*, stroke volume decreased slightly on average to approximately 135 ml per beat at end of exercise (Fig. 3.4D). Thus, cardiac output increased from the *LAT* to peak exercise due to heart rate increase. The arterial, mixed venous, and $C(a - \bar{v})O_2$ oxygen contents are displayed as a function of exercise intensity (Fig. 3.4E). Oxygen pulse, or the amount of oxygen extracted from each heartbeat, increased progressively from the *LAT* to peak exercise (Fig. 3.4F).

The arterial–venous oxygen content difference during exercise is maximized by a small arterial content increase as mixed venous O_2 content decreases with increasing exercise intensity (Fig. 3.4E). Several studies have shown that arterial oxygen content increases approximately 5% to 8% (5,11,12), due to an approximate 1.0 to 1.5 g/dl hemoglobin increase secondary to hemoconcentration above the *LAT*, as described in Chapter 2. Therefore, the oxygen carrying capacity in the arterial blood normally increases from approximately 20.5 ml/100 ml at the start of exercise to 21.5 ml/100 ml (~5%) at the end of exercise (Fig. 3.4E)(12). At the *LAT* (~50% of $\dot{V}O_2$max), the mixed venous blood is approximately 50% to 60% desaturated in normal subjects (oxygen content of 9–10 ml/100 ml, Fig. 3.4E). At the end of exercise (peak $\dot{V}O_2$), the mixed venous oxygen content has decreased to approxi-

mately 5 ml/100 ml, or one-third of the initial mixed venous oxygen content.

Muscle O_2 extraction during leg cycling exercise has been studied in normal subjects by examining arterial–femoral vein O_2 partial pressures and content differences during incremental and constant work rate exercise. The objective was to better understand the effects of muscle metabolism and tissue production of acid (metabolic production of CO_2 and lactic acid) on femoral vein blood gases and oxygen saturation (10,11,13,14). During moderate constant work rate exercise below the lactic acidosis threshold, the fall in pH is initially related to the increase in metabolic production of CO_2 (Fig. 3.5A). Femoral vein oxygen saturation falls from 45% to 22.5 % with a modest decrease in pH (7.35 to 7.2). However, with constant work rate exercise intensity above the LAT, there are two components to this fall in oxyhemoglobin saturation: the early component due to the fall in femoral vein P_{O_2} with a relatively small decrease in pH, and then a decrease in oxyhemoglobin saturation *without* a further fall in femoral vein P_{O_2} (Fig. 3.5B). The latter takes place due to the critical capillary P_{O_2} having been reached, with increased production of H^+ with lactate as the metabolic demand increases. The increased H^+ (decrease in pH) enables O_2 to dissociate from hemoglobin without a decrease in P_{O_2} (Bohr effect) (15). The decrease in

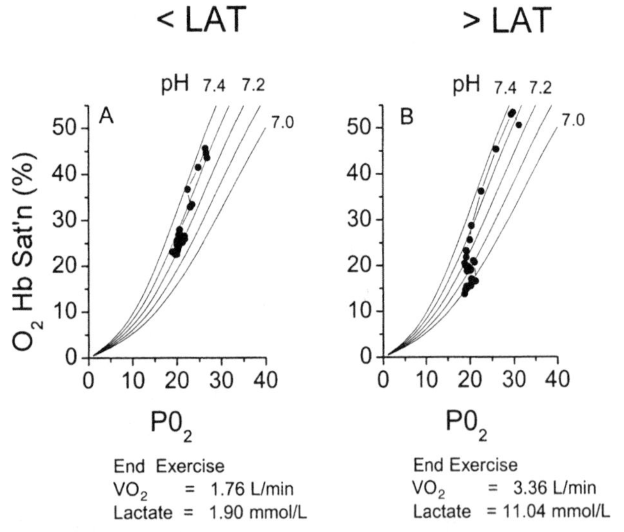

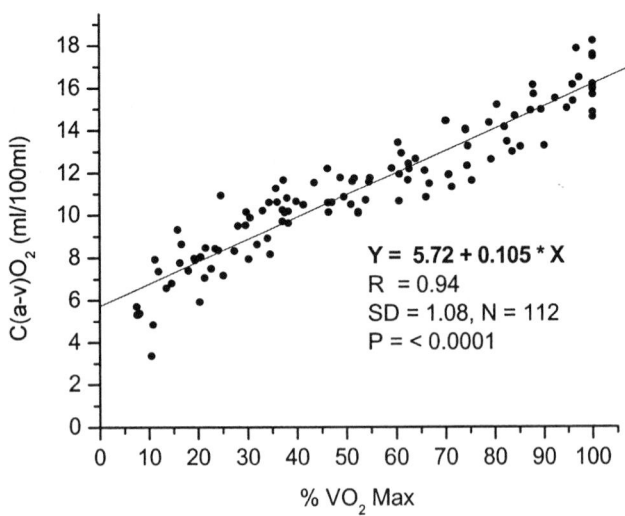

FIGURE 3.5. Femoral vein oxyhemoglobin saturation ($O_2Hb\ Sat'n$) as a function of P_{O_2} during 6 minutes of constant work rate exercise below (<*LAT*) (**A**) and above (>*LAT*) (**B**) the anaerobic threshold (N = 5). pH isopleths for the lower portion of the oxyhemoglobin dissociation curve are superimposed upon the experimental data. The end exercise lactate concentrations and $\dot{V}O_2$ for both exercise bouts are shown beneath the graphs. (From Stringer W, Wasserman K, Casaburi R, et al. Lactic acidosis as a facilitator of oxyhemoglobin dissociation during exercise. *J Appl Physiol* 1994;76:1462–1467, with permission.)

FIGURE 3.6. Arterial–mixed venous oxygen content difference [$C(a - \bar{v})O_2$] as a function of percent $\dot{V}O_2$max during ramp exercise for ten studies on five normal young men. $C(a - \bar{v})O_2$ is linearly correlated with percent $\dot{V}O_2$max: $C(a - \bar{v})O_2 = 5.72 + (0.105 \times \%\dot{V}O_2\text{max})$. (From Stringer W, Hansen J, Wasserman K. Cardiac output estimated non-invasively from oxygen uptake ($\dot{V}O_2$) during exercise. *J Appl Physiol* 1997;82:908–912, with permission.)

oxyhemoglobin saturation from 22.5% to 15% in this study is accounted for by this mechanism (Fig. 3.5A).

Estimating Cardiac Output

The progressive increase in oxygen uptake during exercise is achieved by a combination of increases in both cardiac output and arterial–venous oxygen content differences. The linear relation of $C(a - \bar{v})O_2$ as a function of percent $\dot{V}O_2max$ (Fig. 3.6) allows cardiac output to be estimated with respect to percent $\dot{V}O_2max$ (12). These values compare favorably with directly measured cardiac output using the Fick principle (Fig. 3.7). Cardiac output by the Fick principle (16) can also be calculated from the measured CO_2 output ($\dot{V}CO_2$) and $C(a - \bar{v})CO_2$ content differences during exercise (17). The increased variability of Fick principle–derived CO_2 cardiac output compared with O_2 cardiac output is attributable to the much lower extraction ratio for CO_2 and the greater complexity in calculation of blood CO_2 as compared with O_2 contents. Because of the large variability of results related to estimating cardiac output from direct measurements of $\dot{V}CO_2$ and arterial and mixed venous CO_2 contents, these results raise substantial concerns about the accuracy and precision of estimating cardiac output using CO_2 as the test gas, even in normal subjects (18–27).

CARBON DIOXIDE TRANSPORT

Although CO_2 can bind to hemoglobin and other proteins to create reversible carbamino groups ($RNH_2 + CO_2 \leftrightarrow RNHCOOH \leftrightarrow RNHCOO^- + H^+$)(28), a specific transport protein is not required since CO_2 is more soluble than O_2 in blood and converts, when hydrated, to form a relatively strong acid (carbonic acid, pKi = 3.8)(28–30):

$$H_2O + CO_2 \overset{Kh}{\underset{CA}{\leftrightarrow}} H_2CO_3 \overset{Ki(1)}{\underset{3.8}{\leftrightarrow}} HCO_3^- + H^+ \overset{K_2}{\underset{>10}{\leftrightarrow}} CO_3^{2-} + 2H^+$$

Carbonic anhydrase (CA) in the red blood cells catalyzes the hydration of CO_2 to H_2CO_3.[1]

The log form yields the more familiar equation (Henderson–Hasselbalch equation):

$$pH = pKa' + \log([HCO_3^-]/[s \times P_{CO_2}])$$

where s = 0.0307 mM/Torr at 37°C in human plasma, and pKa' is 6.10 [the apparent dissociation constant, when the hydration and ionization reactions (Kh and Ki) are combined].

The vast majority of CO_2 (88%) is carried as bicarbonate (HCO_3^-) in arterial blood, with physically dissolved and carbamino CO_2 accounting for 5% and 7% of the CO_2 transported, respectively. CO_2 reacts with carbamino groups at two sites: the α-terminal NH_2 group (one per protein chain), and ε-lysine residues in contact with fluid (many per

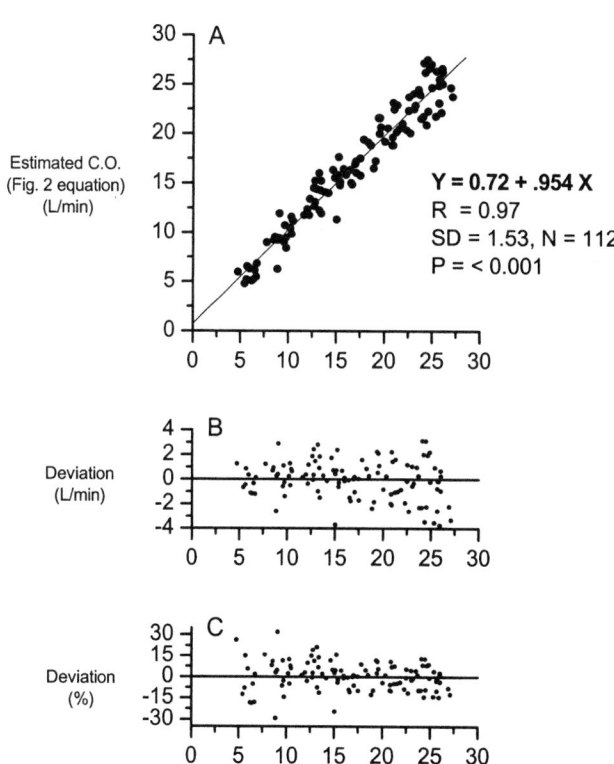

FIGURE 3.7. Estimated cardiac output (C.O.) from measured $\dot{V}O_2$ and estimated $C(a - \bar{v})O_2$ (determined from the equation in Figure 3.6) compared with directly measured Fick C.O. during progressive ramp exercise (A). The estimated and measured values agree well (B), with a 95% confidence limit of ±15% (C). (From Stringer W, Hansen J, Wasserman K. Cardiac output estimated non-invasively from oxygen uptake ($\dot{V}O_2$) during exercise. *J Appl Physiol* 1997;82: 908–912, with permission.)

---

[1]The molecular weight of carbonic anhydrase is approximately 30K, and three isoforms are observed. The red blood cell has two types: I, low activity; II, high activity. A third type (III) is observed in slow-twitch muscle fibers. The active site of all three types contains a zinc ion, and acetazolamide, a drug that inhibits CA enzyme activity, binds to zinc (24). CA is found in red blood cells and the pulmonary endothelium, as well as other sites in the body (e.g., kidney, choroid plexus).

protein chain). About 40% of total carbamino is formed at epsilon sites at pH = 7.40, P_{CO_2} = 40; the remainder is formed on alpha sites.

Although a well-defined titrimetric method for evolution and measurement of the total CO_2 has been developed to assess CO_2 content (31,32), it is rarely used today in clinical medicine. Therefore, we calculate blood CO_2 content based on an equation that uses pH, P_{CO_2}, and hemoglobin (33):

$$\text{Blood } C_{CO_2} = \text{Plasma } C_{CO_2} \times$$

$$\left[1 - \frac{(0.0289 \times [\text{Hb}])}{(3.352 - 0.456 \times S_{O_2}) \times (8.142 - \text{pH})} \right]$$

and

$$\text{Plasma } C_{CO_2} = 2.226 \times s \times \text{Plasma } P_{CO_2} \times$$
$$[1 + 10(\text{pH} - \text{pKa}')]$$

where [Hb] is hemoglobin concentration in g/dl, 2.226 is the conversion factor for mM/L to ml/100 ml, and s and pKa' are as defined above. Oxygen, when it dissociates from hemoglobin, absorbs H^+ ion:

$$\text{Hb } (O_2)_4 + 2.4\, H^+ \leftrightarrow \text{Hb } (H) + 4\, O_2$$

Therefore, the decrease in H^+ manifests as an increase in pH, which increases CO_2 content via increased HCO_3^-.

CO_2 transport during exercise is a very interesting demonstration of the changes in CO_2 content in the various blood compartments as a result of pH and P_{CO_2} perturbations (Fig. 3.8). From rest to the *LAT*, the arterial P_{CO_2} increases slightly, from a mean of 40 mm Hg to a maximum of 43 mm Hg (Fig. 3.8A). As exercise progresses, there is a fall in Pa_{CO_2} to a value below the resting value (37 mm Hg) at end of exercise. Simultaneous values in the mixed venous blood increase in a linear fashion as a function of exercise intensity, from a resting mean value of 47 mm Hg to approximately 80 mm Hg at peak exercise (Fig. 3.8A). CO_2 content in the arterial blood follows a similar contour to the arterial P_{CO_2}. However, the decrease in arterial CO_2 content at end of exercise is greater than the decrease in arterial P_{CO_2} because of the significant fall in arterial pH during exercise (Fig. 3.8B). Resting arterial CO_2 content is 21 mM (or 21 × 2.226 = 46.7 ml/100 ml, where 2.226 is the conversion factor for mM/L to ml/100 ml), and resting mixed venous CO_2 content is 23 mM (or 51.1 ml/100 ml), both of which are more than twice the corresponding resting arte-

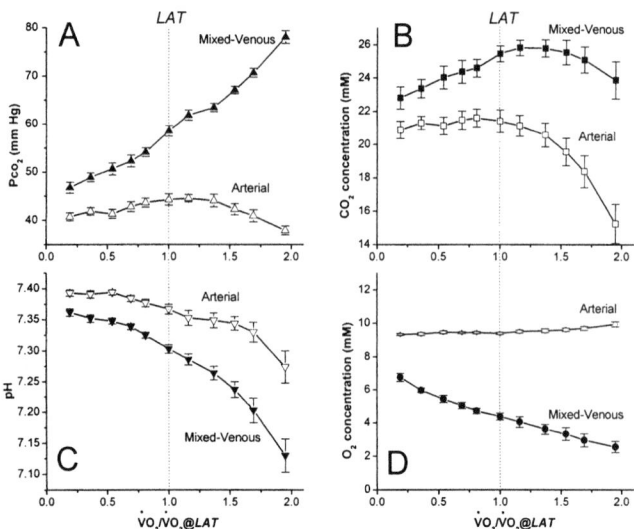

FIGURE 3.8. Arterial and mixed venous P_{CO_2} **(A)**, CO_2 concentration **(B)**, pH **(C)**, and O_2 concentration **(D)** (mean ± standard error of mean) as a function of exercise intensity, below (<1.0) and above (>1.0) the lactic acidosis threshold (*LAT*), where $\dot{V}_{O_2}/(\dot{V}_{O_2}$ at *LAT*) = 1.0. (From Sun XG, Hansen JE, Stringer WW, et al. Carbon dioxide pressure-concentration relationship in arterial and mixed venous blood during exercise. *J Appl Physiol* 2001;90:1798–1810, with permission.)

rial oxygen contents (9.5 mM or 21.1 ml/100 ml, Fig. 3.8D).

The CO_2 content in the mixed venous blood initially increases to maximum values just above the *LAT*. However, as exercise intensity increases further, the CO_2 content falls in the mixed venous blood (despite increasing P_{CO_2}) to a value very similar to the resting mixed venous CO_2 content. This directional change in CO_2 content as compared with P_{CO_2} in mixed venous blood is due to the overriding effect of the fall in pH (Fig. 3.8C). Therefore, the increase in $C(\bar{v} - a)_{CO_2}$ during heavy exercise is primarily due to the decrease in arterial CO_2 content relative to the mixed venous CO_2 content, not due to the increase in mixed venous CO_2 content. This differs from the mechanism of increasing $C(a - \bar{v})_{O_2}$, which is primarily due to the decrease in mixed venous O_2 content and only a small increase in arterial O_2 content.

To better understand the changes in arterial and mixed venous blood CO_2 content with respect to changes in pH, the CO_2 content values have been graphed as a function of P_{CO_2} with pH isopleths (Fig. 3.9). Blood CO_2 content at rest in the arterial blood is approximately 21 mM; in the mixed venous blood, it is approximately 23 mM. Both increase slightly during early exercise due to the increase in P_{CO_2}. As the *LAT* is reached, arterial blood CO_2 content progressively falls to very low values,

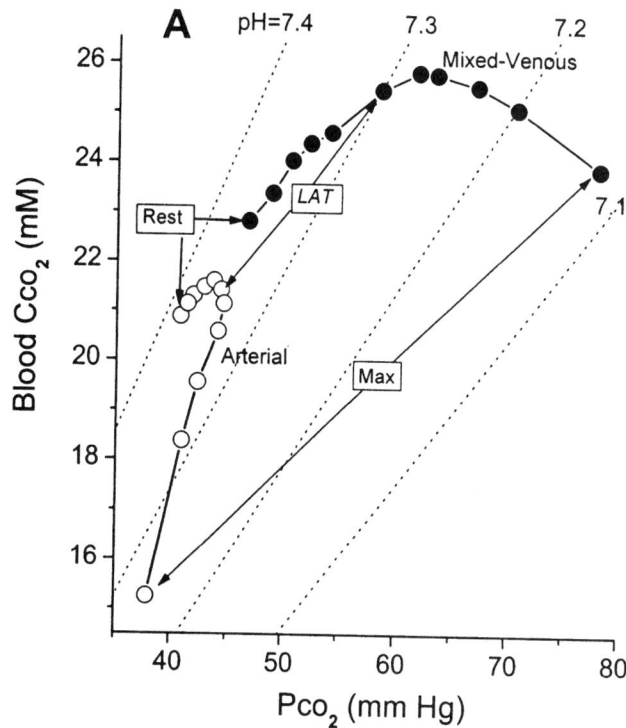

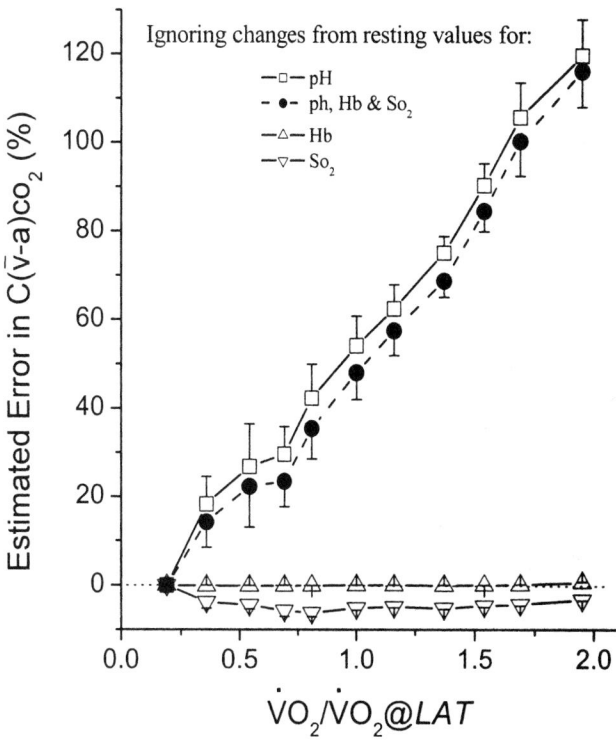

FIGURE 3.9. Arterial and mixed venous blood CO_2 concentration during incremental ramp exercise as related to P_{CO_2} and pH. Above the lactic acidosis threshold (*LAT*), despite the continuing increase in $P_{v_{CO_2}}$, the major mechanism accounting for increasing $C(\bar{v} - a)$ CO_2 was the decrease in $P_{a_{CO_2}}$ and $C_{a_{CO_2}}$. (From Sun XG, Hansen JE, Stringer WW, et al. Carbon dioxide pressure-concentration relationship in arterial and mixed venous blood during exercise. *J Appl Physiol* 2001;90:1798–1810, with permission.)

FIGURE 3.10. Relative contributions for the estimated error caused by ignoring changes from rest to exercise of pH, hemoglobin (Hb), oxyhemoglobin saturation (S_{O_2}), and the three combined to the $C(\bar{v} - a)_{CO_2}$ during exercise. The *x*-axis units are the same as Figure 3.8. Clearly, pH has the dominant effect on carbon dioxide content. (From Sun XG, Hansen JE, Stringer WW, et al. Carbon dioxide pressure-concentration relationship in arterial and mixed venous blood during exercise. *J Appl Physiol* 2001;90:1798–1810, with permission.)

and the mixed venous value returns very close to its resting value. The marked fall in pH is related primarily to lactic acidosis that develops above the *LAT*. Thus, the increase in $C(\bar{v} - a)_{CO_2}$ difference at work levels below the *LAT* is primarily due to an increase in mixed venous blood CO_2 content, with little change in arterial values. In contrast, as exercise proceeds above the *LAT*, the arterial blood CO_2 content is progressively driven downward, primarily accounting for the increase in $C(\bar{v} - a)_{CO_2}$ difference at maximal exercise.

The effects of changes in pH, [Hb], and oxygen saturation on CO_2 content have been compared during exercise (34). The changes in CO_2 content during exercise are essentially fully explained by the changes related to pH (Fig. 3.10), since the changes related to [Hb] and S_{O_2} are very small. The changes in relative proportions of forms of CO_2 carriage (HCO_3^-, carbamino, and free CO_2) during exercise are shown in Figure 3.11. HCO_3^- is the dominant form in which CO_2 is transported and accounts for the major increase in $C(\bar{v} - a)_{CO_2}$ at peak exercise.

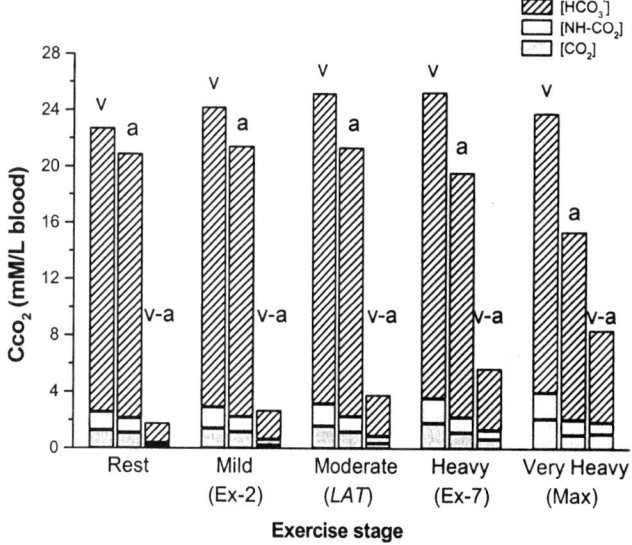

FIGURE 3.11. Blood CO_2 content (HCO_3^-, carbamino, and free CO_2) in the mixed venous ($\bar{v}$), arterial (a), and venous–arterial (v − a) difference as a function of exercise intensity (rest, mild, moderate, heavy, and very heavy exercise). (From Sun XG, Hansen JE, Stringer WW, et al. Carbon dioxide pressure-concentration relationship in arterial and mixed venous blood during exercise. *J Appl Physiol* 2001; 90:1798–1810, with permission.)

SUMMARY

Mechanisms of oxygen and carbon dioxide transport are important physiological concepts that assist our understanding of the physiology of exercise. Oxygen transport optimization must occur during exercise to maximize aerobic energy production, since anaerobic sources cannot sustain exercise. To achieve maximum O_2 transport, arterial oxygenation, hemoglobin concentration, cardiac performance, and blood flow distribution must be functioning optimally. Cardiac performance can be evaluated using the Fick principle [using measured oxygen uptake during exercise and the recognized pattern of change for $C(a - \bar{v})O_2$]. O_2 transport takes place in tandem with CO_2 transport, rather than independently. Both are affected by the pH change accompanying lactate accumulation. Thus, while oxyhemoglobin dissociates more readily when H^+ is formed with lactate, HCO_3^- decreases due to it serving as the buffer of the H^+. Consequently, venous HCO_3^- and PCO_2 do not change in the same direction above the LAT. Optimal exercise performance depends on the effects of pH on oxygen and carbon dioxide transport.

References

1. Finch C, Lenfant C. Oxygen transport in man. *N Engl J Med* 1973;286:407–415.
2. Hill EP, Power GG, Longo LD. Mathematical simulation of pulmonary O_2 and CO_2 exchange. *J Appl Physiol* 1973;224:904–917.
3. Carlson LA, Pernow B. Studies on the peripheral circulation and metabolism in man. I. Oxygen utilization and lactate-pyruvate formation in the legs at rest and during exercise in healthy subjects. *Acta Physiol Scand* 1961;52:328–342.
4. Donald KW, Wormald PN, Taylor SH, Bishop JM. Changes in the oxygen content of femoral venous blood and leg blood flow during leg exercise in relation to cardiac output response. *Clin Sci* 1957;16: 567–591.
5. Hartley LH, Grimby G, Kilbrom A, Nilsson NJ, Astrand I, Bjure J, Ekblom B, Saltin B. Physical training in sedentary middle-aged and older men. II. Cardiac output and gas exchange at submaximal and maximal exercise. *Scand J Clin Lab Invest* 1969;24:335–344.
6. Hartley L, Vogel J, Landowne M. Central, femoral, and brachial circulation during exercise in hypoxia. *J Appl Physiol* 1973;34:87–90.
7. Knuttgen HG, Saltin B. Muscle metabolites and oxygen uptake in short-term submaximal exercise in man. *J Appl Physiol* 1972;32:690–694.
8. Linnarsson D. Dynamics of pulmonary gas exchange and heart rate changes at start and end of exercise. *Acta Physiol Scand* 1974;415(Suppl 1):5–68.
9. Linnarsson D, Karlsson J, Fagraeus L, Saltin B. Muscle metabolites and oxygen deficit with exercise in hypoxia and hyperoxia. *J Appl Physiol* 1974;36:399–402.
10. Poole DC, Schaffartzik W, Knight DR, Derion T, Kennedy B, Guy HJ, Prediletto R, Wagner PD. Contribution of exercising legs to the slow component of oxygen uptake kinetics in humans. *J Appl Physiol* 1991;71:1245–1253.
11. Stringer W, Wasserman K, Casaburi R, Porszasz J, Maehara K, French W. Lactic acidosis as a facilitator of oxyhemoglobin dissociation during exercise. *J Appl Physiol* 1994;76:1462–1467.
12. Stringer W, Hansen J, Wasserman K. Cardiac output estimated non-invasively from oxygen uptake ($\dot{V}O_2$) during exercise. *J Appl Physiol* 1997;82:908–912.
13. Agusti AG, Roca J, Barbera JA, Casademont J, Rodriguez-Roisin R, Wagner PD. Effect of sampling site on femoral venous blood gas values. *J Appl Physiol* 1994;77:2018–2022.
14. Knight DR, Schaffartzik W, Poole DC, Hogan MC, Bebout DE, Wagner PD. Effects of hyperoxia on maximal leg O_2 supply and utilization in men. *J Appl Physiol* 1993;75:2586–2594.
15. Boning D, Hollnagel C, Boecker A, Goke S. Bohr shift by lactic acid and the supply of O_2 to skeletal muscle. *Respir Physiol* 1966;85:231–243.
16. Fick A. The output of the heart. *Phys-Med Gesellschaft* 1870;2:16.
17. Sun XG, Hansen JE, Ting H, Chuang ML, Stringer WW, Adame D, Wasserman K. Comparison of exercise cardiac output by the Fick principle using oxygen and carbon dioxide. *Chest* 2000;118:631–640.
18. Ashton CH, McHardy GJR. A rebreathing method for determining mixed venous PCO_2 during exercise. *J Appl Physiol* 1963;18:668–671.
19. Clausen JP, Larsen OA, Trap-Jensen J. Cardiac output in middle-aged patients determined with CO_2 rebreathing method. *J Appl Physiol* 1970;28:337–342.
20. Coates AL. Measurement of cardiac output during exercise. *Chest* 1992;102:985–986.
21. Collier CR. Determination of mixed venous CO_2 tensions by rebreathing. *J Appl Physiol* 1956;9:25–29.
22. DaSilva GA, El-Manshawi A, Heigenhauser GJF, Jones NL. Measurement of mixed venous carbon dioxide pressure by rebreathing during exercise. *Respir Physiol* 1985;59:379–392.
23. Defares JG. Determination of $PvCO_2$ from the exponential CO_2 rise during rebreathing. *J Appl Physiol* 1958;13:159–164.
24. Ferguson RJ, Faulkner JA, Julius S, Conway J. Comparison of cardiac output determined by CO_2 re-

breathing and dye-dilution methods. *J Appl Physiol* 1968;25:450–454.

25. Godfrey S. Manipulation of the indirect Fick principle by a digital computer program for the calculation of exercise physiology results. *Respiration* 1970;27:513–532.

26. Godfrey S, Wolf E. An evaluation of rebreathing methods for measuring mixed venous P_{CO_2} during exercise. *Clin Sci* 1972;42:345–353.

27. Hamilton WF. Measurement of the cardiac output. In: Fenn WO, Rahn H, eds. *Handbook of physiology*. Washington, DC: American Physiological Society, 1964: 551–584.

28. Klocke RA. Carbon dioxide transport. In: Farhi LE, Tenney SM, eds. *Handbook of physiology*. Washington, DC: American Physiological Society, 1987:173–197.

29. Christiansen J, Douglas CG, Haldane JS. The absorption and dissociation of carbon dioxide by human blood. *J Physiol* 1914;48:244–271.

30. Christiansen J, Douglas CG, Haldane JS. The dissociation of CO_2 by human blood. *J Appl Physiol* 1913;47:ii.

31. Lustgarten D. Evaluation of contemporary methods for serum CO_2. *Clin Chem* 1976;22:374–378.

32. Siggard-Andersen O. The van Slyke equation. *Scand J Clin Lab Invest* 1977;37:15–20.

33. Douglas AR, Jones NL, Reed JW. Calculation of whole blood CO_2 content. *J Appl Physiol* 1988;65:473–477.

34. Sun XG, Hansen JE, Stringer WW, Ting H, Wasserman K. Carbon dioxide pressure-concentration relationship in arterial and mixed venous blood during exercise. *J Appl Physiol* 2001;90:1798–1810.

Measurements During Integrative Cardiopulmonary Exercise Testing

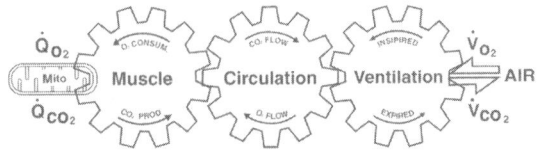

CARDIOPULMONARY EXERCISE TESTING (CPET) permits simultaneous evaluation of the ability of the cardiovascular and respiratory systems to perform their major function, that is, gas exchange between the cells and the environment. Because exercise requires an integrative cardiopulmonary response to support the increase in muscle respiration required to perform exercise, gas exchange measurements are fundamental to understanding the mechanism(s) of exercise limitation. It is evident from the scheme shown in Figure 1.3 that a reduction in $\dot{V}O_2$max (peak $\dot{V}O_2$) can be caused by any disease process affecting skeletal muscle function or the organ systems needed to transport O_2 and CO_2 between the air and the muscle cell. Use of CPET to determine only $\dot{V}O_2$max or peak $\dot{V}O_2$, as is commonly done, fails to employ this laboratory test for its unique capability: to define the pathophysiology of exercise limitation. This chapter describes measurements obtained from CPET that are useful when assessing the responses of each of the organ systems coupling external respiration (O_2 uptake and CO_2 output at the airway) to cellular respiration (O_2 consumption and CO_2 production of the cells) during exercise.

WHAT IS AN INTEGRATIVE CARDIOPULMONARY EXERCISE TEST?

The primary function of the cardiovascular and pulmonary systems is to support cellular respiration. The success of these organ systems in meeting this function is reflected in the O_2 uptake and CO_2 output in response to a specific work rate and their relation to heart rate, ventilation, and one another. An integrative cardiopulmonary exercise test can address many more questions than an exercise test that only assesses the electrocardiogram (ECG) to address the presence or absence of myocardial ischemia. While also employing electrocardiographic measurements, CPET addresses a large number of questions about other disorders as well. These questions are listed in Table 4.1, along with the measurements that can be used to address each question. Because the questions that can be addressed by integrative CPET are so comprehensive, testing at the beginning of a workup of a case of exercise limitation, from any cause, would likely reduce the cost and time required to diagnose disorders of exercise intolerance.

WHEN SHOULD CARDIOPULMONARY EXERCISE TESTING BE USED?

Cardiopulmonary exercise testing is useful in the following situations:

1. *Differential diagnosis.* When the cause of dyspnea or exercise limitation is uncertain (i.e., for differential diagnosis), integrative CPET can serve to define the specific organ system limiting gas transport. This enables a more specific further workup.
2. *Disability evaluation.* By providing an objective assessment of exercise capacity and degree of impairment, CPET is of considerable, if not essential, value in disability evaluation (1).
3. *Rehabilitation.* CPET provides information concerning the level of exercise that the patient can perform without undue stress. Thus, the test results guide the physician regarding exercise prescription in physical rehabilitation. It also furnishes quantitative evidence of the benefit of a rehabilitation program as well as the mechanism(s) of benefit. Improvement in exercise tolerance cannot be objectively assessed without CPET (2).
4. *Assessing preoperative risk.* CPET is of value for preoperative evaluation of risk for patients about to undergo major surgery (3,4); such testing enables the examiner to evaluate the stress that the cardiopulmonary system can undergo before anaerobic *ATP* production, with resulting lactic acidosis, is recruited to complement aerobic *ATP* production. Predictably, CPET provides much more information about cardiovascular and pulmonary reserve during metabolic stress than measurements of cardiovascular and ventilatory function at rest.
5. *Grading severity of heart failure.* Peak $\dot{V}O_2$ has been found to be the best predictor of survival time in patients with chronic heart failure (5,6). To that has been added $\dot{V}E$ versus $\dot{V}CO_2$ (7,8) and anaerobic threshold (9). A given heart lesion may have a different functional significance in two different patients because of a difference in how the peripheral circulation adapts to the cardiac abnormality. Because CPET addresses the body's global physiological adaptation to exercise, including compensatory mechanisms for the abnormal cardiac function, it has been valuable in the prediction of survival time. Therefore

TABLE 4.1.   Questions Addressed by Cardiopulmonary Exercise Testing

Question	Disorder	Markers of Abnormality[a]
1. Is exercise capacity reduced?	Any disorder	Maximal $\dot{V}_{O_2}$ (panel 3)
2. Is the metabolic requirement for exercise increased?	Obesity	$\dot{V}_{O_2}$–WR relationship (panel 3)
3. Is exercise limited by impaired O_2 flow?	Ischemic, myopathic, valvular, congenital heart disease	ECG; AT; $\Delta\dot{V}_{O_2}/\Delta WR$; $\dot{V}_{O_2}$/HR (panels 2, 3, 5)
	Pulmonary vascular disease	$\Delta\dot{V}_{O_2}/\Delta WR$; AT; $\dot{V}_{O_2}$/HR; $\dot{V}_E/\dot{V}_{CO_2}$ (panels 2, 3, 5, 6)
	Peripheral arterial disease	BP; $\Delta\dot{V}_{O_2}/\Delta WR$; $\Delta\dot{V}_{CO_2}/\Delta WR$ (panels 3, 5)
	Anemia, hypoxemia, elevated COHb, AT	$\dot{V}_{O_2}$/HR (panels 2, 3, 5)
4. Is exercise limited by reduced ventilatory capacity?	Lung; chest wall	BR; ventilatory response (panels 1, 7, 9)
5. Is there an abnormal degree of $\dot{V}/\dot{Q}$ mismatching?	Lung disease; pulmonary vascular disease; heart failure	$P(A - a)_{O_2}$; $P(a - {ET})_{CO_2}$; V_D/V_T; $\dot{V}_E/\dot{V}_{CO_2}$ @AT (panels 4, 6, 9)
6. Is there a defect in muscle utilization of O_2 or substrate?	Muscle glycolytic or mitochondrial enzyme defect	AT, R, $\dot{V}_{CO_2}$; HR vs. $\dot{V}_{O_2}$; lactate; lactate/pyruvate ratio (panels 3, 5, 8)
7. Is exercise limited by a behavioral problem?	Psychogenic dyspnea; hysteria	Breathing pattern (panels 7–9)
8. Is work output reduced because of poor effort?	Poor effort with secondary gain.	Increased HRR; increased BR; peak R < 1.0; normal AT, $P(A - a)_{O_2}$ and $P(a - {ET})_{CO_2}$ (panels 2, 5, 7, 8)

Peak $\dot{V}_{O_2}$, highest O_2 uptake measured; WR, work rate; AT, anaerobic threshold; $\Delta\dot{V}_{O_2}/\Delta WR$, increase in $\dot{V}_{O_2}$ relative to increase in work rate; $\dot{V}_{O_2}$/HR, O_2 pulse; $\dot{V}_E/\dot{V}_{CO_2}$ @AT, ventilatory equivalent for CO_2 at anaerobic threshold; BR (breathing reserve), maximum voluntary ventilation minus ventilation at maximum exercise; $P(A - a)_{O_2}$, alveolar–arterial P_{O_2} difference; $P(a - {ET})_{CO_2}$, arterial–end tidal P_{CO_2} difference; V_D/V_T, physiological dead space/tidal volume ratio; R, respiratory exchange ratio ($\dot{V}_{CO_2}/\dot{V}_{O_2}$); HRR (heart rate reserve), predicted maximum heart rate minus maximum exercise heart rate; COHb, carboxyhemoglobin.
[a]Panel numbers refer to Figure 4.30.

it is an essential component in the evaluation of patients with chronic heart failure and in prioritizing patients for heart transplantation (10).

6. *Grading prognosis in chronic obstructive pulmonary disease.* Oga et al. (11) showed that peak O_2 uptake was a better predictor of survival in patients with chronic obstructive pulmonary disease (COPD) than the FEV_1 measurement. The recently completed National Emphysema Treatment Trials (12) also showed that death rate was highest in those patients with a reduced work rate, and that the latter was the critical determinant as to who might benefit from lung volume reduction surgery.

7. *Effectiveness of therapy.* Measurement of gas exchange has also been useful in evaluating functional improvement resulting from pacemakers in patients with heart block (13) and in objectively assessing various forms of medical therapy in patients with a variety of disorders (14,15).

The measurements and functions that integrative CPET assesses are summarized in Table 4.2. Fortunately, most are noninvasive and can be performed in modern cardiopulmonary function laboratories. The gas exchange variables that provide the most valuable information are described in this chapter, whereas the methods of measurement, calculations,

and calibration and the method to assess accuracy are described in Appendix C and Chapter 6.

CPET is useful because it enables the examiner to (a) quantify the level of the subject's exercise limitation, (b) assess the adequacy of the performance of various components in the coupling of pulmonary to cellular gas exchange, (c) determine the organ system limiting exercise, and (d) determine the $\dot{V}_{O_2}$ at which exercise limitation occurs. These evaluations can be addressed during short (approximately 10-minute), progressive, non-steady-state exercise tests, rather than during a more prolonged exercise test with steps of relatively long duration. Prolonged testing is more likely to delay recovery of the patient, thereby making it more difficult for the investigator to repeat exercise testing, if required.

MEASUREMENTS

Electrocardiogram

Myocardial ischemia results from an inadequate O_2 supply to the myocardium to meet the O_2 needed in support of increased cardiac work. When the heart muscle contracts without adequate O_2, lactic acid production increases and the muscle cells alter their ionic permeability. Thus, the rate of reestab-

TABLE 4.2.   Assessing Function with Physiologic Measurements

Measurements	Function
Electrocardiogram	Myocardial O_2 availability–requirement balance
$\dot{V}O_2$	Cardiac output × C(a − $\bar{v}$)O_2
Peak $\dot{V}O_2$	Highest $\dot{V}O_2$ achieved during presumed maximal effort for an incremental exercise test (specific for type of work); may or may not equal $\dot{V}O_2$max
$\dot{V}O_2$max	Highest $\dot{V}O_2$ achievable as evidenced by failure for $\dot{V}O_2$ to increase despite increasing work rate (specific for type of work); highest cardiac output × C(a − $\bar{v}$)O_2
$\Delta\dot{V}O_2/\Delta WR$	Aerobic contribution to exercise (low value suggests high anaerobic contribution); normally 10 ml/min/w
Cardiac output	Useful when evaluating hemodynamics
Anaerobic threshold (AT)	Highest $\dot{V}O_2$ that can be sustained without developing a lactic acidosis; important determinant of potential for endurance work (specific for form of work)
O_2 pulse	Product of SV and C(a − $\bar{v}$)O_2; under conditions when SV is constant, change in O_2 pulse is proportional to change in C(a − $\bar{v}$)O_2
Heart rate reserve (HRR)	Difference between predicted and measured heart rate at peak $\dot{V}O_2$
Arterial pressure	Detecting systemic hypertension, ventricular outflow obstruction, or myocardial failure (pulsus alternans or decreasing pressure with increasing WR).
$\dot{V}E = \dot{V}A + \dot{V}D$	$\dot{V}D$ is increased due to mismatching of $\dot{V}A$ to $\dot{Q}$. $\dot{V}A$ is increased inversely with decrease in $PaCO_2$, whether caused by a low CO_2 set point, metabolic acidosis, or hypoxemia.
BR = MVV − $\dot{V}E$ at max. exercise, or (MVV − $\dot{V}E$ at max. exercise)/MVV	Breathing reserve; theoretical additional $\dot{V}E$ available at cessation of exercise.
Exercise VD/VT	Measure of mismatching of ventilation and perfusion.
P(a − ET)CO_2	Detects high $\dot{V}A/\dot{Q}$ components of lung with mismatching of $\dot{V}A/\dot{Q}$.
P(A − a)O_2	Increased in presence of mismatching of $\dot{V}A/\dot{Q}$, diffusion defect, or right-to-left shunt.
Expired flow pattern	Useful for indicating presence of significant airflow obstruction.
VT/IC	Fraction of the inspiratory capacity used in breathing
Immediate $\dot{V}O_2$ increase (phase I) in response to constant WR	Ability to increase pulmonary blood flow at start of exercise (phase I)
$\Delta\dot{V}O_2$ (6 − 3)	Proportional to lactate increase; positive if work rate is above LT.
Decrease in $\dot{V}E$ during abrupt switch to 100% O_2 breathing	Contribution of the carotid body to ventilatory drive.

WR, work rate; $\dot{V}E$, minute ventilation; HR, heart rate; VD, physiological dead space; SV, stroke volume; BR, breathing reserve; C(a − $\bar{v}$)O_2 arterial–mixed venous O_2 content difference; MVV, maximal voluntary ventilation; VT, tidal volume; $\dot{V}D$, physiological dead space ventilation per minute; IC, inspiratory capacity; $\dot{V}A$, alveolar ventilation per minute; $\Delta\dot{V}O_2$ (6 − 3), difference between $\dot{V}O_2$ at 6 and 3 minutes during constant work rate exercise.

lishing the electrical membrane potential during repolarization is slowed in the ischemic areas of the myocardium. This causes the T wave and ST segments to change acutely when the O_2 requirement for the increased cardiac work of exercise exceeds the availability of O_2 (Table 4.3). Because exercise causes the heart rate to increase and diastolic time to shorten, the time for coronary perfusion is decreased. Thus, coronary artery disease is more likely to be detected during exercise, when heart rate and the pressure–rate product is increasing, than at rest (16–18).

An increased frequency of ectopic beats as the work rate increases is also suggestive of myocardial ischemia. However, some subjects manifest occasional premature ventricular or atrial contractions at rest that disappear or become less frequent during exercise. Such ectopic beats appear to be benign and unrelated to a disturbance in the balance between myocardial O_2 availability and require-

ment, because they are overridden by the sinus tachycardia of exercise.

In many instances, false-positive and borderline changes occur in the ECG when one relies solely on changes in the T wave and ST segments to detect myocardial ischemia. When these ECG changes are accompanied by myocardial dyskinesis, however, $\dot{V}O_2$ may fail to rise appropriately for the increasing work rate (WR). Thus, a reduction in $\Delta\dot{V}O_2/\Delta WR$ accompanied by ECG changes consistent with myocardial ischemia, with or without angina, strengthens the diagnosis of coronary artery disease involv-

TABLE 4.3.   Electrocardiographic Evidence of Myocardial Ischemia During Exercise

ST segment changes
T wave changes
Premature ventricular contractions that appear during exercise

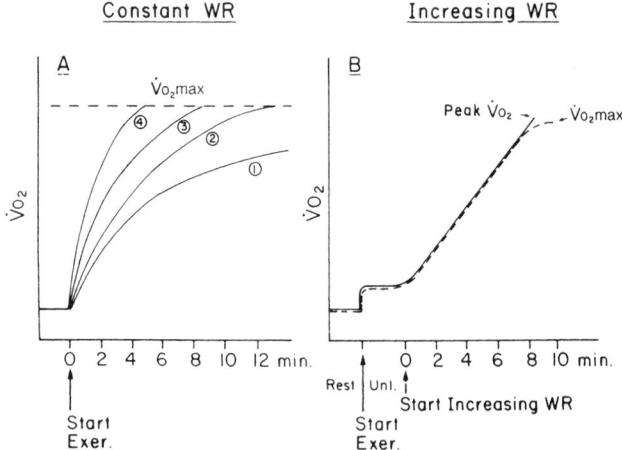

FIGURE 4.1.   **A:** Determining the maximal $\dot{V}O_2$ ($\dot{V}O_2$max) from supramaximal work rate tests. The time course of $\dot{V}O_2$ following the onset of exercise is shown for progressively higher work rates. For work rate 1, the $\dot{V}O_2$ asymptote is below $\dot{V}O_2$max. Work rate 2 reaches a $\dot{V}O_2$ that is the same as the highest $\dot{V}O_2$ reached by work rates 3 and 4. Because the maximum $\dot{V}O_2$ for work rates 2, 3, and 4 is the same, despite increasing work rate, this identifies $\dot{V}O_2$max for the form of exercise studied. **B:** Distinguishing between $\dot{V}O_2$max and "peak" or "maximum" $\dot{V}O_2$ from a maximal-effort incremental exercise test. When the subject's maximum tolerable work rate results in a flattening of the $\dot{V}O_2$–work rate slope, this is the subject's maximal $\dot{V}O_2$, or $\dot{V}O_2$max. When the $\dot{V}O_2$ does not slow its rate of rise with increasing work rate, but the subject has reached his or her maximum tolerable work rate, this is the peak (or maximum) $\dot{V}O_2$ during the test.

ing a significant mass of myocardium. The diagnosis of ischemic heart disease is further supported if systemic blood pressure decreases in the presence of ECG changes characteristic of myocardial ischemia during exercise.

Maximal Oxygen Uptake ($\dot{V}O_2$max) and Maximum Oxygen Uptake (Peak $\dot{V}O_2$)

The body clearly has an upper limit for O_2 utilization at a particular state of fitness or training. This is usually determined by the maximal cardiac output (19), the arterial O_2 content, the fractional distribution of the cardiac output to the exercising muscle (20), and the ability of the muscle to extract O_2 (21). The ventilatory capacity determines the upper limit of $\dot{V}O_2$ only when ventilation is insufficient to eliminate the CO_2 produced by aerobic metabolism and the bicarbonate buffering of lactic acid (22).

Maximal aerobic power (i.e., maximal $\dot{V}O_2$, or $\dot{V}O_2$max) was originally defined as the $\dot{V}O_2$ at which performance of increasing levels of constant work rate exercise failed to increase $\dot{V}O_2$ by 150 ml/min, despite increasing work rate (19). This is illustrated in Figure 4.1A and shown experimentally in Figure

2.6. However, this definition has shortcomings because it is dependent on the exercise protocol and because 150 ml/min is a large fraction of the highest $\dot{V}O_2$ obtained in many patients.

The maximal $\dot{V}O_2$ may also be determined in a progressively increasing exercise test by observing that $\dot{V}O_2$ fails to increase normally relative to the increase in work rate (<10 ml/min/watt) just before the subject fatigues. However, for incremental exercise tests, flattening of the $\dot{V}O_2$–work rate relationship, as peak $\dot{V}O_2$ is approached, is often not seen. This highest $\dot{V}O_2$ is called the *peak* $\dot{V}O_2$. Thus, the maximal $\dot{V}O_2$ represents the *highest* $\dot{V}O_2$, averaged over a 20- to 30-second period, attainable for a given form of exercise, as evidenced by a failure of $\dot{V}O_2$ to increase further despite an increase in work rate. This $\dot{V}O_2$ is contrasted with the peak $\dot{V}O_2$ obtained during a progressively increasing work rate test, defined as the highest $\dot{V}O_2$, averaged over a 20- to 30-second period, achieved for a presumed maximal exercise effort. Although the *peak* $\dot{V}O_2$ does not satisfy the definition of the *maximal* $\dot{V}O_2$ determined from repeated constant work rate tests, it is usually equal to the actual $\dot{V}O_2$max in normal subjects. The distinction between $\dot{V}O_2$max and peak $\dot{V}O_2$ is diagrammed in Figure 4.1.

A plateau in $\dot{V}O_2$ during a series of supramaximal constant work rate tests or progressively increasing work rate tests shows that a maximal $\dot{V}O_2$ has, in fact, been attained. In studies in normal subjects performing progressively increasing exercise to the point of fatigue or dyspnea, only about one-third of normal subjects making maximal effort reach a plateau in $\dot{V}O_2$ (Fig. 4.2). After reaching their peak $\dot{V}O_2$, many subjects cannot endure the discomfort long enough to achieve a work rate–related plateau in $\dot{V}O_2$. Nevertheless, the regression equations and scaling factors of those who did not reach a plateau were indistinguishable from those who reached a plateau (23).

A plateau in $\dot{V}O_2$ may also fail to occur during a progressively increasing work rate test when the subject stops exercising because of leg or chest pain, shortness of breath, mechanical limitation to breathing, or lack of motivation. In these instances, the peak $\dot{V}O_2$ will not satisfy the definition of $\dot{V}O_2$max.

Note that, at high-intensity exercise, the $\dot{V}O_2$ does not reflect all the high-energy phosphate expended by the subject. It does not account for the energy generated when high-energy phosphate is split from phosphocreatine (*PCr*) or for the *ATP* generated from anaerobic glycolysis, resulting in a net increase in lactate. The latter becomes increas-

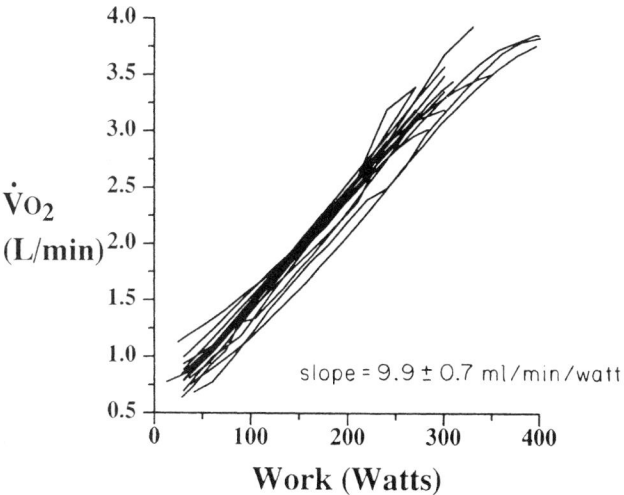

FIGURE 4.2.   The effect of work rate on oxygen uptake ($\dot{V}O_2$) during progressively increasing work rate cycle ergometer exercise for 17 normal subjects. The average regression slope and standard deviation for the subject population are given in the equation in the figure. The slope is consistent among subjects but is displaced upward depending on body weight, as shown in Figure 2.7. (From Wasserman K, Sue DY. Coupling of external to cellular respiration. In: Wasserman K, ed. *Exercise gas exchange in heart disease.* Armonk, NY: Futura, 1996:1–15, with permission.)

ingly important as an energy source as work rate increases above the anaerobic threshold (24).

A progressively increasing work rate exercise test, as illustrated in Figure 4.1B, has several advantages: (a) The test starts out at a relatively low work rate, so that it does not require the abrupt application of great muscle force or a sudden, large cardiorespiratory stress; (b) the $\dot{V}O_2$max or peak $\dot{V}O_2$ can be determined from an exercise test in which the period of increasing work rate lasts only 8 to 12 minutes; (c) the subject is stressed for only a few minutes at relatively high work rates; and (d) the $\dot{V}O_2$–work rate relationship can be determined if the cycle is the form of ergometry. To obtain the best data for interpreting the measured responses to a progressively increasing work rate exercise test, the work rate increments should be uniform in magnitude and duration. This means that the ergometer must be linear and accurately calibrated.

The peak $\dot{V}O_2$ is the first measurement to be examined because it establishes whether the patient's physiologic responses allow normal maximal aerobic function. Other measurements are then used to differentiate the cause of exercise limitation whether or not the subject reaches his or her predicted peak $\dot{V}O_2$.

Oxygen Uptake and Work Rate

Although $\dot{V}O_2$ measurements are made from respired gas measured at the mouth, the increase in $\dot{V}O_2$ reflects O_2 utilization by the muscle cells performing the work of exercise. The $\dot{V}O_2$–work rate relation describes how much O_2 is utilized by the exercising subject in relation to the quantity of external work performed. Because it gives important information concerning the coupling of external to cellular respiration, we find it valuable to graph $\dot{V}O_2$ as a function of work rate.

Pattern of Work Rate Increase and the $\dot{V}O_2$ Response

$\dot{V}O_2$ increases smoothly when cycle ergometer work rate is increased in a continuous ramp pattern or in equal steps of 1-minute duration (Fig. 4.3). This type of protocol has advantages in the ease with which the patient perceives the addition of work rate during testing. Increasing work rate in 2- or 3-minute steps results in relatively large abrupt changes in work rate, and the increase in $\dot{V}O_2$ at each interval is a step pattern (Fig. 4.3) (25). Because the time constant for $\dot{V}O_2$ at work intensities below the anaerobic threshold is 35 to 45 seconds in healthy subjects, steps at 1-minute increments give smooth increases in $\dot{V}O_2$. Thus, the slope of increase in $\dot{V}O_2$ as a function of work rate can be calculated with either the ramp or 1-minute step increase (25).

For 3-minute step increases in work rate, the step appearance in $\dot{V}O_2$ is damped at the higher work intensity because of the slowing of $\dot{V}O_2$ kinetics as the subject approaches $\dot{V}O_2$max (26). The loss of the step change in $\dot{V}O_2$ depends on fitness (Fig. 4.4).

Upward Displacement of $\dot{V}O_2$ as a Function of Work Rate

The position of the $\dot{V}O_2$–work rate relation depends on body weight (Fig. 4.5A). Obese subjects require increased $\dot{V}O_2$ to do a given amount of external work (see the section "Oxygen Cost of Work" in Chapter 2). Compared with a nonobese individual, the increase in $\dot{V}O_2$ during exercise is considerably greater than the increase in $\dot{V}O_2$ at rest in obese subjects. The reason is the added O_2 cost to move the limbs during cycling ergometry and the cost of moving the entire body during treadmill exercise. Based on two separate studies of cycle ergometer exercise on adults, the $\dot{V}O_2$ was found to be displaced upward by approximately 5.8 ml/min per kilogram of body weight (27,28) during unloaded cycling at 60 rpm. Although upwardly displaced, the $\dot{V}O_2$–work rate relation in obesity parallels that of the normal-weight subject during cycle ergometry.

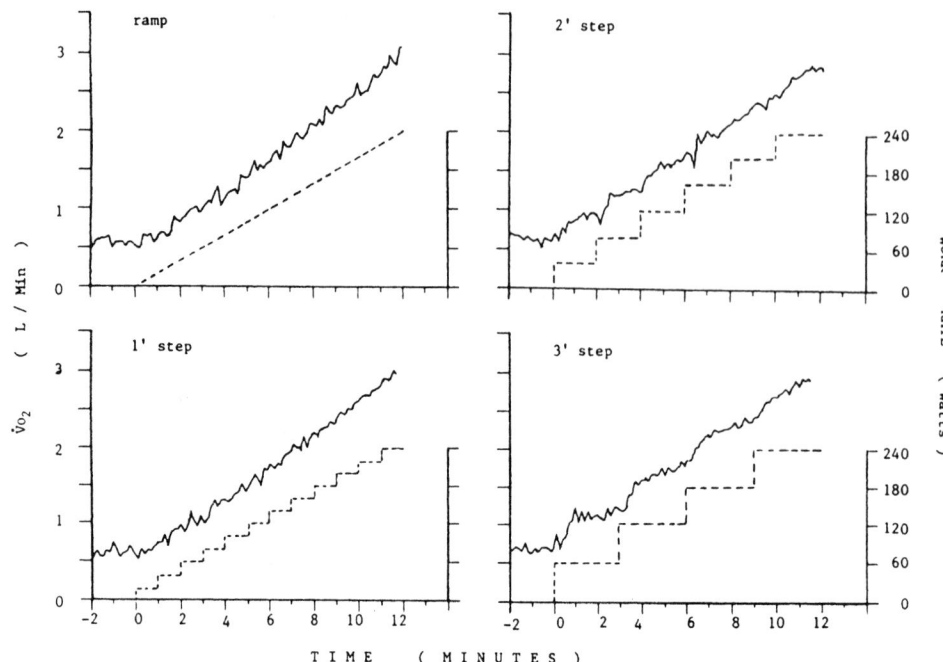

FIGURE 4.3. $\dot{V}O_2$ response in a single subject to four different protocols: ramp and 1-, 2-, and 3-minute steps. The dashed lines show the administered work rate and pattern of work rate increase with time. The $\dot{V}O_2$ data are the average of 9-second periods. (From Zhang YY, Johnson MC, Chow N, et al. Effect of exercise testing protocol on parameters of aerobic function. *Med Sci Sports Exerc* 1991; 23:625–630, with permission.)

For treadmill exercise, a predictable adjustment for body weight is not possible because of complex mechanical factors such as varying center of gravity as the angle of the treadmill is changed, the variable length of the stride as the speed and grade are altered, and the tendency of the subject to hold on to stationary objects for support or balance during the test. These variables make it difficult to estimate the subject's actual power output during treadmill ergometry.

Slope of $\dot{V}O_2$ as a Function of Work Rate

The slope of $\dot{V}O_2$ as a function of work rate is important because it measures the aerobic work efficiency. The slope for the ramp or 1-minute incremental cycle ergometer progressively increasing work rate test was found to be 10.2 ± 1.0 ml O_2/min/watt (W) for normal subjects by Hansen et al. (27) and 9.9 ± 0.7 ml/min/W by Wasserman and Sue (29) (Fig. 4.2). These values are similar to the 10.1 ml O_2/min/W value previously obtained from steady-state measurements in sedentary subjects (28). In 12 trained cyclists, Riley et al. (30) obtained an average slope of 11.5 ml O_2/min/W with a standard deviation of 0.78,

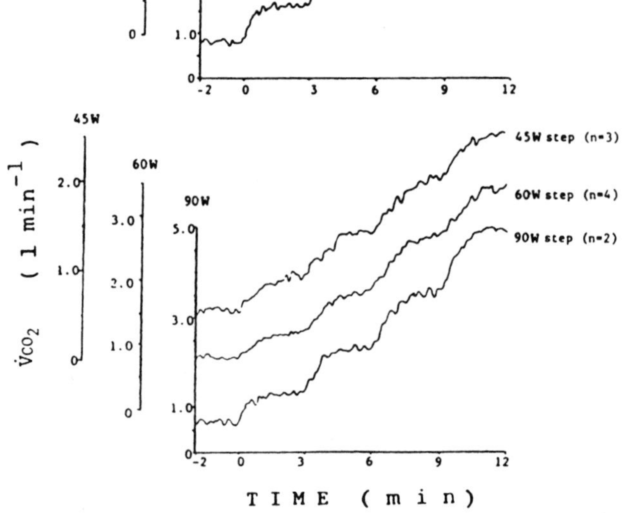

FIGURE 4.4. The average time course of $\dot{V}O_2$ and $\dot{V}CO_2$ for each quarter of a subject's work capacity, assessed in 3-minute work rate steps, is shown for normal subjects at three fitness levels. The greater the size of the step increase in work rate (90-, 60-, or 45-W steps), the greater the subject's fitness ($\dot{V}O_2$peak). At higher work rates, the gas exchange kinetics slow and thereby appear to be more damped. Because the subjects with the larger step increases are more fit, their kinetics are faster and there is less damping of gas exchange. (From Zhang YY, Johnson MC, Chow N, et al. The role of fitness on $\dot{V}O_2$ and $\dot{V}CO_2$ kinetics in response to proportional step increases in work rate. *Eur J Appl Physiol* 1991;63:94–100, with permission.)

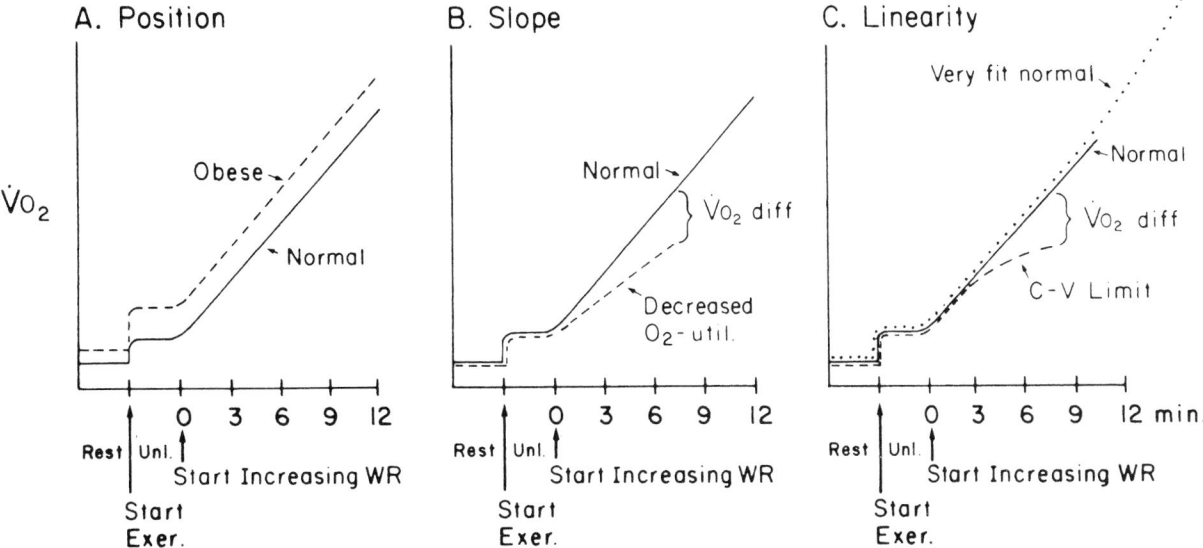

FIGURE 4.5.   Position displacement (A), slope (B), and linearity (C) of the $\dot{V}O_2$–work rate relationship. Obesity displaces the $\dot{V}O_2$–work rate relationship upward, but the slope is unchanged (A). A decreased slope of the $\dot{V}O_2$–work rate relationship (B) reflects inadequate O_2 availability to the exercising muscles, such as when peripheral blood flow is impaired. The linearity of the $\dot{V}O_2$–work rate relationship (C) can be altered in patients with cardiovascular diseases (slope becomes more shallow) because of impaired O_2 flow to the exercising muscles, or in very fit people (slope becomes steeper; see text). The difference between the expected $\dot{V}O_2$ for the work rate performed and the actual $\dot{V}O_2$ at the maximum work rate of the subject is referred to as the $\dot{V}O_2$ difference.

suggesting that athletes may have a slightly higher $\Delta\dot{V}O_2/\Delta WR$ than nonathletes.

If the muscles are unable to extract the O_2 required to perform the exercise, then the slope will be shallower than normal (Fig. 4.5B) and the predicted peak $\dot{V}O_2$ will not be reached. Although there may be several reasons for this slope to be reduced, a reduction is most commonly due to conditions that impair O_2 flow to the exercising extremities, such as heart disease, pulmonary vascular disease, or peripheral arterial occlusive disease. In peripheral arterial occlusive disease, the fixed stenosis prevents the normal increase in blood flow and $\dot{V}O_2$, resulting in a linear but relatively shallow increase in $\dot{V}O_2$ such as shown in Figure 4.5B. In contrast to other cardiovascular disorders, the slope of $\dot{V}CO_2$ relative to work rate increase is also relatively shallow (31).

Linearity of $\dot{V}O_2$ as a Function of Work Rate

Because O_2 uptake kinetics are a more complex function of work rate than a single exponential at work rates above the anaerobic threshold (AT) (32,33), the slope of the $\dot{V}O_2$–work rate relationship is not necessarily the same above the AT as below the AT (Fig. 4.5C). If the rate of increase in work rate is rapid relative to the subject's degree of fitness, then a relatively large proportion of energy generated is from anaerobic sources and the slope would

be expected to become more shallow (60 W/min; see Fig. 2.26). In contrast, when the rate of increase in work rate is slow, several factors may account for an augmented O_2 uptake and thereby cause the $\dot{V}O_2$–work rate slope to steepen above the AT. These can include (a) the use of additional muscle groups when performing heavy exercise (e.g., pulling on cycle handlebars during leg cycling to brace the trunk on the ergometer as the pedals get harder to turn), (b) a nonlinear increase in the work of breathing as high levels of ventilation are reached, (c) the O_2 cost of lactate conversion to glycogen (Cori cycle) by tissues actively involved in gluconeogenesis (liver), and (d) the recruitment of less efficient muscle fibers (type IIx) at high work rates.

In view of the foregoing considerations, the finding of a deviation in the $\dot{V}O_2$–work rate slope above the AT, such as illustrated in Figure 2.26, is understandable. If the rate of the work rate increase were relatively slow for a fit subject, then the four factors noted previously would make a greater contribution to $\dot{V}O_2$ relative to work rate (33,34) than that observed below the AT. In contrast, rapid increases in work rate result in a sizable fraction of anaerobic work above the AT (as assessed by a high rate of lactate increase), and $\dot{V}O_2$ would therefore increase more slowly relative to the work rate increase in the above-AT range of work (35). Thus, in the same subject, the $\dot{V}O_2$–work rate relationship above the AT can be more steep (slow work rate increase) or less steep (rapid work rate increase) than the relation below the *AT*, which is not affected by the rate of work rate increase (see Fig. 2.26). Regardless of the rate of work rate increase, however, the peak $\dot{V}O_2$ is not affected to an appreciable degree. In general, work rate increments of 15 to 25 W per minute in normal men and 10 to 20 W in normal women give a similar rate of rise in $\dot{V}O_2$ both above and below the *AT*. A method for selecting the work rate increment for progressively increasing work rate exercise testing of normal subjects and patients is described in Chapter 6.

In disorders of the cardiovascular system, the linearity of the $\dot{V}O_2$–work rate relationship is commonly abnormal regardless of the rate at which work rate is increased (Fig. 4.5C). The $\dot{V}O_2$ may increase normally as the work rate is increased at low levels, but $\dot{V}O_2$ may slow its rate of increase as the maximum $\dot{V}O_2$ is approached. The nonlinear slowing of the rate of rise in the slope of the $\dot{V}O_2$–work rate relationship in heart disease (Fig. 4.5C) is usually accompanied by a persistently steep $\dot{V}CO_2$–work rate slope. This reflects the CO_2 released from the HCO_3^- buffering of simultaneously generated lactic acid (36,37). In these situations, the subject's peak $\dot{V}O_2$ is clearly reduced.

Can $\dot{V}O_2$ or Mets Be Predicted from the Work Rate?

Some laboratories estimate $\dot{V}O_2$ from work rate during exercise rather than measuring $\dot{V}O_2$ directly. This practice is potentially inaccurate and should be discouraged. A unit called a *met* was derived from the average resting $\dot{V}O_2$ for a 70-kg, 40-year-old man. It is equal to 3.5 ml/min per kilogram of body weight. By assuming a fixed relation between the ergometer work rate and the $\dot{V}O_2$, some laboratories report an *estimate* of $\dot{V}O_2$ from the ergometer work rate. After obtaining this estimated $\dot{V}O_2$ and expressing it per kilogram of body weight, the $\dot{V}O_2$ per kilogram is divided by 3.5 to obtain the number of mets performed by the subject.

However, under many conditions, $\dot{V}O_2$ cannot be accurately predicted from the estimated work rate for the reasons summarized in Table 4.4. If $\dot{V}O_2$ does not increase linearly with increasing work rate, as is common in patients with cardiovascular diseases, $\dot{V}O_2$ cannot be estimated from work rate (38) (see Fig. 4.5C and the cardiovascular cases in Chapter 10). Thus, using work rate to calculate $\dot{V}O_2$ or mets will usually lead to overestimates in these patients.

In addition, work rate fails to predict $\dot{V}O_2$ if the obesity factor is not taken into account. This factor is often ignored, or incorrect estimates of the effect

TABLE 4.4. Conditions in Which Work Rate Fails to Predict $\dot{V}O_2$

$\dot{V}O_2$ fails to increase linearly with work rate
Obesity
Valvular heart disease
Coronary artery disease
Cardiomyopathy
Peripheral arterial disease
Pulmonary vascular disease
Faulty ergometer calibration

of body weight are used. The $\dot{V}O_2$ to perform a given amount of external work will be higher in an obese than in a lean subject because of the need to expend additional energy to move a large body when effecting external work. For cycle ergometer work, we have found that the O_2 cost of cycling an unloaded ergometer at 60 rpm is an additional 5.8 ml/min for each kilogram body weight (27,28).

Furthermore, analysis of the $\dot{V}O_2$–work rate relation is of value only if the ergometer and the measurement system are accurately calibrated. Unfortunately, many cycle ergometers are not accurate, particularly over the low work rate range. The reader should review Chapter 6 on how to obviate flywheel inertia at the start of exercise. Appendix C and Chapter 6 should also be reviewed for methods of assuring accuracy in gas exchange measurements.

Cardiac Output and Stroke Volume

Cardiac output measurement may be useful when trying to assess whether the patient's reduced O_2 uptake is due to reduced O_2 transport or failure of the muscles to extract O_2 for whatever cause. However, cardiac output measurement by itself, even if accurate, may not reveal whether cardiac output is adequate for the work rate performed. The major concern of exercise testing should be to determine whether the heart is capable of providing the exercise-stressed muscles with enough oxygen. To answer this important question, measurement of the *AT* and $\Delta\dot{V}O_2/\Delta WR$ during a progressively increasing work rate test, and measurement of the $\dot{V}O_2$ and $\dot{V}CO_2$ kinetics during a constant work rate test, may be more useful. Because all of these measurements are made noninvasively with cardiopulmonary exercise testing, they can be repeated easily.

Cardiac Output Measurement

Direct Fick Method. From the measurement of $\dot{V}O_2$ and the simultaneous measurement of arterial and mixed venous O_2 content, cardiac output can be determined from the direct Fick equation:

$$\text{Cardiac output} = \dot{V}O_2 / C(a - \bar{v})O_2$$

Mixed venous ($\bar{v}$) O_2 content is determined from a catheter in the pulmonary artery, and systemic arterial (a) O_2 content is determined from an arterial catheter. This method represents the gold standard for cardiac output measurement. Sun et al. (39) compared the direct Fick method using O_2 as the test gas with that using CO_2. The cardiac outputs were very similar, on average, although the variability in the measurements was greater using CO_2 as the test gas than when using O_2.

Indirect Fick Method Using $\dot{V}CO_2$ and Estimated $C\bar{v}CO_2$.
Estimates of cardiac output during exercise are sometimes made with the indirect Fick method,

$$\text{Cardiac output} = \dot{V}CO_2 / C(a - \bar{v})CO_2$$

from a measurement of $\dot{V}CO_2$ and an estimate of arterial PCO_2 ($PaCO_2$) from end-tidal PCO_2 ($PETCO_2$) and mixed venous PCO_2 by the CO_2 rebreathing method (40). (See Appendix A for definitions of symbols and Appendix C for a description of the rebreathing method.)

This approach has many potential errors. First, estimation of $PaCO_2$ from $PETCO_2$ measurements, as commonly done, is unreliable, especially in patients (41,42). $PETCO_2$ is less than $PaCO_2$ in patients with lung disease, heart failure, and pulmonary vascular disease and greater than $PaCO_2$ in normal subjects (see Chapter 5). Second, the assumption is made that mixed venous CO_2 content can be determined accurately from mixed venous PCO_2 using a standard CO_2 dissociation curve in which blood CO_2 content is plotted as a function of blood PCO_2. If the work is above the AT, however, the CO_2 content will be decreased for the same mixed venous PCO_2 as that below the AT (43) because of a shift downward in the subject's CO_2 dissociation curve. This shift downward results from the decrease in CO_2 content for a given PCO_2 of blood when HCO_3^- buffers lactic acid. Third, the assumption is made that the CO_2 dissociation curve is linear, although in reality it gets less steep the higher the PCO_2.

Sun et al. (44) determined the PCO_2 and CO_2 content of mixed venous blood at all levels of exercise and found that CO_2 content increased, although nonlinearly with work rate, up to the AT (see Chapter 3). Above the AT, $P\bar{v}CO_2$ rose steeply but CO_2 content decreased. This is due to the

buffering of lactic acid by HCO_3^- (the pH effect). This effect cannot be estimated without direct mixed venous blood gas and pH measurements. Because of this phenomenon, the CO_2 rebreathing method for determining mixed venous CO_2 content, particularly above the AT, cannot be accurate.

Thermodilution

If a thermistor-tipped catheter is introduced into the pulmonary artery, the cardiac output can be determined from a thermodilution curve after the injection of iced saline into the lumen of the catheter that opens into the right atrium. From this curve and the volume of iced saline injected, blood flow through the right atrium can be calculated (45).

Measuring $\dot{V}O_2$ and Estimating $C(a - \bar{v})O_2$

Stringer et al. (46) pointed out that cardiac output can be calculated during exercise, noninvasively, by the direct Fick principle with a reliability as good as generally reported by other methods. The calculation is made from the $\dot{V}O_2$ measurement alone, at work rates at which $C(a - \bar{v})O_2$ can be estimated with relative accuracy. It was shown that in normal subjects, as in patients with heart failure (47), $C(a - \bar{v})O_2$ increases relatively linearly to peak $\dot{V}O_2$, achieving a value of approximately 15 ml/dl. Agostoni et al. (48) found that patients with chronic heart failure, on average, had higher values for $C(a - \bar{v})O_2$ at the AT the worse the exercise tolerance. However, they had similar values to normal subjects at peak $\dot{V}O_2$ (Table 4.5). From the shape of the $\dot{V}O_2$ curves shown in Figure 4.6, variability in the $C(a - \bar{v})O_2$ has less influence on the cardiac output determination, in absolute terms, as $C(a - \bar{v})O_2$ increases and as $\dot{V}O_2$ decreases.

Normal young men had a standard deviation for $C(a - \bar{v})O_2$ of 7.6% and 7.4% and for extraction ratio of 7.5% and 9.4% at the AT and peak $\dot{V}O_2$, respectively (Table 4.5) (46). Patients with heart failure had a standard deviation for an extraction ratio at AT and peak $\dot{V}O_2$ of 13% and 9%, respectively (Table 4.5) (48). The standard deviation for $C(a - \bar{v})O_2$ at the AT for the patients was higher than that for normal subjects because these values tended to increase the worse the heart failure (Fig. 4.6). However, no values were below 10 ml/min.

In Figure 4.6, Fick cardiac outputs are plotted as a function of $C(a - \bar{v})O_2$ at the AT in normal subjects and in patients with stable chronic heart failure, taken from the work of Stringer et al. (46) and Agostoni et al. (48), respectively. For the heart failure subjects, the higher $C(a - \bar{v})O_2$ values in the

TABLE 4.5. Arteriovenous O_2 Difference and Extraction Ratio ± Standard Deviation at Rest, Anaerobic Threshold (*AT*), and Peak $\dot{V}O_2$

	$\dot{V}O_2$ (L/min)	Arteriovenous O_2 Difference (ml/dl)	Extraction Ratio[a]
Normal men[b]			
Rest		6.14 ± 1.7	0.30 ± 0.09
AT	1.84 ± 0.36	11.3 ± 0.87	0.53 ± 0.04
Peak $\dot{V}O_2$	3.77 ± 0.61	16.2 ± 1.2	0.74 ± 0.07
Chronic heart failure[c]			
Rest	0.28 ± 0.07	7.8 ± 2.6	0.43 ± 0.11
AT	0.83 ± 0.25	13.0 ± 2.4	0.68 ± 0.09
Peak $\dot{V}O_2$	1.26 ± 0.39	15.0 ± 2.7	0.77 ± 0.07

[a]Extraction ratio equals fractional difference between Ca_{O_2} and $C\bar{v}_{O_2}$.
[b]Data from Stringer W, Hansen J, Wasserman K. Cardiac output estimated non-invasively from oxygen uptake ($\dot{V}O_2$) during exercise. *J Appl Physiol* 1997;82:908–912.
[c]Data from Agostoni PG, Wasserman K, Perego G, et al. Stroke volume (SV) measured, non-invasively at anaerobic threshold (AT) in heart failure (HF). *Am J Respir Crit Care Med* 1997;155:A171.

distribution are dominated by the more exercise-limited patients. From Figure 4.6, it is evident that the variability in $C(a - \bar{v})O_2$ has a relatively small effect on estimating exercise cardiac output at the *AT*, particularly in patients with low *AT* values.

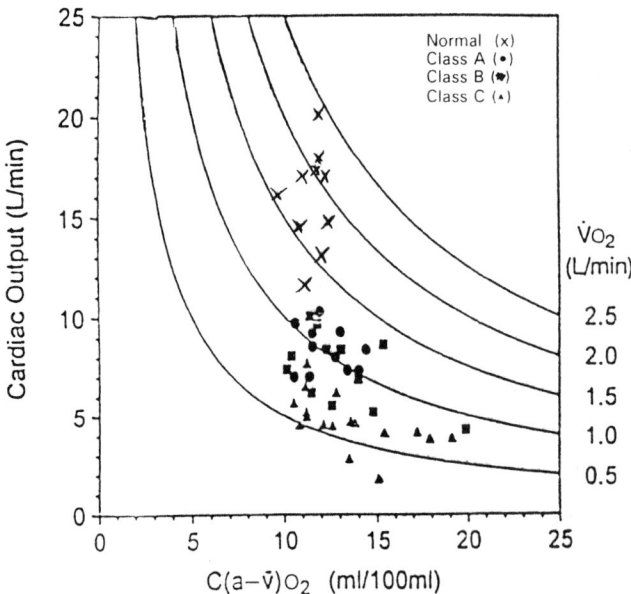

FIGURE 4.6. Cardiac output (calculated by the direct Fick method) is plotted as a function of arteriovenous O_2 difference [$C(a - \bar{v})O_2$] at the anaerobic threshold (*AT*) for normal and heart failure subjects in physiological class A (peak $\dot{V}O_2$ > 20 ml/min/kg), B (peak $\dot{V}O_2$ = 15–20 ml/min/kg), and C (peak $\dot{V}O_2$ = 10–15 ml/min/kg). Superimposed are $\dot{V}O_2$ isopleths. See the text for further discussion of the application of these plots in estimating cardiac output. (Data taken from Stringer W, Hansen J, Wasserman K. Cardiac output estimated non-invasively from oxygen uptake ($\dot{V}O_2$) during exercise. *J Appl Physiol* 1997;82:908–912 and from Agostoni PG, Wasserman K, Perego G, et al. Stroke volume (SV) measured non-invasively at anaerobic threshold (*AT*) in heart failure (HF). *Am J Respir Crit Care Med* 1997;155:A171.)

Whether using a value for $C(a - \bar{v})O_2$ at *AT* or peak $\dot{V}O_2$ for a given population, the stroke volumes derived from the respective cardiac outputs and heart rates should be similar.

In application of this method, the hemoglobin concentration and the arterial oxyhemoglobin saturation must be taken into account as described for the method of measuring peak cardiac output noninvasively during exercise (see Chapter 9; see also "Oxygen Pulse and Stroke Volume" in this chapter).

Anaerobic, Lactate, and Lactic Acidosis Thresholds

The *AT* is defined as the level of exercise $\dot{V}O_2$ above which aerobic energy production is supplemented by anaerobic mechanisms and is reflected by an increase in lactate and lactate-to-pyruvate (L/P) ratio in muscle (49) and arterial blood (see Figs. 2.11 and 2.12). The biochemical and physiological foundations of the *AT* hypothesis and their relation to lactate increase and the development of lactic acidosis are described in Chapter 2. The underlying mechanism for the *AT* measurement depends on the onset of anaerobic glycolysis leading to a net increase in lactic acid production (see Pathway B of Fig. 2.1). At work rates below the *AT*, the muscle (50,51) and blood (52) L/P ratio is the same as at rest, and no metabolic acidosis develops. Above the *AT*, a lactic acidosis develops. Thus, the threshold can be defined physiologically as the $\dot{V}O_2$ above which the critical capillary P_{O_2} has been reached and production of *ATP* through anaerobic glycolysis supplements the aerobic *ATP* production. It can also be defined in terms of changing redox state

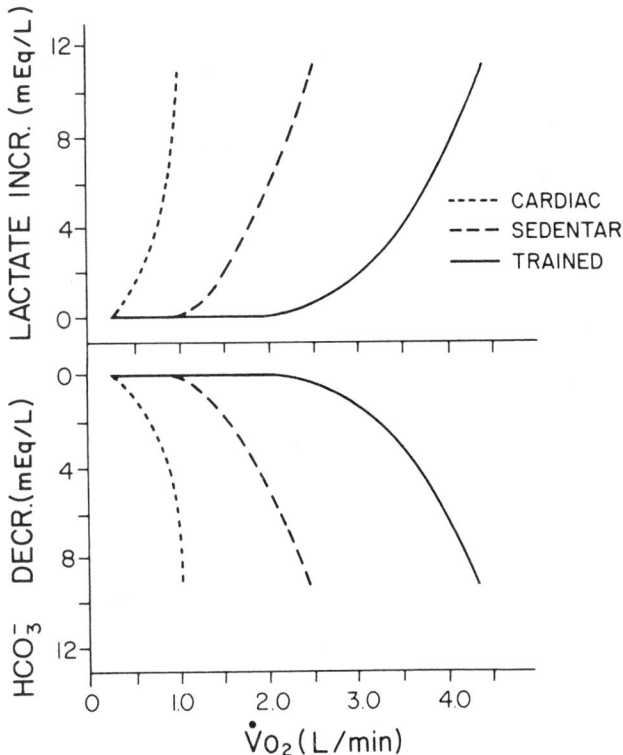

FIGURE 4.7.   Lactate increase and bicarbonate decrease during incremental exercise in trained and sedentary normal subjects and in patients with primary cardiac disease of class II to III severity as defined by the New York Heart Association Classification. (Modified from Wasserman K, Whipp BJ. Exercise physiology in health and disease (state of the art). *Am Rev Respir Dis* 1975;112:219–249.)

within the cell, as the $\dot{V}O_2$ at which lactate and L/P ratio increase (lactate threshold, *LT*); or in terms of acid–base balance change, as the $\dot{V}O_2$ at which lactic acidosis develops (lactic acidosis threshold, *LAT*). Like the $\dot{V}O_2$max, the threshold measurement is influenced by the size of the muscle groups involved in the activity.

Major Physiological Effects

In Chapter 2, the significance of the *AT* and the major changes that take place during the performance of exercise above as compared to below the *AT* were discussed. These include the development of metabolic acidosis with a sustained increase in blood lactate and L/P ratio. Plasma bicarbonate decreases inversely to the lactate increase, at a $\dot{V}O_2$ that depends on the level of fitness and wellness for aerobic work, as shown in Figure 4.7.

The *AT* also demarcates the exercise $\dot{V}O_2$ above which $\dot{V}O_2$ kinetics slow and above which exercise can no longer be performed in a true steady state. Above the *AT*, ventilatory drive is stimulated by the metabolic acidosis resulting from lactate accumula-

tion. The rate of increase in $\dot{V}E$, which is primarily due to an increase in breathing frequency, depends on the magnitude of the lactic acidosis and the work rate (see Fig. 2.43). Importantly, endurance time in the performance of a specific work task is reduced above the *AT* in proportion to the increase in lactate evoked by the exercise (see Fig. 2.10). The higher the lactate concentration, the shorter the endurance time and the steeper the rate of increase of $\dot{V}O_2$ during phase III of constant work rate exercise (53). Other changes in physiological responses to exercise above the *AT* are described in Table 2.2.

Methods of Measurement

H^+ production is increased when lactate concentration is increased in the cell. At the pH of cell water, virtually all of the increase in H^+ production must be buffered. The H^+ produced with the first 0.5 mmol/L increase in lactate appears to be buffered by non-HCO_3^- buffering mechanisms (37,54,55), primarily by the alkaline reaction resulting from hydrolysis of phosphocreatine in muscle during early exercise (55). Above this initial increase in lactate, HCO_3^- buffers the newly produced H^+ stoichiometrically (37,54,56). Thus, at work rates above the threshold, an obligatory increase in CO_2 production above that produced by aerobic metabolism occurs. It is relatively easy to detect the development of cellular lactic acidosis by measuring the rate of increase in $\dot{V}CO_2$ relative to that of $\dot{V}O_2$ during a progressively increasing exercise test. Beaver et al. (36) used a statistical regression method. Sue et al. (57) simplified the method, observing that the $\dot{V}CO_2$ versus $\dot{V}O_2$ relation below the threshold had a slope consistently at or slightly less than 1.0, and that the slope changed to a value greater than 1.0 above the threshold.

A relatively short, progressive work rate test can rapidly determine the $\dot{V}O_2$ at which lactic acidosis develops when gas exchange is measured breath by breath, or as the average of several breaths. The reason gas exchange is so effective in detecting the development of cellular metabolic acidosis is that the time delay between the HCO_3^- buffering of lactic acid in the cell and the increase in CO_2 from this buffering is only a few seconds. A flow diagram describing the sequence of gas exchange and ventilation changes in response to developing lactic acidosis for a progressively increasing work rate exercise test is shown in Figure 4.8. The changes in gas exchange that take place above the *AT* are illustrated in Figure 4.9.

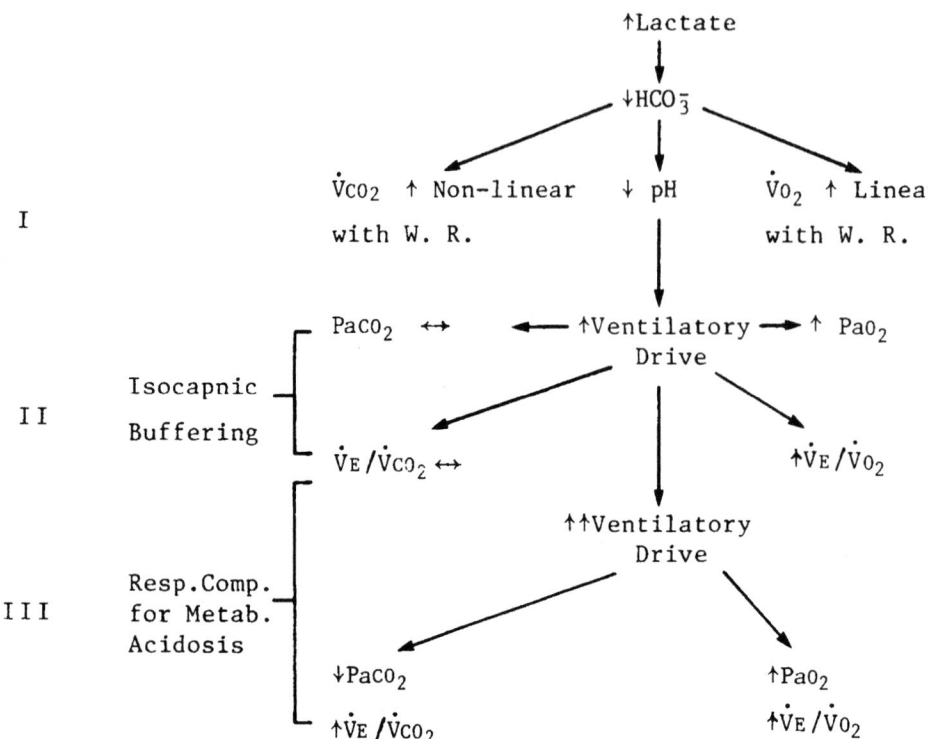

FIGURE 4.8. Diagram of effect of increasing lactate on gas exchange during a progressively increasing work rate exercise test. Small arrows directed upward indicate increases, small arrows directed downward indicate decreases, and horizontal arrows indicate no change. Mechanism I describes gas exchange that results solely from buffering of newly formed lactic acid (lower left panel of Figure 4.9). Mechanism II describes changes in arterial and end-tidal P_{CO_2} and P_{O_2} and ventilatory equivalents for O_2 and CO_2 that result from increased ventilatory drive consequent to CO_2 generated by buffering reaction (right upper and lower panels of Figure 4.9). Mechanism III describes changes caused by further increase in ventilatory drive consequent to respiratory compensation for metabolic acidosis (changes to the right of *AT* lines in right upper and lower panels of Figure 4.9).

V-Slope Method (Fig. 4.8, Mechanism I). When the net increase in lactate accumulation produces an acidosis, $\dot{V}_{CO_2}$ accelerates relative to $\dot{V}_{O_2}$. When these variables are plotted against each other, the relationship is composed of two apparently linear components, the lower of which (S_1) has a slope of slightly less than 1.0, whereas the upper component (S_2) has a slope steeper than 1.0 (see Fig. 2.31). The intercept of these two slopes is the *AT* as measured by gas exchange (Fig. 4.9, lower left panel). The buffering of lactic acid causes an obligatory increase in $\dot{V}_{CO_2}$ relative to $\dot{V}_{O_2}$ from the CO_2 produced when HCO_3^- buffers lactic acid. This technique is referred to as the *V-slope method* because it relates the increase in volume of CO_2 output to volume of O_2 uptake. As shown in Figure 2.31, S_1 and S_2 can be determined from statistically derived regression slopes of $\dot{V}_{CO_2}$ versus $\dot{V}_{O_2}$ in the respective regions of interest. The break point or intercept of the two slopes can be selected by a computer program that defines the $\dot{V}_{O_2}$ above which $\dot{V}_{CO_2}$ increases faster than $\dot{V}_{O_2}$, without hyperventilation. The values obtained by this method agree closely with the lactate threshold and, more precisely, the [HCO_3^-] threshold (36, 57). If a patient develops a lactic acidosis with only minimal exercise, the $\dot{V}_{CO_2}$–$\dot{V}_{O_2}$ plot may become steeper than 1.0 immediately after the start of un-

loaded exercise, and therefore the *AT* will be less than the lowest measured exercise $\dot{V}_{O_2}$.

Sue et al. (57) pointed out that because S_1 must have a slope value of 1.0 or less and S_2 a slope value of greater than 1.0 using the V-slope method, the break-point representing the *AT* can be determined by placing a 45-degree right triangle on the $\dot{V}_{CO_2}$ versus $\dot{V}_{O_2}$ plot (plotted on equal scales). The $\dot{V}_{O_2}$ at which the data points start to increase at an angle greater than 45 degrees (slope > 1.0) is the *AT*.

Whereas this method uses simultaneous measurements of $\dot{V}_{CO_2}$ and $\dot{V}_{O_2}$, it is independent of the subject's ventilatory response and insensitive to irregularities in breathing. Thus, it is useful for measuring the *AT* even in patients who do not develop ventilatory compensation for the exercise lactic acidosis, such as in patients with obesity syndrome or severe chronic obstructive pulmonary disease. Despite its independence of the ventilatory response to exercise, some investigators erroneously refer to the V-slope method as the "ventilatory threshold." This is clearly wrong, because $\dot{V}_E$ is an equal factor on both the x- and y-axes and therefore cannot account for the break point in the V-slope plot. The V-slope plot is actually a plot of moles of CO_2 output to moles of O_2 uptake. It is also the same as a plot of cardiac output $\times$ C(a − v̄)$_{CO_2}$ versus cardiac out-

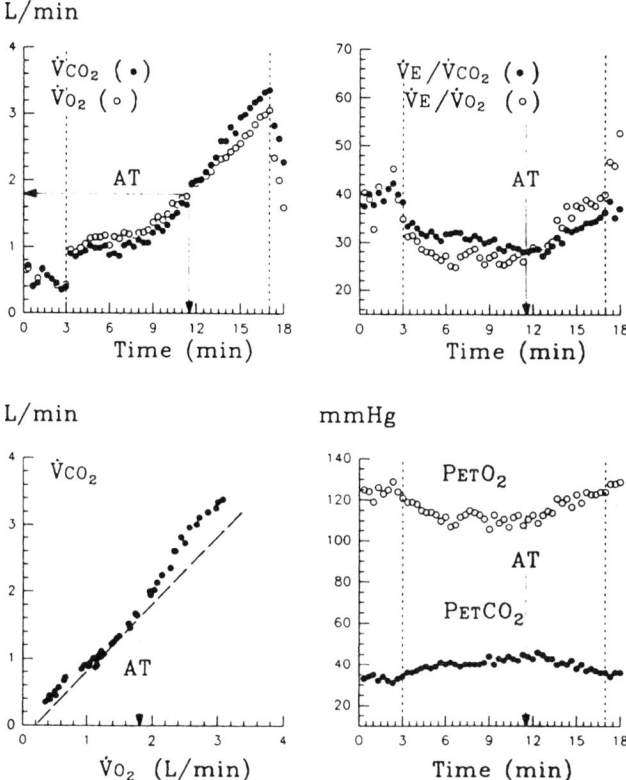

FIGURE 4.9.   Gas exchange for a normal subject during a progressively increasing work rate exercise test to illustrate the gas exchange changes that take place at the anaerobic threshold (*AT*). The far-left vertical dashed line, in the three panels with time as the *x*-axis, indicates the start of unloading cycling. After 3 minutes of unloaded cycling, the work rate was increased 25 watts/min. The right vertical dashed line indicates the end of exercise. The V-slope plot of $\dot{V}_{CO_2}$ versus $\dot{V}_{O_2}$ is shown in the lower left panel. The diagonal line is at 45 degrees, or a slope of 1. The *AT* is where the $\dot{V}_{CO_2}$ starts to increase faster than $\dot{V}_{O_2}$, so the slope of the plot becomes steeper than 1. This is shown as the vertical dashed arrow marked *AT*. The *AT* can also be located where the $\dot{V}_E/\dot{V}_{O_2}$ curve **(right upper panel)** inflects upward (*vertical dashed arrow labeled AT*). The nadir of the $\dot{V}_E/\dot{V}_{O_2}$ curve occurs at a higher work rate and reflects the start of ventilatory compensation for the metabolic acidosis. Because of the hyperventilation with respect to O_2, P_{ETO_2} increases at the *AT* **(right lower panel)**, whereas P_{ETCO_2} does not start to decrease systematically until approximately 2 minutes later, coinciding with the increased ventilatory drive that serves to partially compensate for the decrease in arterial pH.

put $\times$ C($a - \bar{v}$)O_2. Therefore the threshold is due to an increase in C($a - \bar{v}$)CO_2 relative to C($a - \bar{v}$)O_2 as a result of the addition of CO_2 to the venous blood, as shown in Figures 2.20 and 2.32.

Ventilatory Equivalent Method (Fig. 4.8, Mechanism II).

As the work rate is increased in a progressive exercise test (ramp or 1-minute steps), the linear pattern of increase in $\dot{V}_{CO_2}$ and $\dot{V}_E$ seen at low work rates (see Fig. 2.29) changes to a curvilinear

pattern at high work rates, while $\dot{V}_{O_2}$ continues to increase relatively linearly. $\dot{V}_E$ and $\dot{V}_{CO_2}$ initially accelerate in proportion above the *AT*. Therefore, $\dot{V}_E/\dot{V}_{O_2}$ and P_{ETO_2} increase, whereas $\dot{V}_E/\dot{V}_{CO_2}$ and P_{ETCO_2} remain constant for a brief period (isocapnic buffering; see Figs. 2.29 and 4.9). Thus, hyperventilation occurs with respect to O_2 but not CO_2 as the *AT* is exceeded. This isocapnic buffering period normally lasts about 2 minutes during incremental exercise tests. It is referred to as the *isocapnic buffering period* because of the lack of ventilatory compensation for the developing metabolic acidosis (58).

The increase in $\dot{V}_E/\dot{V}_{O_2}$ without an increase in $\dot{V}_E/\dot{V}_{CO_2}$ can only be caused by HCO_3^- buffering metabolic acid. It cannot be caused by other factors that increase ventilation out of proportion to $\dot{V}_{O_2}$ (e.g., hypoxemia, pain, or psychogenic hyperventilation), since these would cause $\dot{V}_E/\dot{V}_{CO_2}$ to increase as well as $\dot{V}_E/\dot{V}_{O_2}$. When $\dot{V}_E/\dot{V}_{O_2}$ increases without a simultaneous increase in $\dot{V}_E/\dot{V}_{CO_2}$ during a progressively increasing work rate test, it is a specific gas exchange demonstration that the *AT* has been surpassed (Fig. 4.8).

One reason for increasing work rate relatively rapidly during the progressively increasing work rate test is to take advantage of the finding that the CO_2 contribution from buffering is observed only during the buffering process (the period of decreasing bicarbonate) and not after the lactate has been buffered. Thus, CO_2 generated from buffering is evident in the expired gas only when lactate and HCO_3^- are changing, not after they have already changed. Increasing the work rate at a relatively fast rate will result in a higher rate of lactate accumulation and steeper S_2 above the *AT* than when the rate of increase in work rate is relatively slow (59).

As the work rate is increased further above the *AT*, the carotid bodies respond to the decreasing pH, and ventilatory stimulation is intensified (see Fig. 4.8, mechanism III, and Figs. 2.29 and 4.9). This causes P_{aCO_2} to decrease, preventing pH from falling as much as would be predicted by the addition of lactic acid to a closed system. This ventilatory compensation for the lactic acidosis is reflected in an increase in $\dot{V}_E/\dot{V}_{CO_2}$ and a decrease in P_{aCO_2} and P_{ETCO_2}, as well as by further increases in $\dot{V}_E/\dot{V}_{O_2}$ and P_{ETO_2} (see Figs. 2.29 and 4.9). When ventilatory compensation for metabolic acidosis starts, the $\dot{V}_{O_2}$ is well above the *AT*, *LT*, or *LAT*. This $\dot{V}_{O_2}$ is referred to as the *ventilatory compensation (VC) point*.

The *AT* is measured as a metabolic stress, that is, in units of O_2 uptake, not work rate. In contrast to the VC point, the *AT* is unaffected by the rate at which the work rate is incremented (60,61) or by metabolic substrate (59,62,63).

Improving Estimation of the Anaerobic Threshold

Occasionally, the *AT* cannot be reliably detected by the ventilatory equivalent method (Fig. 4.8, mechanism II) because of irregular breathing, an inappropriate rate of increase in work rate, suboptimal plotting scales, or a poor ventilatory response by the patient to the metabolic acidosis. To obviate these problems, one can measure blood lactate or standard bicarbonate directly. Beaver et al. (64) found that the *LT* during exercise can be most reliably selected by plotting log blood lactate against $\log \dot{V}O_2$. Similarly, the start of the $[HCO_3^-]$ fall, indicating the start of developing lactic acidosis (*LAT*), can be most reliably detected from a plot of log standard $[HCO_3^-]$ against $\log \dot{V}O_2$ (54). A slight difference exists in the $\dot{V}O_2$ for these thresholds. *LT* precedes *LAT*, because of non-HCO_3^- buffering of the initial lactic acid increase (37). Although we distinguish between *LT* and *LAT* for scientific correctness, the distinction is not of clinical significance.

When the break-point between S_1 and S_2 is not clear using the V-slope method, it is likely that the rate of CO_2 released from HCO_3^- buffering of lactic acid is slow because the rate of increase in work rate is slow relative to the subject's fitness during the progressively increasing work rate test (65). Alternatively, the patient may not produce lactic acid, such as in muscle phosphorylase deficiency (McArdle's syndrome) (66). In the former instance, the test should be repeated with a faster rate of increase in work rate. If the break-point ($\dot{V}CO_2$ increasing faster than $\dot{V}O_2$) is still not observed, the possibility should be investigated that the patient is unable to raise blood lactate levels.

Heart Rate–Oxygen Uptake Relationship and Heart Rate Reserve

Both cardiac output and heart rate normally increase linearly with $\dot{V}O_2$ during increasing work rate exercise (67) (Fig. 4.10). In many types of heart disease, the heart rate increase is relatively steep for the increase in $\dot{V}O_2$ because the stroke volume is low. In addition, $\dot{V}O_2$ commonly slows its rate of increase with work rate when the myocardium becomes ischemic in patients with coronary artery disease. Because heart rate typically continues to

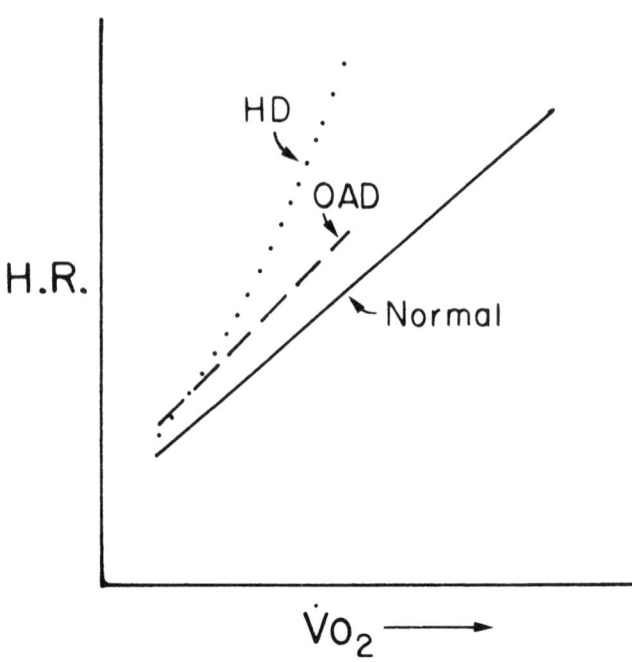

FIGURE 4.10. Characteristic changes in heart rate (HR) relative to $\dot{V}O_2$ for normal subjects, for patients with chronic obstructive airway disease (OAD), and for those with heart disease (HD) without chronotropic incompetence. The steeper heart rate–$\dot{V}O_2$ relationship for the patient with obstructive airway disease may reflect relative unfitness or reduced stroke volume secondary to disturbed lung mechanics or pulmonary vascular occlusion. In contrast, the relatively low maximum heart rate reflects respiratory limitation to the maximum level of exercise. The steepening heart rate–$\dot{V}O_2$ relationship seen in some patients with heart disease reflects the failure of $\dot{V}O_2$ to increase, normally, in response to the increasing work rate, as illustrated in Figure 4.5C.

increase in these patients, the rate of increase in heart rate relative to $\dot{V}O_2$ becomes steeper, deviating from the linearity established at lower work rates (Fig. 4.10). This implies that stroke volume is decreasing and that cardiac output may not be increasing in pace with the O_2 requirement. Although this curvilinear increase in the heart rate–$\dot{V}O_2$ relationship is not uniformly seen in patients with heart disease, it is a useful diagnostic observation and suggests a significant worsening in left ventricular function with increasing work rate (68).

Pulmonary vascular disease is also associated with a steep heart rate response because venous return to the left side of the heart and therefore left ventricular output are low in this disorder.

Patients with airflow obstruction (Fig. 4.10) commonly have a moderately elevated heart rate response at a given $\dot{V}O_2$ due to a reduced stroke volume. The latter results from a restriction in cardiac filling (69) due to high intrathoracic pressure during exhalation or to encroachment of the lung on the cardiac fossa, or both. Heart rate increases lin-

TABLE 4.6. Disorders Associated with Increased Heart Rate Reserve

Claudication limiting exercise
Angina limiting exercise
"Sick sinus" syndrome
β-Adrenergic blockade
Lung disease with impaired ventilatory mechanics
Poor effort

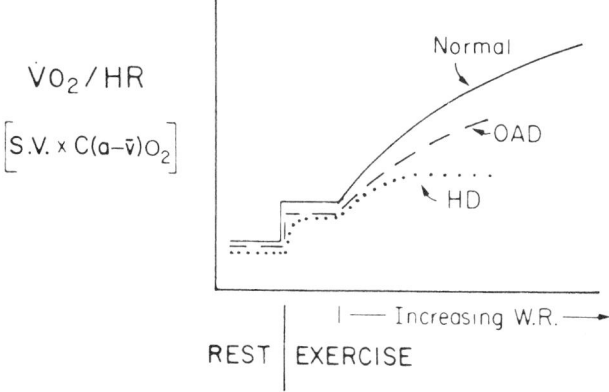

FIGURE 4.11. Characteristic changes in $\dot{V}o_2$/heart rate (HR) or stroke volume times $C(a - \bar{v})o_2$ (O_2 pulse) as related to increase in work rate (W.R.). Thus, patients with low stroke volumes [e.g., heart disease (HD)] will tend to have low O_2 pulse values at maximal exercise. In contrast, patients with obstructive airway disease (OAD) have a pattern similar to that in normal subjects, although the values are lower at each work rate, reflecting the relatively low stroke volume in these patients.

early with $\dot{V}o_2$ in this disorder. The maximum heart rate in the patient with ventilatory limitation is usually below the predicted value for the normal subject because the patient becomes ventilatory limited before the cardiovascular system is maximally stressed (70).

The estimated *heart rate reserve* is a measure of the difference between the predicted maximal heart rate, based on age, and the measured heart rate at peak $\dot{V}o_2$. See the section on maximal heart rate and heart rate reserve in Chapter 7, for normal values.

Although the predicted maximal heart rate has considerable variation, as determined from population studies, the heart rate reserve is still a useful concept for differential diagnosis. Table 4.6 lists disorders in which the heart rate reserve may be increased. Normally, the heart rate reserve is relatively small (less than 15 beats/min). It is also usually normal in patients with silent myocardial ischemia and valvular heart disease and in patients with disorders of the pulmonary circulation. In contrast, patients with peripheral arterial disease and patients with chronic obstructive pulmonary disease become symptom-limited before the predicted maximal heart rate is reached. Patients with disorders of the conducting system of the heart, or sinoatrial node, may also have a low maximum heart rate. Patients who take β-adrenergic blocking drugs or patients who are limited in exercise because of heart block or sick sinus syndrome have a large heart rate reserve. Finally, those patients who make a poor effort have an increased heart rate reserve because they fail to maximally stress their cardiovascular system at the time they stop exercising.

Oxygen Pulse and Stroke Volume

The O_2 pulse is calculated by dividing the $\dot{V}o_2$ by the simultaneously measured heart rate. It is the volume of O_2 taken up by the pulmonary blood during the period of a heartbeat and depends on the volume of O_2 extracted by the peripheral tissues. This

measurement is useful because it equals the product of stroke volume and the arterial–mixed venous O_2 difference [$C(a - \bar{v})o_2$]. The immediate increase in O_2 pulse at the start of exercise depends primarily on the increase in stroke volume. As the work rate is increased, the O_2 pulse increases (Fig. 4.11), primarily because of an increasing $C(a - \bar{v})o_2$. If the stroke volume is reduced, the $C(a - \bar{v})o_2$ and, therefore, the O_2 pulse reach maximal values at a relatively low work rate. In this situation, the O_2 pulse has a low asymptote (70) [see the heart disease (HD) curve in Fig. 4.11]. The O_2 pulse is also low in subjects with anemia, high levels of carboxyhemoglobin, or severe arterial hypoxemia, all because of reduced arterial O_2 content and therefore a reduced $C(a - \bar{v})o_2$ at maximal exercise.

When arterial O_2 content and therefore $C(a - \bar{v})o_2$ at maximal exercise can be assumed to be normal (approximately 15 ml/dl when hemoglobin equals 15 g/dl), stroke volume (SV) can be estimated from the O_2 pulse by the following equation:

$$SV = (O_2 \text{ pulse}/15) \times 100$$

where SV is in ml and O_2 pulse is in ml/beat. The denominator of 15 should be changed to whatever is the hemoglobin concentration (see the section on estimating peak cardiac output during exercise in Chapter 9).

The O_2 pulse measured breath-by-breath in the transition from rest to exercise and from exercise to recovery is also informative. The increase in O_2

pulse at the start of exercise depends on the size of the stroke volume increase and the increase in $C(a - \bar{v})_{O_2}$. It will be low in patients who cannot increase their stroke volume in response to exercise. Whereas the O_2 pulse promptly decreases in the normal subject when stopping exercise, as expected, it often transiently increases in patients with left ventricular failure and exercise-induced myocardial ischemia. The explanation for this paradoxical response is that the afterload of the left ventricle is abruptly decreased when stopping exercise because of the immediate decrease in systemic arterial blood pressure. This allows improved ventricular ejection and increased stroke volume as the patient with the failing heart stops exercising (71). The increase in stroke volume allows capillary blood flow to move more rapidly through the lung during the period of a heartbeat, thereby absorbing more O_2.

Arterial Blood Pressure

Arterial pressure measurements, particularly when directly measured, are helpful diagnostically as well as for patient safety. The normal responses of systolic, diastolic, and pulse pressures are described in Chapter 7 (in the section "Brachial Artery Blood Pressure"). Normally, the systolic pressure increases to a much greater degree than the diastolic pressure and in proportion to the work rate increase. A decrease in systolic and pulse pressures with increasing work rate suggests important cardiac dysfunction and indicates that the exercise test should stop. The direct arterial pressure tracing (made at a fast recorder speed) showing a slow rise in arterial pressure may provide evidence for ventricular outflow obstruction, such as seen with aortic stenosis or hypertrophic cardiomyopathy.

Breathing Reserve

The breathing reserve is expressed as either the difference between the maximal voluntary ventilation (MVV) and the maximum exercise ventilation in absolute terms or this difference as a fraction of the MVV (Table 4.2; Fig. 4.12). Except in extremely fit individuals who can attain high levels of $\dot{V}_E$, normal males have a breathing reserve of at least 11 L/min, or 10% to 40% of the MVV (Fig. 4.13) (72). A low breathing reserve is characteristic of patients with primary lung disease who have ventilatory limitation. The breathing reserve is high when cardiovascular or other diseases limit exercise performance.

Expiratory Flow Pattern

The expiratory flow pattern can be useful in detecting airway obstruction during exercise. The peak expiratory flow rate is near the middle of the expiratory phase of respiration in normal subjects and has an appearance of a half sine wave. In contrast, the expiratory flow pattern of the patient with obstructive airway disease has an early peak and appears trapezoidal because exhalation effort is sustained until the next inspiration is initiated with an abrupt termination of expiration (Fig. 4.14). This

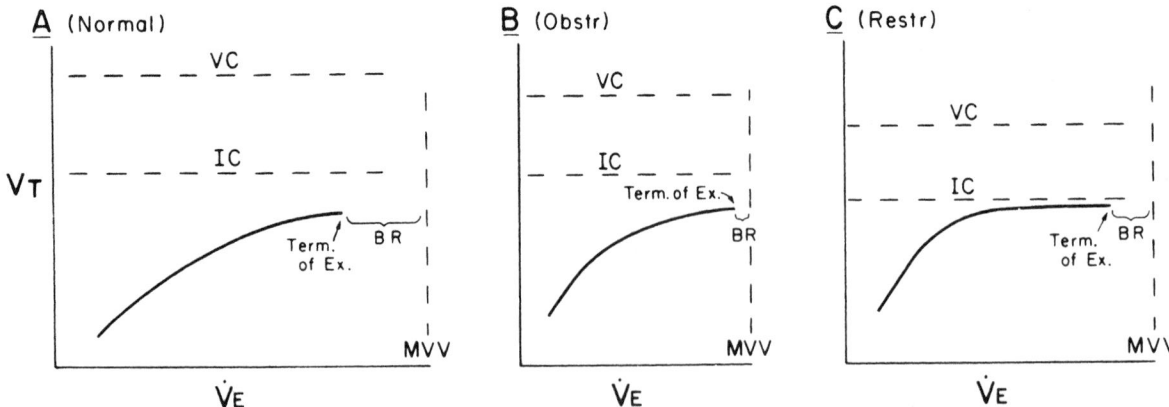

FIGURE 4.12.   Examples of tidal volume change as related to minute ventilation during incremental exercise testing in a normal subject (A) and in patients with obstructive (B) and restrictive (C) lung diseases. The curve ends at the subject's maximal exercise ventilation. The vertical dashed line indicates the subject's maximum voluntary ventilation (MVV). The horizontal dashed lines show the vital capacity (VC) and inspiratory capacity (IC) on the *y*-axis. The distance between the highest $\dot{V}_E$ and MVV on the *x*-axis is the subject's breathing reserve (BR). In the case of patients with obstructive lung disease, the BR is quite small. In restrictive lung diseases, the IC is reduced and V_T closely approximates the IC near and at peak exercise.

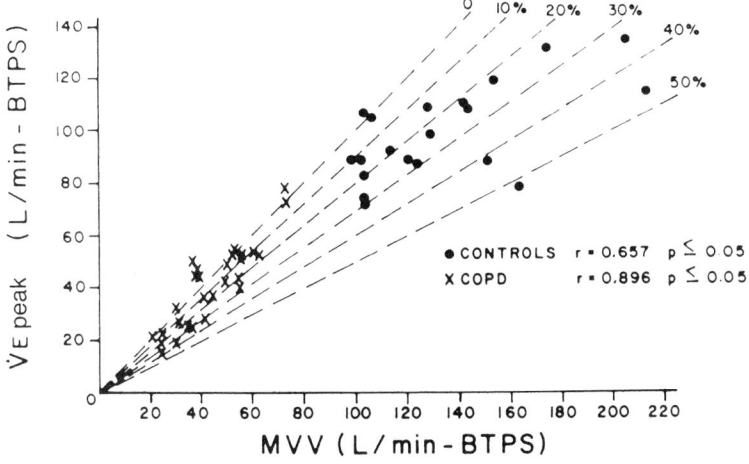

FIGURE 4.13. Maximum exercise ventilation ($\dot{V}_E$ peak) as related to maximum voluntary ventilation (MVV) in patients with chronic obstructive pulmonary disease (COPD) and in normal subjects. The dashed-line isopleths indicate the percentage of breathing reserve [(MVV − $\dot{V}_E$ peak)/(MVV × 100)]. The *r* values are the correlation coefficients for the control and the COPD groups.

pattern can acutely normalize in asthmatic patients after the use of inhaled bronchodilators (Fig. 4.14). Although the expiratory flow pattern gives only qualitative evidence of airflow obstruction during exercise, it is obtained simply by recording expired airflow, breath by breath. Flow–volume analysis (73,74) can give similar information to that of the flow–time analysis.

Inspiratory Capacity

It has long been recognized that functional residual capacity (FRC) increases in many patients with chronic obstructive pulmonary diseases (75). O'Donnell et al. (76) emphasized the value of the reduction in inspiratory capacity (IC) during exercise consequent to the development of hyperinflation and increase in FRC during exercise in patients with COPD. In normal subjects, the IC is maintained or slightly increases during exercise (77), reflecting a decrease in functional residual capacity. In contrast, the IC decreases during exercise in COPD, reflecting hyperinflation and air trapping as the respiratory rate increases. This reduction in IC

in COPD has been used to assess severity of disease. The increase in IC has been used to evaluate the therapeutic efficacy of O_2 breathing (78) and bronchodilators (76) in COPD.

Tests of Uneven $\dot{V}_A/\dot{Q}$

Wasted Ventilation and Dead Space/Tidal Volume Ratio

Alveolar ventilation ($\dot{V}_A$) is the theoretical ventilation participating in pulmonary gas exchange if the ventilation–perfusion ratios of all alveolar units were the same. This is the "ideal" alveolar ventilation for a given $\dot{V}_{CO_2}$. In the ideal lung, the mean alveolar P_{CO_2} equals the arterial P_{CO_2}. However, the lung usually does not have ideal properties, and the actual minute ventilation includes ventilation to non-gas-exchange conducting airways and alveoli that may not be ideally perfused. The difference between the actual minute ventilation and the ideal alveolar ventilation is the physiological dead space ventilation (which includes the anatomical dead space). A valuable estimate of the degree of mismatching of ventilation to perfusion during exercise is the physiological dead space/tidal volume ratio (V_D/V_T). The V_D/V_T is lowest when alveolar ventilation relative to perfusion is uniform.

At rest, the physiological dead space volume is normally about one-third of the tidal volume. During exercise, it is reduced to about one-fifth of the tidal volume (79), with the major decrement occurring at the lowest work rates. In patients with airway disorders, ventilation–perfusion relationships are uneven primarily because of nonuniform ventilation. In patients with pulmonary vascular disease, ventilation–perfusion relationships are uneven pri-

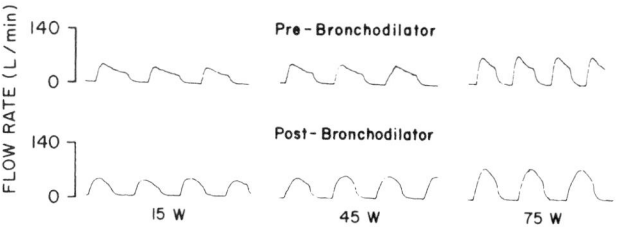

FIGURE 4.14. Expiratory flow pattern in an asthmatic subject at increasing work rates before and after acute bronchodilator therapy. (From Brown HV, Wasserman K, Whipp BJ. Strategies of exercise testing in chronic lung disease. *Bull Eur Physiopathol Resp* 1977;13: 409–423, with permission.)

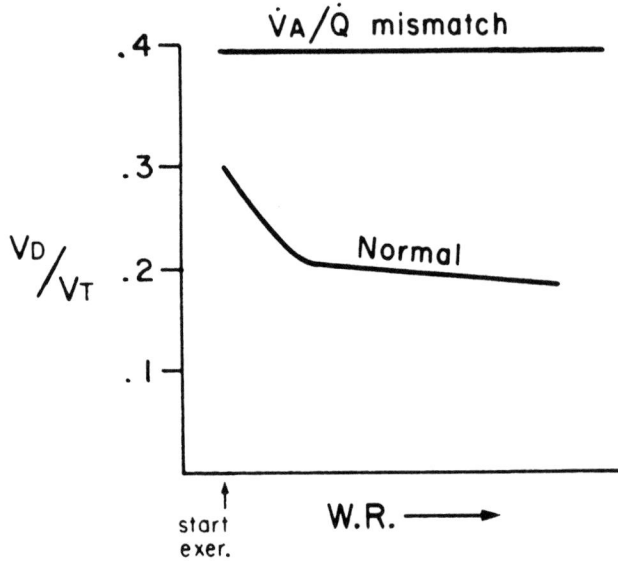

FIGURE 4.15. Example of the change in the ratio of physiologic dead space to tidal volume (VD/VT) during rest and at increasing work rate (W.R.) for a normal subject and a patient with ventilation-perfusion (V̇A/Q̇) mismatch.

marily because of nonuniform perfusion of ventilated lung. In both disorders, VD/VT is higher, particularly during exercise, because the VD/VT is increased at rest and fails to decrease during exercise.

The VD/VT is a valuable measurement because it is typically abnormal in patients with primary pulmonary vascular disease or pulmonary vascular disease secondary to obstructive or interstitial lung disease and patients with heart failure. This is discussed in greater detail in the chapter on pathophysiology of disease (Chapter 5). An elevated VD/VT is sometimes the only gas exchange abnormality evident during exercise testing (42). Figure 4.15 illustrates the pattern of change in VD/VT as the work rate is increased in the normal individual and in patients with nonuniform alveolar ventilation–perfusion ratio (V̇A/Q̇) resulting from lung or pulmonary vascular diseases. In patients with nonuniform V̇A/Q̇, the VD/VT may be only slightly elevated at rest, but it remains relatively unchanged during exercise or even increases if a right-to-left

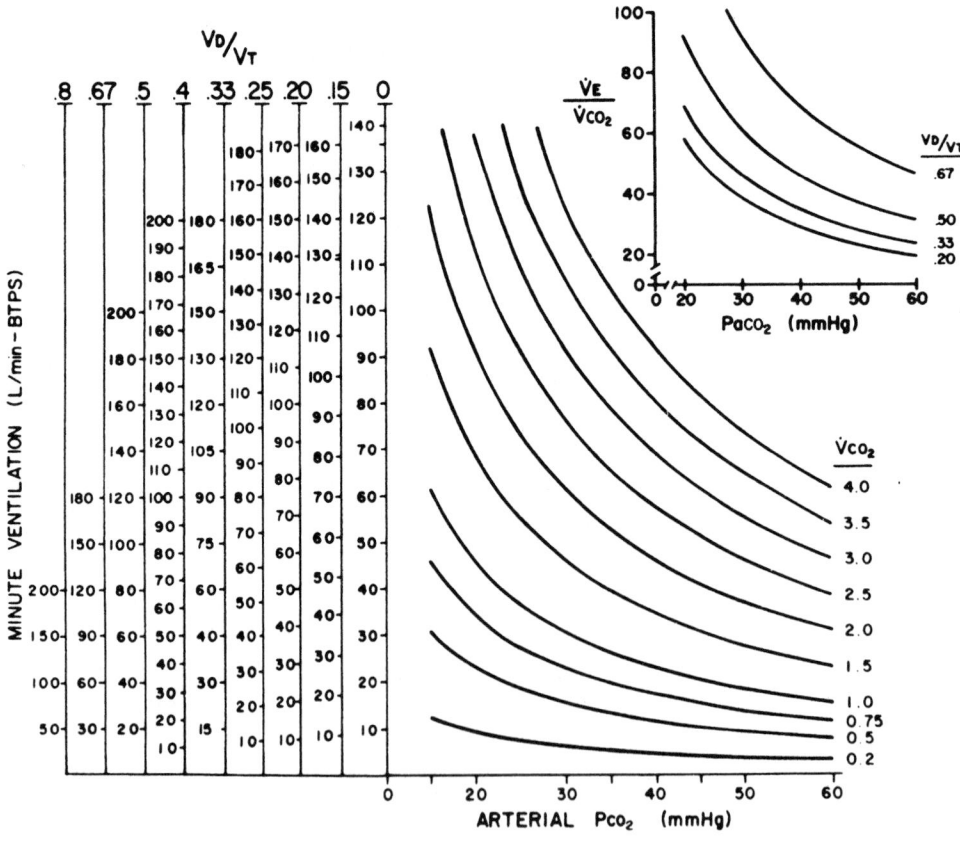

FIGURE 4.16. Minute ventilation (V̇E) required for various values of V̇CO₂, as related to arterial PCO₂ (PaCO₂) for various physiologic dead space/tidal volume (VD/VT) fractions (y-axes). If any three of the foregoing values are known, the fourth can be determined. For instance, if V̇E, V̇CO₂, and PaCO₂ are measured, then VD/VT can be determined from the ordinate that agrees with the measured V̇E. The inset shows the effect of changing PaCO₂ on the V̇E/V̇CO₂ ratio during exercise with a given VD/VT. (From Wasserman K, Whipp BJ. Exercise physiology in health and disease (state of the art). *Am Rev Respir Dis* 1975;112:219–249, with permission.)

shunt develops during exercise (opening a foramen ovale). Thus, exercise brings out the abnormality in ventilation–perfusion relationships.

When V_D/V_T is increased, $\dot{V}_E$ is typically inordinately high for the work rate performed. $\dot{V}_E$ may also be high in conditions in which the $PaCO_2$ is relatively low (low CO_2 set point), such as with a chronic metabolic acidosis. In this setting, V_D/V_T will be normal if the lungs are normal, and arterial blood gas analysis will reveal a low $PaCO_2$ (hyperventilation). Therefore, a high $\dot{V}_E$ at a given work rate (high $\dot{V}_E/\dot{V}CO_2$) is indicative of either high V_D/V_T or hyperventilation. The two pathophysiologic mechanisms can be differentiated by simultaneously measuring gas exchange and arterial blood gases.

Figure 4.16 shows the $\dot{V}_E$ required for various metabolic rates ($\dot{V}CO_2$) for designated values of $PaCO_2$ and V_D/V_T. This plot is useful for demonstrating the relations among $\dot{V}_E$, $PaCO_2$, $\dot{V}CO_2$, and V_D/V_T. It also serves as a nomogram to determine V_D/V_T when the three other variables are known.

Arterial PO_2 and Alveolar–Arterial PO_2 Difference

Normally, PaO_2 does not decrease during exercise, and the $P(A - a)O_2$ remains under 20 to 30 mm Hg (Fig. 4.17A) (27,79,80). In patients with airway disease, a reduced PaO_2 and an increased $P(A - a)O_2$ during progressively increasing work rate exercise testing (Fig. 4.17B) typically result from underventilation of regions of lung relative to their perfusion, that is, lung units with low alveolar ventilation-to-perfusion ratios (79,81). During exercise, when cardiac output increases, causing more desaturated

blood to flow through low-$\dot{V}A/\dot{Q}$ areas of the lungs, arterial hypoxemia becomes more marked. Fortunately, the blood vessels in the poorly ventilated low-$\dot{V}A/\dot{Q}$ areas of the lung normally constrict under the influence of decreasing alveolar PO_2 (82). This diversion of blood flow to areas of relatively good ventilation is a protective mechanism in that it reduces the degree of hypoxemia that would otherwise occur. This mechanism prevents progressive hypoxemia as the work rate is increased in COPD patients (Fig. 4.17B).

Exercise hypoxemia may also develop in patients with pulmonary fibrosis or pulmonary vascular disease who have a reduced pulmonary capillary bed. Because all recruitable pulmonary blood vessels are functioning at rest in these patients, when cardiac output increases, no additional pulmonary capillaries are available to be recruited to accommodate the increase in pulmonary blood flow during exercise. Thus, the red cell transit time must increase at rest and further increase during exercise, resulting in reduced time for diffusion equilibrium between alveolar O_2 and red cell O_2. This pattern of decreasing PaO_2 and increasing $P(A - a)O_2$ with increasing work rate reflects a decrease in residence time of red cells in the pulmonary capillaries when the pulmonary capillary blood volume is critically reduced. Consequently, reduced pulmonary capillary blood volume disorders are accompanied by exercise-induced hypoxemia, which becomes more pronounced as the work rate and pulmonary blood flow increase (Fig. 4.17C).

PaO_2 also decreases as the work rate is increased in conditions in which the alveoli are filled with material in which O_2 is relatively insoluble (e.g., as in pulmonary alveolar proteinosis). When the perfusion increases in these lung units, O_2 in the gas space fails to equilibrate with O_2 in the red cell, and hypoxemia becomes more marked as the blood flow increases (a diffusion defect). At rest, however, when pulmonary blood flow is low, PaO_2 may be normal because red cell residence time in the pulmonary capillary is long enough (>0.3 second) to reach diffusion equilibrium.

Hypoxemia will worsen in patients with lung disease when a potentially patent foramen ovale opens as right atrial pressure exceeds left atrial pressure. This causes part of the venous return to shunt from right to left at the atrial level. A simple, sensitive test to diagnose a right-to-left shunt that develops during exercise uses 100% O_2 breathing. For example, when breathing 100% O_2, the PaO_2 is reduced approximately 100 mm Hg below normal

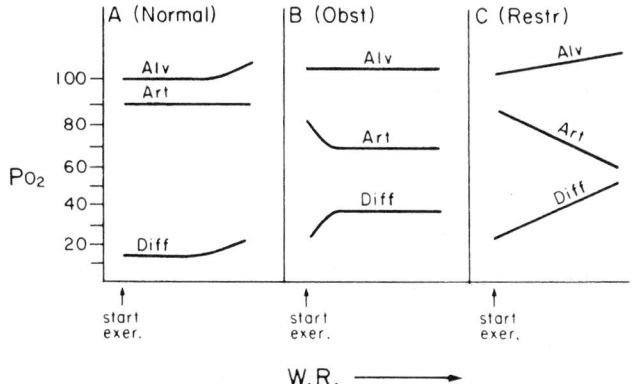

FIGURE 4.17.   General pattern of arterial and alveolar PO_2 and alveolar–arterial PO_2 differences in normal subjects (A) and in patients with obstructive (B) and restrictive (C) lung diseases as related to increasing work rate (WR).

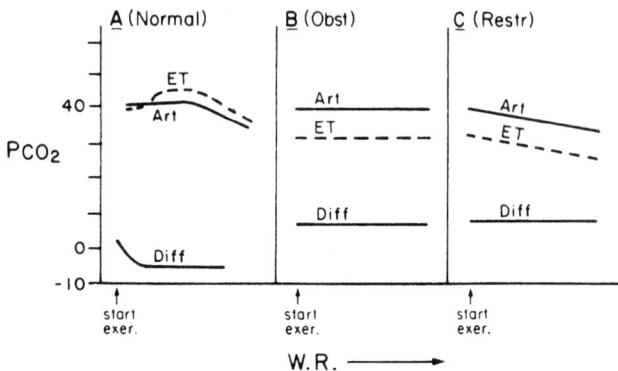

FIGURE 4.18. Pattern of change in arterial and end-tidal (ET) P_{CO_2} and arterial–end-tidal P_{CO_2} difference in normal subjects (A) and in patients with obstructive (B) and restrictive (C) lung diseases for increasing work rate exercise. All have normal resting Pa_{CO_2} values.

(600 mm Hg) for each approximate 5% right-to-left shunt until the Pa_{O_2} reaches a low value of 150 mm Hg. The decrease in Pa_{O_2} is then smaller for a given shunt size.

When a patient hyperventilates, Pa_{O_2} may appear to be normal even in patients with pulmonary disease. Calculation of $P(A - a)_{O_2}$ may reveal abnormalities in blood oxygenation masked by hyperventilation. An abnormally elevated $P(A - a)_{O_2}$ is indicative of uneven $\dot{V}_A/\dot{Q}$, a diffusion defect, and/or a right-to-left shunt.

Arterial–End-Tidal P_{CO_2} Difference

Alveoli that are underperfused or unperfused have a low CO_2 concentration. The ventilation of these alveoli is wasted (alveolar dead space), since these alveoli cannot participate fully in gas exchange. Thus the mixed expired and end-tidal P_{CO_2} values are reduced relative to the Pa_{CO_2}. By measuring the arterial–end-tidal P_{CO_2} difference [$P(a - ET)_{CO_2}$], we have another measurement that can be used as evidence of increased alveolar dead space or uneven $\dot{V}_A/\dot{Q}$ (41,42,79) (Fig. 4.18).

In the healthy lung, Pa_{CO_2} is approximately 2 mm Hg greater than P_{ETCO_2} at rest. During exercise, however, P_{ETCO_2} increases relative to Pa_{CO_2} and

normally exceeds it (Fig. 4.18A and data in Chapter 7). The mechanism for this is relatively straightforward. Because of the increased rate of CO_2 delivery to the lung associated with the high rate of CO_2 production during exercise, alveolar P_{CO_2} continues to increase during exhalation. P_{ETCO_2} is the highest alveolar P_{CO_2} during the respiratory cycle, approaching the mixed venous value. On the other hand, the Pa_{CO_2} is determined by the alveolar P_{CO_2} during the entire respiratory cycle. Therefore, provided that the functioning alveoli are relatively uniformly perfused, the end-of-breath P_{CO_2} (P_{ETCO_2}) will exceed the average of the changing alveolar P_{CO_2} (Pa_{CO_2}) during the respiratory cycle.

Direct measurements of continuously measured P_{CO_2} in the expired air and Pa_{CO_2} are shown in Figure 4.19. The slope of instantaneously measured exhaled P_{CO_2} during the alveolar phase of the breath increases as work rate increases. Because the P_{ETCO_2} is the highest P_{CO_2} in the alveolus during the respiratory cycle, and the arterial P_{CO_2} represents the average alveolar P_{CO_2}, P_{ETCO_2} exceeds Pa_{CO_2} during exercise and $P(a - ET)_{CO_2}$ is normally negative by about 4 mm Hg. The slower the breathing rate, the closer P_{ETCO_2} would be to mixed venous P_{CO_2}, making $P(a - ET)_{CO_2}$ even more negative.

If the $P(a - ET)_{CO_2}$ remains positive during exercise, this is evidence for decreased perfusion to ventilated alveoli (uneven $\dot{V}_A/\dot{Q}$ with high-$\dot{V}_A/\dot{Q}$ units) (Fig. 4.18B, C). An extreme situation may be seen when CO_2-rich venous blood is diverted to the left side of the circulation without passing through the lungs during exercise (right-to-left shunt). In this case, Pa_{CO_2} is much higher than P_{ETCO_2} because the blood perfusing the lung is hyperventilated to compensate for the CO_2 load entering the arterial circulation through the shunt (44,83). In this situation, $P(a - ET)_{CO_2}$ is markedly positive because of a decreased P_{ETCO_2} during exercise. The magnitude of the increased $P(a - ET)_{CO_2}$ depends on the size of the right-to-left shunt.

Sue et al. (42) compared the resting diffusing capacity of the lung for carbon monoxide (D_{LCO}) with

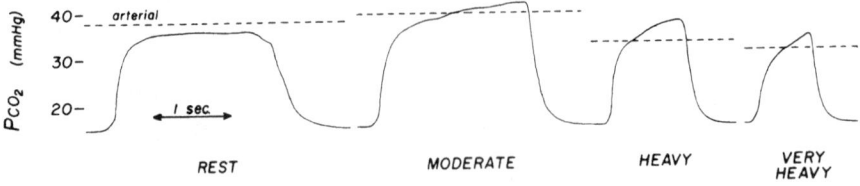

FIGURE 4.19. Arterial (*dashed lines*) compared to instantaneous airway (*solid lines*) P_{CO_2} for the resting state and increasing intensities of exercise. The end-tidal P_{CO_2} is less than Pa_{CO_2} at rest but greater than Pa_{CO_2} during exercise. (From Wasserman K, Van Kessel A, Burton GG. Interaction of physiological mechanisms during exercise. *J Appl Physiol* 1967;22:71–85, with permission.)

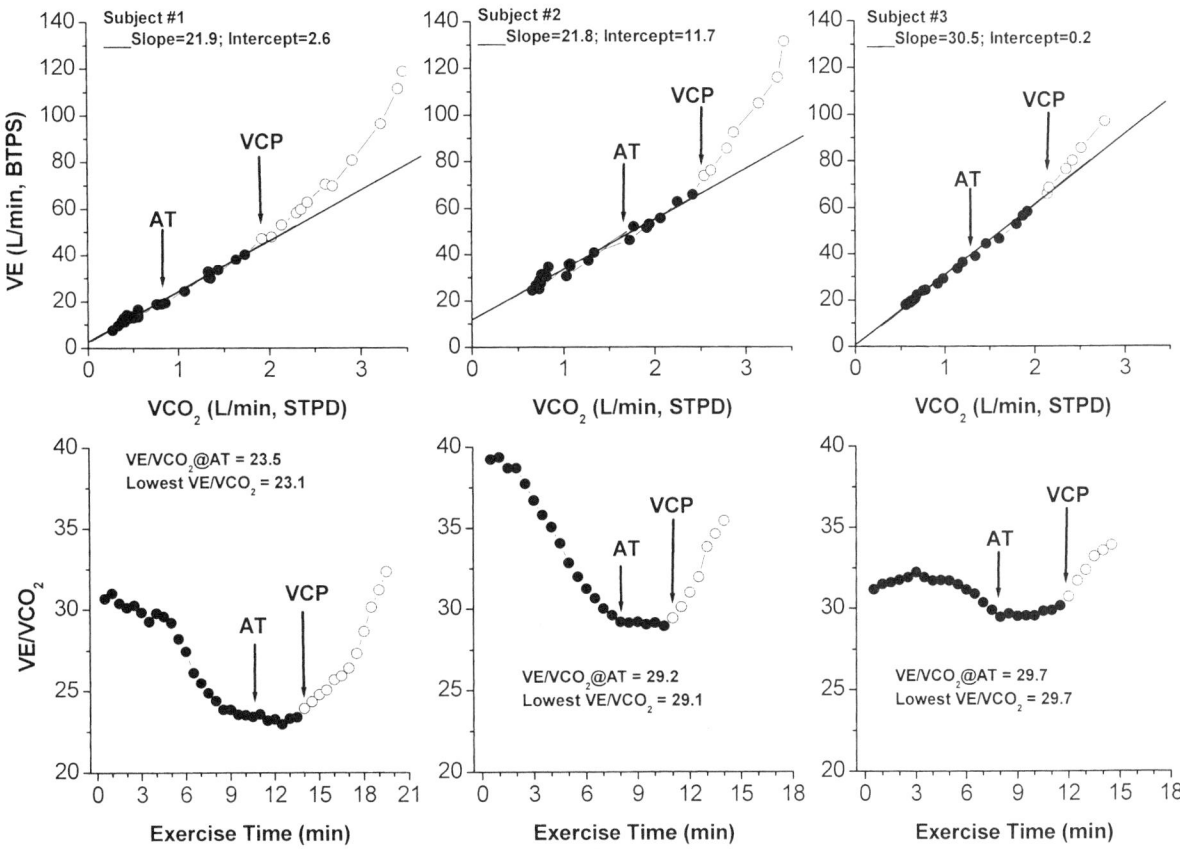

FIGURE 4.20.   Comparison of $\dot{V}E$-versus-$\dot{V}CO_2$ slopes in three normal subjects (**upper panels**) and the $\dot{V}E/\dot{V}CO_2$ ratios as related to time in the same three studies (**lower panels**). Data points are shown every 0.5 minute during progressively increasing cycle ergometer exercise. The open symbols occur above the ventilatory compensation points (VCP) and are not used for calculation of the slopes (*straight solid lines*) and intercepts of $\dot{V}E$ versus $\dot{V}CO_2$. The $\dot{V}E/\dot{V}CO_2$ values (**lower panels**) reach a nearly constant nadir between the anaerobic threshold (*AT*) and VCP arrows. Subject 1 is typical of an average response, subject 2 has an unusually large positive intercept for $\dot{V}E$-versus-$\dot{V}CO_2$ slope, and subject 3 has an intercept close to zero. Although the $\dot{V}E$-versus-$\dot{V}CO_2$ slopes for subjects 1 and 2 are similar, their y-axis intercepts differ; thus, the $\dot{V}E/\dot{V}CO_2$ at *AT* of subject 1 differs considerably from that of subject 2. For subjects 2 and 3, although the $\dot{V}E/\dot{V}CO_2$ at *AT* ratios are similar, the $\dot{V}E$-versus-$\dot{V}CO_2$ slopes differ markedly. If $\dot{V}E$ versus $\dot{V}CO_2$ has an intercept at zero on the y-axis (subject 3), the $\dot{V}E$-versus-$\dot{V}CO_2$ slope is equal to the $\dot{V}E/\dot{V}CO_2$ at *AT*. (From Sun X-G, Hansen JE, Garatachea N, et al. Ventilatory efficiency during exercise in healthy subjects. *Am J Respir Crit Care Med* 2002;166:1443–1448, with permission.)

arterial blood gases during maximal exercise in 276 male shipyard workers. Fourteen of 16 subjects with D_{LCO} less than 70% had abnormal gas exchange, measured as an increase in $P(A - a)_{O_2}$, V_D/V_T, or $P(a - ET)_{CO_2}$, during exercise. However, 88 subjects had abnormal exercise gas exchange with a normal D_{LCO}. Increases in V_D/V_T and $P(a - ET)_{CO_2}$ occurred when there was a major component of uneven, high-$\dot{V}A/\dot{Q}$ lung units. Both were abnormal in the same subjects. In contrast, an increase in $P(A - a)_{O_2}$ was abnormal when there was a major component of uneven, low-$\dot{V}A/\dot{Q}$ lung units. An increased $P(a - ET)_{CO_2}$ and V_D/V_T occurred more frequently than an increased $P(A - a)_{O_2}$. When $P(A - a)_{O_2}$ was increased, $P(a - ET)_{CO_2}$ and V_D/V_T were also increased. In many instances, however, only $P(a - ET)_{CO_2}$ and V_D/V_T were abnormal, without $P(A - a)_{O_2}$ being abnormal.

Ventilatory Equivalents as Indices of Uneven $\dot{V}A/\dot{Q}$. As described previously, the measurements of V_D/V_T, $P(a - ET)_{CO_2}$, and $P(A - a)_{O_2}$ quantify the degree of $\dot{V}A/\dot{Q}$ mismatching and, thereby, inefficient gas exchange. To obtain these measurements, arterial blood gas sampling is required. Because the consequence of inefficient gas exchange dictates an increased ventilatory requirement to eliminate a given amount of CO_2 from the body, two noninvasive techniques have been used to measure $\dot{V}A/\dot{Q}$ mismatching: the slope of $\dot{V}E$ as a function of $\dot{V}CO_2$ in the range of exercise below the ventilatory compensation point (*VCP*) (7,8,44,84,85), and the nadir of the ventilatory equivalent for CO_2 at, and shortly after, the *AT*. (44).

Figure 4.20 shows the difference between these two measurements in three normal subjects. Although the difference between these two measurements is small, the slope of $\dot{V}_E$ versus $\dot{V}_{CO_2}$, measured below the VCP, is usually slightly less than $\dot{V}_E/\dot{V}_{CO_2}$ at the *AT*, depending on the size of the positive intercept on the *y*-axis (44). A small positive intercept is generally present in normal subjects when $\dot{V}_E$ is plotted against $\dot{V}_{CO_2}$, starting from the lowest level of exercise. The intercept is positive if the VD/VT decreases as work rate increases and/or there is early hyperventilation that gradually dissipates as work rate increases (subject 2 of Fig. 4.20). In contrast, if the intercept of the $\dot{V}_E$ versus $\dot{V}_{CO_2}$ plot is at or near zero (no early hyperventilation and no large decrease in VD/VT), the slope of $\dot{V}_E$ versus $\dot{V}_{CO_2}$ below the VCP and the $\dot{V}_E/\dot{V}_{CO_2}$ in the range of the *AT* and VCP are approximately equal (subject 3, Fig. 4.20). Typically, there is a small positive intercept in most normal subjects below the VCP, making the slope a little less than the ratio of $\dot{V}_E/\dot{V}_{CO_2}$ at the *AT* and VCP (subject 1, Fig. 4.20). However, the $\dot{V}_E/\dot{V}_{CO_2}$ slope commonly intercepts at zero in pulmonary vascular disease because these patients cannot decrease their VD/VT during exercise. Therefore, in these patients, the slope and ratio would be similar.

Because the $\dot{V}_E/\dot{V}_{CO_2}$ ratio at the *AT* is slightly less variable (less influenced by early hyperventilation) than the slope of $\dot{V}_E$ versus $\dot{V}_{CO_2}$ below the VCP, we prefer the ratio of $\dot{V}_E/\dot{V}_{CO_2}$ in the range of the *AT* and VCP. No special calculation is required to obtain this ratio, in contrast to the regression slope through a selected range of values below the VCP as in the case of $\dot{V}_E$ versus $\dot{V}_{CO_2}$ (panel 4 of the nine-panel plot). The $\dot{V}_E/\dot{V}_{CO_2}$ is read directly from panel 6 of the nine-panel plot of exercise physiological data. Because the *AT* is determined in virtually every study, we routinely report the $\dot{V}_E/\dot{V}_{CO_2}$ at the *AT* ($\dot{V}_E/\dot{V}_{CO_2}$ @ *AT*), recognizing that it is also approximately the $\dot{V}_E/\dot{V}_{CO_2}$ @ VCP and the lowest value during exercise, that is, that value least affected by anxiety hyperventilation and the H^+ stimulus to the carotid bodies caused by the exercise lactic acidosis.

The range of normal values for the slope of $\dot{V}_E$ versus $\dot{V}_{CO_2}$ below the VCP and $\dot{V}_E/\dot{V}_{CO_2}$ @ *AT*, as related to age and gender, is described in Chapter 7. The values are the same for cycle and treadmill exercise. Although small in most systems, the breathing valve dead space is variable from system to system and therefore should be subtracted from $\dot{V}_E$ to obtain a value that could allow the measurement to be interrelated among all systems. Elevated ventilatory equivalent values at the *AT* (Fig. 4.21B, C) reflect either hyperventilation or an increase in VD/VT (uneven $\dot{V}_A/\dot{Q}$). Acute hyperventilation is supported by a respiratory exchange ratio greater than 1. To distinguish between chronic hyperventilation and increased VD/VT as a cause of high ventilatory equivalents, it is necessary to measure Pa_{CO_2} with respiratory gas exchange during exercise (Fig. 4.16).

Patients with chronic obstructive lung disease (Fig. 4.21B), restrictive lung disease, left ventricular failure, and pulmonary vascular occlusive disease (Fig. 4.21C) usually have uneven $\dot{V}_A/\dot{Q}$. Therefore, their $\dot{V}_E/\dot{V}_{CO_2}$ is often high. Because of mechanical limitation to breathing, patients with severe COPD usually do not hyperventilate or increase $\dot{V}_E/\dot{V}_{CO_2}$ in response to metabolic acidosis, in contrast to the disorders of $\dot{V}_A/\dot{Q}$ without a breathing limitation.

Although the $\dot{V}_E/\dot{V}_{CO_2}$ normally increases from the nadir (isocapnic buffering period) to maximal exercise, with the amount depending on the magnitude of the lactic acidosis, it fails to increase above the *AT* if the chemoreceptors for detecting increased H^+ are insensitive or the work of breathing is high, such as with extreme obesity or severe COPD (Fig. 4.21).

Arterial Bicarbonate and Acid–Base Response

Subjects making a maximal effort during a progressively increasing work rate exercise test normally develop a significant metabolic acidosis by the time

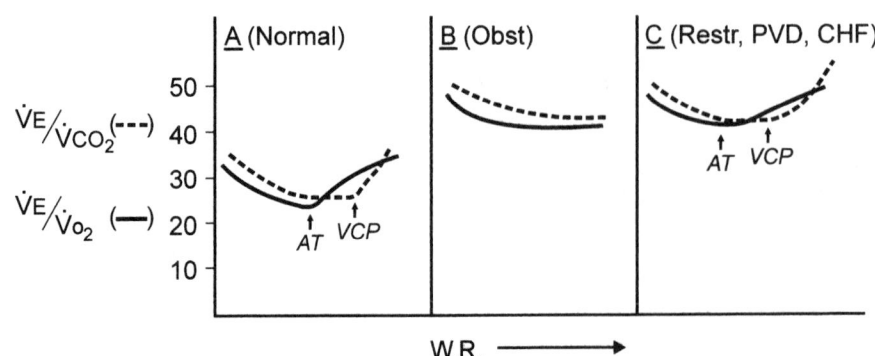

FIGURE 4.21. Typical changes during increasing work rate (WR) in ventilatory equivalent for CO_2 ($\dot{V}_E/\dot{V}_{CO_2}$) and O_2 ($\dot{V}_E/\dot{V}_{O_2}$) for a normal subject (**A**) and for patients with obstructive (**B**) and restrictive lung or pulmonary vascular disease (**C**). The nadir in $\dot{V}_E/\dot{V}_{O_2}$ reflects the anaerobic threshold (*AT*), and the nadir of the $\dot{V}_E/\dot{V}_{CO_2}$ curve occurs between the *AT* and the ventilatory compensation point (VCP).

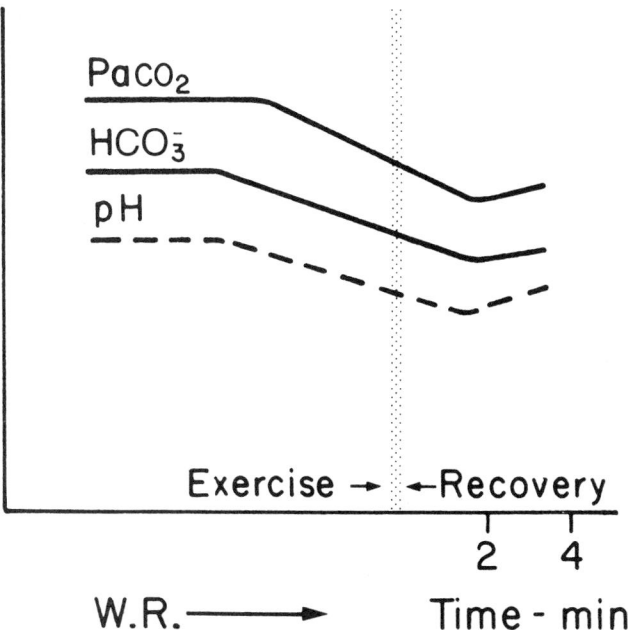

FIGURE 4.22. Normal pattern of change in arterial P_{CO_2}, bicarbonate, and pH as related to increasing work rate and recovery. The stippled vertical bar indicates the point at which exercise stops. Note that the decrease in Pa_{CO_2} is delayed relative to the decrease in $[HCO_3^-]$ and pH (the period of isocapnic buffering). The arterial P_{CO_2}, $[HCO_3^-]$, and pH continue to decrease in the recovery period, before starting to increase back toward normal.

the terminal work rate is reached. This is observed even for an increasing work rate exercise test protocol of relatively short duration (8 to 12 minutes) (Fig. 4.22; also see Figs. 2.21 and 2.29). The greatest increase in arterial lactate and reductions in arterial $[HCO_3^-]$ and pH are noted about 2 minutes into recovery (Fig. 4.22; see Chapters 7 and 10). We find that the 2-minute recovery $[HCO_3^-]$ decreases by at least 6 mmol/L below the resting value if the effort is good and the patient is not limited by a ventilatory or mechanical disorder.

Tidal Volume/Inspiratory Capacity Ratio

Normally, V_T increases during exercise, but it rarely exceeds 80% of the inspiratory capacity (IC), measured during standard resting pulmonary function tests. This ratio may become abnormal during exercise in patients with interstitial lung diseases. Such patients have a reduced IC and limited ability to increase their V_T in response to exercise (Fig. 4.12). Thus, as the work rate increases, the V_T/IC ratio reaches a value close to 1.0 at a relatively low work rate. Because a reduced V_T requires a high breathing rate to achieve the $\dot{V}_E$ needed for CO_2 elimina-

tion, we routinely relate V_T to the IC as well as the ventilatory capacity (VC; see Chapter 10). We find the V_T/IC ratio to be more helpful than the V_T/VC ratio because it is very unusual for V_T to exceed IC, even in severe restrictive lung disease.

Measurements Unique to Constant Work Rate Exercise Testing

Whereas the absolute $\dot{V}_{O_2}$ required to perform a given work rate should be predictable from the work rate, as described in Chapter 2, the ability to supply the O_2 needed to satisfy the O_2 requirement depends on the cardiovascular response. In addition, the increase in $\dot{V}_{CO_2}$ depends on the rate of aerobic metabolism measured as $\dot{V}_{O_2}$ times the muscle substrate RQ, as well as the rate of buffering of lactic acid by HCO_3^- (see Figs. 1.4 and 2.35).

Constant work rate tests permit the study of physiological responses by specific organ systems that transport O_2 and CO_2. They also facilitate investigation of control mechanisms. If the constant rate at which work is performed is above the AT, then $\dot{V}_{O_2}$ kinetics are slowed and the relation between $\dot{V}_{O_2}$ and $\dot{V}_{CO_2}$ kinetics changes relative to the kinetics for below-AT exercise (see Figs. 1.4 and 2.35). These changes reflect the patient's cardiovascular status during exercise at the specific work rate studied (see Fig. 2.55). The following are useful measurements that can be obtained from the time course of the response to the onset of a constant work rate exercise:

Increase in $\dot{V}_{O_2}$ During Phase I

Normally, oxygen uptake abruptly increases at the start of exercise (phase I) during upright exercise because of the immediate increase in flow of venous blood through the lungs resulting from the increased venous return. The latter is enhanced at the start of exercise by increased cardiac inotropy, compression of veins by contracting muscles, and increased heart rate (see Figs. 2.48, 2.50, and 2.53). Increased pulmonary blood flow is the predominant mechanism accounting for the increase in $\dot{V}_{O_2}$ during the first 15 seconds of exercise. Under conditions in which pulmonary blood flow fails to increase abruptly at the start of exercise, the phase I increase in oxygen uptake is attenuated (86–89). A reduced phase I increase in oxygen uptake is found in disorders that limit the increase in pulmonary blood flow at the start of exercise (87–89). A reduced ventilatory response in phase I does not discernibly mask the normal rapid increase in $\dot{V}_{O_2}$ (90).

It should be noted that the phase I increase in $\dot{V}O_2$ is reduced in normal subjects when starting exercise in the supine position (86), because of the lesser increase in stroke volume.

Oxygen Uptake Kinetics Above or Below the Anaerobic Threshold

After the phase I immediate (first 15 seconds of exercise) increase in $\dot{V}O_2$ and $\dot{V}CO_2$ in a constant work rate test, $\dot{V}O_2$ and $\dot{V}CO_2$ increase as exponential functions (phase II). Because of this, their rates of rise have been described by time constants, that is, the time for 63% of the final response to be reached. Although this single-exponential approach has been used by some investigators (24,32,34,91,92), it is not a totally accurate measurement because $\dot{V}O_2$ has first-order exponential kinetics only for work rates below the AT. Above the AT, the $\dot{V}O_2$ kinetics must be defined by at least two exponential functions, the second becoming more prominent the higher the work above the AT (91,92).

Figure 4.23 shows the pattern of oxygen uptake kinetics as related to fitness for a normal subject and a patient with COPD. For the same relatively low work rate (40-W cycling work), the $\dot{V}O_2$ for the

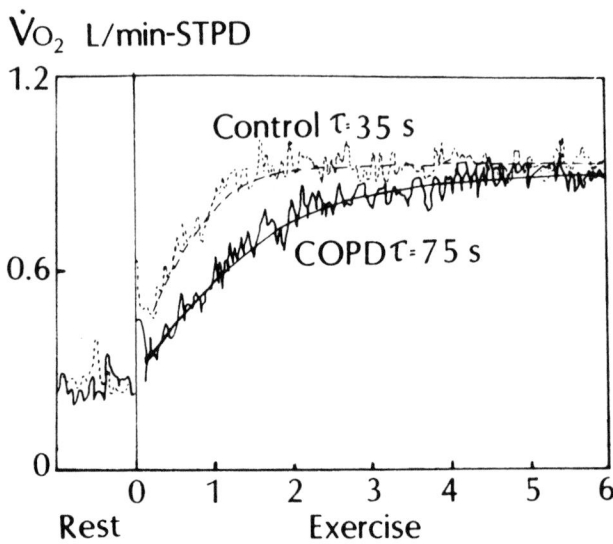

$\dot{V}O_2$ L/min-STPD

FIGURE 4.23. Pattern of oxygen uptake ($\dot{V}O_2$) in a patient with chronic obstructive pulmonary disease (COPD) and a matched normal subject during the performance of a constant 40-W cycle ergometer exercise. Note that $\dot{V}O_2$ during phase I (the first 15 seconds of exercise) is less and the rate of rise of $\dot{V}O_2$ to its asymptote during phase II is slower in the COPD patient. The latter is reflected in the longer time constant (τ), as compared with a normal control subject. (Data from Nery LE, Wasserman K, Andrews JD, et al. Ventilatory and gas exchange kinetics during exercise in chronic airways obstruction. *J Appl Physiol* 1982;53:1594–1602.)

patient with COPD had a longer time constant than that of the normal subject (matched for age and gender). When compared with the time constants for normal subjects at 50 W in Figure 2.55, the increase in oxygen consumption by the exercising muscles is slower in the patient with COPD. This indicates an increased O_2 deficit and implies that a lactic acidosis developed.

Increase in $\dot{V}O_2$ Between Three and Six Minutes of Exercise

When the exercise work rate is below the subject's AT (i.e., the subject is in metabolic steady state), the $\dot{V}O_2$ after 3 minutes (phase III) is constant. However, for work rates above the AT, $\dot{V}O_2$ increases after 3 minutes in proportion to the increase in lactate (53,91,93,94). The increase in $\dot{V}O_2$ between 3 and 6 minutes of exercise [$\Delta\dot{V}O_2$ (6 − 3)] can be determined by linear regression of the $\dot{V}O_2$ between 3 and 6 minutes of exercise (Fig. 4.24). When $\Delta\dot{V}O_2$ (6 − 3) is correlated with the increase in lactate above rest, a good correlation is found for both chronic heart failure patients and normal subjects (Fig. 4.25). The regression of the relationship goes through the origin, suggesting that confounding factors do not override the importance of lactate increase in the development of this slow component in $\dot{V}O_2$ when performing constant work rate exercise above the AT.

Mean Response Time

Sietsema et al. (95) performed multiple 6-minute constant work rate tests in normal subjects at work rates ranging from unloaded cycling to 150 W. These investigators assumed single-exponential kinetics and calculated a *mean response time* (MRT) for the data. The MRT measurement at the higher work rates allowed discrimination of the subject's fitness to perform a progressively increasing work rate test. Thus, the subjects with the highest $\dot{V}O_2$max per kilogram body weight had the lowest MRTs for the 75-, 100-, and 150-W work rates (see Fig. 2.55).

Combining $\dot{V}O_2$ and $\dot{V}CO_2$ Kinetics for Detecting Anaerobic Metabolism and Lactic Acid Buffering

For above-AT constant work rate exercise, $\dot{V}CO_2$ increases more rapidly than $\dot{V}O_2$ after about 1 to 2 minutes (see Fig. 1.4). This is primarily due to the buffering of newly formed lactic acid by HCO_3^-.

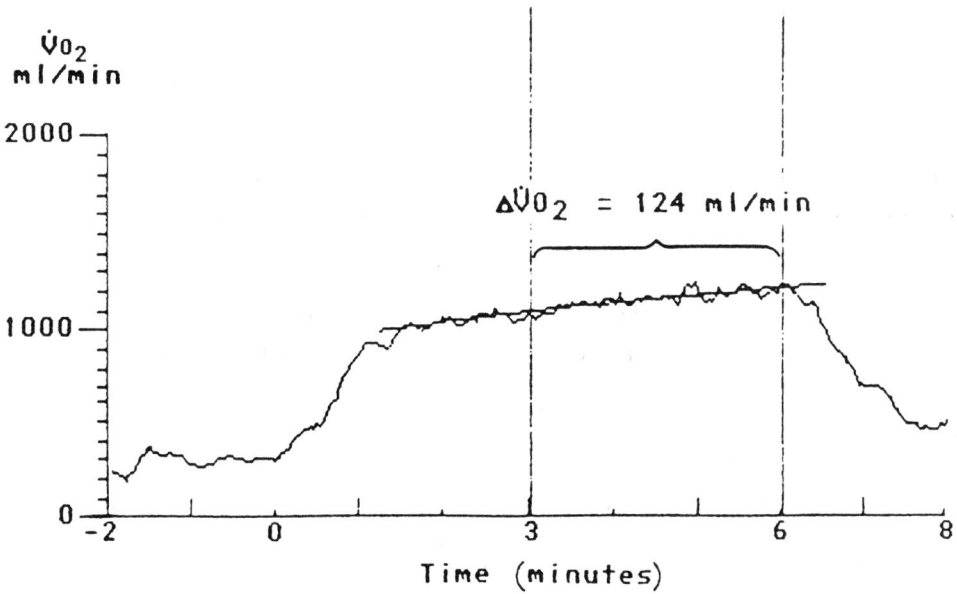

FIGURE 4.24. Method illustrating the measurement of the difference in oxygen uptake ($\dot{V}_{O_2}$) between 3 and 6 minutes [$\Delta\dot{V}_{O_2}$ (6 − 3)] of constant work rate exercise (70 W) in a patient with cardiac disease. The straight line drawn on the plot between 3 and 6 minutes was determined by the best least square fit for the breath-by-breath data. The difference in $\dot{V}_{O_2}$ at the 6- and 3-minute points is calculated from the 3- and 6-minute intercepts of the linear regression of the data between 3 and 6 minutes.

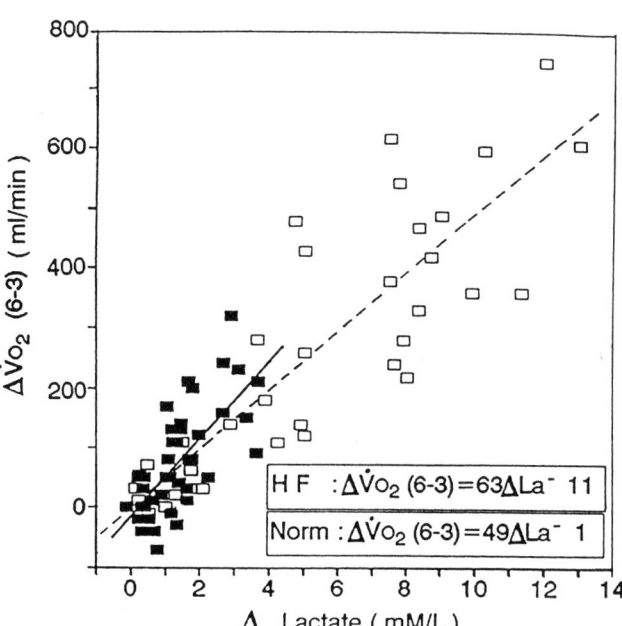

FIGURE 4.25. Degree of unsteady-state in oxygen uptake ($\dot{V}_{O_2}$), expressed as the increase in $\dot{V}_{O_2}$ between 3 and 6 minutes [$\dot{V}_{O_2}$ (6 − 3)], as a function of the increase in blood lactate above rest in normal subjects (*open squares*) and in patients with heart failure (*solid squares*). The blood was sampled from the antecubital vein at rest and at 2 minutes of recovery. Neither the slopes nor the intercepts of the regression equations differed significantly between the two groups. (From Roston WL, Whipp BJ, Davis JA, et al. Oxygen uptake kinetics and lactate concentration during exercise in man. *Am Rev Respir Dis* 1987; 135:1080–1084 and Zhang YY, Wasserman K, Sietsema KE, et al. O₂ uptake kinetics in response to exercise: A measure of tissue anaerobiosis in heart failure. *Chest* 1993;103:735–741, with permission.)

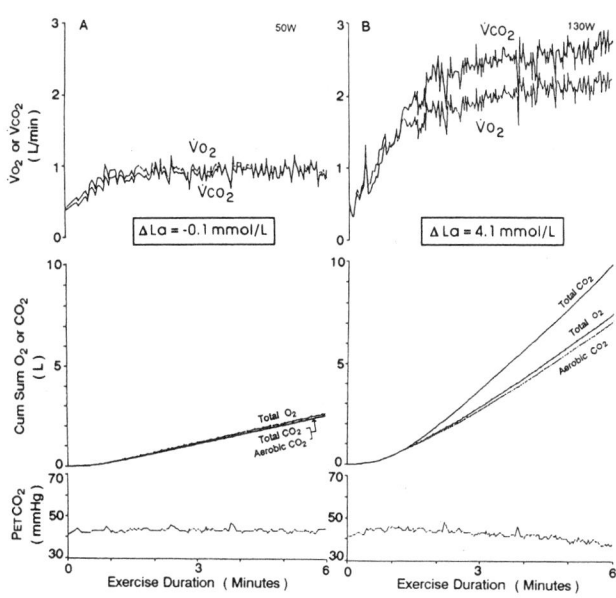

FIGURE 4.26. Breath-by-breath changes in $\dot{V}_{O_2}$, $\dot{V}_{CO_2}$, total or accumulated O_2 uptake (Cum Sum O_2), total or accumulated CO_2 output (Cum Sum CO_2), aerobic CO_2 output ($\dot{V}_{O_2}$ × 0.95), and $P_{ET}CO_2$ in response to 50-W (**A**) and 130-W (**B**) work rate tests for one subject. The difference between the accumulated total CO_2 output and aerobic CO_2 output is the accumulated buffer CO_2 output. In panel **A**, the total and aerobic Cum Sum CO_2 curves overlap and cannot be distinguished. The increase in antecubital vein lactate at the end of 6 minutes of exercise for each study is shown. (From Zhang YY, Sietsema KE, Sullivan CS, et al. A method for estimating bicarbonate buffering of lactic acid during constant work rate exercise. *Eur J Appl Physiol* 1994;69:309–315, with permission.)

Thus, from the simultaneous analysis of $\dot{V}CO_2$ and $\dot{V}O_2$, it is possible to determine whether the work rate is accompanied by a lactic acidosis.

By measuring CO_2 output and O_2 uptake breath-by-breath for work above unloaded cycling exercise, Zhang et al. (96) demonstrated that the cumulative output of CO_2 progressively increases relative to the cumulative increase in O_2 uptake for constant work rate exercise associated with a lactic acidosis, in contrast to work for which a lactic acidosis was not present (Fig. 4.26). By multiplying $\dot{V}O_2$ by the muscle substrate respiratory quotient (on average approximately 0.95), the aerobic CO_2 production was calculated. The difference between the total CO_2 output and the aerobic CO_2 output should represent the CO_2 output from buffering lactic acid plus CO_2 from hyperventilation, if any (Fig. 4.26). The latter accounted for only about 6% of the excess CO_2 over that derived from aerobic metabolism in subjects who hyperventilated in response to the exercise-induced lactic acidosis at 6 minutes of exercise. When the number of millimoles of CO_2 output derived from the buffering of lactic acid at 6 minutes of constant work rate exercise was calculated, this quantity correlated closely with the lactate concentration increase determined from antecubital vein blood sampled 2 minutes into recovery (Fig. 4.27). This method, therefore, describes a noninvasive estimate of the *magnitude* of HCO_3^- decrease or lactate increase at the end of 6 minutes of constant work rate exercise. The slope of the regression line defines the volume of distribution of lactate (25 liters, or about one-third body weight for the population of adult subjects studied).

In a steady state below the *AT*, no anaerobic mechanisms support bioenergetics, and the O_2 debt has reached a maximum (97). However, constant work rate exercise performed above the *AT* results in a delay or an inability to reach a constant $\dot{V}O_2$ (see Figs. 2.35 and 2.36). Thus, $\dot{V}O_2$ continues to increase for exercise above *AT* after 3 minutes, the rate of increase depending on the fractional distance between *AT* and $\dot{V}O_2$max (Fig. 4.28). To determine if a specific work rate is above the *AT*, measurement of $\dot{V}O_2$ at 3 and 6 minutes during a 6-minute constant work rate test is helpful. Measurement of $\dot{V}CO_2$ simultaneously with $\dot{V}O_2$ provides confirmation that the work rate is above the *AT*.

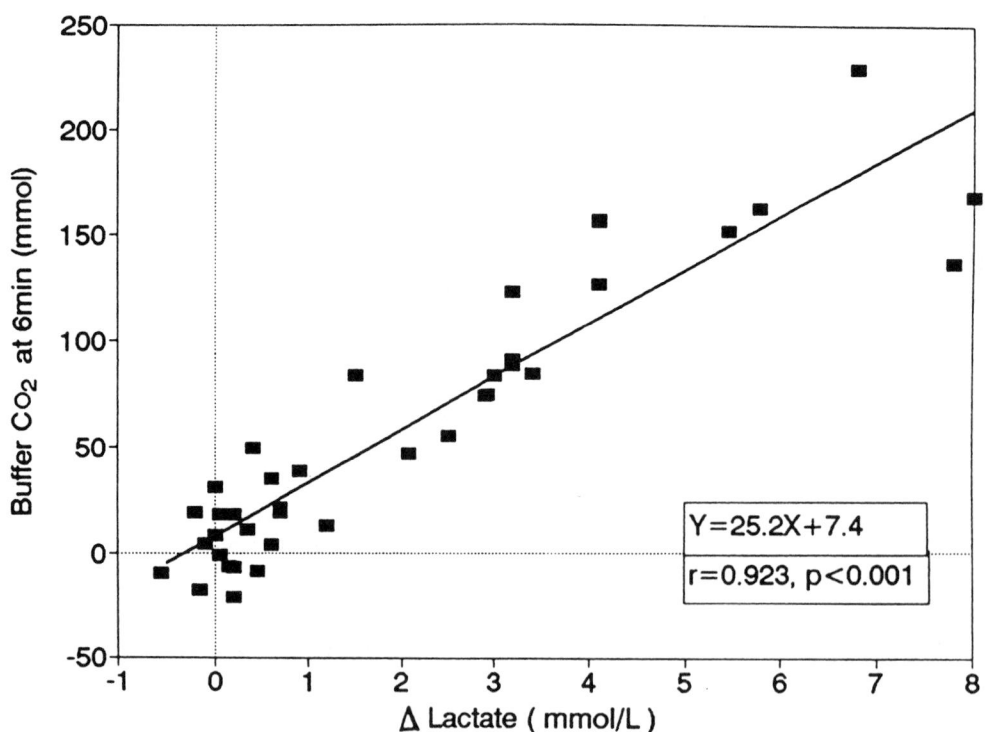

FIGURE 4.27.   Buffer CO_2 (mmol) as a function of the increase in blood lactate concentration (La^-) at the end of 6 minutes of exercise. The correlation coefficient, significance of the correlation, and the equation for the regression are shown. (From Zhang YY, Sietsema KE, Sullivan CS, et al. A method for estimating bicarbonate buffering of lactic acid during constant work rate exercise. *Eur J Appl Physiol* 1994;69:309–315, with permission.)

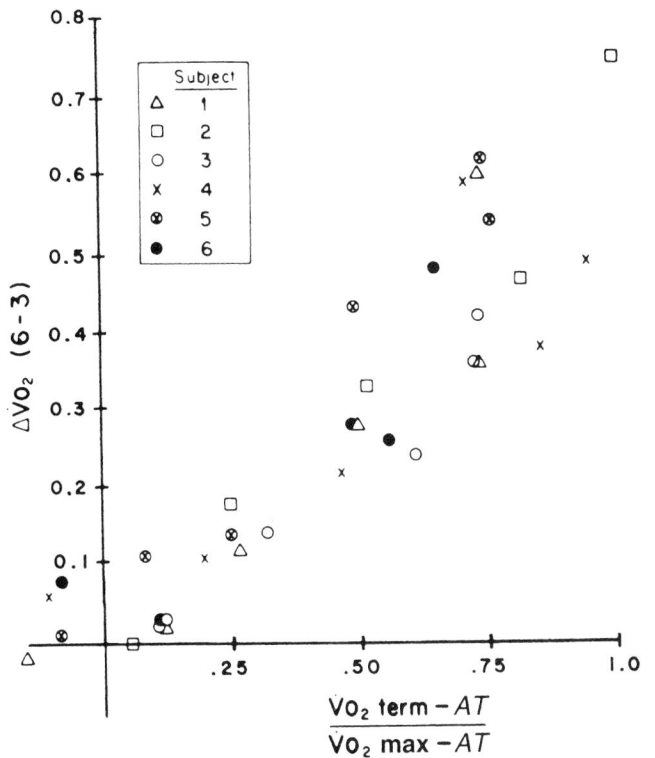

FIGURE 4.28.   Difference between 6- and 3-minute $\dot{V}O_2$ for constant work rate exercise [$\Delta\dot{V}O_2$ (6 − 3)] as related to the ratio of the difference between the $\dot{V}O_2$ asymptote at the termination of exercise ($\dot{V}CO_2$ term) and the anaerobic threshold (AT) and the differences between the $\dot{V}O_2$max and the AT in six normal subjects. (Modified from Roston WL, Whipp BJ, Davis JA, et al. Oxygen uptake kinetics and lactate concentration during exercise in man. *Am Rev Respir Dis* 1987;135:1080–1084.)

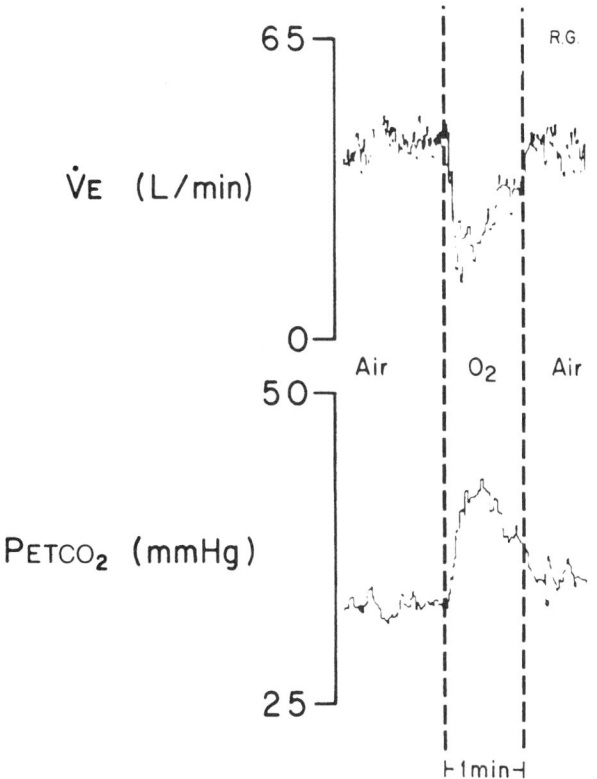

FIGURE 4.29.   Illustration of a safe test for assessing carotid body contribution to ventilation during exercise. The study is that of a patient with pulmonary alveolar proteinosis with a PaO_2 of 54 during exercise. A work rate is selected at which the patient can perform without difficulty and for which a steady state in ventilation is reached by 4 to 5 minutes. When $\dot{V}E$ is constant, the inspired gas is switched from air to 100% oxygen for 1 minute. $\dot{V}E$ decreases to a nadir within several breaths, and, as a consequence, $PETCO_2$ rises. After 15 seconds, $\dot{V}E$ spontaneously starts to rebound toward the air-breathing value, presumably because of CO_2 stimulation of central chemoreceptors. By 45 seconds, $\dot{V}E$ becomes relatively constant at a reduced value, and $PETCO_2$ levels off at an elevated value as compared to the control period. Thus, three phases in ventilation are observed when switching to 100% oxygen breathing: the first 15 seconds, when the carotid bodies are attenuated maximally; the period between 15 and 45 seconds, which shows a rebound in $\dot{V}E$ presumably caused by the increase in arterial PCO_2; and the period after 45 seconds, when $\dot{V}E$ and $PETCO_2$ reach constant values. The abrupt changes in $\dot{V}E$ in response to the O_2 switch and return to air breathing reflect the rapid control exerted by the carotid bodies in the regulation of ventilation. (From Wasserman K, Whipp BJ, Davis JA. Respiratory physiology of exercise: metabolism, gas exchange, and ventilatory control. In: Widdicombe JG, ed. *International review of physiology III.* Baltimore: University Park Press, 1981:149–211, with permission.)

Carotid Body Contribution to Ventilation

Several techniques (98,99) have been proposed to determine the contribution of the carotid bodies to the exercise ventilatory response. A modified Dejours test (100), performed during moderate constant work rate exercise (101,102), is informative and applicable to patients with lung diseases (Fig. 4.29). One hundred percent O_2 attenuates the carotid body output (103). Therefore, in the steady-state of an air breathing exercise test, the surreptitious switch to 100% oxygen results in an almost immediate decrease in ventilation (within one or two breaths) if the carotid bodies actively contribute to ventilatory drive. This decrease reflects the carotid body contribution to the ventilatory drive and can be expressed as a percentage of the pre–O_2 breathing ventilation. Ventilation decreases to a nadir by 15 seconds. Once the nadir is reached, ventilation starts increasing back toward, but not completely to, its control value despite continued breathing of 100% O_2. The most likely stimulus for

this rebound in $\dot{V}E$ is the increase in $PaCO_2$ caused by the abrupt decrease in $\dot{V}E$ resulting from O_2 breathing. Whereas hyperoxia continues to inhibit carotid body drive to ventilation, the increase in $PaCO_2$ resulting from the inhibition stimulates the central chemoreceptors, partially masking the carotid body ventilatory drive. If ventilation is not measured breath-by-breath, the magnitude of the carotid body contribution to the exercise ventilatory stimulus is inadequately quantified.

The advantages of this test are its brevity, its applicability at work rates below or above the *AT*, and its safety, in contrast to breathing hypoxic gas mixtures to stimulate the carotid bodies (100).

DATA DISPLAY AND INTERPRETATION

CPET studies have taught us that different defects in the coupling of external (airway) to cellular (mitochondrial) respiration will affect gas exchange in different ways. Thus, the pattern of gas exchange at the airway can be used to diagnose pathophysiology and to support or refute the correctness of a clinical diagnosis. With an appropriate display of the data, it is possible to noninvasively determine the functional status of the cardiovascular system and the ventilatory system, and the uniformity of matching of ventilation to perfusion. Because graphical displays are much easier to interpret than tabular displays, we transform the CPET data into a graphical display of nine panels on a single page containing 15 graphs. These graphs are systematically arranged to assess cardiovascular, ventilatory, ventilation–perfusion matching, and metabolic responses to exercise (Fig. 4.30). In addition, parameters of pulmonary function and target values such as predicted $\dot{V}O_2$max and maximum heart rate are displayed on relevant plots. Normal values for all the measurements in the nine-panel graphical array are summarized in Chapter 7 and are reported in summary tables in the cases of Chapter 10. The systematic approach, using flowcharts leading to interpretation and specific diagnoses, is described in Chapter 8.

Evaluation of Systemic Function from the Nine-Panel Graphical Array

The questions that can be asked of progressively increasing work rate exercise tests are shown in Table 4.1. Using Figure 4.30 to illustrate the use of the nine-panel graphical array, the answer to the first question relating to exercise capacity is addressed in panel 3 from the measurement of maximal (peak) $\dot{V}O_2$. If peak $\dot{V}O_2$ is reduced, we ask if the reduction is due to a cardiovascular limitation (panels 2, 3, and 5), ventilatory limitation (panels 1, 3, 4, and 7), ventilation–perfusion mismatching (panels 3, 4, 6, and 9), or abnormality in use of metabolic substrate

(panels 3 and 8). The nine panels illustrated in Figure 4.30 describe the following physiology:

- *Panel 1:* $\dot{V}E$ versus time and work rate. This plot normally becomes curvilinear as work rate is increased above the anaerobic threshold, except when $\dot{V}E$ is limited by obesity or obstructive lung disease.
- *Panel 2:* Heart rate (HR) and $\dot{V}O_2$/HR (O_2 pulse or stroke volume $\times$ arteriovenous O_2 difference) versus time and work rate. HR is high and $\dot{V}O_2$/HR is low for a given work rate in patients with certain cardiovascular defects. With chronotropic incompetence or β-adrenergic blockade without systolic or diastolic dysfunction, the O_2 pulse could be normal or high.
- *Panel 3:* $\dot{V}O_2$ and $\dot{V}CO_2$ versus time and work rate, and slope showing predicted rate of increase in $\dot{V}O_2$ for the work rate increase (diagonal line). This is the first panel to address when interpreting if a patient is limited in exercise performance, because this plot gives a global assessment of the presence of exercise limitation. The $\Delta\dot{V}O_2/\Delta WR$ is commonly abnormal in patients with cardiovascular disease, with the pattern varying with the defect (e.g., heart disease, peripheral arterial disease, pulmonary vascular disease). The different patterns are described in Chapter 9. The $\dot{V}CO_2$ increases faster than the $\dot{V}O_2$ above the *AT* even when the rate of $\dot{V}O_2$ increase is reduced.
- *Panel 4:* $\dot{V}E$ versus $\dot{V}CO_2$ plotted on a scale of 30:1. This plot yields a linear relation until ventilatory compensation for metabolic acidosis steepens the plot. The slope of the linear part is steeper than normal with hyperventilation or an increase in the exercise physiological dead space/tidal volume ratio.
- *Panel 5:* HR versus $\dot{V}O_2$, and $\dot{V}CO_2$ versus $\dot{V}O_2$. In normal subjects, HR increases linearly with $\dot{V}O_2$ to their predicted maximums (indicated with an *x*). In patients with heart failure, without chronotropic incompetence, the increase is steep. The relationship may lose its linearity, with HR increasing progressively more rapidly than $\dot{V}O_2$ in patients with myocardial ischemia. The patient's O_2 pulse can be determined from the intersection of the patient's data with plots of HR–$\dot{V}O_2$ isopleths through the origin.

In the second graph in this panel, $\dot{V}CO_2$ increases linearly with $\dot{V}O_2$ with a slope of 1, or slightly less than 1, up to the *AT*. Then $\dot{V}CO_2$ increases more rapidly, with the steepening of the slope depending on the rate of buffering of lactic

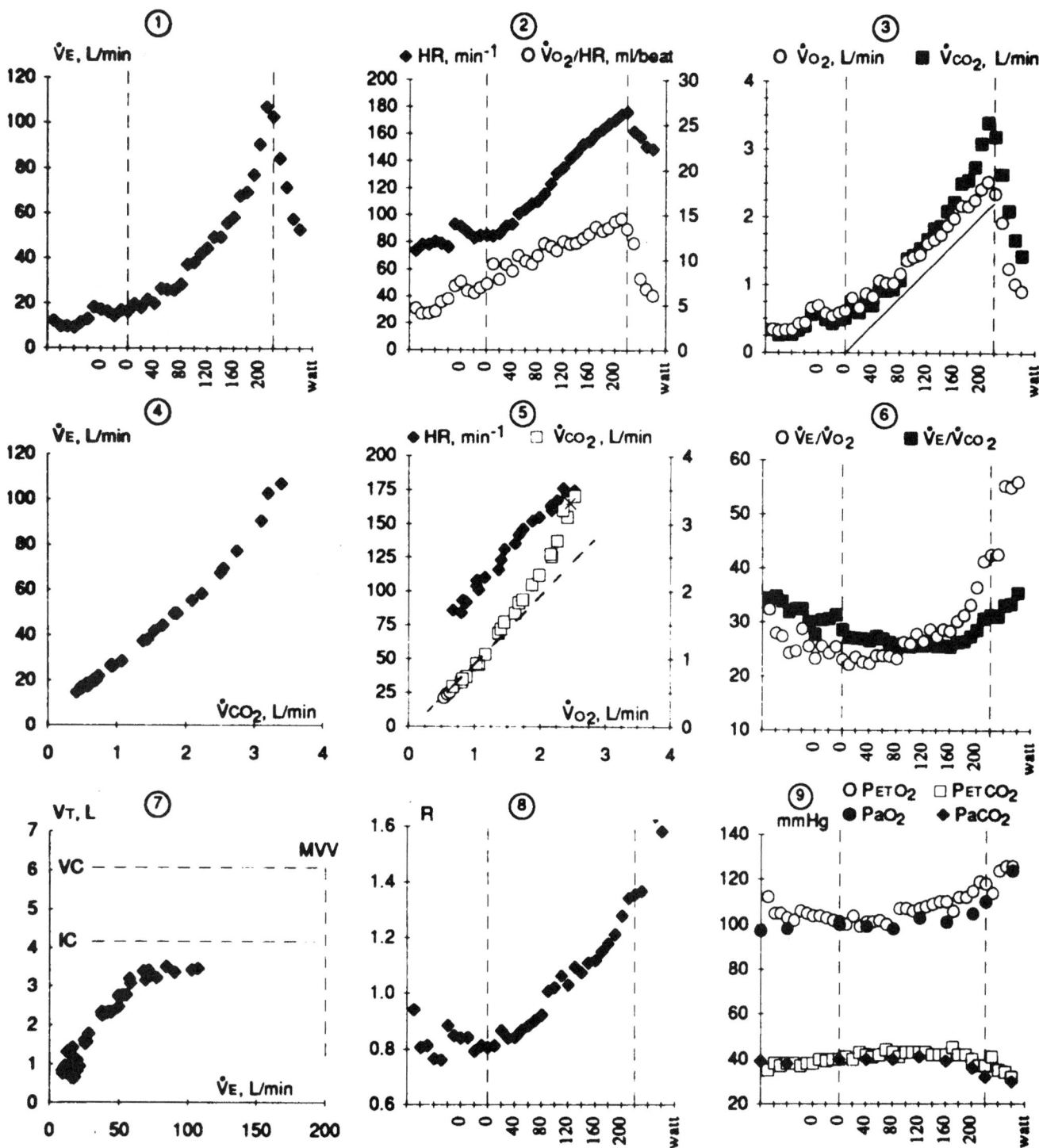

FIGURE 4.30.   Nine-panel graphical array used to describe the cardiovascular, ventilatory, ventilation-perfusion matching and metabolic responses to exercise. The study is from a 55-year-old male patient. The responses are normal. The diagonal line drawn on panel 3 is the slope of the normal increase in $\dot{V}O_2$ for the work rate increase (10 ml/min/watt). The x in panel 5 is the predicted peak $\dot{V}O_2$ and predicted peak heart rate (HR). $\dot{V}E$, minute ventilation; watt, unit of power output (work rate); $\dot{V}O_2/HR$, O_2 pulse; MVV, maximal voluntary ventilation; IC, inspiratory capacity; VC, vital capacity; R, respiratory exchange ratio ($\dot{V}CO_2/\dot{V}O_2$); $PETO_2$, end-tidal PO_2; $PETCO_2$, end-tidal PCO_2; PaO_2, arterial PO_2; $PaCO_2$, arterial PCO_2. (Modified from Case 1 in Chapter 10.)

acid. The break point describes the *AT*. This is the V-slope method for determining *AT* (36). It is low in patients with poor cardiovascular function.

- *Panel 6:* Ventilatory equivalent for O_2 and CO_2 ($\dot{V}E/\dot{V}O_2$ and $\dot{V}E/\dot{V}CO_2$) versus time and work rate. $\dot{V}E/\dot{V}O_2$ decreases to a nadir at the *AT*. $\dot{V}E/\dot{V}CO_2$ decreases to a nadir in the period between the *AT* and the ventilatory compensation point. Both values are high in diseases with uneven ventilation–perfusion relationships (increased $\dot{V}D/\dot{V}T$).
- *Panel 7:* Tidal volume ($\dot{V}T$) versus $\dot{V}E$. The patient's vital capacity (VC) and inspiratory capacity (IC) are shown on the vertical axis, and actually measured maximum voluntary ventilation (MVV) or FEV_1 times 40 is shown on the horizontal axis. Ventilatory frequency can be plotted as isopleths through the origin. With airflow limitation, maximal exercise $\dot{V}E$ approximates the MVV, resulting in a low breathing reserve (MVV − $\dot{V}E$) at maximal exercise. The breathing reserve cannot be predicted from resting pulmonary function measurements alone. With restrictive lung disease, $\dot{V}T$ may approximate the IC at low work rates, and respiratory rate may increase to 50 or 60, in contrast to the values seen in patients with COPD.
- *Panel 8:* Respiratory exchange ratio ($\dot{V}CO_2/\dot{V}O_2$, R) versus time and work rate. This plot usually starts at approximately 0.8 and increases to values higher than 1.0 above the *AT*. Inability or failure to produce an exercise lactic acidosis would mitigate an increase in R to values above 1.0, except when accompanied by acute hyperventilation (decreased $PaCO_2$). Acute hyperventilation at rest or low work rates, as reflected by a decreasing $PETCO_2$, yields an R greater than 1.0.
- *Panel 9:* $PETCO_2$, $PETO_2$, and SpO_2 (arterial oxyhemoglobin saturation determined with a pulse oximeter) versus time and work rate. Low $PETCO_2$ signals either hyperventilation or high $\dot{V}A/\dot{Q}$ mismatching. R (panel 8) reveals if hyperventilation is acute. Arterial blood gases or knowledge of plasma HCO_3^- differentiates chronic hyperventilation from $\dot{V}A/\dot{Q}$ abnormality in patients with a low $PETCO_2$. Arterial blood gases are plotted on this graph to detect the presence of high and low $\dot{V}A/\dot{Q}$ mismatching.

Factors Confounding Interpretation of Cardiopulmonary Exercise Testing

Three physiological derangements, not usually considered as diseases of the cardiorespiratory system, may contribute significantly to exercise intolerance. These physiological derangements are obesity, anemia, and carboxyhemoglobinemia secondary to cigarette smoking.

Obesity adds to the O_2 and cardiac output cost of exercise. It may also restrict the ventilatory system and increase the work of breathing. The restriction of ventilatory capacity caused by obesity is more marked as the $\dot{V}E$ requirement increases, possibly leading to hypercapnia.

Anemia reduces the arterial O_2 content and the maximal arteriovenous O_2 content difference. Therefore, to achieve a given $\dot{V}O_2$, a greater cardiac output is required than if anemia were not present. Also, because the O_2 content of the arterial blood is reduced, the capillary PO_2 decreases to its critical value, inducing anaerobic metabolism and lactic acidosis at a lower than normal work rate and $\dot{V}O_2$.

The carboxyhemoglobin level in the blood of the heavy cigarette smoker may reach 10% to 12%. This not only reduces the arterial O_2 content to a level that would be normally found with an arterial PO_2 of about 50 to 55 mm Hg, but also shifts the oxyhemoglobin dissociation curve to the left, making it more difficult for O_2 to dissociate from hemoglobin at a given PO_2. Thus, the capillary PO_2 falls more rapidly to its critical value, resulting in a lactic acidosis at a reduced level of work (104).

The net effect of each of these complicating factors is a reduction in the amount of external work that the patient can accomplish. However, in moderate obesity, the maximal $\dot{V}O_2$ and *AT* might be normal or high when referenced to the patient's ideal body weight. In contrast, the maximal $\dot{V}O_2$, *AT*, and peak work rate are reduced in patients with anemia and increased carboxyhemoglobinemia.

SUMMARY

Changes in O_2 uptake and CO_2 output by the lungs reflect changes in cell respiration induced by exercise. Although the source of the increased gas exchange with exercise is the increase in cell respiration, cardiac output and ventilation modulate the gas exchange at the airway. Thus, diseases of the cardiovascular and ventilatory systems will affect the gas exchange pattern at the airway, depending on the disease pathophysiology. Measurements that assess these functions following controlled work rate perturbations define the physiologic state of the organ systems that participate in gas transport. Defects in the coupling of external to internal respiration result in gas exchange abnormalities characteristic of the limiting organ system. For example, whereas diseases of the heart, the lungs, and the peripheral and pulmonary circulations all result in demonstrable abnormalities in gas exchange, each type of disorder manifests specific and relatively unique abnormalities that are amplified by exercise testing. The effects of various disease states on these measurements are described in Chapter 5.

References

1. Oren A, Sue DY, Hansen JE, Torrance DJ, Wasserman K. The role of exercise testing in impairment evaluation. *Am Rev Respir Dis* 1987;135:230–235.
2. Wensel R, Opitz CF, Ewert R, Bruch L, Kleber FX. Effects of Iloprost inhalation on exercise capacity and ventilatory efficiency in patients with primary pulmonary hypertension. *Circulation* 2000;101:2388–2392.
3. Older P, Smith R, Courtney P, Hone R. Preoperative evaluation of cardiac failure and ischemia in elderly patients by cardiopulmonary exercise testing. *Chest* 1993;104:701–704.
4. Smith TP, Kinasewitz GT, Tucker WY, Spillers WP, George RB. Exercise capacity as a predictor of postthoracotomy morbidity. *Am Rev Respir Dis* 1984;129: 730–734.
5. Mancini D, Eisen H, Kussmaul W, Mull R, Edmunds L, Wilson J. Value of peak exercise oxygen consumption for optimal timing of cardiac transplantation of ambulatory patients with heart failure. *Circulation* 1991;83:778–786.
6. Stevenson LW. Role of exercise testing in the evaluation of candidates for cardiac transplantation. In: Wasserman K, ed. *Exercise gas exchange in heart disease.* Armonk, NY: Futura Publishing, 1996:271–286.
7. Chua TP, Ponikowski P, Harrington D, Anker SD, Webb-Peploe K, Clark AL, Poole-Wilson PA, Coats AJ. Clinical correlates and prognostic significance of the ventilatory response to exercise in chronic heart failure. *J Am Coll Cardiol* 1997;29:1585–1590.
8. Kleber FX, Vietzke G, Wernecke KD, Bauer U, Optiz C, Wensel R, Sperfeld A, Glaser S. Impairment of ventilatory efficiency in heart failure: prognostic impact. *Circulation* 2000;101:2803–2809.
9. Gitt AK, Wasserman K, Kilkowski C, Kleeman T, Kilkowski A, Bangert M, Schneider S, Schwartz A, Senges J. Exercise anaerobic threshold and ventilatory efficiency identify heart failure patients for high risk of early death. *Circulation* 2002;106:3079–3084.
10. Mudge GH, Goldstein S, Addonizio LJ, Caplan A, Mancini D, Levine TB, Ritsch ME, Stevenson LW. Task force 3: recipient guidelines/prioritization. *J Am Coll Cardiol* 1993;22:21–26.
11. Oga T, Nishimura K, Tsukino M, Sato S, Hajiro T. Analysis of the factors related to mortality in chronic obstructive pulmonary disease. *Am J Respir Crit Care Med* 2003;167:544–549.
12. Fishman A, Martinez F, Naunheim K, Pianadosi S, Wise R, Ries A, Weinmann Wood DE. National Emphysema Treatment Trial Research Group. A randomized trial comparing lung-volume-reduction surgery with medical therapy for severe emphysema. *N Engl J Med* 2003;348:2059–2073.
13. Treese N, MacCarter D, Akbulut O, Coutinho M, Baez M, Liebrich A, Meyer J. Ventilation and heart rate response during exercise in normals: relevance for rate variable pacing. *Pacing Clin Electrophysiol* 1993;16:1693–1700.
14. Koike A, Itoh H, Doi M, Taniguichi K, Marumo F, Umehara I, Hiroe M. Effects of isosorbide dinitrate on exercise capacity in cardiac patients. Relationship between oxygen uptake responses and hemodynamic effects. *Jpn Circ J* 1990;54:1535–1545.
15. Weber KT. What can we learn from exercise testing beyond the detection of myocardial ischemia? *Clin Cardiol* 1997;20:684–696.
16. Gibbons RJ, Balady GJ, Beasley JW, Bricker T, Duvernoy WFC, Froelicher VF, Mark DB, Marwick TH, McCallister BD, Thompson PO, Winters WL, Yanowitz FG. ACC/AHA guidelines for exercise testing: a report of the American College of Cardiology/American Heart Association Task Force on Practice Guidelines (Committee on Exercise Testing). *J Am Coll Cardiol* 1997;30:260–315.
17. Belardinelli R, Lacalaprice F, Carle F, Minnucci A, Cianci G, Perna G, D'Eusanio G. Exercise-induced myocardial ischaemia detected by cardiopulmonary exercise testing. *Eur Heart J* 2003;24:1–10.
18. Itoh H, Tajima A, Koike A, Osada N, Maeda T, Kato M, Omiya K, Fu LT, Watanabe H, Kato K. Oxygen uptake abnormalities during exercise in coronary artery disease. In: Wasserman K, ed. *Cardiopulmonary exercise testing and cardiovascular health.* Armonk, NY: Futura Publishing, 2002:165–172.
19. Taylor HL, Buskirk E, Henschel A. Maximal oxygen intake as an objective measure of cardiorespiratory performance. *J Appl Physiol* 1955;8:73–80.
20. Anderson P, Saltin B. Maximal perfusion of skeletal muscle in man. *J Appl Physiol* 1985;366:233–249.
21. Vogel JA, Gleser MA. Effect of carbon monoxide on oxygen transport during exercise. *J Appl Physiol* 1972; 32:234–239.
22. Whipp BJ, Ward SA. Coupling of ventilation to pulmonary gas exchange during exercise. In: Whipp BJ, Wasserman K, eds. *Exercise: pulmonary physiology and pathophysiology.* New York: Marcel Dekker, 1991:275.
23. Cooper DM, Weiler-Ravell D, Whipp BJ, Wasserman K. Aerobic parameters of exercise as a function of

body size during growth in children. *J Appl Physiol* 1984;56:628–634.

24. DiPrampero PE. Energetics of muscular exercise. *Rev Physiol Biochem Pharmacol* 1981;89:143–222.

25. Zhang YY, Johnson MC, Chow N, Wasserman K. Effect of exercise testing protocol on parameters of aerobic function. *Med Sci Sports Exerc* 1991;23:625–630.

26. Zhang YY, Johnson MC, Chow N, Wasserman K. The role of fitness on $\dot{V}O_2$ and $\dot{V}CO_2$ kinetics in response to proportional step increases in work rate. *Eur J Appl Physiol* 1991;63:94–100.

27. Hansen JE, Sue DY, Wasserman K. Predicted values for clinical exercise testing. *Am Rev Respir Dis* 1984; 129(Suppl):S49–S55.

28. Wasserman K, Whipp BJ. Exercise physiology in health and disease (state of the art). *Am Rev Respir Dis* 1975;112:219–249.

29. Wasserman K, Sue DY. Coupling of external to cellular respiration. In: Wasserman K, ed. *Exercise gas exchange in heart disease*. Armonk, NY: Futura Publishing, 1996:1–15.

30. Riley M, Wasserman K, Fu PC, Cooper CB. Muscle substrate utilization from alveolar gas exchange in trained cyclist. *Eur J Appl Physiol* 1996;72:341–348.

31. Wasserman K. Diagnosing cardiovascular and lung pathophysiology from exercise gas exchange. *Chest* 1997;112:1091–1101.

32. Linnarsson D. Dynamics of pulmonary gas exchange and heart rate changes at start and end of exercise. *Acta Physiol Scand* 1974;415(Suppl 1):5–68.

33. Whipp BJ, Mahler M. Dynamics of pulmonary gas exchange during exercise. In: West JB, ed. *Pulmonary gas exchange*. New York: Academic Press, 1980:33–96.

34. Hesser CM, Linnarsson D, Bjurstedt H. Cardiorespiratory and metabolic responses to positive, negative and minimum-load dynamic leg exercise. *Respir Physiol* 1977;30:51–67.

35. Haouzi P, Fukuba Y, Casaburi R, Stringer W, Wasserman K. O_2 uptake kinetics above and below the lactic acidosis threshold during sinusoidal exercise. *J Appl Physiol* 1993;75:1644–1650.

36. Beaver WL, Wasserman K, Whipp BJ. A new method for detecting the anaerobic threshold by gas exchange. *J Appl Physiol* 1986;60:2020–2027.

37. Stringer W, Casaburi R, Wasserman K. Acid-base regulation during exercise and recovery in man. *J Appl Physiol* 1992;72:954–961.

38. Koike A, Hiroe M, Adachi H, Yajima T, Nogami A, Ito H, Takamoto T, Taniguchi K. Anaerobic metabolism as an indicator of aerobic function during exercise in cardiac patients. *J Am Coll Cardiol* 1992; 20:120–126.

39. Sun XG, Hansen JE, Ting H, Chuang ML, Stringer WW, Adame D, Wasserman K. Comparison of exercise cardiac output by the Fick principle using oxygen and carbon dioxide. *Chest* 2000;118:631–640.

40. Jones NL, Campbell EJM. *Clinical exercise testing*. Philadelphia: W.B. Saunders, 1982.

41. Jones NL, McHardy GJR, Naimark A, Campbell EJM. Physiological dead space and alveolar-arterial gas pressure differences during exercise. *Clin Sci* 1966;31:19–29.

42. Sue DY, Oren A, Hansen JE, Wasserman K. Diffusing capacity for carbon monoxide as a predictor of gas exchange during exercise. *N Engl J Med* 1987;316: 1301–1306.

43. Rubin SA, Brown HV. Ventilation and gas exchange during exercise in severe chronic heart failure. *Am Rev Respir Dis* 1984;129(Suppl):S63–S64.

44. Sun XG, Hansen JE, Garatachea N, Storer TW, Wasserman K. Ventilatory efficiency during exercise in healthy subjects. *Am J Respir Crit Care Med* 2002; 166:1443–1448.

45. Weisel RD, Berger RL, Hechtman HB. Measurement of cardiac output by thermodilution. *N Engl J Med* 1975;292:682–684.

46. Stringer W, Hansen J, Wasserman K. Cardiac output estimated non-invasively from oxygen uptake ($\dot{V}O_2$) during exercise. *J Appl Physiol* 1997;82:908–912.

47. Weber KT, Janicki JS. Cardiopulmonary exercise (CPX) testing in heart and lung disease. In: *Cardiopulmonary exercise testing: physiologic principles and clinical applications*. Philadelphia: W.B. Saunders, 1986:200.

48. Agostoni PG, Wasserman K, Perego G, Marenzi GC, Cattadori G, Guazzi M, Assanelli E, Lauri G. Stroke volume (SV) measured non-invasively at anaerobic threshold (*AT*) in heart failure. *Am J Respir Crit Care Med* 1997;155:A171.

49. Knuttgen HG, Saltin B. Muscle metabolites and oxygen uptake in short-term submaximal exercise in man. *J Appl Physiol* 1972;32:690–694.

50. Bylund-Fellenius AC, Walker PM, Elander A, Holm S, Holm J, Schersten T. Energy metabolism in relation to oxygen, partial pressure in human skeletal muscle during exercise. *Biochem J* 1981;200:247–255.

51. Sahlin K, Katz A, Henriksson J. Redox state and lactate accumulation in human skeletal muscle during dynamic exercise. *Biochem J* 1987;245:551–556.

52. Wasserman K, Beaver WL, Davis JA, Pu J-Z, Heber D, Whipp BJ. Lactate, pyruvate, and lactate-to-pyruvate ratio during exercise and recovery. *J Appl Physiol* 1985;59:935–940.

53. Roston WL, Whipp BJ, Davis JA, Effros RM, Wasserman K. Oxygen uptake kinetics and lactate concentration during exercise in man. *Am Rev Respir Dis* 1987;135:1080–1084.

54. Beaver WL, Wasserman K, Whipp BJ. Bicarbonate buffering of lactic acid generated during exercise. *J Appl Physiol* 1986;60:472–478.

55. Wasserman K, Stringer W, Casaburi R, Zhang YY. Mechanism of the exercise hyperkalemia: an alternate hypothesis. *J Appl Physiol* 1997;83:631–643.

56. Osnes J-B, Hermansen L. Acid-base balance after maximal exercise of short duration. *J Appl Physiol* 1972;32:59–63.

57. Sue DY, Wasserman K, Moricca RB, Casaburi R. Metabolic acidosis during exercise in patients with chronic obstructive pulmonary disease. *Chest* 1988;94:931–938.

58. Wasserman K. Breathing during exercise. (Physiology in Medicine series). *N Engl J Med* 1978;298:780–785.

59. Cooper CB, Whipp BJ, Cooper DM, Wasserman K. Factors affecting the components of the alveolar CO_2 output-O_2 uptake relationship during incremental exercise in man. *Exp Physiol* 1992;77:51–64.

60. Davis JA, Whipp BJ, Lamarra N, Huntsman DJ, Frank MH, Wasserman K. Effect of ramp slope on determination of aerobic parameters from the ramp exercise test. *Med Sci Sports Exerc* 1982;14:339–343.

61. Buchfuhrer MJ, Hansen JE, Robinson TE, Sue DY, Wasserman K, Whipp BJ. Optimizing the exercise protocol for cardiopulmonary assessment. *J Appl Physiol* 1983;55:1558–1564.

62. Yoshida T. Effect of dietary modifications on lactate threshold and onset of blood lactate accumulation during incremental exercise. *Eur J Appl Physiol* 1984;53:200–205.

63. McClellan TM, Gass GC. The relationship between the ventilation and lactate thresholds following normal, low and high carbohydrate diets. *Eur J Appl Physiol* 1989;58:568–576.

64. Beaver WL, Wasserman K, Whipp BJ. Improved detection of the lactate threshold during exercise using a log-log transformation. *J Appl Physiol* 1985;59:1936–1940.

65. Wasserman K. Determinants and detection of anaerobic threshold and consequences of exercise above it. *Circulation* 1987;81(Suppl VI):29–39.

66. Riley M, Nicholls P, Patterson VH. Anaerobic threshold: the problem of McArdle's disease. *J Appl Physiol* 1993;75:745–754.

67. Donald KW, Bishop JM, Cumming C, Wade OL. The effect of exercise on the cardiac output and central dynamics of normal subjects. *Clin Sci* 1955;14:37–73.

68. Koike A, Itoh H, Taniguichi K, Hiroe M. Detecting abnormalities in left ventricular function during exercise by respiratory measurement. *Circulation* 1989;80:1737–1746.

69. Butler J, Schrijen F, Polu JM, Albert RK. Cause of the raised wedge pressure on exercise in chronic obstructive pulmonary disease. *Am Rev Respir Dis* 1988;138:350–354.

70. Nery LE, Wasserman K, French W, Oren A, Davis JA. Contrasting cardiovascular and respiratory responses to exercise in mitral valve and chronic obstructive pulmonary diseases. *Chest* 1983;83:446–453.

71. Koike A, Itoh H, Doi M, Taniguichi K, Marumo F, Umehara I, Hiroe M. Beat-to-beat evaluation of cardiac function during recovery from upright bicycle exercise in patients with coronary artery disease. *Am Heart J* 1990;120:316–323.

72. Sue DY, Hansen JE. Normal values in adults during exercise testing. *Clin Chest Med* 1984;5:89–97.

73. Gallagher CG. Exercise limitation and clinical exercise testing in chronic obstructive pulmonary disease. *Clin Chest Med-Clin Exerc Testing* 1994;15:305–326.

74. Babb TG, Rodarte JR. Estimation of ventilatory capacity during submaximal exercise. *J Appl Physiol* 1993;74:2016–2022.

75. Babb TG, Rodarte JR. Exercise capacity and breathing mechanics in patients with airflow limitation. *Med Sci Sports Exerc* 1992;24:967–974.

76. O'Donnell DE, Lam M, Webb KA. Spirometric correlates of improvement in exercise performance after anticholinergic therapy in chronic obstructive pulmonary disease. *Am J Respir Crit Care Med* 1999;160:542–549.

77. Whipp BJ, Pardy RL. Breathing during exercise. *Handbook of physiology. The respiratory system III*. Bethesda, MD: American Physiological Society, 1992:605–629.

78. Somfay A, Porszasz J, Lee S-M, Casaburi R. Effect of hyperoxia on gas exchange and lactate kinetics following exercise onset in nonhypoxemic COPD patients. *Chest* 2002;121:393–400.

79. Wasserman K, VanKessel A, Burton GB. Interaction of physiological mechanisms during exercise. *J Appl Physiol* 1967;22:71–85.

80. Whipp BJ, Wasserman K. Alveolar-arterial gas tension differences during graded exercise. *J Appl Physiol* 1969;27:361–365.

81. Farhi LE. Ventilation perfusion relationship and its role in alveolar gas exchange. *Adv Respir Physiol* 1966:177.

82. Fishman AP. Hypoxia on the pulmonary circulation: how and where it acts. *Circ Res* 1976;38:221–231.

83. Sietsema KE, Cooper DM, Perloff SK, Child JS, Rosove MH, Wasserman K, Whipp BJ. Control of ventilation during exercise in patients with central venous-to-systemic arterial shunts. *J Appl Physiol* 1988;64:234–242.

84. Neder JA, Nery LE, Peres C, Whipp BJ. Reference values for dynamic responses to incremental cycle ergometry in males and females aged 20 to 80. *Am J Respir Crit Care Med* 2001;164:1481–1486.

85. Metra M, Dei Cas L, Panina G, Visioli O. Exercise hyperventilation in chronic congestive heart failure, and its relation to functional capacity and hemodynamics. *Am J Cardiol* 1992;70:622–628.

86. Weiler-Ravell D, Whipp BJ, Cooper DM, Wasserman K. The control of breathing at the start of exercise as

influenced by posture. *J Appl Physiol* 1983;55:1460–1466.

87. Nery LE, Wasserman K, Andrews JD, Huntsman DJ, Hansen JE, Whipp BJ. Ventilatory and gas exchange kinetics during exercise in chronic airways obstruction. *J Appl Physiol* 1982;53:1594–1602.

88. Sietsema KE, Cooper DM, Rosove MH, Perloff JK, Child JS, Canobbio MM, Whipp BJ, Wasserman K. Dynamics of oxygen uptake during exercise in adults with cyanotic congenital heart disease. *Circulation* 1986;73:1137–1144.

89. Sietsema K. Oxygen uptake kinetics during exercise in patients with pulmonary vascular disease. *Am Rev Respir Dis* 1992;145:1052–1057.

90. Weissman ML, Jones PW, Oren A, Lamarra N, Whipp BJ, Wasserman K. Cardiac output increase and gas exchange at the start of exercise. *J Appl Physiol* 1982;52:236–244.

91. Whipp BJ, Wasserman K. Oxygen uptake kinetics for various intensities of constant load work. *J Appl Physiol* 1972;33:351–356.

92. Barstow TJ, Casaburi R, Wasserman K. Oxygen uptake kinetics and the O_2 deficit as related to exercise intensity and blood lactate. *J Appl Physiol* 1993;75:755–762.

93. Zhang YY, Wasserman K, Sietsema KE, Barstow TJ, Mizumoto G, Sullivan CS, Ben-Dov I. O_2 uptake kinetics in response to exercise: a measure of tissue anaerobiosis in heart failure. *Chest* 1993;103:735–741.

94. Wasserman K, Casaburi R, Beaver WL, Roston WL, Whipp BJ. Assessing the adequacy of tissue oxygenation during exercise. In: Bryan-Brown CW, Ayres SM, eds. *Oxygen transport and utilization.* Fullerton, CA: Society of Critical Care Medicine, 1987:109–144.

95. Sietsema KE, Daly JA, Wasserman K. Early dynamics of O_2 uptake and heart rate as affected by exercise work rate. *J Appl Physiol* 1989;67:2535–2541.

96. Zhang YY, Sietsema KE, Sullivan S, Wasserman K. A method for estimating bicarbonate buffering of lactic acid during constant work rate exercise. *Eur J Appl Physiol* 1994;69:309–315.

97. Schneider EG, Robinson S, Newton JL. Oxygen debt in aerobic work. *J Appl Physiol* 1968;25:58–62.

98. Rebuck AS, Slutsky AS. Measurement of ventilatory responses to hypercapnia and hypoxia. In: Hornbein TF, ed. *Regulation of breathing.* New York: Marcel Dekker, 1981:745–772.

99. Severinghaus JW. Proposed standard determination of ventilatory responses to hypoxia and hypercapnia in man. *Chest* 1976;70(Suppl):129–131.

100. Dejours P. Control of respiration by arterial chemoreceptors. *Ann NY Acad Sci* 1963;109:682–695.

101. Whipp BJ, Wasserman K. Carotid bodies and ventilatory control dynamics in man. Symposium on recent advances in carotid body physiology. *Fed Proc* 1980;39:2668–2673.

102. Springer C, Cooper DM, Wasserman K. Evidence that maturation of the peripheral chemoreceptors is not complete in childhood. *Respir Physiol* 1988;74:55–64.

103. Wasserman K, Whipp BJ, Casaburi R. Respiratory control during exercise. In: Cherniack NS, Widdicombe G, eds. *Handbook of physiology.* Bethesda: American Physiological Society, 1986:595–619.

104. Koike A, Wasserman K, Taniguichi K, Hiroe M, Marumo F. Critical capillary oxygen partial pressure and lactate threshold in patients with cardiovascular disease. *J Am Coll Cardiol* 1994;23:1644–1650.

Pathophysiology of Disorders Limiting Exercise

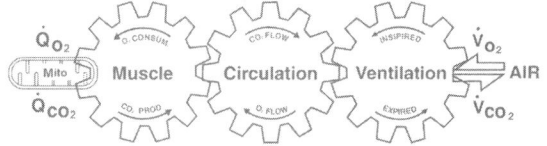

THE COUPLING OF EXTERNAL to cellular respiration to perform exercise involves many organ systems. From Figure 5.1, it is evident that the blood, the peripheral circulation, the heart, the pulmonary circulation, the lungs, the chest wall, respiratory control, and metabolic pathways in bioenergetics influence the normal coupling of external to cellular respiration. Thus, defects of any might limit exercise performance. The objective of this chapter is to describe the changes in external respiration that characterize the pathophysiology brought about by diseases of the organ systems that are required for the support of the exercise bioenergetic mechanisms. These disorders are listed by class in Table 5.1, accompanied by a statement of major pathophysiology and physiological limitation. Individually or in combination, these disorders limit exercise by causing symptoms of dyspnea, fatigue, and/or pain.

OBESITY

Whereas the obese subject has some increase in resting metabolic rate ($\dot{V}O_2$) relative to lean body mass, the increase is more marked during dynamic exercise (see Figs. 2.7 and 4.5; Table 5.2). Additional energy is needed to move heavy legs in leg cycling exercise or a large body mass while ambulating. This adds to the O_2 needed to perform external work (Fig. 5.2) (1,2). Because the metabolic rate is increased to perform a given amount of external work, obese people require an increased cardiorespiratory response to exercise. However, the heart, blood vessels, lungs, and muscles do not usually increase in size commensurate with the subject's added weight. Consequently, for the obese individual to do any amount of physical work, there must be greater than normal cardiovascular and ventilatory responses. Because more O_2 transport than normal is needed to support body movement, less O_2 transport is available for effective external work in obesity.

Constraints are imposed on the maximal exercise performance because of altered cardiovascular and ventilatory mechanics in obesity, especially in the extremely obese subject. Because of the large mass, the resting cardiac output per kilogram of lean body weight is already high. Thus, the cardiac output reserve available to support the increased muscle O_2 requirement for exercise is reduced (3). Furthermore, the added mass on the chest wall and the increased pressure in the abdomen cause increased ventilatory work. In obese subjects, the increased abdominal pressure may constrain diaphragmatic descent during inspiration, reducing the vital capacity. Both the increased abdominal pressure and the added weight to the chest wall effectively "chest strap" (4–7) the patient, causing the resting end-expiratory lung volume (FRC) to be reduced (in extreme cases, close to the residual volume) (8). This

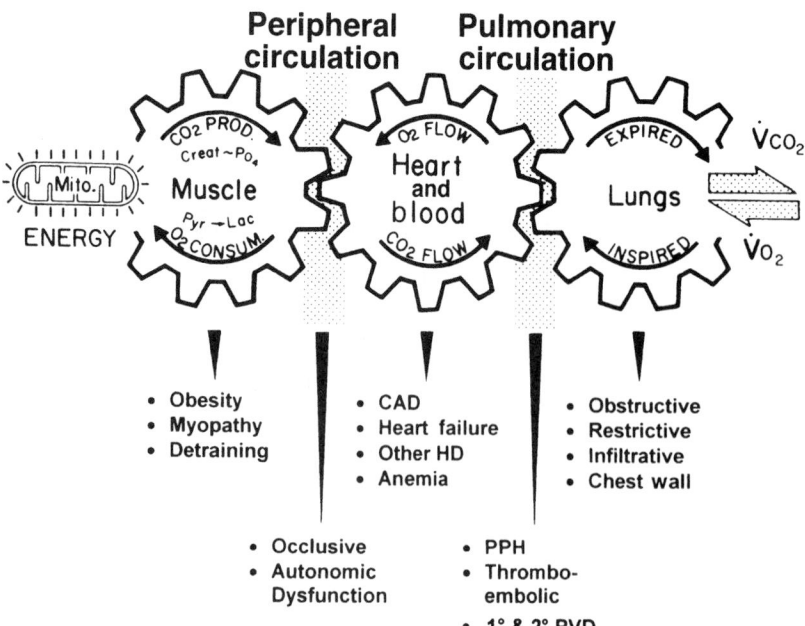

FIGURE 5.1.   Sites of interference in the metabolic-cardiovascular-ventilatory coupling caused by various disease states.

TABLE 5.1.   Disorders and Mechanisms Impairing Work Tolerance

Disorder	Pathophysiology	Primary Limitation
Obesity	Increased metabolic requirement; respiratory restriction	Decreased cardiorespiratory reserve
Peripheral arterial disease	Prevents normal vasodilatation; exercise hypertension	Impaired muscle O_2 supply; increased cardiac work.
Heart diseases	Reduced ability to increase cardiac output (stroke volume); ventilation-perfusion mismatching and lung restriction in heart failure	Reduced tissue O_2 delivery (fatigue); increased ventilatory requirement (dyspnea)
Pulmonary vascular diseases	Limited cardiac output increase; decreased gas exchange efficiency	Impaired tissue O_2 delivery (fatigue); increased ventilatory requirement (dyspnea)
Ventilatory disorders		
Airflow obstruction	Increased airway resistance; abnormal $\dot{V}_A/\dot{Q}$	Reduced ventilatory capacity; increased ventilatory requirement
Restrictive lung disease	Inability to increase pulmonary blood flow; reduced lung distensibility; decreased efficiency of gas exchange; exercise-induced hypoxemia	Reduced tissue O_2 delivery (fatigue); increased drive to breathe (dyspnea)
Chest wall defect	Abnormal rib cage mechanics; respiratory muscle weakness	Reduced ability to breathe (dyspnea)
Defects in hemoglobin content and quality	Reduced blood O_2 content; increased O_2 affinity for hemoglobin (left-shifted HbO_2 dissociation curve)	Impaired tissue O_2 delivery
Smoking	Increased carboxyhemoglobin; hypertension; increased airway resistance	Reduced tissue O_2; increased cardiac output demand; reduced ventilatory capacity
Metabolic acidosis	Reduced buffering capacity; low Pa_{CO_2} set point	Increased ventilatory drive (dyspnea)
Neuromuscular disease	Musculoskeletal coupling inefficiency	Reduced mechanical efficiency; pain
Glycolytic enzyme defect	Deficiency in carbohydrate substrate; inability to regenerate *ATP* by anaerobic metabolism	Muscle pain; reduced aerobic and anaerobic *ATP* regeneration (fatigue)
Electron transport defect	Inability to regenerate *ATP* aerobically	Low work rate metabolic acidosis
Anxiety	Nonphysiological breathing patterns	Shortness of breath
Poor effort or manipulated performance	Secondary gain; chaotic breathing: no or little metabolic acidosis at peak exercise	Self

can lead to atelectasis of peripheral lung units and hypoxemia at rest. In addition, pulmonary vascular resistance may be increased, primarily as a result of pulmonary insufficiency. Thus, cor pulmonale may develop with secondary erythrocytosis, hepatomegaly, peripheral edema, and right ventricular hypertrophy.

TABLE 5.2.   Discriminating Measurements During Exercise in Obesity

High O_2 cost to perform external work
Upward displacement of $\dot{V}_{O_2}$–work rate relationship
Peak $\dot{V}_{O_2}$/body weight and *AT*/body weight values are low
Peak $\dot{V}_{O_2}$/height and *AT*/height values are normal or high (with active lifestyle)
Normal to high O_2 pulse when determined from predicted weight
Low Pa_{O_2} at rest that normalizes during exercise
Normal $\dot{V}_D/\dot{V}_T$
Failure to develop normal ventilatory compensation for metabolic acidosis
$\dot{V}_E$ maintains a linear increase with work rate and $\dot{V}_{CO_2}$

Peak $\dot{V}_{O_2}$, highest O_2 uptake measured; *AT*, anaerobic threshold; $\dot{V}_D$, physiological dead space; $\dot{V}_T$, tidal volume.

The increased O_2 cost of performing mechanical work is predictable and well worked out for cycle ergometer work (1,2). The $\dot{V}_{O_2}$–work rate relationship is displaced upward, depending on the degree of obesity, by 5.8 ml/min/kg (Fig. 5.2). However, obesity causes no discernible change in the slope of the $\dot{V}_{O_2}$–work rate relation (1,2). The effect of adipose tissue distribution in the body (i.e., legs or trunk) on $\dot{V}_{O_2}$ has not been investigated.

The maximum $\dot{V}_{O_2}$ and anaerobic threshold (*AT*) are low when related to actual body weight, but usually normal when related to height (1) or to predicted weight or lean body mass (9). Because of the high metabolic cost of doing even modest levels of exercise, an active, otherwise healthy, obese subject may have good cardiovascular fitness but reduced work capacity. Thus, the actual $\dot{V}_{O_2}$max, based on height or lean body weight, may be greater than that predicted for a normal, sedentary subject.

The hypoxemia commonly present at rest in the obese subject results from atelectasis of peripheral lung units. This usually improves during exercise, because the deep breathing reexpands atelectic lung units. It is the only pulmonary condition in

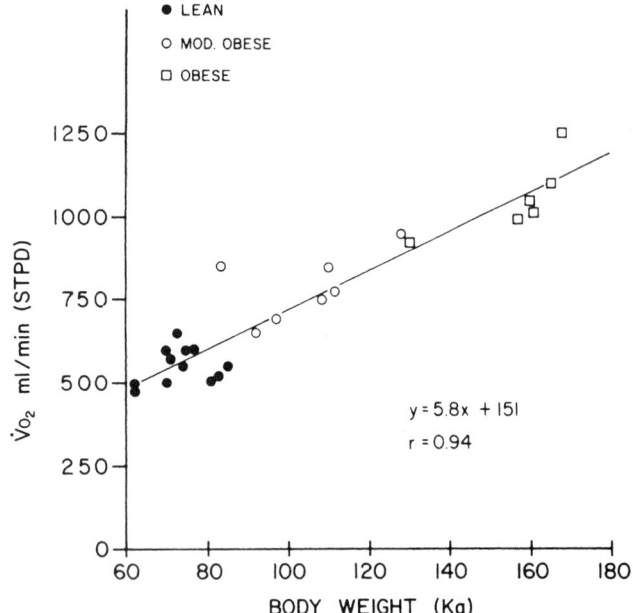

FIGURE 5.2. O_2 cost of performing unloaded cycling as related to body weight. (From Wasserman K, Whipp BJ. Exercise physiology in health and disease (state of the art). *Am Rev Respir Dis* 1975;112: 219–249, with permission.)

which arterial oxygenation improves during exercise. Because ventilation–perfusion relationships usually normalize during exercise in the patient with uncomplicated obesity, exercise V_D/V_T, $P(A − a)O_2$, and $P(a − ET)CO_2$ values are normal.

PERIPHERAL ARTERIAL DISEASES

Because of atherosclerotic changes that reduce the internal diameter of the conducting arteries to the limbs, peripheral arterial diseases prevent the increase in blood flow needed to meet the increased metabolic demand of exercise (Table 5.3). Thus, O_2 flow fails to increase sufficiently to satisfy the O_2 requirement for performing exercise (see Fig. 2.14). The inability to supply sufficient O_2 to the exercis-

TABLE 5.3.   Discriminating Measurements During Exercise in Peripheral Arterial Disease

Low $\Delta\dot{V}O_2/\Delta WR$; low $\Delta\dot{V}CO_2/\Delta WR$
Low maximum $\dot{V}O_2$
Low AT
Leg pain
Exercise-induced hypertension

$\Delta\dot{V}O_2/\Delta WR$, increase in $\dot{V}O_2$ relative to increase in work rate; *AT*, anaerobic threshold.

ing muscles to meet the O_2 requirement is reflected in a reduced $\Delta\dot{V}O_2/\Delta WR$ ratio at low work levels. Although a compensatory increase in mitochondrial number in the ischemic muscle may occur with time, the improved O_2 extraction that this mechanism portends is inadequate to make up for the deficiency in O_2 flow (10). Consequently, the ischemic muscles produce lactic acid at relatively low work rates, with subsequent leg pain and fatigue. Because of slow blood flow through the ischemic leg, relatively little of the lactic acid and the CO_2 released from HCO_3^- buffering of new lactic acid produced in the muscle is readily seen in the lung gas exchange. Thus, $\Delta\dot{V}CO_2/\Delta WR$ may, like $\Delta\dot{V}O_2/\Delta WR$, be relatively shallow. When the lactic acidosis is evident in the central circulation, breathing is further stimulated. If the patient also has lung disease, dyspnea may be an important symptom.

With peripheral arterial disease, the maximum $\dot{V}O_2$ and the lactic acidosis threshold are reduced, although the latter may not be detectable because lactate may enter the central circulation very slowly as a result of reduced muscle perfusion. Thus, the lactic acidosis of the ischemic muscles may not always be obvious from gas exchange.

Patients with peripheral arterial disease have systemic arterial hypertension at the low work rates. The heart rate at maximum exercise is usually relatively low because the patient stops exercise from claudication at a work rate too low to provide maximal heart rate stimulation.

HEART DISEASES

Because gas transport is the major and most immediate role of the cardiovascular system, cardiac dysfunction of all five primary types of heart disease (i.e., rate response, coronary artery, cardiomyopathic, valvular, and congenital defects) will cause changes in the pattern of $\dot{V}O_2$, $\dot{V}CO_2$, and heart rate responses to exercise. Before discussing each major class of heart disease, it is noteworthy to consider features in common with all forms of heart disease.

In nearly all heart defects (heart block excepted), the increase in heart rate (HR) as a function of $\dot{V}O_2$ is steeper than normal. This reflects the increased dependence on heart rate and arteriovenous O_2 extraction to increase the O_2 transport needed to perform exercise. Although the heart rate–$\dot{V}O_2$ relationship is usually relatively steep in heart disease because stroke volume is reduced, exceptions occur when the heart rate response to exercise may be inappropriately low. These include patients taking

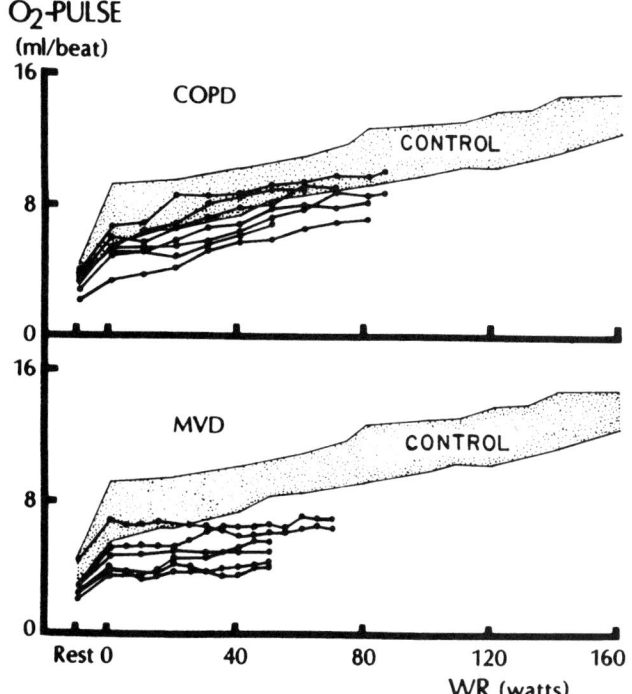

O_2-PULSE (ml/beat)

COPD

CONTROL

MVD

CONTROL

Rest 0   40   80   120   160

WR (watts)

FIGURE 5.3. O_2-pulse response to incremental exercise in patients with chronic obstructive pulmonary disease (COPD) **(upper panel)** and mitral valve disease (MVD) **(lower panel)** compared with the range of values of a control group (*stippled area*). (Modified from Nery LE, Wasserman K, French W, et al. Contrasting cardiovascular and respiratory responses to exercise in mitral valve and chronic obstructive pulmonary diseases. *Chest* 1983;83:446–453.)

β-adrenergic blocking drugs, some patients with cardiomyopathies whose sinoatrial node fails to respond appropriately for the low stroke volume, and patients with heart block.

Because of the relatively low cardiac output response, mixed venous oxygen reaches its lowest value, and the arterial–mixed venous oxygen difference $[C(a - \bar{v})O_2]$ its highest value, at a low work rate (11). Consequently, the O_2 pulse $[C(a - \bar{v})O_2 \times SV]$ reaches a constant value that is abnormally low and occurs at an unusually low work rate compared to normal (Fig. 5.3). The increase in $\dot{V}O_2$ as WR increases commonly becomes smaller near the maximum work rate (see Fig. 4.5C), reflecting an increased contribution of energy from anaerobic metabolism, presumably because of impaired O_2 transport (12) or utilization (13).

A number of studies have shown that patients with chronic left ventricular failure develop mismatching of ventilation relative to pulmonary perfusion, particularly of the high $\dot{V}A/\dot{Q}$ type. This results in an increased VD/VT and a further increase in the breathing requirement to maintain blood pH homeostasis (14–18). The need to maintain pH ho-

meostasis in the presence of the increase in VD/VT is the major factor, along with the increase in $\dot{V}CO_2$ in response to developing lactic acidosis, accounting for the increased ventilatory response to exercise (18), and likely contributes to the symptom of dyspnea in patients with chronic left heart failure.

Patients with heart diseases may develop metabolic acidosis at low work rates (2,19–21); this may become chronic and evident at rest. If accompanied by a low $PaCO_2$ (22), it would necessitate a higher minute ventilation for a given $\dot{V}CO_2$ (see the section "Ventilatory Coupling to Metabolism" in Chapter 2).

Constant work rate tests may be helpful for evaluating the cardiovascular response to specific levels of exercise in heart diseases. If the work rate is above the lactic acidosis threshold, $\dot{V}O_2$ will not reach a steady-state by 3 minutes. The magnitude of the increase in $\dot{V}O_2$ between 3 and 6 minutes $[\Delta \dot{V}O_2 (6 - 3)]$ is correlated to the exercise lactic acidosis (see Fig. 4.25).

Coronary Artery Disease

Although mild coronary artery disease may be difficult to detect, simultaneous gas exchange measurements with the electrocardiogram (ECG) may improve the diagnostic capabilities of an exercise stress test (Table 5.4). Coronary artery disease will usually cause the peak $\dot{V}O_2$ to be reduced. Patients with coronary artery disease may or may not experience chest pain. When the exercise-induced increase in myocardial oxygen requirement is not met by the myocardial oxygen supply, myocardial ischemia may result in ST segment and T wave changes in the ECG, and ventricular ectopic beats may develop with increasing frequency as the work rate is increased. Also, characteristic gas exchange abnormalities may develop during exercise when myocardial ischemia develops.

TABLE 5.4. Discriminating Gas Exchange Measurements During Exercise in Coronary Artery Disease

$\Delta\dot{V}O_2/\Delta WR$ normal at low work rates, but may change to more shallow slope above *AT*

Reduced maximal O_2 pulse

Heart rate–$\dot{V}O_2$ relationship is nonlinear, becoming abnormally steep as peak $\dot{V}O_2$ is approached

High breathing reserve

Metabolic acidosis at end exercise

Occasional immediate postexercise increase in O_2 pulse

$\Delta\dot{V}O_2/\Delta WR$, increase in $\dot{V}O_2$ relative to increase in work rate; *AT*, anaerobic threshold.

The $\Delta\dot{V}O_2/\Delta WR$ ratio is normal at low work rates of an incremental exercise test, but may abruptly decrease when myocardial ischemia prevents the myocardium from contracting with the synchrony required to maintain stroke volume. The ECG usually becomes abnormal, whether or not angina develops, when $\Delta\dot{V}O_2/\Delta WR$ decreases (23,24). Despite a decrease in $\Delta\dot{V}O_2/\Delta WR$ with myocardial ischemia, $\dot{V}CO_2$ continues to increase steeply, creating a large disparity between the increase in $\dot{V}CO_2$ and $\dot{V}O_2$. With myocardial ischemia, heart rate as a function of $\dot{V}O_2$ usually becomes steeper, developing a curvilinear relationship rather than continuing the linear relationship.

The O_2 pulse fails to increase to its normal predicted value when myocardial ischemia develops, or it may remain constant (see Cases 16 to 22 in Chapter 10). This is likely due to a decrease in stroke volume secondary to asynchronous contraction of the left ventricular wall in the region of ischemia. The reduced stroke volume may be compensated for by an increase in $C(a - \bar{v})O_2$, thereby maintaining the O_2 pulse during submaximal work.

In normal persons, the O_2 pulse decreases immediately after exercise. However, a paradoxical increase in O_2 pulse commonly occurs in patients who develop myocardial ischemia or heart failure in response to exercise. This paradoxical increase in O_2 pulse may be due to an immediate increase in stroke volume in these patients because of the abrupt decrease in left ventricular afterload when exercise stops (25).

Metabolic acidosis usually develops because of impaired O_2 transport resulting from the failure to increase cardiac output commensurate with the increasing work rate when a significant portion of the left ventricle stops contracting normally. How much metabolic acidosis develops depends on the number of minutes the subject exercises after myocardial ischemia develops and the level of exercise performed.

In patients with coronary artery disease, the breathing reserve is normal or high because the subject is forced to stop exercise from symptoms at a relatively low metabolic rate. The ventilatory equivalents are normal, manifesting relatively uniform ventilation–perfusion relationships in contrast to those observed in patients with chronic stable heart failure.

Myopathic Heart Disease

Because patients with cardiomyopathies have difficulty in transporting oxygen to the skeletal muscles

TABLE 5.5. Discriminating Gas Exchange Measurements During Exercise in Chronic Heart Failure

$\dot{V}O_2$ increase with WR may *gradually* slow near peak $\dot{V}O_2$
Reduced peak $\dot{V}O_2$
Reduced *AT*
Reduced maximal O_2 pulse
Steep HR–$\dot{V}O_2$ relationship with low maximal HR
Possible development of oscillatory breathing and gas exchange pattern of 45- to 90-second periods at low WR; oscillatory pattern is less evident as peak WR is reached
O_2 pulse increases paradoxically immediately postexercise
Slow $\dot{V}O_2$ kinetics and high $\Delta\dot{V}O_2$ (6 − 3) above *AT* during constant work rate test
Increased VD/VT, $\dot{V}E/\dot{V}CO_2$ @*AT*, and slope of $\dot{V}E$ vs. $\dot{V}CO_2$ are related to degree of severity

AT, anaerobic threshold; HR, heart rate; $\Delta\dot{V}O_2$ (6 − 3), difference between $\dot{V}O_2$ at 6 and 3 minutes during constant work rate exercise; VD/VT, physiological dead space/tidal volume ratio; $\dot{V}E$, minute ventilation; $\dot{V}E/\dot{V}CO_2$ @*AT*, ventilatory equivalent for CO_2 at the *AT*.

during exercise, the increase in $\dot{V}O_2$ relative to the increase in work rate is commonly slower than normal (Table 5.5). This slowing, however, is not abrupt, in contrast to the slowing of $\dot{V}O_2$ increase relative to work rate seen in patients who develop acute myocardial ischemia during exercise. The failure to transport O_2 at the rate needed to regenerate the *ATP* used for muscular contraction makes it impossible to sustain muscular contraction; consequently, the muscles fatigue and the subject must stop.

The peak $\dot{V}O_2$ is reduced consequent to the reduced peak cardiac output response to exercise. The *AT* is also commonly reduced (26,27). The peak O_2 pulse is low because of the reduced stroke volume. The heart rate increase is commonly steep relative to the increase in $\dot{V}O_2$. The maximal heart rate may be reduced in patients with heart failure because the cardiomyopathy is accompanied by chronotropic incompetence, or because the subject stops exercise early because of fatigue, or because of iatrogenic β-adrenogenic blockade.

Because of the relatively low cardiac output response to exercise, mixed venous oxygen reaches its lowest value, and $C(a - \bar{v})O_2$ reaches its highest value, at a low work rate (11). Consequently, the O_2 pulse [$(C(a - \bar{v})O_2) \times SV$] reaches a constant value that is low and that occurs at an unusually low work rate compared with normal (Fig. 5.3). As described earlier, $\Delta\dot{V}O_2/\Delta WR$ is often reduced as the maximum work rate is approached. This can be viewed as a reflection of an increased contribution of energy from anaerobic metabolism, presumably because of impaired O_2 transport (12) or utilization (28).

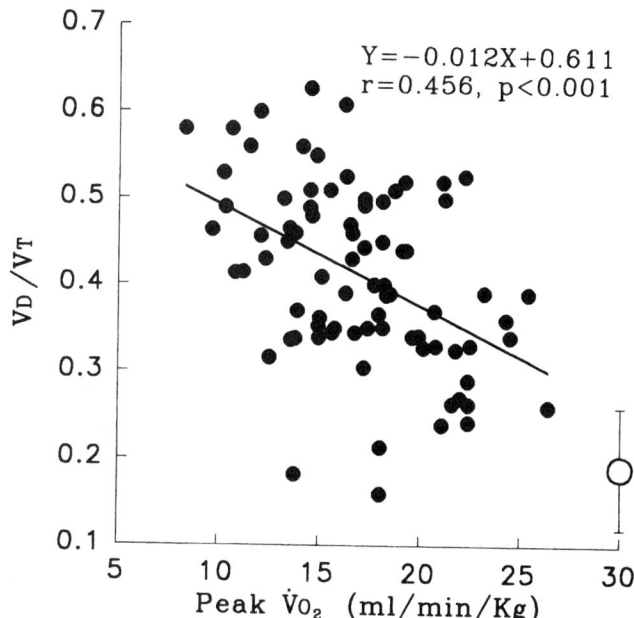

FIGURE 5.4. Ratio of physiological dead space to tidal volume (V_D/V_T) as a function of peak $\dot{V}O_2$ on a cycle ergometer in 78 patients with chronic stable heart failure. The open circle on the right is the mean V_D/V_T ± standard deviation for normal subjects. (From Wasserman K, Zhang YY, Gitt A, et al. Lung function and exercise gas exchange in chronic heart failure. *Am J Respir Crit Care Med* 1997;96:2221–2227, with permission.)

Patients with heart failure have a high ventilatory requirement relative to the metabolic rate of the subject (15,26,29,30). In fact, the ventilatory requirement relative to CO_2 output has been used as a prognosticator of survival (29,30). Three factors contribute to this high ventilatory requirement. Most important, patients with chronic heart failure develop mismatching of ventilation relative to pulmonary perfusion, particularly of the high $\dot{V}A/\dot{Q}$ type, resulting in an increased V_D/V_T. The latter correlates with the degree of functional impairment in exercise performance (Fig. 5.4). This reduced gas exchange efficiency is a major factor accounting for the increased ventilatory drive in heart failure. Second, a metabolic acidosis occurs at lower work rates in patients with heart failure compared with normal (2,20,21); this may become chronic and be evident at rest and be accompanied by a low $PaCO_2$ (22). A low $PaCO_2$ set point will necessitate a high minute ventilation that becomes more marked with exercise (31). Finally, the increase in CO_2 produced at low work rates, because of the buffering of lactic acid by HCO_3^-, increases the acid load to the ventilatory system. All three factors dictate a larger breathing requirement to maintain arterial H^+ homeostasis in response to exercise (18), and likely

contribute to the symptom of dyspnea in patients with chronic heart failure.

A regular oscillatory pattern of breathing in which $\dot{V}O_2$, $\dot{V}CO_2$, $\dot{V}E$, and related variables increase and decrease with a period of approximately 45 to 90 seconds is observed in some patients with chronic heart failure. This oscillatory pattern in gas exchange is more marked at lower work rates and tends to diminish as the subject nears the maximum work rate. During this oscillatory breathing, $\dot{V}O_2$ changes before $\dot{V}CO_2$ and particularly $\dot{V}E$ and is of greater magnitude (32); it is likely that flow through the pulmonary circulation is oscillating. This could account for oscillatory changes in arterial blood gases and pH that, in turn, oscillate ventilation.

These changes in pulmonary blood flow likely reflect the behavior of the failing heart. Cardiac output will change rhythmically in response to the regular rhythmic changes in systemic arterial resistance originating from the vasomotor center (Traube-Hering waves). This behavior contrasts with that of the normal heart, in which the forward output adjusts to changes in the venous return (preload), and is less dependent on changes in systemic arterial resistance (afterload) than someone with a failing heart.

Valvular Heart Disease

Because the stroke volume is reduced in patients with valvular heart disease, the increase in $\dot{V}O_2$ relative to increase in work rate is usually reduced (i.e., low $\Delta\dot{V}O_2/\Delta WR$)(Table 5.6). Both the AT and the peak $\dot{V}O_2$ are reduced. The O_2 pulse is reduced and reaches a plateau value at a relatively low work rate (Fig. 5.3). Heart rate increases steeply relative to $\dot{V}O_2$, with the maximal heart rate achieved at a relatively low work rate. As with other cardiac conditions that lead to heart failure, $\dot{V}O_2$ kinetics are slow.

TABLE 5.6. Discriminating Gas Exchange Measurements in Valvular Heart Disease

$\Delta\dot{V}O/\Delta WR$ commonly low
Low peak $\dot{V}O_2$
Low AT
Low and unchanging O_2 pulse
Steep linear increase in HR–$\dot{V}O_2$ relationship
Slow $\dot{V}O_2$ kinetics and high $\Delta\dot{V}O_2$ (6 − 3) at relatively low constant work rate test

See Table 5.5 for a definition of symbols.

Congenital Heart Disease

Constant work rate tests are of particular value in patients with congenital heart disease (Table 5.7). Because the increases in $\dot{V}_{O_2}$ and $\dot{V}_{CO_2}$ are determined by the increase in flow of O_2-desaturated, CO_2-rich blood through the pulmonary circulation, the pattern of increase in blood flow through the lungs can be measured from the O_2 uptake and CO_2 output kinetics. Thus, patients with pulmonary outflow obstruction (33) or patients with an increase in right-to-left shunt may fail to demonstrate a normal increase in blood flow at the start of exercise, resulting in a reduced or absent phase I increase in $\dot{V}_{O_2}$ and $\dot{V}_{CO_2}$ (34). Phase II kinetics are also inappropriately slow, and the magnitude of phase II becomes a relatively large portion of the total O_2 requirement at low work rates (35). A slowly rising $\dot{V}_{O_2}$ is also evident at relatively low work rates during phase III. Thus, $\Delta\dot{V}_{O_2}$ between 3 and 6 minutes of exercise is increased, indicating that lactate is increasing in response to the exercise. As in other cardiovascular disorders, the peak $\dot{V}_{O_2}$ and AT are reduced.

A markedly elevated ventilatory response is noted at the start of exercise in patients with cyanotic congenital heart disease (36). In this disorder, the blood flowing through the lungs is hyperventilated to compensate for the blood that bypasses the lungs and enters the left side of the circulation through the right-to-left shunt. Hyperventilation of the blood passing through the lungs results in an immediate decrease in P_{ETCO_2}, an increase in P_{ETO_2}, an increase in the respiratory exchange ratio (R), and usually an increase in $\dot{V}_E/\dot{V}_{O_2}$ and $\dot{V}_E/\dot{V}_{CO_2}$ at the start of exercise; this decrease is sustained until the start of recovery. Pa_{CO_2} and pH remain relatively unchanged in patients with a right-to-left shunt, whereas the Pa_{O_2} decreases (36). The relatively unchanged acid–base status suggests that the respiratory control mechanism is sensitive to the regulation of arterial [H⁺] and is not greatly influenced by the high pulmonary artery pressures in this population of patients. In congenital heart diseases accompanied by a left-to-right shunt—for example, a patent ductus arteriosis (Case 34 in Chapter 10)—or in dialysis patients with an a-v fistula, peak $\dot{V}_{O_2}$ and AT are reduced because of the diversion of a sizable part of the cardiac output through the low-resistance shunt (Table 5.7).

PULMONARY VASCULAR DISEASES
Causes of Increased Ventilation

Diseases of the pulmonary circulation, such as pulmonary emboli, idiopathic pulmonary fibrosis, and idiopathic pulmonary vasculopathy (primary pulmonary hypertension), are accompanied by reduced perfusion to ventilated alveoli, particularly during exercise (Table 5.8). Consequently, alveoli with nonoccluded capillaries must accept a greater than normal perfusion and must be ventilated to a proportionately greater degree than normal to remove the metabolic CO_2 and to maintain Pa_{CO_2}, Pa_{O_2}, and pH at appropriate levels. The overventilation of the poorly perfused alveoli is wasted (alveolar dead space). Because of the increase in physio-

---

TABLE 5.7.   Discriminating Gas Exchange Measurements During Exercise in Congenital Heart Disease

Right-to-left shunt
  Low peak $\dot{V}_{O_2}$
  Low *AT*
  Increased $\dot{V}_E/\dot{V}_{CO_2}$ *@AT*
  Phase I $\dot{V}_{O_2}$ reduced when accompanied by increased pulmonary vascular or valvular resistance
  Slow $\dot{V}_{O_2}$ kinetics and high $\Delta\dot{V}_{O_2}$ (6 − 3) during constant work rate test
  Immediate hyperpnea and decrease in P_{ETCO_2} in cyanotic type; magnitude of increase in $\dot{V}_E$ and decrease in P_{ETCO_2} related to size of right-to-left shunt
  Worsening arterial hypoxemia with exercise
Left-to-right shunt
  Low peak $\dot{V}_{O_2}$
  Low *AT*
  Normal $\dot{V}_E/\dot{V}_{CO_2}$ *@AT*
  Normal arterial oxygenation during exercise

AT, anaerobic threshold; $\dot{V}_E/\dot{V}_{CO_2}$ *@AT*, ventilatory equivalent for CO_2 at anaerobic threshold; $\Delta\dot{V}_{O_2}$ (6 − 3), difference between $\dot{V}_{O_2}$ at 6 and 3 minutes during constant work rate exercise; $\dot{V}_E$, minute ventilation.

TABLE 5.8.   Gas Exchange Abnormalities During Exercise in Diseases of the Pulmonary Circulation

High $\dot{V}_E$ at submaximal work rates
High V_D/V_T
Positive $P(a − ET)_{CO_2}$ during exercise
Pa_{O_2} decreases as WR is increased
$P(A − a)_{O_2}$ increases with increasing WR
Low peak $\dot{V}_{O_2}$
Low *AT*
$\Delta\dot{V}_{O_2}/\Delta$WR more shallow toward maximum WR
Low O_2 pulse

$\dot{V}_E$, minute ventilation; V_D/V_T, physiologic dead space/tidal volume ratio; $P(a − ET)_{CO_2}$, arterial–end tidal P_{CO_2} difference; $P(A − a)_{O_2}$, alveolar–arterial P_{O_2} difference; $\Delta\dot{V}_{O_2}/\Delta$WR, increase in $\dot{V}_{O_2}$ relative to increase in work rate.

logical dead space ventilation, minute ventilation is increased in patients with pulmonary vascular diseases at rest and to a greater degree during exercise. The increased dead space ventilation results in a high V_D/V_T and a persistently positive $P(a - ET)CO_2$ during exercise. If a right-to-left shunt develops during exercise, V_D/V_T and $P(a - ET)CO_2$ will increase further as the size of the shunt increases.

An additional cause of increased ventilatory drive during exercise in patients with pulmonary vascular occlusive disease is arterial hypoxemia, which gets worse during exercise. The decrease in PaO_2 stimulates the carotid bodies, the chemoreceptors that stimulate ventilation in the presence of arterial hypoxemia (37).

Causes of Exercise Arterial Hypoxemia

PaO_2 may be near normal at rest but there may be striking arterial oxyhemoglobin desaturation during exercise. Several mechanisms may play a role. First, the time available for diffusion equilibrium of O_2, already shortened at rest by the reduced size of the functional capillary bed, is further shortened by the exercise-induced increase in pulmonary blood flow. In the normal capillary bed, the red cell residence time is about 0.8 second at rest (38). Despite increasing cardiac output as much as fourfold at maximal exercise in the fit normal subject, the red cell residence time is still above 0.3 second (the time required for O_2 equilibration between capillary and alveolar space in a normal lung unit) because of recruitment of pulmonary capillaries (approximately doubling the resting capillary blood volume). However, in the presence of pulmonary vascular occlusive disease, the functional capillary bed is destroyed and the capillary bed reserved for recruitment to perform exercise is already recruited at rest. These phenomena necessarily result in shortened transit times in the pulmonary capillaries during exercise. Consequently, the desaturated red cell arriving from the systemic venous circulation cannot remain in the reduced pulmonary capillary bed long enough for diffusion equilibrium of O_2 between the alveolar gas and red cell to occur, especially if pulmonary capillary blood velocity has increased in response to exercise. This pathophysiological state is a common cause of worsening arterial hypoxemia as VO_2 increases during exercise in patients with pulmonary vascular occlusive disease.

Another cause of hypoxemia during exercise in patients with increased pulmonary vascular resistance is the development of a right-to-left shunt resulting from the opening of a potentially patent foramen ovale. Approximately 35% of the normal population is thought to have an "unsealed" foramen ovale. In the healthy subject, this is of no importance because left atrial pressure is normally higher than right atrial pressure and blood does not shunt in either direction. However, if pulmonary vascular resistance is increased so that the right ventricle cannot pump the venous return into the pulmonary circulation as fast as it is delivered (right ventricular failure), right ventricular end-diastolic pressure and, therefore, right atrial pressure will increase. If the right atrial pressure exceeds that of the left atrium, some of the right atrial flow will pass through the unsealed foramen ovale, creating a right-to-left shunt. This can cause marked exercise hypoxemia and be only evident during exercise (39). The development of a right-to-left shunt can easily be identified by the abrupt increase in $PETO_2$, abrupt decrease in $PETCO_2$, and a sustained increase in R to a value of approximately 1.0, often accompanied by increases in VE/VO_2 and VE/VCO_2 at the start of exercise. Repeating the exercise test while the subject breathes 100% oxygen clearly confirms and quantifies a right-to-left shunt. If the shunt develops, the arterial PO_2 should decrease well below that predicted during O_2 breathing (>550 mm Hg). The PaO_2 will decrease approximately 100 mm Hg for every 3% to 5% of cardiac output passing through the right-to-left shunt.

While arterial hypoxemia from low-VA/Q lung units is common in acute pulmonary embolism, low-VA/Q lung units are a less important cause of arterial hypoxemia in patients with chronic pulmonary vascular occlusive disease. High-VA/Q lung units predominate in chronic pulmonary vascular occlusive disease in patients without airway disease.

Effect on Systemic Hemodynamics

Pulmonary vascular occlusive disease causes a hemodynamic stenosis in the central circulation, making it difficult for the right ventricle to deliver blood to the left atrium at a rate sufficient to meet the increased cardiac output needed for exercise. Because the cardiac output increase in response to exercise is reduced, the *AT* and peak VO_2 and O_2 pulse are reduced in patients with pulmonary vascular disease, similar to that seen in patients with left heart failure. In both conditions, the V_D/V_T and VE/VCO_2 at the *AT* and the VE versus VCO_2 slope are increased. However, the arterial oxyhemoglobin desaturation helps distinguish the pathophysiology of pulmonary vascular occlusive disease from chronic left ventricular failure. Oxygenation is normal in patients with left ventricular failure, but usually decreased in patients with pulmonary vascular occlusive disease. As described earlier, because the capillary blood volume is reduced in the latter condition, the transit time of red cells through the pulmonary capillary bed is abnormally rapid, shortening the time available for O_2 to equilibrate between the alveolar gas and the red cell; shunting through a patent foramen ovale may also occur. In contrast, in left ventricular failure, the circulation of blood through the lung is slower than normal, allowing increased time for diffusion equilibrium of O_2 between the alveolus and red cell.

Because the heart commonly enlarges in patients with left ventricular failure, the vital capacity tends to be reduced more than with pulmonary vascular diseases. Thus, a lesser decline in vital capacity and worsened arterial oxygenation can differentiate primary pulmonary vascular occlusive disease from left ventricular failure in patients with steep ventilatory responses to exercise.

VENTILATORY DISORDERS

Obstructive Lung Diseases

Patients with chronic obstructive pulmonary diseases (COPD), including emphysema, chronic bronchitis, bronchial asthma, and mixtures of these disease entities, are usually limited during exercise by dyspnea or fatigue (Table 5.9). Dyspnea generally results from difficulty in achieving the ventilation and possibly, the O_2 cost of ventilation needed to eliminate the additional CO_2 generated during exercise at the level of Pa_{CO_2} regulated by the patient (the patient's P_{CO_2} set point) (Table 5.10). Also, many of these patients are

TABLE 5.9. Discriminating Measurements During Exercise in Patients with Obstructive Lung Disease

Low peak $\dot{V}_{O_2}$
Low breathing reserve
High heart rate reserve
High V_D/V_T
Increased $P(a - _{ET})_{CO_2}$ during exercise
Usually high $P(_A - a)_{O_2}$
Increased O_2 cost of work
Failure to develop respiratory compensation for exercise metabolic acidosis
Decreased IC with exercise (air trapping)
Abnormal expiratory flow pattern

V_D/V_T, physiological dead space/tidal volume ratio; $P(a - _{ET})_{CO_2}$, arterial–end tidal P_{CO_2} difference; $P(_A - a)_{O_2}$, alveolar–arterial P_{O_2} difference; IC, inspiratory capacity.

highly sedentary and develop a lactic acidosis at a relatively low work rate. The added CO_2 load resulting from the HCO_3^- buffering of lactic acid and the H^+ provide additional chemical stimuli to an inefficient gas-exchanging lung.

Ventilatory Capacity–Ventilatory Requirement Imbalance

Figure 5.5 conceptualizes the pathophysiologic features leading to dyspnea in patients with COPD. The two major contributing factors are the decreased ventilatory capacity and the increased ventilatory requirement. In emphysema, the decreased ventilatory capacity is due to increased airflow obstruction combined with reduced lung elastic recoil, whereas in chronic bronchitis and asthma, the decreased ventilatory capacity is due to increased airway resistance.

The increased ventilatory requirement in patients with COPD is primarily due to inefficient ventilation of the lungs consequent to the mismatching of ven-

TABLE 5.10. Effect of Airway Obstruction Due to Emphysema on Average Blood Lactate Concentration, Minute Ventilation, and Work Rate at an O_2 Consumption of Approximately 1.0 L/min

FEV_1 (L)	$\dot{V}_{O_2}$ (L/min, STPD)	WR (watts)	$\dot{V}_E$ (L/min, BTPS)	$\dot{V}_E/\dot{V}_{O_2}$	La⁻ (mmol/L)	La⁻/$\dot{V}_{O_2}$
1.02	0.90	35	35	39	3.03	3.37[a]
1.80	1.05	34	36	34	2.95	2.80[b]
Normal	~1.0	50	25	25	<1.0	1.0[c]

[a]Mean data from Cooper CB, Daly JA, Burns MR, et al. Lactic acidosis contributes to the production of dyspnea in chronic obstructive pulmonary disease. *Am Rev Respir Dis* 1991;143:A80.
[b]Mean data from Casaburi R, Patessio A, Ioli F, et al. Reductions in exercise lactic acidosis and ventilation as a result of exercise training in patients with obstructive lung disease. *Am Rev Respir Dis* 1991;143:9–18.
[c]Mean data from Chapter 2.
FEV_1, forced expiratory volume in 1 second; WR, work rate; $\dot{V}_E$, minute ventilation; La⁻, blood lactate concentration; STPD, standard temperature and pressure, dry; BTPS = body temperature, ambient pressure, saturated.

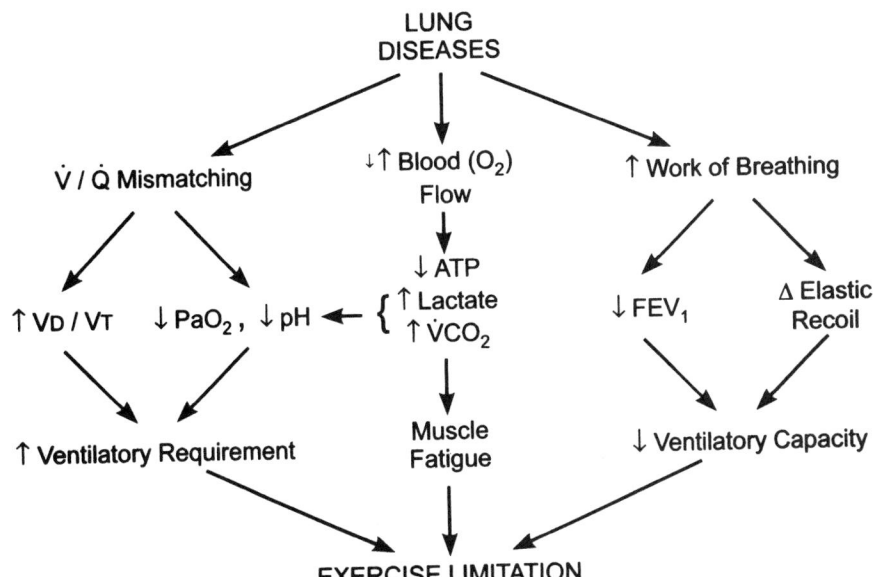

FIGURE 5.5. Factors that play a role in exercise limitation and dyspnea in patients with chronic obstructive pulmonary disease (COPD). These patients have both an increase in ventilatory requirement to perform exercise and a reduction in ventilatory capacity. See text for a detailed discussion of each of the factors shown. $\dot{V}/\dot{Q}$, ventilation-perfusion ratio; V_D/V_T, dead space-to-tidal volume ratio.

tilation to perfusion; that is, certain regions of the lungs are hypoventilated, whereas others are hyperventilated. This has the effect of increasing the fraction of the breath that is wasted (increased V_D/V_T), thereby requiring an increased ventilation to eliminate the CO_2 produced by the patient to maintain the arterial P_{CO_2} at its set point (see Fig. 2.38).

As shown in Figure 5.6, ambulatory patients with stable obstructive lung disease regulate Pa_{CO_2} at a reasonably constant level despite increasing work rates. However, ventilatory compensation for the exercise-induced lactic acidosis rarely occurs in these patients (see Fig. 4.20B and cases of patients with COPD in Chapter 10). With severe airway obstruction, Pa_{CO_2} often increases during exercise because of the increased work of breathing, thereby worsening the exercise acidosis (22). Hypoxemia results from the underventilation of perfused lung units. Despite increasing ventilatory drive through the carotid body chemoreceptors (37), the hypoxic stimulus is insufficient to induce a respiratory alkalosis in patients with COPD. Although regulation of Pa_{O_2} is less precise than Pa_{CO_2} in these patients (Fig. 5.7), Pa_{O_2} usually does not fall to extremely low levels, even at the patient's maximum work rate.

The $P(A - a)O_2$ is usually increased as a consequence of the perfusion of relatively poorly ventilated airspaces. The increase in $P(A - a)O_2$ is usually not systematic with increasing work rate, in contrast to patients with primary pulmonary vascular diseases or pulmonary fibrosis. $P(a - ET)CO_2$ is also increased, reflecting overventilation relative to perfusion. Thus, $P(a - ET)CO_2$ remains relatively constant and elevated as work rate is increased, rather than decreasing and becoming negative as in normal subjects (see Chapter 7).

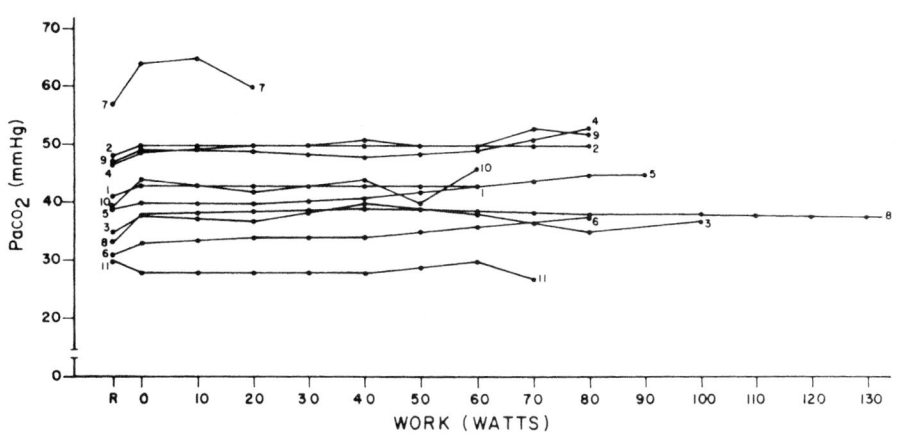

FIGURE 5.6. Pa_{CO_2} as related to work rate in 11 patients with stable chronic airflow obstruction (each point is a different work rate). The numbers on each curve identify the patient.

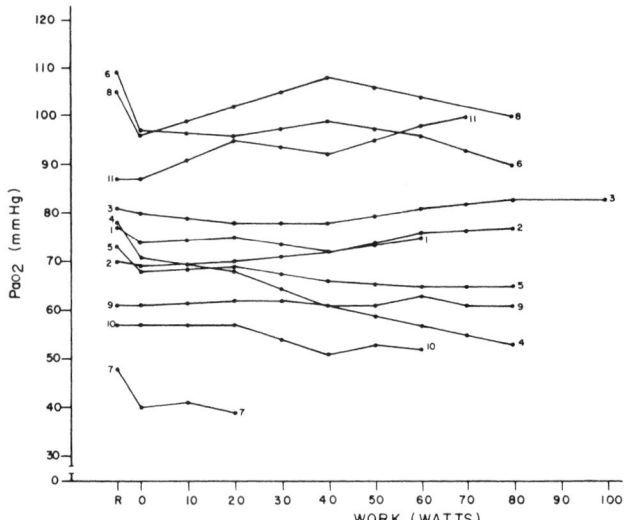

FIGURE 5.7. PaO_2 as related to increase in work rate for the same 11 patients shown in Figure 5.6 (each point is a different work rate). The numbers on each curve identify the patient and allow cross-correlation with each patient's $PaCO_2$, shown in Figure 5.6.

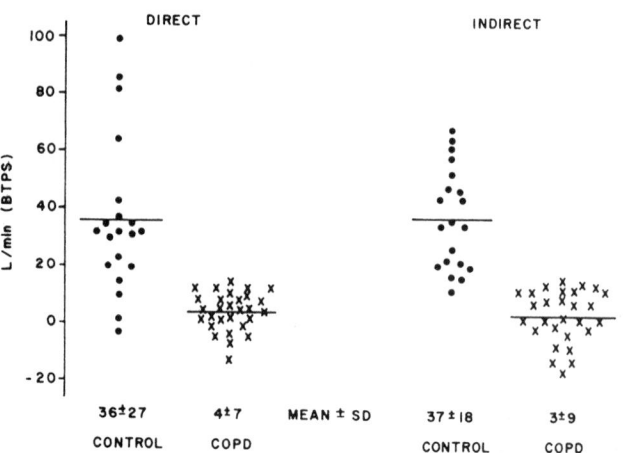

FIGURE 5.8.   Breathing reserve (MVV − max $\dot{V}E$) for a group of normal subjects and a group of patients with stable chronic obstructive pulmonary disease (COPD). The values under each column show the mean ± standard deviation. Measurements are made using the directly measured MVV and the indirectly measured MVV calculated by multiplying FEV_1 by 40. Note that the breathing reserve in patients with COPD is small and the standard deviation is narrow, reflecting the importance of airflow limitation in determining exercise intolerance.

Although one may predict that the O_2 cost of breathing will be increased in patients with COPD, this has been difficult to demonstrate. That these patients do have an increased metabolic cost becomes evident, however, when one examines the external work that can be performed for a given $\dot{V}O_2$ (Table 5.10). We found that the work output was reduced at a $\dot{V}O_2$ of 1 L/min in two studies of patients with COPD. Moreover, patients with COPD may develop a lactic acidosis at a relatively low work rate (40,41). This is most likely due to the sedentary lifestyle of these patients. After training these patients, the lactate level for a given work rate and the ventilatory requirement for exercise decreased (40).

Dyspnea depends on a balance between how much air *must* be breathed to keep pace with metabolism and how much *can* be breathed. Patients with COPD, because of their increase in VD/VT, low work rate lactic acidosis, and hypoxemia, must breathe more to maintain blood gases and pH, but their peak ventilation is less than normal. Although many approaches have been taken to determine if patients with COPD are ventilatory limited, the breathing reserve has served this role very well. The maximal voluntary ventilation (MVV) measured at rest is a reasonable measure of the patient's ventilatory capacity. Work tasks requiring ventilation rates in excess of this value cannot be sustained. Thus, the breathing reserve, defined as the difference between the MVV and $\dot{V}E$ at the maximum level of exercise that the subject could perform, is decreased to values close to zero in patients with

COPD (Fig. 5.8). This contrasts with the large ventilatory reserve at the end of exercise found in most normal subjects (42–44) and, particularly, in patients with heart disease.

Examining the expiratory flow pattern can be useful in documenting airflow limitation. Typically, as shown in Figure 4.14, the pattern has an early expiratory peak and then a sustained expiratory flow until the point of inhalation, giving a trapezoidal appearance to the recorded pattern. No apneic pause occurs at the end of exhalation, in contrast to the finding in normal subjects when work rate is not excessively high. After effective bronchodilatation, the expiratory flow pattern normalizes, with the peak flow moving to the middle of the expiratory phase of respiration (see Fig. 4.14).

When patients develop air trapping with exercise, the FRC increases, as evidenced by a reduction in the inspiratory capacity (Table 5.9). The inspiratory capacity can be measured during exercise by instructing the patient to take a maximum breath after a normal exhalation. This can be done without difficulty after a little practice in patients with obstructive lung disease and normal subjects. In contrast to the decrease in inspiratory capacity in patients with airflow obstruction, normal subjects have an increase in inspiratory capacity, suggesting that their FRC had decreased during exercise.

Whereas the peak $\dot{V}O_2$ is reduced in patients with uncomplicated obstructive lung disease, the $\dot{V}O_2$ usually does not decrease its rate of rise as work rate is increased in response to a progressively increasing work rate test, in contrast to this frequent finding in patients with circulatory limitation. This is because ambulatory patients with stable obstructive lung disease are usually more limited in their ability to eliminate CO_2 (ventilatory limitation) than in their ability to make O_2 available to the mitochondria.

Often, patients with COPD develop a lactic acidosis at relatively low work rates because of their relatively untrained state (Table 5.10). Other patients with very severe airflow obstruction may not be able to exercise sufficiently to reach their AT and develop a lactic acidosis during exercise. Those patients who develop a significant lactic acidosis at a relatively low work rate should benefit most from skeletal muscle training, because they have the potential to decrease the lactic acidosis stimulus to ventilatory drive.

The heart rate at maximum work rate is generally low (high heart rate reserve) (Fig. 5.9), but maximum heart rate can be increased if the patient's maximum work rate can be improved through O_2 breathing or bronchodilatation. In contrast to car-

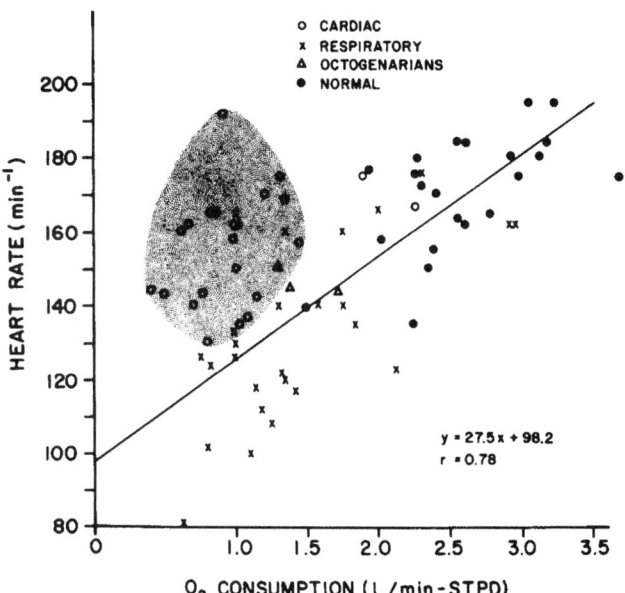

FIGURE 5.9.   Heart rate at maximal exercise for normal subjects, octogenarians, and patients with chronic respiratory disease or cardiac disease. The normal subjects reach a higher maximum heart rate and $\dot{V}O_2$. Note that the octogenarians fall on the same slope as the younger normal subjects, although their maximum heart rate and maximum oxygen uptake are less. Similarly, the patients with respiratory defects have a still lower maximum oxygen uptake and heart rate. The cardiac patients (*stippled area*) have a higher maximum heart rate relative to the maximum O_2 uptake than that of the other subjects. (From Wasserman K, Whipp BJ. Exercise physiology in health and disease (state of the art). *Am Rev Respir Dis* 1975;112: 219–249, with permission.)

diac disorders, O_2 pulse continues to increase normally with increasing work rate, although the final absolute values are usually reduced at peak exercise (Fig. 5.3).

Oxygen Transport–Oxygen Requirement Imbalance

To sustain exercise, *ATP* must be regenerated aerobically. Failure of the left ventricular output to meet the muscle O_2 demand for *ATP* regeneration at the rate required for the increasing work rate will force the patient to stop exercise due to muscular fatigue. An imbalance between the circulatory transport of O_2 to muscles and its requirement will be reflected in a decreased peak $\dot{V}O_2$ and AT and a reduced rate of increase in $\dot{V}O_2$ as work rate increases. The following mechanisms underlie the failure of left ventricular output to keep pace with the increased O_2 requirement of a progressively increasing work rate test in patients with COPD:

1. *Positive intrathoracic pressure.* Large positive pressures develop in the chest during exhalation in patients with poor lung elastic recoil and hyperinflation (patients with emphysema). Thus, right atrial filling and stroke volume will not be able to increase normally during exercise, as expiratory muscles contract to accelerate exhaling respired gases (partial Valsalva maneuver). This process becomes more marked as breathing rate increases to maintain arterial blood gas homeostasis. This impediment to venous return to the heart probably accounts for the relatively low cardiac outputs and stroke volumes observed in emphysema patients during exercise.

2. *Increased pulmonary vascular resistance.* Increased pulmonary vascular resistance might also cause left ventricular output to be inadequate to meet the increased O_2 needed for aerobic regeneration of *ATP* during exercise. Many patients with emphysema have significantly elevated pulmonary vascular resistance that, although not limiting at rest, might prevent the right ventricle from increasing blood flow through the pulmonary circulation at the rate needed to meet the muscle O_2 requirement during exercise.

3. *Coexistent factors, such as primary heart disease and reduced arterial oxygen content.* Patients with lung diseases might also have primary heart disease that limits the ability of the circulation to increase O_2 transport at the rate needed to perform exer-

cise. Other mechanisms that contribute to the impairment of O_2 flow to the muscles, such as reduced arterial O_2 content due to reduced PaO_2, anemia, and carboxyhemoglobinemia, when combined with the pathophysiology of COPD, might cause severe symptoms in patients with only moderate or even mild disease.

Physiological Markers of Inadequate Oxygen Transport

Although respiratory mechanics are significantly impaired in patients with COPD, it is imperative to evaluate exercise gas exchange in these patients in order to determine if reduced O_2 transport is caused by impaired ventilatory mechanics or by metabolic changes with increased ventilatory drive characteristic of heart failure. The increased ventilatory drive in these patients results from the increased H^+ accompanying the increased lactate as well as the CO_2 released by the increased rate of buffering lactic acid. Thus, in the presence of reduced O_2 transport, the AT and $\Delta\dot{V}O_2/\Delta WR$ as well as the peak $\dot{V}O_2$ are likely to be reduced. $\Delta\dot{V}O_2/\Delta WR$ will be below the expected rate of 10 ml/min/W.

TABLE 5.11. Discriminating Measurements During Exercise in Patients with Restrictive Lung Diseases

Low peak $\dot{V}O_2$
High V_T/IC
Breathing frequency >50 at max WR
Low breathing reserve
High V_D/V_T
High $P(a - ET)CO_2$
High $\dot{V}E/\dot{V}CO_2$ @AT
PaO_2 decreases and $P(A - a)O_2$ increases as WR is increased
$\Delta\dot{V}O_2/\Delta WR$ is reduced

IC, inspiratory capacity; WR, work rate; $P(a - ET)CO_2$, arterial–end tidal PCO_2 difference; $\dot{V}E/\dot{V}CO_2$ @AT, ventilatory equivalent for CO_2 at anaerobic threshold; $P(A - a)O_2$, alveolar–arterial PO_2 difference; $\Delta\dot{V}O_2/\Delta WR$, increase in $\dot{V}O_2$ relative to increase in work rate.

Restrictive Lung Diseases

Patients with pulmonary fibrosis generally are exercise limited because of dyspnea or fatigue or both (Table 5.11). Study of the pathophysiology of these patients reveals that they have disturbed lung mechanics and a reduction in the functional pulmonary capillary bed (Fig. 5.10). Hansen and Wasserman (45), in a study of a population of patients with interstitial lung diseases of mixed etiology, found

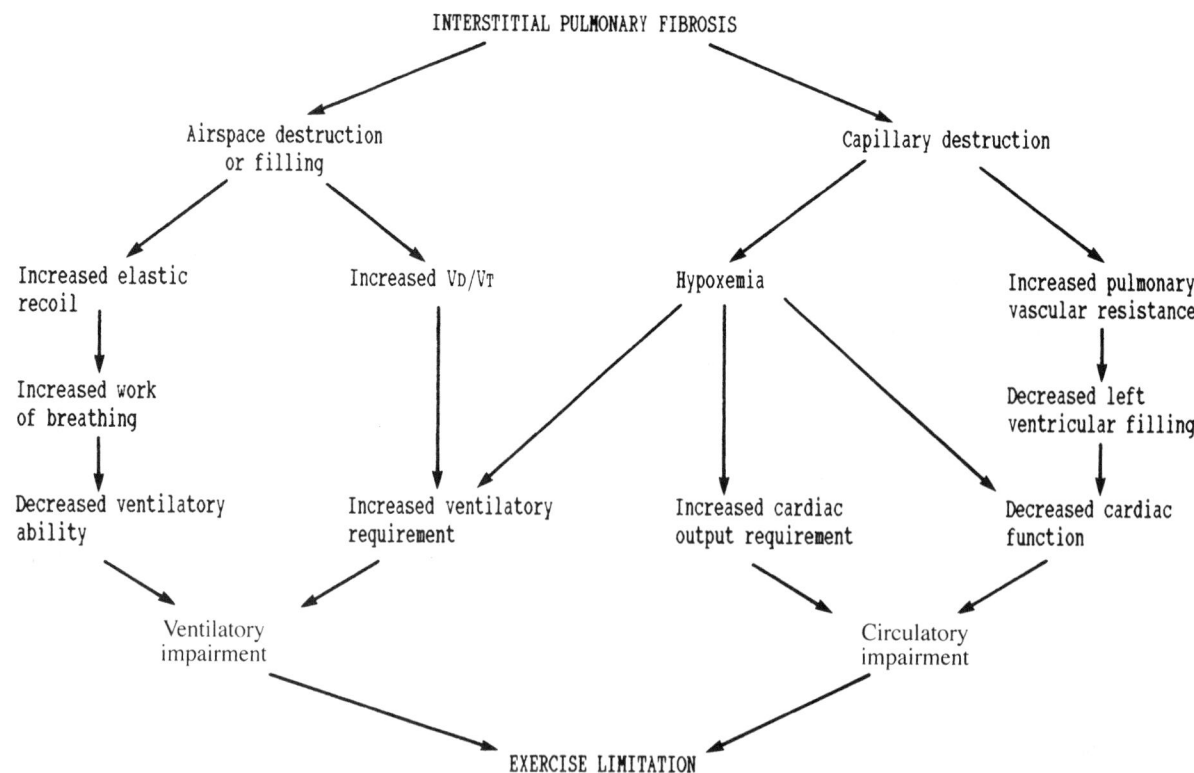

FIGURE 5.10. Pathophysiology of exercise limitation in patients with interstitial lung disease and idiopathic pulmonary fibrosis. (From Hansen JE, Wasserman K. Pathophysiology of activity limitation in patients with interstitial lung disease. *Chest* 1996;109:1566–1576, with permission.)

that most of the patients were limited by their inability to increase pulmonary blood flow adequately in response to exercise (Fig. 5.10, right pathway leading to exercise limitation). Not only did their patients have a reduced peak $\dot{V}O_2$, but also the *AT* was usually reduced. In contrast to COPD patients, $\Delta\dot{V}O_2/\Delta WR$ was reduced, with the slope of the relation becoming more shallow as peak $\dot{V}O_2$ was approached.

Pulmonary fibrosis of the idiopathic type (IPF) develops from chronic lung inflammation (46). The pathologic features are usually nonuniform, so some acini, including their blood supply, are completely replaced by scar tissue. In contrast, neighboring units that are less involved or uninvolved may undergo compensatory hyperinflation. From the point of view of lung mechanics, the net effect of the pathophysiology of IPF is a reduction in the total number of functioning acini and, consequently, a relatively poorly compliant, small lung (47). Whereas both the total lung capacity and its subcompartments are reduced, the predominant reduction is that of the inspiratory capacity. Thus, the extent to which the tidal volume can increase with exercise is limited, and the patient must increase breathing frequency to a value higher than normal to meet the ventilatory requirement for exercise. Consequently, the V_T/IC ratio is high and approaches 1, and the breathing frequency at maximum exercise often exceeds 50 breaths per minute, considerably higher than in patients with COPD. Ventilation at the maximum work rate may approach the MVV if the patient is not limited by inability to increase cardiac output earlier because of the restricted pulmonary capillary bed. However, often the pathophysiological picture is mixed, reflecting both a failure to increase $\dot{V}O_2$ appropriate for the work rate performed and an increased ventilatory response due to exercise lactic acidosis, hypoxemia, and ventilation–perfusion mismatching (increased V_D/V_T).

Early in the pathophysiologic development of interstitial lung diseases, it appears as though the pulmonary capillary bed is functionally reduced and normal recruitment of more capillary bed in response to exercise fails to occur. This restricted capillary bed results in a shortened red cell transit time in the pulmonary capillaries as the exercise work rate is increased. The progressive reduction of the red cell residence time in the pulmonary capillary as work rate and cardiac output increase results in a systematic decrease in PaO_2 as $\dot{V}O_2$ increases, similar to that seen in pulmonary vascular occlusive dis-

ease. This systematic decrease in PaO_2 is usually not seen if pulmonary blood flow ($\dot{V}O_2$) fails to increase and in COPD (Fig. 5.6). Low $\dot{V}A/\dot{Q}$ ratios might also contribute to the hypoxemia in patients with pulmonary fibrosis (46). The ventilatory response of patients with pulmonary fibrosis is steep, partly because of a reduced $PaCO_2$ set point in some subjects, but mainly because of an increased V_D/V_T in all subjects. Worsening hypoxemia as work rate is increased, elevated dead space ventilation caused by nonuniform ventilation–perfusion ratios, increased lactic acidosis from impaired systemic CO_2 transport, and a reduced ability to expand the lungs leading to rapid, shallow breathing contribute to dyspnea in these patients (Fig. 5.10). In addition, exercise fatigue might be brought about by the inability to provide O_2 to the muscles at a rate sufficient for the exercise work rate to be performed aerobically.

Pulmonary alveolar proteinosis is a good example of exercise hypoxemia that is primarily due to a diffusion defect (48). This disease results in alveolar filling by a semisolid proteinaceous material. Pulmonary fibrosis is minimal or nonexistent. Frequently, the vital capacity and total lung capacity are only slightly reduced, and FEV_1 is normal. Because the mean path length from lung gas to lung capillaries is increased considerably in this disorder by a medium unfavorable for O_2 diffusion, this diffusion barrier limits the mass flow of O_2 into the pulmonary capillaries. During exercise, when red cell transit time in the capillary bed is reduced and its residence time shortened, less time is available for diffusion equilibrium. Thus, the major findings in this disorder are a systematic decrease in PaO_2 and an increase in $P(A - a)O_2$ with increasing work rate (49).

Chest Wall (Respiratory Pump) Disorders

Disorders of the respiratory pump include muscle weakness, chest deformities, rigidity of the thoracic cage (as in ankylosing spondylitis), muscle and motor nerve disorders, and extreme obesity. Patients with these disorders, like those with restrictive pulmonary disorders, have a limited ability to increase V_T (Table 5.12). Although their lungs are essentially normal, the maximal intrapleural pressure available to expand the lungs is insufficient to allow V_T to increase normally as work rate is increased. Therefore, to obtain the increase in $\dot{V}E$ required for exercise, these patients must predominantly increase breathing frequency.

TABLE 5.12. Discriminating Measurements During Exercise in Patients with Chest Wall Disorders

Low peak $\dot{V}O_2$
High VT/IC
High breathing frequency
Low breathing reserve
High heart rate reserve

VT, tidal volume; IC, inspiratory capacity.

The reduced maximum $\dot{V}O_2$ defines the degree of exercise limitation. The $\dot{V}O_2$ increases normally with increasing work rate. Because the lung parenchyma is essentially normal, PaO_2 is usually normal and does not decrease as the work rate is increased. The breathing reserve is low when symptom-limited exercise is reached (usually due to dyspnea). Because of the impaired ventilatory mechanics, these patients usually do not develop normal ventilatory compensation for the lactic acidosis of exercise. Heart rate reserve is high at the maximal exercise tolerated because the cardiovascular system is not fully stressed due to the breathing limitation.

DEFECTS IN HEMOGLOBIN CONTENT AND QUALITY

As shown in Figure 1.3, a considerable increase in O_2 flow from the atmosphere to the mitochondria is essential for the normal exercise response. This function is critically dependent on the ability of the circulation to transport O_2 from the lungs to the exercising muscles. Therefore, it is appropriate to consider how changes in the properties of blood might impair O_2 delivery to the mitochondria and thereby reduce exercise capacity (Table 5.13).

TABLE 5.13. Discriminating Measurements During Exercise in Patients with Anemia, Increased Carboxyhemoglobin, or Hemoglobinopathies

Low peak $\dot{V}O_2$
Low *AT*
Low O_2 pulse
Normal VD/VT, P(a − ET)CO_2, and P(A − a)O_2
Tachycardia and relatively high cardiac output

AT, anaerobic threshold; VD/VT, physiological dead space/tidal volume ratio; P(a − ET)CO_2, arterial–end tidal PCO_2 difference; P(A − a)O_2, alveolar–arterial PO_2 difference.

Because cardiac output and heart rate during exercise are determined by the O_2 requirement, patients with a reduced blood O_2 carrying capacity commonly have a relatively high cardiac output and heart rate for a given work rate (i.e., a relative tachycardia). The stroke volume is normal or even increased, in contrast to patients with cardiac diseases and disorders of the pulmonary circulation. Because the arterial O_2 content is low, the potential for the arterial–venous O_2 difference to increase in response to exercise is reduced. Consequently, the maximum O_2 pulse [product of stroke volume and $C(a − \bar{v})O_2$] is reduced in patients with reduced arterial O_2 content. As in other disorders of reduced maximal O_2 flow, the maximum $\dot{V}O_2$ and *AT* are also reduced. Table 9.2 describes the reduction in maximal $C(a − \bar{v})O_2$ as related to reduced hemoglobin concentration. From this and peak $\dot{V}O_2$, the cardiac output and stroke volume can be estimated at peak exercise. Specific mechanisms of reduced arterial O_2 content are described in the following sections.

Anemia

Because anemia results in a reduced blood O_2 carrying capacity, it compromises O_2 delivery to the mitochondria (Fig. 5.1). With anemia, the systemic capillary PO_2 falls more rapidly than normal during the transit of blood from artery to vein (see Fig. 2.14). Thus, the diffusion gradient of O_2 from the blood to the mitochondria decreases more rapidly than in non-anemic conditions. Consequently, a critically low capillary PO_2 may be reached at a lower $\dot{V}O_2$ than normal, necessitating anaerobic mechanisms for *ATP* generation, with increasing lactate concentrations and metabolic acidosis (see Fig. 2.1).

Subjects with anemia commonly experience breathlessness with increased ventilatory drive during exercise. Whereas the arterial O_2 content is low, the arterial PO_2 is not reduced. Because the carotid bodies respond to arterial PO_2 and not O_2 content, the reduced O_2 content is not itself the cause of the increased ventilatory drive and therefore cannot account for the symptom of breathlessness. More likely, the breathlessness and increased ventilatory drive with exercise in the more anemic patient are due to the metabolic acidosis that accompanies the patient's low anaerobic threshold. The acidemia results in an increased ventilatory drive (mediated by the carotid bodies) and a relatively high minute ventilation at a low maximum work rate.

Left-Shifted Oxyhemoglobin Dissociation Curve

Conditions that cause a leftward shift in the oxyhemoglobin dissociation curve (reduced P_{50}), such as some hemoglobinopathies, a decrease in 2,3-DPG due to a defect in red cell metabolism, an increase in carboxyhemoglobin, or increased glycosylated hemoglobin found in poorly controlled diabetic patients, should cause the capillary blood P_{O_2} to decrease more rapidly than normal for a given O_2 extraction across the circulation (50). Thus, at a reduced work rate, the P_{O_2} difference between capillary and mitochondrion may reach a critical value, below which it cannot fall despite an increased bioenergetic demand for O_2. Consequently, O_2 flow through the exercising muscle does not provide all the O_2 needed by the mitochondria to support *ATP* regeneration aerobically. Thus, anaerobic regeneration of *ATP* is needed to support the energy requirement at a relatively low work rate. Exercise studies on patients with a left-shifted hemoglobinopathy support the concept that these disorders lead to anaerobic glycolysis and increased net lactate production at reduced work rates (51).

Carboxyhemoglobinemia and Cigarette Smoking

Carboxyhemoglobinemia from exposure to carbon monoxide results in a reduced O_2 carrying capacity without the reduced blood viscosity found in anemia. When the carboxyhemoglobin level is increased, arterial oxygen content is reduced. In addition, carbon monoxide causes a leftward shift in the oxyhemoglobin dissociation curve. This reduces the peak $\dot{V}_{O_2}$ and *AT* (52–54).

Cigarette smoking adversely affects exercise tolerance by its effects on the blood, the cardiovascular system, and the lungs. Heart rate, blood pressure, and the double product (heart rate times systolic blood pressure) are increased when one performs exercise immediately after smoking (52). Ventilation–perfusion relations become abnormal, as evident from the increased $P(a - ET)_{CO_2}$ during exercise. Short-term cigarette smoking did not have an immediate effect on airway resistance in normal young male subjects. However, it did cause acute cardiovascular changes and changes consistent with worsened $\dot{V}_A/\dot{Q}$ matching immediately after cigarette smoking (52).

CHRONIC METABOLIC ACIDOSIS

Chronic metabolic acidosis, with a reduced blood $[HCO_3^-]$, can result from poorly controlled diabetes, chronic renal failure, renal tubular acidosis, or from certain drugs, such as a carbonic anhydrase inhibitor (acetazolamide) used in the treatment of glaucoma (Table 5.14). To restore normal arterial blood and central chemoreceptor pH, ventilation is stimulated by H^+ until arterial P_{CO_2} is reduced to a new lower P_{CO_2} set point, bringing pH close to 7.4 (31,55). The magnitude of the increase in ventilation is approximately proportional to the reduction in $[HCO_3^-]$ and Pa_{CO_2}.

However, during exercise, to maintain the lower Pa_{CO_2}, the $\dot{V}_{CO_2}$ and ventilation must increase hyperbolically (see Fig. 2.42). The higher the work rate is, the higher the additional ventilation. The higher ventilatory requirement needed to maintain the arterial pH when $[HCO_3^-]$ is reduced leads to an apparent increase in "sensitivity" of the respiratory control mechanisms.

The presence of a chronic metabolic acidosis before exercise begins is evident from the resting arterial blood gases. The $[HCO_3^-]$ and Pa_{CO_2} are reduced, and pH is only slightly reduced or normal. During exercise, $\dot{V}_E$ increases proportionally with the increase in CO_2 production (Fig. 2.43). Because the slope of the $\dot{V}_E$–$\dot{V}_{CO_2}$ relation is steeper the lower the Pa_{CO_2}, the effect of the metabolic acidosis is to amplify the ventilatory response as work rate is increased (see Fig. 4.16). Without measuring arterial blood gases, a relatively steep slope relationship between $\dot{V}_E$ and $\dot{V}_{CO}$ during exercise, with R in the normal range, signifies either chronic hyperventilation or increased V_D/V_T. Arterial blood gas and pH measurements differentiate these two potential causes of a high ventilatory response.

By itself, chronic metabolic acidosis is not a prominent cause of dyspnea, but in conjunction

TABLE 5.14. Discriminating Measurements During Exercise in Patients with a Chronic Metabolic Acidosis

---

Low $[HCO_3^-]$
Steep $\dot{V}_E/\dot{V}_{CO_2}$ relation
Normal $P(A - a)_{O_2}$ and $P(a - ET)_{CO_2}$
Normal V_D/V_T
Low breathing reserve

$P(A - a)_{O_2}$, alveolar–arterial P_{O_2} difference; $P(a - ET)_{CO_2}$, arterial–end tidal P_{CO_2} difference; V_D/V_T, physiological dead space/tidal volume ratio.

with other diseases such as obstructive airways disease, it may lower the CO_2 set point to such a marked degree that the ventilatory requirement to perform a given work rate may exceed the subject's MVV. In this case, the sensation of dyspnea would be high. Correction of the metabolic acidosis might reduce the ventilatory requirement below the subject's MVV and relieve the sensation of dyspnea.

MUSCLE DISORDERS AND ENDOCRINE ABNORMALITIES

Little information is available concerning the metabolic cost of exercise in patients with primary muscle disorders. Because of reduced motor efficiency, patients with neuromuscular disorders with accompanying spasticities and motor incoordination presumably have an increased O_2 requirement for performing physical work. We have not had the opportunity to evaluate many of these patients in the exercise laboratory.

Certain muscle enzyme deficiencies limit exercise performance. For example, patients with inability to use muscle glycogen because of myophosphorylase deficiency (McArdle's syndrome) (56) or other disease of the glycolytic pathway (57) are unable to exercise to work levels that normally require anaerobic mechanisms to supplement the energy generated by aerobic mechanisms. These patients experience severe muscle pain and the release of myoglobin and creatine kinase from muscle when attempting to exercise at levels that normally induce a lactic acidosis. The $\dot{V}O_2$–work rate relationship (work efficiency) appears to be normal for work rates below the level that induces pain in these patients (58). The maximum work capacity of these patients is limited to work rates near the anaerobic threshold of normal sedentary subjects. Thus, their peak $\dot{V}O_2$ is on the order of 1 L/min. Their ventilatory response to exercise is generally normal (59), although it has also been reported to be high (60). The heart rate and cardiac output responses of these patients are inordinately high for the metabolic rate, and the arterial–venous O_2 difference at maximal work rate is low (61), due to the failure to extract O_2 normally secondary to the failure of muscles to produce lactic acid. The reduced production of H^+ ions does not allow the full rightward shift in the oxyhemoglobin dissociation curve and normal O_2 unloading from hemoglobin (Bohr effect) in the capillary bed. The Bohr effect is needed for the normal maximal O_2 extraction from blood during exercise (62).

Patients with mitochondrial electron transport chain defects develop lactic acidosis at exceptionally low work rates (63,64). In contrast with myophosphorylase-deficient patients, however, the gas exchange abnormalities accompanying these metabolic defects have not been well studied. Nevertheless, it is recognized that the gas exchange abnormalities likely differ from those seen with defects in the glycolytic pathway and resemble those found in patients with heart failure, demonstrating increased CO_2 output relative to O_2 uptake (63).

Diabetes mellitus affects large arteries (atherosclerosis), small blood vessels, and capillaries. When the disease is poorly controlled, diabetic patients also have a leftward shift in the oxyhemoglobin dissociation curve (glycosylated hemoglobin). Any one of these abnormalities could cause a reduction in AT and peak $\dot{V}O_2$ (65). Studies in diabetic children suggest that the AT and peak $\dot{V}O_2$ are reduced even when the patient's diabetes is under good control (66–68).

Poorly regulated diabetic patients increase their use of fatty acids for energy. During exercise, use of fatty acids by muscle, in contrast to the normally preferred carbohydrate, should make the poorly controlled patient require slightly more O_2 for the same energy production. Figure 2.3 illustrates the effect of the proportion of carbohydrate to fatty acid substrate on metabolic efficiency with respect to O_2 consumption and energy yield.

The ventilatory response to exercise has been demonstrated to be increased and the $PaCO_2$ reduced in women during the progestational phase of the menstrual cycle. The effect of this increased ventilatory drive on maximal exercise performance in women is unknown.

PSYCHOGENIC CAUSES OF EXERCISE LIMITATION AND DYSPNEA

Anxiety Reactions

Anxiety reactions occasionally cause dyspnea during exercise. One manifestation of anxiety is intense hyperventilation with development of acute respiratory alkalosis. The hyperventilation pattern is unique in that the breathing frequency is quite regular. In addition, the tachypnea starts abruptly, as though switched on, rather than gradually, as is normally seen during progressive exercise. Hyperventilation might actually start at rest, in anticipation of the exercise. Psychogenic dyspnea might also be evident as rapid and unusually shallow breathing.

Another manifestation of an anxiety reaction described as shortness of breath may, in fact, be irregular breathing or breath holding. Observing the behavior pattern and the patient's facial expression may be helpful in detecting this problem.

Poor Effort and Manipulated Exercise Performance

It is important to distinguish manipulated exercise performance for secondary gain from other disorders. An exercise test in which both heart rate reserve (see panel 2, Fig. 4.30) and breathing reserve (see panel 7, Fig. 4.30) are high and the *AT* is not reached (see panel 5, Fig. 4.30) strongly suggests poor effort. However, inadequate effort may also be evident when the *AT* is normal, accompanied by a high heart rate reserve and breathing reserve without the normal increase in R expected during a progressively increasing work rate test (panel 8, Fig. 4.30).

A chaotic breathing pattern, evident in panel 7 of the nine-panel graphical array, supports manipulation of the exercise test. Normally, ventilation, tidal volume, and breathing frequency increase in a distinct systematic pattern. A chaotic breathing pattern and psychogenic dyspnea are most readily diagnosed during exercise when gas exchange is monitored breath by breath.

Before stating that a claimant for disability is not impaired on a pulmonary basis, it is often necessary to sample arterial blood sequentially for measurement of lactate increase, as well as to confirm a normal $P(A - a)O_2$, $P(a - ET)CO_2$, and V_D/V_T during exercise. Also, arterial blood gas and pH measurements are needed to document whether they change in response to exercise as would be expected in a normal person, a person with disease, or a person who is manipulating ventilation. Variable and inconsistent changes in breath-by-breath measurements of P_{ETCO_2} and P_{ETO_2} provide evidence for manipulated exercise performance (see panel 9, Fig. 4.30).

Combinations of Defects

A patient's symptoms may be more marked than predicted from the nonexercise assessment of the severity of the patient's disease. This might be noted particularly when the primary disease is combined with a complicating problem, for example, cigarette smoking or use of a drug that affects ventilatory drive directly or indirectly through a metabolite (e.g., H^+). Thus, patients with coronary artery disease who have hypertension or who smoke might be less symptomatic and have improved exercise tolerance if their blood pressure were under adequate control or if they did not smoke. Patients with chronic airflow obstruction may be more symptomatic if they also have chronic metabolic acidosis or are obese. Because coronary artery disease and chronic airflow obstruction are so common, both defects may be present in the same patient and may therefore make the patient's symptoms more pronounced than if the two diseases did not coexist. When more than one disease is present that can cause the same symptom(s) during exercise, a cardiopulmonary exercise test is probably the best way to identify which disease is the primary contributor to the patient's symptoms, as well as to provide a noninvasive, relatively inexpensive method to assess the efficacy of therapy.

SUMMARY

The major function of the cardiovascular and ventilatory systems is gas exchange between the cells and the atmosphere. Therefore, impairments in cardiovascular and respiratory function are most apparent during exercise because cell respiration is stimulated and defects are amplified. Because each component of the gas transport system that couples external to internal respiration has a different role, the pattern of the gas exchange abnormality differs according to the pathophysiology. Recognition of these differences allows the examiner to distinguish which organ system in the patient most likely accounts for his or her exercise limitation. Thus, whereas primary heart disease and primary lung disease both cause a reduction in work capacity, the pattern of the gas exchange responses differs. By making measurements that address the gas transport function at each site in the coupling of external to cellular respiration, it is possible to deduce the physiological state of each component.

References

1. Hansen JE, Sue DY, Wasserman K. Predicted values for clinical exercise testing. *Am Rev Respir Dis* 1984; 129(Suppl):S49–S55.

2. Wasserman K, Whipp BJ. Exercise physiology in health and disease (state of the art). *Am Rev Respir Dis* 1975; 112:219–249.

3. Alexander JK, Amad KH, Colebatch HJH. Observations on some clinical features of extreme obesity, with particular reference to circulatory effect. *Am J Med* 1962;32:512–524.

4. Bates DV, Macklem PT, Christie RJ. *Respiratory function in disease*. Vol. 2. Philadelphia: W.B. Saunders, 1971:100–101.

5. Cherniack RM. Respiratory effects of obesity. *Can Med Assoc J* 1959;80:613–616.

6. Gilbert R, Sipple JH, Auchincloss JH. Respiratory control and work or breathing in obese subjects. *J Appl Physiol* 1961;16:21–26.

7. Sharp JG, Henry JP, Sweany SK, Meadows WR, Pietras RJ. The total work of breathing in normal and obese men. *J Clin Invest* 1964;43:728–739.

8. Ray CS, Sue DY, Bray G, Hansen JE, Wasserman K. Effects of obesity on respiratory function. *Am Rev Respir Dis* 1983;128:501–506.

9. Buskirk E, Taylor HL. Maximal oxygen intake and its relation to body composition, with special reference to chronic physical activity and obesity. *J Appl Physiol* 1957;11:72–78.

10. Bylund-Fellenius AC, Walker PM, Elander A, Holm S, Holm J, Schersten T. Energy metabolism in relation to oxygen, partial pressure in human skeletal muscle during exercise. *Biochem J* 1981;200:247–255.

11. Weber KT, Janicki JS. *Cardiopulmonary exercise testing: physiological principles and clinical applications*. Philadelphia: W.B. Saunders, 1986:238–243.

12. Wasserman K, Stringer W. Critical capillary P_{O_2}, net lactate production, and oxyhemoglobin dissociation: effects on exercise gas exchange. In: Wasserman K, ed. *Exercise gas exchange in heart disease*. Armonk, NY: Futura Publishing, 1996:157–181.

13. Sullivan MJ, Duscha B, Slentz AC. Peripheral determinants of exercise intolerance in patients with chronic heart failure. In: Wasserman K, ed. *Exercise gas exchange in heart disease*. Armonk, NY: Futura Publishing, 1996:209–227.

14. Kobayashi T, Itoh H, Kato K. The role of increased dead space in the augmented ventilation of cardiac patients. In: Wasserman K, ed. *Exercise gas exchange in heart disease*. Armonk, NY: Futura Publishing, 1996: 145–156.

15. Metra M, Raccagni D, Carini G, Orzan F, Papa A, Nodari S, Cody RJ, Dejours P. Ventilatory and arterial blood gas changes during exercise in heart failure. In: Wasserman K, ed. *Exercise gas exchange in heart disease*. Armonk, NY: Futura Publishing, 1996:125–143.

16. Rubin SA, Brown HV. Ventilation and gas exchange during exercise in severe chronic heart failure. *Am Rev Respir Dis* 1984;129(Suppl):S63–S64.

17. Sullivan MJ, Higginbotham MB, Cobb FR. Increased exercise ventilation in patients with chronic heart failure: intact ventilatory control despite hemodynamic and pulmonary abnormalities. *Circulation* 1988;77: 552–559.

18. Wasserman K, Zhang YY, Gitt A, Belardinelli R, Koike A, Lubarsky L, Agostoni PG. Lung function and exercise gas exchange in chronic heart failure. *Circulation* 1997;96:2221–2227.

19. Kitzman DW, Higginbotham MB, Cobb FR, Sheikh KH, Sullivan MJ. Exercise intolerance in patients with heart failure and preserved left ventricular systolic function: failure of the Frank-Starling mechanism. *J Am Coll Cardiol* 1991;17:1065–1072.

20. Sullivan MJ, Cobb FR. Relation between central and peripheral hemodynamics during exercise in patients with chronic heart failure. *Circulation* 1989;80:769–781.

21. Wilson JR, Martin JL, Schwartz D, Ferraro N. Exercise intolerance in patients with chronic heart failure: role of impaired nutritive flow to skeletal muscle. *Circulation* 1984;69:1079–1087.

22. Nery LE, Wasserman K, French W, Oren A, Davis JA. Contrasting cardiovascular and respiratory responses to exercise in mitral valve and chronic obstructive pulmonary diseases. *Chest* 1983;83:446–453.

23. Itoh H, Tajima A, Koike A, Osada N, Maeda T, Kato M, Omiya K, Fu LT, Watanabe H, Kato K. Oxygen uptake abnormalities during exercise in coronary artery disease. In: Wasserman K, ed. *Cardiopulmonary exercise testing and cardiovascular health*. Armonk, NY: Futura Publishing, 2002:165–172.

24. Belardinelli R, Lacalaprice F, Carle F, Minnucci A, Cianci G, Perna G, D'Eusanio G. Exercise-induced myocardial ischaemia detected by cardiopulmonary exercise testing. *Eur Heart J* 2003;24:1304–1313.

25. Koike A, Itoh H, Doi M, Taniguichi K, Marumo F, Umehara I, Hiroe M. Beat-to-beat evaluation of cardiac function during recovery from upright bicycle exercise in patients with coronary artery disease. *Am Heart J* 1990;120:316–323.

26. Gitt AK, Wasserman K, Kilkowski C, Kleemann T, Kilkowski A, Bangert M, Schneider S, Schwarz A, Senges J. Exercise anaerobic threshold and ventilatory efficiency identify heart failure patients for high risk of early death. *Circulation* 2002;106:3079–3084.

27. Weber KT. Cardiopulmonary exercise testing and the evaluation of systolic dysfunction. In: Wasserman K, ed. *Exercise gas exchange in heart disease*. Armonk, NY: Futura Publishing, 1996:55–62.

28. Sullivan MJ, Green HJ, Cobb FR. Altered skeletal muscle metabolic response to exercise in chronic heart failure: relation to skeletal muscle aerobic enzyme activity. *Circulation* 1991;84:1597–1607.

29. Chua TP, Ponikowski P, Harrington D, Anker SD, Webb-Peploe K, Clark AL, Poole-Wilson PA, Coats AJ.

Clinical correlates and prognostic significance of the ventilatory response to exercise in chronic heart failure. *J Am Coll Cardiol* 1997;29:1585–1590.

30. Kleber FX, Vietzke G, Wernecke KD, Bauer U, Opitz C, Wensel R, Sperfeld A, Glaser S. Impairment of ventilatory efficiency in heart failure: prognostic impact. *Circulation* 2000;101:2803–2809.

31. Oren A, Wasserman K, Davis JA, Whipp BJ. Effect of CO_2 set point on ventilatory response to exercise. *J Appl Physiol* 1981;51:185–189.

32. Ben-Dov I, Sietsema K, Casaburi R, Wasserman K. Evidence that circulatory oscillations accompany ventilatory oscillations during exercise in patients with heart failure. *Am Rev Respir Dis* 1992;145:776–781.

33. Sietsema K. Oxygen uptake kinetics during exercise in patients with pulmonary vascular disease. *Am Rev Respir Dis* 1992;145:1052–1057.

34. Sietsema KE, Cooper DM, Rosove MH, Perloff JK, Child JS, Canobbio MM, Whipp BJ, Wasserman K. Dynamics of oxygen uptake during exercise in adults with cyanotic congenital heart disease. *Circulation* 1986;73:1137–1144.

35. Wasserman K. New concepts in assessing cardiovascular function. The Dickinson W. Richards Lecture. *Circulation* 1988;78:1060–1071.

36. Sietsema KE, Cooper DM, Perloff SK, Child JS, Rosove MH, Wasserman K, Whipp BJ. Control of ventilation during exercise in patients with central venous-to-systemic arterial shunts. *J Appl Physiol* 1988; 64:234–242.

37. Comroe JH. *Handbook of physiology. Section 3: Respiration.* Washington DC: American Physiological Society, 1964:557–583.

38. Comroe JH Jr, Forster RE II, Dubois MD, Briscoe WA, Carlsen E. Diffusion. In: *The lung: clinical physiology and pulmonary function test.* Chicago: Year Book, 1962: 125–133.

39. Sun X-G, Hansen JE, Oudiz R, Wasserman K. Gas exchange detection of exercise-induced right-to-left shunt in patients with primary pulmonary hypertension. *Circulation* 2002;105:54–60.

40. Casaburi R, Patessio A, Ioli F, Zanaboni S, Donner C, Wasserman K. Reductions in exercise lactic acidosis and ventilation as a result of exercise training in patients with obstructive lung disease. *Am Rev Respir Dis* 1991;143:9–18.

41. Cooper CB, Daly JA, Burns MR, et al. Lactic acidosis contributes to the production of dyspnea in chronic obstructive pulmonary disease. *Am Rev Respir Dis* 1991;143:A80.

42. Bye PTP, Farkas GA, Roussos CH. Respiratory factors limiting exercise. *Am Rev Physiol* 1983;45:439–451.

43. Pierce AK, Luterman D, Loundermilk J, Blomquist G, Johnson RL, Jr. Exercise ventilatory patterns in normal subjects and patients with airway obstruction. *J Appl Physiol* 1968;25:249–254.

44. Wasserman K, Brown HV. Exercise performance in chronic obstructive pulmonary diseases. *Med Clin North Am* 1981;65:525–547.

45. Hansen JE, Wasserman K. Pathophysiology of activity limitation in patients with interstitial lung disease. *Chest* 1996;109:1566–1576.

46. Fulmer JD. An introduction to the interstitial lung diseases. *Clin Chest Med* 1982;3:457–473.

47. Keogh BA, Lakatos E, Price D, Crystal RG. Importance of the lower respiratory tract in oxygen transfer. *Am Rev Respir Dis* 1984;129(Suppl):S76–S80.

48. Wagner PD, Dantzker DR, Dueck R, de Polo JR. Distribution of ventilation-perfusion ratios in patients with interstitial lung disease. *Chest* 1976;69:256–257.

49. Wasserman K, Mason GR. Pulmonary alveolar proteinosis. In: Murray JF, Nadel JA, eds. *Textbook of respiratory medicine.* Philadelphia: W.B. Saunders, 1988: 1535–1548.

50. Bunn HF, Forget BG. *Hemoglobin: molecular, genetic and clinical aspects.* Philadelphia: W.B. Saunders, 1986: 595–616.

51. Butler WM, Spratling LS, Kark JA, Shoomaker EB. Hemoglobin Osler: report of a new family with exercise studies before and after phlebotomy. *Am J Hematol* 1982;13:293–301.

52. Hirsch GL, Sue DY, Wasserman K, Robinson TE, Hansen JE. Immediate effects of cigarette smoking on cardiorespiratory responses to exercise. *J Appl Physiol* 1985;58:1975–1981.

53. Pirnay S, Dujardin J, Deroanne R, Petit JM. Muscular exercise during intoxication by carbon monoxide. *J Appl Physiol* 1971;31:573–575.

54. Vogel JA, Gleser MA. Effect of carbon monoxide on oxygen transport during exercise. *J Appl Physiol* 1972; 32:234–239.

55. Jones NL, Sutton JR, Taylor R, Toews CJ. Effect of pH on cardiorespiratory and metabolic responses to exercise. *J Appl Physiol* 1977;43:959–964.

56. McArdle B. Myopathy due to a defect in muscle glycogen breakdown. *Clin Sci* 1951;10:13–35.

57. Lewis SF, Vora S, Haller RG. Abnormal oxidative metabolism and O_2 transport in muscle phosphofructokinase deficiency. *J Appl Physiol* 1991;70:391–398.

58. Davis JA, Wasserman K, Anderson T. O_2 consumption as related to work-rate in McArdle's syndrome. Unpublished observations.

59. Riley M, Nugent A, Steele IC, Bell N, Trimble ER, Nicholls DP, Patterson VH. Gas exchange during exercise in McArdle's disease. *J Appl Physiol* 1993;75:745–754.

60. Haller RG, Lewis SF. Abnormal ventilation during exercise in McArdle's syndrome: modulation by substrate availability. *Radiology* 1986;36:716–719.

61. Lewis SF, Haller RG. The pathophysiology of McArdle's disease: clues to regulation in exercise and fatigue. *J Appl Physiol* 1986;61:391–401.

62. Wasserman K, Hansen JE, Sue DY. Facilitation of oxygen consumption by lactic acidosis during exercise. *News Physiol Sci* 1991;6:29–34.

63. Bogaard JM, Scholte HR, Busch FM, Stam H, Versprille A. Anaerobic threshold as detected from ventilatory and metabolic exercise responses in patients with mitochondrial respiratory chain defect. In: Tavassi L, DiPrampero PE, eds. *The anaerobic threshold: physiological and clinical significance*. Advances in Cardiology. Basel: Karger, 1986:135–145.

64. Haller RG, Lewis SF, Estabrook RW, DiMauro S, Servidei S, Foster DW. Exercise intolerance, lactic acidosis, and abnormal cardiopulmonary regulation in exercise associated with adult skeletal muscle cytochrome c oxidase deficiency. *J Clin Invest* 1989;84:155–161.

65. Lau AC-W, Lo MK-W, Leung GT-C, Choi FP-T, Yam LY-C, Wasserman K. Altered exercise gas exchange as related to albuminuria in type 2 diabetic patients. *Chest* 2004;125:1292–1298.

66. Berger M, Berchtold P, Cuppers HJ, Drost H, Kley HK, Muller WA, Wiegelmann W, Zimmerman H. Metabolic and hormonal effects of muscular exercise in juvenile type diabetics. *Diabetologia* 1977;13:355–365.

67. Rubler S, Arvan S. Exercise testing in young symptomatic diabetic patients. *Angiology* 1976;27:539–548.

68. Storstein L, Jervell J. Response to bicycle exercise testing in long-standing juvenile diabetes. *Acta Med Scand* 1979;205:277–280.

CHAPTER 6

Clinical Exercise Testing

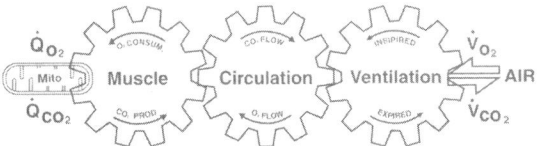

EXERCISE LABORATORY AND EQUIPMENT

General Laboratory Environment

The proper interpretation of exercise test data depends on accurate data collection and correct calculations. Useful exercise testing can be performed with little or no equipment. A measured course, stairway, or hallway can provide a reproducible and functional exercise stress. After review of symptoms and physical examination, information collected might include heart and ventilatory rate and blood pressure at the conclusion of exercise. However, a properly equipped laboratory, with gas exchange measurement, blood pressure, and electrocardiographic capability, provides a site for more complete data collection. The patient can be relatively stationary on an ergometer during a controlled and reproducible stress while measurements are continuously monitored, and blood may be sampled. Figure 6.1 diagrams the devices and measurements that are generally available in a modern exercise laboratory.

The laboratory should be air-conditioned and regulated at a comfortable temperature and humidity. The patient's view should be pleasant and not cluttered with tubing, wires, or a bulletin board with distracting papers. If blood is to be sampled, the syringes should be prepared and placed in a convenient location to avoid confusion or extra motion during the time of the study. The number of people in the laboratory should be limited to those needed for making the measurements and for patient safety. Finally, extra sounds should be kept to a minimum. Soft background music helps to dampen noise but does not interfere with communication between the examiner and the technician. In summary, a pleasant, professional environment is needed to obtain the maximum confidence and therefore performance by the patient.

Gas Exchange Measurement

Although exercise testing can be performed with little or no equipment, the more sophisticated and potentially useful analysis of cardiopulmonary function during exercise necessitates gas exchange measurement. A variety of systems, measuring devices, recorders, and other equipment have been put together for these purposes, and there are commercial systems that determine gas exchange using either a gas mixing chamber or breath-by-breath analysis of respired gas.

Mixing Chambers

In systems using a mixing chamber, expired ventilation is determined using a flow or volume measurement device, while expired gas is passed into a fixed or variable-sized mixing chamber from which

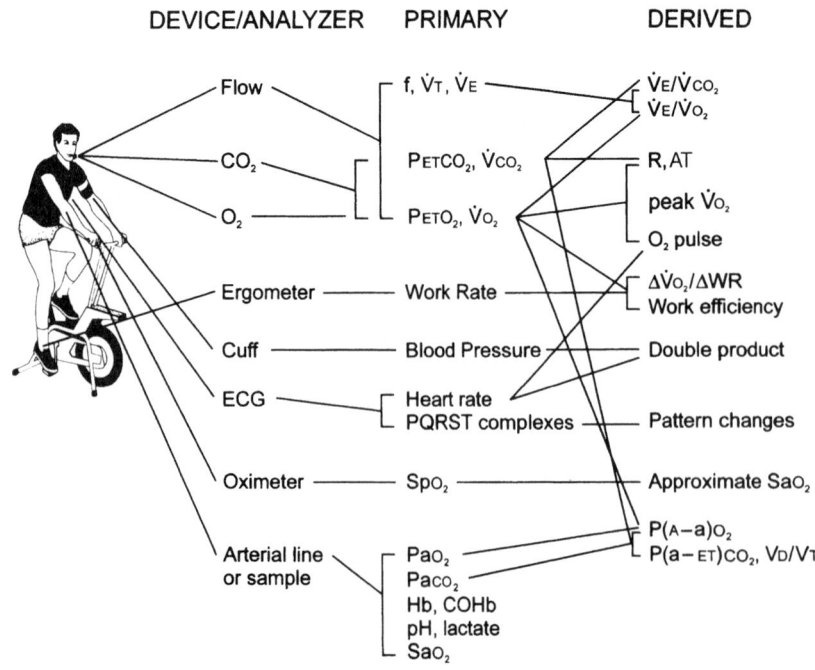

FIGURE 6.1. Devices and analyzers used to measure variables during exercise on a cycle ergometer. Devices and analyzers individually or collectively may measure a single or several primary variables. The variables in the right-hand column are usually calculated from two or more primary variables.

gas is sampled and analyzed for O_2 and CO_2 concentrations. With proper mixing of expired gas from each breath, differences in O_2 and CO_2 concentration from the beginning to the end of each breath are minimized, and the resultant O_2 and CO_2 concentrations are equal to the volume-weighted average or "mixed expired" concentrations. These are equivalent to the O_2 and CO_2 concentrations that would have been obtained by collecting all of the expired gas in a bag.

In an ideal mixing chamber, with instantaneous and complete mixing, the introduction of a constant flow of a given gas eventually results in the mixing chamber having a composition identical to that of this gas. The time course by which the concentration in the mixing chamber approaches that of the input gas is approximately exponential. For an ideal chamber, the mixing characteristics can be described by a time constant equal to $V_{mc}/\dot{V}$, where V_{mc} is the volume of the mixing chamber and $\dot{V}$ is the constant flow of gas into and out of the chamber. A large gas flow (or minute ventilation) or a mixing chamber of small size has a short time constant. Under these conditions, this chamber would respond rapidly to a change in gas concentration; however, the small volume means that a subject with a large tidal volume will produce marked fluctuations in gas concentrations in the chamber. On the other hand, too large a mixing chamber volume compared with tidal volume results in an impracticably long time to reach any new equilibrium, making the mixing chamber poorly responsive to changes in gas concentration. A fixed-volume mixing chamber may be satisfactory during exercise in which $\dot{V}_E$, $FECO_2$ and FEO_2 change slowly, but may not be satisfactory when rapid changes are expected. If ventilation is continuously measured, a time or volume adjustment must be made to match the correct mixed expired gas concentrations with the correct ventilation.

Breath-by-Breath System

A breath-by-breath system measures airflow or volume continuously and simultaneously determines instantaneous expired CO_2 and O_2 concentrations. The CO_2 output and O_2 uptake during each breath are calculated, and the cumulated totals of all breaths over a measured time period are reported as $\dot{V}CO_2$ and $\dot{V}O_2$. To make accurate measurements, ventilation and gas concentrations must be determined as near to continuously as possible. We have used breath-by-breath systems for both research applications and for evaluation of patients (1–3). Commer-

cially available systems make it possible to determine gas exchange rapidly and accurately under many conditions. By interpolating breath-by-breath expired volume, O_2 uptake, and CO_2 output, second by second, it is possible to reduce the variability in breath-by-breath measurements. If necessary, replicate studies with time averaging of the second-by-second values can be performed (1–3) to enhance the measurement of physiological responses to rapid changes in work rate.

Measurement of Volume, Flow Rate, or Ventilation

Several methods of measuring respired gas volume and flow rates during exercise are used. Whereas expired flow is usually measured and integrated into volume, physiological variables can also be calculated from inspired volume or flow with the appropriate adjustments. Devices for measuring volume or flows may be used directly as part of the breathing circuit, or they may be used to measure volumes from a collecting container. If the device is used directly, then flow resistance, linearity, and frequency response may be important considerations (4). Commercially used flow devices include pneumotachographs, Pitot tubes, turbines, and hot-wire anemometers. Volume can be measured directly using a gas meter, spirometer, or volume transducer.

Pneumotachographs consist of a number of parallel tubes (Fleisch type) that offer a small resistance to gas flow. Gas flow is directly proportional to pressure drop across the resistance when flow is laminar, and the relation is given by Poiseuille's law. When flow becomes nonlaminar or turbulent, the relation between flow and pressure becomes nonlinear. In a Fleisch pneumotachograph, laminar flow is encouraged by small flow channels and low gas velocities. Small flexible plastic tubes are connected at each end of the resistance element, and these two tubes are connected to a differential pressure transducer.

For exercise testing in adults, flows encountered generally indicate that a size no. 3 Fleisch pneumotachograph is appropriate (4). Compensation for documented nonlinearities in the pressure–flow relation can be made by altering the output of the differential pressure transducer either electrically or mathematically, using a computer. In commercial systems, empiric calibration curves may be used to optimize pneumotachograph performance.

Because expired gas is usually warmer and contains more water vapor than ambient air, contact of warm expired gas with an ambient-temperature pneumotachograph could result in condensation and obstruction of the pneumotachograph resistance elements. Pneumotachographs, therefore, are often used with an electric heater to warm the pneumotachograph to a temperature slightly above expired gas. However, a heated pneumotachograph not only warms and increases the volume of the expired gas, but also warms it by a variable amount depending on the flow. Whereas theoretic methods can be used to estimate the degree of warming, two practical methods may eliminate the problem. In the first method the expired gas is kept warm, and the temperature of the pneumotachograph is only slightly warmer (0.5°C) than the temperature of the gas passing through it. Another way is to distance the pneumotachograph from the mouth so that it can be kept at ambient temperature and the expired gas allowed to cool.

Pitot tubes (5) measure the difference in pressure at an opening placed directly facing the fluid stream compared with the pressure at an opening perpendicular to the fluid stream (static pressure). From Bernoulli's law, the velocity of fluid movement is proportional to the square root of the pressure difference; from the cross-sectional area of the device, the flow can be calculated. The Pitot tube has the advantage of being nonresistive and dependent on turbulent flow rather than on laminar flow conditions. A flowmeter suitable for exercise gas exchange measurements based on the Pitot tube principle uses a differential pressure transducer to determine the pressure difference between the static and midstream ports. A suitable algorithm calculates the flow from the pressure signal and also corrects for nonlinearities over the flow measurement range. Advantages of such a device include low resistance, lack of a requirement for laminar flow, and minimal problems with heating or cooling of inspired or expired gas.

Turbine flowmeters and hot-wire anemometers (6,7) can also be used to measure the mass or flow of gas. The latter device determines the change in amount of electrical current, compared with baseline, needed to maintain a constant temperature of a wire placed in the air stream. The wire material is selected so the wire resistance is strongly influenced by the wire temperature. The rate of mass movement of gas and its thermal capacity relate to the current change; by using an appropriate model, the flow of gas can be calculated. Although this method is inherently nonlinear, digital computer algorithms can correct this nonlinearity.

Breathing Valves, Mouthpieces, and Masks

Some gas exchange measurement systems require the use of a breathing valve to separate inspired from expired gas flows so expired gas can be collected and analyzed. The ideal valve prevents contamination of either inspired or expired gas flow by the other, has no resistance to breathing, has low rebreathed volume (low valve dead space), is of minimal weight and size, is easily cleaned and sterilized, is low cost, does not generate turbulence, and operates silently.

Dead space for the valve plus attached mouthpiece can be determined by measuring the volume of water it can hold. Valve resistance can be determined during constant airflow using a pressure transducer and flowmeter. Valves may develop back-leaks, especially when subjected to high flows and pressures during heavy exercise. These leaks should be suspected for any valve, but especially after prolonged use, excessive secretions, or damage to component parts. Errors in ventilation or gas exchange measurements may be important clues to a leaking breathing valve. If a leak is suspected, simultaneous recording of inspiratory and expiratory flow during exercise may reveal the presence and location of the leak.

Traditionally, patients have used nose clips so that all inspired and expired gases are routed through rubber or soft plastic mouthpieces. Now, comfortable face masks of differing sizes and shapes to cover the patient's nose and mouth are available. The dead space is usually only slightly more than with a mouthpiece and nose clip.

Gas Analyzers

For gas exchange measurements, the concentration of O_2 and CO_2 in the expired gas can be determined by several devices. Mass spectrometers convert sampled gases to positively charged ions with an electron beam. Then, in a near vacuum, the ions are accelerated by an electric field and are then subjected to a magnetic field. The direction that the ions take in the magnetic field is dependent on their mass-to-charge ratios. The different ions representing different gases are detected by appropriately located detectors that each produce a voltage output proportional to the number of ions that strike the collector per unit time. Because the total voltage is dependent on the sum of the individual detector voltages, any gas for which there is no detector does not contribute to the total. For respiratory mass spectrometry, detectors for O_2, CO_2, and N_2 are typically used; however, there are no detectors for water vapor, argon, or other inert gases present in trace amounts in air. Thus, the O_2, CO_2, and N_2 concentrations given by a mass spectrometer are concentrations relative to a dry gas whether or not water vapor was a component of the originally sampled gas.

Carbon dioxide analyzers measure absorption by CO_2 of appropriate wavelengths of infrared light. Infrared light is passed through a cell containing the gas to be measured, and the amount of light transmitted is compared with a reference value. Absorption is proportional to the fractional CO_2 concentration. The measurement cell must be kept clean and free of water condensation.

Oxygen analyzers use several different principles. The paramagnetic analyzer measures the change in a magnetic field introduced by differences in oxygen concentration. Because other respiratory gases have little paramagnetic susceptibility, these will not affect the magnetic field. The more commonly used electrochemical O_2 analyzer depends on chemical reactions between O_2 and a substrate that generates a small electrical current. This current is proportional to the rate of O_2 molecules reacting with the substrate and thus to the concentration of O_2.

These latter CO_2 and O_2 analyzers measure partial pressure of the gas and are affected by water vapor, pressure in the sampling systems, and changes in barometric pressure and altitude. Thus, for a given fractional concentration of gas, changes in any of these conditions at the sensor location will erroneously result in different measured gas fractions. Because the sample flow rate delivering gas to the analyzer is held constant, a change in sampling site pressure may result from changes in resistance of the delivery tubing. Using a high-pressure suction pump and a large resistance in the connection between the analyzer and the pump can minimize this effect. Care must be taken to ensure that sample tube resistance is identical during calibration and measurement, and that water condensation, saliva, or foreign bodies are not trapped in the delivery tubing.

Both CO_2 and O_2 analyzers report the fraction of CO_2 or O_2 in the total gas, including any water vapor present. This is especially important to consider during calibration because ambient air usually contains some water vapor. Expired gas is saturated with water vapor at the lowest temperature that it reaches before being analyzed. Because temperature determines the partial pressure of water in a saturated gas, this temperature must be accurately known or estimated if expired CO_2 and O_2 are to be accurately determined. Tubing has been developed that allows equilibration of the water vapor partial pressure within the tube with that of ambient air, so that the water vapor partial pressure of the gas delivered to the analyzer is equal to that of ambient air and is not influenced by the temperature of the gas at the point of sampling. Additional discussion of the significance of water vapor can be found in Appendix C.

Ergometers: Treadmills and Cycles

Treadmill

Treadmills allow subjects to walk, jog, or run at measured speeds and grades of incline. A variety of protocols for increasing work performed have been designed, and both low and high work rates may be obtained. Treadmills have some advantages over cycle ergometers. A subject performing on a treadmill generally has a peak $\dot{V}O_2$ approximately 5% to 10% higher than on a cycle ergometer, and some subjects and patients are simply not able to cycle because of problems of coordination or inexperience. On the other hand, treadmills may introduce movement artifacts in measurement of ventilation, pulmonary gas exchange, and blood pressure.

Of greatest importance is the fact that if the subject holds on to any part of the treadmill, such as a hand railing, or to the arm of a technician or physician, the amount of work performed by the patient is reduced, thus interfering with the accurate determination of the $\dot{V}O_2$–work rate relationship and work efficiency.

Cycle Ergometer

Cycle ergometers enable a precise estimation of the work rate. Leg cycling may be performed sitting or supine. Advantages of the cycle ergometer over the treadmill include the ability to vary the work rate in step, incremental, or ramp fashion; the ability to determine work efficiency; potentially greater safety because the subject is supported at all times; and less movement artifact on measurements. Some patients, however, may not be able to pedal the cycle because of lack of coordination and experience, and the seat may become uncomfortable during a long study.

When the patient is seated in the upright position, seat height should be adjusted so that the leg is almost completely extended at the lowest point of the pedaling cycle. It is useful to record the seat height in the subject's records so future studies may be done identically. Subjects should be asked to wear shoes suitable for the types of pedals on the cycle. Toe clips may or may not be used, as desired. Because subjects should cycle at a relatively constant rate, a metronome or tachometer should be used to assist subjects' performance.

Two types of cycle ergometers are in general use. Mechanically braked devices use an adjustable brake to increase or decrease contact of a friction belt with a moving flywheel attached to the pedals. The work rate achieved is proportional to the cycling frequency or speed of the flywheel, but a particular work rate is only achieved if the subject cycles within a narrow range of pedaling rate. An electrically braked cycle ergometer uses a variable electromagnetic field to produce a resistance to pedaling that varies with flywheel speed, changing the resistance to cycling to maintain work rate at the set level regardless of pedaling speed. A work rate set on this type of cycle ergometer is thereby present over a wider range of cycling speeds. The work rate on the electrically braked devices may be set by a remote controller, or it may be adjusted automatically by a digital computer controller.

When a subject pedals on the cycle with "no resistance added" or "unloaded," some work is obviously being performed. In addition to the work rate necessary to move the legs, the work rate needed to keep the cycle flywheel in motion can be 5 to 15 watts (W) for electromagnetically braked ergometers, but it may be as much as 20 to 30 W for mechanically braked cycle ergometers. Particularly for the latter, it will vary considerably with pedaling rate. This low work rate may exceed the maximal capacity of some severely limited patients. Manufacturer's specifications may provide information on the work rate of "unloaded cycling," but users should make this determination for themselves. We have used a special protocol (see "Selecting the Rate of Work Rate Increase," later in this chapter) that uses an accessory motor attached to the cycle flywheel that keeps it spinning at a rate sufficient to remove the inertial energy needed by the subject to start cycling while simultaneously minimizing the "unloaded" work rate (virtually zero watts above the power output needed for moving the legs at the assigned pedaling rate).

Cycle Versus Treadmill

Whether the treadmill or the cycle ergometer is the preferable mode of exercise for exercise testing has

TABLE 6.1. Comparison of Treadmill and Cycle Ergometers for Exercise Testing

Feature	Treadmill	Cycle
Higher maximum $\dot{V}O_2$ and maximum O_2 pulse	+	
Similar maximum heart rate and maximum $\dot{V}E$	+	+
Familiarity of exercise	++	+
Quantitation of external work	−−	++
Freedom from artifacts in ECG, airflow, and pressure tracing	−−	++
Ease of obtaining arterial blood specimens	−−	++
Safety (fewer musculoskeletal injuries)		+
Usefulness in supine position		+
Greater experience in the United States	+	
Greater experience in Europe		+

More important advantage (++) or disadvantage (−−); less important advantage (+) or disadvantage (−).

been a subject of considerable debate (Table 6.1). The treadmill has been in common use for decades. It allows one to exercise most ambulatory patients except those who are severely dyspneic, uncoordinated, or confused, or those who have significant lower extremity musculoskeletal disease. Length of stride as speed or grade is changed, shift of center of gravity, and change from walking to jogging all can affect the patient's metabolic requirement. Repeated experience on the treadmill may lead to some increase in the efficiency of walking.

Probably the greatest disadvantage of the treadmill is the difficulty in quantifying work rate. Any connection between the patient and the treadmill, except that between the patient's shoes and the treadmill belt, decreases the expected energy requirement for body movement at that grade and speed. Thus, railings, arm boards, mouthpieces, blood pressure measuring devices, and steadying hands all have the potential to reduce the patient's actual work rate. For treadmill exercise, we only allow patients to touch the back of their hand against the handrail for balance; we do not allow the subject to grasp or hold on to the handrails.

Even the most athletic patients require several minutes of practice in starting and ending the treadmill exercise before beginning measurement. Although injuries are rarely reported, careful surveillance is necessary. Because patients can lose their balance on the moving belts, it is wise to have additional help immediately available on the sideboard of the treadmill, particularly for elderly patients.

The cycle ergometer allows a more accurate quantifying of external work rate than the treadmill and can be used when patients are in the supine or upright position. A minor disadvantage is that most individuals have a lower peak $\dot{V}O_2$ and anaerobic threshold (*AT*) on the cycle than on the treadmill, even though their maximum heart rate (HR), maximum $\dot{V}E$, and maximum blood lactate are similar on both ergometers. In eight studies of male subjects, the mean peak $\dot{V}O_2$ on the cycle varied from 89% to 95% of treadmill values (8).

None of our patients has been injured using the cycle or treadmill, but we believe that the cycle is safer for those patients who are less well coordinated or who have cardiovascular disease. With the cycle, the subject can stop exercise on his or her own volition, independent of the examiner's action, as soon as he or she feels symptomatic to the point that he or she wishes to stop exercise. With the treadmill, the patient must signal the examiner, and then the examiner must respond by turning off the treadmill. Thus, stopping the exercise is dependent not only on the patient but also on the reaction time of the examiner controlling the treadmill switch.

Because there is less arm and torso movement on the cycle than on the treadmill, one finds fewer artifacts in ventilatory and circulatory measurements. Also, obtaining blood samples can be done with greater ease on the cycle.

Because the tubular post supporting our cycle seat once buckled while being used by a very obese patient, we now use a stainless steel rod to support a conventional bicycle seat (covered with sheepskin or gel) or a platform-type seat. "Seat pain" can be a problem with prolonged repeated testing, but it is uncommon with the short clinical protocols described herein. In agreement with Astrand (9), we prefer the cycle to the treadmill for clinical testing because we can accurately quantify external work rate and thereby establish the patient's work rate–$\dot{V}O_2$ relationship, a critical measurement in assessing cardiovascular function.

Work and Work Rate (Power)

In basic physical units, force (kg-m/sec^2 or newton) equals mass (kg) times acceleration (m/sec^2). When this force is applied over a distance, work is performed. Thus, work (kg-m^2/sec^2 or newton-m or joule) equals force (kg-m/sec^2 or newton) times distance (m). However, we are most often interested in the *rate* of work or *power*, which equals work (kg-m^2/sec^2 or newton-m or joule) per second. The unit of power is the watt, and 1 watt (W) is defined as 1 joule/sec = 1 newton-m/sec = 1 kg-m^2/ sec^3.

During exercise against the resistance of a cycle ergometer, the work rate is the distance traveled by a point on the circumference of the wheel × the rotational frequency of the flywheel × the restraining force. This restraining force can be expressed as newtons or, commonly, as kiloponds, where 1 kilopond (kp) = 1 kg × 9.81 m/sec^2. In practice, cycle ergometer work rate (power) is expressed as watts or kilopond-m/min. To convert from kp-m/min to W, divide the former by 6.12. For example, a work rate of 612 kp-m/min equals 100 W.

Electrocardiogram and Systemic Blood Pressure

Exercise Electrocardiogram

Silver or silver chloride electrocardiogram (ECG) electrodes with circumferential adhesive provide good electrical contact and minimize movement artifacts. These are similar to those used in the intensive care unit (ICU) for ECG monitoring. The skin is shaved if necessary and is rubbed with alcohol before the patches are applied on areas of the body that will not be subject to great motion during exercise. A net vest may reduce artifacts due to movement.

We use 12-lead ECGs for all patients, as shown in Figure 6.2. The arm electrodes are placed on the back above the scapulae; the leg electrodes are placed on the low back above the iliac crests to minimize movement artifact. The chest electrodes (V_1–V_6) are positioned in standard locations on the anterolateral chest. Some systems require additional leads for separate transmission of the heart rate signal to the computer. Commercial systems allow computer processing of summarized signals to reduce motion artifacts. However, if the signals are noisy, we record 12-lead ECGs at least every minute so that heart rates are accurately known throughout the study.

Systemic Blood Pressure

Blood pressure should be measured frequently during exercise to be aware of extreme hypertension or to detect impending hypotension. Blood pressure can also be measured and recorded using several commercial devices: (a) mechanically controlled or automated inflatable cuffs and auscultation, (b) pulse oximeters, or (c) pressure transducers placed over the radial artery. Such devices should be validated against sphygmomanometer measurements made in the opposite arm. Indwelling arterial catheters allow nearly continuous direct measurement of systemic arterial blood pressure and wave contours, and afford optimal patient safety. The pressure trans-

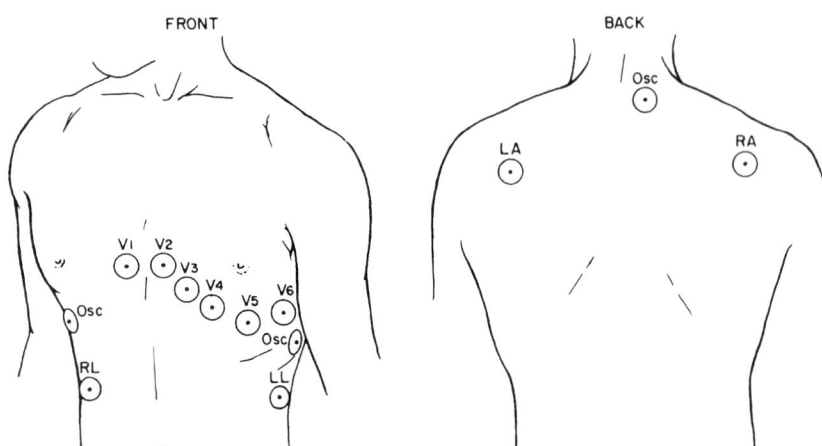

FIGURE 6.2. Electrocardiographic lead placement for upright ergometry. The V_1 and V_2 electrodes are placed more caudad than usually done for supine tracings, whereas V_3, V_4, V_5, and V_6 are in their usual locations. The "arm" electrodes (*LA* and *RA*) are placed posterior to the shoulders, whereas the "leg" electrodes (*LL* and *RL*) are placed anterolaterally near the lower rib margins. The three oscilloscope (*Osc*) electrodes are placed separately to minimize electrical interference.

ducer should be located at the level of the left atrium (approximately the fourth intercostal space at the midaxillary line in the upright position) and the transducer carefully calibrated. More commonly, blood pressure is measured with an anaeroid manometer, inflatable arm cuff, and auscultation.

Oximetry, Blood Sampling, and Arterial Catheters

Valid measurements of PaO_2, $PaCO_2$, or pH for calculation or measurement of SaO_2, $P(A - a)O_2$, $P(a - ET)CO_2$, or VD/VT are very useful for the interpretation of clinical exercise tests. However, on many occasions correct diagnoses and interpretations can be made using less invasive measurements.

Pulse Oximetry

Pulse oximetry estimates arterial blood oxygen saturation using pulsatile changes in light absorption. Since the late 1970s, the principle of pulse oximetry has been widely used (10). This technique estimates arterial oxygen saturation derived from a combination of spectrophotometry and pulse plethysmography. These devices use two wavelengths of light produced by light-emitting diodes, one in the red and one in the infrared spectrum, and a detector that measures transmitted or reflected light from the ear lobe, fingertip, or forehead. Differential absorption of light at these two wavelengths provides enough information to determine the ratio of oxyhemoglobin to total hemoglobin, assuming that all the pulsatile change is due to the effects of arterial blood. Pulse oximetry is theoretically independent of skin pigmentation and the thickness of the ear lobe or finger; however, some studies have shown that dark skin pigmentation may affect results (11,12).

Pulse oximeters cannot distinguish carboxyhemoglobin and methemoglobin from oxyhemoglobin; it may be convenient to think of the percentage of oxygen saturation reported from a pulse oximeter as being equal to (100 − percentage of deoxyhemoglobin). In general, pulse oximetry becomes less accurate when oxygen saturation is less than 75% (10).

During exercise, movement artifact and stray incidental light may interfere with pulse oximeter accuracy. Although some studies have found acceptable accuracy of pulse oximeters during exercise (11–14), Hansen and Casaburi (15) have shown that overestimation and underestimation of arterial blood oxygen saturation may occur near the patient's maximum work rate. Reasons for this may include dependence of the pulse oximeter on sufficient blood flow to the vascular bed measured, a change in the shape of the arterial pulse waveform, a change in empirically determined calibration factors, movement artifact, or other problems. Newer-generation pulse oximeters have improved algorithms that allow the devices to cope better with motion artifacts, reduced perfusion, and changes in pulsatile waveforms. These have been tested in critically ill patients and to a lesser extent in the exercise laboratory (16,17). Fewer motion artifacts may be encountered if a reflectance oximeter probe is placed on the forehead (16) or other less vigorously moving part of the body.

The major disadvantage of pulse oximetry is that arterial oxyhemoglobin saturation rather than arterial PO_2 is measured and that measurements of dead space ventilation cannot be made. Thus, although the correlation between measured arterial O_2 saturation and pulse oximetry O_2 saturation is good, significant decreases in PaO_2 when above 60 mm Hg result in only small decreases in O_2 saturation. For patients whose PaO_2 decreases to below 60 mm Hg during exercise, pulse oximetry proves useful. For other patients whose resting and exercise PaO_2 are greater than 60 mm Hg but who are suspected of significant decreases in PaO_2 during exercise, one approach is to use pulse oximetry during a preliminary test. If arterial oxygen saturation decreases by more than 3% to 5%, then blood samples for direct measurement of PaO_2 and $P(A - a)O_2$ during a repeat exercise study may be necessary to confirm whether or not arterial hypoxemia developed.

Single Samples of Arterial Blood

Arterial blood samples allow direct measurement of SaO_2, PaO_2, $PaCO_2$, pH, lactate, V_D/V_T, $P(a - ET)CO_2$, and other important values. Often, a single sample of arterial blood is obtained during an exercise test to assess blood gases. If this is done, the sample must be obtained before the end of the exercise rather than during recovery because rapid changes in PaO_2 occur immediately when the patient begins to recover from exercise (18–20). Each sample should be drawn over a specific 10- to 20-second period, so that it can be well matched with concurrent gas exchange measurements involving several breaths. The radial artery is the more common site for a single sample; local anesthesia to that site administered before exercise reduces patient discomfort.

Some investigators use free-flowing ear capillary blood or heated hand vein blood as a substitute for arterial blood. Blood values from these sites are likely to approximate arterial PCO_2 values for measurement of V_D/V_T but are less likely to approximate arterial PO_2 values.

Systemic Arterial Catheter

An indwelling arterial catheter makes repeated sampling of arterial blood for blood gases simple and fast, and it provides continuous monitoring of blood pressure during exercise as well. The most common insertion sites are the brachial and radial arteries, and the same kinds of small-bore catheters used in the ICU for arterial catheterization can be used. The radial artery site has the theoretic advantage that the ulnar artery can supply blood to the hand if the radial artery is blocked, whereas the brachial artery is the sole blood supply of the lower arm. With meticulous care, however, we have never had a serious complication of brachial artery catheterization in several thousand insertions over a 30-year period. A disadvantage of the radial artery site is that it may interfere with gripping of the

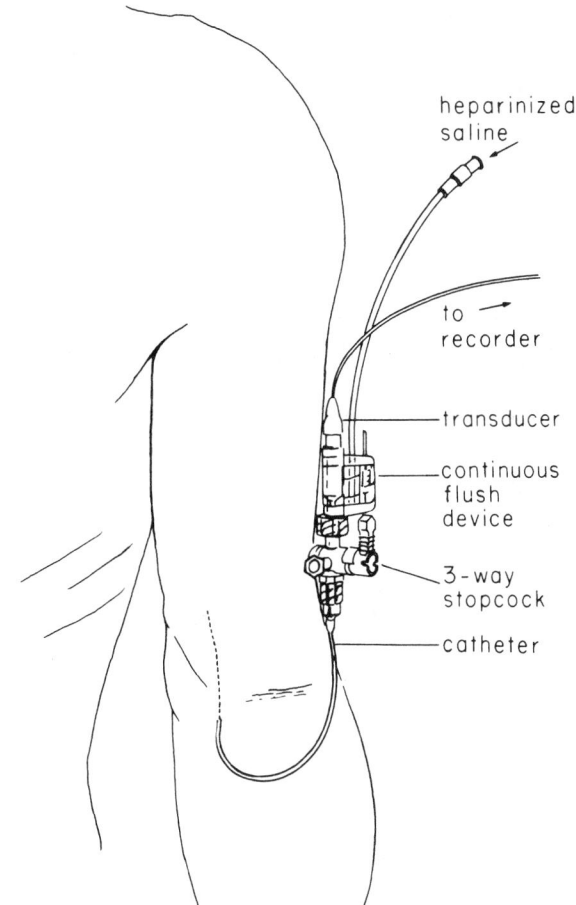

FIGURE 6.3. Brachial artery catheter placement. A 25-cm polyvinyl catheter has been placed percutaneously in the left brachial artery. The dressings have been removed to show catheter placement. The hub of the catheter connects to a continuous-flush device, a three-way stopcock, and a transducer, the last located parallel to the fourth intercostal space in the midclavicular line (at the midatrial level in the sitting position).

cycle ergometer handlebars; in addition, referring direct blood pressure measurements to the left atrial level may be more difficult. Figure 6.3 demonstrates the brachial artery catheter in place, and Appendix D describes its insertion.

Arterial punctures and catheterization are rarely complicated by bleeding, arterial spasm, distal arterial thromboembolism, thrombosis, or infection, or by significant pain or discomfort. Most frequently, subjects complain of mild discomfort and discoloration from bleeding following puncture. Arterial catheters should be used with special care or avoided in patients with known peripheral arterial disease and in patients with bleeding disorders.

Pulmonary Artery Catheter

For some patients, a pulmonary artery catheter can add valuable information during exercise testing.

For example, it may be useful in selected patients with suspected primary or secondary pulmonary hypertension in whom resting pulmonary artery (PA) pressures are borderline elevated. But because of the failure to recruit pulmonary capillary bed during exercise in patients with a pulmonary vasculopathy, the PA pressure can increase strikingly even with a relatively small increase in blood flow induced by exercise. In patients with cardiac disease, PA pressure, PA wedge pressure, mixed venous blood gases, and cardiac output can be measured.

The Swan-Ganz pulmonary artery catheter is balloon tipped and flow directed, and a physician can pass it through a large vein in the arm through the right atrium, right ventricle, and into the pulmonary artery with or without fluoroscopic guidance. Because arrhythmias and heart block potentially occur during placement, insertion should be done only with ECG monitoring and appropriate resuscitation equipment and medications standing by, if needed. For pressure measurements, a calibrated transducer and recorder are used. During exercise, especially with patients with lung disease, large swings in intrathoracic pressure with respiration may be transmitted to the pulmonary artery and wedge pressures, and pressure measurements will be subject to large variation with breathing. Intravascular pressures at end exhalation are selected by convention and are usually most relevant. Blood samples can be drawn from the pulmonary artery distal port to be analyzed for mixed venous P_{O_2} and O_2 content needed for the calculation of cardiac output using the Fick equation, or calculation of venous admixture.

Cardiac output can also be determined by thermodilution, that is, by rapidly injecting a bolus of isotonic fluid (usually 5% dextrose in water) of known volume, temperature (usually 0°C), specific heat, and specific gravity into the right atrial port of the pulmonary artery catheter and measuring the temperature change with a thermistor or temperature sensor at the catheter tip in the pulmonary artery. The temperature change downstream reflects the volume of dilution of the bolus, and cardiac output can be calculated using an automated system. The integral of temperature over time is inversely proportional to cardiac output. Stetz et al. (21) reviewed several studies and concluded that values of cardiac output determined by thermodilution in catheterization laboratories and intensive care units were of comparable accuracy to those determined by Fick or dye-dilution methods. These authors suggested, however, that a 20% to 26% difference in cardiac output should be found before concluding that two single determinations were different. Advantages of thermodilution include safety, speed, and repeatability.

Disadvantages of using a pulmonary artery catheter include increased risks, costs, and preparation time. Uncommon complications can include arrhythmia; heart block; bleeding; perforation of the vein being catheterized or of the right ventricle or pulmonary artery; and infections. Under specific circumstances, however, the benefits gained from the diagnoses obtained from these catheters outweigh the risks.

Data Sampling and Computation

Automated exercise gas exchange systems make intensive use of computers to control data collection, perform calculations, store results, and display information. The speed and capability of computerized calculations can correct data from nonlinear analyzers and make adjustments for different environmental or subject characteristics. The computer can also be used to control the ergometer using preprogrammed protocols. Many commercial cardiopulmonary exercise testing systems come with a variety of data displays and printed tables and graphs capable of showing the results of exercise testing, similar to those shown in Chapter 10 of this book. These tools serve most needs for clinical cardiopulmonary exercise testing. Systems also allow reports to be customized and data to be transferred to database and spreadsheet applications.

Typically, data sampled from a flowmeter transducer, gas analyzer, pulse oximeter, heart rate monitor, or other device undergo analog-to-digital conversion under computer control. Accurate calculations require a sufficiently high sampling rate; for most gas exchange data, a sampling rate in the range of 50 to 100 Hz appears to be adequate. This is easily in the range of available analog-to-digital converters and computer systems.

Quality Control, Validation, and Maintenance

Flowmeter validation is essential for confidence in the ability of the device to measure accurately and reproducibly under testing conditions. Large-volume syringes of 1 to 4 L that can deliver known inspiratory and expiratory volumes at very slow to very rapid flow rates are commonly used to calibrate flow devices. If the flow signals are further processed by analog or digital means, the results will be subject to the response characteristics and calculation methods of these instruments (22). The accuracy of flow and volume can also be determined using a calibrated pump calibrator.

Gas analyzers should be checked for accuracy and linearity within the range of needed values. This can be done by using gases of known concentration of O_2 and CO_2. The Scholander and Haldane methods for gas analysis are accurate, but time-consuming, tedious, and now uncommonly used (23). They may be useful for initial calibration of gas analyzers and primary analysis of stored gases used for calibration purposes. Alternatively, gas having O_2 and CO_2 concentrations of acceptable precision can be obtained from a reliable gas supplier. Such high-precision gases are expensive, but such a tank may be kept for years and used only periodically to assay less expensive gases used for day-to-day calibration. After long storage, it is best to roll tanks to avoid gas stratification.

If an analyzer is nonlinear, a calibration curve can be constructed by observing the analyzer output at several gas concentrations (24). The analyzers should be warmed up for sufficient time to ensure against electrical drift. Once linearity has been established, a two-point calibration can be used. Room air is often used as one calibration point, assuming an O_2 concentration of 20.93% and CO_2 concentration of 0.04%. A calibration gas of approximately 15% O_2, 5% CO_2, and balance N_2 (but whose actual values are accurately known) is appropriate for the second point because these concentrations are near the expected expired gas concentrations.

For the breath-by-breath calculation of $\dot{V}O_2$ and $\dot{V}CO_2$, the gas transport delay time and the response time of each analyzer to the detection of a new gas concentration are important to know. How these play a role in the calculation is further addressed in Appendix C.

Treadmill speed and grade should be routinely checked for accuracy and reproducibility. Grade may be determined by using a plumb line and tape measure. Speed can be accurately determined by using a stopwatch to time the movement of a mark made on the treadmill belt.

Cycle calibration is highly desirable both during initial setup of the laboratory and periodically thereafter. Manufacturers' specifications and calibration procedures should be followed. Commercially available or specially built devices that generate known amounts of power can act as standards for calibration and verification (25). Other methods

have been devised to provide for cycle calibration and validation (26–28).

In the past, systems of analyzers and computers for determination of gas exchange during exercise were developed and assembled in individual laboratories. Validation often comprised the majority of the time required for development of these systems. Now, many good commercial exercise systems are available. They should also undergo validation and have periodic monitoring for accuracy and reproducibility of results.

Validation can be performed by simultaneous collection of mixed expired gas while the exercise system is collecting data (1,2,29). For mixing chamber and breath-by-breath systems, extremes of tidal volume and flow are particularly challenging. It is easiest to collect expired gas during the steady-state of constant work exercise, but such validation may not provide evidence of accurate measurement during rapidly changing exercise protocols or when the major focus is on the short-term time course of gas exchange.

A particularly useful device is an automated calibrator that simulates gas exchange at a known and reproducible rate. One type of simulator uses a sinusoidal pump of known volume and measurable frequency to provide an accurate "expired minute ventilation" (30). Gas exchange (O_2 uptake and CO_2 output) is simulated by the introduction of a gas mixture containing 21% CO_2 in N_2 into a reservoir bag that mixes with room air pumped into the gas exchange measurement system. $\dot{V}O_2$ and $\dot{V}CO_2$ measured by the system should be equal to 0.21 × the flow rate of the 21% CO_2 in N_2 flowing into the reservoir bag of the pump calibrator. The respiratory gas exchange ratio should equal 1.00; however, adjustment of the exercise system algorithms may be necessary to accommodate the nearly dry, room-temperature gas delivered by the calibrator to the gas exchange measuring device that is set up to measure body-temperature, saturated expirate. The pump calibrator has been demonstrated to provide an accurate simulation of gas exchange that can be used for validation and for detection of the source of instrument or algorithm error when an erroneous value is detected. In addition, the device is useful for routine periodic checks of reproducibility. If an error (or change) in measured minute ventilation, $\dot{V}O_2$, or $\dot{V}CO_2$ is found, analysis of the differences in the measurements may also suggest the nature of the problem.

An inexpensive and relatively simple way to test the validity of the entire system is for an individual to cycle at two constant mild to moderate work intensities, such as 20 W and 70 W, for 6 minutes each. On such tests the $\dot{V}O_2$ after 3 minutes should be in a steady state and within 5% to 10% of previously measured values (approximately 0.7 L/min for an individual of average size exercising at 20 W and 1.2 L/min at 70 W, with a difference of 0.5 ± 0.05 L/min). Values significantly deviant from prior tests suggest errors in flow, gas analyzer, or delay measurements or errors in ergometer calibration. If the tested individual can control his or her breathing frequency appropriately, there should be less than 5% difference in $\dot{V}O_2$ whether breathing at a frequency of 15, 30, or 60 breaths per minute. This is an excellent test of the validity of transit delay times and the rapidity of gas analyzer responses. Greater variation in $\dot{V}O_2$ values at higher breathing frequencies suggests errors in delay or response times in the gas analyzers.

Many commercial systems have an option to print a listing of the current status of gas analyzers, environmental conditions, calibration gas concentrations, temperature, and other important system variables. These and validation and reproducibility data should be kept in a laboratory notebook for future reference. This information can be helpful in identifying and resolving problems with the help of the manufacturer.

PREPARING FOR THE EXERCISE TEST

The objective of a clinical exercise test should be to learn the maximum about the patient's pathophysiological causes of exercise limitation (a) with the greatest accuracy, (b) with the least stress to the patient, and (c) in the shortest period of time. The optimal examination allows the simultaneous evaluation of the adequacy of the muscles, heart, lungs, and the peripheral and pulmonary circulations to meet the gas exchange requirements of exercise. The test should enable the investigator to distinguish disorders in these systems from inadequate effort, obesity, anxiety, or unfitness.

For the differential diagnosis of exercise limitation caused by cardiovascular or respiratory disease, relatively complete gas exchange measurements should be made. Exercise with large muscle groups is needed to stimulate internal respiration sufficiently to stress the cardiovascular and pulmonary systems adequately. Therefore, either a cycle ergometer or a treadmill should be used to stimulate large muscle groups for testing. Isometric exercise is of limited value because it is largely anaerobic, providing little information about the ability of the cardiovascular and respiratory systems to support the energy requirements of exercise. The protocol selected for exercise testing depends on the purpose of the test.

Requesting the Test and Notifying the Patient

We use a preprinted request form for exercise tests. On this form, the referring physician gives us the following information:

1. Patient's name, address, and telephone number
2. Patient's weight, height, gender, and age
3. Tentative diagnosis and the reason for the study
4. Type of test requested and special requirements

Optimally, the exercise test should be discussed with the referring physician so the type of test and the reason for doing it are clear beforehand. In addition, the discussion helps one to decide whether the cycle or treadmill is the preferable form of ergometry, whether an arterial catheter is desired, and whether supplemental O_2 should be given during the exercise test. This is also a time at which the patient's medications, results of previous studies, special needs or limitations, and other details can be discussed. Other important information includes the specific complaints of the patient during exertion, and potential risks and contraindications to exercise.

At the time the exercise test is scheduled, the patient is advised to wear comfortable clothes and low heeled or athletic shoes, adhere to his or her usual medical regimen, eat a light meal 2 or more hours before arrival, and avoid cigarettes and coffee for at least 2 hours. The patient is given a brief description of the exercise test and told how long it will take and what to expect.

The Patient in the Exercise Laboratory

Preliminary Tests

Because spirometric data are used in the final report, the vital capacity (VC), inspiratory capacity (IC), forced expiratory volume in 1 second (FEV_1), and maximal voluntary ventilation (MVV) should be obtained when the patient arrives at the exercise laboratory (31). In patients with stable obstructive airway disease, recent spirometric values may be used. The direct MVV is calculated from a 12-second maneuver of rapid and deep breathing; the indirect

MVV is calculated by multiplying the FEV_1 by 40 (32). The MVV values are needed for determination of the exercise breathing reserve. In patients with inspiratory obstruction, neuromuscular disorders, and severe obesity, the direct MVV should be used even if it is considerably less than the indirect MVV. In other patients with poor spirometric efforts, the indirect MVV is usually a more reliable measure of ventilatory capacity.

The hemoglobin and carboxyhemoglobin levels should be known or measured and the DLCO measured in those patients with lung disease or dyspnea. An accurate shoeless height and weight are obtained.

Physician Evaluation

The physician should obtain relevant clinical information from the patient, with particular emphasis on medications, tobacco and recreational drug use, accustomed activity level, and the presence of angina pectoris or other exercise-induced symptoms. The physician should perform a focused examination with particular attention to the heart, lungs, peripheral pulses, and musculoskeletal system. The physician determines the type of exercise test and protocol on the basis of the exercise request, the clinical evaluation, review of the current ECG and other preliminary tests, and any other special considerations.

Informed consent for the exercise test must be obtained. The patient is told what to expect and that he or she will be asked to make a maximal effort (for most studies), but is advised that exercise can be stopped at any time. The patient is warned of potential discomfort and risks associated with the procedure, the kinds of information that will be obtained, and how this may benefit the patient. Finally, the patient is encouraged to ask questions about the testing before giving consent.

Equipment Familiarization

We find it particularly useful to familiarize the patient with the exercise testing equipment before starting the actual test. If the treadmill is used, time is provided for practice trials so the patient can get on and off the moving treadmill belt with confidence. If the cycle is used, the seat height is adjusted so the legs are nearly completely extended when the pedals are at their lowest point.

The mask or mouthpiece and nose clip are tried before the actual test. The patient is advised that it is acceptable to swallow with the mouthpiece in place or moisten the inside of the mouth with the tongue. We explain the importance of having a good seal of the lips around the mouthpiece or the mask about the face.

Ending the Exercise

We advise patients that they are in charge and can stop exercise if they feel distressed. Alternatively, we stop the exercise if we note important abnormalities. Because a mouthpiece or mask interferes with the ability of the patient to communicate verbally in response to questions regarding symptoms, the patient is taught to use the signal "thumb up" if everything is satisfactory and "thumb down" if he or she is experiencing any difficulty but does not wish to stop. The patient is advised to point to the site of discomfort (e.g., chest or leg).

Arterial Blood Sampling and Use of Catheter

If the study requires repeated arterial blood sampling, a catheter is inserted into a radial or brachial artery (see Appendix D for detailed description of how to place the catheter) (33). It is important to check radial and ulnar artery pulsations before and after catheter insertion. The catheter is attached to a stopcock and a blood pressure transducer via a continuous-flush device that provides a slow infusion of a heparin-containing solution (10 units/ml). When one uses a brachial artery catheter, the catheter should be long enough (20–25 cm) so that its hub can be brought around to the lateral aspect of the lower part of the upper arm (Fig. 6.3). The transducer is positioned on the upper arm at a height corresponding to the fourth interspace of the midclavicular line (midatrial level when the patient is upright). To avoid spurious dilution of the blood specimen with heparin-containing solution, about 0.5 ml of fluid is discarded before collecting each arterial blood sample (usually by letting the blood flow into gauze under arterial pressure before the syringe is connected to the stopcock). Each sample is collected over 10 to 20 seconds so that the gas tensions are representative of the mean arterial value and minimally influenced by respiratory variations in alveolar gas tensions. Immediately after sampling, the catheter lumen is flushed with heparinized saline. We usually sample blood at rest, at the end of 3 minutes of unloaded cycling or lowest-level treadmill exercise, every 2 minutes during the period of increasing work rate, and at 2 minutes of recovery.

After use, the arterial catheter is removed while keeping direct pressure over the puncture site for at least 5 to 10 minutes. When the pressure is removed, the site is inspected carefully for evidence of bleeding. With adequate pressure and observation after removal of the catheter, hematomas can be avoided. With any evidence of extravascular bleeding, pressure is continued for at least another 3 minutes. A light dressing covered with a firm elastic bandage is then applied over the puncture site, and the peripheral pulses are checked. The bandage should not be so tight as to obliterate the radial pulse (in the case of brachial artery punctures) or to make the hand colder than the contralateral hand (in the case of radial artery catheters). The patient is advised not to use that arm for heavy exercise for the next 24 hours. The dressing and elastic bandage can be removed by the patient at home after several hours have elapsed.

After an exercise test with blood sampling, it is advisable to review the blood gas results before discarding any remaining blood in the sampling syringes. This makes it possible to reanalyze samples in which the results are questionable.

PERFORMING THE EXERCISE TEST

The following sections describe several different protocols that are used for addressing various clinical questions. Most often, we use a maximum (symptom-limited) incremental exercise test on a cycle ergometer; this protocol is described in detail here. It addresses most clinical and fitness issues. However, if the patient is being evaluated for reasons such as detection of exercise-induced bronchospasm, value of oxygen supplementation in exercise, or other reasons, then other protocols may be appropriate.

Incremental Exercise Test to Symptom-Limited Maximum

In this protocol, the patient exercises on a cycle ergometer (or a treadmill) while measurements of gas exchange are made at rest, during 3 minutes of very low level exercise, and then while the work rate is increased each minute or continuously (ramp pattern). In general, the patient is encouraged by the technician and physician in attendance to continue as long as safely possible. Merely telling subjects that they are in control of how long they exercise, but further advising them that it is important for them to exercise to their maximum level, is suffi-

cient for most patients to go to their reproducible peak $\dot{V}_{O_2}$ or the level of exercise at which $\dot{V}_{O_2}$ no longer increases normally at 10 ml/min/ watt.

Selecting the Rate of Work Rate Increase

We select the rate of work rate increase after considering the patient's history (especially the amount and intensity of his or her daily activity), physical examination (notably obesity and evidence of cardiac or respiratory disease), and pulmonary function evaluation (particularly the FEV_1 and MVV). If we expect the patient to reach a near-normal power output, we estimate the $\dot{V}_{O_2}$ at unloaded pedaling from the patient's body weight and estimate the peak $\dot{V}_{O_2}$ from the patient's age and height. We then calculate the work rate increment necessary to reach the patient's estimated peak $\dot{V}_{O_2}$ in 10 minutes. The steps that we use to approximate the correct increment for the cycle are as follows.

1. $\dot{V}_{O_2}$ unloaded in ml per minute = 150 + (6 × weight in kg)
2. Peak $\dot{V}_{O_2}$ in ml per minute = (height in cm − age in years) × 20 for sedentary men and × 14 for sedentary women
3. Work rate increment per minute in watts = (peak $\dot{V}_{O_2}$ in ml/min − $\dot{V}_{O_2}$ unloaded in ml/min)/100

For example, given an apparently healthy sedentary man 180 cm in height, 100 kg in weight, and 50 years of age, his anticipated $\dot{V}_{O_2}$ unloaded in ml/min = 150 + 6 × 100 kg = 750 ml/min; his anticipated peak $\dot{V}_{O_2}$ = (180 − 50) × 20 = 2,600 ml/min. To achieve an incremental test duration of 10 minutes, we would use a work rate increment of (2,600 − 750)/100 = 18.5 W per minute. Practically, we would select an increment of 20 W per minute and expect the test duration to be slightly less than 10 minutes.

If we know that the patient has an MVV, FEV_1, or DLCO less than 80% of that predicted, we would consider reducing the expected peak $\dot{V}_{O_2}$ proportionally. For example, an MVV or DLCO that is 50% of predicted will reduce the expected peak $\dot{V}_{O_2}$ to roughly one-half to two-thirds of normal. If the patient has resting tachycardia, symptoms suggestive of angina, or evidence of chronic heart failure, we also reduce the expected peak $\dot{V}_{O_2}$, the amount being judged by our pre-exercise assessment of impairment. In each case we reduce the size of the work rate increment in an attempt to keep the total incremental exercise time at about 10 minutes.

Given a choice, however, we would rather overestimate than underestimate the work rate increment. With too large an increment, the test will be too brief, but the patient will recover quickly, an advantage if retesting is necessary. With too small an increment, however, the patient may stop for ambiguous reasons and may feel too fatigued for retesting. At this point, it is important to stress that we do not concern ourselves with hitting the duration of exercise right on the target of 10 minutes. We prefer it shorter rather than longer than the 10 minutes because we are likely to get a more reproducible and easier test for interpretation. For instance, selection of the *AT* will be more discrete. Exercise tests as short as 5 minutes can be satisfactorily interpreted.

Under very rare circumstances, when we expect patients to have extremely severe exercise limitation, we might use a special protocol in which, after the rest period, the external workload is incremented less rapidly than usual in the initial portion of the test. With this protocol, for the first 3 minutes of unloaded pedaling, the patient cycles at 20 rpm; for the fourth minute, at 40 rpm; and for the fifth minute, at 60 rpm. Throughout this portion of the test, an accessory motor attached to the cycle rotates the cycle flywheel at a speed of slightly over 60 rpm so that the exercise performed is truly unloaded exercise—that is, the energy required for just moving the legs. At the sixth minute, the accessory motor is turned off while the patient continues pedaling at 60 rpm, giving a slight load to the cycle. Starting with the seventh minute, the work rate is increased by 5 to 10 W per minute. This protocol allows the accumulation of more data at a very low metabolic rate, and frequently allows delineation of very low *AT* values that are otherwise unmeasurable. This problem may be found in patients with very obese legs, in whom unloaded pedaling at 60 rpm may cause the $\dot{V}_{O_2}$ to exceed 1.0 L per minute, and/or in patients with very severe cardiovascular or pulmonary disease. Using this protocol, we do not insist that the patient cycle smoothly at 20 and 40 rpm.

Resting Measures

A 12-lead ECG is obtained with the patient in the supine position. If an arterial catheter is placed, we obtain a blood specimen in the supine and sitting positions, before the patient breathes through the mouthpiece, to determine the effect of the mouthpiece on the breathing pattern and blood gases.

After the patient mounts the cycle or treadmill and is made comfortable, a nose clip is placed and checked for leaks, and the mouthpiece is inserted.

Heart rate (HR), breathing frequency (f), $\dot{V}_E$, $\dot{V}_{O_2}$, $\dot{V}_{CO_2}$, R, P_{ETO_2}, P_{ETCO_2}, and O_2 pulse ($\dot{V}_{O_2}$/HR) are printed out breath-by-breath every 10 seconds, or every quarter to half minute by averaging an integral number of whole breaths. HR, $\dot{V}_E$, $\dot{V}_{O_2}$, and $\dot{V}_{CO_2}$ are viewed on a screen as the data are collected. Alternatively, averaging can be done of second-by-second interpolation of breath-by-breath data. The measured and calculated variables are plotted after the test, as shown in Chapter 10. With an arterial catheter, arterial blood pressure is recorded continuously and arterial blood is sampled for blood gases, pH, lactate, cooximetry, and hemoglobin values at rest. If an arterial catheter is not used, blood pressure is obtained with a pressure cuff, and pulse oximeter values are recorded.

Unloaded Exercise and Cycling Rate

To overcome the inertia of the cycle flywheel with an electromagnetically braked cycle, an accessory motor (34) can be used to rotate the flywheel at a rate of slightly over 60 rpm while the patient's feet are motionless on the pedals. This unloads the cycle and eliminates the inertial force needed to start the flywheel rotating and reach the desired speed. This is particularly helpful for testing patients with limited strength in their legs. At a verbal signal, the patient begins 3 minutes of unloaded pedaling. The patient is advised to look at the rpm meter and to maintain a cycling speed of 60 rpm, or listen to the cadence of a metronome to establish the pedaling speed. Sometime after the patient has established the cycling rhythm, the motor controlling the flywheel speed is turned off so that the patient is now controlling the speed of the unloaded flywheel. A 12-lead ECG, blood pressure measurement, and, if the patient has an arterial catheter, a blood sample are obtained near the end of the 3 minutes of unloaded pedaling.

Incremental Exercise

Measurements are continued while the work rate is increased continuously (ramp) (35) or by a uniform amount each minute until the patient is limited by symptoms or the examiner believes that exercise cannot be continued safely (Fig. 6.4). An increment rate is selected depending on the expected performance of the patient. A 12-lead ECG and arterial samples for blood gas and pH measurement are or-

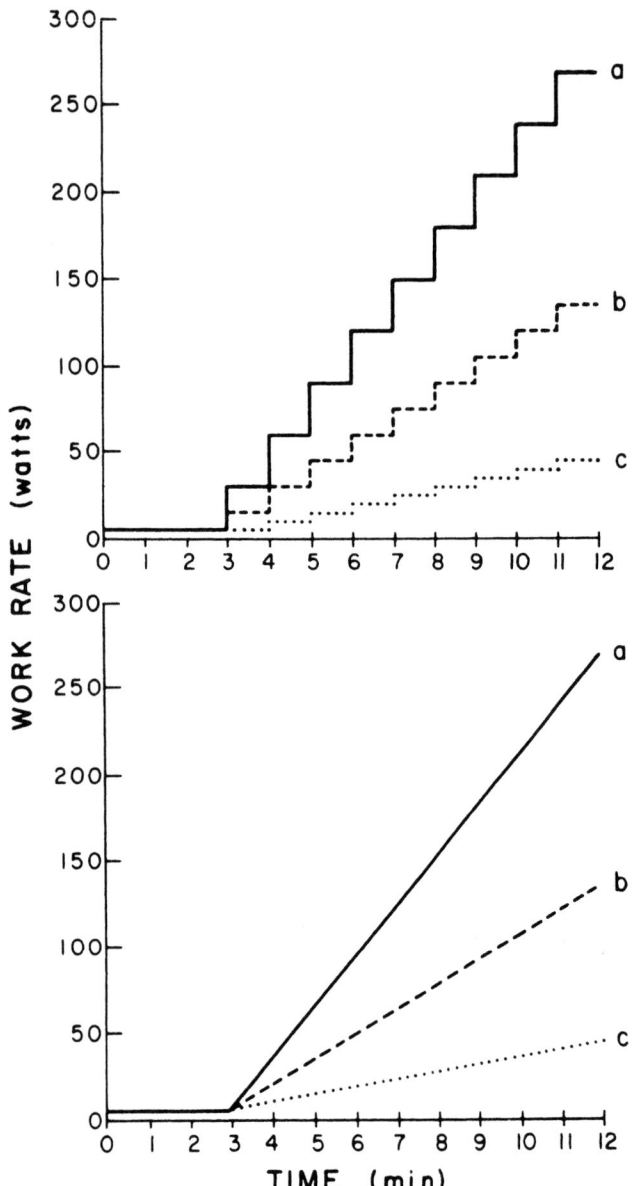

FIGURE 6.4.   One-minute incremental **(upper)** and ramp incremental **(lower)** protocols for cycle ergometry. In both cases, the subject initially cycles for 3 minutes of unloaded pedaling. In the example shown, the work rate is incremented 30 (*a*), 15 (*b*), or 5 (*c*) W per minute depending on the height, age, gender, and health of the subject. The increment is added at the start of each minute for the 1-minute test, whereas the increment is completed at the end of each minute for the ramp test. Larger or intermediate increments can also be used. The cycle is returned to the unloaded setting when the cycling frequency cannot be maintained over 40 rpm or when the physician or subject decides to terminate the incremental exercise.

dinarily obtained every 2 minutes. The technician and physician work cooperatively in observing the patient's facial expression, checking the blood pressure and ECG recordings for untoward changes and arrhythmia, looking for nose or mouthpiece leaks, observing for signals of distress from the pa-

tient, and quietly encouraging the patient to maximize his or her performance. This is done by commenting on the satisfactory nature of the study, and encouraging patients to do their best, but to stop when they feel that they must. The resistance of the cycle is removed if the patient evidences distress, if there is a fall in systolic or mean blood pressure greater than 10 mm Hg, if a significant arrhythmia develops, or if the patient has ST segment depression of 3 mm or greater. The exercise is also terminated if the patient is unable to maintain cycling frequency above 40 rpm. If practical and indicated, an arterial blood sample is obtained during the last half minute of exercise.

Recovery

We ask the patient to continue to breathe through the mouthpiece during at least 2 minutes of recovery. In the immediate postexercise period, the patient is advised to continue to pedal at a slow frequency without a load on the ergometer. This prevents the precipitous fall in blood pressure and light-headedness that are often experienced and the increases in arrhythmias that may occur when vigorous exercise is abruptly terminated. If arterial blood is being sampled, a final sample is obtained at 2 minutes of recovery.

Postexercise Questioning and Review

At the conclusion of the test and soon after removal of the mouthpiece (after at least 2 minutes of recovery gas exchange measurements), the physician should question the patient in a nonleading fashion about what symptoms caused him or her to stop exercise. A series of questions may be required to assess just what the patient means by his or her limiting symptoms. For example, it is important to differentiate calf from thigh pain and to determine the exact character of any chest discomfort. In particular, it is always worthwhile to find out if the symptoms reproduce the complaints of exertional dyspnea or exertional chest pain or other discomfort experienced by the patient outside the laboratory.

If, on review of the data, it appears that a symptom-limited test was terminated prematurely because of inadequate patient effort, a repeat test after a recovery period of 30 to 45 minutes may be indicated. For instance, if the patient made an insufficient effort, as suggested by the combination of high breathing and heart rate reserves, a low R, and only a slight fall in arterial bicarbonate, measured directly or from the V-slope plot, the test bears repeating with greater encouragement from the examiner. In these repeat tests, the reproducibility of the patient's performance should be examined.

Critique of Incremental Tests

Balke and colleagues introduced the use of 1-minute incremental treadmill tests for the study of fitness in a large military population (36,37). Although Balke initially used a 1% increment in grade per minute with a constant treadmill speed of 3.3 mph, he also used a 2% increment in grade every minute. Several investigators, including Consolazio et al. (38), Jones (39), and Spiro (40), used the cycle ergometer with the work rate incremented an equal amount every minute or half minute. Increments of 8, 15, 17, or 25 W per minute, 10 W per half minute, or 4 W every 15 seconds have been reported (41). We introduced the use of a continuously incrementing (ramp-pattern) exercise protocol (35,42) and have used it extensively in adults and children (43).

In comparing the ramp test with 1-, 2-, and 3-minute step increments at the same overall average work rate increase, Zhang et al. (44) have shown that no significant differences were found in the $\dot{V}O_2$max, *AT*, peak $\dot{V}E$, peak HR, $\Delta\dot{V}O_2/\Delta WR$, or exercise duration among the four protocols in healthy subjects. Step patterns in some measures could be seen in the 2- and 3-minute step protocols, however (see Fig. 4.3). Thus, although any of these protocols might be used, either the ramp or the 1-minute incremental test seems practical and preferable for patients, because they do not feel sudden increases in work rate.

Several investigators (45,46) have stressed the desirability of adjusting the work rate increment according to the patient's cardiorespiratory status. Tests that are too brief (i.e., with the work rate increased too rapidly) may not allow a sufficient quantity of data to be accumulated. Tests that are too long (i.e., with too small a work rate increase) are likely to be terminated prematurely because of boredom or "seat discomfort." We found that tests in which the incremental part of the protocol is completed between 6 and 12 minutes give the highest peak $\dot{V}O_2$ in normal subjects (47). Longer or shorter tests are likely to give slightly lower values. We know of no similar study in patients with heart or lung disease; we assume that the findings would be similar in such patients. Therefore, we attempt to select a work rate increment that will result in termination of the incremental part of the exercise test

in 8 to 10 minutes, but tests as short as 6 minutes are acceptable.

Some investigators have expressed concern as to whether the peak $\dot{V}O_2$ is as high in continuous incremental protocols as in discontinuous protocols and whether the highest $\dot{V}O_2$ reached (peak $\dot{V}O_2$) should be identified as the $\dot{V}O_2$max. Taylor et al. (48) defined the $\dot{V}O_2$max from a series of progressively higher constant work rate tests. They defined the $\dot{V}O_2$max as the $\dot{V}O_2$ when an increase in work rate resulted in an increase of $\dot{V}O_2$ of less than 150 ml per minute above the $\dot{V}O_2$ from the previous lower work rate. This criterion is appropriate for tests in fit subjects using large work rate increments, such as a 2.5% grade change at a treadmill speed of 7 mph. In tests featuring a 15 W per minute increase in work rate, however, the rate of increase in $\dot{V}O_2$ is normally only 150 ml per minute. Therefore, at increments of 15 W per minute or less, it is invalid to use the criterion of Taylor et al. to determine whether the peak $\dot{V}O_2$ is indeed the $\dot{V}O_2$max.

A single study (49) reported an approximately 10% lower peak $\dot{V}O_2$ using a continuous rather than a discontinuous graded work rate test; however, the long duration (20 to 30 minutes) of these continuous tests could have accounted for the reduction (46). In contrast, Maksud (50), Wyndham (51), and McArdle (52) and their associates found no difference in peak $\dot{V}O_2$ measured in continuous incremental tests compared with discontinuous constant work rate treadmill tests. Pollack and colleagues (53) found a plateau in $\dot{V}O_2$ in 59% to 69% of the continuous incremental treadmill tests they administered. We found a similar peak $\dot{V}O_2$ in normal men using a ramp-pattern increase in cycle ergometer tests, whether the increase was 20, 30, or 50 W per minute (42). Thus, we believe that the $\dot{V}O_2$max can be approximated with continuous incremental protocols of the proper duration.

Using the ramp-pattern test, we also found that the *AT*, time constant for $\dot{V}O_2$, work efficiency, maximum $\dot{V}E$, and maximum HR were comparable to values found with constant work rate tests (35,42). Because we were concerned that non-steady-state incremental exercise tests might give different values for $\dot{V}E$, $\dot{V}O_2$, $\dot{V}CO_2$, $P(A - a)O_2$, $P(a - ET)CO_2$, and HR as compared to steady state, we studied 23 men (11 normal, 9 with obstructive lung disease, and 3 with restrictive lung disease) during steady-state constant work rate and 1-minute incremental exercise tests (Table 6.2) (54). The steady-state exercise $P(A - a)O_2$ values ranged from 1 to 43 mm Hg, and the VD/VT values ranged from 0.12 to 0.44. We found

TABLE 6.2.   Effect of Protocol on Measurements of Pao_2, P(A − a)o_2, and VD/VT During Cycling at the Same Mean V̇o_2 (0.92 ± 0.03 L/min)

		Pao_2, mm Hg		P(A − a)o_2, mm Hg		VD/VT	
	N	Incr.[a]	Constant[b]	Incr.	Constant	Incr.	Constant
Normal	11	89	94	14	13	0.26	0.25
Restrictive lung disease	3	87	89	18	21	0.21	0.19
Obstructive lung disease	9	79	83	25	22	0.32	0.32
All subjects	23	85[c]	89	19	17	0.27	0.28

[a]1-minute incremental exercise protocol.
[b]Constant work rate protocol; measurements were made at 6 minutes.
[c]Indicates significant difference between 1-minute incremental (Incr.) and constant work rate test at $p < 0.05$ by paired t-test; other measurements are not significantly different.
Data are from Furuike AN, Sue DY, Hansen JE, et al. Comparison of physiologic dead space/tidal volume ratio and alveolar-arterial Po_2 difference during incremental and constant work exercise. *Am Rev Respir Dis* 1982;126:579–583.

that V̇co_2, V̇E, Pao_2, and R were slightly lower during incremental exercise than constant work rate exercise at the same V̇o_2. These differences were anticipated and can be fully explained by the differences in kinetics of V̇o_2, V̇co_2, and V̇E in incremental versus constant work exercise. The P(A − a)o_2, P(a − ET)co_2, Paco_2, V̇E/V̇co_2, and VD/VT values were in close agreement in both protocols for both the normal subjects and the patients, however. Thus, it is possible to make measurements of gas exchange and ventilation–perfusion matching equally well during incremental or steady-state exercise.

With rapid incremental tests, frequent and accurate measurements are needed. Blood pressure and HR are not difficult to measure. Accurate measurement of V̇E, V̇co_2, and V̇o_2 requires special thought and understanding of the properties of the measuring devices. The reader is referred to Beaver et al. (1,55) and Sue et al. (2) for an analysis of potential errors.

Constant Work Rate Exercise Tests

Exercise tests performed with the patient or subject exercising at a constant work rate may be useful in particular situations. The selection of the appropriate work rate depends on the question being addressed and the number of different work rates that are chosen. Constant work rate exercise tests may be helpful in determining V̇$o_2$max or the lactic acidosis threshold, measuring gas exchange kinetics, diagnosing exercise-induced bronchospasm, and assessing the contribution of the carotid bodies to exercise hyperpnea.

Determining V̇$o_2$max

Historically, discontinuous constant work rate tests, each with a large increase in work rate with intervening rest periods, were used to measure V̇$o_2$max (56). The advantages of determining V̇$o_2$max from progressively greater constant work rate tests are as follows: (a) The higher-intensity work rates selected can be based on the patient's cardiovascular and ventilatory responses to the lower work rate tests; (b) timed manual bag collection of mixed expired gas for measurement of V̇co_2 and V̇o_2 near the end of each exercise does not require rapidly responding gas analyzers; and (c) failure of the V̇o_2 to increase despite an increase in work rate provides unequivocal identification of V̇$o_2$max. The disadvantages are the following: (a) The repeated tests take considerable time for patient, physician, and technician; (b) these tests are exhausting and may be more likely to result in injury to the patient; and (c) although such tests are often considered "steady-state" tests, this cannot be true at work rates at or above that necessary to ensure a V̇$o_2$max, and likely at any work rate accompanied by a significant lactic acidosis.

Measuring Gas Exchange Kinetics

Constant work rate tests are ideal for measuring cardiovascular, ventilatory, and gas exchange kinetics. Measurement of these variables, especially V̇o_2, during the transition from rest to low-level exercise or between two levels of exercise using breath-by-breath analysis allows measurements of time constants or half-times of response (57). Averaging the data obtained from several breath-by-breath tests may be necessary for adequate precision (58,59).

Sietsema et al. (3) used such a protocol to demonstrate striking reductions in the $\dot{V}O_2$ increase during the first 20 seconds after exercise onset in patients with cyanotic congenital heart disease. In normal subjects, the magnitude and mean response time (MRT) of $\dot{V}O_2$ correlated well with the fitness (peak $\dot{V}O_2/kg$) of the individual; the lower the peak $\dot{V}O_2/kg$, the longer the MRT for constant work rates of 100 W or higher (60). Similarly, Ben-Dov et al. (61) demonstrated significantly lower increases in $\dot{V}O_2$ in the first 20 seconds of constant work rate exercise in hyperthyroidism, despite the overall higher metabolic requirement of the disease. At higher constant work rates, Koike et al. (62) demonstrated the lengthening of the $\dot{V}O_2$ time constant as carboxyhemoglobin levels were increased.

Determining Anaerobic Threshold

The measurement of $\dot{V}O_2$ kinetics over a 6-minute period of constant work rate can also be useful. If the *AT* is uncertain after incremental testing, a constant work rate test can be performed at a work level expected to approximate the individual's *AT*. If the work rate turns out to be above the individual's *AT*, the $\dot{V}O_2$ will not plateau by the end of the third minute, but will continue to rise (63). The degree of rise will be greater the further the work level is above the *AT* and correlates highly with the extent of the developed lactic acidosis (see Figs. 2.51 and 4.25) (64,65). Repeated testing at one or two other constant work rate levels should allow an accurate determination of the *AT*.

Several studies have shown the utility of precisely assessing the *AT* and the $\Delta\dot{V}O_2$ (6 − 3) to disorders in O_2 transport. Casaburi et al. (66) showed the advantage of training patients with chronic obstructive pulmonary disease with constant work rates above rather than below their *AT*s. Koike et al. (62) demonstrated increases in the $\Delta\dot{V}O_2$ (6 − 3) with reductions in hemoglobin availability for transport of O_2, while Zhang et al. (67) showed a positive correlation between the $\Delta\dot{V}O_2$ (6 − 3) and the severity of heart failure in patients with chronic stable heart failure.

Detecting Exercise-Induced Bronchospasm

Although exercise-induced bronchospasm can often be demonstrated after the usual incremental testing in the afflicted individual, it may be more evident after 6 minutes of near-maximal constant-load exercise (68). It is necessary to obtain good baseline measurements of FEV_1 or some other index of airway obstruction immediately before exercise. Most investigators prefer the treadmill to the cycle ergometer for inducing postexercise bronchospasm, although we have used both successfully. To induce postexercise bronchospasm, it is our practice to increase the work rate to approximately 80% of the predicted maximal work rate after a 1-minute warm-up at a lower work rate. The patient inspires dry air from a bag filled from a tank of compressed air rather than room air because, according to current concepts, dry air aids in the induction of bronchospasm and reduces day-to-day variability if repeated tests are necessary (69). After 6 minutes of heavy exercise, the mouthpiece is immediately removed. Spirometric tracings are obtained as soon as possible and at 3, 6, 10, 15, and 20 minutes after exercise.

Measuring Carotid Body Contribution to Exercise Ventilation

The effect of carotid body input to the medullary respiratory centers can be assessed by altering the PO_2 of the blood reaching the carotid bodies (70). Normally, if the carotid bodies are contributing significantly to ventilatory drive, a rise in carotid artery PO_2 will immediately reduce the carotid body neural outflow and depress ventilation transiently. This can be detected by an immediate fall in $\dot{V}E$, V_T, and f and a rise in $PETCO_2$ approximately 6 to 10 seconds after an unobtrusive switch of inspiratory gas from room air to 100% O_2 (see Fig. 4.29). After 1 minute of 100% O_2 breathing, a switch back to room air results in a return to baseline $\dot{V}E$ and $PETCO_2$ values. Online recording of V_T, f, and gas concentrations, breath by breath, is desirable.

Because ventilation is less variable during exercise than at rest, we prefer to perform these measurements during constant work rate exercise of moderate intensity. Steady-state levels of $\dot{V}E$ at moderate exercise are usually attained in less than 5 minutes. Thus, the effect of the change in FIO_2 can be more clearly detected and quantified during exercise. Maximal inhibitory effect is usually seen with an increase in PaO_2 to 250 mm Hg or more. Usually, with normal arterial O_2 saturation, $\dot{V}E$ will decrease transiently by about 15%. If a pneumotachograph is used to determine ventilation, an adjustment must be made in calculating the ventilatory decrease to account for the 11% higher gas viscosity of 100% O_2 than air. The flowmeters of some commercial systems automatically correct for this difference in gas viscosity with changing O_2 concentration. This can be documented by calibrating with a known volume of air and O_2 and determining if there is a difference in recorded volume.

Treadmill Test for Detecting Myocardial Ischemia

Protocols

Bruce (71), Ellestad (72), Naughton (73), and their colleagues and other cardiologists have developed and popularized several incremental treadmill protocols for inducing and detecting ECG changes consistent with myocardial ischemia.

The Bruce protocol (Fig. 6.5C) begins with 3-minute stages of walking at 1.7 mph at 0%, 5%, or 10% grade (71). The 0% and 5% grades are omitted in more fit individuals. Thereafter, the grade is incremented 2% every 3 minutes and the speed is incremented 0.8 mph every 3 minutes until the treadmill reaches 18% grade and 5 mph. After this, the speed is increased by 0.5 mph every 3 minutes.

Ellestad's protocol (Fig. 6.5E) uses seven periods, each of 2 or 3 minutes' duration, at progressively increasing speeds of 1.7, 3, 4, 5, 6, 7, and 8 mph. The grade is 10% for the first four periods, with durations of 3, 2, 2, and 3 minutes, respectively, and 15% grade for the last three periods, each of 2 minutes' duration (72).

Naughton's protocol (Fig. 6.5A) uses ten exercise periods of 3 minutes' duration, each separated by rest periods of 3 minutes (73). The grade and speed of each period are as follows: 0% and 1 mph; 0% and 1.5 mph; 0% and 2 mph; 3.5% and 2 mph; 7% and 2 mph; 5% and 3 mph; 7.5% and 3 mph; 10% and 12.5% and 3 mph; and 15% and 3 mph.

In each of the foregoing treadmill protocols, blood pressure is measured and a multiple-lead ECG is recorded at each work rate and during recovery. The patient is carefully observed, and the test is terminated at the physician's discretion (e.g., for decline in blood pressure, significant ventricular arrhythmia, progressive ST segment changes, or attainment of a given HR) or by the patient's symptoms.

Itoh et al. (74) and Belardinelli et al. (75) have advanced the application of the exercise ECG in diagnosing myocardial ischemia by combining it with gas exchange measurements. They found that accompanying changes in the ECG, the $\dot{V}O_2$–work rate relation becomes more shallow, providing evidence of myocardial dyskinesis.

Critique

These treadmill tests have the advantage of extensive clinical use. A survey in 1977 concluded that the complication rate for such "exercise stress testing" was 3.6 myocardial infarctions, 4.8 serious arrhythmias, and 0.5 deaths per 10,000 tests (76). In this survey, the treadmill was the ergometer used most often (71%), and the favorite protocol (65%) was that of Bruce.

The peak $\dot{V}O_2$ is generally 5% to 11% higher with treadmill as compared with cycle ergometer testing (1), whereas maximum HR is similar. As usually performed, $\dot{V}E$, breathing pattern, $\dot{V}O_2$, and gas exchange are not measured during these tests, so other important information on cardiovascular and pulmonary system function is not available. Bruce et al. have shown a high correlation of maximum $\dot{V}O_2$ and duration of treadmill exercise in their normal population (77). Nevertheless, it is invalid to consider the duration of exercise a measure of peak $\dot{V}O_2$ in patients suspected of having cardiovascular disease. The unequal duration of increment and variability in increment size are disadvantages of these tests, although interpretation is usually not based on measurements of $\dot{V}O_2$. In addition, HR itself is a poor measure of exercise intensity in many patients with heart disease. Administration of β-adrenergic blocking drugs also modifies the HR–work rate relationship and must be taken into account when interpreting the results of exercise tests.

Rather than using the foregoing protocol for treadmill testing, Jones (39) and we (47) have used constant treadmill speed and have incremented the grade by a constant amount each minute for the entire study. After 3 minutes of warm-up at zero grade and a comfortable walking speed (which may range from 0.8 to 4.5 mph, depending on our assessment of the patient's fitness), we use a constant grade increment of 1%, 2%, or 3% each minute to the patient's maximum tolerance. We scale speed and grade so the test will end approximately 10 minutes after we begin to increment the treadmill grade (Fig. 6.4F).

We have successfully used protocols recommended by Porszasz et al. (78) designed to linearize the increase in work rate. These protocols initially use a slower speed and grade for the 3 minutes of "warm-up," followed by a ramp or minute-by-minute increment in either speed or grade, or both, to maximal toleration. We, of course, also make measurements of $\dot{V}E$, $\dot{V}CO_2$, and $\dot{V}O_2$. Following an initial delay of about 45 seconds after the increment be-

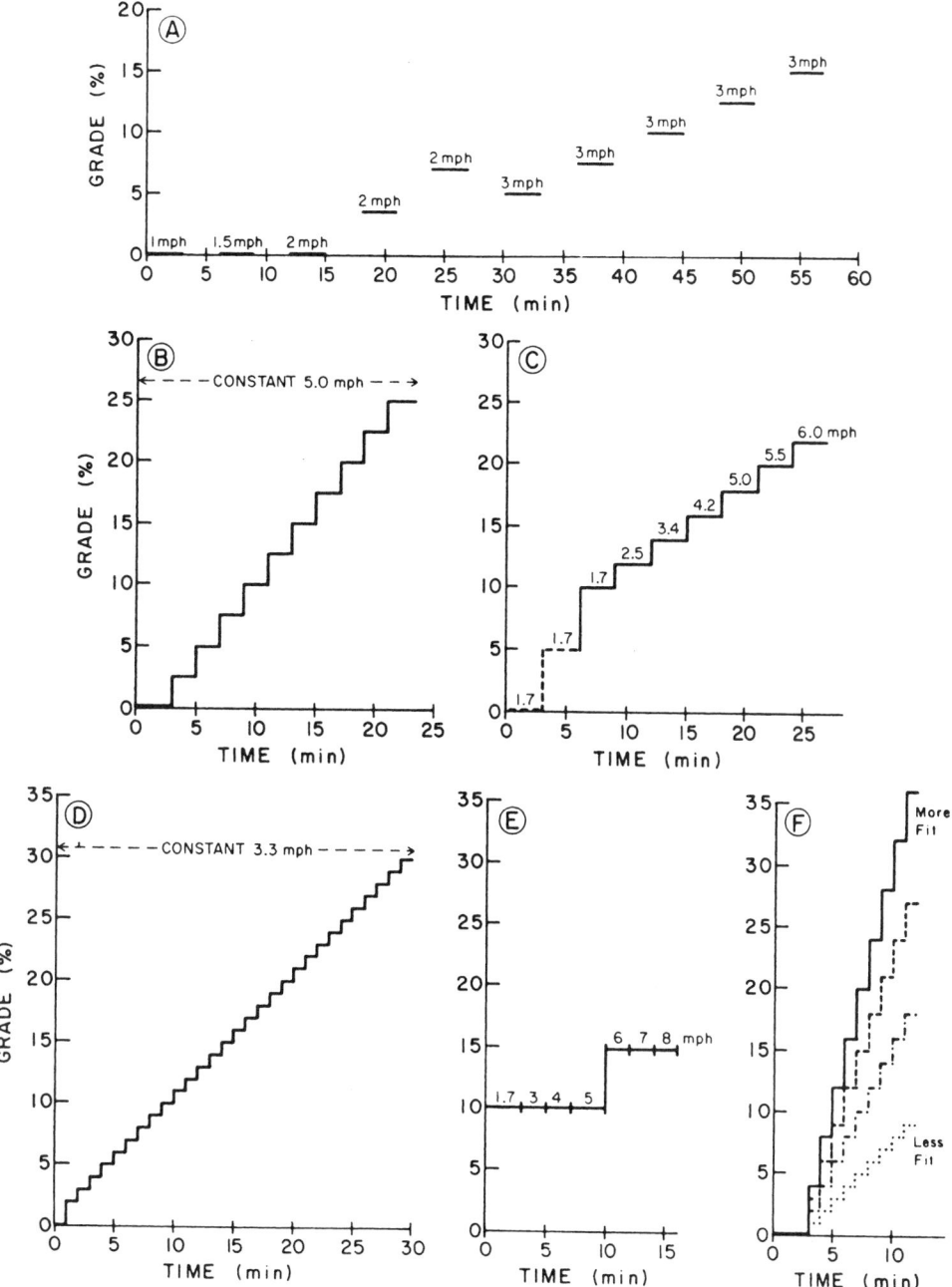

FIGURE 6.5. Several treadmill protocols. **A:** Naughton protocol. Three-minute exercise periods of increasing work rate alternate with 3-minute rest periods. The exercise periods vary in grade and speed. **B:** Astrand protocol. The speed is constant at 5 mph. After 3 minutes at 0% grade, the grade is increased 2.5% every 2 minutes. **C:** Bruce protocol. Grade and speed are changed every 3 minutes. The 0% and 5% grades are omitted in healthier subjects. **D:** Balke protocol. After 1 minute at 0% grade and 1 minute at 2% grade, the grade is increased 1% per minute, all at a speed of 3.3 mph. **E:** Ellestad protocol. The initial grade is 10% and the later grade is 15%, while the speed is increased every 2 or 3 minutes. **F:** Harbor protocol. After 3 minutes of walking at a comfortable speed, the grade is increased at a constant preselected amount each minute—1%, 2%, or 3%—so that the subject reaches his or her peak $\dot{V}O_2$ in approximately 10 minutes.

gins, the above protocols give a relatively linear increase in $\dot{V}O_2$ in normal subjects. The additional measurements allow us to calculate values such as peak $\dot{V}O_2$, *AT*, R, maximum $\dot{V}E/MVV$, $\dot{V}E/\dot{V}O_2$, $\dot{V}E/\dot{V}CO_2$, and O_2 pulse, thus adding considerable insight into gas exchange, ventilatory, and cardiovascular function.

Arm Ergometry

Method

Arm exercise protocols similar to those for lower extremity exercise are usually done because of dysfunction of the lower extremities. The usual technique is to use a converted cycle ergometer with the axle placed at or below the level of the shoulders while the subject sits or stands and moves the pedals so the arms are alternately fully extended. The most common frequency is 50 rpm. Occasionally, upper extremity exercise is performed using wheelchair wheels coupled to a cycle ergometer or by rowing, paddling, or swimming. These modes may be particularly useful for paraplegics, oarsmen, or athletes. To obtain maximal cardiovascular and respiratory stress, arm cycling must be done concurrently with lower extremity exercise.

If the person performing the test is healthy and has not undergone specific upper extremity training, the peak $\dot{V}O_2$ for arm cycling will approximate 50% to 70% of that for leg cycling (79–82). The *AT* for most healthy subjects is also lower. Maximum $\dot{V}E$ is similarly reduced, whereas maximum HR is only 2% to 12% less than with leg cycle exercise. Thus, the maximum O_2 pulse is less with arm than with leg cycling.

Critique

Although arm cycling exercise has occasional uses, it does not stress the cardiovascular and respiratory systems as much as leg cycling or treadmill exercise. As such, it is a poor substitute when one assesses the cardiovascular and respiratory systems, except when lower extremity exercise is impossible.

Other Tests Suitable for Fitness or Serial Evaluations

A variety of tests have been used to evaluate individuals or groups without attempting to ascertain whether a particular system (e.g., cardiovascular, respiratory, or musculoskeletal) or the motivation of the performer is limiting exercise. Such tests are likely to be used for children, young adults, military personnel, or laborers exposed to environmental stress or pollutants (Fig. 6.5B, D). These tests are often considered measures of cardiovascular fitness and may allow division of the population studied into several levels of fitness, but they can also be used to serially evaluate patients with known disorders. Formerly, these tests could be repeated frequently only with simple equipment. Now, gas exchange measurements with telemetry are possible.

Harvard Step Test and Modifications

The original Harvard step test consisted of having the subject step up and down at a uniform rate of 30 step-ups per minute onto a platform 20 inches

high for a period of 5 minutes, if possible, with measurements of pulse rate for 30 seconds after 1 minute of recovery (23). Modifications include (a) the addition of backpacks that add approximately one-third to the subject's weight, (b) reduction in the duration of the test to 3 minutes, (c) reduction in the step height to 17 inches for women, (d) measurement of HR during exercise, (e) change in the time of measurement of recovery pulse, (f) change in test scoring, and (g) use of a gradational step in which the height of the platform can be raised 2 cm every minute or 4.5 cm every 2 minutes (23,83,84).

Six-Hundred-Yard Run-Walk

The 600-yard run-walk requires that the subject cover a 600-yard level distance in the shortest possible time (85). He or she may intersperse running with walking but must try to finish as quickly as possible. A properly marked track or football field is suitable. For 87 male university staff and faculty members, time for completion showed a moderately good correlation ($r = 0.644$) with their peak $\dot{V}O_2$ measured by an incremental cycle ergometer test (which ranged from 25 to 50 ml/min/kg).

Twelve-Minute Field Test

In the 12-minute field performance test, the subjects, dressed in running attire, cover as much distance as possible by running or walking (86). The distance covered was shown to correlate well ($r = 0.897$) with $\dot{V}O_2$max measured during an intermittent incremental treadmill test in 115 military personnel ($\dot{V}O_2$max range of 30 to 60 ml/min/kg) (86).

Twelve-Minute Walk Test

The distance covered in 12 minutes of walking (equivalent to the original 12-minute field test described by Cooper) has been used for assessing disability in patients with chronic bronchitis (87). Each patient is instructed to cover as much distance as possible on foot in 12 minutes, for example, walking over a marked course in a hospital corridor. The patient is told to try to keep going, but not to be concerned if he or she has to slow down or stop to rest. The aim is for the patient to feel that at the end of the test, he or she could not have covered more ground in the time given. A physician or therapist accompanies the patient, acting as timekeeper and giving encouragement as necessary.

Daily repetitions of the 12-minute test in 12 hospital in-patients on three different days showed a significant improvement in distance on day 2 over day 1, but not on day 3 over day 2 (61). In 35 patients with lung disease, the distance correlated significantly with peak $\dot{V}O_2$ ($r = 0.52$), maximum exercise $\dot{V}E$ ($r = 0.53$), and FVC ($r = 0.406$), but not with FEV_1 ($r = 0.283$) (87).

Six-Minute Walk Test

The 6-minute walk test evolved in the 1980s as a less strenuous test than the 12-minute walk test, suitable for patients with heart and lung disorders (88). It is a relatively simple self-paced test useful for measuring the response to interventions in patients with known disease. It requires a flat, hard surface, such as a long indoor hallway at least 100 feet in length, over which the patient travels back and forth as rapidly as he or she can with fixed encouragement by a monitor. Testing should be performed only where a rapid response to an emergency is possible. Patients with unstable angina or recent myocardial infarctions should not be tested (88).

TABLE 6.3.   Recommendations for Final Report on an Exercise Test Patient

Recommendation for the Report	Example
A. Patient and Pretest Information	
Patient's exercise-related complaint or the limitation being addressed by the exercise test	"Patient experiences shortness of breath while walking up hills."
The specific question being addressed by the requested exercise test (often raised by a referring physician)	"What is the degree of exercise limitation?" "Can my patient tolerate a pneumonectomy?" "Should oxygen be prescribed for my patient during exercise?" "Has the new medication improved exercise capacity?"
Pertinent clinical information that may be helpful in relating to the interpretation	Type of exercise limitation noted by the patient (fatigue, chest pain, dyspnea). Level of physical activity in a normal day's routine. Medications. Occupational history.
Findings from a focused physical examination	Blood pressure, chest and heart examination. Patient's actual height and weight.
Results of other studies relevant to exercise capacity, especially if they contribute to developing the interpretation and conclusions	Resting electrocardiograms, chest roentgenograms, pulmonary function tests, echocardiograms.
Recent information	Recent food or medications? VC, IC, FEV_1, MVV on day of testing.
Pretest diagnosis	COPD, coronary artery disease, asthma, claudication.
B. Information About the Exercise Laboratory	
Exercise laboratory equipment	Type of ergometer used. Measurements made.
Exercise protocol	Progressive or constant work rate. Was oxygen supplementation used?
Documentation of other procedures performed in the laboratory, if any	Arterial catheter, pulmonary artery catheter, pulse oximetry, electrocardiograms, postexercise spirometry, noninvasive blood pressure measurements.
C. Observations During and After the Exercise Test	
Patient's effort during exercise test	Good effort.
Reason(s) for stopping exercise	Why did the patient stop? Was the test stopped by the patient or the physician? Ask whether the symptoms duplicated the symptoms that ordinarily limit exercise.
Data displays	Graphs and tables of data obtained during exercise test. Summary tables of most important information.
D. Exercise Test Interpretation	
Maximum exercise capacity	Absolute $\dot{V}O_2$ (ml/min), $\dot{V}O_2$ relative to size (ml/min/kg) and relative to normal subject (% predicted).
Comment on cardiovascular function, ventilation–perfusion mismatching, and breathing pattern and reserve, from the data presented in the nine-panel graphical array	Which functions are abnormal? Does $\dot{V}O_2$ increase normally as related to work rate? Is ventilatory efficiency normal? Was breathing pattern chaotic or ordered?
Link symptom when stopping to pathophysiology, and link pathophysiology to a clinical diagnosis	"The $\dot{V}O_2$ abruptly stopped increasing normally when the ST segments of Std II and III and V_4–V_6 of the ECG started to become depressed. Ventilatory efficiency and breathing reserve were normal. These findings are supportive of myocardial ischemia during exercise at the level of work that the patient stopped exercise because of body fatigue."

COPD, chronic obstructive pulmonary disease; FEV_1, forced expired volume in 1 second; IC, inspiratory capacity; MVV, maximal voluntary ventilation; VC, vital capacity.

The distance covered correlates reasonably well with gas exchange measures of peak $\dot{V}O_2$ measured during incremental tests (89), and even better when the weight of the patient is factored into the distance covered (90). In a large trial of patients with chronic obstructive pulmonary disease, the distance covered during the tests on the day after the first test improved by 7% ± 15%, indicating a significant learning effect (91). The test does not discriminate between the different organ systems that may limit activity, and is therefore not a diagnostic test. However, it has been successfully used in evaluating patients with lung resection, pulmonary rehabilitation, heart failure, pulmonary hypertension, cystic fibrosis, peripheral vascular disease, and obstructive lung disease (88).

PREPARING THE REPORT

In our laboratory, after entry of blood gas and blood pressure values, the computer system produces graphical and tabular displays of the results of the exercise study similar to those shown in Chapter 10. Consistency of format facilitates interpretation. The layout of the nine-panel graphical array allows one to quickly review the cardiovascular and ventilatory systems, ventilation–perfusion relations, and exercise metabolism. The addition of ECG and blood pressure data usually leads to a pathophysiological diagnosis.

The textual report we prepare includes brief summaries of relevant clinical information and medications, specific exercise-related complaints, pulmonary function test results, a brief description of the methods and procedure, a table of key gas exchange variables, and a narrative analysis and interpretation. We also include a glossary of terms found on the report that may be unfamiliar to some referring physicians. Our recommendations regarding information to be included in the final report are listed in Table 6.3.

SUMMARY

Numerous exercise devices, protocols, and physiological measuring systems are available for the safe and economical evaluation of normal individuals, athletes, or patients suspected of having (or known to have) respiratory, cardiovascular, or neuromuscular disease. The specific exercise performed can be tailored to the diagnostic or therapeutic questions being asked and the facilities and technical and professional expertise available. Ordinarily, a maximum amount of information can be obtained by making ventilatory, gas exchange, ECG, blood pressure, and blood gas measurements during a cycle or treadmill test that includes measurements sitting or standing at rest, followed by unloaded cycling or treadmill walking for 3 minutes, further followed by ramp or 1-minute incremental exercise with an increment size enabling the subject to reach his or her maximally tolerated work rate in about 10 minutes, and finally ending in a 2- to 3-minute recovery period. Less frequently, constant work rate tests, arm ergometry, or timed walking tests may be useful.

References

1. Beaver WL, Wasserman K, Whipp BJ. On-line computer analysis and breath-by-breath graphical display of exercise function tests. *J Appl Physiol* 1973;34:128–132.
2. Sue DY, Hansen JE, Blais M, Wasserman K. Measurement and analysis of gas exchange during exercise using a programmable calculator. *J Appl Physiol* 1980; 49:456–461.
3. Sietsema KE, Cooper DM, Rosove MH, Perloff JK, Child JS, Canobbio MM, Whipp BJ, Wasserman K. Dynamics of oxygen uptake during exercise in adults with cyanotic congenital heart disease. *Circulation* 1986;73:1137–1144.
4. Finucane KE, Egan BA, Dawson SV. Linearity and frequency response of pneumotachographs. *J Appl Physiol* 1972;32:121–126.
5. Porszasz J, Barstow T, Wasserman K. Evaluation of a symmetrically disposed Pitot tube flowmeter for measuring gas flow during exercise. *J Appl Physiol* 1994; 77:2659–2665.
6. Yoshiya I, Nakajima T, Nagai I, Jitsukawa S. A bidirectional respiratory flowmeter using the hot-wire principle. *J Appl Physiol* 1975;38:360–365.
7. Yoshiya I, Shimada Y, Tanaka K. Evaluation of a hot-wire respiratory flowmeter for clinical applicability. *J Appl Physiol* 1979;47:1131–1135.
8. Hansen JE. Exercise instruments, schemes, and protocols for evaluating the dyspneic patient. *Am Rev Respir Dis* 1984;129(Suppl):S25–S27.
9. Astrand I. Aerobic work capacity in men and women with special reference to age. *Acta Physiol Scand* 1960; 49(Suppl 169):1–9.
10. Clark JS, Votteri B, Arriagno RL, Cheung P, Eichhorn JH, Fallat RJ, Lee SE, Newth CJL, Sue DY. Noninvasive assessment of blood gases. *Am Rev Respir Dis* 1992;145:220–232.
11. Zeballos RJ, Weisman IM. Reliability of ear oximetry during exercise and hypoxia in black subjects. *Chest* 1989;96:162S.

12. Smyth RJ, D'Urzo AD, Slutsky AS, Galdo BM, Rebuck AS. Ear oximetry during combined hypoxia and exercise. *J Appl Physiol* 1986;60:716–719.

13. Ries AL, Farrow JT, Clausen JL. Accuracy of two ear oximeters at rest and during exercise in pulmonary patients. *Am Rev Respir Dis* 1985;132:685–689.

14. Powers SK, Dodd S, Freeman J, Ayers GD, Samson H, McKnight T. Accuracy of pulse oximetry to estimate HbO_2 fraction of total Hb during exercise. *J Appl Physiol* 1989;67:300–304.

15. Hansen JE, Casaburi R. Validity of ear oximetry in clinical exercise testing. *Chest* 1987;91:333–337.

16. Yamaya Y, Bogaard HJ, Wagner PD, Niizeki K, Hopkins SR. Validity of pulse oximetry during maximal exercise in normoxia, hypoxia, and hyperoxia. *J Appl Physiol* 2002;92:162–168.

17. Gehring H, Hornberger C, Matz H. The effects of motion artifact and low perfusion on the performance of a new generation of pulse oximeters in volunteers undergoing hypoxemia. *Respir Care* 2002; 47:48–60.

18. Ries AL, Fedullo PF, Clausen JL. Rapid changes in arterial blood gas levels after exercise in pulmonary patients. *Chest* 1983;83:454–456.

19. Frye M, DiBenedetto R, Lain D, Morgan K. Single arterial puncture vs. arterial cannula for arterial gas analysis after exercise. *Chest* 1988;93:294–299.

20. O'Neill AV, Johnson DC. Transition from exercise to rest. Ventilatory and arterial blood gas responses. *Chest* 1991;99:1145–1150.

21. Stetz CW, Miller RG, Kelly GE, Raffin RA. Reliability of the thermodilution method in the determination of cardiac output in clinical practice. *Am Rev Respir Dis* 1982;126:1001–1004.

22. Jackson AC, Vinegar A. A technique for measuring frequency response of pressure, volume, and flow transducers. *J Appl Physiol* 1979;47:462–467.

23. Consolazio CF, Johnson RE, Pecora LI. *Physiological measurements of metabolic function in man.* New York: McGraw-Hill, 1963:368–401.

24. Gabel RA. Calibration of nonlinear gas analyzers using exponential washout and polynomial curve fitting. *J Appl Physiol* 1973;34:400–401.

25. Clark JH, Greenleaf JE. Electronic bicycle ergometer: a simple calibration procedure. *J Appl Physiol* 1971;30: 440–442.

26. Van Praagh E, Bedu M, Roddier P, Coudert J. A simple calibration method for mechanically braked cycle ergometers. *Int J Sports Med* 1992;13:27–30.

27. Russell JC, Dale JD. Dynamic torquemeter calibration of bicycle ergometers. *J Appl Physiol* 1986;61:1217–1220.

28. Giezendanner D, Di Prampero PE, Cerretelli P. A programmable electrically braked ergometer. *J Appl Physiol* 1983;55:578–582.

29. Versteeg PG, Kippersluis GJ. Automated systems for measurement of oxygen uptake during exercise testing. *Int J Sports Med* 1989;10:107–112.

30. Huszczuk A, Whipp BJ, Wasserman K. A respiratory gas exchange simulator for routine calibration in metabolic studies. *Eur Respir J* 1990;3:465–468.

31. American Thoracic Society. Standardization of spirometry. *Am Rev Respir Dis* 1987;136:1285–1307.

32. Campbell SC. A comparison of the maximum volume ventilation with forced expiratory volume in one second: an assessment of subject cooperation. *J Occup Med* 1982;24:531–533.

33. Seldinger SI. Catheter replacement of the needle in percutaneous arteriography: a new technique. *Acta Radiol* 1953;39:368–376.

34. Huszczuk A. Personal communication, 1985.

35. Whipp BJ, Davis JA, Torres F, Wasserman K. A test to determine parameters of aerobic function during exercise. *J Appl Physiol* 1981;50:217–221.

36. Balke B. *Correlation of static and physical endurance. 1. A test of physical performance based on the cardiovascular and respiratory response to gradually increased work.* Project No. 21–32–004, Report No. 1 (San Antonio, TX: United States Air Force School of Aviation Medicine, 1952).

37. Balke B, Ware RW. An experimental study of "physical fitness" of Air Force personnel. *U S Armed Forces Med J* 1959;10:675–688.

38. Consolazio CF, Nelson RA, Matoush LO, Hansen JE. Energy metabolism at high altitude (3,475). *J Appl Physiol* 1966;21:1732–1740.

39. Jones NL. *Clinical exercise testing.* 3rd ed. Philadelphia: W.B. Saunders, 1988.

40. Spiro SG. Exercise testing in clinical medicine. *Br J Dis Chest* 1977;71:145–172.

41. Fairshter RD, Walters J, Salvess K, Fox M, Minh VD, Wilson AF. Comparison of incremental exercise test during cycle and treadmill ergometry. *Am Rev Respir Dis* 1982;125(Suppl):254.

42. Davis JA, Whipp BJ, Lamarra N, Huntsman DJ, Frank MH, Wasserman K. Effect of ramp slope on determination of aerobic parameters from the ramp exercise test. *Med Sci Sports Exerc* 1982;14:339–343.

43. Cooper DM, Weiler-Ravell D. Gas exchange response to exercise in children. *Am Rev Respir Dis* 1984; 129(Suppl):S47–S48.

44. Zhang YY, Johnson MC, Chow N, Wasserman K. Effect of exercise testing protocol on parameters of aerobic function. *Med Sci Sports Exerc* 1991;23:625–630.

45. Arstilla M. Pulse-conducted triangular exercise-ECG test. *Acta Med Scand* 1972;529(Suppl):103–109.

46. Redwood DR, Rosing DR, Goldstein AR, Beiser G, Epstein SE. Importance of the design of an exercise protocol in the evaluation of patients with angina pectoris. *Circulation* 1971;43:618–628.

47. Buchfuhrer MJ, Hansen JE, Robinson TE, Sue DY, Wasserman K, Whipp BJ. Optimizing the exercise protocol for cardiopulmonary assessment. *J Appl Physiol* 1983;55:1558–1564.

48. Taylor HL, Buskirk E, Henschel A. Maximal oxygen intake as an objective measure of cardiorespiratory performance. *J Appl Physiol* 1955;8:73–80.

49. Froelicher VF, Brammel H, Davis GD, Noguera I, Stewart A, Lancaster MD. A comparison of three maximal treadmill exercise protocols. *J Appl Physiol* 1974;36:720–725.

50. Maksud MG, Coutts KD. Comparison of a continuous and discontinuous graded treadmill test for maximal oxygen uptake. *Med Sci Sports Exerc* 1971;3:63–65.

51. Wyndham CH, Strydom NB, Leary WP, Williams CG. Studies of the maximum capacity for men for physical effort. *Arbeitsphysiologie* 1966;22:285–295.

52. McArdle WD, Katch FI, Pechar GS. Comparison of continuous and discontinuous treadmill and bicycle tests for max $\dot{V}O_2$. *Med Sci Sports Exerc* 1972;5:156–160.

53. Pollack ML, Bohannon RL, Cooper KM, Ayres J, Ward A, White SR, Linnerud ND. A comparative analysis of four protocols for maximal treadmill stress testing. *Am Heart J* 1976;92:39–46.

54. Furuike AN, Sue DY, Hansen JE, Wasserman K. Comparison of physiologic dead space/tidal volume ratio and alveolar-arterial PO_2 difference during incremental and constant work exercise. *Am Rev Respir Dis* 1982;126:579–583.

55. Beaver WL. Water vapor corrections in oxygen consumption calculation. *J Appl Physiol* 1973;35:928–931.

56. Astrand PO, Rodahl K. *Textbook of work physiology.* 2nd ed. New York: McGraw-Hill, 1977.

57. Nery LE, Wasserman K, Andrews JD, Huntsman DJ, Hansen JE, Whipp BJ. Ventilatory and gas exchange kinetics during exercise in chronic airways obstruction. *J Appl Physiol* 1982;53:1594–1602.

58. Lamarra N, Whipp BJ, Blumenberg M, Wasserman K. Model-order estimation of cardiorespiratory dynamics during moderate exercise. In: Whipp BJ, Wiberg DM, eds. *Modelling and control of breathing.* New York: Elsevier Biomedical, 1983:338–345.

59. Whipp BJ, Ward SA, Lamarra N, Davis JA, Wasserman K. Parameters of ventilatory and gas exchange dynamics during exercise. *J Appl Physiol* 1982;52:1506–1513.

60. Sietsema KE, Daly JA, Wasserman K. Early dynamics of O_2 uptake and heart rate as affected by exercise work rate. *J Appl Physiol* 1989;67:2535–2541.

61. Ben-Dov I, Sietsema KE, Wasserman K. O_2 uptake in hyperthyroidism during constant work rate and incremental exercise. *Eur J Appl Physiol* 1991;62:261–267.

62. Koike A, Wasserman K, McKenzie DK, Zanconato S, Weiler-Ravell D. Evidence that diffusion limitation determines oxygen uptake kinetics during exercise in humans. *J Clin Invest* 1990;86:1698–1706.

63. Whipp BJ, Wasserman K. Oxygen uptake kinetics for various intensities of constant load work. *J Appl Physiol* 1972;33:351–356.

64. Roston WL, Whipp BJ, Davis JA, Effros RM, Wasserman K. Oxygen uptake kinetics and lactate concentration during exercise in man. *Am Rev Respir Dis* 1987;135:1080–1084.

65. Casaburi R, Barstow TJ, Robinson T, Wasserman K. Influence of work rate on ventilatory and gas exchange kinetics. *J Appl Physiol* 1989;67:547–555.

66. Casaburi R, Wasserman K, Patessio A, Ioli F, Zanaboni S, Donner CF. A new perspective in pulmonary rehabilitation; anaerobic threshold as a discriminant in training. *Eur J Respir Dis* 1989;2:618–623.

67. Zhang YY, Wasserman K, Sietsema KE, Barstow TJ, Mizumoto G, Sullivan CS, Ben-Dov I. O_2 uptake kinetics in response to exercise: a measure of tissue anaerobiosis in heart failure. *Chest* 1993;103:735–741.

68. Cropp GIA. The exercise bronchoprovocation test: standardized of procedures and evaluation of response. *J Allergy Clin Immunol* 1979;64:627–633.

69. Deal EC Jr, McFadden ER Jr, Ingram RH, Strauss RH, Jaeger JJ. Role of respiratory heat exchange in production of exercise-induced asthma. *J Appl Physiol* 1979; 46:467–475.

70. Wasserman K. Testing regulation of ventilation with exercise. *Chest* 1976;70(Suppl):173–178.

71. Bruce RA. Exercise testing of patients with coronary artery disease. *Ann Clin Res* 1971;3:323–332.

72. Ellestad MH. *Stress testing.* 2nd ed. Philadelphia: F.A. Davis, 1980.

73. Patterson JA, Naughton J, Pietras RJ, Gumar RN. Treadmill exercise in assessment of patients with cardiac disease. *Am J Cardiol* 1972;30:757–762.

74. Itoh H, Tajima A, Koike A, Osada N, Maeda T, Kato M, Omiya K, Fu LT, Watanabe H, Kato K. Oxygen uptake abnormalities during exercise in coronary artery disease. In: Wasserman K, ed. *Cardiopulmonary exercise testing and cardiovascular health.* Armonk, NY: Futura Publishing, 2002:165–172.

75. Belardinelli R, Lacalaprice F, Carle F, Minnucci A, Cianci G, Perna G, D'Eusanio G. Exercise-induced myocardial ischaemia detected by cardiopulmonary exercise testing. *Eur Heart J* 2003;24:1304–1313.

76. Stuart RJ, Ellestad MH. National survey of exercise stress testing facilities. *Chest* 1980;77:94–97.

77. Bruce RA, Kusumi F, Hosmer D. Maximal oxygen intake and nomographic assessment of functional aerobic impairment in cardiovascular disease. *Am Heart J* 1973;85:546–562.

78. Porszasz J, Casaburi R, Somfay A, Woodhouse L, Whipp B. A treadmill protocol using simultaneous changes in speed and grade. *Med Sci Sports Exerc* 2003;35:1596–1603.

79. Bar-Or O, Zwiren LD. Maximal oxygen consumption test during arm exercise—reliability and validity. *J Appl Physiol* 1975;38:424–426.

80. Vokac Z, Bell H, Bautz-Holter E, Rodahl K. Oxygen uptake/heart rate relationship in leg and arm exercise, sitting and standing. *J Appl Physiol* 1975;39:54–59.

81. Davis JA, Vodak P, Wilmore JH, Vodal J, Kurtz P. Anaerobic threshold and maximal aerobic power for three modes of exercise. *J Appl Physiol* 1976;41:544–550.

82. Casaburi R, Barstow T, Robinson T, Wasserman K. Dynamic and steady-state ventilatory and gas exchange responses to arm exercise. *Med Sci Sports Exerc* 1992; 24:1365–1374.

83. Nagle FJ, Balke B, Naughton JP. Gradational step tests for assessing work capacity. *J Appl Physiol* 1965;21: 745–748.

84. Nagle FJ, Balke B, Baptista G, Alleyia J, Hawley E. Comparability of progressive treadmill, bicycle and step tests based on oxygen uptake responses. *Med Sci Sports Exerc* 1971;3:149–154.

85. Fleishman EA. *The structure and measurement of physical fitness.* Englewood Cliffs, NJ: Prentice-Hall, 1964: 171–172.

86. Cooper KM. A means of assessing maximal oxygen intake. *JAMA* 1968;203:201–204.

87. McGavin CR, Gupta SP, McHardy GJR. Twelve minute walking test for assessing disability in chronic bronchitis. *Br Med J* 1976;1:822–823.

88. American Thoracic Society. ATS statement: guidelines for the six-minute walk test. *Am J Respir Crit Care Med* 2002;166:111–117.

89. Miyamoto S, Nagaya N, Satoh T, Kyotani S, Sakamaki F, Fujita M, Nakanishi N, Miyatake K. Clinical correlates and prognostic significance of six-minute walk test in patients with primary pulmonary hypertension. *Am J Respir Crit Care Med* 2000;161:487–492.

90. Chuang ML, Lin IF, Wasserman K. The body weight–walking distance product as related to lung function, anaerobic threshold and peak $\dot{V}O_2$ in COPD patients. *Respir Med* 2001;95:618–626.

91. Sciurba F, Criner GJ, Lee SM, Mohsenifar Z, Shade D, Slivka W, Wise RA. Six-minute walk distance in chronic obstructive pulmonary disease. *Am J Respir Crit Care Med* 2003;167:1522–1527.

Normal Values

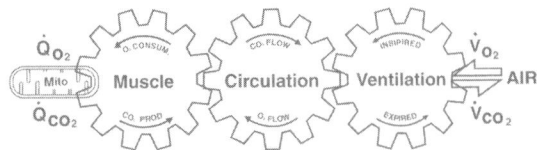

INTERPRETATION OF THE RESULTS of exercise tests requires knowledge of the normal responses. This chapter presents values for important physiological variables that we think represent the best predictive data available for sedentary normal subjects during exercise. In some instances, several sets of normal values for the same measurement are included. When doing so, we have made recommendations as to which to use.

PEAK OXYGEN UPTAKE

The selection of peak $\dot{V}O_2$ predicted values (both mean and at the 95% confidence level) is a challenging problem, especially because the geographic area, body sizes, and activity levels of a specific clinical population may differ from those of reference populations. It is relevant to note that the measurement of $\dot{V}O_2$ during heavy exercise may be technically difficult. Peak $\dot{V}O_2$ in normal subjects during exercise varies with age, gender, body size, lean body mass, level of ordinary activity, and type of exercise. When comparing the peak $\dot{V}O_2$ of an individual to the predicted peak $\dot{V}O_2$, a predicted value generated for the same form of exercise must be used. It is preferable if the population from which the predicting equations were obtained included a large number of individuals with similar characteristics to the patient being tested.

Astrand and Rodahl (1) pointed out that peak $\dot{V}O_2$ expressed as (ml/min) $\times$ kg^{-1} is higher in smaller compared with larger top athletes, even when obesity is not a factor. However, when expressed as (ml/min) $\times$ kg$^{-2/3}$, peak $\dot{V}O_2$ does not differ between smaller and larger athletes. They argued against the practice of using weight as a primary variable in predicting peak $\dot{V}O_2$. Despite their rational explanation and the obvious bias introduced by obesity on peak values when expressed as (ml/min) $\times$ kg^{-1}, many exercise physiologists and clinicians continue to estimate cardiovascular function by comparing actual values to values predicted from age, gender, and weight, even in obese individuals. However, this practice will predict too high a peak $\dot{V}O_2$ in obese individuals. We believe that sufficient evidence now exists to assert that, even though peak $\dot{V}O_2$ values may still be expressed as (ml/min) $\times$ kg^{-1} in many publications, this practice is not optimal for the clinical evaluation of the cardiorespiratory function of patients (2–4).

Age and Gender

Many investigators have reported that peak $\dot{V}O_2$ declines with age and is smaller for women than men

(5–7). Although cross-sectional studies of change in peak $\dot{V}O_2$ with age are easier to perform than longitudinal studies, they may be misleading on account of selection bias. Older subjects included in such a study are more likely to be active, relative to their peers, than their younger counterparts; hence, the peak $\dot{V}O_2$ values in older subjects in cross-sectional studies tend to decrease more slowly than peak $\dot{V}O_2$ values in longitudinal studies (8). In a longitudinal study, Astrand et al. (9) measured $\dot{V}O_2$max during cycling exercise in 66 well-trained, physically active men and women aged 20 to 33 years and studied them again 21 years later. The mean decrease in $\dot{V}O_2$max was 22% for the 35 women and 20% for the 31 men.

Bruce et al. (10) used stepwise multiple regression analysis to identify whether gender, age, physical activity, weight, height, or smoking aided in the prediction of $\dot{V}O_2$max during treadmill exercise in adults. They found that gender and age were the two most important factors. The $\dot{V}O_2$max of women was approximately 77% of the $\dot{V}O_2$max of men when adjusted for body weight and activity. Astrand (11) reported 17% lower $\dot{V}O_2$max for 18 women students compared with 17 male students of comparable size.

Activity Level

Investigators generally agree that values obtained from athletes, physical education teachers, servicemen, or participants in organized exercise groups are not representative as reference values for a clinical population. Balke and Ware (12) found the peak $\dot{V}O_2$ of Air Force personnel to be strongly related to their activity pattern. Drinkwater et al. (6) found that the peak $\dot{V}O_2$ of extremely active women did not decline over two decades despite a gradual increase in body weight. The decline in peak $\dot{V}O_2$ with age is more rapid in habitually inactive men, even allowing for greater weight gain in the inactive group (8). Importantly, even brief periods of physical training can increase peak $\dot{V}O_2$ by 15% to 25% or more (5,13).

Adults of Normal (Predicted) Body Weight

It is logical to assume that physical size would be a factor in peak $\dot{V}O_2$ because the mass of the exercising muscles as well as the dimensions of the cardiovascular and pulmonary systems should determine the maximum quantity of O_2 that can be delivered and used. As previously noted, Astrand and Rodahl (1) found that peak $\dot{V}O_2$ expressed as (ml/min) $\times$ kg^{-1} was higher in smaller than in larger athletes. When expressed as (ml/min) $\times$ kg$^{-2/3}$, however, peak $\dot{V}O_2$ was not different. These data would argue against the traditional practice of using weight as a primary variable in predicting peak $\dot{V}O_2$ or defining fitness.

Despite the variability related to activity levels, relatively good agreement among series exists for mean predicted peak $\dot{V}O_2$ values of nonobese, sedentary populations if one uses age, gender, and height rather than age, gender, and weight. Pulmonologists are accustomed to predicting most respiratory function values using height rather than weight. Jones et al. (4) found that in a population of over 1,000 patients referred to their laboratory, maximum work capacity was best related to gender, height, and age rather than gender, weight, and age. In 204 volunteers between 20 and 70 years of age, Davis et al. (14) found that the prediction of peak $\dot{V}O_2$ of average-sized individuals was not improved by adding weight as a variable to gender, age, and height nor height as a variable to gender, age, and weight. However, variance in that series could be reduced by using fat-free mass as an independent variable.

We have reviewed the similarities and differences in peak $\dot{V}O_2$ in several series of men and women of relatively normal body weight (2,10,14–17). Figures 7.1 and 7.2 show values of three North American, one Japanese (16), and one Brazilian series (17) for sedentary men and women of normal body proportions. For men (Fig. 7.1), all five series show reasonably similar parallel declines with age at all heights. The variability is least at 170 cm and 180 cm (less than 0.6 L/min) and greatest at the extremes of height. Jones's values are lowest at 160 cm and highest at 190 cm. On average, the values in the study of Neder et al. (17) on Brazilian men tend to be lower than others.

The values in the women's series also show reasonably similar parallel declines with age at all heights (Fig. 7.2). The values for Japanese women (16) are generally higher, and for Brazilian women (17) generally lower. The North American series agree remarkably well at a height of 160 cm (Fig. 7.2B). Davis and Bruce–Hansen formulas also agree well at other heights, with the series of Jones et al. (15) having lesser values at shorter heights and greater values for taller women.

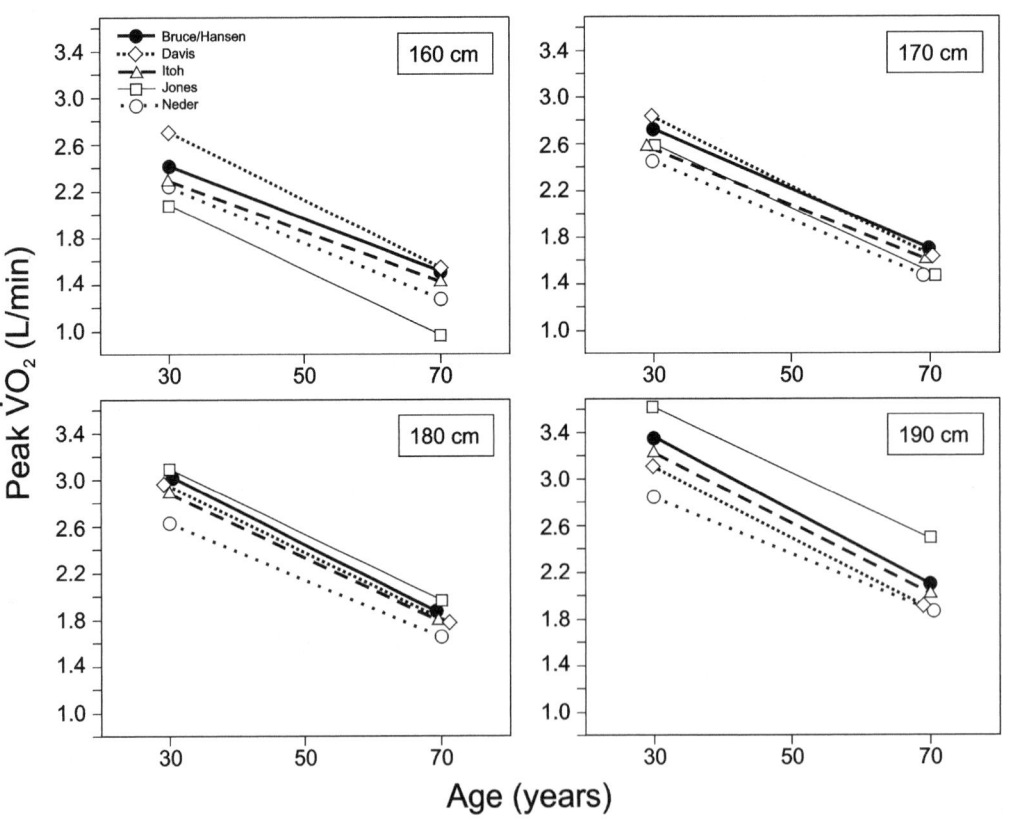

FIGURE 7.1.   Comparison of predicted peak $\dot{V}O_2$ for cycle ergometry of sedentary men with body mass index of 22 calculated from five reference series for ages 30 to 70 for four different heights and weights: 160 cm and 56 kg, 170 cm and 64 kg, 180 cm and 71 kg, and 190 cm and 80 kg. Data are from Jones et al. (15), Bruce et al. (10) as modified by Hansen et al. (2), Itoh et al. (16), Davis (14), and Neder et al. (17).

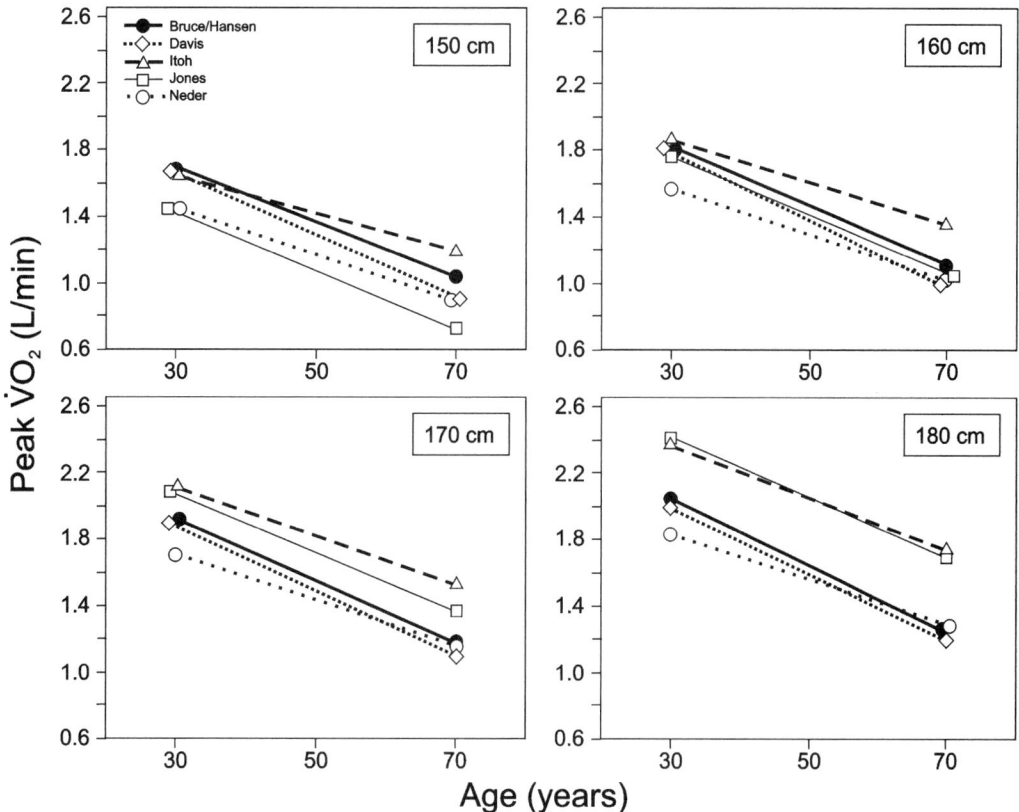

FIGURE 7.2.   Comparison of predicted peak V̇O₂ for cycle ergometry of sedentary women with body mass index of 22 calculated from five reference series for ages 30 to 70 for four different heights and weights: 150 cm and 50 kg, 160 cm and 56 kg, 170 cm and 64 kg, and 180 cm and 71 kg. Data are from Jones et al. (15), Bruce et al. (10) as modified by Hansen et al. (2), Itoh et al. (16), Davis (14), and Neder et al. (17).

For both genders, the close agreement in peak V̇O₂ in North American series at average heights suggests confidence in these values at these heights, with lesser confidence at the extremes of height. We have no clear methodologic or other reasons to justify discarding any of these series. The diversity of values for both genders at different locales suggests differences in physical activity levels or selection criteria. Therefore, it is a good policy for each laboratory to measure peak V̇O₂ in a group of "average" sedentary persons in their vicinity to see how well they match the "normal" values from other series, such as those presented here. This was an approach taken by Stelken et al. (18), who found that after comparing their normal population with that of Jones et al. (15) and with Bruce–Hansen normal values (2), their results agreed more closely with the latter than the former.

Overweight Patients

The selection of an appropriate predicted peak V̇O₂ in the overweight patient is difficult. This is largely because the usual overweight individual is more likely to have predominantly an increase in adipose tissue rather than an increase in potential exercising muscle mass. Thus, it is difficult to envision that peak V̇O₂ increases in direct proportion to increased body weight. Furthermore, neither cardiovascular nor pulmonary function scale with total body weight.

In a cycle ergometer study of 77 middle-aged men (mean age 54 years, range 34 to 74) whom we judged to have normal cardiovascular and respiratory systems and good motivation, we compared peak V̇O₂ with the predicted values for V̇O₂max of Bruce et al. (10), modified for cycle ergometry. There was good agreement for normal-weight subjects, but when a subject was overweight (2,3), there was better agreement using normal weight (weight predicted from height) rather than actual weight. Buskirk and Taylor (19) found that V̇O₂max correlated better with a measure of fat-free body weight ($r = 0.85$) than total body weight ($r = 0.63$) in 43 healthy students and in 13 soldiers performing treadmill exercise.

TABLE 7.1.   Comparison of Physical Characteristics of Three Healthy Reference Populations and a Clinical Population

Series	Number	Age (yr)	Height (cm)	Weight (kg)
Men				
Bruce et al. (10)	138	48.6 ± 11.1	177.5 ± 6.6	78.6 ± 8.6
Jones et al. (4)	732	48.0 ± 12.0	174.0 ± 6.5	81.8 ± 12.6
Davis (14)	103	43.4 ± 14.6	178.7 ± 7.1	82.3 ± 12.1
Harbor-UCLA	750	54.2 ± 11.7	172.8 ± 7.4	83.4 ± 17.1
Women				
Bruce et al. (10)	157	41.4 ± 11.2	166.0 ± 6.3	62.1 ± 9.8
Jones et al. (4)	339	47.0 ± 13.5	162.0 ± 6.2	67.3 ± 12.8
Davis (14)	101	44.6 ± 14.6	164.4 ± 6.6	63.6 ± 10.4
Harbor-UCLA*	240	49.1 ± 13.5	160.5 ± 8.4	71.2 ± 21.6

*The clinical population is the series from Harbor-UCLA. Values are mean ± standard deviation.

Although Jones et al. (4) did not report peak $\dot{V}O_2$ for their 1,000 normal individuals, they found that adding weight as a variable to height, age, and gender did not improve the prediction of cycle ergometry exercise capacity. Thus, weight alone did not appreciably influence external work capacity on the cycle. Yet we know that in healthy individuals, peak $\dot{V}O_2$ correlates highly with maximum external work performed; and at all external work rates on the cycle, those with larger legs have higher measured $\dot{V}O_2$ than those with smaller legs. On average, we estimate that during unloaded cycling, $\dot{V}O_2$ will increase approximately 6 ml/min/kg of extra body weight (20). In addition, overweight individuals can be expected to have slightly higher peak $\dot{V}O_2$ and anaerobic threshold (*AT*) values than others of the same age, gender, and height, probably because in walking similar distances they expend more energy and their muscles become more trained. Thus, body weight can change predicted peak $\dot{V}O_2$ without af-

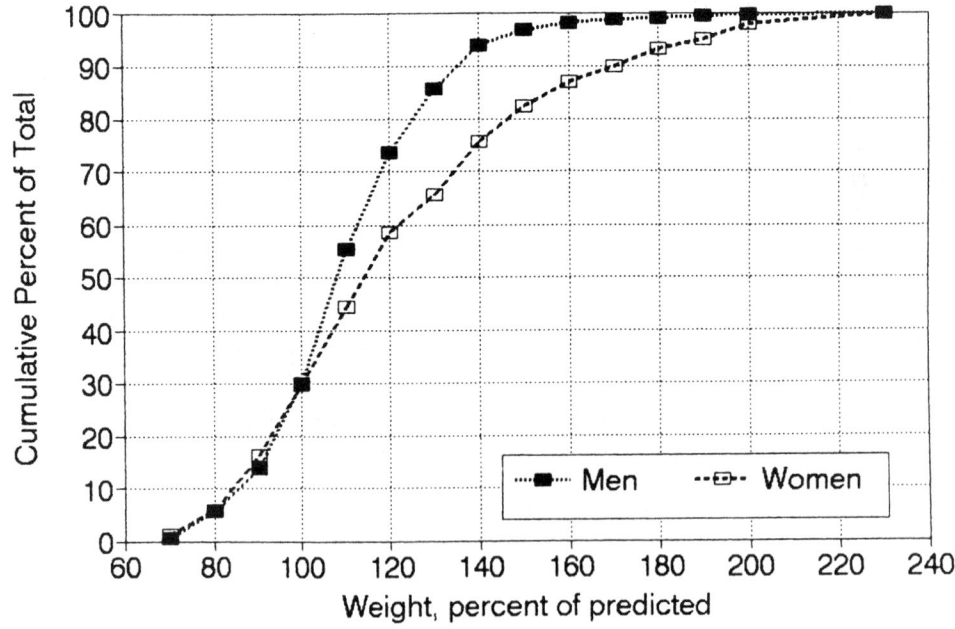

FIGURE 7.3.   Relation of actual with normal (predicted) weight in approximately 1,000 consecutive patients who presented to our laboratory for diagnostic exercise testing. Normal (predicted) weight for men in kilograms = 0.79 × height in centimeters − 60.7, and for women in kilograms = 0.65 × height in centimeters − 42.8. Our patient population can be seen to include a high proportion of overweight individuals. (Formula from Bruce RA, Kusumi F, Hosmer D. Maximal oxygen intake and nomographic assessment of functional aerobic impairment in cardiovascular disease. *Am Heart J* 1973;85:546–562.)

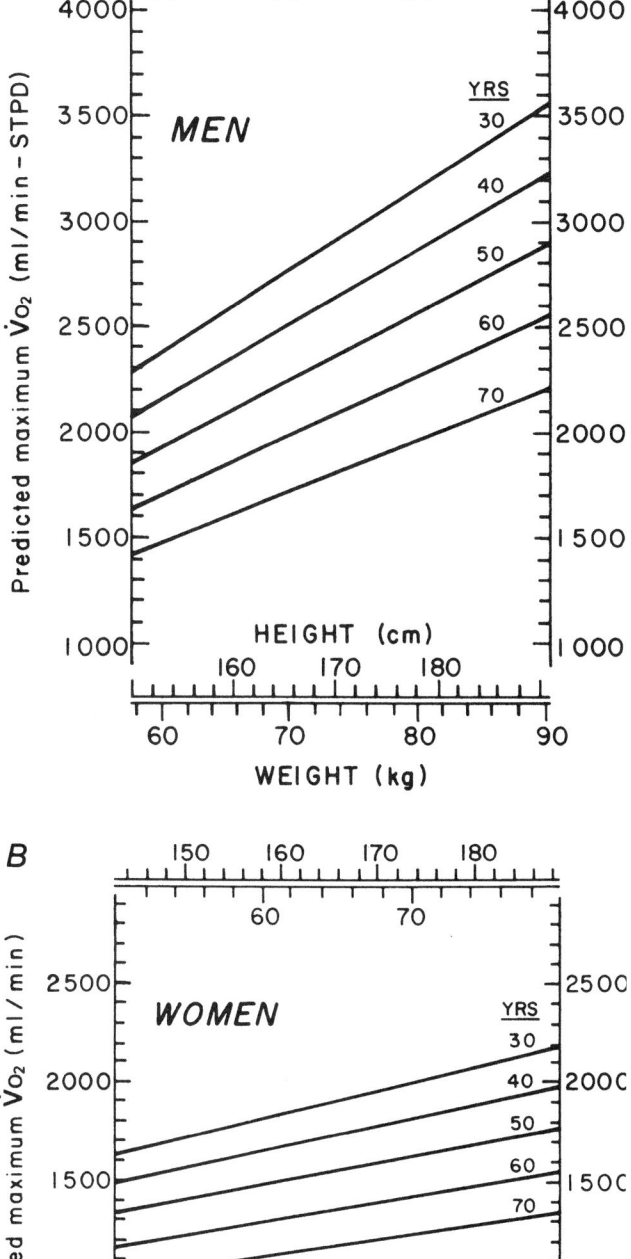

fecting maximum external work capacity on the cycle ergometer.

We recently reviewed our experience of approximately 1,000 clinical cardiopulmonary exercise tests performed in our laboratories. Our clinical population is, on average, shorter, more obese, and more variable in weight than any of the reference populations in standard series of healthy, relatively sedentary North American older adults (Table 7.1, Fig. 7.3). This is especially true of the women tested. For men, 70% exceeded normal (predicted) weight (see Table 7.2 equations), 45% exceeded 110% of normal weight, 26% exceeded 120% of normal weight, 6% exceeded 140% of normal weight, and 2% exceeded 160% of normal weight. For women, 70% exceeded normal weight, 56% exceeded 110% of normal weight, 42% exceeded 120% of normal weight, 25% exceeded 140% of normal weight, and 12% exceeded 160% of normal weight. These findings emphasize the importance of not using predicted peak $\dot{V}O_2$ values expressed as (ml/min) × kg^{-1} in populations of this makeup.

Although it is difficult to be certain of correct predicted values in patients who are overweight, we recommend increasing the predicted peak $\dot{V}O_2$ by 6 ml/min for each kilogram of weight above normal (predicted) weight, whether the cycle or treadmill is used for exercise testing.

In our analysis, it is clear that the predicted peak $\dot{V}O_2$ in obese patients using weight normalized to height will be less than that expected using actual weight. Nevertheless, although an overweight patient may have a "normal" peak $\dot{V}O_2$ value, this does not mean that person is necessarily capable of performing the same amount of external work as a nonoverweight person of the same height, age, and gender. Because a greater proportion of the $\dot{V}O_2$ is needed to move the heavier legs and body of the overweight person, a smaller amount of $\dot{V}O_2$ is

axis and read off the predicted peak $\dot{V}O_2$ in liters per minute STPD. *If the patient is overweight* (i.e., the patient's actual weight is to the right of that directly above the patient's height), draw a line vertically from the height marker to the line that indicates the patient's age. From this intersection draw a line horizontally to the vertical axis and read off the preliminary predicted peak $\dot{V}O_2$ in liters per minute STPD. To obtain the actual predicted peak $\dot{V}O_2$ for the obese patient, add 6 ml/min for each kilogram the patient is overweight. Finally, if the treadmill is used, predicted cycle values should be increased 11%. (Formula from Bruce RA, Kusumi F, Hosmer D. Maximal oxygen intake and nomographic assessment of functional aerobic impairment in cardiovascular disease. *Am Heart J* 1973;85:546–562. Data are from Hansen JE, Sue DY, Wasserman K. Predicted values for clinical exercise testing. *Am Rev Respir Dis* 1984;129(Suppl):S49–S55.)

FIGURE 7.4.   Mean peak $\dot{V}O_2$ values for sedentary men **(A)** and women **(B)** of normal (predicted) weight using the cycle ergometer. To use, locate the patient's height and weight on the horizontal axis. *If the patient is underweight* (i.e., the patient's actual weight is to the left of that directly above the patient's height), draw a line halfway between the marks vertically to the line that indicates the patient's age. From this intersection draw a line horizontally to the vertical

therefore available for performing useful external work. For example, on the cycle ergometer, an overweight and a nonoverweight patient may have the same peak $\dot{V}O_2$, but the work rate at which the nonoverweight patient reaches this peak $\dot{V}O_2$ value will be substantially higher than that for the overweight patient.

Underweight Patients

In the first edition of this book, we suggested decreasing the predicted peak $\dot{V}O_2$ in direct proportion to the decrease in body weight for those patients whose weight was less than normal (as if the loss of weight were due solely to a decrease in muscle mass). Because there is likely to be reduction in fat as well as muscle in most underweight persons, we now prefer to use the average of the actual weight and normal weight to predict peak $\dot{V}O_2$ and in related calculations in underweight patients, as noted in Figure 7.4.

Children

Cooper and colleagues (21,22) reported peak $\dot{V}O_2$ for 109 children, aged 6 to 17 years, who performed cycle ergometry using a continuously increasing work rate protocol (Fig. 7.5). Because these subjects were not obese, peak $\dot{V}O_2$ correlated similarly with

either weight or height. These investigators found, in addition, that their data were similar to those of Astrand (5) for the boys, but that the girls studied by Astrand had a significantly higher $\dot{V}O_2$max versus height relation. Cooper et al. (21) suggested that cultural or societal differences might account for this difference observed in girls.

Exercise Mode

The type of exercise is an important determinant of peak $\dot{V}O_2$. Peak $\dot{V}O_2$ during arm cranking ergometer exercise (which is inappropriate to use in evaluating most patients) is about 70% of that of leg cycling exercise (23) because of the smaller mass of muscle and lower maximum work rate achievable. Many studies (7,24–29) have shown that the peak $\dot{V}O_2$ of leg cycling is approximately 89% to 95% of

TABLE 7.2. Calculation of Predicted Peak $\dot{V}O_2$ (mL/min)

A. Sedentary Men
Cycle factor = 50.72 − 0.372 × A
Step 1. Measure man's weight (*W*, kg) and height (*H*, cm) in light clothes without shoes and record age (*A*, yr).
Step 2. Calculate man's normal (predicted) *W* in kg as follows: Normal (predicted) *W* = 0.79 × *H* − 60.7.
Step 3A. If man's actual *W* equals normal *W*:
    Predicted peak $\dot{V}O_2$ (ml/min) = Actual *W* × Cycle factor.
Step 3B. If patient's actual *W* is less than normal *W*:
    Predicted peak $\dot{V}O_2$ (ml/min) = [(Normal *W* + Actual *W*)/2] × Cycle factor.
Step 3C. If patient's actual *W* exceeds normal *W*:
    Predicted peak $\dot{V}O_2$ (ml/min) = (Normal *W* × Cycle factor) + 6 × (Actual *W* − Normal *W*).
Step 4. If treadmill is used rather than cycle:
    Multiply predicted $\dot{V}O_2$ by 1.11.

B. Sedentary Women
Cycle factor = 22.78 − 0.17 × A
Step 1. Measure woman's weight (*W*, kg) and height (*H*, cm) in light clothes without shoes and record age (*A*, yr).
Step 2. Calculate woman's normal (predicted) *W* in kg as follows: Normal (predicted) *W* = 0.65 × *H* − 42.8.
Step 3A. If woman's actual *W* equals normal *W*:
    Predicted peak $\dot{V}O_2$ (ml/min) = (Actual *W* + 43) × Cycle factor.
Step 3B. If patient's actual *W* is less than normal *W*:
    Predicted peak $\dot{V}O_2$ (ml/min) = [(Normal *W* + Actual *W* + 86)/2] × Cycle factor.
Step 3C. If patient's actual *W* exceeds normal *W*:
    Predicted peak $\dot{V}O_2$ (ml/min) = [(Normal *W* + 43) × Cycle factor] + 6 × (Actual *W* − Normal *W*).
Step 4. If treadmill is used rather than cycle: Multiply predicted peak $\dot{V}O_2$ by 1.11.

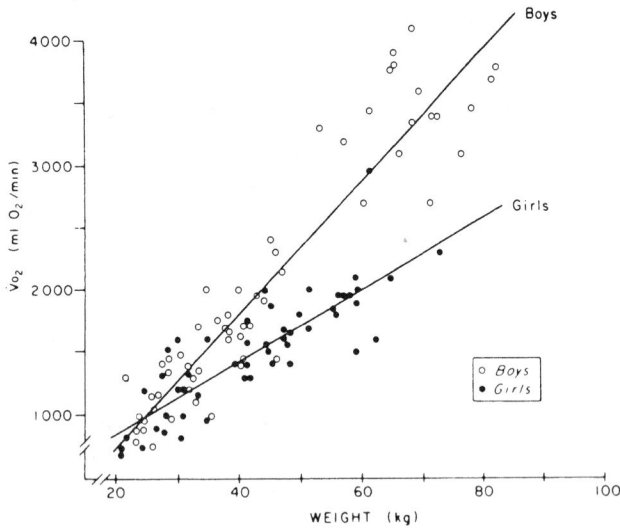

FIGURE 7.5.   Peak $\dot{V}O_2$ of 109 normal North American boys and girls for leg cycling. Regression equations for peak $\dot{V}O_2$ (ml/min) as function of body weight (kg) were as follows: for boys, $\dot{V}O_2$ = 52.8 × weight − 303 (*r* = 0.94); for girls, $\dot{V}O_2$ = 28.5 × weight + 288 (*r* = 0.84). (From Cooper DM, Weiler-Ravell D, Whipp BJ, et al. Aerobic parameters of exercise as a function of body size during growth in children. *J Appl Physiol* 1984;56:628–634, with permission.)

Modified from Hansen JE, Sue DY, Wasserman K. Predicted values for clinical exercise testing. *Am Rev Respir Dis* 1984;129(Suppl):S49–S55 and Bruce RA, Kusumi F, Hosmer D. Maximal oxygen intake and nomographic assessment of functional aerobic impairment in cardiovascular disease. *Am Heart J* 1973; 85:546–562.

TABLE 7.3.   Predicted Peak $\dot{V}O_2$ and Anaerobic Threshold in Normal Children for Cycle Ergometry

	Boys ≤ 13	Boys > 13	Girls ≤ 11	Girls > 11
Number studied	37	21	24	27
Peak $\dot{V}O_2$, ml/min/kg (mean ± SD)	42 ± 6	50 ± 8	38 ± 7	34 ± 4
Lower 95% confidence limit	32	37	26	27
AT, ml/min/kg (mean ± SD)	26 ± 5	27 ± 6	23 ± 4	19 ± 3
Lower 95% confidence limit	18	17	16	14

AT, anaerobic threshold; SD, standard deviation.
From Cooper DM, Weiler-Ravell D. Gas exchange response to exercise in children. *Am Rev Respir Dis* 1984;129(Suppl.):S47–S48, with permission.

the maximal values achieved with treadmill exercise. Thus, the form of ergometry and muscle groups involved must be considered when predicting peak $\dot{V}O_2$.

Recommendations

- Reported peak $\dot{V}O_2$ values may include data recorded before or shortly after the apparent cessation of exercise. Peak $\dot{V}O_2$ should be determined by averaging consecutive breaths over a 20- to 30-second period giving the highest $\dot{V}O_2$ rather than using the $\dot{V}O_2$ value of a single or two consecutive breaths as the peak $\dot{V}O_2$.
- Recommended mean values for peak $\dot{V}O_2$ are given for sedentary men and women (Table 7.2) and children of average activity levels (Table 7.3) performing cycle and, in the case of adults, treadmill exercise. Figure 7.4 gives mean predicted peak $\dot{V}O_2$ values for sedentary men and women of normal (predicted) weight. Figure 7.5 gives mean predicted peak $\dot{V}O_2$ values for leg cycling for children.
- For *overweight patients*, increase the predicted peak $\dot{V}O_2$ by 6 ml/min for each kilogram of weight above normal (predicted) weight.
- In order to separate changes in health status due to cardiovascular dysfunction from those due to obesity, we express ml/min of $\dot{V}O_2$ in "ideal" or "normal" body weight rather than actual body weight. Considering the known relation between height and normal weight in the adult U.S. population, we find advantages in expressing cardiorespiratory function as (ml/min) × (cm − 100)$^{-1}$ rather than (ml/min) × kg^{-1}. The former is the same as normalizing the $\dot{V}O_2$ to predicted body weight or height. An example is given in Box 7.1.
- For *underweight patients*, reduce the predicted peak $\dot{V}O_2$ values for normal-sized persons by using the average of the actual and normal weight for the peak $\dot{V}O_2$. An example is given in Box 7.2.
- Use 83% of mean predicted value as a reasonable approximation for the lower 95% confidence limit in the patient of average height. Patients at extremes in height, weight, or age, especially women, are likely to have an even lower 95% confidence limit. As pointed out by Jones et al. (4), peak exercise values tend to be skewed even in relatively sedentary populations because training increases values above the mean considerably more than inactivity decreases values below the mean.

Box 7.1
Sample Calculation

Find the predicted peak $\dot{V}O_2$ for treadmill exercise for a 60-year-old sedentary man who is 180 cm tall and weighs 110 kg.

Using Table 7.2A, step 2, or the horizontal axis of Figure 7.3A, we ascertain that the patient is overweight, his predicted weight being 81.5 kg (normal $W = 0.79 × 180 − 60.7 = 81.5$ kg). Using Table 7.2A, step 3C, we find his predicted peak $\dot{V}O_2$ for cycle ergometry is [81.5 × (50.72 − 0.372 × 60)] + [6 × (110 − 81.5)] = (81.5 × 28.4) + (6 × 28.5) = 2,486 ml/min. Using step 4, the predicted peak $\dot{V}O_2$ for treadmill ergometry is 2,486 × 1.11 = 2,760 ml/min.

Using Figure 7.4A, by extending a line vertically from 180 cm to the 60-year line, we find that the predicted peak $\dot{V}O_2$ for cycle ergometry is 2,320 ml/min for a nonobese man. This amount, plus 6 ml/kg × 28.5 kg (excess weight over predicted), yields a predicted peak $\dot{V}O_2$ of 2,490 ml/min for cycle ergometry for this patient. This value times 1.11 yields a predicted value of 2,750 ml/min for treadmill ergometry.

Box 7.2
Sample Calculation

Find the predicted peak $\dot{V}_{O_2}$ for cycle ergometry for a 50-year-old sedentary woman who is 160 cm tall and weighs 45 kg.

Using Table 7.2B, step 2, or Figure 7.4B, we find that she is underweight and that her normal weight is 61.2 kg (normal $W = 0.65 \times 160 - 43 = 61.2$). Using Table 7.2B, step 3B, her predicted peak $\dot{V}_{O_2}$ is $[(61.2 + 45 + 86)/2] \times (22.78 - 0.17 \times 50) = 1,372$ ml/min.

Using Figure 7.4B, by extending a line vertically from 53 kg (which is the average of her actual and normal weight) to the 50-year line, we find that the predicted peak $\dot{V}_{O_2}$ is 1,350 ml/min.

PEAK HEART RATE AND HEART RATE RESERVE

The maximum or peak heart rate (HR) achieved declines with age in all studies. No consistent differences have been found between men and women or among the types of exercise used (i.e., leg cycling, stepping, inclined treadmill, walking, or running).

The two most common formulas for predicting peak HR in adults are as follows: 220 − Age (years) and 210 − 0.65 × Age (years) (30). Data from this laboratory fit the former equation slightly better. The standard deviation for each formula is 10 beats per minute. As reported by Sheffield et al. (31) and Astrand and Rodahl (1), the peak heart rates derived from fit individuals approximate either formula reasonably well. The study of K. H. Cooper et al. (32) shows a lower peak HR in the less fit than the fit individual of the same age. Our finding that the peak HR was reduced in obese men is consistent with the suggestion that a sedentary existence may reduce peak HR even in well-motivated subjects (2).

Scandinavian children were found to have an average peak HR of 205 beats per minute (1), whereas North American children aged 8 to 18 years had an average peak heart rate of 187 beats per minute, with a lower 95% confidence limit of 160 (33).

The concept of heart rate reserve (HRR) can be useful for estimating the relative stress of the cardiovascular system during exercise, but it should be used with caution. A normal HRR is zero. The mean predicted peak HR may not be reached because of normal population variability, poor motivation, medications such as β-adrenergic blockers, or because of heart, peripheral vascular, lung, endocrine, or musculoskeletal diseases.

Recommendations

Peak heart rate values should be measured and averaged at the same time as the peak $\dot{V}_{O_2}$ values. The following equations can be used to estimate the predicted peak heart rate and the heart rate reserve for adults and children:

- Maximum heart rate (beats/min) = 220 − Age (years)
- Heart rate reserve = Predicted peak HR − Observed peak HR

RELATIONSHIP OF OXYGEN UPTAKE AND HEART RATE: THE PEAK OXYGEN PULSE

In a given individual, a consistent relationship exists between $\dot{V}_{O_2}$ and HR during exercise (see Fig. 4.10). The quotient of the $\dot{V}_{O_2}$ and HR is the O_2 pulse (see Fig. 4.11); its values are dependent on the stroke volume and the difference between the arterial and mixed venous blood O_2 content. The arteriovenous O_2 difference is, in turn, dependent on the availability of hemoglobin, blood oxygenation in the lung, and extraction of oxygen in the periphery.

Examples of normal and abnormal $\dot{V}_{O_2}$ versus HR responses and O_2 pulse responses are shown in Figure 7.6. The normal relationship of $\dot{V}_{O_2}$ with HR (patients 1 and 2) is linear over a wide range, with a positive intercept on the HR axis. Although sedentary patients 1 and 2 differ considerably in their predicted peak values (because they differ in age and gender or size), both have normal responses. An exercise response with a higher $\dot{V}_{O_2}$/HR than predicted indicates better than average cardiorespiratory function, whereas a response with a lower $\dot{V}_{O_2}$/HR indicates poorer than average cardiorespiratory function (patient 3). In our clinical population, this latter response is most commonly due to low stroke volume, but it could be due to anemia or carboxyhemoglobinemia, poor blood oxygenation in the lung, right-to-left shunt, or (rarely) low peripheral oxygen extraction. In patient 4, the increasing slope of the HR versus $\dot{V}_{O_2}$ relation for the last several minutes of exercise is abnormal, indicating that the rise in HR is disproportionately faster than

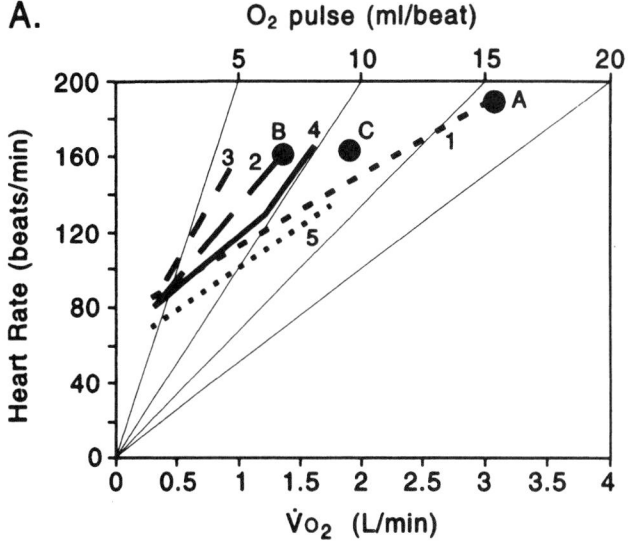

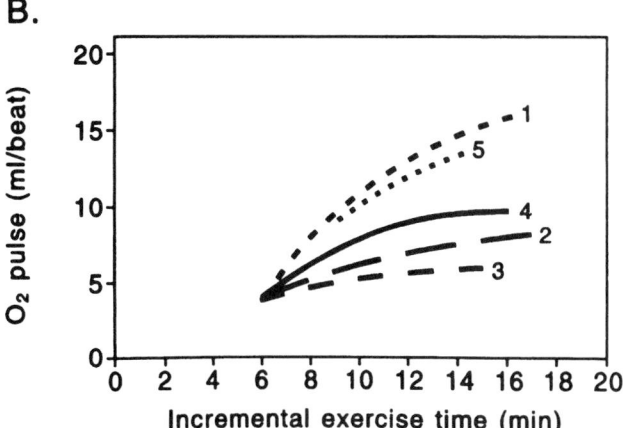

FIGURE 7.6. Values of $\dot{V}_{O_2}$, heart rate, and O_2 pulse for five individuals during incremental cycle ergometer tests. For clarity, the resting, unloaded pedaling, and recovery data are not shown. The upper figure (**A**) has isopleths for O_2 pulse at 5, 10, 15, and 20 ml/beat. The three large solid circles are maximal exercise target values (each of which depends on each patient's age, gender, size, activity level, and exercise mode) and are labeled *A* for patients 1 and 5, *B* for patients 2 and 3, and *C* for patient 4. The responses for patients 1 and 2 are normal. Patient 3 had decreased cardiovascular function throughout the test and would not have reached target values even if able to exercise longer. Patient 4 manifested decreased cardiovascular function about 2 minutes before the cessation of exercise. Patient 5 stopped exercise prematurely for other than cardiovascular causes. **B:** Plots of the same O_2 pulse data against time for the five patients. Patients 1 and 2 reach their target values, whereas patients 3, 4, and 5 do not. The plateau in O_2 pulse seen for patient 4 is abnormal.

$\dot{V}_{O_2}$ as work rate increases. In patient 5, the rate of rise of the HR versus $\dot{V}_{O_2}$ is normal, but exercise ends at a relatively low work rate. If the cessation of incremental exercise is due to pain, musculoskeletal disease, ventilatory insufficiency, or other such factors, these factors (rather than circulatory disease) may be the cause of an abnormally low maximum O_2 pulse.

These differing responses can be seen in Figure 7.6A, in which HR is plotted as a function of $\dot{V}_{O_2}$ with O_2 pulse isopleths. Figure 7.6B plots the O_2 pulse versus time for the same responses. Normally, the rate of increase in O_2 pulse declines gradually as the O_2 pulse approaches maximum values. (This is a necessary consequence of a linear

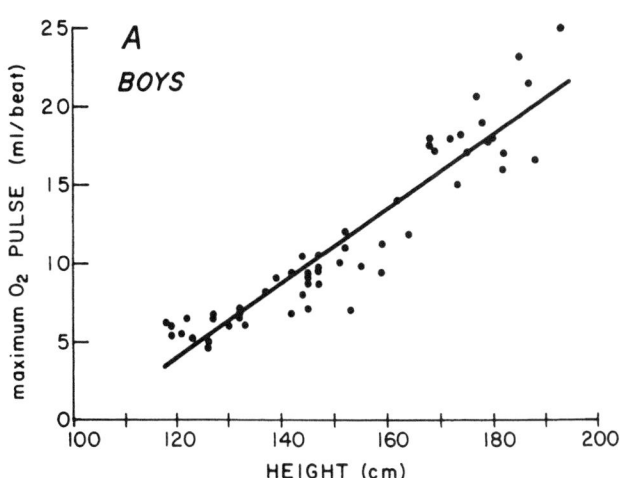

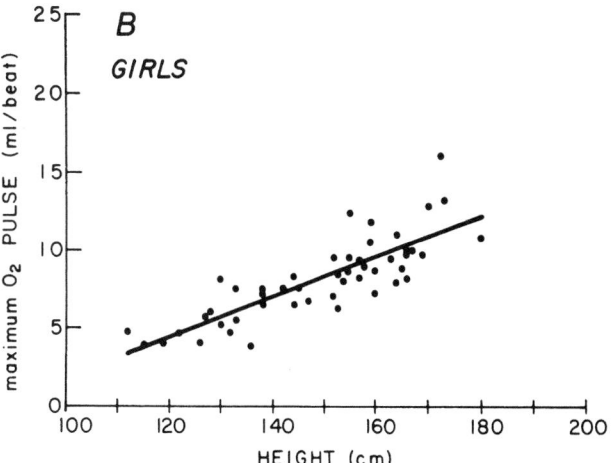

FIGURE 7.7. Maximum O_2 pulse for normal North American boys (**A**) and girls (**B**). For boys, the best-fit regression line is O_2 pulse (ml/beat) = 0.23 × height (cm) − 24.4. The lower 95% confidence limit is 3.8 ml/beat below the regression line. For girls, the equation is O_2 pulse (ml/beat) = 0.128 × height (cm) − 10.9 with a lower 95% confidence limit of 3.0 ml/beat below the regression line. (Modified from Cooper DM, Weiler-Ravell D, Whipp BJ, et al. Growth-related changes in oxygen uptake and heart rate during progressive exercise in children. *Pediatr Res* 1984;18:845–851.)

$\dot{V}O_2$ versus HR response with a positive intercept on the HR axis.) This curvilinear response of the O_2 pulse during incremental exercise is clearly demonstrated in Figure 7.6B. Thus, both the peak values and the patterns of change of $\dot{V}O_2$, HR, and O_2 pulse may vary importantly in various diseases.

The predicted peak O_2 pulse at any given work rate is strongly dependent on the individual's body size, gender, age, degree of fitness, and hemoglobin concentration. Normal values for the predicted peak O_2 pulse on the cycle ergometer range from approximately 5 ml/beat in a 7-year-old child to 8 ml/beat in a 150-cm, 70-year-old woman to 17 ml/beat in a 190-cm, 30-year-old man. The actual peak O_2 pulse may be considerably higher than predicted in the cardiovascularly fit person or in the patient receiving β-adrenergic blocking drugs.

Recommendations

- Predicted peak O_2 pulse (ml/beat) = Predicted peak $\dot{V}O_2$ (ml/min)/Predicted peak HR (beats/min).
- Both the pattern of change as well as the absolute values of O_2 pulse should be considered.
- Mean values, confidence limits, and graphic data for children are given in Figure 7.7.

BRACHIAL ARTERY BLOOD PRESSURE

Blood pressure can be measured by auscultation during exercise by skilled technicians or physicians, but assessing the fourth Korotkoff phase diastolic pressure (muffling of sound) and the fifth Korotkoff phase diastolic pressure (disappearance of sound) may be difficult because of the background noise of the ergometer. An American Heart Association statement (34) addresses the problems related to the measurement of blood pressure by sphygmomanometry. However, intraarterial pressures can be accurately and continuously measured by means of a pressure transducer attached to an indwelling catheter whenever arterial blood specimens are not being drawn through the catheter.

Jones et al. (15) reported an average increase of 19 mm Hg in systolic pressure as cycle work increased from 50 to 100 W. The blood pressure measurements recorded in Table 7.4 are from a predominantly cigarette-smoking, sedentary normal population (2,35). Values may be lower in non-smoking, more active individuals. Noteworthy are the striking rise in systolic (by both cuff and direct intraarterial recording) and mean pressures, the considerable rise in intraarterial diastolic pressures, the modest rise in fourth-phase cuff diastolic pressures, and the gradual decline in fifth-phase cuff diastolic pressures during incremental exercise. Although resting pressures are higher in older men, the mean maximum exercise systolic and diastolic pressures are similar in both groups. Note that the true mean arterial pressure closely approximates the diastolic pressure plus half the pulse pressure, rather than one-third the pulse pressure during exercise when using a cuff (35).

Accurate intraarterial blood pressure values are more difficult to obtain during treadmill ergometry because of movement artifacts. When the subject is

TABLE 7.4. Blood Pressure During One-Minute Incremental Cycle Exercise Measured Directly from Catheter in Brachial Artery and in Opposite Arm by Cuff

	Prior Exam, at Rest	Rest on Cycle	Exercise Near AT	Exercise Near Maximum
Sedentary, Nonhypertensive Men, Ages 34 to 74				
Systolic intra-arterial		142 ± 18	182 ± 23	207 ± 27
Systolic cuff	124 ± 11	131	171	200
Diastolic intra-arterial		86 ± 10	92 ± 11	99 ± 12
Diastolic fourth phase	79 ± 7	84	86	88
Diastolic fifth phase		81	80	77
Mean intra-arterial		107	128	142
Sedentary, Nonhypertensive Men, Ages 19 to 24				
Systolic intra-arterial		129		203
Diastolic intra-arterial		78		106
Mean intra-arterial		96		141

Values are mean or mean ± standard deviation in mm Hg. AT, anaerobic threshold.
Data are from Hansen JE, Sue DY, Wasserman K. Predicted values for clinical exercise testing. *Am Rev Respir Dis* 1984;129(Suppl):S49–S55 and Robinson TR, Sue DY, Huszczuk A, et al. Intra-arterial and cuff blood pressure responses during incremental cycle ergometry. *Med Sci Sports Exerc* 1988;20:142–149.

using the cycle, the hand on the handlebar stabilizes the arm and transducer, but tight gripping should be avoided to minimize the hypertensive effect of isometric exercise.

Recommendations

The brachial artery blood pressure values of nonhypertensive men, measured directly (intraarterially) or by cuff and sphygmomanometer during 1-minute incremental exercise, are given in Table 7.4.

ANAEROBIC THRESHOLD

The anaerobic threshold (*AT*) is expressed in units of O_2 uptake, but it can also be related to the predicted peak $\dot{V}O_2$. The $\dot{V}O_2$ at which the blood lactate level begins to rise has been used to define the *AT* in normal subjects (36,37) and noninvasively is best measured by the V-slope method (38–40). A useful way to define abnormality is to multiply the lower 95% confidence limit of the ratio of predicted *AT* to predicted peak $\dot{V}O_2$ (Table 7.5) by the predicted peak $\dot{V}O_2$ of the subject. Thus, although the mean *AT* for men ranged between 49% and 63% of peak $\dot{V}O_2$ in several series (13,41–43), the lowest value in our study of 77 middle-aged (34 to 74 years) normal sedentary men was 40% of peak $\dot{V}O_2$ (2). This lower limit of normal agrees well with the lowest value for *AT* in normal men suggested by Wasserman et al. (41) of 1 L/min of $\dot{V}O_2$, approximately the cost of maintaining a moderate walking pace.

Jones et al. (15) and Davis et al. (44) have studied the effect of age on *AT*. The ratios of *AT* to peak $\dot{V}O_2$

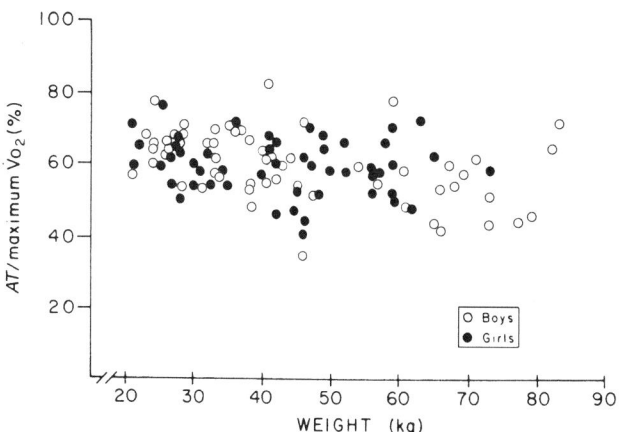

FIGURE 7.8.   The ratio of anaerobic threshold to peak $\dot{V}O_2$ (*AT*/maximum $\dot{V}O_2$), as a percentage, for 109 normal North American boys and girls. (From Cooper DM, Weiler-Ravell D, Whipp BJ, et al. Aerobic parameters of exercise as a function of body size during growth in children. *J Appl Physiol* 1984;56:628–634, with permission.)

found by Jones et al. are slightly higher than those of Davis et al. Though different *AT* detection methods were used (Jones et al. used ventilatory equivalents and Davis et al. used V-slope), both groups found that the absolute *AT* declines with age in both sexes, but less than the decrease in predicted peak $\dot{V}O_2$; thus, the ratio of predicted *AT* to predicted peak $\dot{V}O_2$ tends to increase with age. In addition to the gradual increase in the ratio with age, the ratios tend to be higher in women than men.

Cooper et al. (22) tested 51 girls and 58 boys between the ages of 6 and 17 years. The subjects were healthy and nonobese, but did not participate in vigorous sports. Mean *AT* was 58% of peak $\dot{V}O_2$, and the lower limit of normal for this sample of normal children was approximately 44% of peak $\dot{V}O_2$ (Fig. 7.8).

The mode of exercise may affect the value of *AT* in normal subjects. Davis et al. (45) studied 39 healthy college-aged men. Mean $\dot{V}O_2$ at the *AT* was 46% ± 9% of peak $\dot{V}O_2$ for arm cycling, 64% ± 9% of peak $\dot{V}O_2$ for leg cycling, and 59% ± 6% of peak $\dot{V}O_2$ for treadmill exercise. A substantial difference was noted between the *AT* during arm cycling and either form of leg exercise, but no significant difference existed between the *AT* obtained from cycle exercise and that obtained from treadmill exercise. Buchfuhrer et al. (46) found similar ratios of *AT* to peak $\dot{V}O_2$ for treadmill and for cycle exercise: 50% ± 9% and 47% ± 11%, respectively. Withers et al. (47), however, comparing highly trained cyclists and runners, found a higher *AT* for the total group on the treadmill (mean 76% of peak $\dot{V}O_2$) than on the cycle (mean 64% of peak $\dot{V}O_2$), with the cyclists reach-

TABLE 7.5.   Mean and Lower 95% Confidence Limits for Ratio of Predicted Anaerobic Threshold to Predicted Peak $\dot{V}O_2$ in Adults, as a Percentage

Age (yr)	Men		Women	
	Mean	Lower 95% Limit	Mean	Lower 95% Limit
20	53	42	52	41
30	54	43	55	44
40	55	44	58	47
50	56	45	60	49
60	57	46	63	52
70	58	47	65	54

Data are from Jones NL, Makrides L, Hitchcock C, et al. Normal standards for an incremental progressive cycle ergometer test. *Am Rev Respir Dis* 1985; 131:700–708 and Davis JA, Storer TW, Caiozzo VJ. Prediction of normal values for lactate threshold estimated by gas exchange in men and women. *J Appl Cardiol* 1997;76:157–164.

ing higher *AT* and *AT*/peak $\dot{V}O_2$ on the cycle and runners reaching higher *AT* and *AT*/peak$\dot{V}O_2$ on the treadmill.

Recommendations

- The mean values and confidence limits for the predicted *AT* in normal children are given in Table 7.3, with the ratios of predicted *AT* to predicted peak $\dot{V}O_2$ in Figure 7.8. It can be seen in the latter that the lower 95% confidence limit for the ratio of predicted *AT* to predicted peak$\dot{V}O_2$ is about 44%.
- Table 7.5 gives the mean and lower 95% confidence limit for the ratio of predicted *AT* to predicted peak $\dot{V}O_2$ in normal adult men and women.

OXYGEN UPTAKE–WORK RATE RELATIONSHIP

When a progressively increasing work rate test is initiated, a delay occurs before oxygen uptake begins to increase in a linear fashion. This delay must be considered in the calculation of the overall value of the oxygen uptake–work rate relationship ($\Delta\dot{V}O_2$/ΔWR). This kinetic delay is equal to the time constant of $\dot{V}O_2$ following a stepwise increase, is accounted for by the kinetics of muscle O_2 utilization, and is normally between one-half and three-quarters of a minute. Thus, the formula used to calculate $\Delta\dot{V}O_2$/ΔWR is

$$\Delta\dot{V}O_2/\Delta WR = (\text{Peak}\,\dot{V}O_2 - \text{Unloaded}\,\dot{V}O_2)/[(T - 0.75) \times S]$$

where $\dot{V}O_2$ is measured in ml per minute, *T* is the time of incremental exercise, and *S* is the slope of work rate increment in watts per minute (48).

The overall $\Delta\dot{V}O_2$/ΔWR during incremental cycle ergometer exercise varies modestly with the slope of work rate increase, the cardiovascular fitness of the individual, and the duration of the test (48,49). In ten normal young men, tests of approximately 15 minutes' duration (15-W/min increment) gave higher $\Delta\dot{V}O_2$/ΔWR values (11.2 ± 0.15 ml/min/W) than tests of approximately 5 minutes' duration (60-W/min increment) (8.8 ± 0.15 ml/min/W). In tests of long duration, a lower fraction of the total energy cost of the work is supported from body stores of oxygen and anaerobic sources (e.g., lactate production), and a larger fraction is supported by oxygen extracted from the inspired air. Thus, $\Delta\dot{V}O_2$/ΔWR is slightly greater for the slower increasing work rate test (see Fig. 2.26). The reverse allocation of energy support occurs in maximal tests of short duration. In tests of intermediate duration, however, the mean ± the standard error of $\Delta\dot{V}O_2$/ΔWR found in ten normal young men was 10.2 ± 0.16 ml/min/W (49), and in 54 older sedentary normal men the mean ± the standard deviation (SD) was 10.3 ± 1.0 ml/min/W (48). The mean ± SD of 17 normal men was 9.9 ± 0.7 ml/min/W (see Fig. 4.2). Jones et al. (15) also found a $\Delta\dot{V}O_2$/ΔWR of 10.3 ml/min/W in 100 healthy adult men and women. This range is small enough that the $\Delta\dot{V}O_2$/ΔWR is clinically useful in identifying patients with circulatory disorders.

Most patients with circulatory disorders have a significantly reduced $\Delta\dot{V}O_2$/ΔWR (48). In patients with circulatory disease (pulmonary, cardiac, or peripheral), the $\Delta\dot{V}O_2$/ΔWR may be reduced because of either abnormally slow O_2 extraction kinetics at the muscle or the inability to raise muscle blood flow appropriately to provide oxygen rapidly enough to satisfy muscle requirements (48,50,51). Many persons with coronary artery disease manifest a low $\Delta\dot{V}O_2$/ΔWR relation during the latter portion of their maximal exercise test because of an inability to increase cardiac output.

We have not analyzed data to describe the mean and range of $\Delta\dot{V}O_2$/ΔWR for normal children, but we have seen that many athletes have a higher than average $\Delta\dot{V}O_2$/ΔWR (in the range of 11 to 12 ml/min/W) when cycling, perhaps due to their tendency to involve arm, chest, abdominal, and back musculature more than nonathletes.

Recommendations

For incremental cycle ergometry exercise of 6 to 12 minutes' duration, the $\Delta\dot{V}O_2$/ΔWR for sedentary adults is 10.0 ml/min/W, with a standard deviation of 1.0 ml/min/W and a lower limit of normal at the 95% confidence level of 8.4 ml/min/W.

BREATHING RESERVE, TIDAL VOLUME, AND BREATHING FREQUENCY AT MAXIMUM EXERCISE

Exercise Ventilation and Breathing Reserve

Maximum exercise ventilation (maximum exercise $\dot{V}E$) is similar for leg cycling, treadmill walking, and running (7,46), but is less for arm cycling (45) because the maximal metabolic rate is lower when smaller muscle groups are used. The breathing reserve relates the ventilatory response during such maximum exercise to the maximum ability to breathe. Because normal, untrained subjects do not ordinarily have ventilatory limitations in their ability to perform work (20), some ability to increase ventilation further is usually present during maximal exercise. This potential increase in ventilation is generally estimated from the maximal voluntary ventilation (MVV), a test performed at rest. The MVV is highly dependent on the subject's motivation and effort. Normal values for MVV tests lasting 12 and 15 seconds are available (52,53). The difference between the measured MVV and the maximum $\dot{V}E$ during exercise is used as a measure of the ventilatory or breathing reserve. A low breathing reserve suggests that a subject's exercise capacity may be limited by his or her ventilatory capacity. The breathing reserve is usually reduced in patients with moderate to severe restrictive or obstructive lung disease (see Fig. 5.8).

Many investigators have examined the normal relation between the MVV and the maximum exercise $\dot{V}E$. Maximum exercise $\dot{V}E$ averages 50% to 80% of the 12- or 15-second MVV, indicating a breathing reserve of 20% to 50% of the MVV. Because the MVV is dependent on the subject's cooperation, effort, and technique of performance, the MVV is sometimes indirectly estimated from the FEV_1 or $FEV_{0.75}$. Gandevia and Hugh-Jones (54) suggested that the indirect MVV could be estimated as $FEV_1 \times 35$, whereas Cotes (55) suggested $FEV_{0.75} \times 40$ or $(36.8 \times FEV_1 - 2.8)$. Miller and colleagues (56) found that $FEV_1 \times 41$ or $FEV_{0.75} \times 46$ best estimated MVV.

Our data (2) and those of Campbell (57) indicate that $FEV_1 \times 40$ provides an optimal estimate of the direct MVV both in normal subjects and in patients with obstructive lung disease. If the directly measured MVV is less than the indirectly measured MVV ($FEV_1 \times 40$), poor cooperation or understanding in the performance of the maneuver, extreme obesity, neurologic disorders, or inspiratory obstruction may be possible causes. If one is uncertain regarding a discrepancy between the direct MVV and the indirect MVV, or if the patient has variable obstruction, it may be necessary to have the patient repeat the direct MVV before performing the exercise test. We believe it preferable to use the indirect MVV ($FEV_1 \times 40$) rather than the direct MVV for calculation of the breathing reserve in patients with interstitial disease who use inordinately high frequencies (e.g., over 100 breaths per minute) in the MVV maneuver, frequencies that are unrealistic for the patient to maintain during exercise.

In 77 normal middle-aged subjects during an incremental cycle ergometer exercise test (2,3), the mean direct MVV was 131 ± 23.6 L/min (range 81–203 L/min). The mean maximum exercise $\dot{V}E$/MVV was 71.5% ± 14.6%; only 13 subjects had a value greater than 80%. When we used $FEV_1 \times 40$ as an indirect estimate of the MVV, the mean maximum exercise $\dot{V}E$/indirect MVV was 71.5% ± 15.3%, that is, the same percentage as for the directly measured MVV. Expressing breathing reserve as MVV minus maximum exercise $\dot{V}E$, we obtain an average of 38.1 ± 22.0 L/min using the directly measured MVV and 38.0 ± 21.5 L/min for the indirect MVV. We consider it likely that the patient is ventilatory limited when the breathing reserve is less than 11 L/min.

Tidal Volume and Breathing Frequency

We consider that patients have ventilatory limitation if the exercise tidal volume (V_T) reaches the resting inspiratory capacity (IC), particularly early during a progressively increasing work rate test, or if the breathing frequency exceeds 50 breaths per minute (bpm). The expected maximum exercise V_T, like ventilatory capacity (VC) and other resting pulmonary function measurements, depends on the subject's height, age, and gender. In addition, the dead space or rebreathed volume of the breathing apparatus influences ventilation (58–60).

Hey et al. (61) recommended that V_T be related to $\dot{V}E$ to analyze the breathing pattern, such as is shown in Figure 4.12. At low exercise intensity, the increase in $\dot{V}E$ is accomplished primarily by an increase in V_T. After the V_T reaches approximately 50% to 60% of the VC, further increases in $\dot{V}E$ are accomplished primarily by increasing breathing frequency (f) (55,62). Thus, f is a curvilinear function of $\dot{V}E$. Spiro et al. (62) found that the maximum V_T reached in normal subjects was approximately 55% of VC in normal men and 45% in normal women, whereas Cotes (55) suggested that maximum V_T is about 50% of VC for VC values between 2.0 and 5.0 L in normal men and women of European descent. Astrand (1) found that at maximal exercise the V_T averaged between 1.9 and 2.0 L, or 52% to 58% of the VC, whereas f at maximal exercise ranged between 34 and 46 bpm. Little difference in V_T/VC was noted among age groups, but f was lower in the older subjects studied.

Wasserman and Whipp (20) compared exercise V_T to IC. They found that V_T does not usually exceed approximately 70% of the IC during exercise, but it increases to a value approaching 100% in patients with restrictive lung disease, suggesting that the IC may limit the increase in V_T (see Fig. 4.12). In a series of 77 healthy middle-aged men, the mean resting V_T of 0.71 ± 0.26 L increased to 1.44 ± 0.43 L at the AT and 2.28 ± 0.43 L at maximum exercise (2,3). Maximum f was 41.6 ± 9.6 min^{-1}. Maximum V_T averaged 70.0% ± 10.7% of the IC and 55.0% ± 8.7% of the VC. No one had a maximum exercise V_T greater than his resting IC, and only three had a maximal exercise breathing frequency greater than 60 min^{-1}.

Partitioning the duration of the ventilatory cycle (T_{TOT}) into inspiratory (T_I) and expiratory (T_E) components may also prove useful, but to date this measurement is not commonplace in clinical exercise testing. T_I/T_{TOT} should be quite low for patients with chronic obstructive pulmonary disease (COPD) compared with other patients.

Recommendations

Resting spirometry values must be reliable. At maximum work rates, the following values (mean ± SD) have been found for normal adult men, aged 34 to 74, for cycle ergometry using a breathing valve with a dead space of 64 ml (2,3).

- Maximum exercise $\dot{V}_E$/maximum voluntary ventilation (MVV) = 72% ± 15%.
- Breathing reserve = (MVV − maximum exercise $\dot{V}_E$) = 38 ± 22 L/min; lower limit of normal = 11 L/min.
- Maximum tidal volume (maximum V_T) is less than inspiratory capacity (IC) in all subjects.
- Maximum breathing frequency (f) is less than 55 bpm in over 95% of all subjects.

VENTILATORY EFFICIENCY

Because ventilation is more closely linked to CO_2 output than O_2 uptake, ventilatory efficiency is best defined by the relationship of the liters of ventilation required to eliminate a liter of CO_2. Mathematically, this relationship can be expressed either as a ratio or a slope (see Fig. 4.20), with the only factors being dead space volume–tidal volume ratio, Pa_{CO_2}, $\dot{V}_{CO_2}$, $\dot{V}_E$, and a constant:

$$\dot{V}_E/\dot{V}_{CO_2} = k/[Pa_{CO_2} \times (1 - V_D/V_T)]$$

Practically, the efficiency or inefficiency of elimination of CO_2 can be affected by many factors, including anxiety, the pattern of breathing, the metabolic demand, the matching of ventilation to perfusion in the lung, the arterial or mixed alveolar P_{CO_2}, and the intensities of H^+, CO_2, and O_2 stimulation of the carotid bodies and the responsiveness of ventilatory control mechanisms. Because these factors, in turn, are strongly affected by the presence, absence, or changes caused by both lung and heart diseases, the measurements of ventilatory efficiency can be clinically very useful.

Measurement of the slope of $\dot{V}_E$ (BTPS) versus $\dot{V}_{CO_2}$ (STPD) during incremental exercise below the ventilatory compensation point (VCP) (i.e., before acidemia increases ventilatory drive; see Fig. 4.20) is often favored by cardiologists (63–66) because it is influenced by the changes in V_D/V_T occurring with heart failure (67). Measurement of the ratio of $\dot{V}_E/\dot{V}_{CO_2}$ is often favored by others (see Fig. 4.20) because it is slightly less variable than the slope in a normal population, the pattern of its changes during an exercise test may be distinctive, and it is very stable at and immediately above the anaerobic threshold ($\dot{V}_E/\dot{V}_{CO_2}$ @ AT) (68). Furthermore, the $\dot{V}_E/\dot{V}_{CO_2}$ @ AT is similar to the lowest $\dot{V}_E/\dot{V}_{CO_2}$ ratio when the AT is indeterminate. Stability occurs at this time during exercise because psychological factors affecting breathing patterns are minimal and ventilation has not yet been further stimulated by the acidemia of heavy exercise (69). Using normal apparatus, the $\dot{V}_E$ versus $\dot{V}_{CO_2}$ slope is trivially affected by the gas exchange system dead space apparatus. When calculating $\dot{V}_E/\dot{V}_{CO_2}$ ratios, the apparatus dead space ventilation (volume times frequency of breathing) should be subtracted from the total ventilation.

In normal young adult men performing mild to moderate exercise, $\dot{V}_E$ can be predicted from the following equation (70):

$$\dot{V}_E \text{ (L/min, BTPS)} = 24.6 \times \dot{V}_{CO_2} \text{ (L/min, STPD)} + 3.2; \text{ standard error of estimate (SEE) of 2.4 L/min}$$

Fairbarn et al. (73) found this relation to change with age as follows: $\dot{V}_E$ (L/min, BTPS) = 22.6 × $\dot{V}_{CO_2}$ (L/min, STPD) + 4.4 with an SEE of 5.3 L/min at age 30, $\dot{V}_E$ = 25.8 × $\dot{V}_{CO_2}$ + 4.3 with an SEE of 5.0 at mean age 55, and $\dot{V}_E$ = 29.5 × $\dot{V}_{CO_2}$ + 4.3 with an SEE of 7.5 at mean age 75. Cotes also found the $\dot{V}_E/\dot{V}_{CO_2}$ to increase approximately 1.0 for each decade of age (55).

TABLE 7.6. Ventilatory Efficiency During Exercise for Men*

Age (yr)	N	$\dot{V}E$ vs. $\dot{V}CO_2$ Slope	Lowest $\dot{V}E/\dot{V}CO_2$
<20	46	22.9 ± 2.8	23.5 ± 2.0
21–30	90	23.6 ± 2.8	23.9 ± 2.1
31–40	49	23.9 ± 3.1	25.0 ± 2.7
41–50	37	25.2 ± 2.9	26.1 ± 2.2
51–60	54	27.2 ± 3.0	28.0 ± 2.9
>60	34	27.5 ± 3.1	29.4 ± 2.3

*To determine values for women, add 1 to the values shown for men.

Selected normal and upper 95% confidence limit values for $\dot{V}E$ versus $\dot{V}CO_2$, and $\dot{V}E/\dot{V}CO_2$ at the *AT*, and lowest $\dot{V}E/\dot{V}CO_2$ for a large population of normal adults at sea level are given in Table 7.6 (68).

It is clear from the formula given at the start of this section that $\dot{V}E/\dot{V}CO_2$ will be higher than normal when the physiological dead space–tidal volume ratio (VD/VT) is high or when the patient hyperventilates (i.e., $PaCO_2$ is lower than normal). VD/VT cannot be calculated unless the $PaCO_2$ is measured. Importantly, $PETCO_2$ cannot be substituted for $PaCO_2$ to calculate VD/VT. $PETCO_2$ is lower than $PaCO_2$ in diseases with ventilation–perfusion mismatching. A low $PETCO_2$ does not necessarily indicate hyperventilation because it also can be seen with a normal $PaCO_2$ combined with a high VD/VT. $PETCO_2$ is higher than $PaCO_2$ during exercise in normal subjects, and VD/VT can be assumed to be normal when this is found. Thus, when $\dot{V}E/\dot{V}CO_2$ is high and there is no evidence for acute hyperventilation (normal R) or low blood HCO_3^-, it is likely that VD/VT is high.

Recommendations

Normal values (mean ± SD) and upper 95% confidence limits for $\dot{V}E/\dot{V}CO_2$ and $\dot{V}E$ versus $\dot{V}CO_2$ below the respiratory compensation point (with $\dot{V}E$ expressed as L/min BTPS and $\dot{V}CO_2$ as L/min STPD) for cycle or treadmill ergometry are given in Table 7.6.

PHYSIOLOGICAL DEAD SPACE–TIDAL VOLUME RATIO

The physiological dead space (VD) is dependent on anatomic and physiological factors, whereas the physiological dead space–tidal volume ratio (VD/VT) is also dependent, even in normal subjects, on the pattern of breathing. At rest, the VD/VT may be elevated because of rapid shallow breathing or anxiety. Physiological control mechanisms usually stabilize ventilation at a slower and more efficient breathing pattern soon after the onset of exercise unless anxiety is extreme. Calculation of the VD and VD/VT must be carefully performed, making an adjustment for the apparatus dead space (see Appendix C). In addition, gas exchange measurements must be synchronous with arterial blood sampling for measuring $PaCO_2$.

All studies have shown a fall in VD/VT during exercise in normal subjects. Thus, whereas mean VD/VT at rest ranged from 0.28 to 0.35 in several studies of normal subjects, mean VD/VT decreased to between 0.20 and 0.25 near the *AT* and to less than 0.21 at maximum exercise (2,59,69,72).

Figure 7.9 shows the effect of exercise on VD/VT at various levels of cycle exercise in normal young men. As can be seen, the VD/VT stabilizes at a new low value soon after exercise starts and is slightly lower at higher work rates. Cotes (55) suggested that VD (ml) = 140 + 0.07 VT (ml) with an SD = 90 ml in young men during exercise. Jones et al. (59) found the following relation during exercise in 17 normal young men: VD (ml) = 138 + 0.077 VT (ml), with r = 0.69. Lifshay et al. (60) showed that men aged 50 to 81 had a significantly higher VD than men and women aged 18 to 37 years. The prediction equations of Bradley et al. (73) for VD use sex, age, height, $\dot{V}CO_2$, $\dot{V}E$, f, and temperature as factors.

The practice of some manufacturers of offering a calculation of "noninvasive VD/VT" is invalid. This calculation substitutes $PETCO_2$ for $PaCO_2$ in the foregoing alveolar mass balance equation rearranged to allow VD/VT calculations. Because the difference between $PETCO_2$ and $PaCO_2$ is influenced by VD/VT, this calculation involves a heavy dose of circular reasoning.

Recommendations

Normal values for VD/VT at rest and during upright exercise after allowance for valve dead space are as follows.

- For men under age 40: VD/VT (mean ± SD) = 0.29 ± 0.06 at rest, 0.17 ± 0.05 at the *AT*, and 0.16 ± 0.04 at maximum exercise.
- For men over age 40: VD/VT (mean ± SD) = 0.30 ± 0.08 at rest, 0.20 ± 0.07 at the *AT*, and 0.19 ± 0.07 at maximum exercise (2).

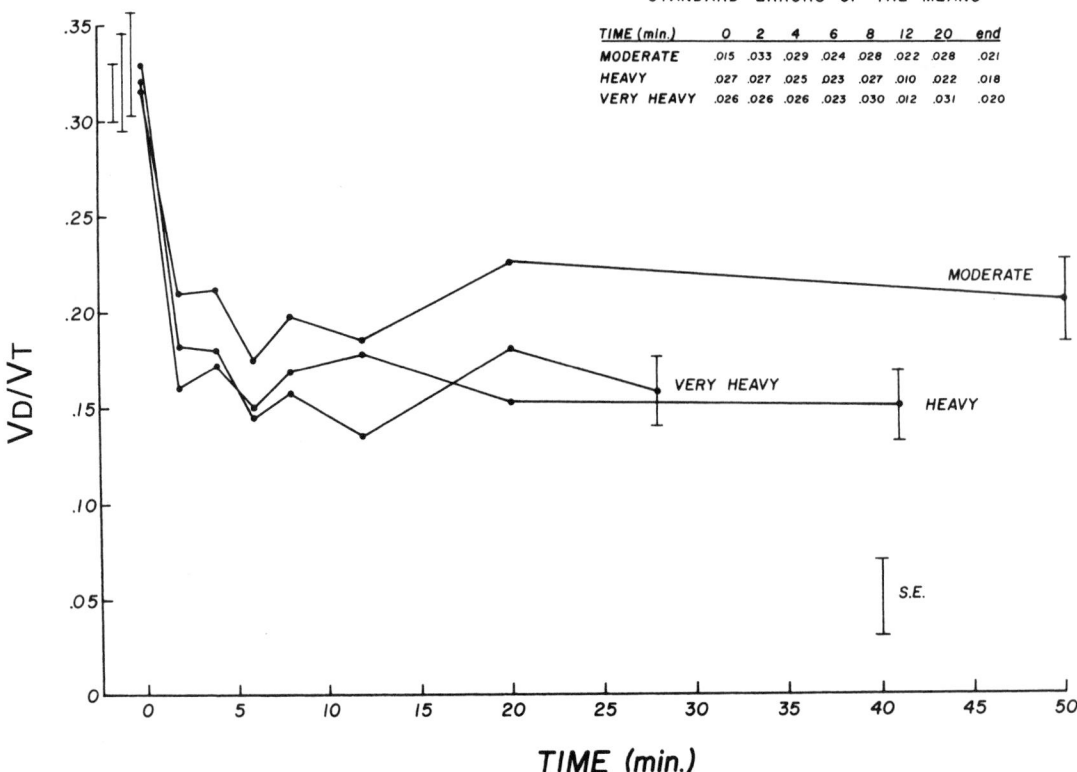

FIGURE 7.9.   The physiological dead space–tidal volume ratio (VD/VT) in ten normal young men at rest and during three intensities of cycle ergometer exercise as related to exercise time. The standard errors of the means (SEM) are given in the table inset. (From Wasserman K,
VanKessel A, Burton GB. Interaction of physiological mechanisms during exercise. *J Appl Physiol* 1967;22:71–85, with permission.)

- Upper 95% confidence limits for men over 40: VD/VT = 0.45 at rest, 0.33 at the *AT*, and 0.30 at maximum exercise (2).

The VD/VT of patients should not be reported using Pa_{CO_2} calculated from expired gas measures such as PET_{CO_2}. Blood P_{CO_2} from a systemic artery or well-heated hand vein must be used.

ARTERIAL AND END-TIDAL CARBON DIOXIDE TENSIONS

Resting PET_{CO_2} and Pa_{CO_2} values are dependent on the degree of apprehension, anxiety, and training of the subject. Many anxious individuals have a strong tendency to hyperventilate, especially while breathing through a mouthpiece and awaiting the signal to begin exercise (Fig. 7.10). Once exercise starts, however, the blood gases and pH are not discernibly different whether the individual is performing the work while breathing through a low-resistance breathing valve or breathing normally without a mouthpiece (74). In more apprehensive

individuals, the Pa_{CO_2} values rise from rest to moderate exercise as physiological control mechanisms suppress psychogenic hyperventilation. In the relaxed individual, Pa_{CO_2} values remain relatively stable at rest and during mild and moderate exercise. Although Pa_{CO_2} values cannot be predicted accurately from PET_{CO_2} values in an individual person, particularly in a patient with lung disease, measurement of PET_{CO_2} is often valuable for following trends in Pa_{CO_2}.

Wasserman et al. (69) found that $P(a - ET)_{CO_2}$ changed from approximately +2.5 mm Hg at rest to −4 mm Hg during heavy work in ten normal men (Fig. 7.11). Jones et al. (59) found that in 17 normal subjects at the highest work rates reached, PET_{CO_2} was always more than 2 mm Hg higher than Pa_{CO_2}. In five normal men, Whipp and Wasserman (72) found that $P(a - ET)_{CO_2}$ was 2.8 ± 1.6 mm Hg at rest and -2.8 ± 0.6 mm Hg at a work rate of 220 W. All $P(a - ET)_{CO_2}$ values were negative for work rates above 115 W. In five normal young men near the *AT*, Jones et al. (75) found that $Pa_{CO_2} = 5.5 + 0.9\ PET_{CO_2} - 0.0021\ VT$ (SE = 1.4). These relations are unlikely to be valid

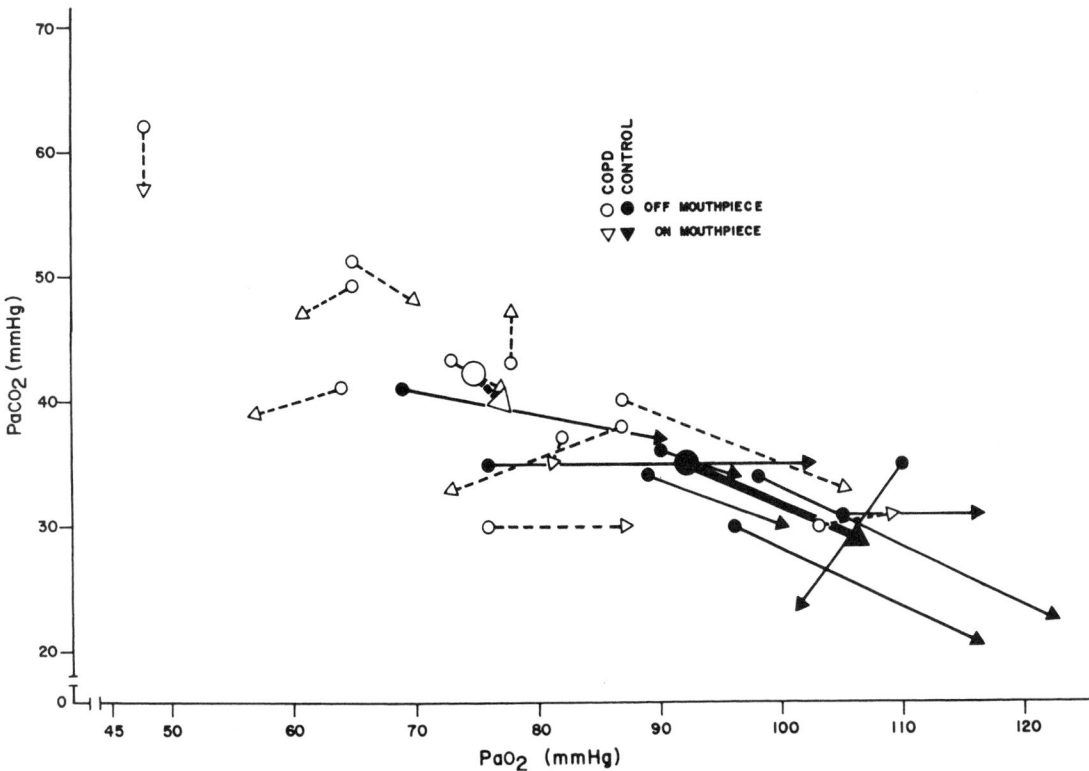

FIGURE 7.10.   Resting arterial partial pressures of CO_2 ($PaCO_2$) and O_2 (PaO_2) in normal control subjects and in patients with chronic obstructive pulmonary disease (COPD) off and acutely on the mouthpiece while awaiting the signal to start cycle ergometer exercise. Small arrows show individual values, and large arrows show mean values. Note the small mean decline in $PaCO_2$ and the increase in PaO_2 in the patients with COPD while breathing on the mouthpiece. In contrast, the controls show a larger decline in $PaCO_2$ and a much larger rise in PaO_2 with the same mouthpiece at rest. (Courtesy of Dr. J. D. Andrews.)

in patients with lung disease or with disorders affecting the ventilation–perfusion relations. In 77 asbestos-exposed healthy men (2, 3), $P(a - ET)CO_2$ at rest was 0.3 ± 2.9 mm Hg (mean $\pm$ SD) and decreased to -4.1 ± 3.2 mm Hg at maximum exercise. At the peak of exercise, a positive $P(a - ET)CO_2$ was rare.

Recommendations

Normal values at sea level during upright exercise in adult men are as follows.

- $PaCO_2$: Resting value = 36 to 42 mm Hg; stable or increasing slightly during mild and moderate exercise, declining with heavy exercise.
- $PETCO_2$: Resting value = 36 to 42 mm Hg; increases normally by 3 to 8 mm Hg during mild and moderate exercise (depending on breathing pattern), and decreases with heavy exercise.
- $P(a - ET)CO_2$ (mean $\pm$ SD) at the AT = -3 ± 3 mm Hg. At maximum exercise the $P(a - ET)CO_2$ = -4 ± 3 mm Hg and is negative ($PETCO_2$ exceeds $PaCO_2$) in more than 95% of normal men.

ARTERIAL, ALVEOLAR, AND END-TIDAL OXYGEN TENSIONS AND ARTERIAL OXYHEMOGLOBIN SATURATION

The normal resting PaO_2 is dependent on age, body position, and nutritional status. Values are lower with increasing age, obesity, fasting, and in the supine position. Nevertheless, sea-level values less than 80 mm Hg are not seen in normal persons younger than 70 years in the sitting position except in those who are quite obese. The $PETO_2$ and PAO_2 (the latter calculated from the alveolar air equation; see Appendix C) are normally similar, but they may differ by 10 or more mm Hg in patients with severe maldistribution of ventilation. The PAO_2 and PaO_2 decrease transiently soon after the start of exercise (because the rise in $\dot{V}E$ is slower than the rise in $\dot{V}O_2$; i.e., R decreases) and then increase back to approximately resting values (see Chapter 2 on O_2 uptake kinetics).

The arterial oxyhemoglobin saturation (SaO_2) normally changes less than 2% from rest to maxi-

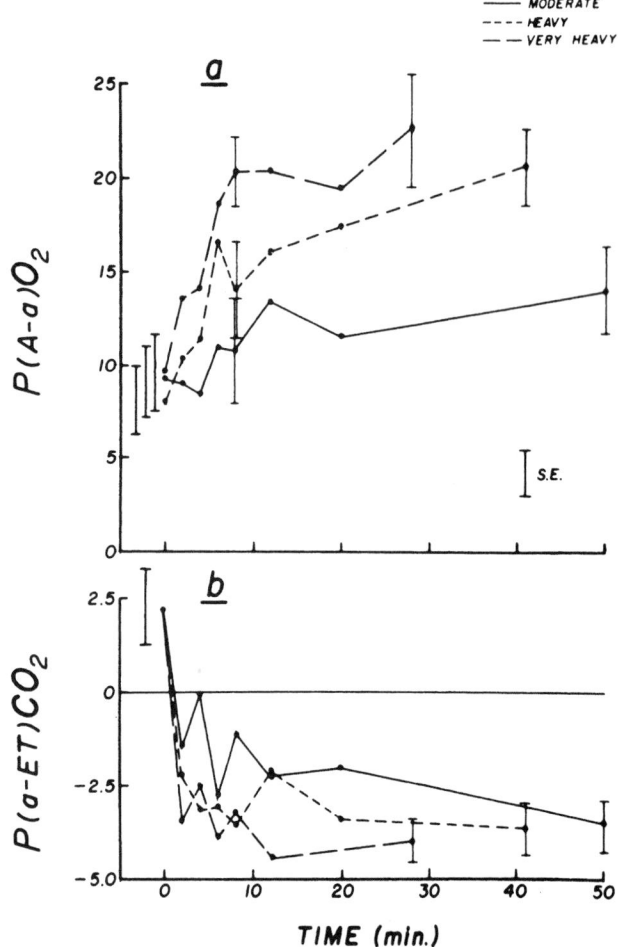

FIGURE 7.11.   The P(A − a)O$_2$ and P(a − ET)CO$_2$ in ten normal young men at rest and during three intensities of cycle ergometer exercise as related to exercise duration. The mean and standard error of the mean (SEM) are depicted. (From Wasserman K, VanKessel A, Burton GB. Interaction of physiological mechanisms during exercise. *J Appl Physiol* 1967;22:71–85, with permission.)

mal exercise. In highly motivated athletes, the SaO$_2$ has been reported to fall below resting values (76), but this is uncommon.

The PETO$_2$ normally increases 10 to 30 mm Hg for exercise above the *AT* because of metabolic acidosis–induced hyperventilation and rising R at maximal exercise.

Many reports show that the P(A − a)O$_2$ increases during heavy exercise in normal subjects. Lilienthal et al. (77) and Asmussen and Nielsen (78) found a mean P(A − a)O$_2$ of 30 mm Hg at high work rates. Jones et al. (59) found, in 17 normal active men not in physical training, a mean P(A − a)O$_2$ of 12 mm Hg at rest, with an increase to approximately 20 mm Hg at work rates with a V̇O$_2$ over 1.5 L/min. Whipp and Wasserman (72) found, in five healthy young men, a P(A − a)O$_2$ of 7.4 ± 4.2 mm Hg (mean ± SD) at rest and 10.8 ± 3.6 mm Hg at heavy exer-

cise. Cruz et al. (79) studied four subjects at rest and at work rates approximating 50%, 75%, and 100% of peak V̇O$_2$ at sea level and found P(A − a)O$_2$ values of 11.5 ± 5.4, 11.0 ± 4.2, 16.3 ± 2.6, and 20 ± 8.8 mm Hg, respectively. Hansen et al. (80) studied 16 healthy young men, aged 18 to 24, during sea-level exercise on a cycle ergometer and found that the mean P(A − a) O$_2$ was 8 mm Hg while sitting at rest, 7 mm Hg during mild exercise, 11 mm Hg during moderate exercise, and 15 mm Hg during maximum exercise.

Similar results were obtained by Wasserman et al. (69) in ten healthy young men; values are shown at rest and at three work intensities as related to time in Figure 7.11. We found, in 77 normal older men (aged 34 to 74 years), P(A − a)O$_2$ values (mean ± SD) of 12.8 ± 7.4 mm Hg at rest and 19.0 ± 8.8 mm Hg at maximum exercise (2,3). At maximum exercise, P(A − a)O$_2$ was greater than 35 mm Hg in only 3 of these 77 men.

Recommendations

The normal arterial blood and PETO$_2$ values at sea level during upright exercise in adult men are as follows.

- PaO$_2$ at rest = 80 mm Hg or greater; usually increases slightly with heavy exercise.
- SaO$_2$ at rest = 95% or greater; no decrease with exercise.
- PETO$_2$ at rest = 90 mm Hg or greater; increases with heavy exercise.
- P(A − a)O$_2$ (mean ± SD) for ages 20 to 39 years: At rest = 8 mm Hg, at the *AT* = 11 mm Hg, and at maximum exercise = 15 mm Hg.
- P(A − a)O$_2$ (mean ±SD) for ages 40 to 69 years: At rest = 13 ± 7 mm Hg, at the *AT* = 17 ± 7 mm Hg, and at maximum exercise = 19 ± 9 mm Hg. The upper limit of normal (95% confidence level) at the *AT* = 28 mm Hg and at maximum exercise = 35 mm Hg.

FEMORAL AND MIXED VENOUS VALUES AND ESTIMATION OF CARDIAC OUTPUT

Muscle blood flow and oxygen extraction both increase strikingly with exercise. At near-maximum leg exercise, femoral vein values in normal subjects reach the following mean ± SE values: PO$_2$ = 20 ± 2 mm Hg, SO$_2$ = 17% ± 3%, pH = 7.00 ± 0.04, PCO$_2$ =

80 ± 5 mm Hg, and lactate = 10 ± 1 mmol/L (81). In patients with heart disease, minimum mean femoral vein values are similar: P_{O_2} = 18 mm Hg and S_{O_2} = 18% to 21% (82,83). Concurrent mixed venous values in the same patients are 2 mm Hg and 4% higher, respectively.

The usual values found for mixed venous S_{O_2} ($S\bar{v}_{O_2}$) at peak treadmill or cycle exercise approximate 25%. In normal subjects, as well as in patients with heart failure, the $S\bar{v}_{O_2}$, $C\bar{v}_{O_2}$, $C(a - \bar{v})_{O_2}$, and O_2 extraction ratio [$C(a - \bar{v})_{O_2}/Ca_{O_2}$] change in relatively linear fashion as $\dot{V}_{O_2}$ changes from rest to peak values. In five normal men, the $C(a - \bar{v})_{O_2}$ values (in ml/100 ml blood) were 5.72 + 0.1 × % peak $\dot{V}_{O_2}$, with a standard deviation of 1.08 ml/100 ml, r = 0.94. Combining the data from three studies (84–86) involving normal subjects and patients with congestive heart failure, the $C(a - \bar{v})_{O_2}$ values (in ml/100 ml blood) were 5.55 + 0.085 × % peak $\dot{V}_{O_2}$, with a standard deviation of 1.09, r = 0.97. Absolute Ca_{O_2} values are dependent on the hemoglobin concentration, which usually rises 5% to 8% at peak exercise in healthy individuals, and the Sa_{O_2}.

Historically, it has been suggested that cardiac output could be measured noninvasively during exercise with the Fick principle by estimating mixed venous CO_2 content using rebreathing techniques (30). This method for estimating cardiac output depends on the premise that mixed venous P_{CO_2} values are highly correlated with mixed venous CO_2 content. This is not the case, as shown in Chapter 3.

Recommendations

- In the normal person and the person with heart disease, femoral vein mean ± standard error (SE) values are P_{O_2} = 19 ± 3 mm Hg and S_{O_2} = 19% ± 3% at maximum leg exercise, when such exercise is not limited by other than cardiovascular factors.

- Concurrent mixed venous values are P_{O_2} = 21 ± 3 mm Hg and S_{O_2} = 23% ± 3%. In such individuals, the $S\bar{v}_{O_2}$, $C\bar{v}_{O_2}$, $C(a - \bar{v})_{O_2}$, and O_2 extraction ratio change in near linear fashion from rest to maximum exercise.

- In the absence of anemia, hypoxemia, or significant carboxyhemoglobinemia, $C(a - \bar{v})_{O_2}$ in ml/100 ml of blood is 5.55 + 0.085 × peak $\dot{V}_{O_2}$ with an SD = 1.1 ml/100 ml blood. These values can be used to estimate cardiac output and stroke volume, especially at maximum exercise (84).

ACID–BASE BALANCE

In the normal individual, an intense metabolic acidosis is induced by heavy exercise (see Chapters 2 and 3). Measurement of the acid–base status at the termination of an incremental exercise test is valuable in deciding whether the subject has made a good effort and performed near maximum. Resting venous and arterial lactate values are normally less than 1 mmol/L and typically rise substantially before the termination of maximal exercise. During exercise, venous lactate values can be dependent on the site of lactate production and the sampling site (87), whereas arterial or mixed venous lactate values give a better indication of the total body lactate burden.

As previously described, the rise in blood lactate during exercise is accompanied by a nearly equimolar decline in bicarbonate and a decrease in pH. This metabolic acidosis stimulates hyperventilation, a decrease in Pa_{CO_2}, and an increase in $\dot{V}_{CO_2}$ beyond that predicted from aerobic metabolism. This is reflected by an increase in R. The arterial lactate and R reach their peak and the pH and bicarbonate reach their nadir at about 2 minutes into recovery. The magnitudes of the lactate and bicarbonate changes indicate the severity of exercise-induced metabolic acidosis.

TABLE 7.7.   Metabolic Acidosis at the End of and During Recovery from Maximum Incremental Cycle Ergometer Exercise in Normal Sedentary Men

	At End of Exercise		2 Minutes into Recovery	
Age (yr)	18–24	34–74	18–24	34–74
Number studied	10	77	10	77
Average exercise duration (min)	18	9	18	9
Arterial lactate increase (mmol/L)[a]	6.6 ± 1.4		7.6 ± 1.8	
Arterial HCO_3^- decrease from rest (mmol/L)[a]	6.2 ± 2.3	4.0 ± 2.5	8.7 ± 2.6	8.5 ± 2.9
Arterial pH[a]	7.31 ± 0.04	7.37 ± 0.04	7.29 ± 0.04	7.33 ± 0.03
Gas exchange ratio (R)[a]		1.21 ± 0.12		1.59 ± 0.19

[a]Values are mean ± standard deviation.
Data are from Hansen JE, Sue DY, Wasserman K. Predicted values for clinical exercise testing. *Am Rev Respir Dis* 1984;129(Suppl):S49–S55 and Beaver WL, Wasserman K, Whipp BJ. Bicarbonate buffering of lactic acid generated during exercise. *J Appl Physiol* 1986;60:472–478.

Normal values for younger (88) and older (2) men for incremental cycle exercise tests are given in Table 7.7. Small changes signify a mild degree of exercise stress secondary to low motivation or disorders that preclude the performance of exercise at a significant level above the *AT*.

Recommendations

- R values (mean ± SD) in normal older men at end of exercise are 1.21 ± 0.12 and are 1.59 ± 0.19 at 2 minutes of recovery. However, the value of R depends on the rate at which lactate increases and HCO_3^- decreases, not on the work rate per se.
- Decline in HCO_3^- and increase in lactate (both in mmol/L) at end of exercise are approximately 6 ± 2 in younger men and 4 ± 2.5 in older men; at 2 minutes of recovery, these are approximately 8.4 ± 2.5 in all men.

SUMMARY

This chapter presented and critiqued normal exercise values for peak $\dot{V}O_2$, *AT*, HR, HRR, O_2 pulse, arterial blood pressure, ventilatory pattern, breathing reserve, ventilatory equivalents, arterial blood gases, $P(A - a)O_2$, $P(a - ET)CO_2$, VD/VT, femoral and mixed venous blood gases, and acid–base balance for use in assessment of patients.

References

1. Astrand PO, Rodahl K. *Textbook of work physiology*. 3rd ed. New York: McGraw-Hill, 1986.
2. Hansen JE, Sue DY, Wasserman K. Predicted values for clinical exercise testing. *Am Rev Respir Dis* 1984; 129(Suppl):S49–S55.
3. Sue DY, Hansen JE. Normal values in adults during exercise testing. *Clin Chest Med* 1984;5:89–97.
4. Jones NL, Summers E, Killian KJ. Influence of age and structure on exercise during incremental cycle ergometry in men and women. *Am Rev Respir Dis* 1989;140: 1373–1380.
5. Astrand I. Aerobic work capacity in men and women with special reference to age. *Acta Physiol Scand* 1960; 49(Suppl 169):1–9.
6. Drinkwater BL, Horvath SM, Wells CL. Aerobic power of females, ages 10 to 68. *Gerontology* 1975;30:385–394.
7. Hermansen L, Saltin B. Oxygen uptake during maximal treadmill and bicycle exercise. *J Appl Physiol* 1969; 26:31–37.
8. Dehn MM, Bruce RA. Longitudinal variations in maximal oxygen intake with age and activity. *J Appl Physiol* 1972;33:805–807.
9. Astrand I, Astrand PO, Hallback I, Kilborn A. Reduction in maximal oxygen uptake with age. *J Appl Physiol* 1973;35:649–654.
10. Bruce RA, Kusumi F, Hosmer D. Maximal oxygen intake and nomographic assessment of functional aerobic impairment in cardiovascular disease. *Am Heart J* 1973;85:546–562.
11. Astrand PO. Human physical fitness with special reference to sex and age. *Physiol Rev* 1956;36:307–335.
12. Balke B, Ware RW. An experimental study of "physical fitness" of Air Force personnel. *U S Armed Forces Med J* 1959;10:675–688.
13. Davis JA, Frank MH, Whipp BJ, Wasserman K. Anaerobic threshold alterations caused by endurance training in middle-aged men. *J Appl Physiol* 1979;46:1039–1046.
14. Davis JA, Storer TW, Caizzo VJ, Pham PH. Lower reference limit for maximal oxygen uptake in men and women. *Clin Physiol Funct Imaging* 2002;22:332–338.
15. Jones NL, Makrides L, Hitchcock C, McCartney N. Normal standards for an incremental progressive cycle ergometer test. *Am Rev Respir Dis* 1985;131:700–708.
16. Itoh H, Koike A, Taniguchi K, Marumo F. Severity and pathophysiology of heart failure on the basis of anaerobic threshold (*AT*) and related parameters. *Jpn Circ J* 1989;53:146–154.
17. Neder JA, Nery LE, Castello A, Sachs A, Silva AC, Whipp BJ. Normal values for clinical exercise testing: a prospective and randomized study. *Am J Respir Crit Care Med* 1998;157:A89.
18. Stelken AM, Younis LT, Jennison SH, Miller DD, Miller LW, Shaw LJ, Kargl D, Chaitman BR. Prognostic value of cardiopulmonary exercise testing using percent achieved of predicted peak oxygen uptake for patients with ischemic and dilated cardiomyopathy. *J Am Coll Cardiol* 1996;27:345–352.
19. Buskirk E, Taylor HL. Maximal oxygen intake and its relation to body composition, with special reference to chronic physical activity and obesity. *J Appl Physiol* 1957;11:72–78.
20. Wasserman K, Whipp BJ. Exercise physiology in health and disease (state of the art). *Am Rev Respir Dis* 1975;112:219–249.
21. Cooper DM, Weiler-Ravell D, Whipp BJ, Wasserman K. Aerobic parameters of exercise as a function of body size during growth in children. *J Appl Physiol* 1984;56:628–634.
22. Cooper DM, Weiler-Ravell D. Gas exchange response to exercise in children. *Am Rev Respir Dis* 1984; 129(Suppl): S47–S48.
23. Astrand PO, Saltin B. Maximal oxygen uptake and heart rate in various types of muscular activity. *J Appl Physiol* 1961;16:977–981.
24. Wyndham CH, Strydom NB, Leary WP, Williams CG. Studies of the maximum capacity for men for physical effort. *Arbeitsphysiologie* 1966;22:285–295.

25. Dempsey JA, Reddan W, Rankin J, Balke B. Alveolar-arterial gas exchange during muscular work in obesity. *J Appl Physiol* 1966;21:1807–1814.

26. Shephard RJ, Allen C, Benade AJS, Davies CTM, DiPrampero PE, Hedman R, Merriman JE, Myhre K, Simmons R. The maximum oxygen intake. *Bull WHO* 1968;38:757–764.

27. Faulkner JA, Roberts DE, Elk RL, Conway J. Cardiovascular responses to submaximum and maximum effort cycling and running. *J Appl Physiol* 1971;30:457–461.

28. McArdle WD, Katch FI, Pechar GS. Comparison of continuous and discontinuous treadmill and bicycle tests for max $\dot{V}_{O_2}$. *Med Sci Sports Exerc* 1972;5:156–160.

29. Davis JA, Kasch FW. Aerobic and anaerobic differences between maximal running and cycling in middle-aged males. *Aust J Sports Med* 1975;7:81–84.

30. Jones NL. *Clinical exercise testing*. 3rd ed. Philadelphia: W.B. Saunders, 1988.

31. Sheffield LT, Maloof JA, Sawyer JA, Roitman D. Maximal heart rate and treadmill performance of healthy women in relation to age. *Circulation* 1978;57:79–84.

32. Cooper KH, Purdy J, White S, Pollack M, Linnerud AC. Age-fitness adjusted maximal heart rates. *Med Sci Sports* 1977;10:78–86.

33. Cooper DM, Weiler-Ravell D, Whipp BJ, Wasserman K. Growth-related changes in oxygen uptake and heart rate during progressive exercise in children. *Pediatr Res* 1984;18:845–851.

34. American Heart Association. Human blood pressure determination by sphygmomanometry. *Circulation* 1993;88:2460–2470.

35. Robinson TR, Sue DY, Huszczuk A, Weiler-Ravell D, Hansen JE. Intra-arterial and cuff blood pressure responses during incremental cycle ergometry. *Med Sci Sports Exerc* 1988;20:142–149.

36. Wasserman K, McIlroy MB. Detecting the threshold of anaerobic metabolism in cardiac patients during exercise. *Am J Cardiol* 1964;14:844–852.

37. Wasserman K. The anaerobic threshold measurement to evaluate exercise performance. *Am Rev Respir Dis* 1984;129(Suppl):535–540.

38. Beaver WL, Wasserman K, Whipp BJ. A new method for detecting the anaerobic threshold by gas exchange. *J Appl Physiol* 1986;60:2020–2027.

39. Sue DY, Wasserman K, Morrica RB, Casaburi R. Measurement of anaerobic threshold by V-slope method in patients with chronic obstructive lung disease. *Chest* 1988;94:931–938.

40. Wasserman K, Beaver WL, Whipp BJ. Gas exchange theory and the lactic acidosis (anaerobic) threshold. *Circulation* 1990;81(Suppl II):II-14–II-30.

41. Wasserman K, Whipp BJ, Koyal S, Beaver WL. Anaerobic threshold and respiratory gas exchange during exercise. *J Appl Physiol* 1973;35:236–243.

42. Nery LE, Wasserman K, French W, Oren A, Davis JA. Contrasting cardiovascular and respiratory responses to exercise in mitral valve and chronic obstructive pulmonary diseases. *Chest* 1983;83:446–453.

43. Orr GW, Green HJ, Hughson RL, Bennett GW. A computer linear regression model to determine ventilatory anaerobic threshold. *J Appl Physiol* 1982;52:1349–1352.

44. Davis JA, Storer TW, Caiozzo VJ. Prediction of normal values for lactate threshold estimated by gas exchange in men and women. *J Appl Cardiol* 1997;76:157–164.

45. Davis JA, Vodak P, Wilmore JH, Vodal J, Kurtz P. Anaerobic threshold and maximal aerobic power for three modes of exercise. *J Appl Physiol* 1976;41:544–550.

46. Buchfuhrer MJ, Hansen JE, Robinson TE, Sue DY, Wasserman K, Whipp BJ. Optimizing the exercise protocol for cardiopulmonary assessment. *J Appl Physiol* 1983;55:1558–1564.

47. Withers RT, Sherman WM, Miller JM, Costillo DL. Specificity of the anaerobic threshold in endurance trained cyclists and runners. *Eur J Appl Physiol* 1981;47:93–101.

48. Hansen JE, Sue DY, Oren A, Wasserman K. Relation of oxygen uptake in low work rate in normal men and men with circulatory disorders. *Am J Cardiol* 1987;59:669–674.

49. Hansen JE, Casaburi R, Cooper DM, Wasserman K. Oxygen uptake as related to work rate increment during cycle ergometer exercise. *Eur J Appl Physiol* 1988;57:140–145.

50. Auchincloss JH, Ashutosh K, Rana S, Peppi D, Johnson LW, Gilbert R. Effect of cardiac, pulmonary, and vascular disease on one-minute oxygen uptake. *Chest* 1976;70:486–493.

51. Sietsema KE, Cooper DM, Rosove MH, Perloff JK, Child JS, Canobbio MM, Whipp BJ, Wasserman K. Dynamics of oxygen uptake during exercise in adults with cyanotic congenital heart disease. *Circulation* 1986;73:1137–1144.

52. Kory RC, Callahan R, Boren NC, Syner JC. The Veterans Administration-Army cooperative study of pulmonary function. 1. Clinical spirometry in normal men. *Am J Med* 1961;30:243–258.

53. Lindall A, Medine A, Grismor JT. A re-evaluation of normal pulmonary function measurements in the adult female. *Am Rev Respir Dis* 1967;95:1061–1064.

54. Gandevia B, Hugh-Jones P. Terminology for measurements of ventilatory capacity. *Thorax* 1957;1:290–293.

55. Cotes JE. *Lung function: assessment and application in medicine*. 3rd ed. Oxford: Blackwell Scientific, 1975.

56. Miller WF, Johnson RL Jr, Wu N. Relationships between maximal breathing capacity and timed expiratory capacities. *J Appl Physiol* 1959;14:510–516.

57. Campbell SC. A comparison of the maximum volume ventilation with forced expiratory volume in one second: an assessment of subject cooperation. *J Occup Med* 1982;24:531–533.

58. Bradley PW, Younes M. Relation between respiratory valve dead space and tidal volume. *J Appl Physiol* 1980;49:528–532.

59. Jones NL, McHardy GJR, Naimark A, Campbell EJM. Physiological dead space and alveolar-arterial gas pressure differences during exercise. *Clin Sci* 1966;31:19–29.

60. Lifshay A, Fast CW, Glazier JB. Effects of changes in respiratory pattern on physiological dead space. *J Appl Physiol* 1971;31:478–483.

61. Hey EN, Lloyd BB, Cunningham DJC, Jukes MGM, Bolton DPG. Effects of various respiratory stimuli on the depth and frequency of breathing in man. *Respir Physiol* 1966;1:193–205.

62. Spiro SC, Juniper E, Bowman P, Edwards RHT. An increasing work rate test for assessing the physiological strain of submaximal exercise. *Clin Sci Molec Med* 1974;46:191–206.

63. Metra M, Raccagni D, Carini G, Orzan F, Papa A, Nodari S, Cody RJ, Dejours P. Ventilatory and arterial blood gas changes during exercise in heart failure. In: Wasserman K, ed. *Exercise gas exchange in heart disease.* Armonk, NY: Futura Publishing, 1996:125–143.

64. Chua TP, Ponikowski P, Harrington D, Anker SD, Webb-Peploe K, Clark AL, Poole-Wilson PA, Coats AJ. Clinical correlates and prognostic significance of the ventilatory response to exercise in chronic heart failure. *J Am Coll Cardiol* 1997;29:1585–1590.

65. Kleber FX, Vietzke G, Wernecke KD, Bauer U, Opitz C, Wensel R, Sperfeld A, Glaser S. Impairment of ventilatory efficiency in heart failure: prognostic impact. *Circulation* 2000;101:2803–2809.

66. Gitt AK, Wasserman K, Kilkowski C, Kleemann T, Kilkowski A, Bangert M, Schneider S, Schwarz A, Senges J. Exercise anaerobic threshold and ventilatory efficiency identify heart failure patients for high risk of early death. *Circulation* 2002;106:3079–3084.

67. Wasserman K, Zhang YY, Gitt A, Belardinelli R, Koike A, Lubarsky L, Agostoni PG. Lung function and exercise gas exchange in chronic heart failure. *Circulation* 1997;96:2221–2227.

68. Sun XG, Hansen JE, Garatachea N, Storer TW, Wasserman K. Ventilatory efficiency during exercise in healthy subjects. *Am J Respir Crit Care Med* 2002;166:1443–1448.

69. Wasserman K, VanKessel A, Burton GB. Interaction of physiological mechanisms during exercise. *J Appl Physiol* 1967;22:71–85.

70. Davis JA, Whipp BJ, Wasserman K. The relation of ventilation to metabolic rate during moderate exercise in man. *Eur J Appl Physiol* 1980;44:97–108.

71. Fairbarn MS. Personal communication, 1998.

72. Whipp BJ, Wasserman K. Alveolar-arterial gas tension differences during graded exercise. *J Appl Physiol* 1969; 27:361–365.

73. Bradley CA, Harris EA, Seelye ER, Whitlock RML. Gas exchange during exercise in healthy people. I. The physiological dead-space volume. *Clin Sci Molec Med* 1976;51:323–333.

74. Ward SA, Wasserman K, Davis JA, Whipp BJ. Breathing-valve encumbrance and arterial blood gas and acid-base homeostasis during incremental exercise. *Fed Proc* 1984;43:634.

75. Jones NL, Robertson DG, Kane JW. Difference between end-tidal and arterial P_{CO_2} in exercise. *J Appl Physiol* 1979;47:954–960.

76. Dempsey JA, Hanson P, Henderson K. Exercise-induced arterial hypoxemia in healthy humans at sea-level. *J Physiol (Lond)* 1984;355:161–175.

77. Lilienthal JL, Riley RL, Proemmel DD, Franke RE. An experimental analysis in man of the oxygen pressure gradient from alveolar air to arterial blood during rest and exercise at sea level and at altitude. *Am J Physiol* 1946;147:199–216.

78. Asmussen E, Nielsen M. Alveolo-arterial gas exchange at rest and during work at different O_2 tensions. *Acta Physiol Scand* 1960;50:153–166.

79. Cruz JC, Hartley LH, Vogel JA. Effect of altitude relocations upon $AaDO_2$ at rest and during exercise. *J Appl Physiol* 1975;39:469–474.

80. Hansen JE, Vogel JA, Stelter GP, Consolazio CF. Oxygen uptake in man during exhaustive work at sea level and high altitude. *J Appl Physiol* 1967;23:511–522.

81. Stringer W, Wasserman K, Casaburi R, Porszasz J, Maehara K, French W. Lactic acidosis as a facilitator of oxyhemoglobin dissociation during exercise. *J Appl Physiol* 1994;76:1462–1467.

82. Agostini PG, Wasserman K, Perego GB, Marenzi GC, Guazzi M, Assanelli E, Lauri G, Guazzi MD. Oxygen transport to muscle during exercise in chronic congestive heart failure secondary to idiopathic dilated cardiomyopathy. *Am J Cardiol* 1997;79:1120–1124.

83. Koike A, Wasserman K, Taniguichi K, Hiroe M, Marumo F. The critical capillary P_{O_2} and the lactate threshold in patients with cardiovascular disease. *J Am Coll Cardiol* 1994;23:1644–1650.

84. Stringer W, Hansen J, Wasserman K. Cardiac output estimated non-invasively from oxygen uptake ($\dot{V}_{O_2}$) during exercise. *J Appl Physiol* 1997;82:908–912.

85. Weber KT, Janicki JS. Cardiopulmonary exercise testing for evaluation of chronic cardiac failure. *Am J Cardiol* 1985;55:22A–31A.

86. Sullivan MJ, Cobb FR. Relation between central and peripheral hemodynamics during exercise in patients with chronic heart failure. *Circulation* 1989;80:769–781.

87. Yoshida T, Nagata A, Maro M, Takeuchi N, Sada Y. The validity of anaerobic threshold determination by a Douglas bag method compared with arterial blood lactate concentration. *Eur J Appl Physiol* 1981;46:423–430.

88. Beaver WL, Wasserman K, Whipp BJ. Bicarbonate buffering of lactic acid generated during exercise. *J Appl Physiol* 1986;60:472–478.

CHAPTER 8

Principles of Interpretation:
A Flowchart Approach

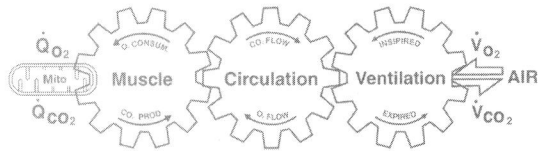

INTRODUCTION TO FLOWCHARTS

When patients complain of exercise intolerance, it is usually because they are unable to accomplish a task that they expect to complete with comparative ease and without unusual effort or undue feelings of fatigue or shortness of breath. Identifying the cause of exercise intolerance is a major objective of integrative cardiopulmonary exercise testing.

The measurements needed for physiological assessment are discussed in Chapter 4, and their patterns of change in response to the pathophysiology of specific diseases are described in Chapter 5 and further in Chapters 9 and 10. Once the optimal exercise protocol is chosen (see Chapter 6) and the predicted values are selected for the discriminating physiological variables (see Chapter 7), the task of identifying the probable cause(s) of the exercise intolerance still remains. This chapter introduces a flowchart strategy to show how the measurements made during exercise may be used to systematically deduce pathophysiology. Although the analytic method presented here is not necessarily ideal in all instances, the flowcharts serve to establish a discipline for interpreting cardiopulmonary exercise tests. The flowcharts are also of considerable value in providing a foundation for reaching a physiologically based interpretation, as well as providing instruction on the pathophysiology of different diseases that limit exercise tolerance.

In the flowcharts, the patient's peak $\dot{V}O_2$ is referred to the predicted peak $\dot{V}O_2$ or $\dot{V}O_2$max values provided in Chapter 7. Thus, a reduced peak $\dot{V}O_2$ identified at the start of flowcharts 3 to 5 means that the value is below the 95% confidence limits of the predicted peak $\dot{V}O_2$.

To facilitate description of each decision based on physiological measurements, each decision branch point is numbered on the flowcharts. The letter R refers to the right branch of the numbered branch point, and L to the left branch. Each final branch point leads to a box containing a diagnosis that can account for the parameters or measurements found in the decision-making process. Under the diagnosis is a list of additional measurements that lend further support to that diagnosis.

Each branch point decision and the choice of which flowchart to use for data analysis should not be regarded as rigid. If the physiological variable addressed at a particular branch point does not strongly favor one or the other branch, or if the measurements described in the diagnosis box do not consistently support that diagnosis, both branches of a branch point should be considered. Similarly, if flowcharts 3 or 4 (see Figs. 8.3 and 8.4) lead the clinician to a conclusion about pathophysiology that appears unwarranted or difficult to support, flowchart 5 (see Fig. 8.5), using an alternative strategy of reasoning, may be used. The flowcharts should always be used with some degree of flexibility and always with consideration of sound physiological principles.

ESTABLISHING THE PATHOPHYSIOLOGICAL BASIS OF EXERCISE INTOLERANCE

The first question to address is whether the peak $\dot{V}O_2$ is normal or decreased. The second question is whether the anaerobic threshold (AT) is normal or decreased. The answers to these two questions put the interpreter into the correct subsequent flowchart. By this time the diagnostic possibilities will be considerably focused. Other measurements then lead to the single pathophysiological state most consistent with the exercise data. From knowledge of the pathophysiological state, anatomical correlates may be sought, if deemed necessary, through other studies.

MAXIMUM EXERCISE CAPACITY AND ANAEROBIC THRESHOLD (FLOWCHART 1)

Analysis of data obtained during the exercise test begins on flowchart 1 (Fig. 8.1), which separates patients based on their measured peak $\dot{V}O_2$ and anaerobic threshold. Patients are divided into those with normal or reduced exercise capacity (normal or reduced peak $\dot{V}O_2$). Patients with a reduced maximum exercise capacity are further divided into those with normal, reduced, or indeterminate AT. The analysis then proceeds to one of four other flowcharts (flowcharts 2 to 5; see Figs. 8.2 to 8.5) for each of these groups.

Only a few conditions are associated with subjective exercise intolerance and normal peak $\dot{V}O_2$; these are considered in flowchart 2 (Fig. 8.2). For those with a low peak $\dot{V}O_2$, a normal AT suggests that O_2 flow at a submaximal exercise level is

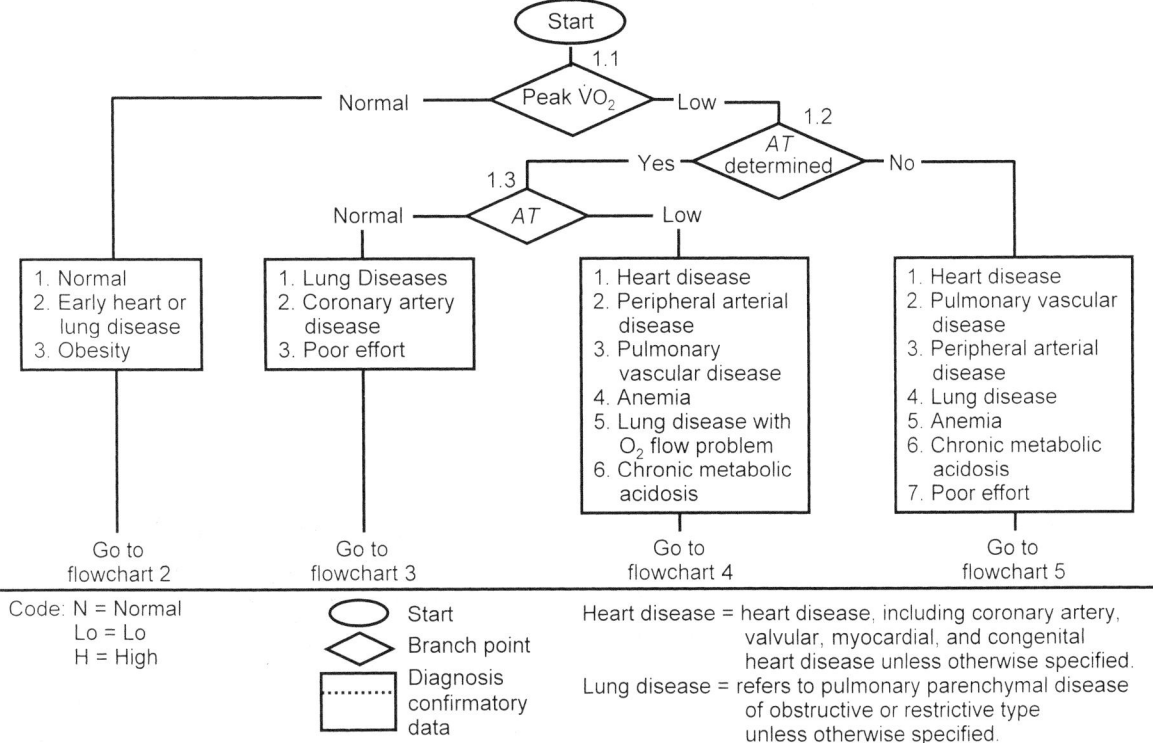

FIGURE 8.1. Flowchart 1, for the differential diagnosis of the cause of exercise limitation. Analysis starts with the measurement of peak $\dot{V}O_2$. Ellipsoids indicate starting points, highlighting a question. The diamonds indicate branch points in the decision logic based on further questions. The boxes provide potential diagnoses (listed above the horizontal line) and measurements that support the diagnosis (below the line). If the supporting measurements do not fit well, try a closely related branch point leading to a different diagnosis in which the supporting measurements fit better. Branch points are numbered to correspond to the text. The codes shown at the bottom of this figure pertain to all five flowcharts.

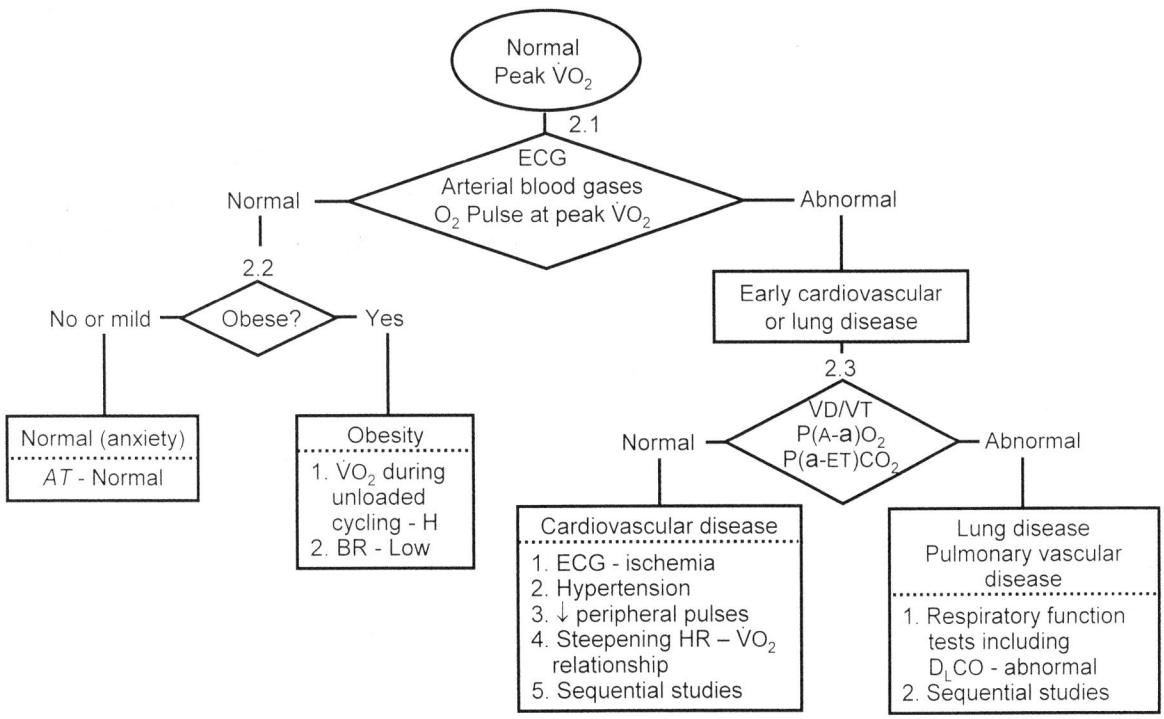

FIGURE 8.2. Flowchart 2, for conditions in which peak $\dot{V}O_2$ is normal but the patient feels limited during exercise. If the supporting measurements do not fit well, try a closely related branch point leading to a different diagnosis in which the confirmatory measurements fit better. Symbols and use of flowchart are as described in "Introduction to Flowcharts" and Figure 8.1.

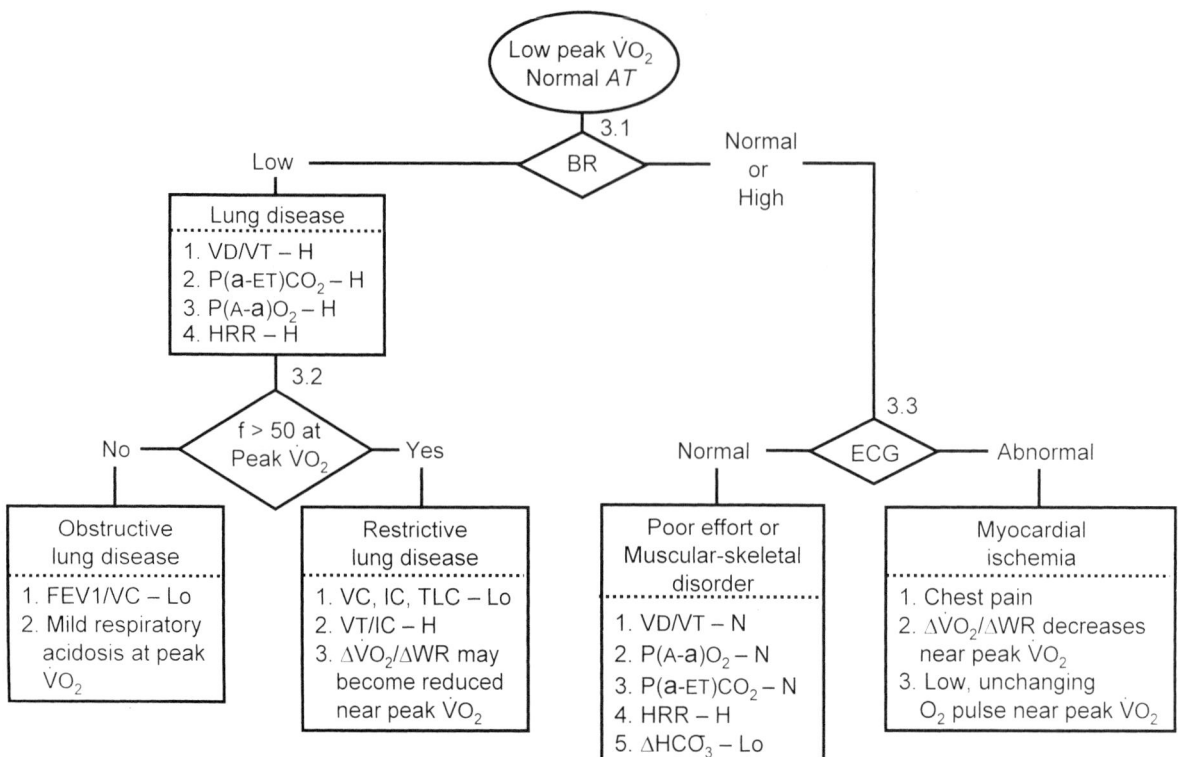

FIGURE 8.3.   Flowchart 3, for conditions in which peak $\dot{V}O_2$ is low but the anaerobic threshold (*AT*) is normal. If the supporting measurements do not fit well, try a closely related branch point leading to a different diagnosis in which the supporting measurements fit better. Symbols and use of flowchart are as described in "Introduction to Flowcharts" and Figure 8.1.

within normal limits but maximum exercise capacity is limited by one of a variety of other causes, as shown in flowchart 3 (Fig. 8.3). The combination of both low peak $\dot{V}O_2$ and *AT* leads to flowchart 4 (Fig. 8.4), in which disorders that limit the capacity to transport oxygen are described. Finally, it is recognized that the *AT* may not always be able to be determined because of poor patient effort, artifacts of measurement, or inappropriate work rate protocol, or, in rare cases, because an enzyme deficiency within the glycolytic pathway precludes development of lactic acidosis from anaerobic metabolism. A diagnostic scheme for these circumstances is described in flowchart 5 (Fig. 8.5).

EXERCISE INTOLERANCE WITH NORMAL PEAK OXYGEN UPTAKE (FLOWCHART 2)

When peak $\dot{V}O_2$ is normal, but the patient complains of exercise intolerance, the diagnostic possibilities are as follows:

1. The patient is actually normal but has anxiety about failing health.
2. The patient is excessively obese, thereby requiring an increased metabolic and cardiopulmonary response to perform minimal activity.
3. The patient, previously fit, has developed early cardiovascular or lung disease. Thus, despite a reduced ability to do the physical work to which he or she is accustomed, the peak $\dot{V}O_2$ still falls within the normal range of the subject's predicted peak $\dot{V}O_2$.

The diagnostic flowchart leading to each of these diagnoses is shown in Figure 8.2.

A normal peak $\dot{V}O_2$ (equal to the predicted peak $\dot{V}O_2$) with a low *AT* is somewhat unusual in normal subjects. However, it might be found in unusually sedentary subjects or patients with very mild disease that compromises O_2 transport to muscle cells.

Normal Individual with Anxiety State (Branch Points 2.1-L and 2.2-L)

People anxious about their health tend to be physically active and try to maintain their general state of

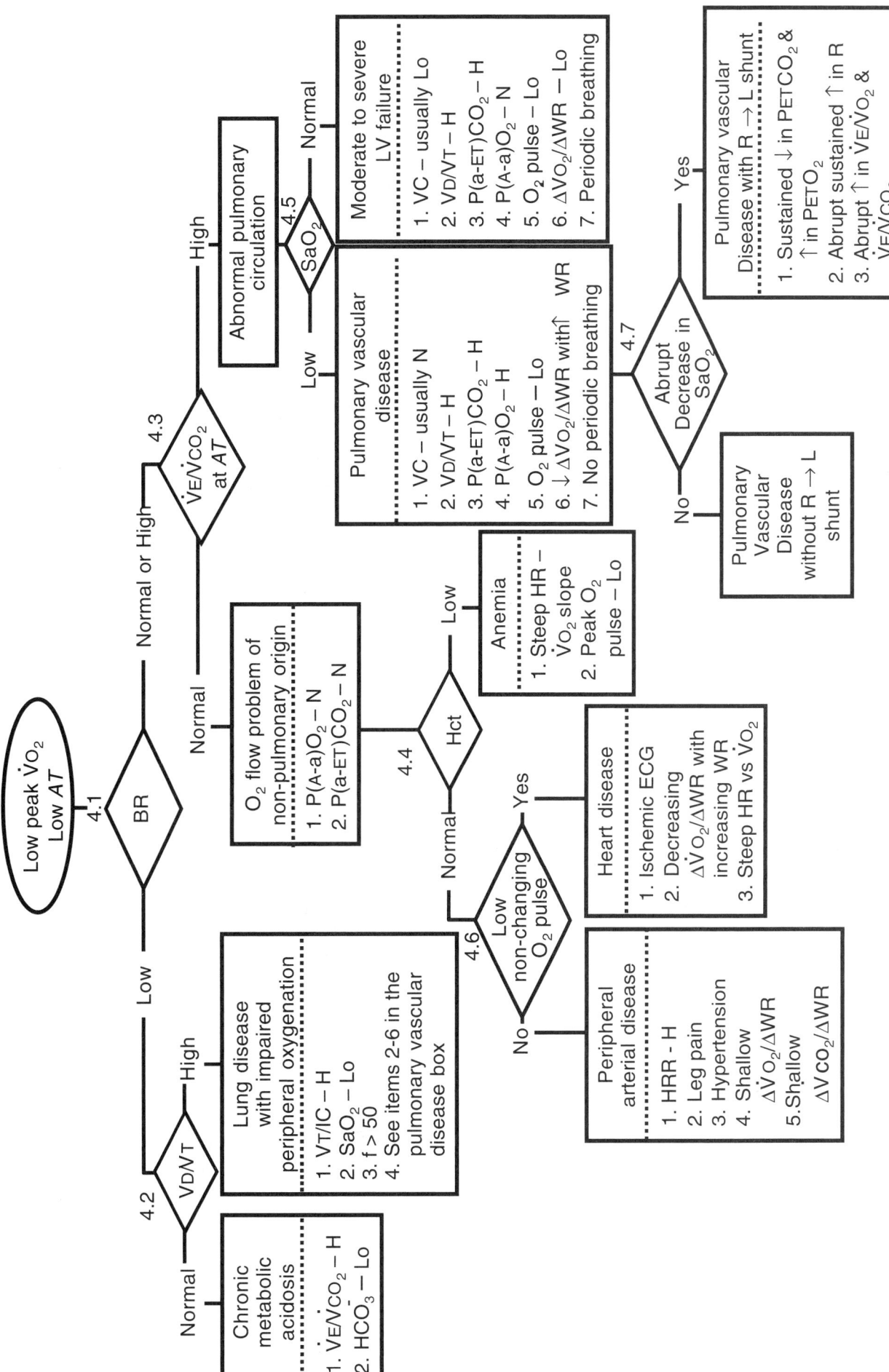

FIGURE 8.4. Flowchart 4, for conditions in which both peak $\dot{V}O_2$ and anaerobic threshold (AT) are low. If the supporting measurements do not fit well, try a closely related branch point leading to a different diagnosis in which the supporting measurements fit better. Symbols and use of flowchart are as described in "Introduction to Flowcharts" and Figure 8.1.

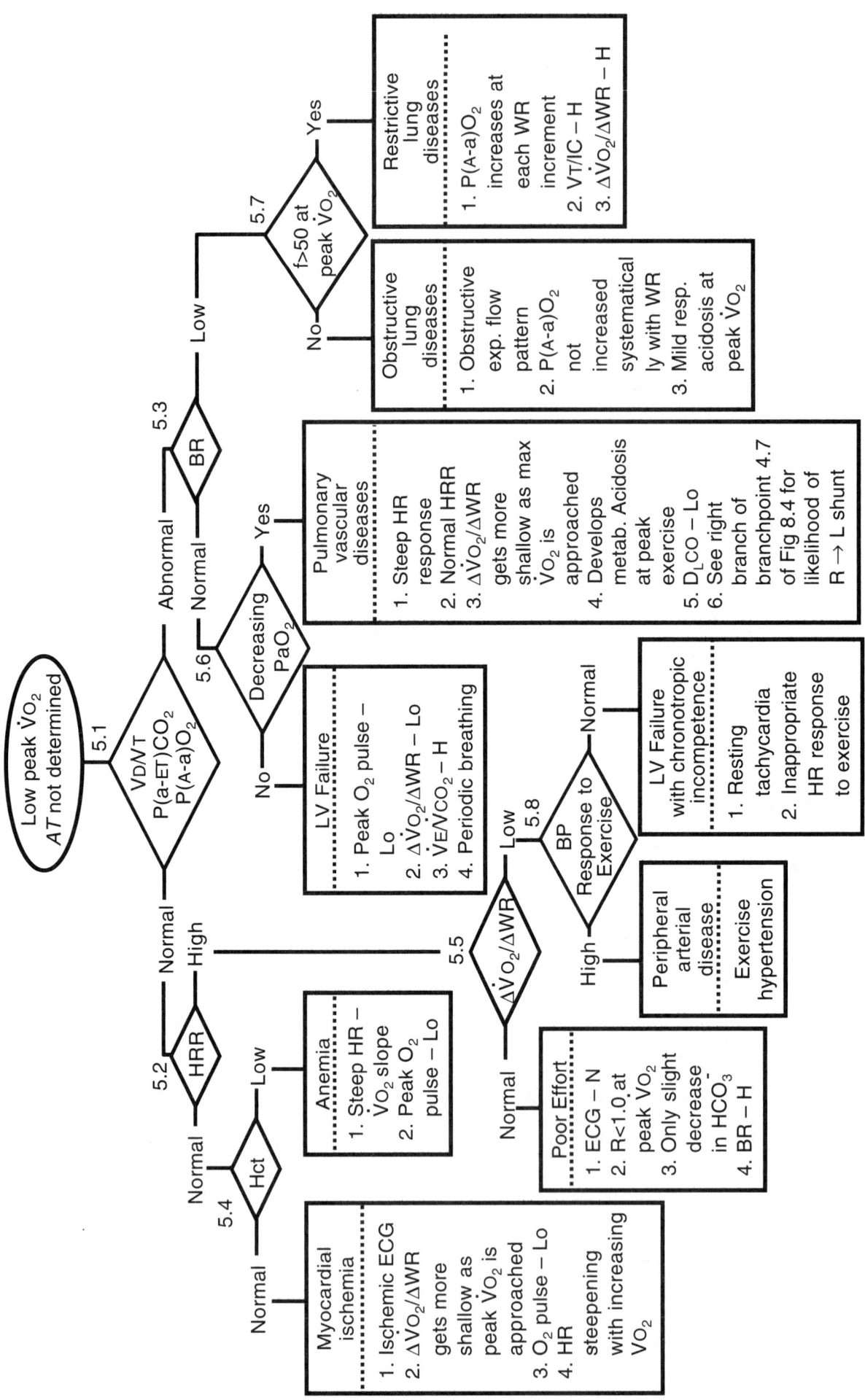

FIGURE 8.5. Flowchart 5, for conditions in which peak $\dot{V}O_2$ is low but the anaerobic threshold (AT) has not been measured or cannot be reliably determined. If the supporting measurements do not fit well, try a closely related branch point leading to a different diagnosis in which the supporting measurements fit better. Symbols and use of flowchart are as described in "Introduction to Flowcharts" and Figure 8.1.

health; otherwise, they would not be concerned. Therefore, their peak $\dot{V}O_2$ is generally on the high side of normal, and they are not obese. If the exercise electrocardiogram (ECG), O_2 pulse, and arterial blood gas values are normal at all work rates, including the maximum, the patient is probably normal. The breathing reserve should also be normal, but it may be on the low side of normal if the subject has a peak $\dot{V}O_2$ that is considerably better than the predicted normal value (i.e., the subject is in good physical condition). A confirmatory measurement is a normal *AT* that is above the mean predicted value. A patient with these findings would benefit from reassurance (see Cases 1 and 13 in Chapter 10).

Obesity (Branch Points 2.1-L and 2.2-R)

Obese subjects require an increased metabolic rate ($\dot{V}O_2$ and $\dot{V}CO_2$) to perform a given physical activity compared with nonobese subjects. The increased metabolic rate mandates increased cardiac output [cardiac output $= \dot{V}O_2/C(a - \bar{v})O_2$] and minute ventilation ($\dot{V}E = \dot{V}CO_2/[(1 - VD/VT) \times (PaCO_2/PB)]$) requirements compared with the nonobese subject for a given level of work. The increased metabolic work due to obesity is confirmed by a higher than expected $\dot{V}O_2$ during unloaded pedaling.

When the obese individual is relatively young, the increased oxygen cost for work caused by the large body mass is generally well tolerated (see Case 15, Chapter 10). When the normal deteriorating effects of aging on maximal ventilatory capacity are combined with the extra ventilatory cost of moving a large body to perform work, however, a reduced breathing reserve results. In addition, because a higher cardiac output is needed to support the increased O_2 to perform work by the obese subject, the cardiac reserve is low. Although the *AT* (when expressed as a percentage of predicted peak $\dot{V}O_2$) is normal, the O_2 cost of walking may be too great to perform this activity without developing a metabolic acidosis. The patient's heart rate reserve is normal at maximal exercise, although the breathing reserve is usually reduced because of ventilatory restriction and increased ventilatory requirement.

Early Cardiovascular or Lung Disease (Branch Points 2.1-R and 2.3)

In early mild cardiovascular or lung disease, the disorder may not be severe enough to cause the

peak $\dot{V}O_2$ to be less than predicted, because the latter is based on a relatively sedentary population. Specific physiological variables may become abnormal, however, depending on the site of the defect in the metabolic-cardiovascular-ventilatory coupling. For example, a patient may have a recently developed mild abnormality of the heart or lungs but still have a peak $\dot{V}O_2$ value that falls within the normal range. It may be difficult to document such a developing abnormality except by sequential studies demonstrating a decreasing peak $\dot{V}O_2$ or *AT* with time. The most common important diagnosis that should be identified or excluded in the middle-aged and elderly patient is ischemic heart disease. Also to be excluded are subtle abnormalities in gas exchange that might suggest pulmonary vascular disease that limits the ability to recruit lung capillary bed in response to exercise. Thus, the most important measures during maximal effort exercise are the ECG and arterial blood gas values, along with analysis of gas exchange.

If the arterial blood gas values are normal (2.3-L), then early heart disease, particularly coronary artery disease, may be present. Examination of the exercise ECG along with gas exchange measurements that relate the increase in $\dot{V}O_2$ and $\dot{V}CO_2$ to the increase in work rate are helpful and may be diagnostic for coronary artery disease. The ECG may provide evidence of myocardial ischemia. When this evidence is accompanied by an abrupt decrease in the rate of $\dot{V}O_2$ increase despite a sustained increase in work rate, strong evidence exists that the ECG changes are associated with abnormalities in ventricular function due to myocardial dyskinesis. In addition, if the heart rate increases proportionally faster than $\dot{V}O_2$ toward the end of exercise, this will result in a flattening of the O_2 pulse at submaximal exercise levels, also suggesting the presence of a reduced stroke volume consistent with heart disease. These changes, associated with evidence of myocardial ischemia on the ECG, make a strong case for the diagnosis of coronary artery disease (2.3-L) (see Case 18, Chapter 10).

Abnormal changes in VD/VT, $P(a - ET)CO_2$, and $P(A - a)O_2$ as work rate is increased to the subject's maximum are the most sensitive markers of lung disease (see Case 46, Chapter 10). Normal values essentially rule out mild or developing pulmonary vascular, lung parenchymal, or airway diseases because these measurements are almost always abnormal in these conditions (2.3-R). Although resting pulmonary function tests, such as vital capacity, FEV_1, total lung capacity, and $DLCO$, may be confirmatory, they may still be within the normal range.

LOW PEAK OXYGEN UPTAKE WITH NORMAL ANAEROBIC THRESHOLD (FLOWCHART 3)

The breathing reserve provides a good first branch point for the differential diagnosis of disorders characterized by a low peak $\dot{V}O_2$ and a normal *AT* (branch point 3.1, Fig. 8.3). Patients with a normal or high breathing reserve (3.1-R) include those making a poor effort, those who are limited by muscular and skeletal diseases, or those who develop myocardial ischemia at work rates above their predicted *AT*. On the other hand, a low breathing reserve in a patient with a normal *AT* (3.1-L) often identifies those patients with lung diseases.

Normal or High Breathing Reserve (Branch Point 3.1-R)

Poor Effort or Musculoskeletal Disorder (Branch Point 3.3-L)

Poor effort should be considered if the exercise ECG is normal. Perhaps for secondary gain, the subject may make a poor effort and may thereby have a low peak $\dot{V}O_2$ during exercise testing. Both the breathing reserve and heart rate reserve are high, indicating that the patient has not used the full potential of either the cardiovascular or the ventilatory system. The absence of metabolic acidosis at the end of exercise is also evidence of poor effort. Normal exercise VD/VT, $P(A - a)O_2$, and $P(a - ET)CO_2$ confirm that the lungs and pulmonary circulation are functionally normal. These demonstrate that the distribution of ventilation relative to perfusion is uniform, virtually ruling out primary lung or pulmonary vascular disease or significant chronic heart failure.

Simultaneous measurement of lactate and arterial blood for assessment of acid–base balance should confirm if an adequate effort was made during the exercise test. Everyone who makes a reasonable maximal effort should develop a significant metabolic acidosis during exercise, with a $[HCO_3^-]$ decrease of at least 4 mmol/L at peak

$\dot{V}O_2$. The rare exceptions are patients who have a defect in one of the skeletal muscle enzymes employed in the process of glycolysis (e.g., myophosphorylase). Also, patients limited during exercise due to severe airflow obstruction may not be able to increase work rate sufficiently to develop a lactic acidosis during exercise. Certain patients with very severe heart failure and thus with very limited blood flow to exercising muscles might not be able to generate high levels of lactate in their central circulation. These latter two groups, however, have quite severe lung or heart disease and would not be confused with a patient making a poor effort.

Optimal cardiovascular and pulmonary evaluation is impossible when arthritis or neuromuscular disease limits exercise. These patients have difficulty in performing enough exercise to stress the cardiovascular or respiratory systems sufficiently to bring out gas exchange abnormalities. Occasionally, however, a patient with exercise limitation has both a musculoskeletal defect and a defect in the cardiovascular or respiratory system. Thus, it is important to distinguish if the exercise-induced lactic acidosis because of a circulatory limitation is driving ventilation beyond the subject's capability or if breathing is so limited that the CO_2 generated from aerobic metabolism cannot be eliminated at a rate compatible with the patient's circulatory competency (see Cases 68 to 70, Chapter 10).

Myocardial Ischemia (Branch Point 3.3-R)

The ECG usually becomes abnormal if the myocardium becomes ischemic as the work rate is increased to the patient's symptom-limited maximum. The ECG abnormality may be evident only at high work rates, and the patient may or may not experience angina. Whereas coronary artery disease is the most frequent cause of myocardial ischemia, it may also occur with aortic stenosis or marked systemic hypertension without significant coronary artery disease (see Cases 21 and 33, Chapter 10). At the $\dot{V}O_2$ at which myocardial ischemia develops, the $\dot{V}O_2$, initially increasing normally with work rate at a rate of 10 ml/min/W, commonly decreases its rate of increase beyond the ischemic point (see Cases 18 and 22, Chapter 10). The most likely explanation is that the stroke volume decreases, resulting in the failure of cardiac output to keep pace with the O_2 requirement despite a continuing increase in heart rate.

Low Breathing Reserve (Branch Point 3.1-L)

Low breathing reserve suggests lung disease. The breathing frequency may be a useful next branch point to determine if obstructive or restrictive lung disease dominates in patients with mixed obstructive and restrictive defects (branch point 3.2).

Obstructive Lung Diseases (Branch Point 3.2-L)

Although the peak $\dot{V}O_2$ achieved during incremental exercise testing is low in this disorder, the AT is often normal. The normal AT suggests that the patient does not have a problem with oxygen transport to the tissues at these submaximal work rates (see Case 37, Chapter 10). Characteristically, these patients have abnormalities in PaO_2, VD/VT, $P(a - ET)CO_2$, and $P(A - a)O_2$ during exercise consequent to ventilation–perfusion mismatching. Decreases in PaO_2 commonly occur in a single step at low work rates, with little further change as the work rate is increased (see Fig. 5.7). This is probably because the increased perfusion during exercise goes predominantly to normal and high $\dot{V}A/\dot{Q}$ regions of the lungs. Except in mild obstructive lung disease, the breathing reserve is decreased, indicating a ventilatory limitation during exercise. In contrast to O_2 flow–limiting disorders, $\dot{V}O_2$ continues to increase linearly as the work rate is increased to the patient's peak $\dot{V}O_2$; that is, there is no decrease in $\Delta\dot{V}O_2/\Delta WR$ as the peak $\dot{V}O_2$ is approached. The heart rate reserve is commonly increased because the cardiovascular capacity cannot be fully challenged as a result of the breathing limitation. Finally, expiratory flow frequently has an obstructive pattern (trapezoidal in appearance, with an early peak), as illustrated in Figure 4.14.

In patients with marked airflow obstruction, the AT measured by gas exchange must be determined by the V-slope method rather than methods that rely on the increase in ventilation, such as the ventilatory equivalent for O_2. Although CO_2 output will increase when HCO_3^- buffers lactic acid, the ventilatory response to the increased CO_2 load from buffering is often poor in patients with chronic obstructive pulmonary disease (COPD), and the ven-

tilatory equivalent for O_2 usually does not increase measurably at the AT (see Cases 40 and 42, Chapter 10).

Restrictive Lung Diseases (Branch Point 3.2-R)

The pathophysiological responses seen in restrictive lung diseases have much in common with those of the obstructive lung diseases, but clear differences exist. The VD/VT and $P(a - ET)CO_2$ are increased in both physiological types of lung disorders as reflections of ventilation–perfusion mismatching. In contrast to obstructive lung diseases, however, the $P(A - a)O_2$ usually increases systematically at each work rate during the incremental test. Moreover, the VT increases to its maximum at a relatively low work rate, and the ratio of VT to inspiratory capacity (IC) nears a value of 1. Because VT cannot increase normally in patients with restrictive lung diseases, the ventilatory response to the increasing work rate is achieved primarily by increasing the breathing frequency, commonly exceeding 50 breaths per minute at the end of exercise, in contrast to the much slower breathing rate adopted by patients with airflow limitation due to airway obstruction.

Patients with restrictive lung diseases also commonly manifest an O_2 flow problem (see Cases 49 to 53 in Chapter 10). This is shown by the failure of $\dot{V}O_2$ to increase normally as the work rate progressively increases to the patient's maximum. This may be caused both by the falling arterial O_2 content and narrowing of $C(a - \bar{v})O_2$ and the increased pulmonary vascular resistance (resulting from destruction of pulmonary blood vessels by the fibrosing process). This limits the rate of increase in cardiac output in response to exercise. These patients, therefore, have a reduced AT with a low peak $\dot{V}O_2$. This diagnosis is analyzed in greater detail in flowchart 4 (Fig. 8.4).

LOW PEAK OXYGEN UPTAKE WITH LOW ANAEROBIC THRESHOLD (FLOWCHART 4)

The breathing reserve serves as a good primary branch point (4.1) for the differential diagnosis of disorders having a low peak $\dot{V}O_2$ and low AT, as shown in flowchart 4 (Fig. 8.4), but further questions about pathophysiology need to be addressed to distinguish among the various conditions that cause a low *AT*. The $\Delta \dot{V}O_2/\Delta WR$ is a good second branch point (4.2) for the conditions that have a low breathing reserve; $\dot{V}E/\dot{V}CO_2$ at the *AT* is a useful second branch point (4.3) for the conditions with a normal or high breathing reserve.

Normal or High Breathing Reserve (Branch Point 4.1-R)

Normal $\dot{V}E/\dot{V}CO_2$ at the Anaerobic Threshold (Branch Point 4.3-L)

If the breathing reserve is normal or high and the $\dot{V}E/\dot{V}CO_2$ at the *AT* is normal (4.3-L), then we must consider an O_2 flow problem of nonpulmonary vascular disease origin. This is because there is little evidence of lung or pulmonary vascular disease, i.e., the normal breathing reserve and $\dot{V}E/\dot{V}CO_2$ at the *AT* are normal. Myocardial ischemia, low-grade cardiomyopathy, valvular heart disease, peripheral arterial disease, and anemia or hemoglobinopathy are diagnoses that should be seriously considered because they can result in reduced O_2 flow during exercise. Hematocrit (branch point 4.4) and O_2 pulse ($\dot{V}O_2/HR$; branch point 4.6) help distinguish these diagnoses.

Anemia (Branch Point 4.4-R). Because of the reduced O_2 carrying capacity of the blood, the *AT* and lactic acidosis occur at a lower than normal work rate. Anemia decreases the oxygen content of the arterial blood, leading to decreased maximal C(a − $\bar{v}$)O_2. Thus, the maximal O_2 pulse is reduced, reflecting the decreased maximal C(a − $\bar{v}$)O_2. A high cardiac output and heart rate are required to meet the tissue O_2 requirement. It should be noted that the arterial blood gas tensions and the VD/VT are normal in anemia, even at maximal exercise (see Case 76, Chapter 10).

Heart Disease (Branch Point 4.6-R). Patients with primary heart disease (myocardial ischemia secondary to coronary artery disease, cardiomyopathy secondary to any cause, and valvular heart disease) usually have a low peak $\dot{V}O_2$ with a low *AT*. In these disorders, the rate of rise of $\dot{V}O_2$ is slow relative to the increase in work rate as the peak $\dot{V}O_2$ is approached (see Cases 16 to 28 in Chapter 10). However, the pattern of slowing differs according to diagnosis. The contrasting patterns of change are described in Chapter 9. The

heart rate often continues to increase as the work rate is increased despite the slower increase of $\dot{V}O_2$, resulting in a steepening of the heart rate–$\dot{V}O_2$ relation as the maximum work rate is approached. Also, the O_2 pulse reaches a constant value at subnormal values (see Fig. 4.11). Changes in the ECG consistent with myocardial ischemia during exercise, combined with concurrent failure of $\dot{V}O_2$ to increase normally, provide support for the diagnosis of exercise-induced myocardial ischemia (see Table 5.4).

In mild to moderate forms of heart failure, regardless of cause, acute metabolic acidosis occurs at relatively low levels of exercise. In more severe heart failure (New York Heart Association classes 3 to 4), VD/VT becomes elevated because of ventilation–perfusion mismatching. In such patients, the $\dot{V}E/\dot{V}CO_2$ is increased at the *AT*, and the flowchart leads to the right at branch point 4.3. Consequently, chronic stable advanced heart failure is accompanied by pulmonary vascular changes that must be distinguished from diseases in which the pulmonary circulation is the primary site of disease (see Tables 5.5 and 5.8).

Peripheral Arterial Disease (Branch Point 4.6-L). In contrast to primary heart diseases, the heart rate reserve is generally high in this condition since the patient stops exercising because of leg pain before the heart can be maximally stressed. Because of narrowing of major conducting arteries, the normal decrease in peripheral vascular resistance in response to exercise cannot take place. Thus, systemic arterial hypertension develops beyond that expected with exercise. The increase in $\dot{V}O_2$ relative to the increase in work rate is expected to be reduced, resulting in a relatively shallow slope for the $\dot{V}O_2$–work rate relation (low $\Delta \dot{V}O_2/\Delta WR$). In contrast to other cardiovascular disorders, the $\dot{V}CO_2$– work rate relation is also shallow. Finally, in the absence of concomitant lung disease, measurements of VD/VT, P(a − ET)CO_2, and P(A − a)O_2, which reflect the distribution of ventilation relative to perfusion, are normal (see Cases 30 and 31, Chapter 10).

High $\dot{V}E/\dot{V}CO_2$ at the Anaerobic Threshold or Ventilatory Compensation Point (Branch Point 4.3-R)

If the breathing reserve is normal or high (4.1-R) but the $\dot{V}E/\dot{V}CO_2$ at the *AT* or ventilatory compensation point (VCP, see Fig. 4.20) is high (4.3-R), then the most likely disorders are diseases originating in the pulmonary circulation or moderate to severe left ventricular failure. Both manifest abnormalities in the pulmonary circulation.

Pulmonary Vascular Disease Originating in the Pulmonary Circulation (Branch Point 4.5-L).

What most commonly distinguishes patients with pulmonary vascular disorders originating in the pulmonary circulation from pulmonary vascular changes that accompany left ventricular failure is the arterial oxyhemoglobin saturation (SaO_2) at peak exercise (branch point 4.5). Patients with primary pulmonary arterial occlusive diseases commonly develop arterial hypoxemia during exercise, although SaO_2 might be normal at rest. These disorders include pulmonary thromboembolic disease, primary pulmonary hypertension, and diseases that cause pulmonary vasculitis, such as various connective tissue diseases. Because of the loss of capillary bed, the red cell residence time is shortened during exercise as cardiac output increases. This reduces the time for the PO_2 in the alveolus to equilibrate with that of the red cell during its shortened transit through the restricted pulmonary capillary bed. Thus, arterial oxygenation decreases as work rate increases. The decrease in SaO_2 is even more marked during exercise if the increase in right atrial pressure exceeds the left atrial pressure, causing systemic venous blood to flow directly into the left atrium through a patent foramen ovale, present in about one-third of patients. This exercise-induced abnormality of lung gas exchange is seen as a reduced PaO_2 and increased $P(A - a)O_2$, or as a decreased SaO_2 detected with a pulse oximeter.

If the pulmonary circulation, interposed between the right and left sides of the heart, does not dilate or recruit pulmonary blood vessels during exercise, the increased venous return that accompanies exercise cannot be readily transmitted to the left ventricle, and cardiac output cannot respond appropriately to the exercise stimulus. Because cardiac output does not increase normally, the increase in $\dot{V}O_2$ relative to increase in work rate progressively slows below the normal rate of increase of 10 ml/min/W. In addition to abnormal slowing in the rate of rise in $\dot{V}O_2$, the AT and peak $\dot{V}O_2$ are reduced. Because the increase in $\dot{V}O_2$ with work rate slows but heart rate continues to increase with work rate, heart rate increases steeply relative to $\dot{V}O_2$ and gets steeper as the peak $\dot{V}O_2$ is approached. Thus, the O_2 pulse fails to increase as the work rate is increased and is reduced at the maximum work rate.

Patients with all forms of pulmonary vascular disease have a high VD/VT and a positive value for $P(a - ET)CO_2$, evidence of poor perfusion of ventilated air spaces. Moreover, the $P(A - a)O_2$ increases to abnormally high values as work rate is increased, probably because of the shortened red cell transit time due to a reduced capillary bed, as described in Chapter 5. Although these changes may be seen in patients with interstitial lung diseases (ILD), other measurements made during exercise distinguish these disorders. For instance, the breathing reserve is normal in patients with a primary pulmonary vasculopathy, whereas restrictive lung mechanics are present in patients with ILD. In addition, metabolic acidosis develops during exercise in patients with pulmonary vascular diseases, rather than the respiratory acidosis that commonly accompanies severe obstructive lung diseases in response to exercise when the mechanics of ventilation are severely affected (see Cases 40, 42, 43, and 45 in Chapter 10).

Primary lung diseases can cause major disturbances in function of the pulmonary circulation, which may become the dominant pathophysiological feature limiting exercise (see Cases 41, 44, and 53, Chapter 10). In such instances, the abnormalities noted in the "Pulmonary Vascular Disease" diagnostic box of flowchart 4 (Fig. 8.4) become evident during exercise testing. Limitations in exercise caused by the pulmonary circulation cannot be reliably predicted from resting measurements (see Chapters 5 and 9).

Pulmonary Vascular Disease with a Right-to-Left Shunt, or Cyanotic Congenital Heart Disease (Branch Point 4.7-R).

Patients with pulmonary vascular disease who open a potentially patent foramen ovale or who have congenital heart disease with a right-to-left shunt may demonstrate marked reductions in PaO_2 during air and O_2 breathing in response to exercise (see Case 51, Chapter 10). The VD/VT, $P(a - ET)CO_2$, and $P(A - a)O_2$ values become exceptionally abnormal in response to exercise depending on the degree of pulmonary hypoperfusion relative to ventilation, the latter depending on the size of the right-to-left shunt. These values generally become more abnormal as the work rate is increased. Patients with these disorders can be distinguished from those with other pulmonary vascular diseases by an abrupt and sustained decrease in $PETCO_2$ and increase in $PETO_2$, sustained increases in R, $\dot{V}E/\dot{V}O_2$, and $\dot{V}E/\dot{V}CO_2$, and a decrease in arterial O_2 saturation as soon as exercise begins. O_2 pulse is low because of the reduced $C(a - \bar{v})O_2$ resulting from arterial hypoxemia. $\Delta\dot{V}O_2/\Delta WR$ is usually reduced, with the rate of $\dot{V}CO_2$ increasing faster than the rate of $\dot{V}O_2$ increase at low work rates, reflecting a low *AT*.

Repeating the exercise test while the patient breathes 100% O_2 is particularly helpful in distinguishing a right-to-left shunt from other causes of hypoxemia. With no shunt, the arterial PaO_2 will be in the range of 550 to 650 mm Hg at rest and at all levels of exercise with 100% O_2 breathing. If a right-to-left shunt develops during exercise, PaO_2 will fall precipitously. It can be calculated that the arterial PaO_2 will decrease by approximately 100 mm Hg for each 3% to 5% of the venous return that shunts from right to left while breathing 100% O_2 until PaO_2 falls to about 150 mm Hg. This represents the reduction of physically dissolved O_2 in the arterial blood caused by the shunt. Shunting below a PaO_2 of 150 mm Hg results in a lesser fall in PaO_2 because the shunted blood decreases both oxyhemoglobin concentration as well as physically dissolved O_2.

Pulmonary Vascular Changes Secondary to Moderate to Severe Left Ventricular Failure (Branch Point 4.5-R).

Patients with moderate to severe left ventricular failure have an increase in VD/VT and increase in $P(a - ET)CO_2$, but without hypoxemia (normal SaO_2) or an increase in $P(A - a)O_2$ at peak $\dot{V}O_2$ (see Chapter 5). This increase in VD/VT and in $P(a - ET)CO_2$ indicates that ventilation–perfusion relations are mismatched, but with high-$\dot{V}A/\dot{Q}$ lung units and without low-$\dot{V}A/\dot{Q}$ lung units. This disparity between the abnormality in VD/VT [and increase in $P(a - ET)CO_2$] without a decrease in SaO_2 [and increase in $P(A - a)O_2$ is presumably accounted for by the slow pulmonary blood flow in left ventricular heart failure. The slow pulmonary blood flow of left ventricular failure allows adequate time for alveolar PO_2 to come into diffusion equilibrium with the red cell PO_2, in contrast to the situation seen in primary pulmonary vascular occlusive diseases. The normal PaO_2 and $P(A - a)O_2$ values at peak $\dot{V}O_2$ distinguish left ventricular failure from pulmonary vascular disease

originating in the pulmonary circulation. Because of the increase in VD/VT, the slope of $\dot{V}E$ versus $\dot{V}CO_2$ is abnormally steep in left ventricular failure, as it is in primary pulmonary vascular disease. These increases in VD/VT and slope of $\dot{V}E$ versus $\dot{V}CO_2$ may not be present in more mild forms of left ventricular failure.

Low Breathing Reserve (Branch Point 4.1-L)

In the category of patients with a low peak $\dot{V}O_2$ and low AT accompanied by a low breathing reserve and a high VD/VT (4.2-R), the most likely disorder is a primary lung disease such as pulmonary fibrosis (restrictive lung disease) or COPD in a sedentary patient. In contrast, a low breathing reserve with a normal VD/VT can be caused by diseases associated with a chronic metabolic acidosis with hyperventilation or a normal person adapted to high altitude (4.2-L). The following sections describe the pathophysiology that characterizes each of these disorders.

Lung Disease with Impaired Peripheral Oxygenation (Branch Point 4.2-R)

In certain pulmonary patients the *AT* as well as the peak $\dot{V}O_2$ are reduced. Moreover, $\Delta\dot{V}O_2/\Delta WR$ may be reduced as work rate is increased. These are usually pulmonary patients with severe interstitial lung disease or COPD patients in whom the pulmonary circulation is markedly impaired (see Table 5.11). Oxyhemoglobin desaturation may, but not necessarily, contribute to the impairment in O_2 flow to the exercising muscles. Commonly, the reduced $\Delta\dot{V}O_2/\Delta WR$ is accompanied by a gradual reduction in the rate of increase in $\dot{V}O_2$ as work rate is increased. The physiological explanation for this finding is that patients with restrictive lung diseases have a significant loss of pulmonary capillary bed caused by the disease process. Thus, the pulmonary capillary bed is already maximally recruited at rest, and blood flow can increase to satisfy the increase in O_2 required for exercise only if pulmonary artery pressure increases sufficiently to achieve a pulmonary blood flow adequate to meet the tissue O_2 requirement. However, the degree of pulmonary hypertension may be insufficient to increase pulmonary blood flow (cardiac output) enough to support the O_2 required by the exercising muscle. Because the dominant pathophysiology in patients with restrictive lung diseases usually resides in the pulmonary circulation, the abnormalities described in the "Pulmonary Vascular Disease" box of flowchart 4 (Fig. 8.4) also apply to these lung diseases (see Cases 51 and 53, Chapter 10).

Low Pa_{CO_2} Set Point (Branch Point 4.2-L)

Chronic metabolic acidosis characterizes patients with chronic renal failure, renal tubular acidosis, or poorly controlled diabetes mellitus with partially compensated metabolic acidosis, or patients taking acetazolamide (e.g., patients with glaucoma). Because ventilatory compensation occurs in these conditions (low Pa_{CO_2} set point), exercise alveolar and minute ventilation are higher than normal. The higher alveolar ventilation is needed to clear the increased metabolic CO_2 generated during exercise (see Fig. 2.42) at a lower Pa_{CO_2}. Similarly, the Pa_{CO_2} set point is low in people who reside at high altitude. The low Pa_{CO_2} causes the ventilatory equivalents for O_2 and CO_2 to be high (increased ventilatory drive), thereby decreasing the breathing reserve at maximum exercise. Because of the high ventilatory requirement, these patients may experience exertional dyspnea before reaching their predicted peak $\dot{V}_{O_2}$ and AT. Exertional dyspnea is especially likely to occur in patients with a low Pa_{CO_2} when accompanied by lung or heart disease, anemia, or obesity. A low Pa_{CO_2} set point state is easily identified from arterial blood gas and pH measurements.

LOW PEAK OXYGEN UPTAKE WITH ANAEROBIC THRESHOLD NOT DETERMINED (FLOWCHART 5)

The importance of the *AT* in deciding the cause of exercise limitation is demonstrated in the previous flowcharts. However, in some patients, the *AT* may not be determined or the interpreter may feel that the *AT* is unreliable because of breathing irregularity after reviewing an exercise test. Failure to identify an *AT* may also result from the patient stopping exercise before the *AT* was reached. The interpreter then knows that the *AT* is greater than the peak $\dot{V}_{O_2}$ of the study.

An alternative strategy to using the *AT* as the second major branch point in the decision-making process (flowchart 1) is described in flowchart 5 (Fig. 8.5). Given a reduced peak $\dot{V}_{O_2}$, tests that detect mismatching of ventilation to perfusion make it possible to distinguish disorders associated with inefficiency of lung gas exchange from disorders associated with normal lung function and pulmonary circulation. Thus, branch point 5.1 uses arterial blood gas and pulmonary gas exchange measurements to identify the presence of mismatching of ventilation and perfusion. Diseases associated with abnormal ventilation–perfusion relations include restrictive lung diseases, obstructive lung diseases, pulmonary vascular diseases, and moderately severe left heart failure. Patients with acute coronary syndromes without chronic heart failure, mild left ventricular failure, congenital heart disease without a right-to-left shunt, anemia, peripheral arterial disease, and poor effort have normal ventilation–perfusion relations.

The simplest and cheapest way to detect the presence of ventilation–perfusion mismatching reliably is the measurement of V_D/V_T, $P(a - _{ET})_{CO_2}$, and $P(_A - a)_{O_2}$ during exercise. In the absence of arterial blood, an alternative is to approximate Pa_{CO_2} from venous blood drawn from a superficial vein of a warmed hand or from capillary blood from an ear lobe. From these measurements, V_D/V_T and $P(a - _{ET})_{CO_2}$ can be calculated.

But strong suspicion of abnormal lung gas exchange can be obtained noninvasively from measurement of $\dot{V}_E/\dot{V}_{CO_2}$ at the *AT* and $P_{ET}_{CO_2}$ at the *AT* (see Chapters 4, 7, and 9), because these measurements have a very narrow normal range and are characteristically abnormal in conditions in which ventilation–perfusion relations become nonuniform. Therefore, if these noninvasive (surrogate) variables are abnormal, we can say that $\dot{V}_A/\dot{Q}$ is nonuniform with reasonable but not absolute confidence. As shown in flowchart 5 (Fig. 8.5), if V_D/V_T, $P(a - _{ET})_{CO_2}$, and $P(_A - a)_{O_2}$ (or the surrogate measurements for $\dot{V}_A/\dot{Q}$ mismatch just mentioned) are normal (5.1-L), we examine the heart rate reserve (HRR) (5.2); if V_D/V_T, $P(a - _{ET})_{CO_2}$, and $P(_A - a)_{O_2}$ values (or $\dot{V}_E/\dot{V}_{CO_2}$ at the AT and $P_{ET}_{CO_2}$ at the *AT*) are abnormal (5.1-R), we examine the breathing reserve (5.3). The possible diagnoses at each of these branch points separate into two major groups depending on whether the heart rate reserve is normal or high or the breathing reserve is normal or low.

Normal V_D/V_T, $P(a - ET)CO_2$, and $P(A - a)O_2$ (Branch Point 5.1-L)

Heart disease, anemia, poor effort, and peripheral arterial disease are all associated with a low peak $\dot{V}O_2$ but have normal indices of gas exchange efficiency [V_D/V_T, $P(a - ET)CO_2$, and $P(A - a)O_2$]. The HRR allows this group to be further subdivided into those with a normal HRR (5.2-L) (heart disease or anemia) or a high HRR (5.2-R) (poor effort, peripheral arterial disease, and heart failure with chronotropic incompetence).

Anemia can be distinguished from the heart disorders with a low peak $\dot{V}O_2$, uniform $\dot{V}A/\dot{Q}$, and normal HRR (5.2-L) by a low hematocrit (5.4). Ischemic, valvular, cardiomyopathic, or noncyanotic congenital heart diseases are usually characterized by a greater rise in heart rate and lesser rise in $\dot{V}O_2$ than expected for the work rate performed.

Poor effort, peripheral arterial disease, and mild to moderate chronic heart failure with chronotropic incompetence are associated with a low peak $\dot{V}O_2$, uniform $\dot{V}A/\dot{Q}$, and high HRR (5.2-R). The $\Delta\dot{V}O_2/\Delta WR$ (5.5) is a useful branch point to distinguish poor effort (normal $\Delta\dot{V}O_2/\Delta WR$) from peripheral arterial disease and chronic heart failure with chronotropic incompetence (low $\Delta\dot{V}O_2/\Delta WR$). Poor effort can be confirmed by other measurements, including a high breathing reserve, failure to develop a significant metabolic acidosis at end of exercise, an R less than 1.0 at the peak $\dot{V}O_2$, a normal ECG, and possibly a very irregular breathing pattern.

Patients with peripheral arterial disease and those with left ventricular failure with chronotropic incompetence usually have a low $\Delta\dot{V}O_2/\Delta WR$ (5.5-R). Further distinguishing these diagnoses is a pronounced systolic hypertension in response to exercise in the former, but normal or low systolic pressure response in the latter (branch point 5.8).

Abnormal V_D/V_T, $P(a - ET)CO_2$, and $P(A - a)O_2$ (Branch Point 5.1-R)

Pulmonary vascular diseases, moderately severe chronic left ventricular heart failure, and obstructive and restrictive lung diseases are associated with a low peak $\dot{V}O_2$ and abnormal indices of gas exchange efficiency (nonuniform $\dot{V}A/\dot{Q}$). The breathing reserve (branch point 5.3) subdivides these patients into those with a normal breathing reserve (heart failure and pulmonary vascular diseases) and those with a low breathing reserve (obstructive and restrictive lung diseases).

The two disorders with a low peak $\dot{V}O_2$ and nonuniform $\dot{V}A/\dot{Q}$ but a normal breathing reserve (5.3-L) can usually be distinguished by the PaO_2 or arterial oxyhemoglobin (O_2Hb) saturation in response to exercise (5.6). The patient with pulmonary vascular disease usually has a normal PaO_2 or arterial O_2Hb saturation at rest that decreases progressively as the work rate increases (5.6-R). If pulmonary vascular disease is accompanied by a right-to-left shunt, such as in cyanotic congenital heart disease or the opening of an unsealed foramen ovale, then the decrement in PaO_2 at the start of exercise will be marked. Item 6 in the diagnostic box for pulmonary vascular diseases (Fig. 8.5) describes simple measurements that can support the development of a right-to-left shunt during exercise. The patient with moderately severe left ventricular failure will have a normal PaO_2 and arterial O_2Hb saturation, even at maximum exercise, although V_D/V_T will be elevated as with primary pulmonary vasculopathies (5.6-L).

Both obstructive and restrictive lung diseases have a low peak $\dot{V}O_2$, nonuniform $\dot{V}A/\dot{Q}$, and low breathing reserve (5.3-R), but can generally be distinguished by the breathing frequency and the measurements listed in the respective diagnostic boxes for obstructive and restrictive lung diseases. A breathing frequency higher than 50 at the patient's peak $\dot{V}O_2$ is commonly associated with restrictive lung disease (5.7-R), whereas a breathing frequency less than 50 at the peak $\dot{V}O_2$ is characteristic of the patient with obstructive lung disease (5.7-L). Although the distinction between obstructive and restrictive lung disease is generally evident from standard pulmonary function measurements, the question addressed by exercise testing is whether or not the resting pulmonary function abnormalities account for the patient's exercise intolerance.

SUMMARY

To determine the likely pathophysiological causes of exercise limitation, we found that a logical approach can be developed and displayed in five flowcharts. Each flowchart starts with a question as to whether the peak $\dot{V}O_2$ and AT are normal or abnormal. Other physiological measurements relating breathing reserve, heart rate and $\dot{V}O_2$, ventilation and perfusion, and $\dot{V}O_2$ and work rate are then used to define the pathophysiological sites in the gas transport coupling of muscle metabolism to ventilation. The pathophysiology identified can be used to establish the likely clinical diagnosis.

The first flowchart separates four major categories of patients. The second addresses the cause of exercise limitation in patients with a normal peak $\dot{V}O_2$. The third considers the diagnosis in patients with a reduced peak $\dot{V}O_2$ but with a normal *AT*. The fourth considers the diagnosis in patients with a reduced peak $\dot{V}O_2$ and reduced *AT*. The fifth addresses the diagnosis of the patient with a reduced peak $\dot{V}O_2$ but with the *AT* not determined. These flowcharts usually enable the examiner to make a specific organ-related physiological diagnosis. The flowcharts are designed as guides to an orderly decision-making process. The final judgment must be made by the examiner.

CHAPTER 9

Clinical Applications of Cardiopulmonary Exercise Testing

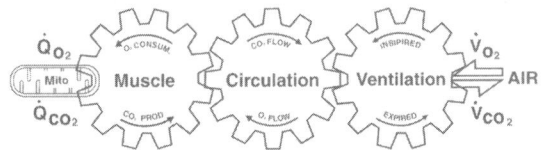

DIFFERENTIAL DIAGNOSIS OF DISORDERS
CAUSING EXERCISE INTOLERANCE

PATHOPHYSIOLOGICAL RESPONSES IN
COMMON DISORDERS

Oxygen Uptake and Carbon Dioxide Output as
Related to Work Rate

Heart Rate and Carbon Dioxide Output as a Function
of Oxygen Uptake

Heart Rate and Oxygen Pulse as a Function of Work
Rate

Tidal Volume as a Function of Exercise Minute
Ventilation

Exercise Minute Ventilation as a Function of Carbon
Dioxide Output

Ventilatory Equivalents for Oxygen and Carbon Dioxide

End-Tidal Oxygen and Carbon Dioxide

DIAGNOSES UNIQUELY MADE BY
CARDIOPULMONARY EXERCISE
TESTING

Development of Myocardial Dyskinesis with
Myocardia Ischemia During Exercise

Chronic Heart Failure Due to Diastolic Dysfunction

Pulmonary Vascular Occlusive Disease Without
Pulmonary Hypertension (Pulmonary
Vasculopathy)

Patent Foramen Ovale with Development of a Right-
to-Left Shunt During Exercise

Pulmonary Vascular Disease Limiting Exercise in
Chronic Obstructive Pulmonary Disease

Impaired Muscle Bioenergetic Function

Psychogenic Dyspnea and Behavioral Causes of
Exercise Intolerance

GRADING SEVERITY OF HEART DISEASE

ESTIMATING PEAK CARDIAC OUTPUT
DURING EXERCISE FROM OXYGEN
UPTAKE AT PEAK WORK RATE

Cardiac Output Estimated from Oxygen Uptake
Applying the Fick Principle

Behavior of Changing Arterial–Venous Oxygen
Difference During Exercise

Estimating Arterial–Venous Oxygen Difference

Shortcut Estimate of Stroke Volume from Oxygen Pulse

CARDIOPULMONARY EXERCISE TESTING
FOR PROGNOSTIC EVALUATION

Prognosis in Heart Failure and Prioritizing Patients for
Heart Transplantation

Prognosis in Primary Pulmonary Hypertension and
Prioritizing Patients for Lung Transplantation

Prognosis in Chronic Obstructive Pulmonary Disease
and Prioritizing Emphysema Patients for Lung
Reduction Surgery

PREOPERATIVE EVALUATION OF SURGICAL
RISK

Thoracic Surgery

Abdominal Surgery

Who Should Undergo Cardiopulmonary Exercise
Testing Preoperatively?

MEASURING IMPAIRMENT FOR DISABILITY
EVALUATION

Impairment and Disability

Problems in Assessing Impairment from Only Resting
Measures

Exercise Testing and Impairment Evaluation

Oxygen Cost of Work

EXERCISE REHABILITATION

Physiological Basis of Exercise Rehabilitation

Exercise Rehabilitation in Heart Disease

Exercise Rehabilitation in Chronic Obstructive
Pulmonary Disease

ASSESSING THE EFFECTIVENESS OF
TREATMENT

SCREENING FOR DEVELOPMENT OF
DISEASE IN HIGH-RISK PATIENTS

GRADED EXERCISE TESTING AND THE
ATHLETE

SUMMARY

THE INCREASING NUMBER of applications for which cardiopulmonary exercise testing (CPET) is currently employed attests to the growing recognition of its importance in medicine. This chapter describes applications of CPET. In some instances, these applications are well established. In others, the applications are inadequately recognized and appreciated. These applications are of great value in patient care and have the potential to reduce health care costs by streamlining diagnosis and facilitating treatment decisions.

DIFFERENTIAL DIAGNOSIS OF DISORDERS CAUSING EXERCISE INTOLERANCE

The physician is sometimes at a loss to determine and understand the pathophysiological mechanism(s) causing exercise intolerance; therefore, the disease that accounts for the patient's symptom(s)— usually those of fatigue, dyspnea, or pain—goes undiagnosed. Different defects in the coupling of external (airway) to cellular respiration affect gas exchange in different ways (see Fig. 5.1), with the gas exchange responses to CPET differing according to the defect. Thus, the pattern of gas exchange at the airway can be used to identify pathophysiology and also to support or refute the correctness of a specific clinical diagnosis. With an appropriate display of gas exchange data obtained during exercise testing, it is possible to determine the functional status of the cardiovascular and ventilatory systems.

There are also certain diagnoses for which CPET is a unique diagnostic tool. That is, these diagnoses cannot be made very easily with other diagnostic modalities, but can be inferred from the gas exchange responses to exercise. These include exercise intolerance due to silent myocardial ischemia; chronic heart failure due to diastolic dysfunction; pulmonary vascular occlusive disease without overt pulmonary hypertension; the development of a right-to-left shunt during exercise; pulmonary vascular disease limiting exercise in chronic obstructive pulmonary disease (COPD); disorders of muscle that impair muscle bioenergetic function; and psychogenic dyspnea and behavioral causes of exercise intolerance, such as anxiety or malingering. In addition, there is no faster or more inexpensive way of confirming a normal cardiovascular and ventilatory physiological state than cardiopul-

monary exercise testing because it simultaneously confirms a normal cardiac output, ventilation–perfusion matching, breathing pattern, and breathing response to exercise.

A graphical display of CPET data of the essential physiological responses is easier to read than a tabular display, and so it is advantageous to transform the data into graphs that describe the essential physiological responses to exercise. We find it particularly useful to assemble these data into the form of nine strategically positioned panels containing 15 graphs on a single page (see Fig. 4.30). These graphs enable the examiner who is knowledgeable in the physiology and pathophysiology of exercise to systematically assess the cardiovascular, ventilatory, ventilation–perfusion, and metabolic responses to exercise. Armed with this information, the cause of exercise intolerance can usually be determined with a high degree of certainty.

A major reason why the patterns of data for different diseases can be recognized on the nine-panel graphical display is that gas exchange responses are very uniform in healthy subjects. For example, the increase in $\dot{V}O_2$ as related to work rate is normally approximately 10 ml/min/watt with relatively small standard deviation (± 0.7). Because the heart rate normally increases linearly with $\dot{V}O_2$, the heart rate–$\dot{V}O_2$ and the O_2 pulse responses are highly predictable. Because of the relative uniformity of $PaCO_2$ and VD/VT values in normal subjects and the tight regulation of arterial H^+ concentration (see Chapter 7), the normal ventilatory response to exercise is closely coupled to $\dot{V}CO_2$, with small variation (see Table 7.6). (Normal values for all measurements on the nine-panel graphical display are summarized in Chapter 7.)

Chapter 8 discussed how a diagnosis is reached using a deductive reasoning strategy. After it is determined, for example, that peak $\dot{V}O_2$ is reduced, a systematic series of questions is asked about other physiological measurements. In the following section, specific panels from the nine-panel graphical display are used to contrast the responses seen in several common disorders. By contrasting the response patterns of a set of variables in eight different diseases to the normal pattern, it will become clearer how CPET helps in the differential diagnosis of disorders limiting exercise. However, it must be stressed that a diagnosis is not made by examining one panel or variable alone; a specific diagnosis usually depends on abnormalities in certain panels, with normal responses in others.

PATHOPHYSIOLOGICAL RESPONSES IN COMMON DISORDERS

Oxygen Uptake and Carbon Dioxide Output as Related to Work Rate

The basic requirement to sustain muscular exercise is an increase in cellular respiration for regeneration of the adenosine triphosphate (*ATP*) used to fuel the muscular contractions. To support the increase in cellular respiration, O_2 and CO_2 transport between the cells and the environment must match the rate of cellular respiration (except for transient lags allowed by the capacitance in the transport system). The increases in O_2 and CO_2 transport are functions of the peripheral circulation, heart, pulmonary circulation, blood, lungs, and respiratory muscles. Any defect in this interactive system could result in failure of the muscle to take up and use the O_2 needed for aerobic regeneration of *ATP*. On the nine-panel graphical display (see Fig. 4.30 and Chapter 10), $\dot{V}O_2$ and $\dot{V}CO_2$ are plotted against work rate (WR) and time in panel 3 (upper right), and the slope of $\Delta\dot{V}O_2/\Delta WR$ can be seen (Fig. 9.1).

Figure 9.1 contrasts the characteristic findings of $\dot{V}O_2$ and $\dot{V}CO_2$ plotted against WR for a normal subject with those of eight patients with different disorders. The age and gender of each subject, case number of the subject in Chapter 10, and predicted $\dot{V}O_2$ are shown in the respective panel. The smaller number under the age is the case number. Figure 9.1a (Case 1 of Chapter 10) shows the responses of a 55-year-old man who was diagnosed as normal. This is the only subject shown in Figure 9.1 with a normal peak $\dot{V}O_2$, $\dot{V}CO_2$ response, and $\Delta\dot{V}O_2/\Delta WR$. The $\Delta\dot{V}O_2/\Delta WR$ can be compared with the normal response by contrasting the slope of $\dot{V}O_2$ increase versus work rate with the diagonal line drawn with a slope of 10 ml/min/watt, the predicted normal slope.

Figure 9.1b shows a 47-year-old man who developed depressed ST segments on the electrocardiogram (ECG) starting at the work rate where $\dot{V}O_2$ stopped increasing normally. The failure of $\dot{V}O_2$ to increase normally with increasing work rate, despite the increase being normal at lower work rates, is not uncommon when myocardial ischemia impairs the heart's ability to increase cardiac output normally (1,2).

Figure 9.1c displays the data for a 65-year-old male diabetic and cigarette smoker with peripheral arterial disease. Both the $\dot{V}O_2$ and $\dot{V}CO_2$ increase linearly, but more slowly than normal, from the lowest work rate, as might be predicted for someone with a fixed stenosis of the conducting arteries to exercising extremities.

The study shown in Figure 9.1d is of a 55-year-old woman with dilated cardiomyopathy. She had a significantly reduced peak $\dot{V}O_2$ and a very low anaerobic threshold (*AT*) reflected by a relatively high CO_2 output at low work rates. Reduced gas exchange efficiency in chronic left ventricular failure is reflected in Figure 9.6d.

The study shown in Figure 9.1e is of a 54-year-old male with vasculitis that primarily affected his pulmonary circulation. The rate of rise in $\dot{V}O_2$ decreases progressively as the peak $\dot{V}O_2$ is approached. Thus, the average $\Delta\dot{V}O_2/\Delta WR$ is quite low. The abnormal gas exchange efficiency accompanying this pulmonary vasculitis is addressed in Figures 9.5 and 9.6.

The high O_2 cost of exercise during treadmill walking in an obese subject can be seen in Figure 9.1f, which demonstrates the large increase in $\dot{V}O_2$ following the onset of walking at zero grade at 3 miles per hour. Because the actual work rate performed on a treadmill is very difficult to determine, $\Delta\dot{V}O_2/\Delta WR$ cannot be readily calculated.

The data in Figure 9.1g are those of a 50-year-old man with COPD. The $\Delta\dot{V}O_2/\Delta WR$ is normal, but the peak $\dot{V}O_2$ is reduced. Abnormal ventilatory mechanics and reduced gas exchange efficiency contribute to his exercise limitation, as shown in Figures 9.4g and 9.6g, respectively.

Exercise data from a 29-year-old man with sarcoidosis resulting in severe pulmonary hypertension are shown in Figure 9.1h. The low peak $\dot{V}O_2$ and reduced $\Delta\dot{V}O_2/\Delta WR$ place him in the severely impaired category.

Finally, the study shown in Figure 9.1i is of a 20-year-old man with severe interstitial pulmonary fibrosis (IPF), but without pulmonary hypertension. His failure to increase $\dot{V}O_2$ despite increasing work rate reflects his inability to increase pulmonary blood flow and the maximizing of $C(a - \bar{v})O_2$ at a very low work rate. This finding represents very severe disease and a loss of ability to sustain even mild exercise. The lack of pulmonary hypertension

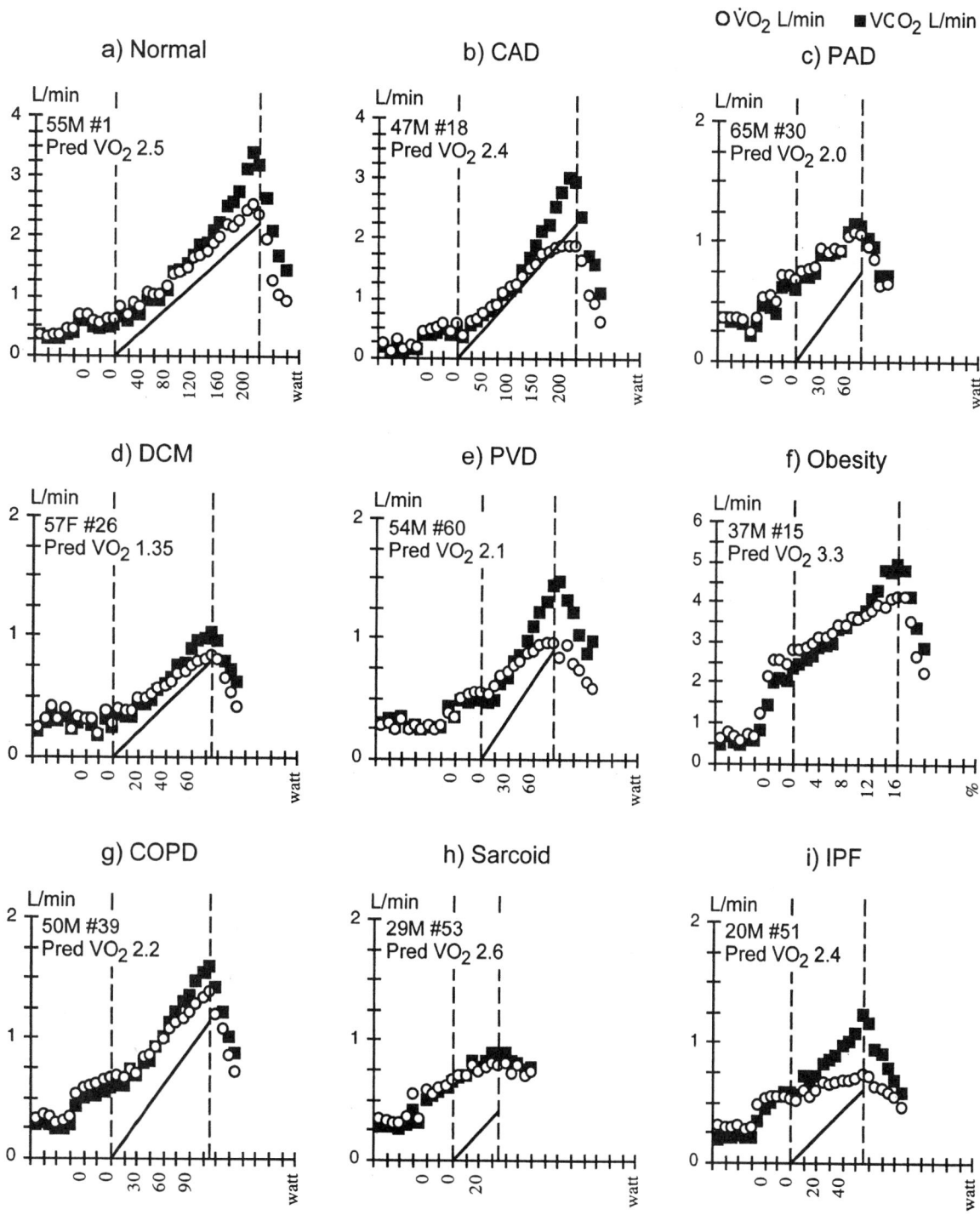

FIGURE 9.1.   Plot of V̇o₂ and V̇co₂ (STPD) as a function of work rate (watts) and time (1 minute between tick marks on x-axis) for patients with normal exercise performance (a), coronary artery disease (b), peripheral arterial disease (c), dilated cardiomyopathy (d), pulmonary vascular disease (e), obesity (abscissa is % treadmill grade) (f), chronic obstructive pulmonary disease (g), sarcoidosis (h), and interstitial pulmonary fibrosis (i). The data to the left of the first "0" are from the rest period. "0" work rate is unloaded cycling. The period of increasing work rate starts at the left vertical dashed line and ends at the right vertical dashed line. The diagonal line between the vertical dashed lines is the normal rate of rise for V̇o₂ against work rate with a slope of 10 ml/min/W. The predicted peak V̇o₂ is shown in the upper left of each panel. Just above the predicted peak V̇o₂ are the age and gender of the patient, and the case number of the subject in Chapter 10. Further history and data can be found for each patient in Chapter 10.

in this patient is due to failure of the right ventricle to hypertrophy and does not connote the absence of severe loss of pulmonary vascular bed. The high $\dot{V}CO_2$ relative to $\dot{V}O_2$ reflects the substantial lactic acidosis that the patient developed during this short exercise test.

Heart Rate and Carbon Dioxide Output as a Function of Oxygen Uptake

Panel 5 of the nine-panel graphical display (see Fig. 4.30) shows heart rate (solid squares) and $\dot{V}CO_2$ (open squares) as functions of $\dot{V}O_2$. These relations are shown in Figure 9.2 for the same nine patients depicted in Figure 9.1. Heart rate normally increases linearly with $\dot{V}O_2$ to the predicted maximum values for both variables, as indicated by the X in the figure and illustrated in Figure 9.2a (Case 1 of Chapter 10). The heart rate–$\dot{V}O_2$ slope is steeper than normal and often becomes nonlinear in the patients with cardiovascular diseases (Figs. 9.2b, d), including those in which the diseases affect the pulmonary circulation, such as pulmonary vasculitis (Fig. 9.2e), sarcoidosis (Fig. 9.2h), and IPF (Fig. 9.2i).

$\dot{V}CO_2$ normally increases as a function of $\dot{V}O_2$ with a slope of approximately 1 until the *AT* is reached (Fig. 9.2a). Above that point, $\dot{V}CO_2$ increases more steeply than $\dot{V}O_2$ in all of the patients except in the patient with peripheral arterial disease (Fig. 9.2c), presumably due to trapping of CO_2 in the muscle because of the relatively small contribution of blood flow coming from the ischemic lower limbs. In the patient with coronary artery disease (CAD) (Fig. 9.2b), the obese patient (Fig. 9.2f), and the COPD patient (Fig. 9.2g), the *AT* is normal. In the patient with heart failure (Fig. 9.2d) and the three other patients (vasculitis, Fig. 9.2e; sarcoidosis, Fig. 9.2h; and IPF, Fig. 9.2i), the *AT* is significantly below the 95% confidence limit for normal.

Heart Rate and Oxygen Pulse as a Function of Work Rate

Panel 2 of the nine-panel graphic display (see Fig. 4.30) shows the heart rate (solid squares) and O_2 pulse (open circles) plotted against work rate and time. Figure 9.3 shows panel 2 for the same nine patients included in Figure 9.1. Heart rate normally increases abruptly at the start of unloaded cycling

and then increases approximately linearly with work rate to the predicted maximal heart rate (Fig. 9.3a). Deviation from the normal heart rate response is seen in patients with chronotropic incompetence (Fig. 9.3d) or when the patient is stopped in the performance of exercise because of noncardiac or nonpulmonary vascular disease problems. The latter is exemplified by the patients with peripheral arterial disease (Fig. 9.3c) and COPD (Fig. 9.3g).

The O_2 pulse, the product of stroke volume and arteriovenous O_2 difference, also shown in panel 2, normally increases with a gradually decreasing rate of rise to the predicted normal value (Fig. 9.3a). However, O_2 pulse fails to increase normally in patients with CAD in which myocardial ischemia reduces stroke volume and, therefore, exercise capacity (Fig. 9.3b). The O_2 pulse also fails to increase normally in heart failure (Fig. 9.3d), as well as in the three patients in whom the pulmonary circulation is seriously deranged (pulmonary vasculitis, sarcoidosis, and IPF). As shown in Figures 9.3e, 9.3h, and 9.3i, the value of peak O_2 pulse during exercise is abnormally low in these patients.

As noted in Chapter 7, the O_2 pulse can also be discerned from the panels shown in Figure 9.2. The O_2 pulse is low when the extension of the slope of the heart rate–$\dot{V}O_2$ relation projects to the left of the target X (e.g., Fig. 9.2b–e, h, and i).

Tidal Volume as a Function of Exercise Minute Ventilation

Tidal volume (V_T) is plotted as a function of $\dot{V}E$ in panel 7 of the nine-panel graphical display (see Fig. 4.30). Figure 9.4 shows panel 7 for the same nine patients illustrated in Figure 9.1. Tidal volume normally increases preferentially to breathing frequency during low- and moderate-intensity exercise to account for the early increase in $\dot{V}E$ in normal subjects (Fig. 9.4a). Above the *AT*, breathing frequency is the primary factor accounting for the increase in $\dot{V}E$. At peak exercise, there is normally a breathing reserve of greater than 10 to 15 L/min, the latter calculated as the difference between the maximal voluntary ventilation (MVV) and the peak exercise $\dot{V}E$. The tidal volume may increase to the inspiratory capacity (IC), but not above it.

However, patients limited in their exercise tolerance by lung mechanics characteristically have

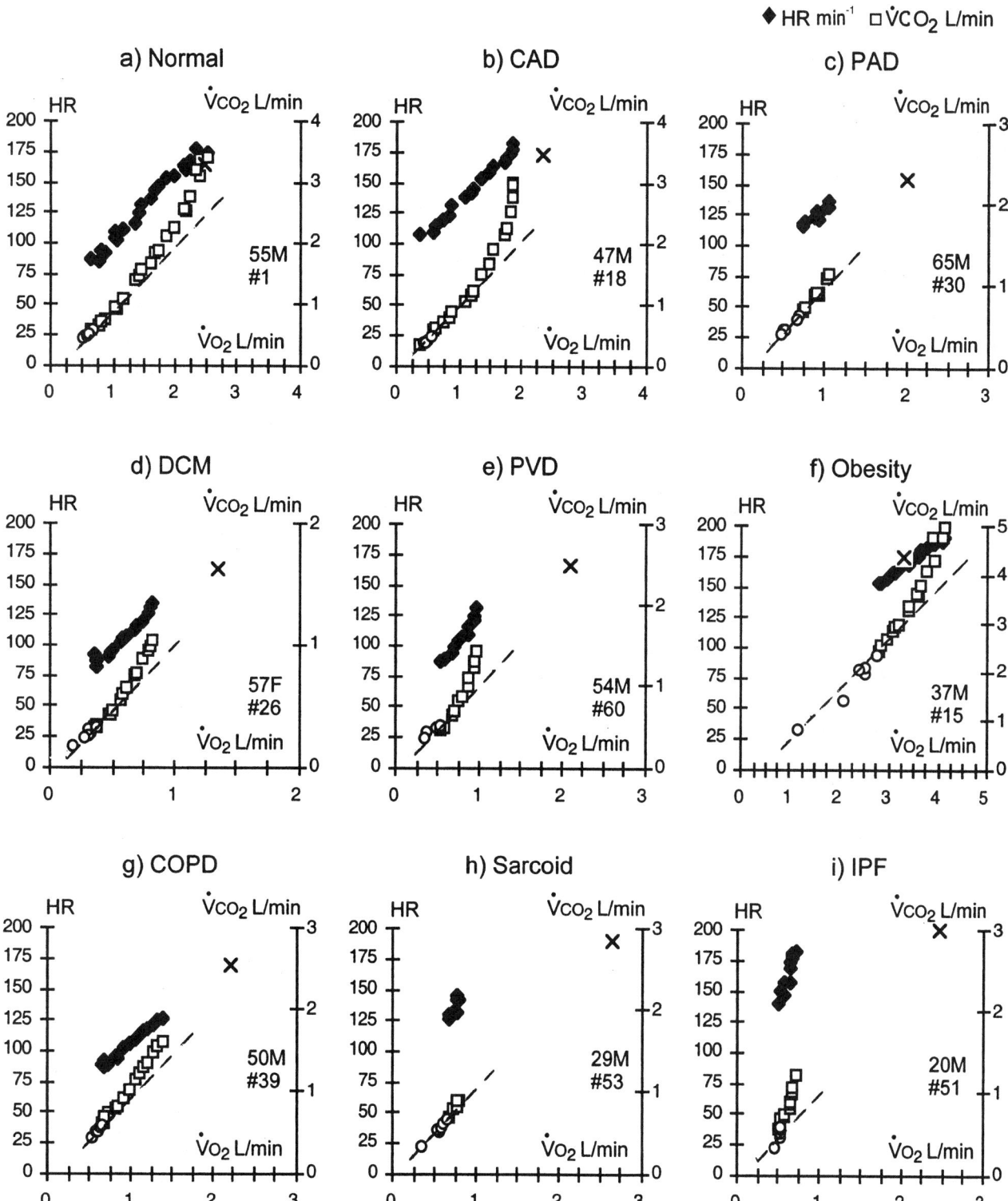

FIGURE 9.2.   Heart rate and $\dot{V}_{CO_2}$ plotted as functions of $\dot{V}_{O_2}$ for the same nine patients shown in Figure 9.1. Age, gender, and case number (Chapter 10) are shown at lower right. The diagonal dashed line has a slope of 1. The anaerobic threshold (*AT*) is read as the $\dot{V}_{O_2}$ at which $\dot{V}_{CO_2}$ starts increasing at a slope greater than 1.

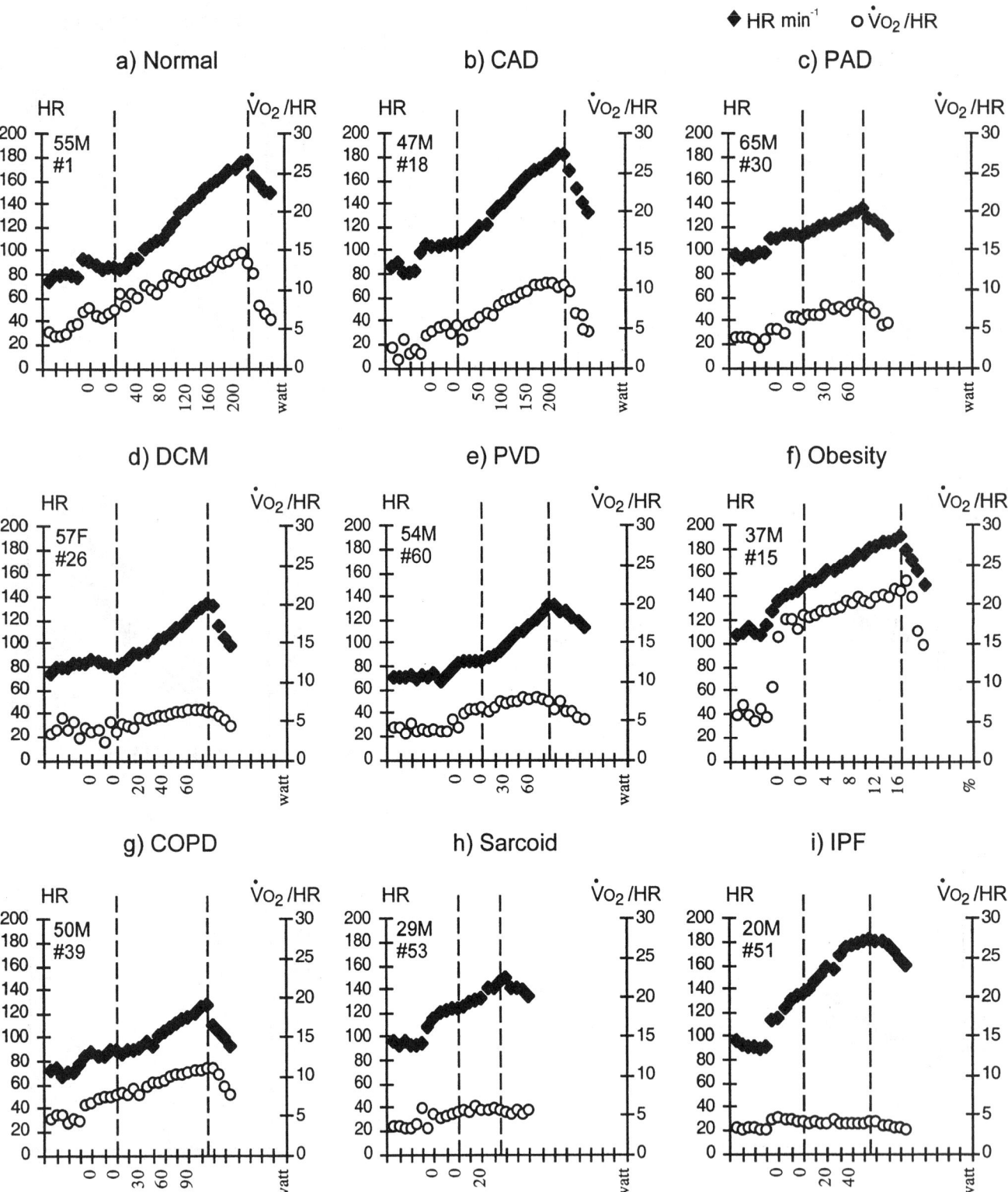

FIGURE 9.3.   Heart rate (HR) and O$_2$ pulse ($\dot{V}O_2$/HR) plotted as functions of work rate (watts) and time (1 minute between tick marks on *x*-axis) for the same nine patients shown in Figure 9.1. The period of increasing work rate starts at the left vertical dashed line and ends at the right vertical dashed line. Age, gender, and case number (Chapter 10) are shown at upper left.

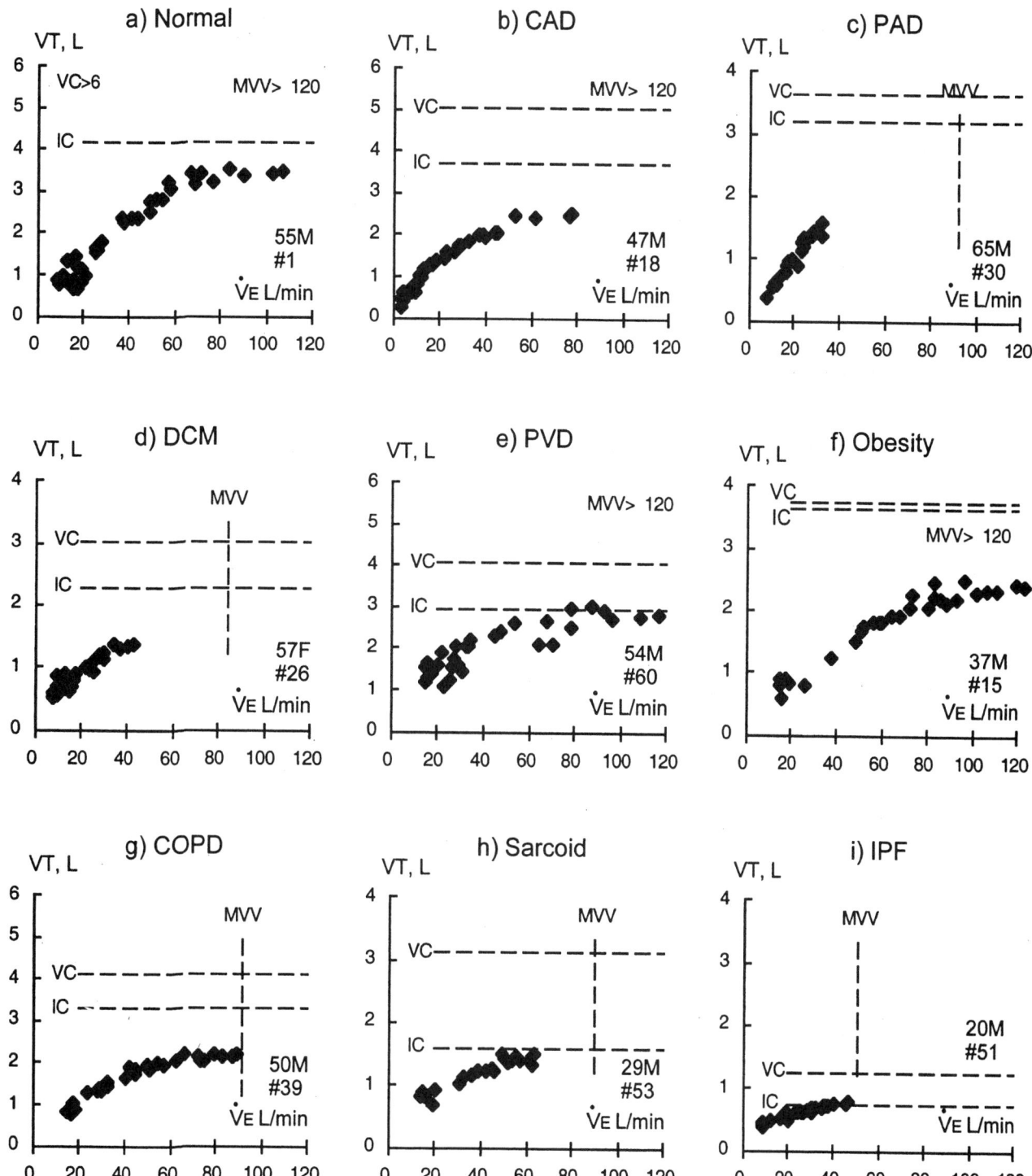

FIGURE 9.4.   Exercise tidal volume plotted as a function of minute ventilation ($\dot{V}E$) for the same nine patients shown in Figure 9.1. Age, gender, and case number (Chapter 10) are shown at lower right. Also shown are the subject's maximal voluntary ventilation (MVV) on the abscissa (*vertical dashed line*) and the subject's resting inspiratory capacity (IC) and vital capacity (VC) on the ordinate (*horizontal dashed lines*) unless above scale.

no or a very small breathing reserve (<10 L/min). Thus, despite only a moderate reduction in MVV, the patient with COPD commonly has no breathing reserve when ventilatory limited due to a combination of poor gas exchange efficiency and reduced ventilatory capacity (Fig. 9.4g). This is also true of the patient with IPF (Fig. 9.4i). Further, the patient with IPF has a tidal volume that reaches inspiratory capacity early in exercise, characteristic of restrictive lung disease. The breathing reserves in the other patients in Figure 9.4 are normal.

Exercise Minute Ventilation as a Function of Carbon Dioxide Output

$\dot{V}E$ is plotted as a function of $\dot{V}CO_2$ in panel 4 of the nine-panel graphical display (see Fig. 4.30). Figure 9.5 shows panel 4 for the nine patients illustrated in Figure 9.1. $\dot{V}E$ normally increases linearly with $\dot{V}CO_2$ with a slope of 23 to 28 (see Table 7.6) in normal subjects up to the point where ventilatory compensation for the developing lactic acidosis starts (Fig. 9.5a). This slope is not increased in patients with CAD (Fig. 9.5b), peripheral arterial disease (Fig. 9.5c), and obesity (Fig. 9.5f). However, it is usually increased in patients with chronic heart failure (Fig. 9.5d) (3–7), pulmonary vasculitis (Fig. 9.5e), COPD (Fig. 9.5g), sarcoidosis (Fig. 9.5h), and IPF (Fig. 9.5i), diseases associated with an increase in VD/VT (6,8–10) or a reduced arterial PCO_2, or both. The slope of the linear component of the plot of $\dot{V}E$ versus $\dot{V}CO_2$ is steeper the more extensive the disease.

Ventilatory Equivalents for Oxygen and Carbon Dioxide

$\dot{V}E/\dot{V}O_2$ and $\dot{V}E/\dot{V}CO_2$ are plotted against work rate and time in panel 6 of the nine-panel graphic display (see Fig. 4.30). Figure 9.6 shows panel 6 for the nine patients illustrated in Figure 9.1. When VD/VT and $PaCO_2$ are normal, $\dot{V}E/\dot{V}O_2$ decreases and reaches a nadir at the *AT* with a value less than 28, and $\dot{V}E/\dot{V}CO_2$ decreases to a nadir at the ventilatory compensation point with a value less than 32, as shown in Figure 9.6a. The nadir values of $\dot{V}E/\dot{V}O_2$ and $\dot{V}E/\dot{V}CO_2$ are normal for patients with CAD (Fig. 9.6b), peripheral arterial disease (Fig. 9.6c), and obesity (Fig. 9.6f), but increased for patients with chronic heart failure (Fig. 9.6d), pulmonary vasculitis (Fig. 9.6e), COPD (Fig. 9.6g), sarcoidosis (Fig. 9.6h), and IPF (Fig. 9.6i), diseases associated

with an increase in VD/VT. The more severe the disease or the lower the $PaCO_2$, the higher the values of $\dot{V}E/\dot{V}O_2$ and $\dot{V}E/\dot{V}CO_2$.

End-Tidal Oxygen and Carbon Dioxide

$PETO_2$ and $PETCO_2$—and, when available, PaO_2 and $PaCO_2$—are plotted against work rate and time in panel 9 of the nine-panel graphical display (see Fig. 4.30). Figure 9.7 shows panel 9 for the nine patients illustrated in Figure 9.1. Normally, $PETO_2$ and $PETCO_2$ track their arterial blood counterparts (Fig. 9.7a). Normally, $PaCO_2$ is higher than $PETCO_2$ at rest, but $PETCO_2$ increases approximately 4 mm Hg above $PaCO_2$ during exercise (Fig. 9.7a). Thus, $PETCO_2$ during exercise is slightly above 40 mm Hg at sea-level altitudes. $PETCO_2$ increases with exercise when the pulmonary circulation is normal, such as shown in the cases of the patients with coronary artery disease (Fig. 9.7b), peripheral arterial disease (Fig. 9.7.c), and obesity (Fig. 9.7f).

The increase in $PETCO_2$ during exercise is greater than normal in many obese patients because the mechanical restriction caused by the excessively heavy chest wall and abdomen prevents ventilation from keeping a precise pace with the increase in CO_2 production (Fig. 9.7f).

In severe heart failure (Fig. 9.7d), $PETCO_2$ is reduced because blood flow is slow relative to ventilation in regional lung units. At rest and low work rates, $PETCO_2$ might be quite variable in left ventricular failure because of the periodic breathing that these patients commonly develop (see Case 26 in Chapter 10). This is reflected in panel 9 of the nine-panel plot as a regular oscillatory change in $PETCO_2$ and $PETO_2$ at rest and low work rates (Fig. 9.7d). Consequently, at rest and low work rate exercise, two sets of values appear, as shown in Figure 9.7d.

$PETCO_2$ is reduced in pulmonary vascular occlusive disease (Fig. 9.7e) because of lack of perfusion of ventilated lung. The underperfused acini function as dead space because they contain little CO_2 as compared with the ideal alveolar or arterial PCO_2. Thus, the mixed end-tidal gas is relatively dilute in CO_2, and $PETCO_2$ is less than $PaCO_2$, in contrast to the pattern seen in normal subjects (Fig. 9.7a).

In COPD patients, the $PETCO_2$ is reduced relative to $PaCO_2$ because the high-$\dot{V}A/\dot{Q}$ lung units account for most of the subject's ventilation (Fig. 9.7g). If airway obstruction is quite severe, $PETCO_2$ might increase in response to exercise.

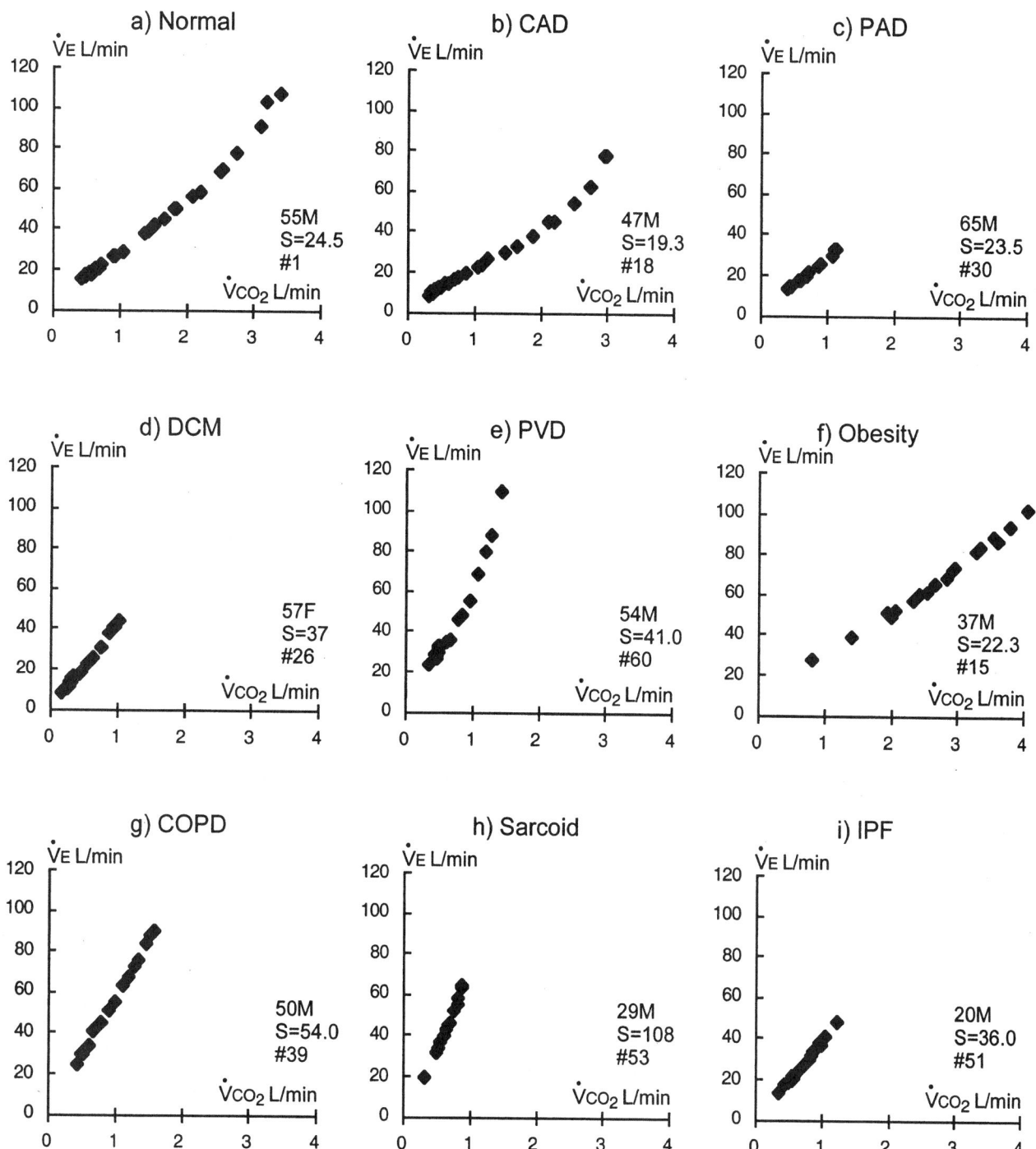

FIGURE 9.5.   Exercise minute ventilation (V̇E) plotted as a function of CO_2 output (V̇CO_2) for the same nine patients shown in Figure 9.1. At lower right in each panel is the slope (S) of the linear component of the V̇E versus V̇CO_2 relation. The age, gender, and case number, as presented in Chapter 10, are shown below the slope values.

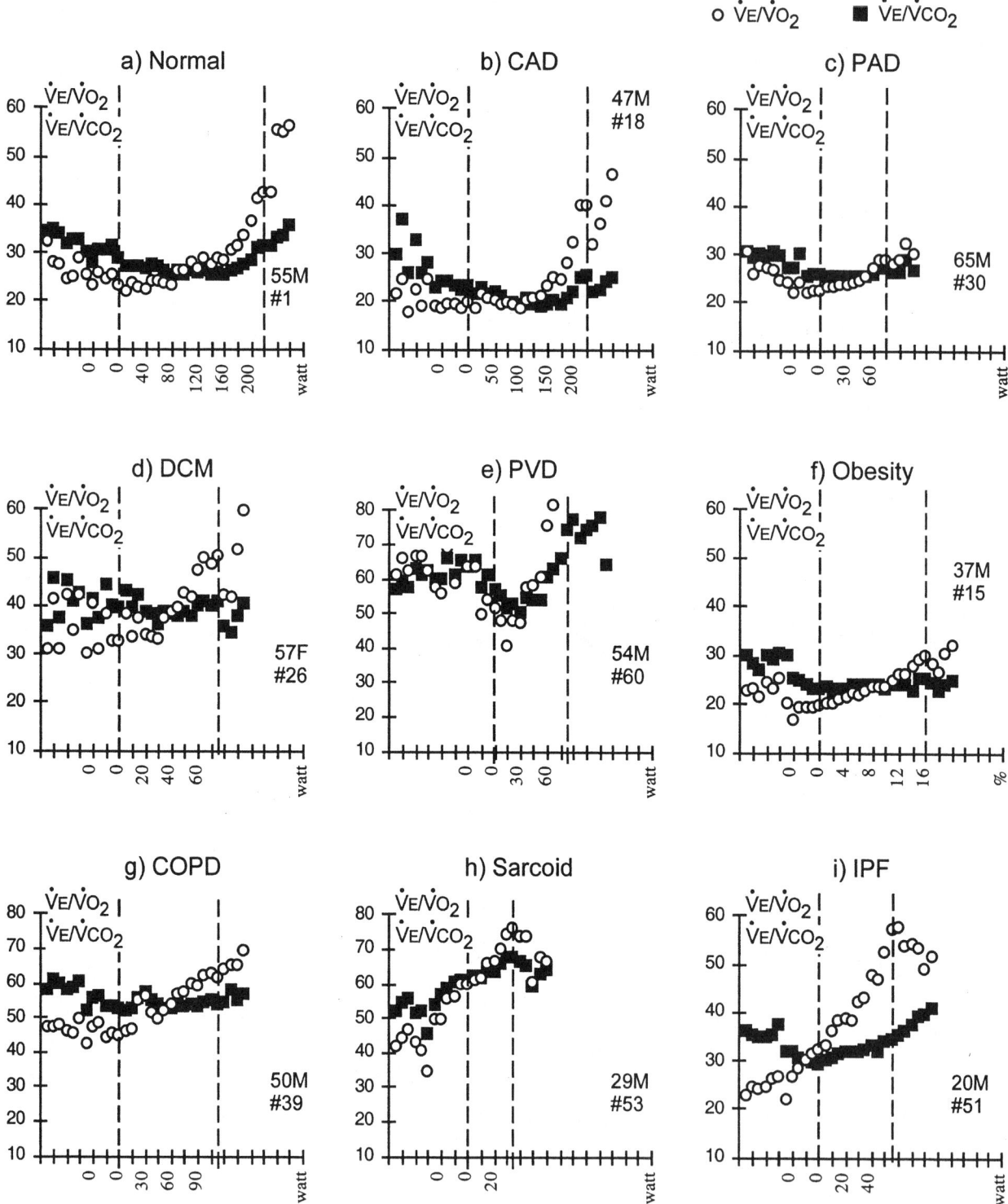

FIGURE 9.6.   Plot of ventilatory equivalent for O_2 ($\dot{V}E/\dot{V}O_2$) (*open circles*) and CO_2 ($\dot{V}E/\dot{V}CO_2$) (*closed squares*) as functions of work rate (watts) and time (1 minute between tick marks on *x*-axis) for the same nine patients shown in Figure 9.1. The age, gender, and case number, as presented in Chapter 10, are shown in the lower right in each panel. The period of increasing work rate starts at the left vertical dashed line and ends at the right vertical dashed line.

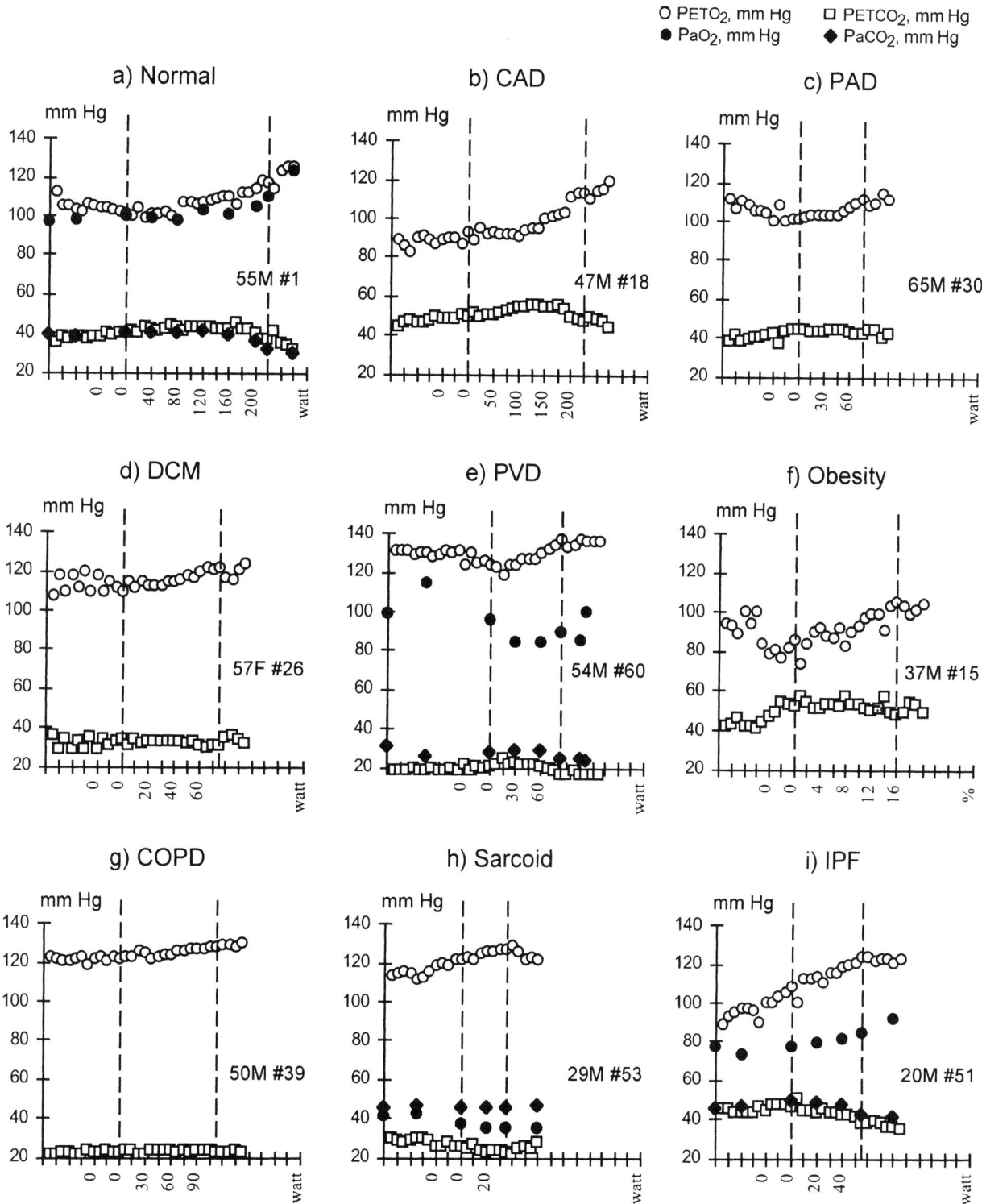

FIGURE 9.7.   Plot of PETO$_2$ and PETCO$_2$, and in four cases, the corresponding arterial values, as functions of work rate (watts) and time (1 minute between tick marks on x-axis) for the same nine patients shown in Figure 9.1. The age, gender, and case number, as presented in Chapter 10, are shown in the lower right in each panel. The period of increasing work rate starts at the left vertical dashed line and ends at the right vertical dashed line.

Figure 9.7h shows a case of a young man with severe sarcoidosis. In this disorder, the pulmonary circulation may be greatly affected, reducing the size of the pulmonary vascular bed. Thus, $P_{ET}CO_2$ is markedly reduced relative to $PaCO_2$ (Fig. 9.7h). PaO_2 might also be markedly reduced, as in Figure 9.7h, particularly if the foramen ovale opens during exercise, causing a right-to-left shunt.

$P_{ET}CO_2$ decreases below $PaCO_2$ in idiopathic pulmonary fibrosis. Normally, $PaCO_2$ is regulated near normal if the lung mechanics are not too severely affected. However, if lung mechanics are severely impaired, hypercapnia may take place during exercise (Fig. 9.7i).

In subjects with good chemosensitivity, $\dot{V}E$ increases at the AT, reducing the extraction of O_2 from the respired air, causing $P_{ET}O_2$ to increase without a decrease in $P_{ET}CO_2$ (isocapnic buffering) (Fig. 9.7a–f, h, i). Thus, panel 9 can be used as a method for detecting the AT. However, it is not as reliable a method as the V-slope method because the former depends on good chemoreceptor sensitivity. This is not a requirement of the latter method. (Compare the AT determined from Fig. 9.7 with that of Fig. 9.2.)

The abrupt change in $P_{ET}O_2$ and $P_{ET}CO_2$ may also be used as noninvasive evidence of the opening of a right-to-left shunt at the start of exercise. As an example of the changes in $P_{ET}O_2$ and $P_{ET}CO_2$ with development of a right-to-left shunt at the start of exercise, see Case 80 in Chapter 10.

The patterns of change of $\dot{V}E$ and R as a function of work rate (panels 1 and 8, respectively, of Fig. 4.30) are not presented for the nine cases selected here in the interest of space and because these changes can be reviewed in Chapter 10. They provide important correlative data needed to properly interpret the changes in gas exchange accompanying the diseases, already described. All of the panels have greater meaning when reviewed in relation to each other.

DIAGNOSES UNIQUELY MADE BY CARDIOPULMONARY EXERCISE TESTING

Development of Myocardial Dyskinesis with Myocardial Ischemia During Exercise

The normal contraction of the myocardium depends on the ability of all the myofibrils of the heart muscle to contract synchronously in response to the electrical depolarization set off by the sinoatrial pacemaker. With each heartbeat, ATP is primarily consumed by the heart during systole and regenerated in diastole when the myocardium is resupplied with oxygenated blood. For normal regeneration of ATP, the O_2 supply must be adequate. Since the diastolic period shortens as heart rate increases, exercise is a useful way to precipitate myocardial ischemia in regions of the heart that have impaired ability to increase blood flow commensurate with the increased myocardial O_2 demand. In addition, the increase in cardiac output during exercise induces an increase in myocardial work because the left ventricle must contract against a higher systemic arterial pressure.

Asynchronous contraction of the myocardium could result in a reduction in stroke volume and a consequent failure of $\dot{V}O_2$ to increase in proportion to the work rate, as illustrated in Cases 16 to 22 in Chapter 10. The slowing or failure of $\dot{V}O_2$ to increase with increasing work rate indicates that cardiac output is not increasing appropriately. When $\dot{V}O_2$ reaches a plateau despite increasing work rate, cardiac output has reached a maximum. When heart rate continues to increase even though cardiac output has apparently stopped increasing (Cases 16–22), stroke volume must be decreasing, reflecting the myocardial dyskinesis of ischemia.

In patients with ST segment depression (with or without chest pain), simultaneous flattening in $\Delta\dot{V}O_2/\Delta WR$ and flattening of the O_2 pulse response with increasing work rate confirm the development of myocardial ischemia during exercise. ECG changes suggestive of myocardial ischemia without chest pain and without gas exchange responses that are characteristic of myocardial dyskinesis make the diagnosis of myocardial ischemia questionable. By measuring gas exchange, the physician can confirm that myocardial dyskinesis did occur and also the $\dot{V}O_2$ and heart rate at which it occurred.

Chronic Heart Failure Due to Diastolic Dysfunction

Systolic dysfunction resulting in heart failure is usually easily diagnosed by the finding of a low ejection fraction and cardiomegaly. On the other hand, detecting heart failure due to diastolic dysfunction—a problem not uncommon in the elderly, patients with myocardial ischemia, heart transplant recipient patients, and patients with hypertrophic cardiomyopathy (11)—is difficult because heart size and ejection fraction are normal. Without the clue provided by cardiopulmonary exercise testing, the cardiologist is unlikely to make the critical objective measurements necessary to establish the diagnosis of diastolic dysfunction.

On the other hand, in patients with chronic heart failure (whether due to systolic or diastolic dysfunction), noninvasive CPET can identify a reduced peak $\dot{V}O_2$ and *AT*, reflecting reduced O_2 transport, and when dysfunction is moderate to severe, an increase in $\dot{V}E/\dot{V}CO_2$ (decreased gas exchange efficiency). Because the increase in $\dot{V}E/\dot{V}CO_2$ is due to an increased VD/VT in proportion to the reduction in exercise tolerance and is not accompanied by hypoxemia, Wasserman et al. (8) pointed out that these findings must reflect decreased perfusion of ventilated lung and not airway dysfunction. Thus, CPET with gas exchange measurements is a test especially suited for making the diagnosis of chronic heart failure secondary to either systolic or diastolic dysfunction.

Pulmonary Vascular Occlusive Disease Without Pulmonary Hypertension (Pulmonary Vasculopathy)

Most patients limited in exercise because of pulmonary vascular disease (pulmonary vasculopathy) have exertional dyspnea well before they have signs of pulmonary hypertension at rest. Once signs of pulmonary hypertension are present, the patient has recruited all the pulmonary blood vessels normally reserved for recruitment during exercise. By this time, the clinical condition has seriously deteriorated, and the opportunity to intervene at an early stage of the disease with some potential pulmonary vasodilator or anti-inflammatory treatments may be lost.

There is no diagnostic method in medicine other than exercise gas exchange, and possibly ventilation–perfusion scans, that is capable of identifying a patient with abnormal pulmonary circulation in an early stage of the disease (i.e., when a patient is symptomatic but before pulmonary hypertension develops). This is because the patient's symptoms are present only during exercise, not at rest. Although the pulmonary blood flow may be adequate at rest, these patients have difficulty in increasing pulmonary blood flow appropriately in response to exercise, when they have their symptoms.

In patients with pulmonary vascular disease, $\dot{V}O_2$ usually does not continue to increase with a normal slope of 10 ml/min/watt with progressive increases in work rate. Rather, the rate of rise gradually decreases (Fig. 9.1e) up to the point where continuation of exercise becomes intolerable, usually because of dyspnea or fatigue or both. $\dot{V}E$ relative to $\dot{V}CO_2$ is characteristically significantly elevated in patients with pulmonary vascular disease (Figs. 9.5e and 9.6e).

The peak $\dot{V}O_2$ (panel 3) and *AT* (panel 5), $\dot{V}E$–$\dot{V}CO_2$ relationship (panels 4 and 6), and $PETCO_2$ at the *AT* (panel 9) probably best quantify the severity of the illness (12,13) and may well prove to be the best guides in the selection of patients with pulmonary vascular disease for lung transplantation. The steep heart rate rise and low O_2 pulse (likely reflecting a low stroke volume) will be evident in panels 2 and 5. The slope of $\dot{V}E$ plotted as a function of $\dot{V}CO_2$ (panel 4), which is about 25 in the normal individual, will be much higher in patients with pulmonary vascular disease (Fig. 9.5e, g–i). This increase depends on the increase in VD/VT and low $PaCO_2$ set point (9,14). Panel 6 shows high values for $\dot{V}E/\dot{V}CO_2$ at the *AT* or lowest $\dot{V}E/\dot{V}CO_2$, reflecting decreased perfusion to ventilated lung (high $VA/\dot{Q}$) and quantitatively related to the degree of pulmonary vascular occlusion. Arterial blood gases, displayed on panel 9, along with end-tidal O_2 and CO_2 and calculation of VD/VT, further characterize the abnormal physiological state of the pulmonary circulation.

Patent Foramen Ovale with Development of a Right-to-Left Shunt During Exercise

About 25% of the population has a potentially patent foramen ovale (15), but this phenomenon is functionally unimportant unless right atrial pressure exceeds left atrial pressure. However, this situation can develop during exercise in patients with primary pulmonary vascular disease (e.g., primary pulmonary hypertension) or pulmonary vascular disease secondary to lung or connective tissue diseases. It must be kept in mind that attempts at detecting a patent foramen ovale at rest may be unsuccessful because the patient may only shunt right atrial blood into the left atrium during exercise.

If, during exercise, the increase in venous return exceeds the rate at which the right ventricle can pump blood into the pulmonary circulation, right ventricular end-diastolic pressure and right atrial pressure will rise. Simultaneously, because of the resistance to blood flow in the lungs, right atrial may exceed left atrial pressure. The presence of a potentially patent foramen ovale allows venous return to flow from the right to the left atrium when right atrial exceeds left atrial pressure. The rapid decrease in systemic arterial P_{O_2}, and the increase in the CO_2 and H^+ load entering the arterial circulation, stimulate the arterial ventilatory chemoreceptors. This phenomenon can occur despite normal or near-normal arterial oxyhemoglobin saturation at rest (see Case 61, Chapter 10). An exercise test with arterial blood sampling during 100% O_2 breathing allows the confirmation of a diagnosis of an anatomical right-to-left shunt developing during exercise.

The diagnosis of a right-to-left shunt developing during exercise can be suspected from characteristic changes in gas exchange at the start of exercise (16). These include an abrupt decrease in P_{ETCO_2} and increase in P_{ETO_2} (panel 9) at the start of exercise, along with simultaneous abrupt increase in R (panel 8), $\dot{V}_E/\dot{V}_{O_2}$ (panel 6), and $\dot{V}_E/\dot{V}_{CO_2}$ (panel 6), reflecting hyperventilation of the pulmonary blood flow as compensation for the blood flowing through the foramen ovale (see Case 80, Chapter 10). A decrease in arterial O_2 saturation at the start of exercise can usually be documented with a pulse oximeter (panel 9). The state of the shunt during exercise can be followed over time, without sampling of arterial blood for measurement of blood gases, by repeat CPET with particular attention paid to panels 9, 8, and 6.

An example of gas exchange abnormalities revealing the intermittent development of a right-to-left shunt during exercise is shown in Figure 9.8 in a sequential series of studies at 4-month intervals over a 16-month period during treatment with continuous intravenous epoprostenol. When blood begins to shunt from right to left during exercise, $\dot{V}_E$ abruptly increases, with an increase in $\dot{V}_E/\dot{V}_{CO_2}$ (panel 6), rather than the usual decrease seen in normal subjects when exercise starts. The slope of $\dot{V}_E$ as a function of $\dot{V}_{CO_2}$ sharply increases at the work rate at which the blood starts to shunt right to left (see the $\dot{V}_E/\dot{V}_{CO_2}$ versus time and the $\dot{V}_E$ versus $\dot{V}_{CO_2}$ in test 1 of Fig. 9.8). The reason ventilation increases so steeply when the shunt develops is that arterial pH continues to be regulated. Thus, shunting of high CO_2 and H^+ (primary ventilatory stimulants) blood from the venous system into the left side of the circulation bypasses the lungs (17). When the shunted blood reaches the arterial and

subsequently central chemoreceptors, ventilation is stimulated in proportion to the shunted CO_2 and H^+ load.

In test 2 (Fig. 9.8), the shunt no longer develops early in exercise because of a reduction in right atrial pressure, but did develop late in exercise (see S in panel 3 of the second test), forcing the patient to stop exercise soon after the development of the right-to-left shunt. By test 3 (after 8 months of treatment), the pulmonary hypertension was much reduced, peak $\dot{V}_{O_2}$ and O_2 pulse had increased, and the evidence for an exercise-induced right-to-left shunt had disappeared. Now, and in the remaining two tests, $\dot{V}_E/\dot{V}_{CO_2}$ (third panel down) remained relatively constant, although elevated in the transition from rest to exercise, indicating that V_D/V_T was relatively fixed and shunting no longer occurred.

All this information about this patient's pathophysiology and change with treatment or time was obtained noninvasively and could not have been obtained as successfully even with more complicated invasive tests. More invasive and complex tests could not be repeated with the frequency and at the low cost of CPET. In this case, exercise testing with gas exchange measurements allowed the treating physician to recognize that the patient, who was extremely ill when first seen, had improved sufficiently to be taken off the lung transplantation list. The patient was studied for an additional 4 years with CPET-guided therapy. The patient remained at the same level of performance as shown in test 5.

Pulmonary Vascular Disease Limiting Exercise in Chronic Obstructive Pulmonary Disease

Although patients with COPD usually are exercise limited because of abnormal lung mechanics, as reflected by a low exercise breathing reserve, some are limited primarily by a reduced pulmonary capillary bed, which limits the increase in blood flow in response to exercise. In such a patient, lung reduction surgery might improve the lung mechanics but not improve exercise tolerance because pulmonary blood flow cannot increase beyond that achieved before surgery. Case 44 in Chapter 10 is an example of this problem. Exercise testing should therefore be done before lung reduction surgery, with the objective of confirming that impaired lung mechanics that limits CO_2 elimination and pH regulation is the primary cause of exercise

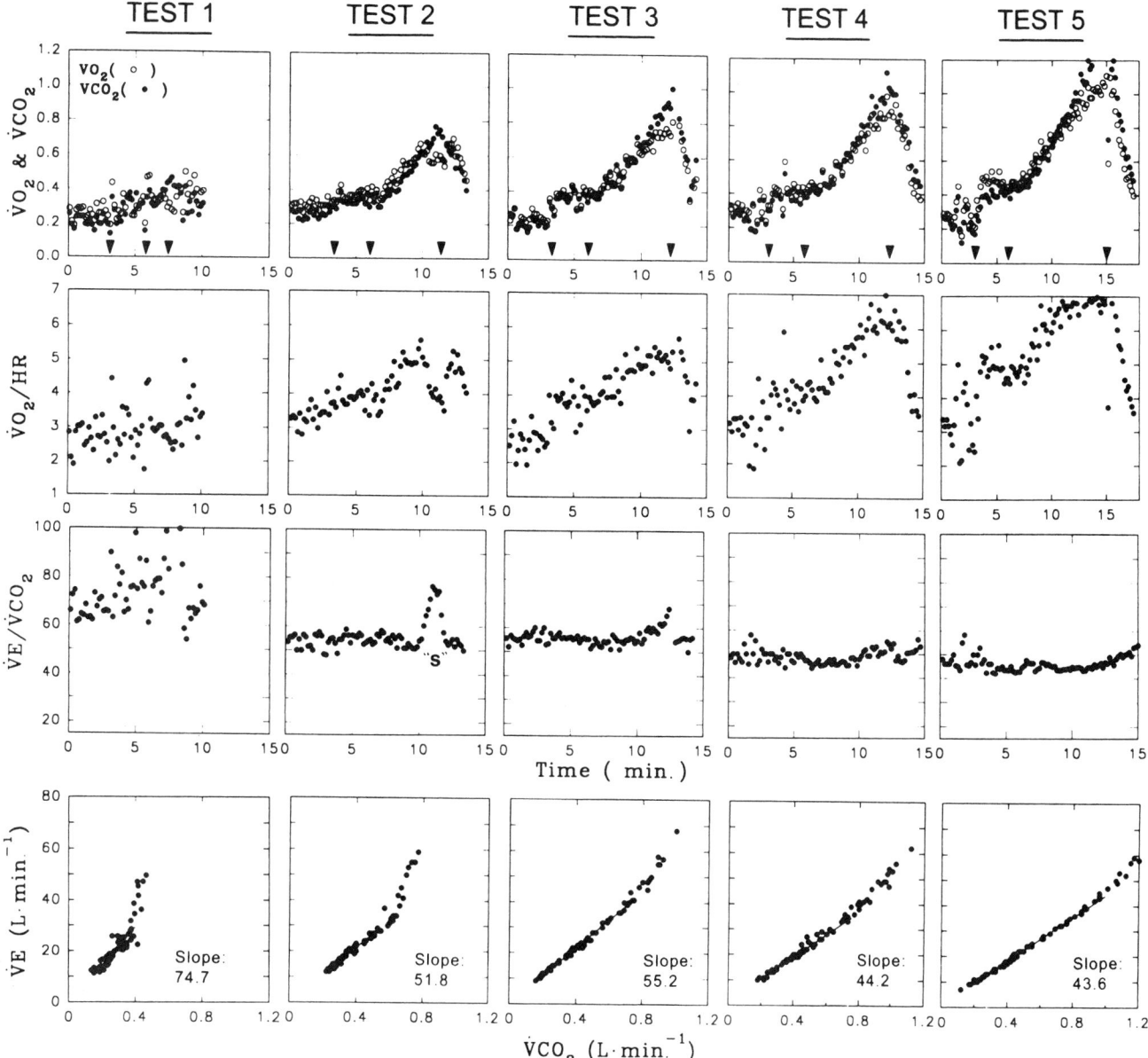

FIGURE 9.8.   Five tests in a patient with primary pulmonary hypertension, each done at 4-month intervals. Test 1 was done as a control before the start of continuous intravenous epoprostenol, a preparation of prostacyclin. Test 2 was done after 4 months of treatment, and test 3 was done 4 months later, and so on, for a total of 16 months. Although the full nine-panel plots were obtained, for ease of comparing the physiological changes with time, only four panels of data are shown for each test. The top panel contains plots of $\dot{V}O_2$ and $\dot{V}CO_2$ (L/min) against time. On the abscissa of this plot are three arrows, the left indicating the transition from rest to unloaded cycling, the middle arrow indicating the start of the increasing exercise period, and the arrow on the right indicating the end of exercise. As is evident from this panel in test 1, the patient was very restricted and could perform very little exercise. At that time, her O_2 pulse (ml/beat) (second panel down) could not increase in response to exercise, indicating that the product of her stroke volume and arteriovenous O_2 difference was fixed. The ventilatory equivalents for CO_2 (third panel down) are very high at rest (first 3 minutes) and increase further after exercise starts due to the opening of a right-to-left shunt, presumably through the foramen ovale. This is reflected in a large change in the slope of $\dot{V}E$ versus $\dot{V}CO_2$ in the fourth panel down. The slope value shown in this panel is that for the lower slope before the diverting of blood through the right-to-left shunt. The slope value of 74.7 is very high (normal being about 25; see Chapter 7). This steep slope primarily reflects the poor perfusion to ventilated lung (increased VD/VT). The abrupt steepening of this slope reflects an increase in right-to-left shunt.

The repeat study 4 months after the start of treatment (test 2) shows a significant increase in peak $\dot{V}O_2$ and O_2 pulse and a reduced ventilatory response as evident from the decrease in $\dot{V}E/\dot{V}CO_2$ and in the lower slope of $\dot{V}E$ versus $\dot{V}CO_2$ (51.8 versus 74.7). The latter two values indicate that perfusion to ventilated lung had become more uniform, although still quite abnormal. Just before the end of exercise, a right-to-left shunt developed, reflected in the abrupt decrease in $\dot{V}O_2$ and O_2 pulse and the increase in $\dot{V}E/\dot{V}CO_2$, designated by "S" in the third panel down, and the abrupt steepening of the slope of $\dot{V}E$ versus $\dot{V}CO_2$ in the fourth panel down.

The next three tests show improvement in all measurements, reaching a plateau response by the fifth test. Additional tests were done over the next 4 years and are not shown because there was no significant change from test 5. Thus, the patient is considerably improved and has become stable, but still has significant inability to increase cardiac output, as reflected by a reduced peak $\dot{V}O_2$ and O_2 pulse (60% and 70% of predicted, respectively) and elevated $\dot{V}E$ versus $\dot{V}CO_2$ slope and $\dot{V}E/\dot{V}CO_2$ at the anaerobic threshold.

limitation, rather than impaired systemic blood flow and O_2 transport.

Impaired Muscle Bioenergetic Function

Skeletal muscle myopathy that affects bioenergetic function has effects on exercise gas exchange that depend on the site of the muscle enzyme defect. Thus, a patient with a myopathy that affects myophosphorylase or one of the glycolytic enzymes (e.g., phosphofructokinase) would have a reduced maximum exercise tolerance because of the inability to develop a lactic acidosis and the benefits therefrom, as described in Chapter 2. This will be reflected in exercise gas exchange, not only because of the reduced peak $\dot{V}O_2$ (18) but also because of the failure to produce extra CO_2 from the buffering of lactic acid, as described by Riley et al. (19). In contrast, enzyme defects in the electron transport chain cause a lactic acidosis at a very low work rate (20), with accompanying gas exchange abnormalities similar to those observed in patients with heart failure (21,22). Exercise studies are a good screening technique for detecting muscle enzyme defects affecting bioenergetics and are useful for objectively assessing therapeutic modalities.

Psychogenic Dyspnea and Behavioral Causes of Exercise Intolerance

How do physicians diagnose psychogenic dyspnea or behavioral causes (volitional or nonvolitional) of exertional intolerance? It is difficult to make these diagnoses reliably unless the patient is studied during CPET with quantitative gas exchange measurements being performed.

It appears that these patients often undergo extensive diagnostic assessment, at great expense, that *indirectly* evaluates the cause of exercise intolerance—usually yielding negative results. Then, rather than performing the *direct* diagnostic assessment, the physician may prescribe an irrelevant drug that only adds to the patient's problem (see Cases 13 and 83 in Chapter 10). Obviously, to diagnose the cause(s) of exercise intolerance, the patient should be studied during exercise, and the essential values that evaluate cellular and external respiration should be measured (see Case 85, Chapter 10). Logically, CPET should be done before

the patient undergoes expensive imaging studies and an extensive invasive workup that searches in a state of rest for an abnormality that takes place during exercise.

Volitional behavioral causes of exercise intolerance also require CPET to make or confirm this diagnosis (see Cases 65 and 66, Chapter 10). Thus, these diagnoses are only available to those physicians who learn how to use CPET and can interpret the results.

GRADING SEVERITY OF HEART DISEASE

Symptoms have been the primary method by which physicians previously graded severity of heart failure. The New York Heart Association (NYHA) provided a valuable classification system based on symptoms, which has been almost universally used for over half of a century (23). It has four functional classifications (classes I to IV) based on the perceived activity level of the patient. Matsumura et al. (24) found that the NYHA classification correlated reasonably well with the anaerobic threshold and peak $\dot{V}O_2$, showing that symptoms and the ability to transport O_2 were correlated. However, the peak $\dot{V}O_2$ and AT had a relatively large range of values within an NYHA class. This is thought to be due to differences in how patients perceive their symptoms and differences in how physicians interpret the severity of patients' described symptoms.

Because of this subjectivity, Weber and Janicki sought a more objective assessment based on peak $\dot{V}O_2$ and AT (25). They established an A through D classification for progressive severity as a function of the decline in peak $\dot{V}O_2$/kg (Table 9.1). They found that this classification for objectively assessing cardiac dysfunction was superior to the NYHA classification. A consensus conference on prioritizing patients with heart failure for heart transplantation based on predicted survival time also agreed with this more objective assessment (26).

Stelken et al. (27) felt that the Weber–Janicki approach, although an advance, would be more satisfactory if it were normalized for age and gender as well as body size. They analyzed the normal predictive values based on size, age, and gender (described in Chapter 7) and found that the percent predicted peak $\dot{V}O_2$ was a good predictor of survival. Stevenson (28) and Gitt et al. (3) assessed prognosis by comparing peak $\dot{V}O_2$/kg with-

TABLE 9.1. Weber's Exercise Functional Classification Based on Maximal Oxygen Uptake and Anaerobic Threshold

Class	$\dot{V}O_2max$ (mL/min/kg)	AT (mL/min/kg)	CImax (L/min/m²)
A	>20	>14	>8
B	16–20	11–14	6–8
C	10–15	8–11	4–6
D	<10	<8	<4

$\dot{V}O_2max$, maximal or peak $\dot{V}O_2$; AT, anaerobic threshold; CImax, maximal exercise cardiac index (cardiac output per square meter of body surface area). From Weber KT. Cardiopulmonary exercise testing and the evaluation of systolic dysfunction. In: Wasserman K, ed. *Exercise gas exchange in heart disease*. Armonk, NY: Futura Publishing, 1996:55–62, with permission.

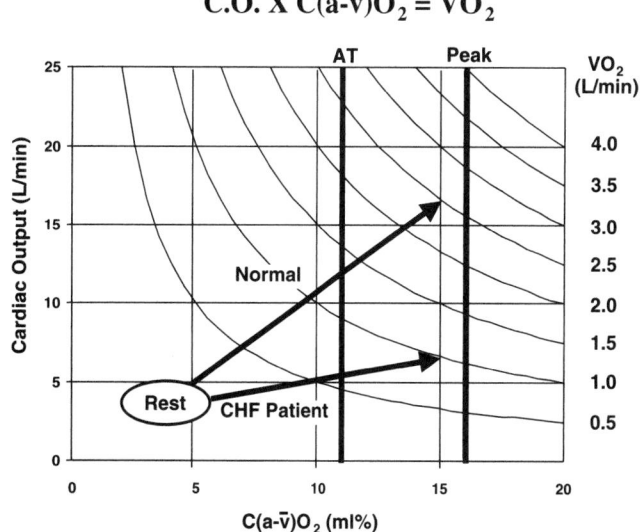

$$C.O. \times C(a-\bar{v})O_2 = VO_2$$

FIGURE 9.9. O_2 uptake guided measurement of cardiac output during exercise. Each $\dot{V}O_2$ isopleth is a product of cardiac output and arterial–mixed venous O_2 difference [$C(a-\bar{v})O_2$]. If $C(a-\bar{v})O_2$ can be estimated, such as at peak $\dot{V}O_2$ or at the anaerobic threshold (*AT*), cardiac output can be estimated at those points. The arrows illustrate how the values of $\dot{V}O_2$ at the *AT* and peak can be used to estimate the subject's cardiac output noninvasively. This graph also illustrates that the *AT* becomes a larger fraction of the peak $\dot{V}O_2$ the lower the peak $\dot{V}O_2$.

out normalizing for age and gender with the percentage of predicted $\dot{V}O_2$, which itself normalizes for age, gender, and height. Both groups found that either method was a good predictor of survival. However, Gitt et al. (3) found that normalizing just to body weight gave a better assessment of prognosis than percent predicted $\dot{V}O_2$. Importantly, the physiological assessment (using peak $\dot{V}O_2$/kg) has been determined to be a more reliable independent predictor of survival than the NYHA symptom classification or measurements of ejection fraction (27,29–31).

ESTIMATING PEAK CARDIAC OUTPUT DURING EXERCISE FROM OXYGEN UPTAKE AT PEAK WORK RATE

Cardiac Output Estimated from Oxygen Uptake Applying the Fick Principle

$\dot{V}O_2$ is equal to the cardiac output × $C(a-\bar{v})O_2$. The relation is illustrated graphically in Figure 9.9. From this figure, it can be seen that exercise performance depends on the ability to extract O_2 from the arterial blood and to increase cardiac output. The ability to increase $C(a-\bar{v})O_2$ depends primarily on the hemoglobin concentration and arterial O_2 content. Given a normal hemoglobin concentration of 15 g/dL and normal arterial oxyhemoglobin saturation and content, the arterial O_2 content is approxi-

mately 20 ml/100 ml. The maximal extraction is about 75% to 80%, resulting in a maximal $C(a-\bar{v})O_2$ at peak exercise of 15 to 16 ml/100 ml. Thus, without increasing cardiac output, the maximum that $\dot{V}O_2$ can increase over resting is threefold. All further increase in exercise $\dot{V}O_2$ depends on increasing cardiac output.

Normal middle-aged subjects who are relatively sedentary have a peak $\dot{V}O_2$ about 10 times resting, and well-trained subjects can have peak $\dot{V}O_2$ values of 20 times resting. Thus, referring to Figure 9.9, peak $\dot{V}O_2$ reveals the magnitude of the increase in cardiac output in response to maximal exercise. If hemoglobin and arterial O_2 content are normal, a peak exercise $\dot{V}O_2$ that is only three times the resting value reveals that the patient is in the category of patients waiting for a heart transplant. In contrast, a sixfold increase reveals that the patient can at least double his or her cardiac output in response to exercise. As the ability to increase cardiac output diminishes, $C(a-\bar{v})O_2$ has a greater influence on the $\dot{V}O_2$ increase in response to exercise. Consequently, measurement of $\dot{V}O_2$ increase in response to exercise provides critical information about the ability of cardiac output to increase.

$C(a - \bar{v})O_2$ changes almost linearly from a predictable low value of 5 ml/100 ml (normal) to 6 ml/100 ml (heart failure) at rest to about 15 to 16 ml/100 ml in fit normal subjects (32) (see Fig. 3.3) and 13 to 16 ml/100 ml in patients with heart failure (25,33,34) at maximal exercise when the hemoglobin concentration is normal. If we knew the change in $C(a - \bar{v})O_2$ over the range of $\dot{V}O_2$ increase from rest to peak, or at specific levels of exercise such as at the anaerobic threshold (see Fig. 4.6) or peak $\dot{V}O_2$, we could estimate cardiac output from the $\dot{V}O_2$ alone. For instance, if the $C(a - \bar{v})O_2$ values were approximately 12 ml/100 ml and 15 ml/100 ml at the *AT* and peak $\dot{V}O_2$, respectively, we could calculate the cardiac output and the stroke volume from the $\dot{V}O_2$ values at these two levels of exercise.

Variation of the relation between $C(a - \bar{v})O_2$ and percent peak $\dot{V}O_2$ is small among normal subjects (32) and among patients with heart failure (25,33, 34) when the hemoglobin is normal. But despite the linear change with respect to percent peak $\dot{V}O_2$ during incremental exercise, the absolute value of $C(a - \bar{v})O_2$ must vary with factors that affect oxyhemoglobin content in arterial and mixed venous blood. These factors are considered next.

Behavior of Changing Arterial–Venous Oxygen Difference During Exercise

As noted in Chapters 3 and 4, cardiac output can be estimated noninvasively at peak exercise and the *AT* by using the Fick principle. Calculation depends on the measurement of peak or *AT* $\dot{V}O_2$ and a con-current estimate of $C(a - \bar{v})O_2$. Stroke volume is estimated by dividing the derived cardiac output by heart rate.

The measurement of $\dot{V}O_2$ and heart rate and estimation of CaO_2 are straightforward. Because $C(a - \bar{v})O_2$ changes in a relatively linear and predictable way from rest to peak $\dot{V}O_2$ (25,32–34), it is possible to estimate $C(a - \bar{v})O_2$ from hemoglobin concentration and arterial oxyhemoglobin saturation given the parameter of 75% to 80% maximal extraction in mixed venous blood ($C\bar{v}O_2$). The assumptions should be valid unless exercise is terminated by other than circulatory factors, such as by ventilatory limitation, musculoskeletal disorders, poor motivation, peripheral arterial disease, or a defect in muscle bioenergetics, in which instances $C\bar{v}O_2$ is abnormally high at maximal exercise and the normal maximal oxygen extraction does not take place.

Estimating Arterial–Venous Oxygen Difference

Estimates of $C(a - \bar{v})O_2$ at peak exercise are shown in Table 9.2. The estimates take into account the resting hemoglobin concentration and assume a hemoconcentration at peak exercise of 5% (see Fig. 2.34), an arterial oxyhemoglobin (O_2Hb) saturation of 96% (normal), a carboxyhemoglobin (COHb) saturation of 1% (normal), and a mixed venous O_2Hb saturation at maximal exercise of 24% (25,32,34). From these values, and recognizing that the hemoglobin O_2 binding capacity is 1.34 ml/g Hb, the $C(a - \bar{v})O_2$ at peak exercise would be the same as the hemoglobin concentration itself (Table 9.2).

TABLE 9.2.   Estimation of Arteriovenous Oxygen Difference [C(a − v̄)O$_2$] at Peak Exercise

Hb (g/100 ml)[a]	O$_2$ Capacity (ml/100 ml)	Arterial O$_2$ Saturation (%)	Mixed Venous O$_2$ Saturation (%)	Arterial O$_2$ Concentration (ml/100 ml)	Mixed Venous O$_2$ Concentration (ml/100)	C(a − v̄)o$_2$ (ml/100 ml)[b]
16	22.5	96	24	21.4	5.4	16.0
15	21.1	96	24	20.0	5.0	15.0
14	19.7	96	24	18.7	4.7	14.0
13	18.3	96	24	17.4	4.4	13.0
12	16.9	96	24	16.0	4.0	12.0
11	15.5	96	24	14.7	3.7	11.0
10	14.1	96	24	13.4	3.4	10.0

[a]The left column identifies the resting hemoglobin concentration. The hemoglobin concentration at peak exercise is considered to be 5% higher than the resting hemoglobin—that is, a fitness factor of 1.05 (see text for definition). The carboxyhemoglobin concentration is assumed to be 1%.
[b]Modifications: (i) If the person is very unfit, decrease the $C(a - \bar{v})O_2$ (right column) by up to 6%; if the person is very fit, increase the $C(a - \bar{v})O_2$ by up to 6%. (ii) Reduce the $C(a - \bar{v})O_2$ by 1% for each 1% increase in carboxyhemoglobin above 1%. (iii) Reduce the $C(a - \bar{v})O_2$ by 1% for each 1% decrease in arterial oxyhemoglobin saturation below 96%.

However, adjustments in maximal $C(a - \bar{v})O_2$ can be made in subjects who are exceptionally fit or have disease. Corrections might be made for how fitness and disease affect (a) hemoconcentration and (b) mixed venous O_2Hb saturation at peak exercise. Also, corrections might be made for the effect of change in arterial O_2Hb content resulting from (c) arterial O_2 desaturation (e.g., patients with lung diseases) and (d) increased COHb (e.g., cigarette smokers).

Exercise Hemoconcentration

The degree of hemoconcentration (up to 10%) varies with the peak $\dot{V}O_2$ or fitness of the subject. The initial estimate shown in Table 9.2 is for a subject of average fitness and hemoconcentration (5%). For an exceptionally fit subject, the $C(a - \bar{v})O_2$ obtained from Table 9.2 should be increased by up to 5%. In contrast, the $C(a - \bar{v})O_2$ should be decreased by up to 5% in the very unfit subject or the patient who has a very low peak $\dot{V}O_2$.

Mixed Venous Oxyhemoglobin Saturation

The $C(a - \bar{v})O_2$ shown in Table 9.2 is calculated for a subject with average fitness whose mixed venous O_2Hb saturation at peak exercise is 24%. However, mixed venous O_2Hb saturation can decrease at peak exercise to as low as 18% in the fit and be as high as 30% in disease. To apply the data in Table 9.2 to patients with different levels of fitness, increase $C(a - \bar{v})O_2$ by up to 6% in the very fit subject and decrease $C(a - \bar{v})O_2$ by up to 6% according to the patient's disease limitation.

Oxyhemoglobin Saturation

If the subject has hypoxemia, the $C(a - \bar{v})O_2$ determined from Table 9.2 should be decreased by 1% for each 1% decrease in arterial O_2Hb saturation below 96%.

Carboxyhemoglobin Saturation

If the subject has a COHb saturation greater than 1%, decrease the $C(a - \bar{v})O_2$ by the percentage of COHb saturation minus 1.

Examples of Estimating Arterial–Venous Oxygen Difference

The following examples illustrate how the initial estimate of $C(a - \bar{v})O_2$ from Table 9.2 is modified to take into account unusual fitness, arterial oxyhemoglobin desaturation, and increased COHb concentration.

Example A. If the resting Hb is 14 g/100 ml of blood, the first estimate of $C(a - \bar{v})O_2$ is 14 ml O_2/100 ml blood (Table 9.2). If we consider the person to be very fit, we might find more hemoconcentration (from 5% to 8%) and a slightly lower $S\bar{v}O_2$ (from 24% to 20%). In this case, the final estimate of $C(a - \bar{v})O_2$ would be $14 \times 1.07 = 15.0$ ml O_2/100 ml blood, instead of the 14 ml O_2/100 ml blood provided by the general relation shown in Table 9.2.

Further, in this example, where the $C(a - \bar{v})O_2$ is 150 ml O_2 per liter of blood and the $\dot{V}O_2$ is 3,500 ml/min and heart rate is 170 beats per minute at peak exercise, the cardiac output at peak exercise is 3,500/150 = 23.3 L/min, and the concurrent stroke volume is 23,300/170 = 137 ml/beat.

Example B. If the resting Hb is 12 g/100 ml of blood, the initial estimate of $C(a - \bar{v})O_2$ is 12 ml O_2/100 ml blood. For an extreme example, if we considered the person to be quite ill, we might estimate that there is less hemoconcentration (from 5% to 3%) and less decline in $S\bar{v}O_2$ (from 24% to 30%). If, in addition, the SaO_2 is only 90% [a 6% decrease in $C(a - \bar{v})O_2$] and the COHb is 5% [a 4% total decrease in $C(a - \bar{v})O_2$], then the final estimate of $C(a - \bar{v})O_2$ is $0.82 \times 12 = 9.8$ ml O_2/100 ml blood.

In this example, where $C(a - \bar{v})O_2$ is 98 ml O_2 per liter and the $\dot{V}O_2$ is 900 ml/min and heart rate is 160 at peak exercise, the cardiac output at peak exercise is 900/98 = 9.2 L/min, and the concurrent stroke volume is 9,200/160 = 58 ml/beat.

By referring to Figure 9.9, one can see the magnitude of the effect on the final estimate of cardiac output of taking into account these corrections of $C(a - \bar{v})O_2$. In general, the effect on the finally derived cardiac output measurement is relatively small, especially when peak $\dot{V}O_2$ is low.

Shortcut Estimate of Stroke Volume from Oxygen Pulse

The O_2 pulse is equal to the product of $C(a - \bar{v})O_2$ and stroke volume (SV). Therefore, stroke volume can be estimated at peak exercise by dividing the O_2 pulse at that time by the concurrent $C(a - \bar{v})O_2$, derived from Table 9.2. Thus, if the arterial oxyhemoglobin saturation is 96% (normal at sea level) and the resting hemoglobin concentration is 15 g/dl, and the maximum O_2 pulse is 15, the maximum stroke volume would be 100 ml (SV = 15/15 × 100). If the O_2 pulse is 25, the stroke volume would be 167 ml (SV = 25/15 × 100). Thus, the maximum O_2 pulse provides a convenient shortcut for estimating the concurrent stroke volume.

Application of Cardiac Output Determined from Oxygen Uptake and the Fick Principle

Because the most reliable work rate domain for cardiac output estimation from $\dot{V}O_2$ appears to be during submaximal work (e.g., near the lactic acidosis threshold), this observation was applied clinically to calculate cardiac output and predict outcomes in patients after anterior myocardial infarction (AMI) (35). Bigi et al. (35) studied 46 patients with AMI [39 male, 7 female patients aged 55 ± 8 years (mean ± SD) with an ejection fraction of 39 ± 7%]. Each subject underwent CPET and coronary angiography following hospital discharge. The estimated cardiac output was calculated using the linear regression of arterial–venous oxygen content against percent $\dot{V}O_2$max (see Fig. 3.6) (32).

Cardiac output at the anaerobic threshold of less than 7.3 L/min was the best cutoff value for identifying multivessel coronary artery disease (relative risk = 3.1). Angiographic scores were significantly higher in patients with a cardiac output at the *AT* of less than 7.3 L/min and were inversely and significantly correlated to cardiac output at the *AT*. Moreover, cardiac output at the *AT* of less than 7.3 L/min was associated with an increased risk of further cardiac events (odds ratio = 5; 95% confidence interval = 1.4–17) and was a significant discriminator of survival for the combined end-point of cardiac death, reinfarction, and clinically driven revascularization.

For cardiac output at the *AT* estimated by this method for normal subjects and patients with left ventricular failure, see Figure 4.6. Cardiac output at the *AT* determined from CPET, appears to be a safe and useful measurement for providing additional diagnostic and prognostic information in patients with coronary artery disease. From the studies reported later in this chapter, this statement could be extended to patients with left ventricular failure, primary pulmonary hypertension, and chronic obstructive pulmonary disease.

CARDIOPULMONARY EXERCISE TESTING FOR PROGNOSTIC EVALUATION

Prognosis in Heart Failure and Prioritizing Patients for Heart Transplantation

Exercise testing makes a variety of contributions to the understanding of exercise impairment and exertional dyspnea in chronic heart failure (36). A number of investigators have found that measurements of cardiac function at rest, both invasive and noninvasive, are poorly predictive of patients' symptoms, exercise capacity, prognosis, or need for heart transplantation. Weber and colleagues (37) compared resting cardiac function with exercise capacity in heart failure patients and found that such variables as cardiac index, left ventricular ejection fraction, wedge pressure, and radiographic heart size correlated poorly with measured peak $\dot{V}O_2$. Neither resting nor exercise pulmonary capillary wedge pressure correlated significantly with peak $\dot{V}O_2$. However, peak $\dot{V}O_2$ did correlate with maximum cardiac output during exercise. Matsumura et al. (38) and Itoh et al. (39) showed that peak $\dot{V}O_2$ and *AT* correlated with symptom scores as measured by NYHA class. Mean *AT* was 90% ± 15%, 77% ± 14%, and 60% ± 12% of the predicted values for NYHA class I, class II, and class III, respectively, in the study of Itoh et al. (39). *AT* correlated only weakly with resting left ventricular ejection fraction measured by echocardiogram or angiography.

Weber and colleagues suggested a classification of heart failure patients based on peak oxygen uptake and anaerobic threshold, as shown in Table 9.1 (37). Koike and colleagues (40) have similarly linked exercise capacity to symptom score. In these patients, peak $\dot{V}O_2$, *AT*, $\Delta\dot{V}O_2/\Delta WR$, and maximum WR decreased as NYHA symptom scores increased. NYHA class III patients had a maximum $\dot{V}O_2$ averaging 17 ± 3 ml/min/kg, *AT* of 11 ± 2 ml/min/kg, $\Delta\dot{V}O_2/\Delta WR$ equal to 6.2 ± 2 ml/min, and maximum work rate of 98 ± 22 watts.

In a study by Rickenbacher et al. (41), 116 consecutive patients with severe but stable congestive heart failure referred for heart transplantation were studied in close follow-up with medical management. This group demonstrated a very good prognosis, with actuarial survival at 1 year of 98% and at 4 years of 84%. The mean peak $\dot{V}O_2$ was 17.4 ± 4.3 ml/kg/min for the group as a whole. These authors concluded that stable symptoms and a relatively high peak exercise $\dot{V}O_2$ identified patients with a favorable prognosis despite a very low resting ejection fraction. In an earlier study (42), patients with peak $\dot{V}O_2$ of less than 10 ml/min/kg had a 77% 1-year mortality; if peak $\dot{V}O_2$ was between 10 and 18 mL/min/kg, mortality at 1 year was only 14%.

Some remarkable clinical trials have led to exercise testing providing the critical criteria in predicting survival and therefore in prioritizing patients for cardiac transplantation (43). A prospective study by Mancini et al. (29) randomized patients referred for heart transplantation into the following groups: (a) those with peak $\dot{V}O_2$ greater than 14 ml/kg/min (considered too well for transplantation), (b) those with peak $\dot{V}O_2$ less than 14 ml/kg/min and accepted for transplantation, and (c) those with peak $\dot{V}O_2$ less than 14 ml/kg/min but not accepted for surgery because of noncardiac reasons. If peak $\dot{V}O_2$ was greater than 14 ml/kg/min, then 1-year survival was 94%, whereas those with peak $\dot{V}O_2$ below 14 ml/kg/min had a 70% 1-year survival with medical management. The prognostic value of these criteria was not appreciably improved when peak $\dot{V}O_2$ was expressed as a percentage of predicted (44). Deaths and complications were also predicted by a peak $\dot{V}O_2$ of less than 14 ml/kg/min in a study by Roul et al. (45).

Osada et al. (46) identified 154 of 500 congestive heart failure patients referred for cardiac transplantation, a peak $\dot{V}O_2$ equal to or less than 14 ml/min/kg. They found that 3-year survival rate was reduced from 83 to 55% in those unable to reach a SBP of 120 mm Hg.

Stevenson et al. (47) presented data on 68 heart transplantation candidates (peak $\dot{V}O_2$ less than 14 ml/min/kg) who had repeat exercise tests at a mean 6 ± 5 months after initial evaluation to examine the possibility of the patient being able to be removed from the transplantation list. Thirty were without "major" improvement, but 38 had an increase in peak $\dot{V}O_2$ of more than 2 ml/min/kg, to a value greater than 12 ml/kg/min. Of these, 7 had no clinical improvement, but 31 were clinically improved. The "major improvement" group also had improved *AT*, peak O_2 pulse, and exercise heart rate reserve, and a decrease in resting heart rate. In the 31 patients removed from the heart transplantation waiting list, the actuarial survival rate was 100%. All of these patients were vigorously treated with diuretics and afterload reduction and were advised to become involved in informal exercise rehabilitation training.

Myers et al. (31) reported the results of studies on 644 patients with chronic heart failure over a 10-year period. They found that peak $\dot{V}O_2$ outperformed right heart catheterization data, exercise time, and the usual clinical variables used to assess heart failure patients in predicting outcome. They concluded that direct measurement of $\dot{V}O_2$ should be done when clinical or surgical decisions need to be made in patients referred for evaluation of heart failure or for consideration of heart transplantation.

Although most studies normalized the peak $\dot{V}O_2$ to body weight and ignored the variables of age and gender, Stelken et al. (27) compared the sensitivity of percentage of predicted peak $\dot{V}O_2$ based on weight, age, and gender, using the predicted values described in Chapter 7. In 181 ambulatory patients with NYHA class II to III symptoms, peak $\dot{V}O_2$, percent predicted peak $\dot{V}O_2$, and *AT* were significantly different for survivors and nonsurvivors when compared at 12 and 24 months. Eighty-nine patients with a peak $\dot{V}O_2$ of less than 50% predicted had 1- and 2-year survival rates of 74% and 43%, respectively, compared with 98% and 90% for the 92 patients who had a peak $\dot{V}O_2$ greater than 50% predicted. Although Stelken et al. (27) found the percent predicted value to be a better predictor of survival than that of $\dot{V}O_2$/kg, Gitt et al. (3), making the same comparison, found that normalizing to body weight was a better predictor. The difference might be due to the relative obesity factor in the two populations and its effect on the $\dot{V}O_2$/kg parameter.

Prognosis Based on Peak Oxygen Uptake, Anaerobic Threshold, and $\dot{V}E$ Versus $\dot{V}CO_2$ Relation

Since the late 1980s, heart transplant cardiologists have appreciated that peak $\dot{V}O_2$ more sensitively predicts prognosis than more classic heart failure risk factors such as left ventricular ejection fraction, NYHA class IV symptoms, and neurohormonal markers (Table 9.3). Increasing experience has confirmed the prognostic value of *peak* $\dot{V}O_2$ in the evaluation of heart failure patients for cardiac transplantation (27–31,46,48,49). The 1993 Bethesda Conference for Cardiac Transplantation (49) listed the indications for heart transplantation shown in Table 9.3. A low peak $\dot{V}O_2$ was the primary criterion provided that anaerobic metabolism (i.e., exercise above the *AT*) when the peak $\dot{V}O_2$ is reached.

Because peak $\dot{V}O_2$ might be underestimated due to reduced patient effort as well as by premature

TABLE 9.3. Bethesda Conference: Indications for Heart Transplantation

I. Accepted Indications for Transplantation
  1. Maximal $\dot{V}O_2$ less than 10 ml/kg per minute with achievement of anaerobic metabolism
  2. Severe ischemia consistently limiting routine activity not amenable to bypass surgery or angioplasty
  3. Recurrent symptomatic ventricular arrhythmias refractory to all accepted therapeutic modalities
II. Probable Indications for Cardiac Transplantation
  1. Maximal $\dot{V}O_2$ less than 14 ml/kg per minute and major limitation of the patient's daily activities
  2. Recurrent unstable ischemia not amenable to bypass surgery or angioplasty
  3. Instability of fluid balance and/or renal function not due to patient noncompliance with regimen of weight monitoring, flexible use of diuretic drugs, and salt restriction
III. Inadequate Indications for Transplantation
  1. Ejection fraction less than 20%
  2. History of functional class III or IV symptoms of heart failure
  3. Previous ventricular arrhythmias
  4. Maximal $\dot{V}O_2$ greater than 15 ml/kg per minute without other indications

From Mudge GH, Goldstein S, Addonizio LJ, et al. Task force 3: recipient guidelines/prioritization. *J Am Coll Cardiol* 1993;22:1–64, with permission.

termination of exercise by the examiner, Gitt et al. (3) studied the submaximal criteria of AT and $\dot{V}E$ versus $\dot{V}CO_2$ slope below the ventilatory compensation point (VCP) compared with peak $\dot{V}O_2$, normalized to both body weight and percent predicted, as measures of heart failure severity based on survival. The AT reflects a sustainable $\dot{V}O_2$ and is an objective parameter of cardiopulmonary exercise capacity. It can be derived from submaximal exercise testing and therefore does not require maximal patient effort. Another submaximal CPET measurement that has been shown to have prognostic value for survival is the $\dot{V}E$ versus $\dot{V}CO_2$ slope below the VCP (see Fig. 4.20) (5,6). Thus, Gitt et al. (3) compared the peak $\dot{V}O_2$ and the submaximal parameters as predictors of 6-month and 24-month patient survival rate in a cohort of 223 patients. Thresholds were peak $\dot{V}O_2$ of less than 14 ml/min/kg; AT of less than 11 ml/min/kg; and $\dot{V}E$ versus $\dot{V}CO_2$ slope below the VCP of more than 35 for high risk. They found that each of these parameters separates the high-risk from the low-risk patients (Fig. 9.10).

Figure 9.11 shows the odds ratio of early death if these parameters are in the high-risk range. The combination of AT and $\dot{V}E$ versus $\dot{V}CO_2$ below the VCP was found to be the best predictor of early death (within 6 months) in patients with left ventricular failure, using the threshold criteria selected

in this study. Because both AT and $\dot{V}E$ versus $\dot{V}CO_2$ below the VCP are determined at submaximal work levels and are not effort dependent, these are exceptionally valuable measurements.

Prognosis in Primary Pulmonary Hypertension and Prioritizing Patients for Lung Transplantation

In patients with primary pulmonary hypertension (PPH) who are unresponsive to pulmonary vasodilator therapy, lung transplantation is the only way of lowering the pulmonary vascular resistance. The decision to remove a patient's lung and replace it with a lung from a cadaver or a living donor is a critical decision. Importantly, it needs objective documentation that the medical pulmonary vasodilator therapy is not working and that the disease is so severe that the patient is at imminent risk of dying without this major surgical intervention (one that will subsequently require lifelong medical immunosuppressive therapy). Thus, reliable quantitative evaluation of the ability to increase pulmonary blood flow under exercise stress is essential. Wensel et al. (13) reported that reduced peak $\dot{V}O_2$ was a prognosticator of early death from pulmonary arterial hypertension. But exercise test parameters that monitor the specific pathophysiology of PPH have not been evaluated as prognostic indicators.

Sun et al. (12) studied the exercise pathophysiology in a cohort of 64 patients with PPH and showed that peak O_2 uptake decreases in proportion to worsening NYHA symptom class. However, symptoms are too variable with respect to function to be relied upon for making the decision to resort to lung transplantation. The physiological measurements, such as peak $\dot{V}O_2$, which is proportional to the peak pulmonary blood flow; the AT, which reflects the maximum sustainable O_2 uptake; the O_2 pulse, which is equal to the stroke volume $\times$ C(a $-$ $\bar{v}$)O_2; the $\Delta\dot{V}O_2/\Delta WR$, which reveals the ability to increase pulmonary blood flow with increasing work rate; and the $\dot{V}E/\dot{V}CO_2$ at the AT, which provides an index of the degree of $\dot{V}A/\dot{Q}$ mismatch, were all highly significantly correlated with symptoms.

Despite the existence of these excellent noninvasive descriptors of the abnormalities found in pulmonary hypertension, they have not been systematically used to prognosticate survival or select patients for lung transplantation. However, we have found that those patients with PPH with the shortest survival tend to have the lowest peak $\dot{V}O_2$, AT, and P_{ETCO_2} at the AT and the highest $\dot{V}E/\dot{V}CO_2$

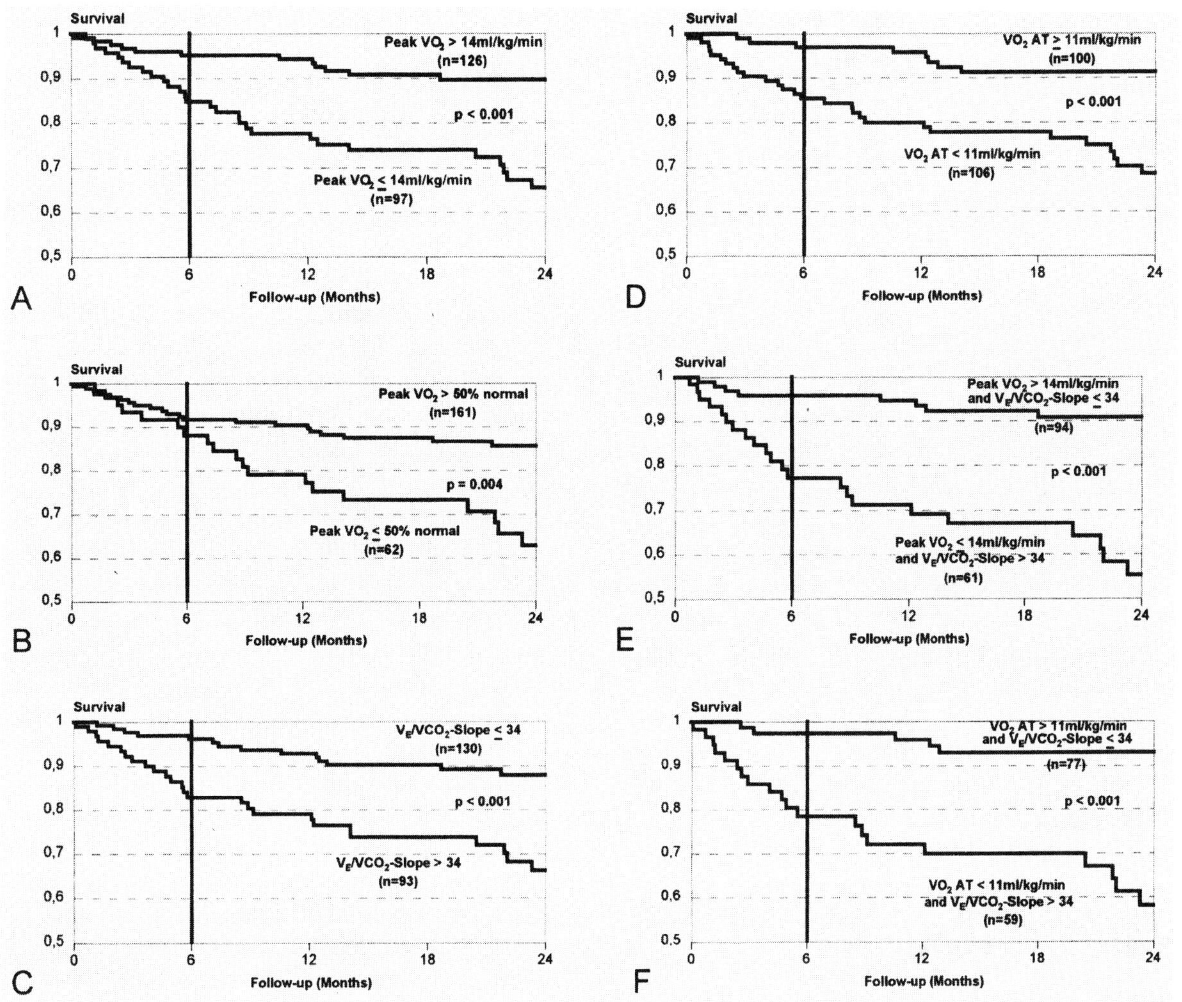

FIGURE 9.10. Kaplan–Meier survival curves using peak $\dot{V}O_2 \le 14$ **(A)**, peak $\dot{V}O_2 < 50\%$ predicted normal **(B)**, $\dot{V}E$ versus $\dot{V}CO_2$ slope > 34 **(C)**, $\dot{V}O_2$ @ AT < 11 mL/kg per minute **(D)**, the combination of peak $\dot{V}O_2 \le 14$ and $\dot{V}E$ versus $\dot{V}CO_2$ slope > 34 **(E)**, as well as $\dot{V}O_2$ @ AT < 11 and $\dot{V}E$ versus $\dot{V}CO_2$ slope > 34 **(F)** as cutoff points. Significant differences in survival were found at 6 months after the initial evaluation in A, C, D, E, and F. (From Gitt AK, Wasserman K, Kilkowski C, et al. Exercise anaerobic threshold and ventilatory efficiency identify heart failure patients for high risk of early death. *Circulation* 2002;106: 3079–3084, with permission.)

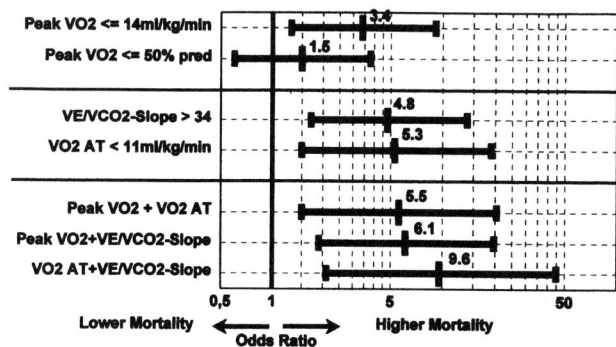

FIGURE 9.11. Cardiopulmonary predictors of early death within 6 months: univariate analysis. Numbers are odd ratios. Bars are 95% confidence interval. (From Gitt AK, Wasserman K, Kilkowski C, et al. Exercise anaerobic threshold and ventilatory efficiency identify heart failure patients for high risk of early death. *Circulation* 2002;106: 3079–3084, with permission.)

at the AT. From this experience and that of Wensel et al., we believe that objective physiological measurements should be used to decide if and when the lung should be transplanted in patients with primary pulmonary hypertension.

Prognosis in Chronic Obstructive Pulmonary Disease and Prioritizing Emphysema Patients for Lung Reduction Surgery

Oga et al. (50) analyzed the relations among exercise capacity, health status, and mortality rate in 150 male patients with stable COPD with a mean post-bronchodilator FEV_1 of 47.4% of predicted. Each patient was studied with pulmonary function testing, progressive cycle ergometry exercise testing with gas exchange, and health status questionnaires (51) at entry into the study. In a 5-year follow-up, 31 had died. Multivariate Cox proportional hazards analysis revealed that the peak oxygen uptake was predictive of mortality independent of FEV_1 and age. Stepwise Cox proportional hazards analysis revealed that the peak oxygen uptake was the most significant predictor of early mortality. Hiraga et al. (52) also studied the relation between physiological parameters (derived from CPET) and prognosis in terms of survival time over a 3- to 5-year period in 120 COPD patients, with similar findings to Oga et al. (50).

The recently concluded National Emphysema Treatment Trial in the United States (53), the focus of which was treatment with pulmonary rehabilitation alone or with rehabilitation and lung reduction surgery, revealed that the only patient group that benefited from the surgery was the group with upper lung field emphysema and reduced exercise tolerance (40 W or less at peak). If the patient did not have reduced exercise tolerance, regardless of the distribution of the emphysema, surgical resection did not improve the prognosis or exercise tolerance of the patient.

PREOPERATIVE EVALUATION OF SURGICAL RISK

Evaluation of perioperative risk has been a topic of considerable interest for application of CPET. Similar demands on the heart, lungs, and the peripheral circulation to support an increased metabolic rate such as that during exercise would likely take place perioperatively. A patient's capacity to increase oxygen delivery during exercise may correlate with capacity to maintain organ system function after surgery. Exercise testing, especially determination of peak $\dot{V}O_2$ and $\dot{V}O_2$ at the anaerobic threshold, might prove useful in identifying high-risk surgical patients, including those judged to have normal cardiopulmonary function by clinical assessments and measurements made at rest. CPET might prove particularly useful in the elderly, those with heart or lung disease that is unsuspected, and those with marginal organ system function.

Thoracic Surgery

Patients being considered for thoracotomy, usually for resection of lung cancer, are at particular risk of postoperative complications. Cardiopulmonary exercise testing has been suggested as a valuable ad-

junct because spirometry, radionuclide scanning, and arterial blood gases have not been completely successful in identifying all high-risk patients and, most important, may miss patients with significant cardiovascular disease (54–60). In addition, because resectional surgery remains the most effective therapy for lung cancer, exercise testing may identify patients who are likely to tolerate resection even though their poor resting lung function would otherwise preclude surgery.

Smith et al. (61) retrospectively reported 22 patients who underwent elective thoracotomy and found 11 who had postoperative respiratory failure, myocardial infarction, arrhythmias, lobar atelectasis, pulmonary embolism, or death. These 11 patients had a significantly lower mean peak $\dot{V}O_2$ than those without complications after surgery; if patients who had a peak $\dot{V}O_2$ during cycle exercise of less than 20 ml/kg/min had not been offered surgery, 91% of patients with complications would have been eliminated. In this study, 6 of 6 patients who had a peak $\dot{V}O_2$ of less than 15 ml/min/kg and 4 of 6 patients who had a peak $\dot{V}O_2$ of 15 to 20 ml/min/kg had complications. Similarly, a peak $\dot{V}O_2$ of less than 10 ml/kg/min identified the 2 patients who died and the majority of postoperative complications among 50 patients reported by Bechard and Wetstein (62).

Bolliger and co-workers (63) found that peak $\dot{V}O_2$, expressed as percent predicted during cycle ergometry, was predictive of postresection complications such as CO_2 retention, prolonged mechanical ventilation, myocardial infarction, pneumonia, pulmonary embolism, and death. In a group of 80 patients, 8 of 9 patients with peak $\dot{V}O_2$ of less than 60% predicted had complications, whereas only 8 of the remaining 71 patients had complications. When patients had a maximum $\dot{V}O_2$ of greater than 75% of predicted, 90% were complication free. The same group (64) found that a peak $\dot{V}O_2$ of less than 10 ml/kg/min was associated with 100% mortality. Patients with complications had a lower mean peak $\dot{V}O_2$ (10.6 ± 3.6 ml/kg/min vs. 14.8 ± 3.5 ml/kg/min).

A prospective study by Morice and co-workers (65) provided additional evidence for the value of exercise testing in "high-risk" patients undergoing thoracotomy. Thirty-seven patients had been considered inoperable because of a low FEV_1 (<40% predicted), an anticipated postsurgical FEV_1 of less than 33% predicted, an abnormal radionuclide scan, or an arterial PCO_2 of more than 45 mm Hg. Thirteen patients who underwent exercise testing had a maximum $\dot{V}O_2$ greater than 15 ml/kg/min. Eight of these patients subsequently had resectional surgery. Although mean FEV_1 was poor in this group (mean 40% of predicted), six of eight patients had an uncomplicated course, and all patients were discharged within 22 days of surgery. This study suggests that even some "high-risk" patients, based on resting lung function, can be more objectively assessed with data from exercise testing.

Abdominal Surgery

Older et al. (66) found, in a retrospective study of elderly patients undergoing major abdominal surgeries, that the *AT* obtained during CPET was particularly valuable in identifying postoperative complications. In 187 patients aged over 60 years, mean $\dot{V}O_2$ at the *AT* averaged 12.4 ± 2.7 ml/min/kg. If the *AT* was less than 11 ml/min/kg (found in 30% of the study patients), mortality from cardiovascular complications was 18%. On the other hand, if the *AT* was greater than 11 ml/min/kg, the cardiovascular death rate in the postoperative period was only 0.8%. Of interest, those patients who manifested evidence of myocardial ischemia in addition to having an *AT* of less than 11 ml/min/kg had a 42% mortality rate.

In a later prospective study of 548 patients over 60 years of age (or younger, if the patient was known to have ischemic heart disease), Older et al. (67) used the *AT* determined during CPET to separate high from low risk for mortality following major surgery. Based on their earlier retrospective study, they used an *AT* of 11 ml/min/kg as the threshold for separating high from low risk. Patients were triaged to the ward for routine care if their *AT* was greater than 11 ml/min/kg, they had no ECG evidence of myocardial ischemia, and their $\dot{V}E/\dot{V}O_2$ at the *AT* was less than 35. This represented 51% of the total population studied. None of these patients died of cardiovascular causes. Twenty-one percent (115 patients) of the population studied had an *AT* greater than 11/ml/min/kg, but also had either ECG evidence of myocardial ischemia or a $\dot{V}E/\dot{V}O_2$ at the *AT* of more than 35, a change found with heart failure. They were admitted to the intermediate care unit. Of this population, 1.7 % (2 patients) died of cardiovascular causes. The remaining 28% (153 patients) of the starting population were identified as high risk based on an *AT* of less than 11 ml/min/kg or aortic or esophageal surgery. These were triaged to the intensive care unit and had a 4.6 % cardiovascular system mortality. Thus, use of CPET to determine the high-risk patient for major surgery proved quite successful, allowing the services to use their high-care units for those people who were most ill and admitting patients at low risk, as assessed by CPET, to the ward.

Who Should Undergo Cardiopulmonary Exercise Testing Preoperatively?

Several questions remain about the use of CPET in preoperative evaluation. First, who are the most suitable candidates? It is unlikely that all patients need to be tested, but patients with suspected cardiopulmonary disease (especially cardiac disease) may be confirmed with testing. It does appear important to offer exercise testing to older patients and those with marginal lung or cardiac function who would otherwise be excluded from major thoracic or abdominal surgery as being at too high a risk for surgical complications. Good exercise capacity may translate into surprisingly low postoperative risk.

Second, there is the question about the type of exercise testing to be performed for preoperative evaluation. Measurements of peak $\dot{V}O_2$ and $\dot{V}O_2$ at the *AT* provide objective data that can be used to identify high- and low-risk populations. But how useful is CPET in comparison with more simple tests with less sophisticated measurements, such as stair-climbing or timed walking tests (68,69)?

Third, there is further need to focus on postoperative complications relating to specific types of surgery and on CPET that reveals the most limiting organ system. Results of exercise testing in patients have been largely used in those undergoing thoracic (lung) and abdominal surgery. The value of exercise testing for predicting complications of other forms of surgery, such as heart or vascular surgery or orthopedic procedures, has not been determined. Finally, there is a need for more evidence that improvement in pre-operative exercise capacity by smoking cessation, medical therapy, exercise training, or other interventions can reduce postoperative risks.

MEASURING IMPAIRMENT FOR DISABILITY EVALUATION

Exercise testing has an important role in impairment and disability evaluation. Sometimes, the focus is on establishing causation of disease from a substance encountered in the workplace; in other cases, the process is to determine the degree of impairment.

Impairment and Disability

Impairment, as used in the United States, is a measurable, objective decrease in functional capacity. *Disability* is an assessment of the impact of impairment on the individual and requires socioeconomic and environmental input, including factors such as age, gender, education, economic and social environment, and energy requirements of the occupation (70). A World Health Organization statement (71) defined impairment as "any loss or abnormality of psychological, physiological, or anatomical structure or function," while disability was defined as "any restriction or lack (resulting from impairment) of ability to perform an activity within the range considered normal for a human being." Physicians are asked to identify and measure impairment, but, although opinions are often sought about a patient's disability, such decisions are usually made through an administrative or legal process. Exercise testing permits objective measurement of physiological function, thereby determining impairment, not disability.

Cardiopulmonary exercise testing is indicated when a precise measurement of work capacity (work rate, peak $\dot{V}O_2$, or the anaerobic threshold) is required, often when symptoms or subjective exercise capacity are inconsistent with resting measurements. The greatest potential advantages may be in evaluating those with disease (heart disease, peripheral arterial disease, etc.) coexisting with lung disease, or those with potentially confounding risk factors such as increased blood carboxyhemoglobin from cigarette smoking or $\dot{V}A/\dot{Q}$ abnormality in whom ventilatory drive is exceptionally high. Thus, mild to moderate defects in ventilatory mechanics might be sufficient to create dyspnea during exercise. In some patients, exercise capacity may be limited by a mechanism other than impairment in ventilatory mechanics detected by resting pulmonary function testing. In others, the sensitivity of exercise-related abnormalities of arterial blood gases, alveolar–arterial PO_2 difference, or dead space–tidal volume ratio may be useful in identifying subtle evidence of respiratory disease as a cause of exercise limitation.

Problems in Assessing Impairment from Only Resting Measures

In 1986, the American Thoracic Society statement on evaluation of impairment and disability sec-

ondary to respiratory disorders recommended a systematic evaluation process (70). The statement was "concerned primarily with impairments related to reduced lung function," and presented a rating system for impairment from lung disease based on forced vital capacity (FVC), forced expiratory volume in 1 second (FEV_1), FEV_1/FVC, and single-breath diffusing capacity for carbon monoxide ($DLCO$). It also implied that there was a well-documented relation between measurements made at rest (e.g., FEV_1 and $DLCO$) and measurements made during exercise (maximum $\dot{V}O_2$ and work capacity). The authors concluded that the majority of subjects undergoing an evaluation for impairment would not require exercise testing.

This conclusion can be challenged, however, by considering whether maximum work capacity can be predicted from resting pulmonary function. In this analysis, begin by assuming that a subject's FEV_1 = 1.5 L. If FEV_1 is used to predict maximum exercise minute ventilation ($\dot{V}E$) by using two reported estimates ($FEV_1 \times 35$ and $FEV_1 \times 40$) (72,73), the maximum $\dot{V}E$ values would range from 52.5 L/min to 60 L/min. Next, assume that dead space–tidal volume ratio (VD/VT) at maximum exercise ranges from a low of 0.15 in a normal subject to 0.40 in someone with moderate ventilation–perfusion mismatching from lung disease. Using this range, the estimated maximum alveolar ventilation [$\dot{V}A = \dot{V}E \times (1 - VD/VT)$] would range from 31.5 to 51 L/min for the maximum $\dot{V}E$ values calculated from the FEV_1 values above. Then, assuming that $PaCO_2$ (PCO_2 set point) is between 25 to 35 mm Hg (not unusual numbers), one could estimate the extremes of $\dot{V}CO_2$ that could be present by the following equation:

$$\dot{V}CO_2 \text{ L/min (STPD)} = PaCO_2 \times \dot{V}A \text{ L/min (BTPS)}/863$$

The estimated $\dot{V}CO_2$, using these example figures, ranges from 0.91 to 2.10 L/min.

Finally, what is the relationship between $\dot{V}CO_2$ and $\dot{V}O_2$? $\dot{V}O_2 = \dot{V}CO_2/R$, and R at maximum exercise ranges from 0.9 to 1.2. Therefore, our hypothetical subject's maximum $\dot{V}O_2$ might be as low as 0.76 L/min or as high as 2.33 L/min for the same FEV_1.

In conclusion, although the *ventilatory capacity* of the respiratory system for ventilation may be successfully predicted from resting FEV_1 (and this, too, is open to question), the *ventilatory requirement* for a given level of work cannot be predicted from the resting pulmonary function measurements.

Exercise Testing and Impairment Evaluation

A number of investigators have emphasized the usefulness of integrative CPET for determination of impairment (74–84). Exercise testing complements clinical evaluation and adds to resting pulmonary function and roentgenographic studies. It increases diagnostic accuracy both quantitatively (measurement of work capacity, peak $\dot{V}O_2$, and sustained work capacity) and qualitatively (identification of the cause of exercise limitation).

For example, during an approximately 3-year period, we had the opportunity to see 490 current or retired shipyard workers (79). Of this population, 348 men who had complaints of exercise limitation or who were suspected of having exercise limitation were studied using 1-minute incremental cycle ergometry exercise with gas exchange measurements. A conclusion was made by the physician referring the patient for exercise studies as to the likelihood of exercise limitation, if any, and the specific organ system limiting exercise. This determination was based on chest roentgenograms, resting pulmonary function tests, resting ECG, medical history, physical examination, and smoking history (Fig. 9.12), but not CPET. Following CPET, another conclusion was made, but this time using all data acquired during the evaluation, including the exercise test (Fig. 9.12).

On the initial assessment, 148 subjects were predicted to have normal work capacity, but 46 of these subjects (31%) turned out to have a peak $\dot{V}O_2$ below the 95% confidence limit. The accuracy of the clinical prediction of a low work capacity was similar: 66 subjects were expected to have low work capacity; of these, only 43 (67%) were correctly categorized. Furthermore, the referring physicians could not judge whether the work capacity was normal or reduced in 134 subjects (38.5% of the total to be evaluated) without CPET.

Following CPET, 60% of the indeterminate group were found to have a normal peak $\dot{V}O_2$, while 37% had an abnormally low peak $\dot{V}O_2$. Although the magnitude of reduction of peak $\dot{V}O_2$ had a significant correlation with resting pulmonary function (VC, FEV_1, DLCO as percent predicted), prediction of reduced work capacity from resting pulmonary function was often unhelpful. Overall, 138 workers had abnormally low peak $\dot{V}O_2$. Of these, 43 were correctly predicted to be impaired without CPET, while a further 46 were incorrectly predicted to be

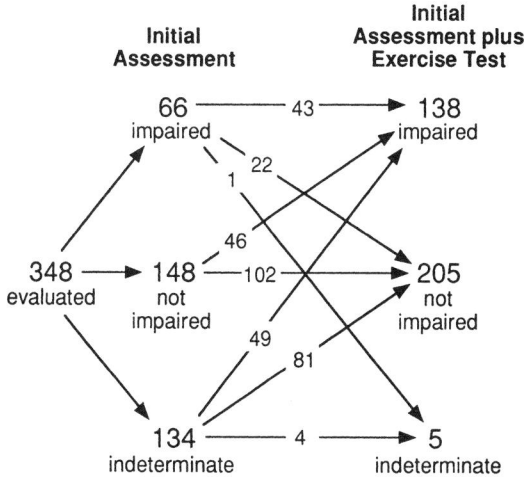

FIGURE 9.12.   The influence of cardiopulmonary exercise testing on the evaluation of work impairment; 348 patients were initially referred for suspicion of functional impairment secondary to asbestos exposure. The initial assessment was done without exercise testing but with all other clinical modalities available to the evaluating physician. This assessment concluded that 66 were impaired, but no decision could be reached on 134 of the 348 patients being evaluated. In the final assessment, cardiopulmonary exercise data were added to the information available to the physician rendering the interpretation. This new information confirmed (cardiopulmonary exercise testing taken as the gold standard) impairment in 43 of the 66, with 22 going into the "not impaired" category and 1 into the indeterminate category. In contrast, 95 subjects were added to the impaired category: 46 from the "not impaired" category and 49 from the indeterminate category; 102 of the 148 subjects thought to be not impaired were confirmed as being not impaired. However, 81 were added to this category from the indeterminate category and 22 from the impaired category, making a total of 205 subjects for whom it was thought that there was no basis on which to conclude that the patient had a physiological impairment in the ability to perform physical work. Only 4 of the 130 subjects whose impairment was uncertain before cardiopulmonary exercise testing remained in this category after the cardiopulmonary exercise test.

normal without CPET, and 49 who had impairment by CPET were indeterminate without it (Fig. 9.12). The sensitivity of resting pulmonary function tests, chest roentgenograms, and other studies for detecting low peak $\dot{V}O_2$ was only about 31%.

The cause of exercise limitation may not be reflected in resting studies, largely because the most often used resting data are the tests of pulmonary function. Among our 138 subjects with low peak $\dot{V}O_2$, only 25 were limited by obstructive or restrictive lung diseases, whereas in 95 (69%) of 138 cases, the exercise limitation was due to cardiovascular diseases (Table 9.4). The presence of a high proportion of cardiovascular disease in this patient population is not unique; Agostoni et al. (75) also found that 37% of 120 asbestos workers had unex-

TABLE 9.4.   Diagnostic Causes (%) of Reduced Work Capacity in 138 Workers with Impairment

69% cardiovascular
   41% cardiac
   28% peripheral arterial or other
14% airway obstruction
   4% restrictive lung disease
11% neurologic or musculoskeletal
2% obesity

Impairment is defined as peak $\dot{V}o_2$ below the 95% confidence limit of predicted.

pected cardiac limitation rather than ventilatory limitation.

Oxygen Cost of Work

In approximate terms, the oxygen cost ($\dot{V}o_2$) for office work might be about 5 to 7 ml/kg/min, for moderate labor about 15 ml/kg/min, and for strenuous labor 20 to 30 ml/kg/min. Some guidelines suggest, in addition, that workers can perform manual labor at a comfortable "work pace" when this was approximately 40% of predicted peak $\dot{V}o_2$, a value interestingly approximating the lactic acidosis threshold in sedentary normal subjects.

Having obtained measurements of peak $\dot{V}o_2$ and the $\dot{V}o_2$ at the *AT*, it might be tempting to relate these to the oxygen cost of specific work tasks. A number of sources of information about specific O_2 costs of various physical activities, occupations, and specific kinds of movements exist, but these are estimates (see Appendix E). These values should be used with caution. For given individuals who differ in age, weight, gender, rate of work, efficiency of movement, or degree of intermittency of the work task, the true metabolic cost of work ($\dot{V}o_2$) may vary greatly. For this reason, we recommend that broad estimates of metabolic cost of exercise be used rather than trying to make precise estimates for very specific tasks.

EXERCISE REHABILITATION

Physiological Basis of Exercise Rehabilitation

Endurance exercise training is commonly used to improve exercise tolerance and quality of life. It has proved useful in healthy subjects (e.g., athletes) and in a number of patient groups. It is widely conceded that an exercise-training regimen is the most beneficial portion of rehabilitation programs. CPET is uniquely suited to gauge the specific benefits of exercise training. In addition, CPET serves to rule out coexisting disease processes that could contraindicate a rigorous exercise program. CPET also helps one to understand the physiological changes induced by exercise training in patients and normal subjects.

The benefits of exercise training may include (a) increasing muscle mass and mitochondrial number; (b) improving the distribution of blood and therefore O_2 flow to the contracting muscle, thereby reducing the cardiac (heart rate) stress; (c) reducing lactic acid production, resulting in a reduction in CO_2 and H^+ production, thereby reducing ventilatory drive at a given work rate; and (d) improving the patient's sense of well-being. The general physiological changes in response to training are discussed in the following sections.

Skeletal Muscle

Skeletal muscles are composed of two major varieties of contractile cells (85). One type of fiber seems designed for prolonged repetitive contraction. These fibers are known as *type I, oxidative,* or *slow-twitch* fibers. The other fiber type has rapid contractile properties but has a limited capacity for prolonged repetitive contraction; these fibers are known as *type II, glycolytic,* or *fast-twitch* fibers. The relative proportion of these two fiber types varies from muscle group to muscle group.

After an effective program of training, subpopulations of type II fibers remodel. Type IIb fibers, which have a very low capacity for oxidative metabolism, remodel into type IIa fibers (86), which have a high oxidative potential—in some ways similar to type I fibers. Type I fibers undergo extensive biochemical and structural modification (85). In these fibers, the mitochondrial number and size increase. The concentrations of a number of enzymes in both the cytosol and the mitochondria increase (87). These enzymatic changes facilitate the Krebs cycle reactions and oxidative phosphorylation so that the capacity to oxidatively metabolize the end product of glycolysis (pyruvate) and fatty acids and ketone bodies is increased (85). In parallel with the increased ability to utilize oxygen, the ability to supply oxygen by improved blood flow to the muscle cells increases. Myoglobin levels in the trained muscle are higher (88); this may contribute to the ability to transport oxygen from the muscle capillary to the site of metabolism. More important, muscle capillaries proliferate (89). The number of capillaries increases out of proportion to the increase in muscle fiber size, so that more capillaries surround a given muscle fiber. Consequent decreases in the diffusion distance from the oxygen source (hemoglobin in the muscle capillary) to the oxygen sink (the mitochondrion in the muscle cell) allow a given level of oxygen consumption to be sustained at a lower capillary P_{O_2}.

These structural and biochemical changes are seen only in the muscle groups involved in the training regimen (90); this is known as the *principle of specificity* (91). For example, walking or running does not induce such changes in the arm muscles. Training on a stationary bicycle will not fully translate into improvements in running performance, because a somewhat different group of muscles is involved.

Changes in organ systems other than the exercising muscles also occur. The cardiovascular system undergoes significant changes as a result of exercise training (91–93). The heart hypertrophies, with increases in both ventricular wall thickness and chamber size. Body composition usually changes as a result of an effective program of endurance training (94,95). Muscle size increases and is reflected by an increase in lean body mass. Body fat often decreases more than muscle mass increases, so that body weight falls (although changes in body weight vary).

Cardiac Output and Heart Rate

After an effective program of training in normal subjects, cardiac output at peak exercise is increased, although cardiac output at rest and at a given work rate is not appreciably altered. However, stroke volume is higher at rest, at any given work rate, and at peak exercise. Consequently, heart rate at rest and at a given level of exercise is distinctly lower after exercise training, although peak heart rate is unchanged. Both systolic and diastolic blood pressure tend to be lower after training, especially in the hypertensive subject. Training tends not to increase cardiac output in patients with heart disease. However, heart rate is reduced at a given work rate after training, presumably due to better blood flow distribution to the working muscles and perhaps improved capillarization of muscle fibers, allowing an increase in O_2 extraction.

Blood Lactate

After an effective program of endurance training, the remodeling of the exercising muscles yields both improved oxygen delivery to the mitochondria

and improved mitochondrial capability for aerobic metabolism. As a result, the onset of anaerobic metabolism is delayed. At any given work rate above the pretraining anaerobic threshold, blood lactate levels are lower after exercise training (96,97) (Fig. 9.13). Sullivan et al. (98) demonstrated that knowledge of peak $\dot{V}_{O_2}$ and *AT* allowed good prediction of an individual's blood lactate level in response to a given level of constant work rate exercise.

Oxygen Uptake

Endurance training increases maximal $\dot{V}_{O_2}$, both because arteriovenous O_2 content difference widens and maximal cardiac output increases (95). In healthy subjects, improvements on the order of 8% to 15% are commonly seen. During incremental exercise tests at below-*AT* work rates, $\dot{V}_{O_2}$ is not altered by training. For above-*AT* work rates, there is a tendency for $\dot{V}_{O_2}$ to decrease at a given work rate after training, although in most cases the differences are difficult to appreciate (the overall $\Delta\dot{V}_{O_2}$/

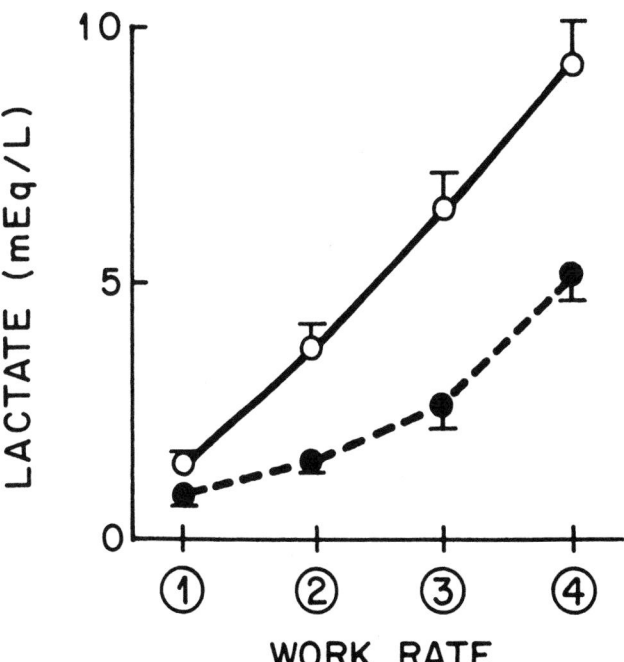

FIGURE 9.13. Effect of endurance training on end-exercise blood lactate levels at four work rates. Values plotted are the average (± standard error) responses of ten subjects before (*solid line*) and after (*dashed line*) endurance training. Subjects exercised for 15 minutes at work rates ranging from moderate (work rate 1) to very heavy intensity (work rate 4). After training, blood lactate levels are lower in response to identical exercise tasks. (From Casaburi R, Storer TW, Ben-Dov I, et al. Effect of endurance training on possible determinants of $\dot{V}_{O_2}$ during heavy exercise. *J Appl Physiol* 1987;62:199–207, with permission.)

ΔWR slope remains approximately 10 ml/min/watt).

Effective exercise training increases phase II $\dot{V}O_2$ kinetics and reduces the size of the slow (phase III) rise in $\dot{V}O_2$ in response to heavy constant work rate exercise. The decrease in the size of the phase III response is in close proportion to the decrease in blood lactate elicited by training (96). Despite this close correlation, the mechanism of the decreased oxygen requirement remains controversial (99).

Ventilation

In both the steady state and during exercise transients, $\dot{V}E$ responds in close proportion to CO_2 output (100). After training, at a given work rate, $\dot{V}E$ is lower in proportion to the decrease in CO_2 output, the latter primarily due to the reduced HCO_3^- buffering of lactic acid. Moreover, because lactic acid production is lower, the hydrogen ion stimulation of the carotid bodies is reduced, resulting in less hyperventilation at a given heavy work rate (97). This means that arterial PCO_2 is higher at a given heavy work rate, above the AT. Figure 9.14 shows the responses to 15 minutes of exercise at four progressively higher work rates before and after a program of endurance training. At higher (above-AT) work rates, there is a dramatically lower ventilatory response to exercise.

Other Physiological Responses

Blood catecholamine responses to a given level of heavy exercise are often dramatically lower after training (101), although the fractional reduction varies appreciably among subjects (96). Other hormonal responses are reduced as well (101,102). The body temperature increase that occurs with exercise is attenuated (96,103). Finally, ratings of perceived exertion for a given work rate are generally reduced (104). Whether this reduction is predominantly linked to improved physiological function or to psychological factors is unclear (105).

Exercise Rehabilitation in Heart Disease

The objective of exercise training is to improve exercise tolerance and quality of life. Because patients with heart disease become physically inactive as a result of reduced ability to deliver blood to the muscles of locomotion, the skeletal muscles undergo change similar to that of detraining. The American Heart Association Committee on Exercise, Rehabilitation, and Prevention (106) wrote a comprehensive statement on the role of exercise in chronic heart failure (HF). The role of exercise training in HF was particularly emphasized. In contrast to the practice up until about 20 years ago,

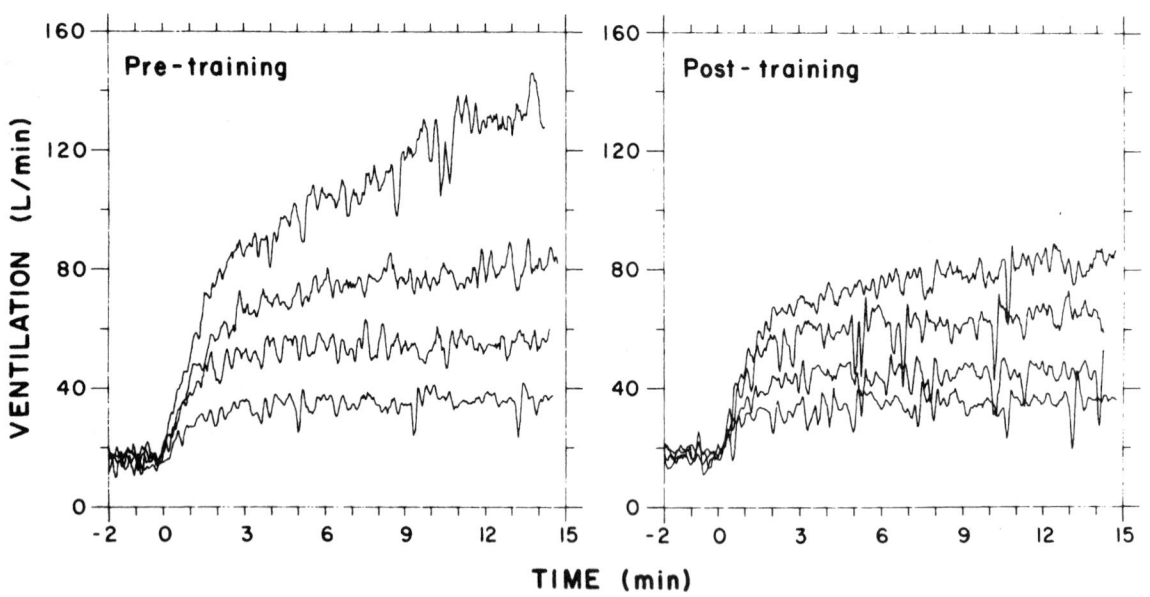

FIGURE 9.14.   Effect of endurance training on the breath-by-breath time course of ventilation following the onset of constant work rate exercise in a healthy subject. **Left:** Pretraining responses to 95, 148, 191, and 233 watts. **Right:** Post-training responses to identical work rates after 8 weeks of endurance training. Note the dramatic decrease in ventilation at the higher work rates after training. (From Casaburi R, Storer TW, Ben-Dov I, et al. Effect of endurance training on possible determinants of $\dot{V}O_2$ during heavy exercise. *J Appl Physiol* 1987;62:199–207, with permission.)

when patients with HF were put to bed to rest their hearts, patients with heart failure are now put on exercise training programs. The statement summarizes many studies showing the benefits of exercise training, in which exercise tolerance and peak $\dot{V}O_2$ are increased, the latter by 12% to 31%, depending on the study. The training effect was correlated with the duration of the program. No significant exercise-related complications were reported. Despite the consistent increase in peak $\dot{V}O_2$ and exercise tolerance with training found in HF patients, no consistent changes are demonstrable with echocardiography.

Although it has not been demonstrated that catecholamines consistently decrease with exercise training in patients with HF, Casaburi et al. (96) demonstrated striking reductions in catecholamines in the pretraining above-AT range of work in normal subjects after training. As in normal subjects (Fig. 9.13), exercise training reduces the lactate response to exercise and its accompanying H^+. Consequently, ventilatory drive is decreased in patients with HF in response to exercise training (107), as seen in normal subjects (Fig. 9.14) (97). However, in contrast to the predominant mechanism for the decrease in $\dot{V}E$ with training in normal subjects, which is attributable to the decrease in lactic acid production, some of the decrease in $\dot{V}E$ in HF might be attributed to a decrease in VD/VT, which can be markedly elevated. Some investigators also attribute the decrease in $\dot{V}E$ to attenuation of an abnormally stimulated ergoreflex originating in skeletal muscle (108).

Exercise training results in a decrease in heart rate in response to a given exercise O_2 uptake. Some of this reduction in heart rate might be due to an increase in stroke volume, as reported in some studies, but most is thought to be due to peripheral changes and better perfusion and extraction of O_2 by the muscles involved in the exercise. When cardiac function and ability to increase cardiac output improve, the changes in muscle that came about due to inactivity might be reversed. Thus, exercise limitation because of muscle atrophy might be rectified with exercise training.

With that logic in mind, Itoh and Kato (109) studied the effect of short-term training after cardiac surgery for valvular heart disease and coronary artery bypass graft surgery. As their training work rate, they used the anaerobic threshold rather than the level of exercise training recommended by the American College of Sports Medicine (110), which is 40% to 85% of the above-rest predicted maxi-

mum heart rate. They found the latter impractical because of the range of heart rate recommended and also because most of the patients with coronary artery bypass graft surgery received β-adrenoreceptor blockade therapy, which limits the heart rate increase. Using peak $\dot{V}O_2$, AT, $\Delta\dot{V}O_2/\Delta WR$, and the time constant for the $\dot{V}O_2$ in response to constant work rate exercise as outcome measures, they found significant improvement in aerobic function in the group of postsurgery patients who underwent exercise training, but did not find improvement in the control group of postsurgical patients who did not undergo exercise training.

Itoh and Kato (109) selected the work rate at the subject's anaerobic threshold because they regarded it as a safe, yet effective work level for exercise training. They reasoned that at the AT, patients are able to supply the O_2 required to perform work because they do not endure a significant lactic acidosis and therefore the heart is not "overstressed." The sympathetic nervous system is not excessively stimulated at this work level, as evidenced by the minor changes in norepinephrine and epinephrine that take place at the AT (see Chapter 2). Also, patients find this training program acceptable because they are able to maintain exercise at the AT over a prolonged period of time.

Using similar logic to Itoh and Kato, Dubach et al. (111) examined the effect of a 2-month endurance exercise training program using a combination of walking and cycling training at a work rate comparable to that which would approximate the subject's anaerobic threshold. Training was started approximately 36 days after myocardial infarction. Myocardial injury, as evaluated by magnetic resonance imaging of the heart, was not extended by the training program. The trained patients increased peak $\dot{V}O_2$ and lactate threshold by 26% and 39%, respectively, whereas there was no detectable improvement in the nontrained control group.

Belardinelli et al. (112) studied the effect of exercise training on left ventricular diastolic filling in patients with dilated cardiomyopathy, using pulsed Doppler echocardiography. They found that exercise training increased the AT and peak $\dot{V}O_2$ in patients with dilated cardiomyopathy and associated impairment of left ventricular relaxation. The basis of the increase in cardiac function was an improvement in peak early filling of the left ventricle.

The key physiological effect of training in the heart disease patient is the reduction in heart rate, thereby allowing more time for blood to flow through the coronary blood vessels and more time for cardiac filling. Also, because of more aerobic and less anaerobic regeneration of *ATP* after training, the lactic acidosis is less severe at a given level of exercise. Thus, there is less ventilatory drive and therefore less breathing stress. Finally, of great importance is a greater sense of well-being in patients as they find that they are becoming physically stronger and more active.

Exercise Rehabilitation in Chronic Obstructive Pulmonary Disease

The National Emphysema Treatment Trial and other randomized trials support the concept that exercise training improves exercise tolerance and reduces dyspnea on exertion in patients with COPD undergoing rehabilitation (113). Cardiopulmonary exercise testing provides unequivocal evidence of the physiological benefits of training in these patients. Although most of the studies have been in patients with COPD, results of exercise programs in patients with cystic fibrosis (114) and asthma (115) have also been published.

Patients with COPD are usually ventilatory limited; that is, their exercise tolerance is limited by the level of ventilation that they can sustain. This occurs both because the level of ventilation that can be sustained is low and because the level of ventilation required for a given level of exercise is high (see Fig. 5.5). The low ventilatory ceiling is related to the impaired lung mechanics demonstrated by a functionally zero breathing reserve when ventilatory capacity is measured by the maximum voluntary ventilation maneuver or $FEV_1 \times 40$ (see Fig. 5.8). Although we can predict that respiratory muscle fatigue is induced by the high work of breathing resulting from high expiratory airway resistance and hyperinflation-induced mechanical disadvantage of the diaphragm and chest wall muscles (116), the evidence for this is not straightforward. The tidal volume usually does not get smaller and $\dot{V}E$ does not decrease as exercise is sustained. However, $PaCO_2$ commonly increases as exercise work rate increases, providing evidence that alveolar ventilation cannot keep pace with the CO_2 load (see Case 42, Chapter 10).

The high ventilatory requirement for a given level of exercise is dictated by inefficient gas exchange (high VD/VT), hypoxic stimulation of ventilation, and H^+ stimulation resulting from the production of CO_2 and lactate (117,118) (see Fig. 5.5).

In some patients, a low work rate lactic acidosis, as a result of detraining, is a contributory factor to the increased ventilatory drive. But the detraining does not reduce the ability of the muscles to extract and utilize O_2 from the blood. Maltais et al. (119) showed that the muscles of patients with COPD are capable of extracting O_2 normally, suggesting that a primary defect in muscle bioenergetics is not limiting exercise tolerance in these patients. Also, the studies of Richardson et al. (120) demonstrate that if the ventilatory and cardiac requirements of exercise are reduced by exercising only one leg at a time, the exercising leg can increase its work capacity as compared with when both legs perform the same form of exercise. These studies suggest that defects in the leg muscles do not limit exercise capacity in COPD.

Because patients with COPD are ventilatory limited, it is logical to turn our attention to modalities that can reduce the abnormal increases in ventilatory drive during exercise in these patients. For example, a low work rate onset of lactic acidosis, arte-

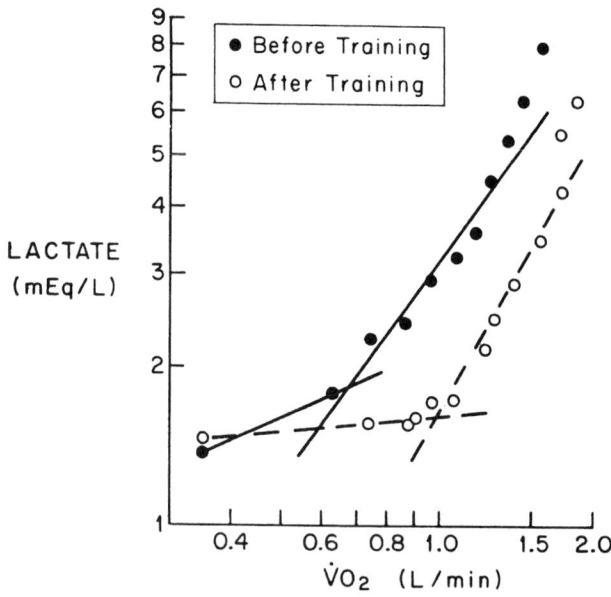

FIGURE 9.15. Blood lactate levels, before and after training, during increasing work rate exercise tests in a patient with chronic obstructive pulmonary disease undergoing rehabilitation. Arterial lactate is plotted versus oxygen uptake on a log-log scale. Closed circles are responses before training; open circles are responses after training. Before training, blood lactate rises very early in exercise. After training, blood lactate rise is delayed, and the lactate threshold (point of intersection of two line segments) occurs at a considerably higher $\dot{V}O_2$, indicating that a physiologic training response has occurred. (From Casaburi R, Patessio A, Ioli F, et al Reductions in exercise lactic acidosis and ventilation as a result of exercise training in patients with obstructive lung disease. *Am Rev Respir Dis* 1991;143:9–18, with permission.)

rial hypoxemia, and decreased oxygen delivery to the tissues, either due to increased pulmonary vascular resistance, decreased cardiac output due to the interference of lung mechanics on cardiac function (121), or inefficient muscle perfusion, all might result in a higher ventilatory requirement than normal. A portion of these abnormalities is likely related to severe deconditioning due to inactivity (118), but a myopathy related to corticosteroid use might also be a factor.

Although it was doubted in the past that COPD patients could gain physiological benefits from a program of exercise training (122), it is now generally accepted as a useful therapeutic modality. New strategies, chief among them the employment of exercise intensities that are a high percentage of peak exercise tolerance (123), have demonstrated that physiological benefits are achievable. Thus, it is possible to decrease the exercise lactic acidosis by exercise training (Fig. 9.15), thereby reducing CO_2 and H^+ production. Cardiopulmonary exercise testing shows that the increased exercise tolerance after a rigorous program of rehabilitative exercise training in COPD patients is associated with a decreased ventilatory requirement at a given level of exercise. In a group of patients with predominantly moderate COPD, training-induced reductions in ventilatory requirement were closely correlated with the reduction in blood lactate levels (Fig. 9.16) (124). In a group of patients with more severe disease, the reduction in ventilatory requirement was associated with the adoption of a more efficient (slower, deeper) breathing pattern (125).

Besides determining the degree (and mechanism) of improvement in exercise tolerance that occurs as a result of an exercise program, CPET has other well-defined uses in the context of pulmonary rehabilitation:

• The contraindications to an exercise training program can be defined.
• Exercise prescription guidelines for the patient can be developed.
• The mechanism(s) of exercise limitation can be clarified.

A further modality to increase exercise tolerance is to provide O_2 during exercise to the patient with COPD, even if there is no significant arterial hypoxemia (126). This maneuver might have four effects. First and most obvious, it inhibits the carotid bodies' responses to hypoxemia and H^+, thereby slowing breathing rate. Second, as a consequence of the slower breathing rate, it allows the COPD patient to have more expiratory time and thereby exhale to

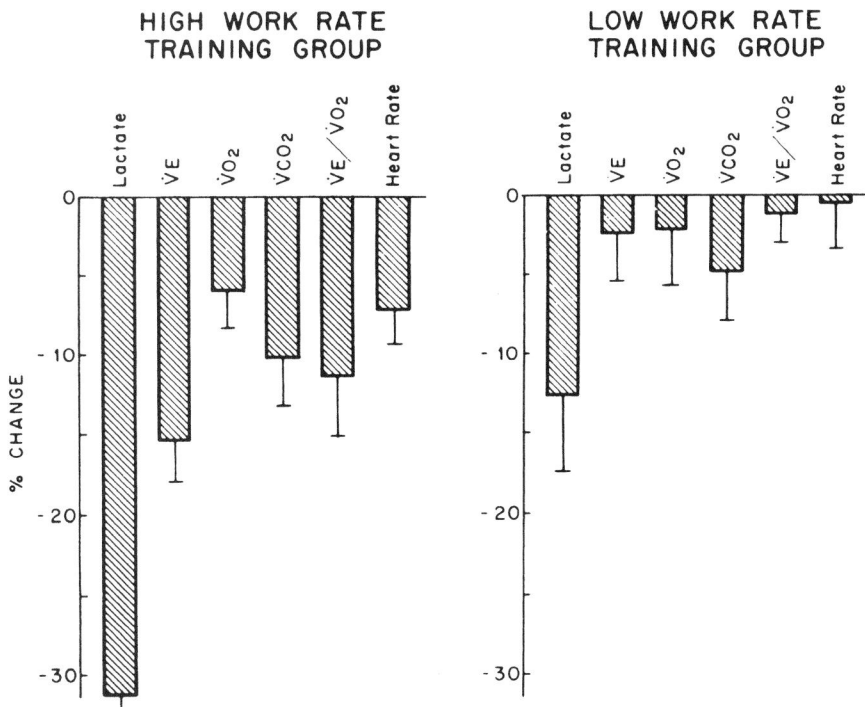

FIGURE 9.16. Changes in physiologic responses to an identical exercise task (high constant work rate test) produced by two exercise training strategies in patients with chronic obstructive pulmonary disease. **Left:** High work rate training group (n = 11). **Right:** Low work rate training group (n = 8). Note that patients performed the same total work in their training program irrespective of group assignment. Percent change is calculated from the average change in response at the time the pretraining study ended. Vertical lines represent 1 standard error of mean. Decreases in blood lactate, ventilation, O_2 uptake, CO_2 output, ventilatory equivalent for O_2, and heart rate are observed for both training regimens, but decreases are appreciably greater for the high work rate training group. (From Casaburi R, Patessio A, Ioli F, et al. Reductions in exercise lactic acidosis and ventilation as a result of exercise training in patients with obstructive lung disease. *Am Rev Respir Dis* 1991;143:9–18, with permission.)

a lower end-expiratory lung volume than during air breathing. Third, O_2 has some bronchodilator action. Fourth, it allows for washout of nitrogen from low-$\dot{V}_A/\dot{Q}$ areas of the lungs, thereby allowing end-expiratory lung volume to adjust downward because some of the O_2 replacing the N_2 will be absorbed.

ASSESSING THE EFFECTIVENESS OF TREATMENT

The major role of the heart, pulmonary and peripheral circulations, lungs, and ventilatory apparatus is to support the respiration of the cells and, specifically during exercise, the increased respiration of the skeletal muscles. Therefore, measurements of respiration in response to exercise should give the most direct global assessment of the function of these organ systems.

To use CPET for the purpose of evaluating therapy, however, it is necessary for the laboratory calibration to be accurate, to use sensitive end-points, and to be consistent in methodology. Based on the experience of the multicenter Vasodilator Heart Failure Trials (V-HeFT II) of the Veterans Affairs Hospitals, Cohn et al. (127) pointed out the need for well-trained technicians and careful calibration of the cardiopulmonary exercise system. Thus, it was of concern that some centers were performing CPET without a good understanding of what constituted a good or poor test. Several centers produced results in which tests of normal subjects (controls) yielded $\Delta\dot{V}_{O_2}/\Delta WR$ values that were either too low or too high to be physiological, i.e., that were considerably outside of the normal range (see Chapter 2). Eventually, the normal control subjects at all centers had appropriate values for $\Delta\dot{V}_{O_2}/\Delta WR$, thereby increasing confidence in the data from the sites. If the leaders at these centers had been trained in cardiopulmonary exercise physiology, they would have recognized immediately that their results were incorrect, rather than recognizing the problem only when experts reviewed the collected data. Knowing that $\Delta\dot{V}_{O_2}/\Delta WR$ should be approximately 10 ml/min/W in all normal subjects for any increasing work rate cycle ergometer exercise test protocol provides an internal calibration for a laboratory and an ability to detect gross errors early.

Figure 4.2 and the cases in Chapter 10 show the consistency of the value of $\Delta\dot{V}_{O_2}/\Delta WR$ in all normal subjects. We obtain the same exercise gas exchange measurements when studying the same subject in any of our three hospital laboratories. All give the same results despite different equipment because of the use of trained technicians and the calibration procedures described in Chapter 6. Accuracy is further validated by use of a metabolic simulator (128).

The physiological responses to exercise are reproducible in patients with relatively stable pathophysiology. Figure 9.17 shows the first and second tests done at 3-month intervals of a young male subject (described in greater detail as Case 81 in Chapter 10, in which a third test is also shown). In the third test, pulmonary artery, femoral vein, and brachial artery catheters were placed for simultaneous sampling of blood gases and lactate during CPET. Despite the fact that these tests were done at different times and in different laboratories, the parameters of aerobic function (i.e., peak $\dot{V}_{O_2}$ and AT) and the cardiovascular and ventilatory changes as related to work rate and metabolism were highly reproducible.

Hansen et al. (129) studied patient performance reproducibility and reader reproducibility in 114 paired tests performed 1 to 3 days apart in 42 exercise-limited patients with pulmonary arterial hypertension. Patient performance reproducibility rates were 5.8%, 6.5%, and 3.3%, and the reader reproducibility rates were 0.6%, 8.5%, and 2.1% for peak $\dot{V}_{O_2}$, AT, and $\dot{V}_E/\dot{V}_{CO_2}$ at the AT, respectively.

Evidence for the value of CPET for assessment of treatment is further provided by the case shown in Figure 9.8. This figure illustrates the wealth of information obtained from both a single exercise test and sequential exercise testing to evaluate the efficacy of epoprostenol treatment in pulmonary arterial hypertension. These studies demonstrate that at the outset of therapy, the patient was totally and critically incapacitated, despite being willing to do cycle ergometry to her best ability. Fortunately, she responded to the therapy in a gratifying way at 4 months (test 2). At 8 months (test 3), based on further improved perfusion to ventilated lung (reduction in $\dot{V}_E/\dot{V}_{CO_2}$ at the AT, and slope of $\dot{V}_E$ versus $\dot{V}_{CO_2}$) and increased O_2 transport (increase in peak $\dot{V}_{O_2}$, AT, and O_2 pulse) during exercise, she was taken off the lung transplantation list. She had no further functional gain past test 5 (16 months) and remained at the same level of function for the subsequent 4 years, the limit of observation. Thus, she was left with an abnormally low peak $\dot{V}_{O_2}$ and O_2 pulse (60% and 70% of predicted, respectively) and high $\dot{V}_E/\dot{V}_{CO_2}$ at the AT (third panel down, Fig. 9.8), but at a level of function that was adequate to pursue most forms of physical activity. These objective

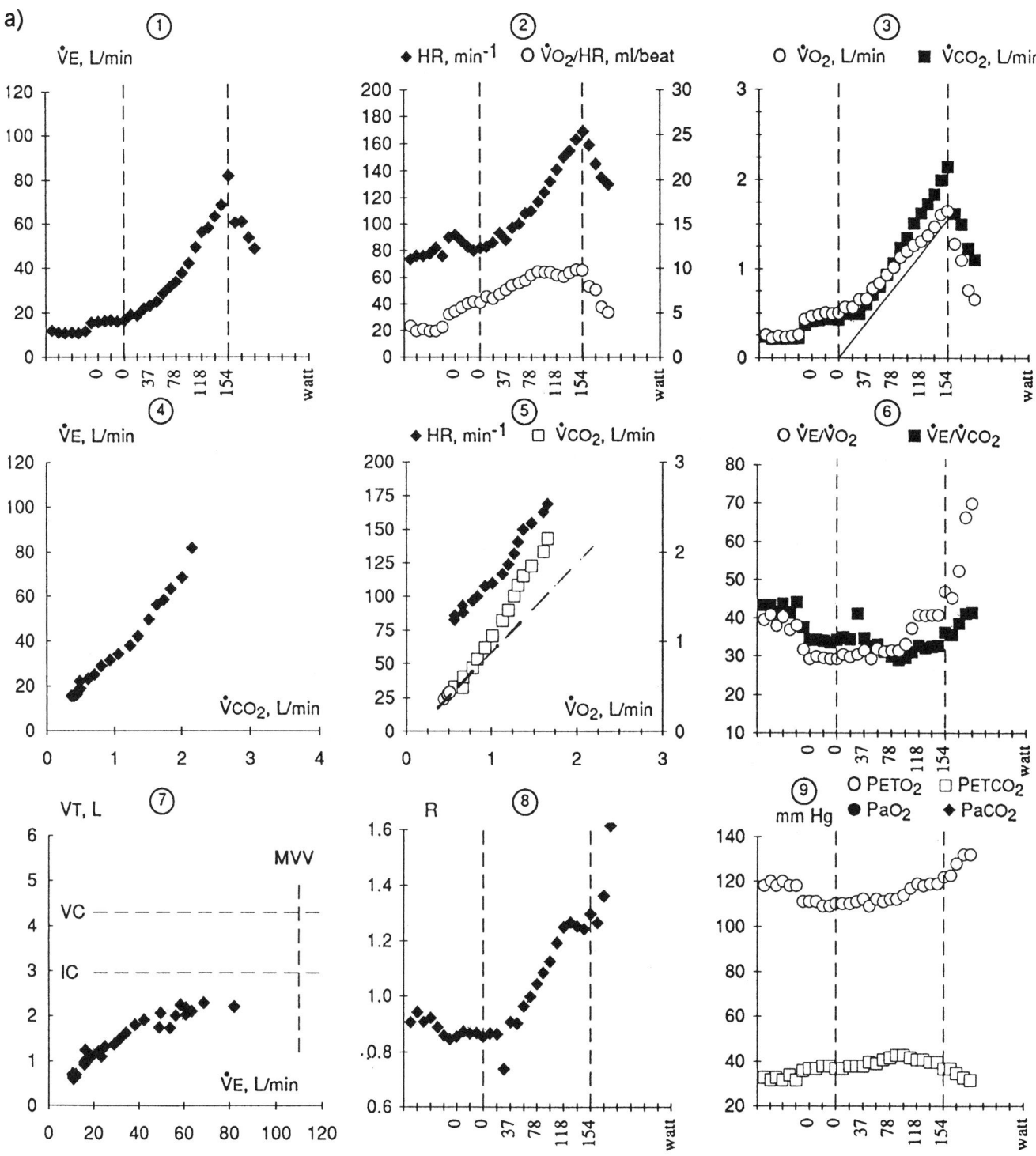

FIGURE 9.17.   Reproducibility of cardiopulmonary exercise testing in the patient presented as Case 81 in Chapter 10. This 29-year-old man, who noted progressive decrease in exercise tolerance over about a year, was studied by us three times over a period of 6 months to confirm a diagnosis made at the time of the first study (**a**). Although he was symptomatic during this period of evaluation, he was stable. Because of skepticism by the consulting cardiologist regarding the diagnosis of cardiomyopathy with diastolic dysfunction suggested by the first evaluation, the second study (**b**) was done 3 months later, this time with arterial blood gas analysis (not shown). As can be seen, despite a 3-month interval between studies a and b, the peak $\dot{V}O_2$ (1.6 L/min) and *AT* (0.8 L/min) were essentially the same and the graphs are almost superimposable. A third test was done 3 months after study b in another exercise laboratory at our institution, this time with right heart catheterization to confirm the low exercise stroke volume of the patient predicted from tests a and b. This third test, with cardiac output and mixed venous and femoral vein blood gases, is shown as Case 81 in Chapter 10. Again, the results of the gas exchange studies of this third test are virtually superimposable on the first two, including very similar peak $\dot{V}O_2$, *AT*, and O_2 pulse values. See Case 81, Chapter 10 for the predicted normal values for this patient.

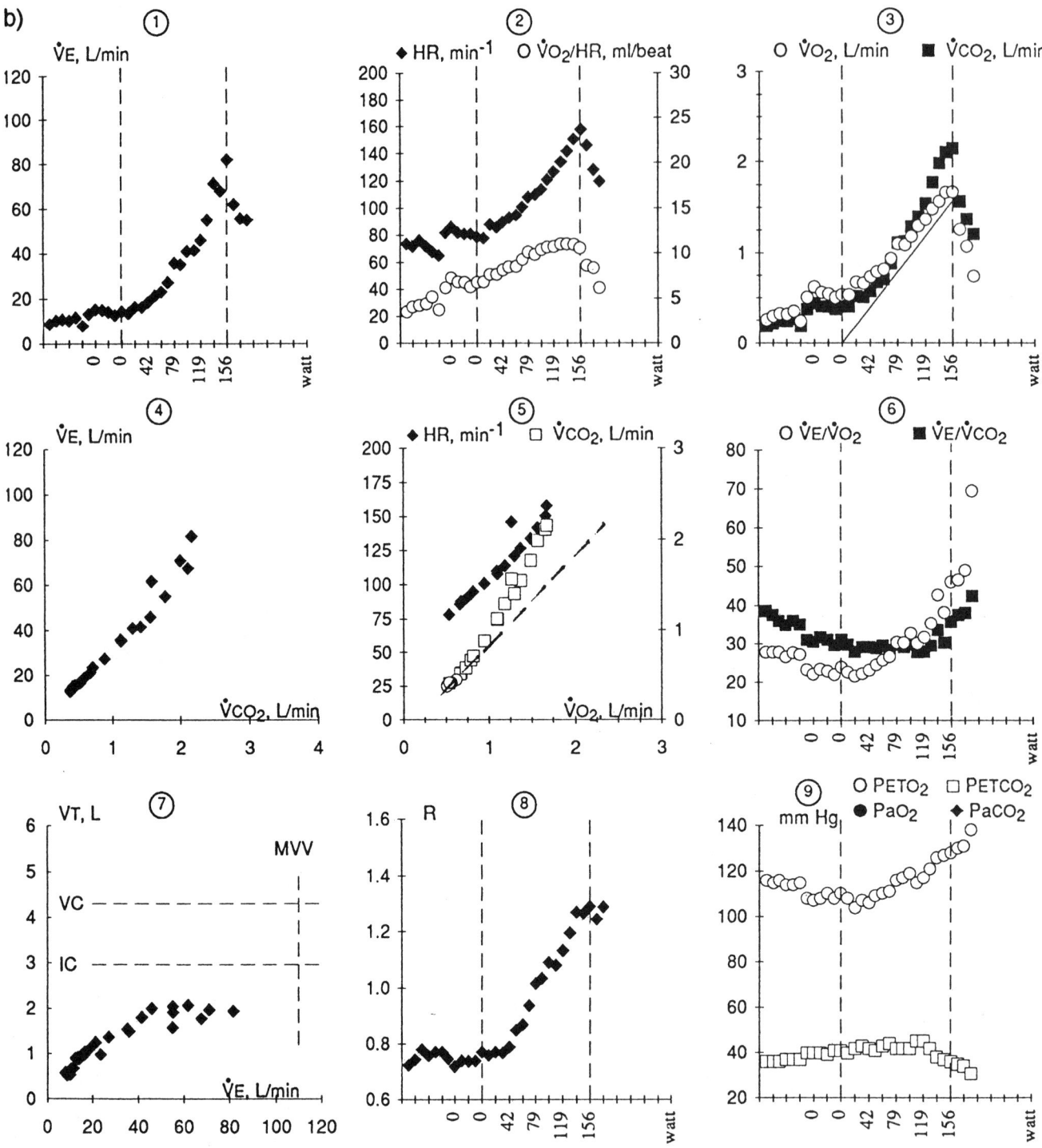

FIGURE 9.17.   *Continued*

assessments allowed her and her physicians to understand her functional disability and capacity much better than without the cardiopulmonary exercise tests.

In Chapter 10, several other cases are presented in which sequential studies helped determine that therapy improved function (Cases 25, 28, 45, 53, 54, and 57) and several in which therapy did not change the exercise pathophysiology (Cases 44, 51, 60). Importantly, the cardiopulmonary exercise tests provide the physician with reproducible and objective information needed to evaluate the clinical course of the patient and the effectiveness of therapeutic interventions.

SCREENING FOR DEVELOPMENT OF DISEASE IN HIGH-RISK PATIENTS

The intimate relationship between O_2 transport and exercise bioenergetics is clear. The normal gas exchange response to exercise is also well defined. Abnormal gas exchange responses to exercise are characteristic for disease in a specific organ system. Thus, to detect disease of impaired coupling of external to cellular respiration at an early stage—and possibly prevent serious progression of the illness—a noninvasive cardiopulmonary exercise test is probably the most sensitive, most comprehensive, and most cost-effective single test available to patients and physicians at this time.

To our knowledge, no investigative studies have been done that take advantage of noninvasive CPET to detect developing disease of the heart, lungs, pulmonary or systemic circulations, or the muscles. A normal peak $\dot{V}O_2$, AT, and $\Delta\dot{V}O_2/\Delta WR$ in response to exercise are required for an individual to function normally. Because these measurements will become abnormal with any functional impairment of the organs coupling pulmonary to cellular respiration, sequential CPET would be expected to be sensitively affected with a developing defect in the coupling. For example, the physician can use CPET measurements to detect deterioration of cardiovascular function with time, such as illustrated by Cases 13, 19, and 82 in Chapter 10. Thus, periodic cardiopulmonary exercise tests measuring $\dot{V}O_2$, AT, and $\Delta\dot{V}O_2/\Delta WR$ might be important to perform in people with strong family histories of coronary artery disease, including silent myocardial ischemia. Similarly, the measurement of the slope of $\dot{V}E$ versus $\dot{V}CO_2$ and $\dot{V}E/\dot{V}CO_2$ at the AT, in view of the uniform predicted values of these measurements, would likely be a sensitive noninvasive method to detect the development of pulmonary vascular disease in patients such as those susceptible to thromboembolic disease and the pulmonary vasculopathy that leads to primary pulmonary hypertension or pulmonary hypertension with connective tissue diseases.

GRADED EXERCISE TESTING AND THE ATHLETE

Training for athletic competition, especially of the endurance kind, owes as much to the accumulated lore of the practices of previously successful athletes as to the application of training strategies based on the results of physiological experimentation. The underlying theme of the various approaches to endurance training, however, is that of stressing the "system" during training beyond the demands of the actual event. How far beyond the power demands of the event and with what patterns of work–rest repetition remain the central issues.

Although many approaches will improve performance, the challenge is to determine the optimum pattern: the one that will achieve the greatest improvement in the available time. Laboratory exercise testing of the graded or incremental kind can provide a basis for establishing such a strategy, ensuring that the chosen strategy is successfully accomplished during the training session, and establishing objective criteria to support the physiological benefits of the training scheme.

This is most clearly evident in considering the extremes of event duration: sprints and marathons (and beyond). It is hard to see how knowledge of a subject's $\dot{V}O_2$max, critical power, anaerobic threshold, and so on can possibly influence the choice of training speeds for a sprinter. Considerations of the recovery kinetics of, for example, muscle or blood lactate (which for the purposes of this discussion we will use as proxy variables for the fatigue-inducing mechanisms) might be beneficial to the choice of interval strategy in the future. Indices of peak and mean power over a short maximum-effort sprint, such as provided by the Wingate test (130), offer more in this regard. For example, if these indices show improvement as a result of the training program but performance at the event does not, this would suggest that the athlete's technique should be the focus of attention.

For events of marathon duration or longer, the glycogen-squandering aspects of anaerobic glycolysis and consequent increased rate of lactate production are detrimental to performance. Consequently, a knowledge of the athlete's speed at the AT, by an appropriate measurement or estimation technique [including perceptual correlates (131)], can serve both as a means of optimizing the rate at which the event is actually performed (132) and as a frame of reference for a strategy for training at some higher speed that will induce a given degree of lactic acidemia (i.e., one that is sustained at some target value aimed at inducing a training effect—in this case, to increase the AT and hence the potential optimum performance rate).

At the intervening "middle distances," knowledge of the subject's profile of aerobic function is likely to be of considerably greater importance. Although Newsholme and Castell (133) have suggested that muscle glycogen depletion can contribute to fatigue at running events as "short" as 10,000 meters, it is likely that in these events fatigue is a result of metabolites increasing inexorably locally within muscle (134) and/or in sites within the brain (133) at a rate that causes them to attain a maximal, and limiting, value at the end of the race.

The upper limit of the work rate at which both $\dot{V}O_2$ and blood lactate can be maintained at a high but constant level has been demonstrated to be the subject's critical power (135). In healthy young subjects, this occurs, on average, at a $\dot{V}O_2$ of approximately 50% of the difference between the *AT* and the peak $\dot{V}O_2$ and at a blood lactate level of approximately 4 to 5 mM. However, these levels vary among subjects; hence, it is important to determine the specific level for a given subject rather than relying on a group mean value to guide training. These profiles will establish whether the training intensity is sufficiently high for the training target and also serve to monitor training-induced improvements. However, it is important to recognize that a particular level of blood lactate, for instance, can be attained either by a relatively low constant-load exercise bout or by work–rest repetitions involving appreciably greater work rates. This allows the recruitment pattern of muscle fibers and the metabolic and acid–base consequences of work to be proportionally manipulated for the training purpose.

Overtraining is also important to the athlete because it can lead to increased risk of infections and depressed immunologic function, in addition to decrements of performance (136). This appears to be a manifestation of prolonged high-intensity training; lower levels can boost immune function. The use of graded exercise testing to establish the upper level of beneficial training intensities and duration should provide insight into the deleterious aspects of inappropriate training.

As more is learned about the physiological mechanisms that trigger "training effects" and how the variables of intensity, duration, and recovery interact to induce the effects (137), laboratory testing will become even more useful in training prescriptions.

SUMMARY

Up until recently, cardiopulmonary exercise testing has not been applied in a general way in medicine because of the apparent complexity and time demands of the methods required to obtain the useful data. However, with the advent of automated gas analyzers, sensitive measuring devices, and computerized methods to calculate and display the massive amount of useful data that can be obtained from cardiopulmonary exercise tests, it is being recognized as an accurate, noninvasive technology with widespread applications at relatively low cost. We have used it most effectively for differential diagnosis, including unique diagnoses that cannot be made objectively without CPET. It takes the guesswork and bias out of differential diagnosis. It also makes impairment evaluation for disability more objective. It has been a very helpful guide in both cardiac and pulmonary rehabilitation for determining both the training work rate and whether improvement in exercise performance has occurred. In recent years, CPET has been shown to be a more accurate predictor of severity of disease and predictor of survival time in patients with heart failure than other techniques currently used by cardiologists for grading severity of chronic heart failure. Thus, it is now used to prioritize patients for heart transplantation, with the predicted insights from the measured peak $\dot{V}O_2$ overriding other cardiologic measurements. It is likely that these same guidelines can be applied to lung transplantation in patients with primary pulmonary hypertension and lung reduction surgery in patients with emphysema.

Cardiopulmonary exercise testing has obvious applications in determining the therapeutic effectiveness of drugs and procedures. Less well documented, but obvious in application, is the use of this quantitative approach to detect disease early in its time course—that is, before it is so advanced that abnormalities develop at rest and before they may be irreversible. The increasing number of applications for which CPET is currently employed attests to the growing recognition of its importance in medicine. It provides the potential to reduce health care costs by streamlining the diagnostic approach to disease and facilitating treatment decisions.

References

1. Belardinelli R, Lacalaprice F, Carle F, Minnucci A Cianci G, Perna G, D'Eusanio G. Exercise-induced myocardial ischaemia detected by cardiopulmonary exercise testing. *Eur Heart J* 2003;24:1304–1313.

2. Itoh H, Tajima A, Koike A, Osada N, Maeda T, Kato M, Omiya K, Fu LT, Watanabe H, Kato K. Oxygen uptake abnormalities during exercise in coronary artery disease. In: Wasserman K, ed. *Cardiopulmonary exercise testing and cardiovascular health*. Armonk, NY: Futura Publishing, 2002:165–172.

3. Gitt AK, Wasserman K, Kilkowski C, Kleeman T, Kilkowski A, Bangert M, Schneider S, Schwarz A,

Senges J. Exercise anaerobic threshold and ventilatory efficiency identify heart failure patients for high risk of early death. *Circulation* 2002;106:3079–3084.

4. Metra M, Raccagni D, Carini G, Orzan F, Papa A, Nodari S, Cody RJ, DeJours P. Ventilatory and arterial blood gas changes during exercise in heart failure. In: Wasserman K, ed. *Exercise gas exchange in heart disease*. Armonk, NY: Futura Publishing, 1996:125–143.

5. Chua TP, Ponikowski P, Harrington D, Anker SD, Webb-Peploe K, Clark AL, Poole-Wilson PA, Coats AJ. Clinical correlates and prognostic significance of the ventilatory response to exercise in chronic heart failure. *J Am Coll Cardiol* 1997;29:1585–1590.

6. Kleber FX, Vietzke G, Wernecke KD, Bauer U, Optiz C, Wensel R, Sperfeld A, Glaser S. Impairment of ventilatory efficiency in heart failure: prognostic impact. *Circulation* 2000;101:2803–2809.

7. Tabet J-Y, Beauvais F, Thabut G, Tartiere J-M, Logeart D, Cohen-Solal A. A critical appraisal of the prognostic value of the V_E/V_{CO_2} slope in chronic heart failure. *Eur J Cardiovasc Rehab* 2003;10:267–272.

8. Wasserman K, Zhang YY, Gitt A, Belardinelli R, Koike A, Lubarsky L, Agostini PG. Lung function and exercise gas exchange in chronic heart failure. *Circulation* 1997;96:2221–2227.

9. Ting H, Sun XG, Chuang ML, Lewis DA, Hansen JE, Wasserman K. A noninvasive assessment of pulmonary perfusion abnormality in patients with primary pulmonary hypertension. *Chest* 2001;119:824–832.

10. Kobayashi T, Itoh H, Kato K. The role of increased dead space in the augmented ventilation of cardiac patients. In: Wasserman K, ed. *Exercise gas exchange in heart disease*. Armonk, NY: Futura Publishing, 1996:145–156.

11. Higginbotham MB. Diastolic dysfunction and exercise gas exchange. In: Wasserman K, ed. *Exercise gas exchange in heart disease*. Armonk, NY: Futura Publishing, 1996:39–54.

12. Sun XG, Hansen JE, Oudiz RJ, Wasserman K. Exercise pathophysiology in patients with primary pulmonary hypertension. *Circulation* 2001;104:429–435.

13. Wensel R, Optiz CF, Anker SD, Winkler J, Hoffken G, Kleber FX, Sharma R, Hummel M, Hetzar R, Ewert R. Assessment of survival in patients with primary pulmonary hypertension. *Circulation* 2002;106:319–324.

14. Waurick PE, Kleber FX. Cardiopulmonary exercise testing in pulmonary vascular disease: arterial and end-tidal CO_2 partial pressures in patients with acute and chronic pulmonary embolism and primary pulmonary hypertension. In: Wasserman K, ed. *Cardiopulmonary exercise testing and cardiovascular health*. Armonk, NY: Futura Publishing, 2003:173–178.

15. Schaeffer JP, ed. *Morris' human anatomy*. Philadelphia: Blakiston Company, 1953.

16. Sun X-G, Hansen JE, Oudiz R, Wasserman K. Gas exchange detection of exercise-induced right-to-left shunt in patients with primary pulmonary hypertension. *Circulation* 2002;105:54–60.

17. Sietsema KE, Cooper DM, Perloff SK, Child JS, Rosove MH, Wasserman K, Whipp BJ. Control of ventilation during exercise in patients with central venous-to-systemic arterial shunts. *J Appl Physiol* 1988;64:234–242.

18. Haller RG, Lewis SF, Estabrook RW, DiMauro S, Servidei S, Foster DW. Exercise intolerance, lactic acidosis, and abnormal cardiopulmonary regulation in exercise associated with adult skeletal muscle cytochrome c oxidase deficiency. *J Clin Invest* 1989;84:155–161.

19. Riley M, Nugent A, Steele IC, Bell N, Trimble ER, Nicholls DP, Patterson VH. Gas exchange during exercise in McArdle's disease. *J Appl Physiol* 1993;75:745–754.

20. Haller RG, Henriksson KG, Jorfeldt L, Hultman E, Wibom R, Sahlin K, Areskog N-H, Gunder M, Ayyad K, Blomquist CG, Hall RE, Thuillier P, Kennaway NG, Lewis SF. Deficiency of skeletal muscle succinate dehydrogenase and aconitase. Pathophysiology of exercise in a novel human muscle oxidative defect. *J Clin Invest* 1991;88:1197–1206.

21. Bogaard JM, Scholte HR, Busch FM, Stam H, Versprille A. Anaerobic threshold as detected from ventilatory and metabolic exercise responses in patients with mitochondrial respiratory chain defect. In: Tavassi L, DiPrampero PE, eds. *The anaerobic threshold: physiological and clinical significance*. Advances in Cardiology. Basel: Karger, 1986:135–145.

22. Bogaard JM, Busch HFM, Scholte HR, Stam H, Versprille A. Exercise responses in patients with an enzyme deficiency in the mitochondrial respiratory chain. *Eur Respir J* 1988;1:445–452.

23. Pardee HEB, DeGraff AG, Della Chapelle CE, Eggleston C, Kossman CE, Maynard E, Schwedel JB, Stewart HJ, Wright IS. Functional capacity classification of patients: In: *Nomenclature and criteria for diagnosis of diseases of the heart and blood vessels*. New York: New York Heart Association, 1953:81.

24. Matsumura N, Nishijima H, Kojima S, Hashimoto F, Minami M, Yasuda H. Determination of anaerobic threshold for assessment of functional state in patients with chronic heart failure. *Circulation* 1983;68:360–367.

25. Weber KT, Janicki JS. Cardiopulmonary exercise testing for evaluation of chronic cardiac failure. *Am J Cardiol* 1985;55:22A–31A.

26. Mudge GH, Goldstein S, Addonizio LJ, Caplan A, Mancini D, Levine TB, Ritsch ME, Stevenson LW. Task force 3: recipient guidelines/prioritization. *J Am Coll Cardiol* 1993;22:21–26.

27. Stelken AM, Younis LT, Jennison SH, Miller DD, Miller LW, Shaw LJ, Kargl D, Chaitman BR. Prognostic value of cardiopulmonary exercise testing

using percent achieved of predicted peak oxygen uptake for patients with ischemic and dilated cardiomyopathy. *J Am Coll Cardiol* 1996;27:345–352.

28. Stevenson LW. Role of exercise testing in the evaluation of candidates for cardiac transplantation. In: Wasserman K, ed. *Exercise gas exchange in heart disease*. Armonk, NY: Futura Publishing, 1996:271–286.

29. Mancini D, Eisen H, Kussmaul W, Mull R, Edmunds L, Wilson J. Value of peak exercise oxygen consumption for optimal timing of cardiac transplantation of ambulatory patients with heart failure. *Circulation* 1991;83:778–786.

30. Likoff MJ, Chandler SL. Clinical determinants of mortality in chronic congestive heart failure secondary to idiopathic dilated or to ischemic cardiomyopathy. *Am J Cardiol* 1987;59:634–638.

31. Myers J, Gullestad L, Vagelos R, Do D, Bellin D, Ross H, Fowler MB. Clinical, hemodynamic, and cardiopulmonary exercise test determinants of survival in patients referred for evaluation of heart failure. *Ann Intern Med* 1998;129:286–293.

32. Stringer W, Hansen J, Wasserman K. Cardiac output estimated non-invasively from oxygen uptake ($\dot{V}O_2$) during exercise. *J Appl Physiol* 1997;82: 908–912.

33. Sullivan MJ, Knight D, Higginbotham MB, Cobb FR. Relation between central and peripheral hemodynamics during exercise in patients with chronic heart failure. Muscle blood flow is reduced with maintenance of arterial perfusion pressure. *Circulation* 1989;80:769–781.

34. Agostoni PG, Wasserman K, Perego GB, Marenzi GC, Guazzi M, Assanelli E, Lauri G, Guazzi MD. Oxygen transport to muscle during exercise in chronic congestive heart failure secondary to idiopathic dilated cardiomyopathy. *Am J Cardiol* 1997;79:1120–1124.

35. Bigi R, Desideri A, Rambaldi R, Cortigiani L, Sponzilli C, Fiorentini C. Angiographic and prognostic correlates of cardiac output by cardiopulmonary exercise testing in patients with anterior myocardial infarction. *Chest* 2001;120:825–833.

36. Sullivan MJ, Hawthorne MH. Exercise intolerance in patients with chronic heart failure. *Prog Cardiovasc Dis* 1995;38:1–22.

37. Weber KT. Cardiopulmonary exercise testing and the evaluation of systolic dysfunction. In: Wasserman K, ed. *Exercise gas exchange in heart disease*. Armonk, NY: Futura Publishing, 1996:55–62.

38. Matsumura N, Nishijima H, Kojima S, Hashimoto F, Minami M, Yasuda H. Determination of anaerobic threshold for assessment of functional state in patients with chronic heart failure. *Circulation* 1983;68:360–367.

39. Itoh H, Taniguchi K, Koike A, Doi M. Evaluation of severity of heart failure using ventilatory gas analysis. *Circulation* 1990;81(Suppl II):II31–II37.

40. Koike A, Hiroe M, Adachi H, Yajima T, Nogami A, Ito H, Takamoto T, Taniguichi K, Marumo F. Anaerobic metabolism as an indicator of aerobic function during exercise in cardiac patients. *J Am Coll Cardiol* 1992;20:120–126.

41. Rickenbacher PR, Trindade PT, Haywood GA, Vagelos RH, Schroeder JS, Willson K, Prikazsky L., Fowler MB. Transplant candidates with severe left ventricular dysfunction managed with medical treatment: characteristics and survival. *J Am Coll Cardiol* 1996; 27:1192–1197.

42. Szlachic J, Massie BM, Kramer BL, Topic N, Tubau J. Correlates and prognostic indication of exercise capacity in chronic congestive heart failure. *Am J Cardiol* 1985;55:1037–1042.

43. Costanzo MR, Augustine S, Bourge R, Bristow M, O'Connell JB, Driscoll D, Rose E. Selection and treatment of candidates for heart transplantation. A statement for health professionals from the Committee on Heart Failure and Cardiac Transplantation of the Council on Clinical Cardiology, American Heart Association. *Circulation* 1995;92:3593–3612.

44. Aaronson KD, Mancini DM. Is percentage of predicted maximal oxygen consumption a better predictor of survival than peak exercise oxygen consumption for patients with severe heart failure? *J Heart Lung Transplant* 1995;14:981–989.

45. Roul G, Moulichon ME, Bareiss P, Gries P, Sacrez J, Germain P, Missard JM, Sacrez A. Exercise peak $\dot{V}O_2$ determination in chronic heart failure: is it still of value? *Eur Heart J* 1994;15:495–502.

46. Osada N, Chaitman BR, Miller LW, Yip D, Cishek MB, Wolford TL, Donohue TJ. Cardiopulmonary exercise testing identifies low risk patients with heart failure and severely impaired exercise capacity considered for heart transplantation. *J Am Coll Cardiol* 1998;31:577–582.

47. Stevenson LW, Steimle AE, Fonarow G, Kermani M, Kermani D, Hamilton MA, Moriguchi JD, Walden J, Tillisch JH, Drinkwater DC, Laks H. Improvement in exercise capacity of candidates awaiting heart transplantation. *J Am Coll Cardiol* 1995;25:163–170.

48. Cohn JN, Johnson GR, Shabetai R, Loeb H, Tristani F, Rector T, Smith R, Fletcher R. Ejection fraction, peak exercise oxygen consumption, cardiothoracic rat ventricular arrhythmias, and plasma norepinephrine as determinants of prognosis in heart failure. The V-HeFT VA Cooperative Studies Group. *Circulation* 1993;87:V15–V16.

49. Mudge GH, Goldstein S, Addonizio LJ, Caplan A, Mancini D, Levine TB, Ritsch ME, Stevenson LW. Task force 3: recipient guidelines/prioritization. *J Am Coll Cardiol* 1993;22:21–26.

50. Oga T, Nishimura K, Tsukino M, Sato S, Hajiro T. Analysis of the factors related to mortality in chronic

obstructive pulmonary disease. *Am J Respir Crit Care Med* 2003;167:544–549.

51. Jones PW. Health status measurements in chronic obstructive pulmonary disease. *Thorax* 2001;56:880–887.

52. Hiraga T, Maekura R, Okuda Y, Okamoto T, Hirotani A, Kitada S, Yoshimura K, Yokota S, Ito M, Ogura T. Prognostic predictors for survival in patients with COPD using cardiopulmonary exercise testing. *Clin Physiol Funct Imaging* 2003;23:324–331.

53. Fishman A, Martinez F, Naunheim K, Pianadosi S, Wise R, Ries A, Weinmann Wood DE, National Emphysema Treatment Trial Research Group. A randomized trial comparing lung-volume-reduction surgery with medical therapy for severe emphysema. *N Engl J Med* 2003;348:2059–2073.

54. Olsen GN, Weiman DS, Bolton JWR, Gass GD, Mclain WC, Schoonover GA, Hornung CA. Submaximal invasive exercise testing and quantitative lung scanning in the evaluation for tolerance of lung resection. *Chest* 1989;95:267–273.

55. Olsen GN. The evolving role of exercise testing prior to lung resection. *Chest* 1989;9:218–225.

56. Olsen GN. Preoperative physiology and lung resection [Editorial]. *Chest* 1992;101:300–301.

57. Miyoshi S, Nakahara K, Ohno K, Monden Y, Kawashima Y. Exercise tolerance in lung cancer patients: the relationship between exercise capacity and postthoracotomy hospital mortality. *Ann Thorac Surg* 1987;44:487–490.

58. Gilbreth EM, Weisman IM. Role of exercise stress testing in preoperative evaluation of patients for lung resection. *Clin Chest Med* 1994;15:389–403.

59. Sue DY, Wasserman K. Impact of integrative cardiopulmonary exercise testing on clinical decision making. *Chest* 1991;99:981–992.

60. Wasserman K. Preoperative evaluation of cardiovascular exercise training on clinical decision making. *Chest* 1993;104:663–664.

61. Smith TP, Kinasewitz GT, Tucker WY, Spillers WP, George WP. Exercise capacity as a predictor of postthoracotomy morbidity. *Am Rev Respir Dis* 1984;129:730–734.

62. Bechard D, Wetstein L. Assessment of exercise oxygen consumption as preoperative criterion for lung resection. *Ann Thorac Surg* 1987;44:344–349.

63. Bolliger CT, Jordan P, Soler M, Stulz P, Gradel E, Skarvan K, Elsasser S, Gonon M, Wyser C, Tamm M. Exercise capacity as a predictor of postoperative complications in lung resection candidates. *Am J Respir Crit Care Med* 1995;151:1472–1480.

64. Bolliger CT, Wyser C, Roser H, Soler M, Perruchoud AP. Lung scanning and exercise testing for the prediction of postoperative performance in lung resection candidates at increased risk for complications. *Chest* 1995;108:341–348.

65. Morice RC, Peters EJ, Ryan MB, Putnam JB, Ali MK, Rith JA. Exercise testing in the evaluation of patients at high risk for complications from lung resection. *Chest* 1992;101:356–361.

66. Older P, Smith R, Courtney P, Hone R. Preoperative evaluation of cardiac failure and ischemia in elderly patients by cardiopulmonary exercise testing. *Chest* 1993;104:701–704.

67. Older P, Hall A, Hader R. Cardiopulmonary exercise testing as a screening test for perioperative management of major surgery in the elderly. *Chest* 1999;116:355–362.

68. Epstein SK, Faling LJ, Daly BD, Celli BR. Predicting complications after pulmonary resection. Preoperative exercise testing vs. a multifactorial cardiopulmonary risk index. *Chest* 1993;104:694–700.

69. Holden DA, Rice TW, Stelmach K, Meeker DP. Exercise testing, 6-min walk, and stair climb in the evaluation of patients at high risk for pulmonary resection. *Chest* 1992;102:1774–1779.

70. Renzetti AD, Bleecker ER, Epler GR, Jones RN, Kanner RE, Repsher LH. Evaluation of impairment/disability secondary to respiratory disorders. *Am Rev Respir Dis* 1986;133:1205–1209.

71. Wood PH. Appreciating the consequences of disease: international classification of impairments, disabilities, and handicaps. *WHO Chronicle* 1980;34:376–380.

72. Campbell SC. A comparison of the maximum volume ventilation with forced expiratory volume in one second: an assessment of subject cooperation. *J Occup Med* 1982;24:531–533.

73. Gandevia B, Hugh-Jones P. Terminology for measurements of ventilatory capacity. *Thorax* 1957;1:290–293.

74. Cotes JE, Zejda J, King B. Lung function impairment as a guide to exercise limitation in work-related lung disorders. *Am Rev Respir Dis* 1988;137:1089–1093.

75. Agostoni P, Smith DD, Schoene RGB, Robertson HT, Butler J. Evaluation of breathlessness in asbestos workers. *Am Rev Respir Dis* 1987;135:812–816.

76. Agusti AG, Roca J, Rodriguez-Roisin R, Xaubet A, Agusti-Vidal A. Different patterns of gas exchange response to exercise in asbestos and idiopathic pulmonary fibrosis. *Eur Respir J* 1988;1:510–516.

77. Howard J, Mohsenifar Z, Brown HV, Koerner SK. Role of exercise testing in assessing functional respiratory impairment due to asbestos exposure. *J Occup Med* 1982;24:685–689.

78. Markos J, Musk AW, Finucane KE. Functional similarities of asbestosis and cryptogenic fibrosing alveolitis. *Thorax* 1988;43:708–714.

79. Oren A, Sue DY, Hansen JE, Torrance DJ, Wasserman K. The role of exercise testing in impairment evaluation. *Am Rev Respir Dis* 1987;135:230–235.

80. Pearle J. Exercise performance and functional impairment in asbestos-exposed workers. *Chest* 1981;80:701–705.

81. Risk C, Epler GR, Gaensler EA. Exercise alveolar-arterial oxygen pressure difference in interstitial lung disease. *Chest* 1984;85:69–74.

82. Sue DY, Oren A, Hansen JE, Wasserman K. Lung function and exercise performance in smoking and non-smoking asbestos-exposed workers. *Am Rev Respir Dis* 1985;132:612–618.

83. Wiedemann HP, Gee JBL, Balmes JR. Exercise testing in occupational lung disease. *Clin Chest Med* 1984;5:157–171.

84. Ortega F, Montemayor T, Sanchez A, Cabello F, Castillo J. Role of cardiopulmonary exercise testing and the criteria used to determine disability in patients with severe chronic obstructive pulmonary disease. *Am J Respir Crit Care Med* 1994;150:747– 751.

85. Saltin B, Gollnick PD. Skeletal muscle adaptability: significance for metabolism and performance. In: *Handbook of Physiology*. Washington DC: American Physiological Society, 1986:555.

86. Anderson P, Henriksson J. Training induced changes in the subgroups of human type II skeletal muscle fibers. *Acta Physiol Scand* 1977;99:123–125.

87. Holloszy JO. Adaptation of skeletal muscle to endurance exercise. *Med Sci Sports* 1975;7:155–164.

88. Pattengale PK, Holloszy JO. Augmentation of skeletal muscle myoglobin by a program of treadmill running. *Am J Physiol* 1967;213:783–785.

89. Saltin B, Henriksson J, Nygaard E, Andersen P, Jansson E. Fiber types and metabolic potentials of skeletal muscles in sedentary men and endurance runners. *Ann N Y Acad Sci* 1977;301:3–29.

90. Henriksson J. Training induced adaptation of skeletal muscle and metabolism during submaximal exercise. *J Physiol* 1977;270:661–675.

91. McArdle WD, Katch FI, Pechar GS. Comparison of continuous and discontinuous treadmill and bicycle tests for max $\dot{V}O_2$. *Med Sci Sports Exerc* 1972;5:156–160.

92. Clausen JP, Klausen K, Rasmussen B, Trap-Jensen J. Central and peripheral circulatory changes after training of the arms and legs. *Am J Physiol* 1973;225:675–682.

93. Saltin B. Cardiovascular and pulmonary adaptation to physical activity. In: Bouchard C, Shephard RJ, Stephens T, Sutton JR, eds. *Exercise, fitness, and health: a consensus of current knowledge*. Champaign, IL: Human Kinetics, 1990:187.

94. Pollock ML, Miller HS, Janeway R. Effects of walking on body composition and cardiovascular function of middle-aged men. *J Appl Physiol* 1971;30:126–130.

95. Pollock ML, Wilmore JH. *Exercise in health and disease*. Philadelphia: Saunders, 1990.

96. Casaburi R, Storer TW, Ben-Dov I, Wasserman K. Effect of endurance training on possible determinants of $\dot{V}O_2$ during heavy exercise. *J Appl Physiol* 1987;62:199–207.

97. Casaburi R, Storer TW, Wasserman K. Mediation of reduced ventilatory response to exercise after endurance training. *J Appl Physiol* 1987;63:1533–1538.

98. Sullivan CS, Casaburi R, Storer TW, Wasserman K. Prediction of blood lactate response to constant power outputs. *Eur J Appl Physiol* 1995;71:349–354.

99. Poole DC, Barstow TJ, Gaesser GA, Willis WT, Whipp BJ. $\dot{V}O_2$ slow component: physiological and functional significance. *Med Sci Sports Exerc* 1994; 26:1354–1358.

100. Casaburi R, Whipp BJ, Wasserman K, Beaver WL, Koyal SN. Ventilatory and gas exchange dynamics in response to sinusoidal work. *J Appl Physiol* 1977;42:300–311.

101. Winder WW, Hickson RC, Hagberg JA, Ehsani AA, McLane JA. Training-induced changes in hormonal and metabolic responses to submaximal exercise. *J Appl Physiol* 1979;46:766–771.

102. Sutton JR, Farrell PS, Harber VJ. Hormonal adaptation to physical activity. In: Bouchard C, Shephard RJ, Stephens T, Sutton JR, eds. *Exercise, fitness, and health: a consensus of current knowledge*. Champaign, IL: Human Kinetics Books, 1990:217.

103. Gisolfi C, Robinson S. Relations between physical training, acclimatization and heat tolerance. *J Appl Physiol* 1969;26:530–534.

104. Hill DW, Cureton KJ, Grisham SC, Collins MA. Effect of training on the rating of perceived exertion at the ventilatory threshold. *Eur J Appl Physiol* 1987; 56:206–211.

105. Haas F, Schicchi JS, Axen K. Desensitization to dyspnea in chronic obstructive pulmonary disease. In: Casaburi R, Petty TL, eds. *Principles and practice of pulmonary rehabilitation*. Philadelphia: Saunders, 1993:241–251.

106. Pina IL, Apstein CS, Balady GJ, Belardinelli R, Chaitman BR, Duscha BD, Fletcher BJ, Fleg JL, Myers JN, Sullivan MJ. Exercise and heart failure. A statement from the American Heart Association Committee on Exercise, Rehabilitation, and Prevention. *Circulation* 2003;107:1210–1225.

107. Reindl I, Kleber FX. Exertional hyperpnea in patients with chronic heart failure is a reversible cause of exercise intolerance. *Basic Res Cardiol* 1996;91:37–41.

108. Ponikowski PP, Chua TP, Francis DP, et al. Muscle ergoreceptor overactivity reflects deterioration in clinical status and cardiorespiratory reflex control in chronic heart failure. *Circulation* 2001;104:2324–2330.

109. Itoh H, Kato K. Short-term exercise training after cardiac surgery. In: Wasserman K, ed. *Exercise gas exchange in heart disease*. Armonk, NY: Futura Publishing, 1996:229–244.

110. American College of Sports Medicine. *ACSM's guidelines for exercise testing and prescription*. Baltimore: Williams & Wilkins, 1995:151–235.

111. Dubach P, Myers J, Dziekan G, Goebbels U, Reinhart W, Vogt P, Ratti R, Muller P, Miettunen R, Buser P. Effect of exercise training on myocardial remodeling in patients with reduced left ventricular function after myocardial infarction. *Circulation* 1997;95:2060–2067.

112. Belardinelli R, Georgiou D, Cianci G, Berman N, Ginzton L, Purcaro A. Exercise training improves left ventricular diastolic filling in patients with dilated cardiomyopathy. *Circulation* 1995;91:2775–2784.

113. Ries AL, Carlin BW, Carrieri-Kohlman V, Casaburi R, Celli BR, Emery CF, Hodgkin JE, Mahler DA, Make B. Pulmonary rehabilitation: evidence based guidelines. *Chest* 1997;112:1363–1396.

114. Orenstein DM, Noyes BE. Cystic fibrosis. In: Casaburi R, Petty TL, eds. *Principles and practice of pulmonary rehabilitation*. Philadelphia: Saunders, 1993:439–458.

115. Clark CJ. The role of physical training in asthma. In: Casaburi R, Petty TL, eds. *Principles and practice of pulmonary rehabilitation*. Philadelphia: Saunders, 1993:424–438.

116. Whipp BJ, Casaburi R. Physical activity, fitness and chronic lung disease. In: Bouchard C, Shephard RJ, Stephens T, eds. *Physical activity, fitness and health*. Champaign IL: Human Kinetics, 1994:749–761.

117. Wasserman K, Sue DY, Moricca RB, Casaburi R. Selection criteria for exercise training in pulmonary rehabilitation. *Eur J Appl Physiol* 1989;2(Suppl 7): S604–S610.

118. Casaburi R. Deconditioning. In: Fishman AP, ed. *Pulmonary rehabilitation*. Lung Biology in Health and Disease Series. New York: Marcel Dekker, 1996: 213–230.

119. Maltais F, Jobin J, Sullivan MJ, Bernard S, Whittom F, Killian KJ, Desmeules M, Belanger M, LeBlanc P. Metabolic and hemodynamic responses of lower limb during exercise in patients with COPD. *J Appl Physiol* 1998;84:1573–1580.

120. Richardson R, Leak B, Haseler L, Gavin T, Sheldon J, Eltin P, Olfert I, Ries A, Wagner P. Normal skeletal muscle function in patients with COPD when exercise is not centrally limited. *Med Sci Sports Exerc* 1999;31:S277.

121. Butler J, Schrijen F, Polu JM, Albert RK. Cause of the raised wedge pressure on exercise in chronic obstructive pulmonary disease. *Am Rev Respir Dis* 1988;138:350–354.

122. Belman MJ. Exercise training in chronic obstructive pulmonary disease. *Clin Chest Med* 1986;7:585–597.

123. Ries AL, Archibald CJ. Endurance exercise training at maximal targets in patients with chronic obstructive pulmonary disease. *J Cardiopulm Rehabil* 1987;7: 594–601.

124. Casaburi R, Patessio A, Ioli F, Zanaboni S, Donner C, Wasserman K. Reductions in exercise lactic acidosis and ventilation as a result of exercise training in patients with obstructive lung disease. *Am Rev Respir Dis* 1991;143:9–18.

125. Casaburi R, Porszasz J, Burns MR, Carithers ER, Chang RSY, Cooper CB. Physiologic benefits of exercise training in rehabilitation of severe COPD patients. *Am J Respir Crit Care Med* 1997;155:1541–1551.

126. Somfay A, Porszasz J, Lee S-M, Casaburi R. Effect of hyperoxia on gas exchange and lactate kinetics following exercise onset in nonhypoxemic COPD patients. *Chest* 2002;121:393–400.

127. Cohn JN, Ziesche S, Johnson G, Cobb F. Use of exercise gas exchange measurements in multicenter drug studies. In: Wasserman K, ed. *Exercise gas exchange in heart disease*. Armonk, NY: Futura Publishing, 1996:245–256.

128. Huszczuk A, Whipp BJ, Wasserman K. A respiratory gas exchange simulator for routine calibration in metabolic studies. *Eur Respir J* 1990;3:465–468.

129. Hansen JE, Sun X-G, Yasunobu Y, Garafano RP, Gates G, Barst RJ, Wasserman K. Reproducibility of cardiopulmonary exercise parameters in patients with pulmonary arterial hypertension. Chest (*in press*, 2004).

130. Bar-Or O. The Wingate test. An update on methodology, reliability and validity. *Sports Med* 1987;4: 381–394.

131. Cafarelli E. Sensory processes and endurance performance. In: Shephard RJ, Astrand PO, eds. *Endurance in sport*. Oxford: Blackwell Scientific, 1992: 261–269.

132. Zoladz JA, Sargeant AJ, Emmerich J, Stoklosa J, Zychowski A. Changes in acid-base status of marathon runners during incremental field test. *Eur J Appl Physiol* 1993;67:71–76.

133. Newsholme E, Castell LM. Can amino acids influence exercise performance in athletes? In: Steinacker J, Ward SA, eds. *The physiology and pathophysiology of exercise tolerance*. New York: Plenum Press, 1996:269–274.

134. Sargeant AJ, Beelen A. Human muscle fatigue in dynamic exercise. In: Sargeant AJ, Kernell D, eds. *Neuromuscular fatigue*. Amsterdam: North Holland Publishers, 1992:81–92.

135. Poole DC, Ward SA, Gardner GW, Whipp BJ. Metabolic and respiratory profile of the upper limit for prolonged exercise in man. *Ergonomics* 1988;31:1265–1279.

136. Hoffman-Goetz L, Pedersen BK. Exercise and the immune system: a model of the stress response? *Immunol Today* 1994;15:382–387.

137. Banister EW, Morton RH, Fitz-Clarke JR. Clinical dose-response effects of exercise. In: Steinacker J, Ward SA, eds. *The physiology and pathophysiology of exercise tolerance*. New York: Plenum Press, 1996: 297–309.

CHAPTER 10

Case Presentations

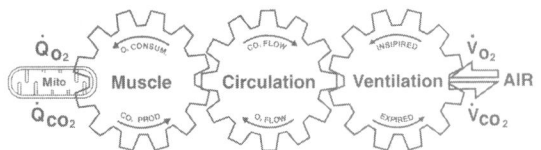

THE CASES PRESENTED in this chapter were selected because they are either representative of specific pathophysiology or teach a unique lesson. They were not selected because they show data from especially cooperative subjects or are pretty records. In fact, these studies were done on typical patients evaluated in our clinical exercise laboratory and therefore include records that range between the best and the worst with respect to appearance. The primary goal of this chapter is to offer a systematic approach to interpretation of exercise performance. It demonstrates how measurements can be used as decision-making branch points for reaching an appropriate diagnosis and how to apply these measurements to a range of abnormalities that lead to exercise intolerance.

The data given in these case presentations are restricted to information needed to interpret the exercise test. When arterial blood gases are presented, two sets of resting values are included. The first is obtained with the subject sitting on the ergometer but before breathing on the mouthpiece (i.e., without accompanying respiratory gas exchange data), and the second is obtained with the subject on the ergometer while breathing on the mouthpiece prior to exercise (i.e., with accompanying gas exchange data). Both sets of data are reported for comparison, when available.

The graphs given with each case display data points every 30 seconds, calculated as the average of whole breath-by-breath measurements over the preceding 15- to 20-second period. The protocol is shown on panels 1, 2, 3, 6, 8, and 9 of the nine-panel plots, in which the abscissa is the work rate and time. After a period of rest (usually 3 minutes) and unloaded pedaling (usually 3 minutes; 0 W), the work rate is increased in equal increments each minute or in a ramp pattern. The time during which the work rate is being progressively increased begins at the left vertical dashed line; the right vertical dashed line indicates the termination of exercise. Two minutes of recovery data are also plotted. In panel 3, work rate is scaled to be one-tenth that of $\dot{V}O_2$. Thus, when the $\dot{V}O_2$ increase exactly parallels the work rate increase, $\Delta\dot{V}O_2/\Delta WR$ equals 10 mL/min/W.

In panel 5 of the nine-panel plots, the mean predicted peak $\dot{V}O_2$ and maximum heart rate (HR) for a sedentary person of the same sex, age, and body size are marked with an x. Moreover, plotted on panel 5 is $\dot{V}CO_2$ as a function of $\dot{V}O_2$. The dashed diagonal line through this plot has a slope of 1. When $\dot{V}CO_2$ versus $\dot{V}O_2$ increases more steeply than this line, CO_2 is being generated from the bicarbonate buffering of lactic acid in addition to that from aerobic metabolism. Thus, higher values of $\dot{V}O_2$ must be above the subject's anaerobic threshold (AT), the latter marked by the break point in the $\dot{V}CO_2$ versus $\dot{V}O_2$ relation where $\dot{V}CO_2$ starts to increase faster than $\dot{V}O_2$. In each case, the data shown in Table 2 are a summary of the data shown in Table 3 (and Table 4, if provided) and the figure(s).

The predicted values given for each case are the mean values taken from Chapter 7. As with any predicted values, there are normal ranges. To the best of our judgment, our interpretations take the range of normal values into account.

Eighty-five cases are presented for interpretation. Practical considerations limited our ability to provide more examples, and of course, there are many disorders of exercise performance that we have not studied directly. Because each category of disease can have perturbations that are instructive to review, we sometimes found it desirable to present more than one case example of a type of disorder. Moreover, patients frequently have more than one abnormality. Thus, we thought it important to present some of these complex cases and to provide the rationale for our conclusions regarding the dominant pathophysiology.

Of the 85 cases, the first 15 are of men and women who we concluded were normal at the time of the initial study. They were selected to show the effects of age, gender, form of ergometry used for testing, O_2 breathing, β-adrenergic blockade, obesity, and cigarette smoking on the test results.

Cases 16 to 29 are examples of coronary artery disease, valvular heart disease, cardiomyopathies, and congenital heart disease. Other examples of heart diseases are provided in the "complex" case category described later. Cases 30 to 35 are examples of peripheral arterial diseases. Again, some ex-

amples are included in the "complex" case category because these disorders are commonly associated with primary heart disease.

Cases 36 to 45 include several types and severities of diseases primarily associated with airflow obstruction. Other examples of obstructive airway disease can be found in the "complex" category. Cases 46 to 58 are examples of pulmonary fibrosis or respiratory restriction of various causes or identified as idiopathic. Two cases show results before and after treatment.

Cases 59 to 64 are examples of chronic pulmonary vascular diseases of several types. Two of the major roles of exercise testing are diagnosis and the noninvasive evaluation of the effect of therapy in these disorders. Other examples of pulmonary vascular diseases are presented in the group of patients with lung diseases.

Cases 65 to 67 are examples of subjects who were classified as having made a poor effort during exercise testing. It was concluded that they did not have evidence of organic disease reducing exercise tolerance.

Examples of disorders of the respiratory pump are presented in Cases 68 to 70. These disorders can be found in many forms, and the three cases presented are representative.

Cases 71 to 79 are among the most challenging in that these are patients with multiple abnormalities (complex cases). We have analyzed these cases with the intent of diagnosing the limiting disorder or disorders.

Case 80 is a woman with primary pulmonary hypertension. This case highlights the abnormalities that can be used to track the progress of the patient's disorder, and shows the changes in gas exchange with effective pulmonary vasodilator therapy.

Cases 81 and 82 are two men with heart disease. The first is a young man with a restrictive cardiomyopathy, the diagnosis of which was made by cardiopulmonary exercise testing and later documented by cardiac catheterization. The second shows a senior citizen who transitioned from a normal state to cardiomyopathy, thought to be based on diastolic dysfunction. Case 83 is an example of psychogenic dyspnea complicated by an impaired ability to increase cardiac output due to heavy β-adrenergic blockade. Case 84 is that of a hypertensive patient treated with β-adrenergic blockade to control her blood pressure. Although inadequate for controlling her arterial blood pressure, it did reduce her exercise tolerance by restricting her heart rate response to exercise. Case 85 is a man with a distant history of myocardial infarction and coronary artery bypass graft surgery. The exercise test was done to evaluate symptoms of decreasing exercise tolerance.

In a few instances, the conclusions we reached in the case analysis will not be obtained easily from the logical sequence suggested by the flowcharts (see Chapter 8). Nevertheless, we started each analysis by applying the flowchart logic. The supporting data listed under each diagnosis in the flowchart are intended to be used to confirm or refute the diagnosis derived from the flowchart analysis.

This chapter is intended to provide examples of cardiorespiratory disorders that reduce exercise tolerance and of the pathophysiology that accompanies each disorder. Cases with arterial blood gas measurements were preferred in the case selection process so that the effect of exercise on arterial blood gases could be illustrated in health and disease. Because of the variety of conditions that can interfere with the coupling of external to cellular respiration, it is not possible to include examples of all conditions that limit exercise. Nevertheless, we hope that the principles taught by the cases selected, and by the earlier chapters, provide the reader with the necessary physiologic background to interpret the many pathophysiologic conditions that lead to exercise intolerance.

Case 1 Normal Man

Clinical Findings

This 55-year-old executive was referred for exercise testing because of his complaint of decreased exercise tolerance. He complained of weakness, fatigue, and some dyspnea after jogging one block, but he could walk 3 miles on the level without difficulty. He had become symptomatic after recovery from an ankle injury 2 years earlier and felt unable to satisfactorily improve his exercise tolerance. He did not report chest pain, syncope, palpitations, coughing, or wheezing. He had smoked half a pack of cigarettes per day for 10 years but had reduced his smoking to three to four cigarettes per week. He took no medications. Physical examination, chest roentgenograms, and resting electrocardiogram (ECG) were normal.

Exercise Findings

The patient performed exercise on a cycle ergometer. He pedaled at 60 rpm without added load for 3 minutes. The work rate was then increased 20 W per minute to his symptom-limited maximum. Arterial blood was sampled every second minute, and intraarterial blood pressure was recorded from a percutaneously placed brachial artery catheter. The patient stopped exercise because of thigh fatigue. Twelve-lead ECG recordings remained normal during exercise.

Interpretation

Comments

The results of the respiratory function studies are within normal limits (Table 10.1.1).

Analysis

Referring to flowchart 1 (Chapter 8), the peak $\dot{V}O_2$ and anaerobic threshold are normal (Table 10.1.2).

See flowchart 2. The ECG and arterial blood gases (Table 10.1.3) are normal throughout exercise; the O_2 pulse at the maximum work rate is normal.

Conclusion

This is a normal man, with a high level of anxiety regarding his physical status.

TABLE 10.1.1.   Selected Respiratory Function Data

Measurement	Predicted	Measured
Age, yr		55
Sex		Male
Height, cm		182
Weight, kg	83	80
Hematocrit, %		41
VC, L	4.75	6.06
IC, L	3.17	4.16
TLC, L	7.08	8.24
FEV_1, L	3.76	4.52
FEV_1/VC, %	79	75
MVV, L/min	151	200
D_LCO, ml/mm Hg/min	28.8	28.3

TABLE 10.1.2.   Selected Exercise Data

Measurement	Predicted	Measured
Peak $\dot{V}O_2$, L/min	2.47	2.53
Maximum HR, beats/min	165	176
Maximum O_2 pulse, ml/beat	15.0	14.5
$\Delta\dot{V}O_2/\Delta WR$, ml/min/W	10.3	9.8
AT, L/min	>1.07	1.2
Blood pressure, mmHg (rest, max)		144/81, 225/87
Maximum $\dot{V}E$, L/min		107
Exercise breathing reserve, L/min	>15	93
PaO_2, mmHg (rest, max ex)		98, 110
$P(A - a)O_2$, mmHg (rest, max ex)		5, 15
$P(a - ET)CO_2$, mmHg (rest, max ex)		0, −5
VD/VT (rest, heavy ex)		0.26, 0.15
HCO_3^-, mEq/L (rest, 2-min recov)		25, 12

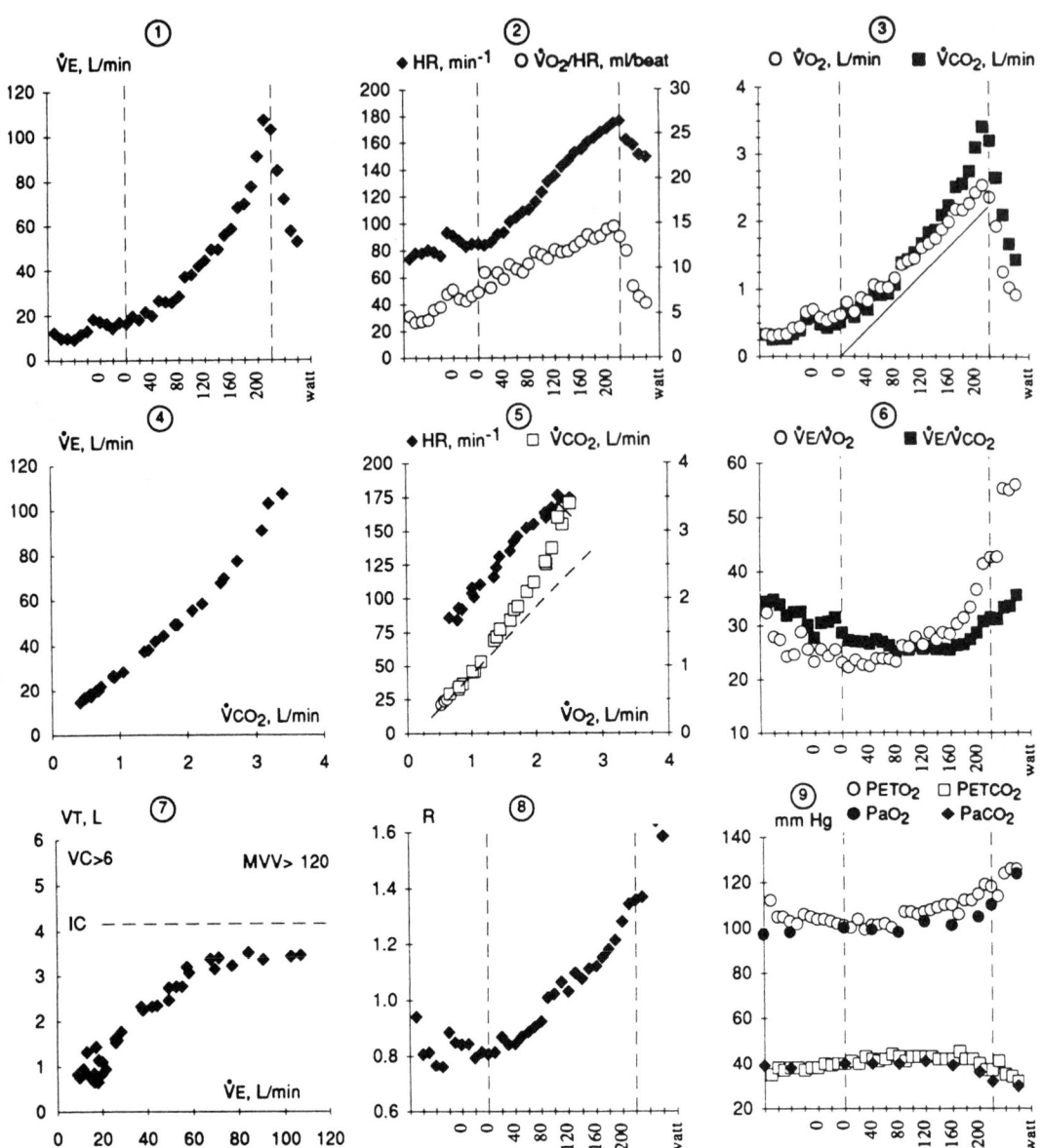

FIGURE 10.1.1.   **1:** Vertical dashed lines in panels 1 to 3 and 6, 8, and 9 indicate the beginning and the end of the increasing work period. **2:** Unloaded cycling is performed for 3 minutes before the left vertical dashed line. **3:** In panel 3, the diagonal line shows the increase of $\dot{V}O_2$ at a slope of 10 ml/min/W. **4:** In panel 5, the diagonal dashed line has a slope of 1; the x in the upper right is the predicted maximum heart rate and $\dot{V}O_2$ for the subject.

TABLE 10.1.3. Air Breathing

Time min	Work rate watts	BP mmHg	HR min⁻¹	f min⁻¹	$\dot{V}_E$ L/min BTPS	$\dot{V}_{CO_2}$ L/min STPD	$\dot{V}_{O_2}$ L/min STPD	$\dot{V}_{O_2}$/HR ml/beat	R	pH	HCO_3^- meq/L	P_{O_2}, mmHg ET	a	(A − a)	P_{CO_2}, mmHg ET	a	(a − ET)	$\dot{V}_E/\dot{V}_{CO_2}$	$\dot{V}_E/\dot{V}_{O_2}$	V_D/V_T
	Rest	153/87								7.42	25		97			39				
	Rest		74	14	12.2	0.32	0.34	4.6	0.94			112			35			34	32	
	Rest		78	13	9.8	0.25	0.31	4.0	0.81			105			38			35	28	
	Rest		78	13	9.9	0.26	0.32	4.1	0.81			105			37			34	27	
	Rest	144/81	80	11	9.2	0.26	0.34	4.3	0.76	7.42	24	103	98	5	38	38	0	32	24	0.26
	Rest		79	12	11.4	0.32	0.42	5.3	0.76			102			38			32	25	
	Rest		76	10	13.2	0.38	0.43	5.7	0.88			106			37			33	29	
	Unloaded		93	16	18.2	0.56	0.66	7.1	0.85			105			38			30	26	
	Unloaded		91	12	17.1	0.58	0.69	7.6	0.84			104			38			28	23	
	Unloaded		87	19	16.2	0.48	0.57	6.6	0.84			104			40			30	26	
	Unloaded		83	19	14.5	0.42	0.53	6.4	0.79			103			39			31	24	
	Unloaded		85	22	16.9	0.48	0.59	6.9	0.81			102			40			31	25	
	Unloaded	171/87	85	25	16.4	0.50	0.62	7.3	0.81	7.41	25	101	100	2	40	40	0	29	23	0.21
0.5	20		84	24	19.7	0.65	0.80	9.5	0.81			100			41			27	22	
1.0	20		86	28	18.1	0.58	0.67	7.8	0.87			104			40			27	23	
1.5	40		92	23	21.6	0.73	0.87	9.5	0.84			99			43			27	23	
2.0	40	183/84	93	18	19.9	0.69	0.82	8.8	0.84	7.40	24	101	99	5	42	40	−2	27	22	0.18
2.5	60		101	17	26.7	0.92	1.06	10.5	0.87			101			41			27	24	
3.0	60		104	17	26.0	0.91	1.03	9.9	0.88			102			42			27	24	
3.5	80		108	16	25.8	0.93	1.03	9.5	0.90			100			44			26	24	
4.0	80	195/81	110	16	28.4	1.07	1.16	10.5	0.92	7.38	23	103	98	9	43	40	−3	25	23	0.14
4.5	100		116	16	37.3	1.38	1.37	11.8	1.01			107			41			26	26	
5.0	100		123	17	38.1	1.44	1.41	11.5	1.02			107			43			25	26	
5.5	120		131	18	42.0	1.54	1.45	11.1	1.06			106			43			26	28	
6.0	120	207/87	135	19	44.5	1.67	1.62	12.0	1.03	7.37	23	107	103	7	43	41	−2	26	26	0.17
6.5	140		142	18	49.4	1.83	1.67	11.8	1.10			108			43			26	29	
7.0	140		146	20	49.4	1.87	1.74	11.9	1.07			109			42			26	27	
7.5	160		152	20	55.5	2.09	1.88	12.4	1.11			110			42			26	29	
8.0	160	213/90	155	19	58.3	2.23	1.99	12.8	1.12	7.35	21	110	101	13	42	39	−3	25	28	0.13
8.5	180		160	20	67.7	2.51	2.18	13.6	1.15			106			45			26	30	
9.0	180		163	22	69.5	2.55	2.16	13.3	1.18			112			42			27	31	
9.5	200		167	24	77.3	2.74	2.26	13.5	1.21			112			42			27	33	
10.0	200	225/87	170	27	90.7	3.10	2.42	14.2	1.28	7.31	18	115	105	15	40	36	−4	29	37	0.16
10.5	220		174	31	107.2	3.40	2.53	14.5	1.34			119			37			31	41	
11.0	220	216/90	176	30	102.9	3.20	2.36	13.4	1.36	7.30	15	118	110	15	37	32	−5	31	43	0.14
	Recovery		162	24	84.3	2.64	1.93	11.9	1.37			114			41			31	43	
	Recovery		158	21	71.5	2.10	1.26	8.0	1.67			124			35			33	55	
	Recovery		151	18	57.6	1.67	1.02	6.8	1.64			126			34			34	55	
	Recovery	165/75	149	19	52.7	1.44	0.91	6.1	1.58	7.22	12	126	124	5	32	30	−2	35	56	0.18

Case 2 Normal Athlete

Clinical Findings

This 31-year-old physiologist was a frequent marathon runner. He had no known health problems and trained several times weekly.

Exercise Findings

The subject performed exercise on a cycle ergometer. He pedaled without added load at 60 rpm for 2 minutes. The work rate was then increased 30 W every minute to his symptom-limited maximum. There were no arrhythmias, and the ECG remained normal.

Interpretation

Comments

This case is presented to illustrate the results of a normal, athletic subject.

Analysis

Referring to flowchart 1, the peak $\dot{V}O_2$ and the anaerobic threshold are considerably above the predicted values (Table 10.2.2). The predicted values are, of course, those for a sedentary population. The results of this study demonstrate how much better an athlete can perform than the average member of the sedentary group. The exceptionally high O_2 pulse at maximum work rate reflects the large stroke volume and $C(a - \bar{v})O_2$ that this subject must have. Assuming that the mixed venous O_2 saturation was as low as 20%, the O_2 pulse of 28.3 mL/beat would indicate that the subject's stroke volume must be approximately 175 mL. The normal ventilatory equivalents for O_2 and CO_2 at the anaerobic threshold (panel 6, Fig. 10.2.1) reflect the ventilation–perfusion matching of a normal subject. The maximum exercise ventilation is approximately equal to his maximum voluntary ventilation (MVV). Thus, his breathing reserve is approximately zero, a common finding in exceptionally fit people.

Conclusion

This is an exceptionally fit, normal subject.

TABLE 10.2.1. Selected Respiratory Function Data

Measurement	Predicted	Measured
Age, yr		31
Sex		Male
Height, cm		182
Weight, kg	83	81
Hematocrit, %		43
VC, L	5.48	6.27
IC, L	3.65	3.56
FEV$_1$, L	4.43	4.51
FEV$_1$/VC, %	81	72
MVV, L/min	182	185

TABLE 10.2.2. Selected Exercise Data

Measurement	Predicted	Measured
Peak $\dot{V}O_2$, L/min	3.22	4.95
Maximum HR, beats/min	189	175
Maximum O_2 pulse, ml/beat	17.0	28.3
$\Delta\dot{V}O_2/\Delta WR$, ml/min/W	10.3	11.5
AT, L/min	>1.32	2.5
Maximum $\dot{V}E$, L/min		186
Exercise breathing reserve, L/min	>15	−1

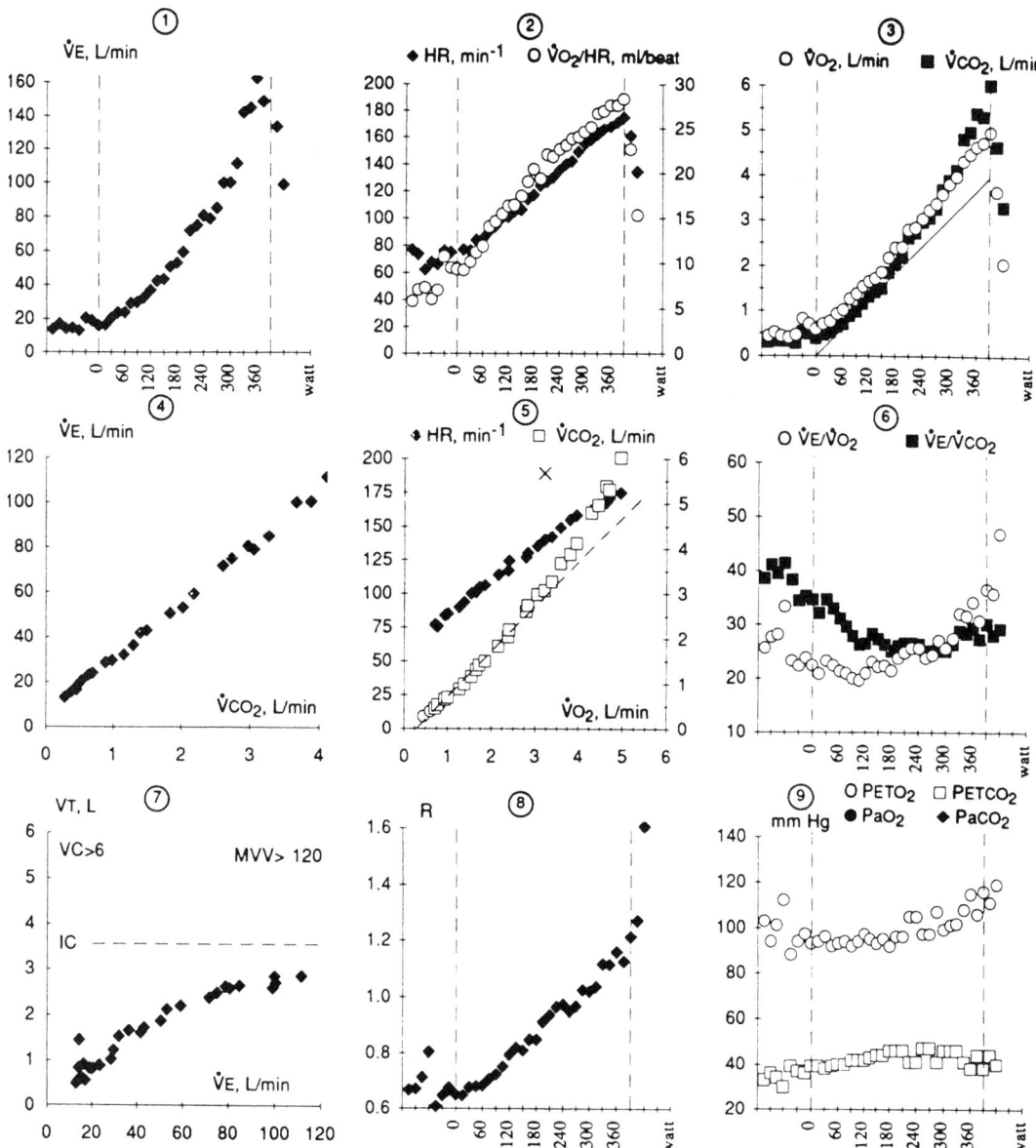

FIGURE 10.2.1. **1:** Vertical dashed lines in panels 1 to 3 and 6, 8, and 9 indicate the beginning and the end of the increasing work period. **2:** Unloaded cycling is performed for 3 minutes before the left vertical dashed line. **3:** In panel 3, the diagonal line shows the increase of $\dot{V}O_2$ at a slope of 10 ml/min/W. **4:** In panel 5, the diagonal dashed line has a slope of 1; the *x* in the upper right is the predicted maximum heart rate and $\dot{V}O_2$ for the subject.

TABLE 10.2.3. Air Breathing

Time min	Work rate watts	BP mmHg	HR min⁻¹	f min⁻¹	V̇E L/min BTPS	V̇CO₂ L/min STPD	V̇O₂ L/min STPD	V̇O₂/HR ml/beat	R	pH	HCO₃⁻ meq/L	PO₂ ET	PO₂ a	PO₂ (A−a)	PCO₂ ET	PCO₂ a	PCO₂ (a−ET)	V̇E/V̇CO₂	V̇E/V̇O₂	VD/VT
	Rest		77	25	13.7	0.30	0.45	5.8	0.67			103			33			39	26	
	Rest		74	31	17.0	0.35	0.52	7.0	0.67			94			36			41	28	
	Rest		62	17	14.1	0.32	0.45	7.3	0.71			101			34			40	28	
	Rest		68	10	14.5	0.33	0.41	6.0	0.80			112			30			41	33	
	Unloaded		66	27	13.0	0.28	0.46	7.0	0.61			88			39			38	23	
	Unloaded		76	25	20.4	0.53	0.82	10.8	0.65			94			37			34	22	
	Unloaded		75	23	18.9	0.48	0.71	9.5	0.68			97			36			35	24	
	Unloaded		64	26	15.7	0.39	0.60	9.4	0.65			93			39			35	22	
0.5	30		77	18	16.3	0.46	0.71	9.2	0.65			94			39			32	21	
1.0	30		76	25	20.1	0.52	0.77	10.1	0.68			96			38			35	23	
1.5	60		84	26	23.3	0.64	0.94	11.2	0.68			92			39			33	22	
2.0	60		85	27	23.8	0.69	1.01	11.9	0.68			93			40			31	21	
2.5	90		90	28	28.7	0.89	1.26	14.0	0.71			94			40			30	21	
3.0	90		94	24	29.6	0.99	1.37	14.6	0.72			92			42			28	20	
3.5	120		100	21	32.2	1.16	1.54	15.4	0.75			94			42			26	20	
4.0	120		101	22	36.5	1.31	1.65	16.3	0.79			97			42			26	21	
4.5	150		105	26	41.9	1.41	1.72	16.4	0.82			95			43			28	23	
5.0	150		106	25	43.1	1.50	1.85	17.5	0.81			93			44			27	22	
5.5	180		114	27	50.6	1.84	2.17	19.0	0.85			95			44			26	22	
6.0	180		117	25	53.2	2.03	2.39	20.4	0.85			92			46			25	21	
6.5	210		124	27	59.3	2.19	2.40	19.4	0.91			96			46			26	24	
7.0	210		127	30	71.7	2.61	2.79	22.0	0.94			96			46			26	25	
7.5	240		130	30	75.0	2.73	2.83	21.8	0.96			105			41			27	26	
8.0	240		135	31	80.6	2.97	3.05	22.6	0.97			105			41			26	26	
8.5	270		140	30	78.9	3.06	3.22	23.0	0.95			97			47			25	24	
9.0	270		142	32	85.0	3.27	3.38	23.8	0.97			97			47			25	24	
9.5	300		149	35	100.0	3.67	3.58	24.0	1.03			107			41			26	27	
10.0	300		155	37	100.4	3.88	3.80	24.5	1.02			99			46			25	26	
10.5	330		158	39	111.6	4.11	3.96	25.1	1.04			101			46			26	27	
11.0	330		162	48	142.4	4.81	4.31	26.6	1.12			102			46			29	32	
11.5	360		166	48	144.8	4.97	4.46	26.9	1.11			108			41			28	32	
12.0	360		168	53	162.6	5.38	4.64	27.6	1.16			115			38			29	34	
12.5	390		171	50	149.1	5.31	4.71	27.5	1.13			106			44			27	31	
13.0	390		175	63	186.0	6.01	4.95	28.3	1.21			116			38			30	36	
	Recovery		161	46	133.7	4.63	3.64	22.6	1.27			111			44			28	36	
	Recovery		134	38	99.1	3.29	2.05	15.3	1.60			119			40			29	47	

Case 3 Normal Man: Air and Oxygen Breathing Studies

Clinical Findings

The patient was a 59-year-old retired shipyard worker with a history of asbestos exposure and a 2-pack/day history of cigarette smoking. He had stopped working 4 years previously. He was asymptomatic at the time of this examination. Physical and laboratory examinations were normal; chest roentgenograms revealed focal pleural plaques with calcification.

Exercise Findings

After we obtained informed consent, the patient participated in a blinded-crossover exercise study on a cycle ergometer, receiving one of two humidified gas mixtures (compressed air or 100% oxygen) just prior to and during each study. He pedaled at 60 rpm without added load for 3 minutes. The work rate was then increased 15 W per minute to his symptom-limited maximum. Arterial blood was sampled every second minute, and intraarterial blood pressure was recorded from a percutaneously placed brachial artery catheter. He rested 1 hour between the two studies and exercised to his maximum tolerance on each occasion. On both occasions, he stopped exercise because of general fatigue. Resting and exercise ECG readings were normal.

Interpretation

Comments

Resting respiratory function is normal (Table 10.3.1). The exercise test was repeated with the patient breathing O_2, as part of an experimental study. At rest, the patient acutely hyperventilated while breathing with the mouthpiece; this ceased as soon as the exercise started. The associated relative hypoventilation noted in the transition from rest to unloaded cycling (panel 9, Fig. 10.3.1) caused a simultaneous marked decrease in R (panel 8, Fig. 10.3.1).

Analysis

Referring to flowchart 1, the peak $\dot{V}O_2$ is normal (Table 10.3.2 and panel 3 of Fig. 10.3.1). Referring to flowchart 2, the ECG and arterial blood gases at peak $\dot{V}O_2$ are normal (branch point 2.1). The subject is not obese (branch point 2.2). Although the patient and we thought that he was volunteering for this study as a normal subject, we noted a resting tachycardia that persisted during exercise, so that he went 31 beats per minute higher than his maximum predicted heart rate at the peak work rate. As a consequence, he had a reduced peak O_2 pulse. Questioning the patient about medication and ex-

TABLE 10.3.1.   Selected Respiratory Function Data

Measurement	Predicted	Measured
Age, yr		59
Sex		Male
Height, cm		155
Weight, kg	62	53
Hematocrit, %		46
VC, L	2.90	3.19
IC, L	1.94	2.12
TLC, L	4.51	4.62
FEV$_1$, L	2.26	2.49
FEV$_1$/VC, %	78	78
MVV, L/min	112	118
D$_L$CO, ml/mm Hg/min	19.9	20.7

TABLE 10.3.2.   Selected Exercise Data

Measurement	Predicted	Air	O_2
Peak $\dot{V}CO_2$, L/min		2.03	1.93
Peak $\dot{V}O_2$, L/min	1.65	1.57	
Maximum HR, beats/min	161	192	188
Maximum O_2 pulse, ml/beat	10.2	8.2	
$\Delta\dot{V}O_2/\Delta WR$, ml/min/W	10.3	9.7	
AT, L/min	>0.73	0.8	
Blood pressure, mmHg (rest, max)		100/56, 213/88	100/63, 231/94
Maximum $\dot{V}E$, L/min		89	72
Exercise breathing reserve, L/min	>15	29	46
PaO$_2$, mmHg (rest, max ex)		102, 101	585, 586
P(A − a)O$_2$, mmHg (rest, max ex)		24, 25	103, 93
P(a − ET)CO$_2$, mmHg (rest, max ex)		−4, −4	1, −2
VD/VT (rest, heavy ex)		0.19, 0.27	0.37, 0.26
HCO$_3^-$ mEq/L (rest, 2-min recov)		23, 12	19, 14

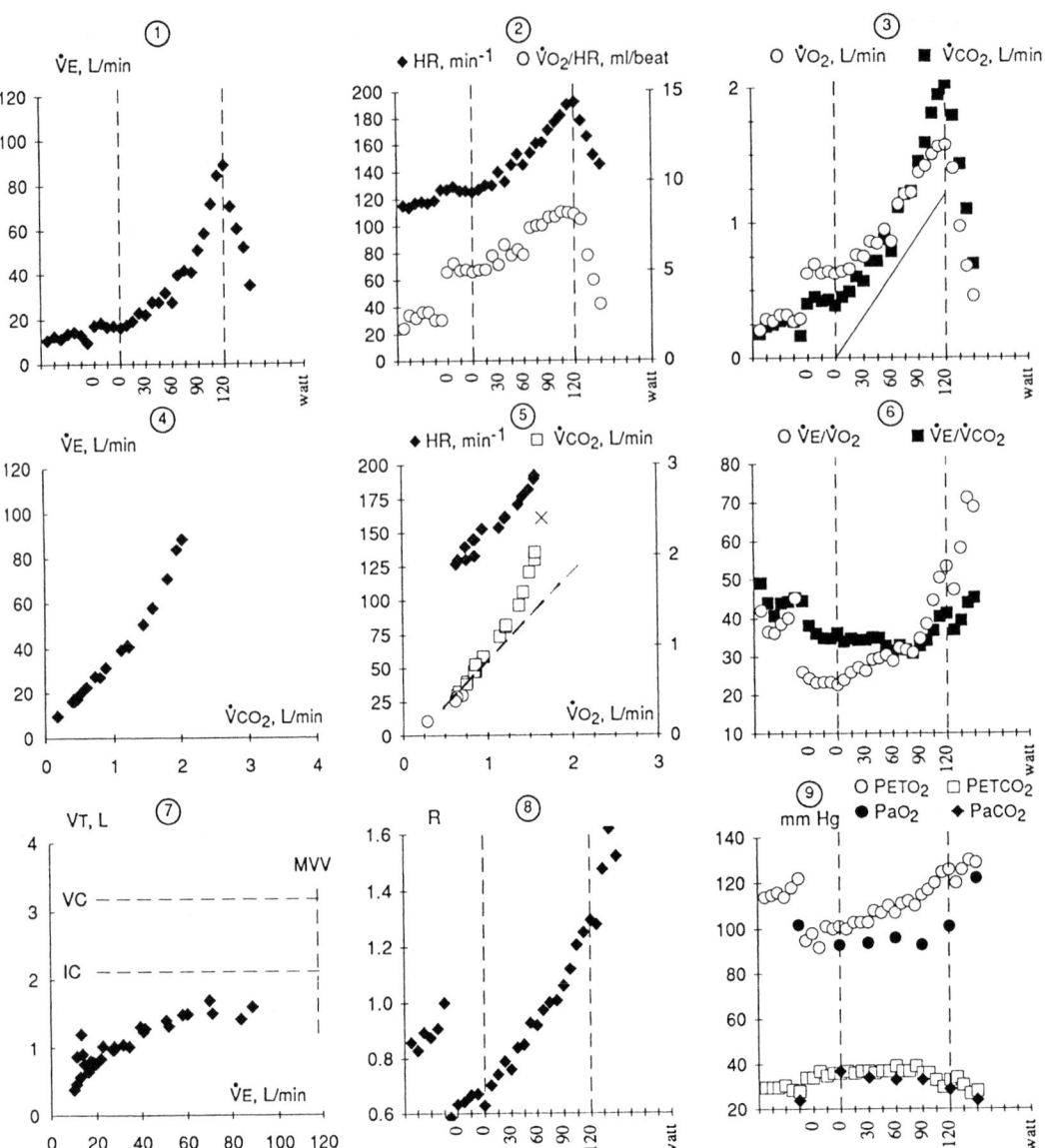

FIGURE 10.3.1.   Air breathing. **1:** Vertical dashed lines in panels 1 to 3 and 6, 8, and 9 indicate the beginning and the end of the increasing work period. **2:** Unloaded cycling is performed for 3 minutes before the left vertical dashed line. **3:** In panel 3, the diagonal line shows the increase of $\dot{V}O_2$ at a slope of 10 mL/min/W. **4:** In panel 5, the diagonal dashed line has a slope of 1; the x in the upper right is the predicted maximum heart rate and $\dot{V}O_2$ for the subject.

amining the patient for hyperthyroidism did not provide us with a satisfactory explanation of his tachycardia. The recommendation was to restudy this subject on another occasion with the request that he take no recreational drugs or medications.

The major difference between the air and O_2 breathing studies is a significantly reduced exercise ventilation in the latter when performing at the same work rate (Tables 10.3.3 and 10.3.4 and panel 1 of Figs. 10.3.1 and 10.3.2). Consistent with this is the higher $PaCO_2$ at maximum exercise during the

O_2 breathing study. Arterial oxygen tension was normal (585 mm Hg) at rest and remained unchanged throughout exercise during the oxygen breathing study, demonstrating the absence of a significant right-to-left shunt.

Conclusion

Probably a normal subject with unexplained tachycardia. Repeat study recommended.

TABLE 10.3.3.   Air Breathing

Time min	Work rate watts	BP mmHg	HR min⁻¹	f min⁻¹	$\dot{V}_E$ L/min BTPS	$\dot{V}_{CO_2}$ L/min STPD	$\dot{V}_{O_2}$ L/min STPD	$\dot{V}_{O_2}$/HR ml/beat	R	pH	HCO_3^- meq/L	P_{O_2} ET	P_{O_2} a	P_{O_2} (A−a)	P_{CO_2} ET	P_{CO_2} a	P_{CO_2} (a−ET)	$\dot{V}_E/\dot{V}_{CO_2}$	$\dot{V}_E/\dot{V}_{O_2}$	V_D/V_T
	Rest		115	23	10.8	0.18	0.21	1.8	0.86			114			30			49	42	
	Rest		114	22	12.5	0.24	0.29	2.5	0.83			115			30			44	37	
	Rest		117	13	11.3	0.25	0.28	2.4	0.89			116			30			41	36	
	Rest		118	15	13.6	0.28	0.32	2.7	0.88			114			31			44	39	
	Rest		117	19	14.5	0.29	0.32	2.7	0.91			118			29			44	40	
	Rest	100/56	119	11	13.2	0.27	0.27	2.3	1.00	7.48	18	122	102	24	28	24	−4	45	45	0.19
	Unloaded		127	25	9.7	0.17	0.29	2.3	0.59			95			34			45	26	
	Unloaded		127	21	17.1	0.40	0.63	5.0	0.63			98			34			38	24	
	Unloaded		129	23	18.2	0.45	0.70	5.4	0.64			92			37			36	23	
	Unloaded		126	23	16.7	0.42	0.63	5.0	0.67			101			35			35	23	
	Unloaded		126	24	17.0	0.43	0.64	5.1	0.67			100			36			35	23	
	Unloaded	150/75	125	25	16.3	0.39	0.62	5.0	0.63	7.41	23	101	93	3	36	37	1	36	23	0.31
0.5	15		127	23	17.3	0.45	0.64	5.0	0.70			100			37			34	24	
1.0	15		130	25	19.2	0.49	0.66	5.1	0.74			103			36			35	26	
1.5	30		130	22	22.6	0.60	0.76	5.8	0.79			103			37			35	27	
2.0	30	163/75	140	26	21.9	0.57	0.75	5.4	0.76	7.40	21	103	94	14	37	34	−3	35	26	0.24
2.5	45		133	27	27.6	0.72	0.86	6.5	0.84			108			36			35	29	
3.0	45		145	28	27.6	0.72	0.85	5.9	0.85			107			37			35	30	
3.5	60		153	30	31.5	0.88	0.95	6.2	0.93			110			37			33	30	
4.0	60	194/81	145	28	27.2	0.79	0.86	5.9	0.92	7.40	20	107	96	19	39	33	−6	31	29	0.15
4.5	75		154	30	39.4	1.11	1.14	7.4	0.97			111			37			33	32	
5.0	75		161	32	41.4	1.21	1.21	7.5	1.00			112			37			32	32	
5.5	90		162	33	40.8	1.23	1.22	7.5	1.01			110			39			31	31	
6.0	90	194/75	171	36	50.8	1.45	1.37	8.0	1.06	7.39	20	115	93	25	36	33	−3	33	35	0.19
6.5	105		177	39	58.0	1.59	1.42	8.0	1.12			117			36			34	39	
7.0	105		182	47	71.0	1.81	1.50	8.2	1.21			120			33			37	45	
7.5	120		190	59	83.9	1.95	1.56	8.2	1.25			125			30			40	51	
8.0	120	213/88	192	55	88.6	2.03	1.57	8.2	1.29	7.37	16	126	101	25	33	29	−4	41	53	0.27
	Recovery		178	41	69.9	1.79	1.40	7.9	1.28			120			34			37	47	
	Recovery		166	40	60.0	1.43	0.97	5.8	1.47			126			31			40	58	
	Recovery		152	39	51.8	1.10	0.68	4.5	1.62			130			27			44	71	
	Recovery	169/63	145	34	34.6	0.70	0.46	3.2	1.52	7.33	12	129	122	11	28	24	−4	45	69	0.19

TABLE 10.3.4.   Oxygen Breathing

Time min	Work rate watts	BP mmHg	HR min^{-1}	f min^{-1}	$\dot{V}_E$ L/min BTPS	$\dot{V}_{CO_2}$ L/min STPD	$\dot{V}_{O_2}$ L/min STPD	$\dot{V}_{O_2}$/HR ml/beat	R	pH	HCO_3^- meq/L	P_{O_2}, mmHg ET	a	(A − a)	P_{CO_2}, mmHg ET	a	(a − ET)	$\dot{V}_E$/$\dot{V}_{CO_2}$	$\dot{V}_E$/$\dot{V}_{O_2}$	V_D/V_T
	Rest		120	14	13.9	0.24									23			52		
	Rest		120	12	13.2	0.23									23			53		
	Rest		119	11	15.1	0.27									22			52		
	Rest		123	22	15.9	0.23									22			61		
	Rest		121	19	17.4	0.27									24			58		
	Rest	100/63	119	15	11.4	0.17				7.49	19		585	103	24	25	1	60		0.37
	Unloaded		128	38	13.6	0.13									29			80		
	Unloaded		125	44	11.9	0.10									32			82		
	Unloaded		119	41	9.8	0.07									35			90		
	Unloaded		121	28	13.9	0.24									35			48		
	Unloaded		123	28	13.9	0.23									36			50		
	Unloaded	163/81	122	22	12.7	0.28									37			39		
0.5	15		129	23	16.1	0.38									37			37		
1.0	15		126	22	16.8	0.40									37			37		
1.5	30		130	23	17.5	0.43									37			36		
2.0	30	181/88	134	26	19.4	0.48				7.40	21		591	87	38	35	−3	36		0.28
2.5	45		134	23	22.2	0.61									39			33		
3.0	45		141	22	22.1	0.64									40			32		
3.5	60		145	22	23.9	0.78									40			28		
4.0	60	206/88	146	25	27.9	0.84				7.38	20		576	103	40	34	−6	31		0.16
4.5	75		152	27	32.3	0.96									40			31		
5.0	75		156	27	34.8	1.05									40			31		
5.5	90		160	29	39.0	1.17									41			31		
6.0	90	225/91	163	34	43.7	1.28				7.37	21		581	95	40	37	−3	32		0.25
6.5	105		174	39	51.6	1.40									38			34		
7.0	105		176	42	56.3	1.55									37			34		
7.5	120		185	42	62.0	1.70									41			34		
8.0	120	231/94	188	45	71.7	1.93				7.35	18		586	93	36	34	−2	35		0.26
	Recovery		173	34	55.3	1.56									38			34		
	Recovery		156	29	46.9	1.25									36			36		
	Recovery		146	27	40.3	0.97									32			39		
	Recovery	219/75	140	30	32.7	0.69				7.33	14		584	102	30	27	−3	44		0.25

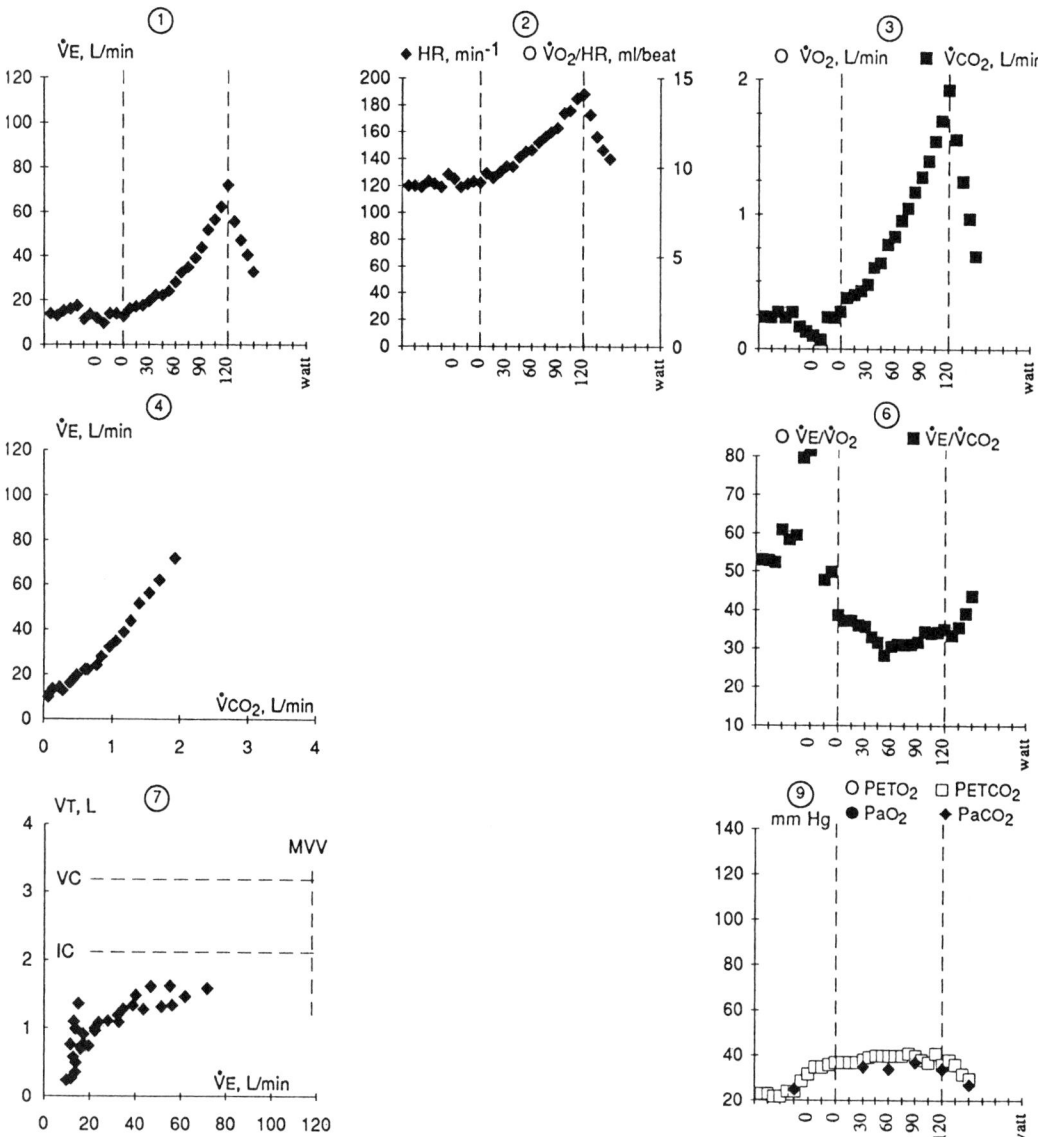

FIGURE 10.3.2.   Oxygen breathing. **1:** Vertical dashed lines in panels 1 to 3 and 6 and 9 indicate the beginning and the end of the increasing work period. **2:** Unloaded cycling is performed for 3 minutes before the left vertical dashed line.

Case 4 Normal Woman: Air and Oxygen Breathing Studies

Clinical Findings

This 45-year-old housewife was referred for evaluation of dyspnea. She had recently begun to increase her activity and felt that she was shorter of breath than she should be. Physical and laboratory examinations revealed no abnormalities.

Exercise Findings

The patient performed exercise on a cycle ergometer. She pedaled at 60 rpm without added load for 3 minutes. The work rate was then increased 10 W per minute to her symptom-limited maximum. Arterial blood was sampled every second minute, and intraarterial blood pressure was recorded from a percutaneously placed brachial artery catheter. A second incremental exercise test was performed with O_2 breathing 1.5 hours after recovery from the first test, with work rate increments of 20 W per minute. She stopped exercise in each case complaining of general fatigue and shortness of breath. Resting and exercise ECGs were normal.

Interpretation

Comments

Resting respiratory function (Table 10.4.1) and ECG are normal.

Analysis

Referring to flowchart 1, the peak $\dot{V}O_2$ and anaerobic threshold are normal (Table 10.4.2). See flowchart 2 for further analysis. There are no ECG abnormalities, and arterial blood gas values and VD/VT are normal throughout exercise (Table 10.4.3) (branch point 2.1). The patient is not obese (Table 10.4.1) (branch point 2.2). Thus, this patient has no limitation to exercise for her age and has no physiologic evidence of cardiovascular or pulmonary disease.

PaO_2 is also normal during 100% O_2 breathing (Table 10.4.4), ruling out a significant right-to-left shunt.

Of special note is that the patient was able to exercise to a higher work rate with a slightly lower heart rate during O_2 breathing instead of air breathing. Moreover, respiratory compensation for the metabolic acidosis (decrease in $PaCO_2$) was less evident during the O_2 breathing study.

TABLE 10.4.1.   Selected Respiratory Function Data

Measurement	Predicted	Measured
Age, yr		45
Sex		Female
Height, cm		165
Weight, kg	64	61
Hematocrit, %		40
VC, L	3.30	3.21
IC, L	2.20	1.99
FEV_1, L	2.68	2.71
FEV_1 VC, %	81	84
MVV, L/min	112	117
$D_L CO$, ml/mmHg/min	24.1	21.1

TABLE 10.4.2.   Selected Exercise Data

Measurement	Predicted	Room Air	O_2
Peak work rate, W		130	160
Peak $\dot{V}O_2$, L/min	1.60	1.71	
Maximum HR, beats/min	175	160	155
Maximum O_2 pulse, ml/beat	9.1	10.7	
$\Delta \dot{V}O_2/\Delta WR$, ml/min/W	10.3	11.9	
AT, L/min	>0.78	0.9	
Blood pressure, mmHg (rest, max)		138/81, 194/81	106/75, 181/88
Maximum $\dot{V}E$, L/min		70	54
Exercise breathing reserve, L/min	>15	47	63
PaO_2, mmHg (rest, max ex)		105, 108	643, 552
$P(A - a)O_2$, mmHg (rest, max ex)		5, 16	33, 117
$P(a - ET)CO_2$, mmHg (rest, max ex)		−1, −6	4, −3
VD/VT (rest, heavy ex)		0.21, 0.11	0.34, 0.18
HCO_3^-, mEq/L (rest, 2-min recov)		25, 13	25, unknown

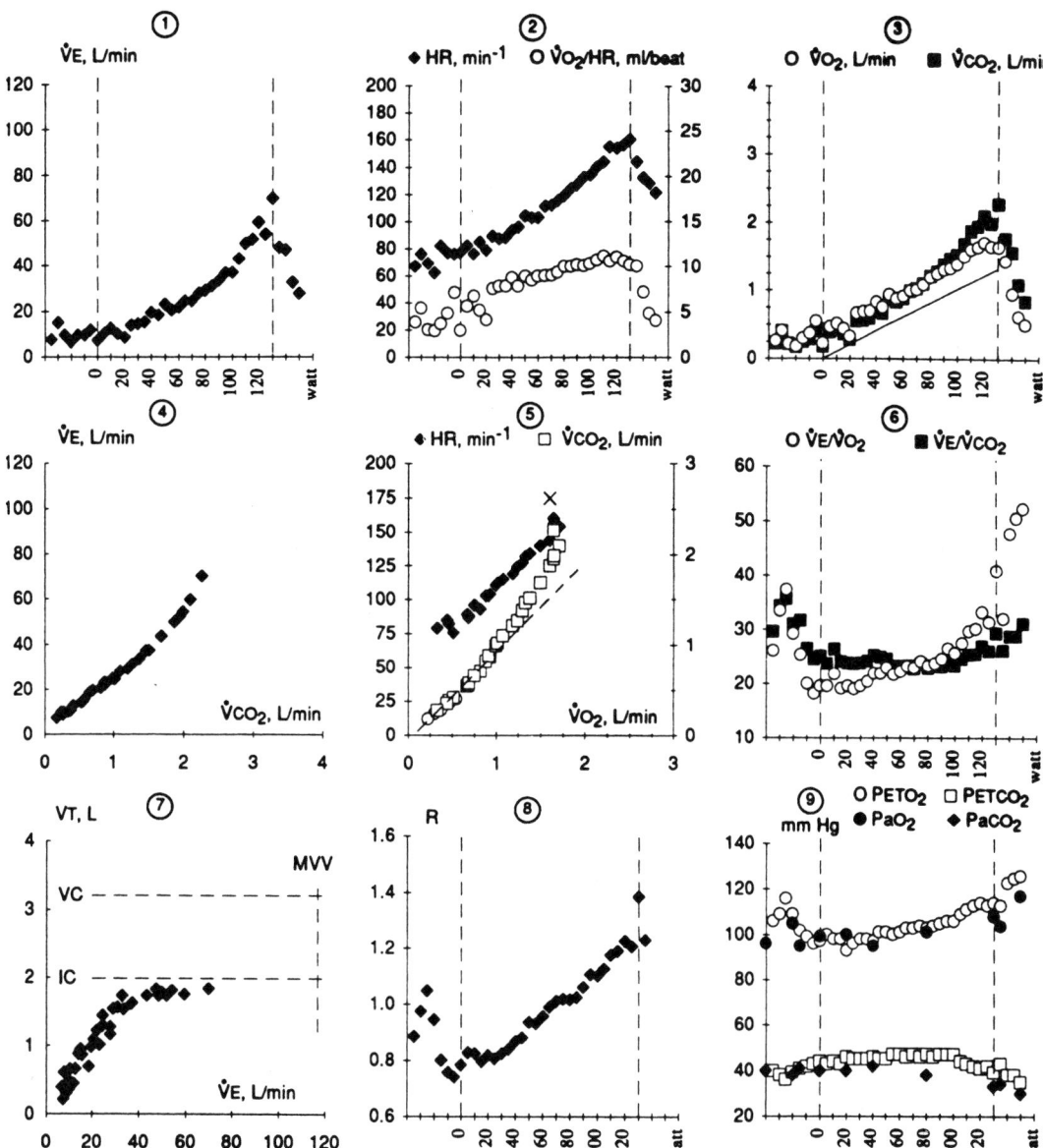

FIGURE 10.4.1.   Air breathing. **1:** Vertical dashed lines in panels 1 to 3 and 6, 8, and 9 indicate the beginning and the end of the increasing work period. **2:** Unloaded cycling is performed for 3 minutes before the left vertical dashed line. **3:** In panel 3, the diagonal line shows the increase of $\dot{V}O_2$ at a slope of 10 ml/min/W. **4:** In panel 5, the diagonal dashed line has a slope of 1; the x in the upper right is the predicted maximum heart rate and $\dot{V}O_2$ for the subject.

Conclusion

Our final assessment is that this patient was normal and her symptoms were the result of anxiety regarding her performance at sports.

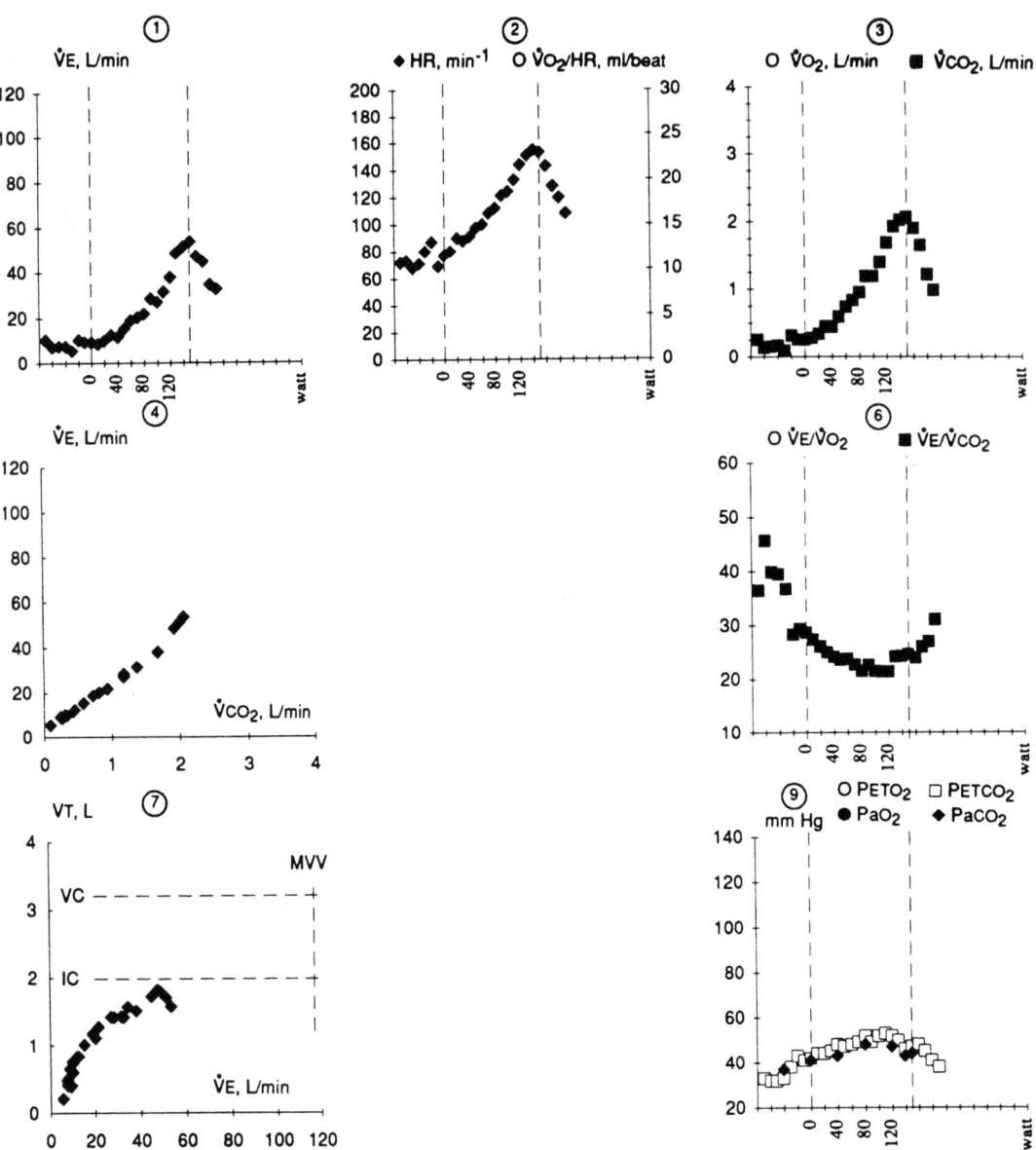

FIGURE 10.4.2.   Oxygen breathing. **1:** Vertical dashed lines in panels 1 to 3 and 6 and 9 indicate the beginning and the end of the increasing work period. **2:** Unloaded cycling is performed for 3 minutes before the left vertical dashed line.

TABLE 10.4.3. Air Breathing

Time min	Work rate watts	BP mmHg	HR min⁻¹	f min⁻¹	V̇E L/min BTPS	V̇CO₂ L/min STPD	V̇O₂ L/min STPD	V̇O₂/HR ml/beat	R	pH	HCO₃⁻ meq/L	PO₂ ET	PO₂ a	PO₂ (A−a)	PCO₂ ET	PCO₂ a	PCO₂ (a−ET)	V̇E/V̇CO₂	V̇E/V̇O₂	VD/VT
	Rest	138/81								7.42	25		96			40				
	Rest		67	13	7.9	0.23	0.26	3.9	0.88			106			40			30	26	
	Rest		76	16	15.1	0.40	0.41	5.4	0.98			109			38			34	34	
	Rest		69	22	9.7	0.22	0.21	3.0	1.05			116			36			36	37	
	Rest	138/75	62	17	6.7	0.17	0.18	2.9	0.94	7.43	25	109	105	5	39	38	−1	31	29	0.21
	Unloaded	138/81	82	27	9.9	0.24	0.30	3.7	0.80	7.41	26	102	95	6	41	41	0	32	25	0.26
	Unloaded		77	28	9.8	0.28	0.37	4.8	0.76			99			42			27	20	
	Unloaded		76	27	12.1	0.40	0.54	7.1	0.74			96			43			25	18	
	Unloaded	144/75	77	34	7.4	0.18	0.23	3.0	0.78	7.41	25	97	99	2	44	40	−4	25	20	0.08
0.5	10		82	16	10.4	0.38	0.46	5.6	0.83			100			43			24	20	
1.0	10		76	19	12.7	0.42	0.51	6.7	0.82			98			44			26	22	
1.5	20		85	21	10.2	0.35	0.44	5.2	0.80			98			43			24	19	
2.0	20	144/75	79	29	8.9	0.27	0.33	4.2	0.82	7.41	25	93	100	3	46	40	−6	24	20	0.07
2.5	30		89	16	14.1	0.54	0.67	7.5	0.81			96			45			24	19	
3.0	30		87	16	14.7	0.56	0.68	7.8	0.82			98			45			24	20	
3.5	40		88	18	15.6	0.58	0.69	7.8	0.84			98			45			24	20	
4.0	40	144/75	93	20	19.6	0.71	0.82	8.8	0.87	7.39	25	97	95	8	46	42	−4	25	22	0.17
4.5	50		96	27	18.7	0.66	0.75	7.8	0.88			101			45			25	22	
5.0	50		104	23	23.3	0.87	0.93	8.9	0.94			101			45			25	23	
5.5	60		103	19	20.7	0.82	0.88	8.5	0.93			100			47			23	22	
6.0	60	156/75	103	18	22.0	0.88	0.92	8.9	0.96			101			47			23	22	
6.5	70		111	19	24.7	0.99	1.01	9.0	0.99			103			46			23	23	
7.0	70		112	17	24.6	1.02	1.01	9.0	1.01			103			47			23	23	
7.5	80		115	24	28.0	1.10	1.08	9.4	1.02			104			46			24	24	
8.0	80	163/75	119	19	29.3	1.21	1.19	10.0	1.02	7.37	22	103	101	11	47	38	−9	23	23	0.01
8.5	90		124	20	31.2	1.27	1.24	10.0	1.02			104			46			23	24	
9.0	90		127	22	33.7	1.38	1.30	10.2	1.06			105			47			23	24	
9.5	100		132	23	37.1	1.47	1.33	10.1	1.11			106			47			24	26	
10.0	100	175/81	134	23	37.4	1.52	1.38	10.3	1.10			106			47			23	26	
10.5	110		140	25	43.5	1.69	1.50	10.7	1.13			109			44			24	28	
11.0	110		144	28	50.0	1.88	1.60	11.1	1.18			111			43			25	30	
11.5	120		155	30	52.1	1.95	1.64	10.6	1.19			113			42			25	30	
12.0	120		154	34	59.6	2.10	1.71	11.1	1.23			114			41			27	33	
12.5	130		156	30	54.3	1.99	1.65	10.6	1.21			113			42			26	31	
13.0	130	194/81	160	38	70.0	2.27	1.64	10.3	1.38	7.31	16	114	108	16	39	33	−6	29	41	0.11
	Recovery	156/69	144	28	48.6	1.77	1.44	10.0	1.23	7.28	16	113	104	17	43	34	−9	26	32	0.03
	Recovery		132	26	47.5	1.57	0.95	7.2	1.65			123			38			29	48	
	Recovery		128	19	33.0	1.09	0.62	4.8	1.76			125			38			29	51	
	Recovery	131/63	121	22	28.0	0.84	0.50	4.1	1.68	7.26	13	126	117	13	35	30	−5	31	52	0.07

TABLE 10.4.4.   Oxygen Breathing

Time min	Work rate watts	BP mmHg	HR min⁻¹	f min⁻¹	$\dot{V}_E$ L/min BTPS	$\dot{V}_{CO_2}$ L/min STPD	$\dot{V}_{O_2}$ L/min STPD	$\dfrac{\dot{V}_{O_2}}{HR}$ ml/beat	R	pH	HCO₃⁻ meq/L	P_{O_2}, mmHg ET	a	(A − a)	P_{CO_2}, mmHg ET	a	(a − ET)	$\dfrac{\dot{V}_E}{\dot{V}_{CO_2}}$	$\dfrac{\dot{V}_E}{\dot{V}_{O_2}}$	$\dfrac{V_D}{V_T}$
	Rest		72	14	10.3	0.25									33			36		
	Rest		73	15	7.2	0.13									32			46		
	Rest		68	18	7.5	0.15									32			40		
	Rest	106/75	71	15	7.6	0.16				7.44	25		643	33	33	37	4	40		0.34
	Unloaded		80	27	5.6	0.09									38			37		
	Unloaded		87	17	10.2	0.31									43			28		
	Unloaded		69	23	9.3	0.25									41			29		
	Unloaded	113/69	77	24	9.2	0.25				7.39	24		605	67	42	41	−1	29		0.21
0.5	20		80	13	8.5	0.27									44			27		
1.0	20		90	13	10.0	0.34									44			26		
1.5	40		88	15	12.5	0.45									45			25		
2.0	40	125/69	91	14	11.6	0.43				7.39	26		595	75	48	43	−5	24		0.15
2.5	60		97	15	15.2	0.59									47			24		
3.0	60		100	16	18.8	0.73									48			24		
3.5	80		108	18	20.1	0.82									49			23		
4.0	80	144/75	112	17	21.7	0.94				7.34	25		601	64	52	48	−4	22		0.15
4.5	100		121	20	28.3	1.18									49			23		
5.0	100		124	19	27.1	1.18									52			22		
5.5	120		133	22	31.5	1.38									53			21		
6.0	120	169/81	144	25	38.0	1.68				7.29	22		587	79	52	47	−5	21		0.13
6.5	140		151	27	48.7	1.92									50			24		
7.0	140	175/81	155	30	51.4	2.01				7.30	21		564	106	46	43	−3	24		0.17
7.5	160	181/88	153	34	53.6	2.06				7.28	20		552	117	47	44	−3	25		0.19
	Recovery		143	26	47.4	1.89									48			24		
	Recovery		128	26	44.8	1.64									45			26		
	Recovery		120	22	34.6	1.21									41			27		
	Recovery		108	23	32.5	0.98									38			31		

Case 5 Normal Woman

Clinical Findings

This nonsmoking occupational therapist was referred for evaluation of dyspnea. She described the sensation as the inability to take a deep breath. She also noted nervousness, dizziness, and shortness of breath while eating. She was usually active in sports, but also noted shortness of breath in these activities. Physical examination was normal except for resting tachycardia and a grade 2/6 systolic ejection murmur. Echocardiogram revealed a mitral valve prolapse. There were no dysrhythmias on 24-hour Holter monitoring. Chest roentgenograms, ECG, and respiratory function tests were normal, except for some reduction in expiratory flow rates attributable to reduced effort.

Exercise Findings

The patient performed exercise on a cycle ergometer. She pedaled at 60 rpm without added load for 3 minutes. The work rate was then increased 15 W per minute to her symptom-limited maximum. Arterial blood was sampled every second minute, and intraarterial blood pressure was recorded from a percutaneously placed brachial artery catheter. She stopped pedaling at 150 W complaining of fatigue and a feeling of palpitations. She felt somewhat short of breath. There were no abnormal ST changes or arrhythmia. No wheezing or diminution of FEV_1 occurred in the postexercise period.

Interpretation

Comments

This young woman, who experienced occasions of dyspnea, has normal lung volumes and flow rates, indicating the absence of restrictive or obstructive lung disease (Table 10.5.1). In addition, her diffusing capacity is normal. Her resting ECG is also normal.

Analysis

Referring to flowchart 1, the peak $\dot{V}O_2$ and anaerobic threshold are normal (Table 10.5.2). Referring to flowchart 2, her ECG and O_2 pulse at maximum exercise are normal, and her arterial blood gases remain normal through exercise (branch point 2.1). This patient is not obese (branch point 2.2). This

TABLE 10.5.1.   Selected Respiratory Function Data

Measurement	Predicted	Measured
Age, yr		24
Sex		Female
Height, cm		159
Weight, kg	61	51
Hematocrit, %		40
VC, L	3.60	3.50
IC, L	2.40	2.11
TLC, L	4.91	4.71
FEV_1, L	3.01	2.55
FEV_1/VC, %	84	73
MVV, L/min	115	118
$D_L co$, ml/mm Hg/min	26.5	29.8

TABLE 10.5.2.   Selected Exercise Data

Measurement	Predicted	Measured
Peak $\dot{V}O_2$, L/min	1.84	1.62
Maximum HR, beats/min	196	198
Maximum O_2 pulse, ml/beat	9.4	8.2
$\Delta\dot{V}O_2/\Delta WR$, ml/min/W	10.3	9.1
AT, L/min	>0.83	1.0
Blood pressure, mmHg (rest, max)		135/84, 177/87
Maximum $\dot{V}E$, L/min		64
Exercise breathing reserve, L/min	>15	54
Pao_2, mmHg (rest, max ex)		95, 100
$P(A - a)O_2$, mmHg (rest, max ex)		14, 17
$P(a - ET)CO_2$, mmHg (rest, max ex)		−1, −3
VD/VT (rest, heavy ex)		0.20, 0.16
HCO_3^-, mEq/L (rest, 2-min recov)		25, 15

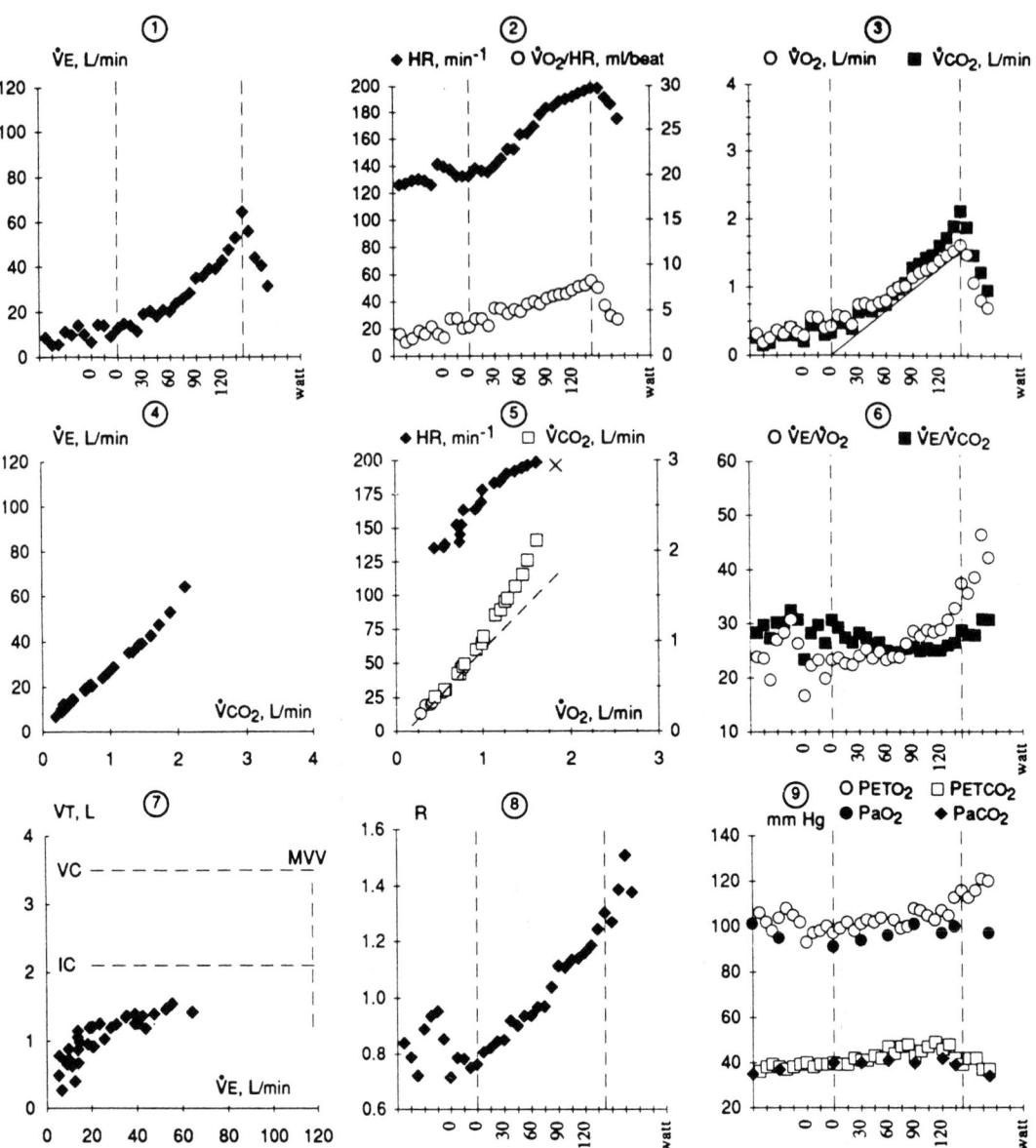

FIGURE 10.5.1.   **1:** Vertical dashed lines in panels 1 to 3 and 6, 8, and 9 indicate the beginning and the end of the increasing work period. **2:** Unloaded cycling is performed for 3 minutes before the left vertical dashed line. **3:** In panel 3, the diagonal line shows the increase of $\dot{V}O_2$ at a slope of 10 ml/min/W. **4:** In panel 5, the diagonal dashed line has a slope of 1; the x in the upper right is the predicted maximum heart rate and $\dot{V}O_2$ for the subject.

leads to the diagnosis of a normal subject with anxiety; however, she has a marked tachycardia at rest and an appropriate heart rate response to exercise. Hyperthyroidism was ruled out, and the tachycardia was not a persistent observation (Holter monitoring), as might be found with vasoregulatory asthenia.

Conclusion

This is a normal young woman with anxiety; however, the sensation of palpitations was not related to a cardiac arrhythmia. The patient deserves follow-up for endocrine disorders or other conditions that might account for her symptoms.

TABLE 10.5.3.   Air Breathing

Time min	Work rate watts	BP mmHg	HR min⁻¹	f min⁻¹	$\dot{V}_E$ L/min BTPS	$\dot{V}_{CO_2}$ L/min STPD	$\dot{V}_{O_2}$ L/min STPD	$\dot{V}_{O_2}$/HR ml/beat	R	pH	HCO₃⁻ meq/L	P_{O_2} ET	P_{O_2} a	(A − a)	P_{CO_2} ET	P_{CO_2} a	(a − ET)	$\dot{V}_E/\dot{V}_{CO_2}$	$\dot{V}_E/\dot{V}_{O_2}$	V_D/V_T
	Rest	135/84								7.47	25		101			35				
	Rest		126	12	8.4	0.26	0.31	2.5	0.84			106			36			28	24	
	Rest		127	11	5.4	0.15	0.19	1.5	0.79			102			38			30	24	
	Rest		129	7	5.5	0.18	0.25	1.9	0.72			98			39			27	20	
	Rest	144/84	130	18	11.2	0.32	0.36	2.8	0.89	7.44	25	104	95	14	38	37	−1	30	27	0.20
	Rest		129	11	9.7	0.29	0.31	2.4	0.94			108			37			30	28	
	Rest		126	13	13.7	0.39	0.41	3.3	0.95			105			38			32	31	
	Unloaded		141	14	10.1	0.29	0.34	2.4	0.85			102			39			31	26	
	Unloaded		139	25	6.8	0.20	0.28	2.0	0.71			93			40			23	17	
	Unloaded		137	21	14.2	0.44	0.56	4.1	0.79			97			38			28	22	
	Unloaded		132	12	13.8	0.43	0.55	4.2	0.78			98			39			30	23	
	Unloaded		132	14	9.1	0.30	0.40	3.0	0.75			100			39			26	20	
	Unloaded	141/81	132	32	12.5	0.32	0.42	3.2	0.76	7.42	25	97	91	9	40	40	0	31	23	0.23
0.5	15		138	15	14.7	0.46	0.57	4.1	0.81			99			39			29	24	
1.0	15		136	16	14.0	0.46	0.56	4.1	0.82			102			39			27	23	
1.5	30		135	17	11.5	0.38	0.45	3.3	0.84			98			42			26	22	
2.0	30	150/84	140	16	19.1	0.63	0.74	5.3	0.85	7.42	25	101	94	10	41	40	−1	28	24	0.22
2.5	45		145	17	20.4	0.69	0.75	5.2	0.92			103			41			27	25	
3.0	45		152	19	18.3	0.64	0.71	4.7	0.90			102			43			26	24	
3.5	60		152	23	21.0	0.72	0.77	5.1	0.94			104			42			26	25	
4.0	60	159/84	163	22	20.3	0.74	0.79	4.8	0.94	7.40	25	96	96	11	47	41	−6	25	23	0.14
4.5	75		164	19	23.8	0.90	0.93	5.7	0.97			103			44			25	24	
5.0	75		169	25	25.9	0.97	1.00	5.9	0.97			99			47			25	24	
5.5	90		178	24	28.6	1.05	1.01	5.7	1.04			100			48			25	26	
6.0	90	171/81	183	26	35.1	1.28	1.15	6.3	1.11	7.38	23	108	101	12	43	40	−3	26	29	0.15
6.5	105		184	26	35.6	1.34	1.21	6.6	1.11			107			45			25	28	
7.0	105		188	31	39.0	1.43	1.26	6.7	1.13			105			47			25	29	
7.5	120		190	28	39.1	1.47	1.29	6.8	1.14			103			49			25	28	
8.0	120	174/87	192	31	42.6	1.60	1.38	7.2	1.16	7.32	21	107	97	16	46	42	−4	25	29	0.17
8.5	135		194	34	47.6	1.73	1.46	7.5	1.18			105			48			26	31	
9.0	135	177/87	196	36	52.8	1.89	1.52	7.8	1.24	7.31	19	113	100	17	42	39	−3	26	33	0.15
9.5	150		198	45	64.2	2.11	1.62	8.2	1.30			116			39			29	37	
	Recovery		198	36	55.6	1.88	1.48	7.5	1.27			113			42			28	36	
	Recovery		191	37	43.9	1.47	1.06	5.5	1.39			116			42			28	38	
	Recovery		186	32	40.3	1.22	0.81	4.4	1.51			121			37			31	46	
	Recovery	153/78	175	25	31.2	0.95	0.69	3.9	1.38	7.27	15	120	97	26	37	34	−3	31	42	0.16

Case 6 Normal Man

Clinical Findings

This 37-year-old shipyard machinist was evaluated because of complaints of dyspnea. He stated that he had been unable to play a full game of baseball for the last 6 years and that he gets out of breath and has to stop after climbing three to four flights of stairs on shipboard. He never smoked. He denied cough, chest pain, edema, or other symptoms. Physical, roentgenographic, and laboratory examinations were normal.

Exercise Findings

The patient performed exercise on a cycle ergometer. He pedaled at 60 rpm without added load for 3 minutes. The work rate was then increased 25 W per minute to his symptom-limited maximum. Arterial blood was sampled every second minute, and intraarterial blood pressure was recorded from a percutaneously placed brachial artery catheter. He stopped exercise because of general fatigue. Resting and exercise ECGs were normal.

Interpretation

Comments

The results of this patient's resting respiratory function studies are normal (Table 10.6.1). The resting ECG is normal.

Analysis

Referring to flowchart 1, peak $\dot{V}O_2$ and the anaerobic threshold are within normal limits (Table 10.6.2). See flowchart 2. ECG, O_2 pulse at peak $\dot{V}O_2$, and arterial blood gases are normal (branch point 2.1). The patient is not obese (branch point 2.2).

Conclusion

This is a normal 37-year-old man. Symptoms probably relate to anxiety and lack of fitness.

TABLE 10.6.1.   Selected Respiratory Function Data

Measurement	Predicted	Measured
Age, yr		37
Sex		Male
Height, cm		157
Weight, kg	63	67
Hematocrit, %		45
VC, L	3.30	4.38
IC, L	2.20	2.80
TLC, L	4.52	5.30
FEV_1, L	2.66	3.52
FEV_1/VC, %	81	80
MVV, L/min	127	124
D_LCO, ml/mm Hg/min	22.4	29.8

TABLE 10.6.2.   Selected Exercise Data

Measurement	Predicted	Measured
Maximum $\dot{V}O_2$, L/min	2.36	2.23
Maximum HR, beats/min	183	188
Maximum O_2 pulse, ml/beat	12.9	11.9
$\Delta\dot{V}O_2/\Delta WR$, ml/min/W	10.3	10.4
AT, L/min	>0.99	1.1
Blood pressure, mmHg (rest, max)		125/75, 188/94
Maximum $\dot{V}E$, L/min		90
Exercise breathing reserve, L/min	>15	34
PaO_2, mmHg (rest, max ex)		84, 114
$P(A - a)O_2$, mmHg (rest, max ex)		7, 2
$P(a - ET)CO_2$, mmHg (rest, max ex)		0, −4
VD/VT (rest, heavy ex)		0.31, 0.16
HCO_3^-, mEq/L (rest, 2-min recov)		24, 16

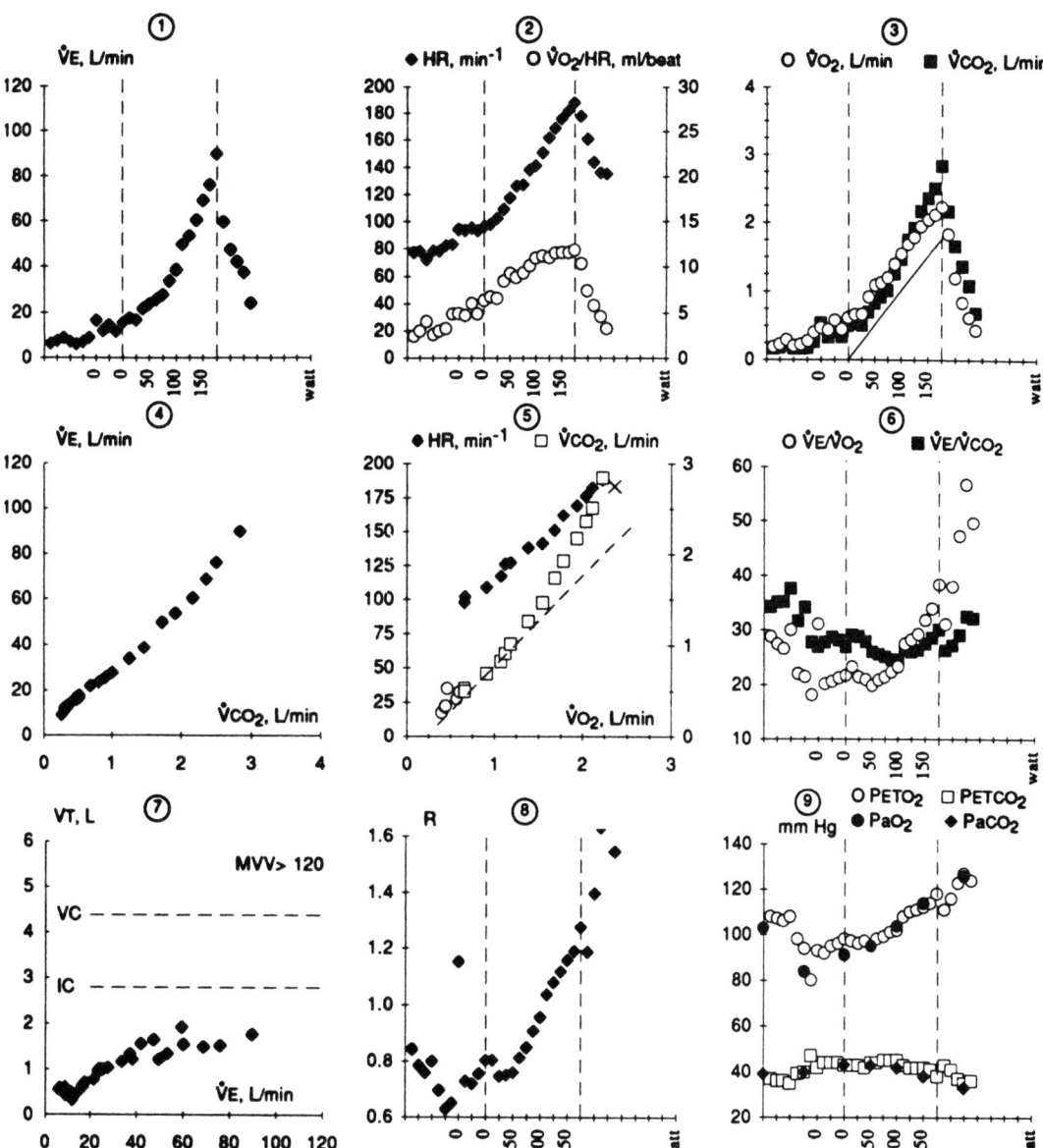

FIGURE 10.6.1.   **1:** Vertical dashed lines in panels 1 to 3 and 6, 8, and 9 indicate the beginning and the end of the increasing work period. **2:** Unloaded cycling is performed for 3 minutes before the left vertical dashed line. **3:** In panel 3, the diagonal line shows the increase of $\dot{V}_{O_2}$ at a slope of 10 ml/min/W. **4:** In panel 5, the diagonal dashed line has a slope of 1; the x in the upper right is the predicted maximum heart rate and $\dot{V}_{O_2}$ for the subject.

TABLE 10.6.3. Air Breathing

Time min	Work rate watts	BP mmHg	HR min⁻¹	f min⁻¹	$\dot{V}_E$ L/min BTPS	$\dot{V}_{CO_2}$ L/min STPD	$\dot{V}_{O_2}$ L/min STPD	$\dfrac{\dot{V}_{O_2}}{HR}$ ml/beat	R	pH	HCO_3^- meq/L	P_{O_2}, mmHg ET	a	(A − a)	P_{CO_2}, mmHg ET	a	(a − ET)	$\dfrac{\dot{V}_E}{\dot{V}_{CO_2}}$	$\dfrac{\dot{V}_E}{\dot{V}_{O_2}}$	$\dfrac{V_D}{V_T}$
	Rest	125/75								7.41	24		103			39				
	Rest		77	11	6.4	0.16	0.29	2.5	0.84			108			37			34	29	
	Rest		78	14	7.5	0.18	0.23	2.9	0.78			107			36			35	27	
	Rest		72	15	9.0	0.22	0.29	4.0	0.76			106			36			35	27	
	Rest		78	13	7.1	0.16	0.20	2.6	0.80			108			35			37	30	
	Rest		78	11	6.0	0.16	0.23	2.9	0.70			98			39			32	22	
	Rest	125/81	82	13	6.9	0.17	0.27	3.3	0.63	7.39	24	94	84	7	40	40	0	34	21	0.31
	Unloaded		83	21	9.0	0.26	0.40	4.8	0.65			80			47			28	18	
	Unloaded		94	28	16.7	0.53	0.46	4.9	1.15			93			42			27	31	
	Unloaded		93	38	12.1	0.32	0.44	4.7	0.73			92			44			28	20	
	Unloaded		95	31	14.4	0.41	0.57	6.0	0.72			95			44			29	21	
	Unloaded		93	23	11.5	0.34	0.45	4.8	0.76			96			44			28	21	
	Unloaded	144/81	96	28	15.6	0.49	0.61	6.4	0.80	7.37	24	98	91	8	43	43	0	27	22	0.22
0.5	25		98	25	17.5	0.53	0.66	6.7	0.80			97			43			29	23	
1.0	25		102	26	16.6	0.50	0.67	6.6	0.75			96			43			29	21	
1.5	50		109	28	21.6	0.69	0.92	8.4	0.75			97			42			28	21	
2.0	50	150/81	117	25	23.5	0.82	1.08	9.2	0.76	7.38	25	95	95	1	44	43	−1	26	20	0.21
2.5	75		126	26	25.5	0.91	1.12	8.9	0.81			98			44			26	21	
3.0	75		127	27	27.7	1.01	1.19	9.4	0.85			99			45			25	21	
3.5	100		138	29	33.6	1.26	1.39	10.1	0.91			101			45			25	22	
4.0	100	181/94	141	32	38.6	1.47	1.54	10.9	0.95	7.37	24	102	104	2	45	42	−3	24	23	0.15
4.5	125		151	41	49.7	1.74	1.68	11.1	1.04			108			43			27	28	
5.0	125		162	40	53.5	1.92	1.78	11.0	1.08			110			42			26	28	
5.5	150		169	39	60.2	2.17	1.94	11.5	1.12			111			42			26	29	
6.0	150	188/94	176	46	68.8	2.36	2.04	11.6	1.16	7.37	22	112	114	2	42	38	−4	27	32	0.16
6.5	175		182	50	76.0	2.51	2.11	11.6	1.19			114			41			29	34	
7.0	175		188	51	89.7	2.84	2.23	11.9	1.27			118			38			30	38	
	Recovery		178	31	59.6	2.17	1.83	10.3	1.19			111			43			26	31	
	Recovery		161	29	47.5	1.66	1.19	7.4	1.39			116			41			27	38	
	Recovery		144	27	42.0	1.37	0.84	5.8	1.63			123			37			29	47	
	Recovery	181/100	136	28	37.5	1.08	0.62	4.6	1.74	7.30	16	127	126	2	35	33	−2	33	57	0.18
	Recovery		135	24	23.9	0.68	0.44	3.3	1.55			124			36			32	50	

Case 7 Normal Man
Clinical Findings

This 74-year-old retired shipyard worker was referred for evaluation and exercise testing because workup at another institution had resulted in a diagnosis of emphysema despite no evidence of airway obstruction. The patient had a mild, nonproductive cough, had smoked approximately 35 years, and continued to smoke. He had no other circulatory or respiratory symptoms, except for shortness of breath from climbing two flights of stairs (but not from walking for 1 mile on the level). Physical examination was normal. Exercise testing was performed to help resolve the difference between clinical impressions.

Exercise Findings

The patient performed exercise on a cycle ergometer. He pedaled at 60 rpm without added load for 3 minutes. The work rate was then increased 15 W per minute to his symptom-limited maximum. Arterial blood was sampled every second minute, and intraarterial blood pressure was recorded from a percutaneously placed brachial artery catheter. The patient stopped exercise because of shortness of breath. Resting and exercise ECGs were normal.

Interpretation
Comments

This patient's resting respiratory function is normal (Table 10.7.1). The resting ECG is normal.

Analysis

In flowchart 1, the maximum $\dot{V}O_2$ is normal. The anaerobic threshold is normal (Table 10.7.2). Referring to flowchart 2, the ECG, O_2 pulse, arterial blood gases, and VD/VT are normal (branch point 2.1). The patient is not obese (branch point 2.2).

Conclusion

This is a normal cardiovascular and respiratory response to exercise. The patient has no evidence of abnormalities consistent with the diagnosis of emphysema given to the patient in a previous examination.

TABLE 10.7.1.   Selected Respiratory Function Data

Measurement	Predicted	Measured
Age, yr		74
Sex		Male
Height, cm		169
Weight, kg	73	82
Hematocrit, %		44
VC, L	3.37	4.88
IC, L	2.25	4.12
TLC, L	5.60	6.05
FEV_1, L	2.58	3.96
FEV_1/VC, %	77	81
MVV, L/min	110	107
$D_L CO$, ml/mm Hg/min	21.6	24.8

TABLE 10.7.2.   Selected Exercise Data

Measurement	Predicted	Measured
Maximum $\dot{V}O_2$, L/min	1.74	1.95
Maximum HR, beats/min	146	132
Maximum O_2 pulse, ml/beat	11.9	14.8
$\Delta\dot{V}O_2/\Delta WR$, ml/min/W	10.3	10.6
AT, L/min	>0.78	1.4
Blood pressure, mmHg (rest, max)		150/84, 177/79
Maximum $\dot{V}E$, L/min		68
Exercise breathing reserve, L/min	>15	39
PaO_2, mmHg (rest, max ex)		97, 101
$P(A-a)O_2$, mmHg (rest, max ex)		20, 16
$P(a-ET)CO_2$, mmHg (rest, max ex)		3, 0
VD/VT (rest, heavy ex)		0.35, 0.22
HCO_3^-, mEq/L (rest, 2-min recov)		20, 15

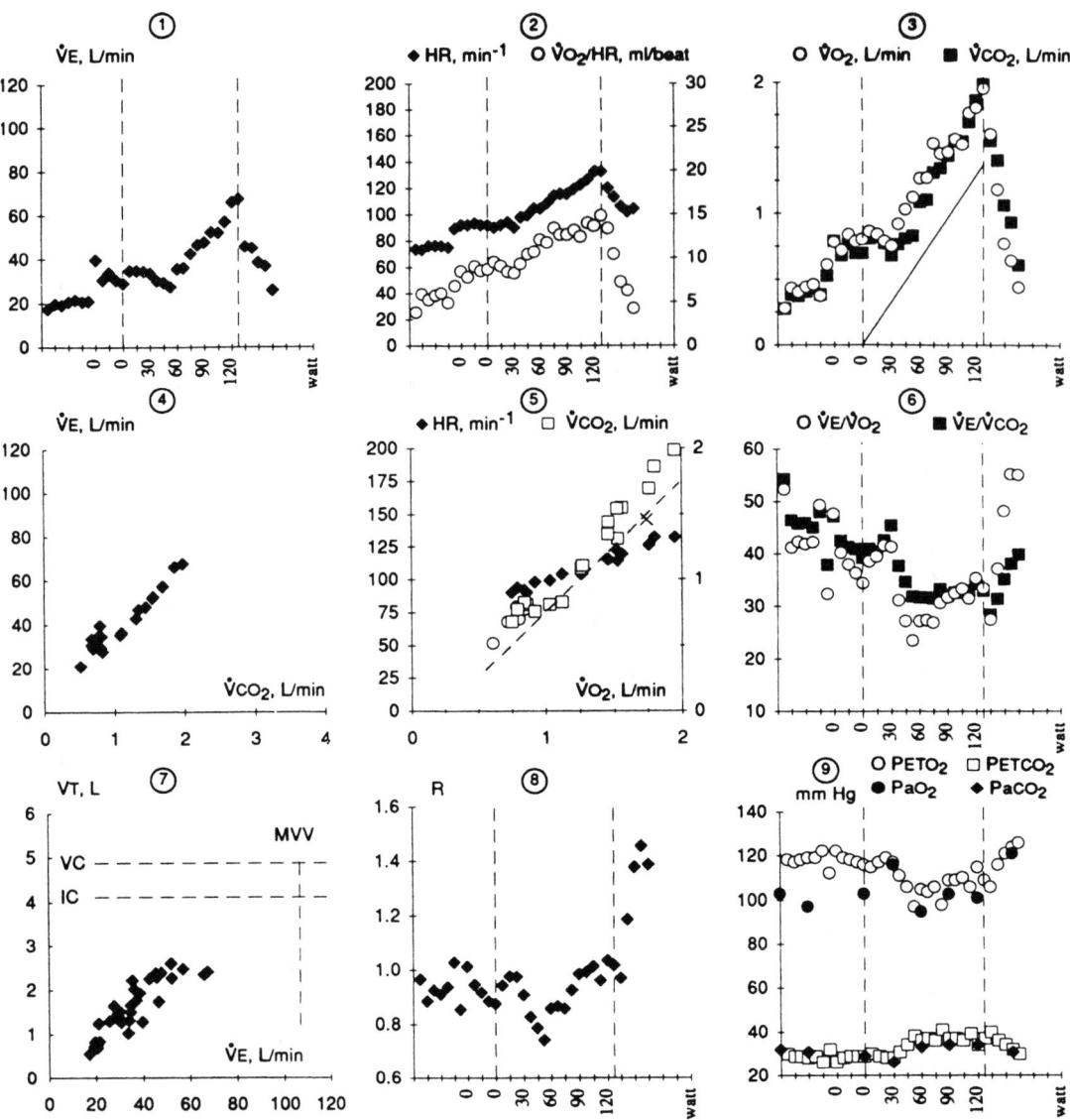

FIGURE 10.7.1. **1:** Vertical dashed lines in panels 1 to 3 and 6, 8, and 9 indicate the beginning and the end of the increasing work period. **2:** Unloaded cycling is performed for 3 minutes before the left vertical dashed line. **3:** In panel 3, the diagonal line shows the increase of $\dot{V}_{O_2}$ at a slope of 10 ml/min/W. **4:** In panel 5, the diagonal dashed line has a slope of 1; the x in the upper right is the predicted maximum heart rate and $\dot{V}_{O_2}$ for the subject.

TABLE 10.7.3.   Air Breathing

Time min	Work rate watts	BP mmHg	HR min⁻¹	f min⁻¹	$\dot{V}_E$ L/min BTPS	$\dot{V}_{CO_2}$ L/min STPD	$\dot{V}_{O_2}$ L/min STPD	$\dfrac{\dot{V}_{O_2}}{HR}$ ml/beat	R	pH	HCO₃⁻ meq/L	P_{O_2}, mmHg ET	a	(A−a)	P_{CO_2}, mmHg ET	a	(a−ET)	$\dfrac{\dot{V}_E}{\dot{V}_{CO_2}}$	$\dfrac{\dot{V}_E}{\dot{V}_{O_2}}$	$\dfrac{V_D}{V_T}$
	Rest	150/82								7.41	20		103			32				
	Rest		74	31	17.3	0.27	0.28	3.8	0.96			118			30			54	52	
	Rest		73	24	19.7	0.38	0.43	5.9	0.88			117			29			46	41	
	Rest	147/84	76	27	19.2	0.37	0.40	5.3	0.93			118			29			46	42	
	Rest		76	27	20.7	0.40	0.44	5.8	0.91	7.42	20	119	97	20	28	31	3	46	42	0.35
	Rest		76	26	21.6	0.43	0.46	6.1	0.93			119			29			45	42	
	Rest		75	30	20.8	0.38	0.37	4.9	1.03			122			26			48	49	
	Unloaded		89	17	21.1	0.52	0.61	6.9	0.85			112			32			38	32	
	Unloaded		92	31	39.8	0.79	0.78	8.5	1.01			122			26			47	48	
	Unloaded		92	23	30.8	0.68	0.72	7.8	0.94			119			28			42	40	
	Unloaded		93	26	34.0	0.77	0.84	9.0	0.92			118			29			41	38	
	Unloaded		92	24	30.7	0.70	0.79	8.6	0.89			117			29			41	36	
	Unloaded	162/84	92	20	29.1	0.70	0.80	8.7	0.88	7.42	18	116	103	15	29	29	0	39	34	0.23
0.5	15		90	21	34.9	0.81	0.86	9.6	0.94			115			30			41	39	
1.0	15		92	21	34.8	0.82	0.84	9.1	0.98			117			29			40	39	
1.5	30		94	23	34.7	0.77	0.79	8.4	0.97			119			28			43	41	
2.0	30	159/81	90	33	33.7	0.68	0.75	8.3	0.91	7.44	17	117	116	6	28	26	−2	45	41	0.25
2.5	45		98	20	30.3	0.76	0.92	9.4	0.83			111			31			38	31	
3.0	45		99	20	29.7	0.81	1.03	10.4	0.79			106			34			35	27	
3.5	60		100	17	27.8	0.83	1.12	10.8	0.74			97			38			32	24	
4.0	60	168/84	104	16	35.6	1.08	1.26	12.1	0.86	7.37	19	105	95	18	36	33	−3	32	27	0.17
4.5	75		108	18	36.4	1.10	1.27	11.8	0.87			104			37			32	27	
5.0	75		114	19	42.8	1.31	1.53	13.4	0.86			106			36			31	27	
5.5	90		115	27	46.8	1.34	1.45	12.6	0.92			98			41			33	31	
6.0	90	186/90	115	20	47.9	1.44	1.46	12.7	0.99	7.36	19	109	103	13	37	34	−3	32	32	0.20
6.5	105		119	23	52.5	1.55	1.56	13.1	0.99			109			37			33	32	
7.0	105		122	20	52.2	1.54	1.52	12.5	1.01			110			36			33	33	
7.5	120		126	23	57.2	1.69	1.76	14.0	0.96			106			39			33	31	
8.0	120	177/79	132	28	66.1	1.86	1.80	13.6	1.03	7.33	18	115	101	16	34	34	0	34	35	0.25
8.5	135		132	28	67.5	1.98	1.95	14.8	1.02			109			37			33	33	
	Recovery		120	20	45.8	1.55	1.60	13.3	0.97			106			40			28	28	
	Recovery		113	19	45.4	1.40	1.18	10.4	1.19			116			36			31	37	
	Recovery		106	20	38.8	1.06	0.77	7.3	1.38			121			34			35	48	
	Recovery	168/78	102	21	37.1	0.93	0.64	6.3	1.45	7.31	15	124	121	6	32	31	−1	38	55	0.25
	Recovery		104	20	25.9	0.61	0.44	4.2	1.39			126			30			40	55	

Case 8 Normal Man with Ventilatory Chemoreflex Insensitivity

Clinical Findings

This 67-year-old retired man had worked for 30 years in the shipyards. He had never smoked. Three months previously, he was diagnosed with hypertension, for which he was treated with triamterene and hydrochlorothiazide. He noted shortness of breath after climbing two flights of stairs and frequent mild substernal pressure not related to exertion, meals, body position, or stress. Physical examination, roentgenographic, laboratory, and ECG results were normal.

Exercise Findings

The patient performed exercise on a cycle ergometer. He pedaled at 60 rpm without added load for 3 minutes. The work rate was then increased 20 W per minute to his symptom-limited maximum. Arterial blood was sampled every second minute, and intraarterial blood pressure was recorded from a percutaneously placed brachial artery catheter. He stopped exercise with shortness of breath, but without chest pain or pressure. ECG pattern remained normal.

Interpretation

Comments

Results of the resting respiratory function studies are normal (Table 10.8.1). The resting ECG is normal.

Analysis

Referring to flowchart 1, the peak $\dot{V}O_2$ and anaerobic threshold are normal (Table 10.8.2). See flowchart 2. The exercise ECG, arterial blood gases, VD/VT, and O_2 pulse at peak $\dot{V}O_2$ are normal (branch point 2.1). The patient is not obese (branch point 2.2). Although the arterial CO_2 tension is normal at rest, the increase in ventilation lagged the increase in CO_2 production, causing arterial PCO_2 to rise gradually during exercise (panel 9, Fig. 10.8.1; Table 10.8.3). This is occasionally seen when the ventila-

tory chemoreflex is relatively insensitive to the exercise metabolic acidosis. Because the CO_2 stores are increasing in the body as a consequence of the rising $PaCO_2$, CO_2 output does not rise as steeply as it otherwise might, particularly above the AT. Thus, $\dot{V}E/\dot{V}CO_2$ at the termination of work is not increased over that at the AT (panel 6, Fig. 10.8.1), and there is no steepening in the $\dot{V}E$–work rate relation (panels 1 and 4, Fig. 10.8.1).

Conclusion

This is normal cardiovascular and respiratory function in a patient likely to have a ventilatory chemoreflex that is relatively insensitive to pH decrease.

TABLE 10.8.1.   Selected Respiratory Function Data

Measurement	Predicted	Measured
Age, yr		67
Sex		Male
Height, cm		173
Weight, kg	76	80
Hematocrit, %		48
VC, L	3.82	3.86
IC, L	2.55	2.42
TLC, L	6.06	6.04
FEV_1, L	2.97	3.07
FEV_1/VC, %	78	80
MVV, L/min	124	121
D_LCO, ml/mm Hg/min	26.3	32.3

TABLE 10.8.2.   Selected Exercise Data

Measurement	Predicted	Measured
Peak $\dot{V}O_2$, L/min	1.98	1.94
Maximum HR, beats/min	153	142
Maximum O_2 pulse, ml/beat	13.0	13.7
$\Delta\dot{V}O_2/\Delta WR$, ml/min/W	10.3	9.9
AT, L/min	>0.89	1.5
Blood pressure, mmHg (rest, max)		176/92, 215/92
Maximum $\dot{V}E$, L/min		56
Exercise breathing reserve, L/min	>15	65
PaO_2, mmHg (rest, max ex)		96, 81
$P(A - a)O_2$, mmHg (rest, max ex)		8, 22
$P(a - ET)CO_2$, mmHg (rest, max ex)		1, −6
VD/VT (rest, heavy ex)		0.39, 0.26
HCO_3^-, mEq/L (rest, 2-min recov)		27, 22

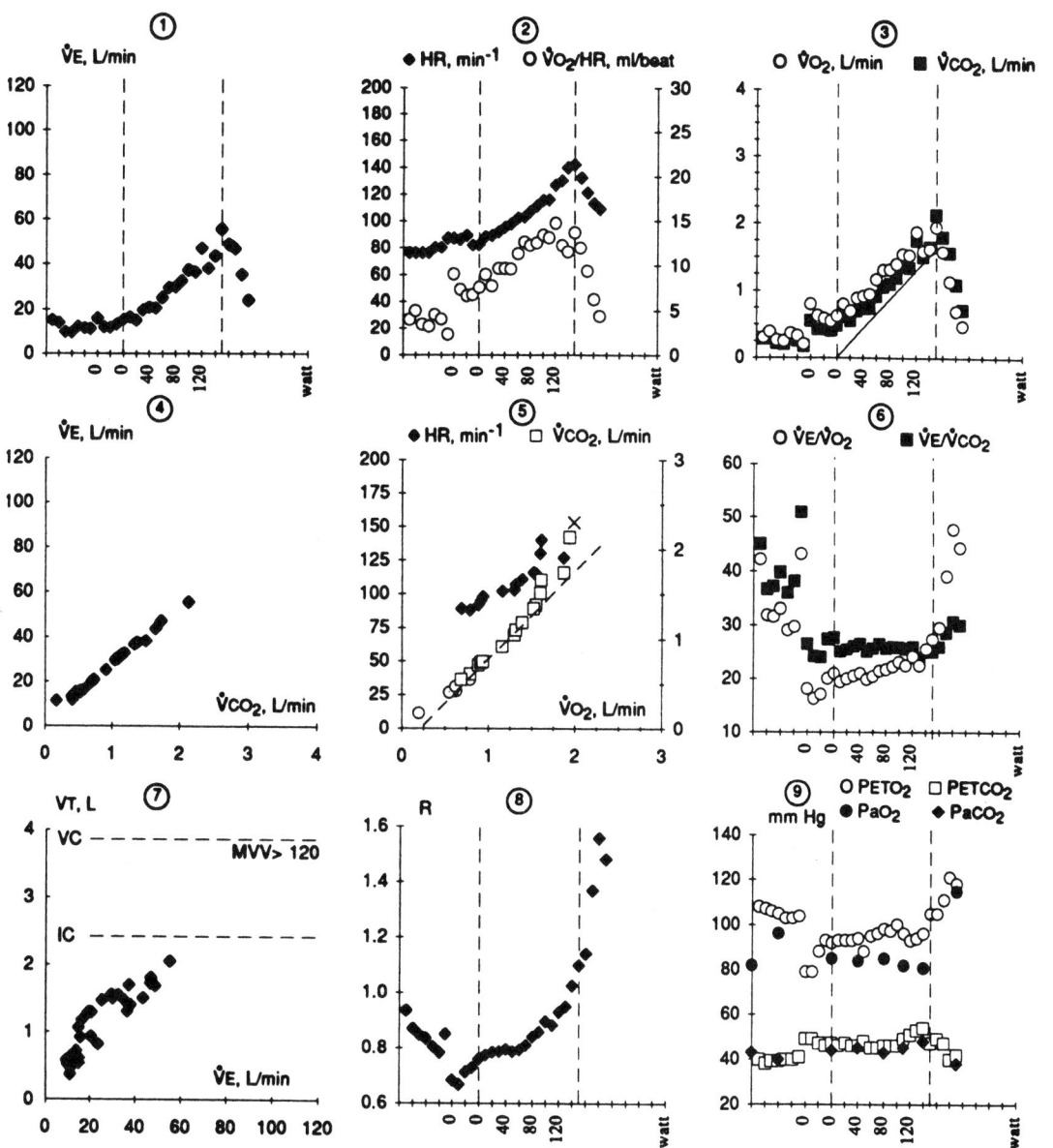

FIGURE 10.8.1.   **1:** Vertical dashed lines in panels 1 to 3 and 6, 8, and 9 indicate the beginning and the end of the increasing work period. **2:** Unloaded cycling is performed for 3 minutes before the left vertical dashed line. **3:** In panel 3, the diagonal line shows the increase of $\dot{V}O_2$ at a slope of 10 ml/min/W. **4:** In panel 5, the diagonal dashed line has a slope of 1; the x in the upper right is the predicted maximum heart rate and $\dot{V}O_2$ for the subject.

TABLE 10.8.3. Air Breathing

Time min	Work rate watts	BP mmHg	HR min⁻¹	f min⁻¹	$\dot{V}E$ L/min BTPS	$\dot{V}CO_2$ L/min STPD	$\dot{V}O_2$ L/min STPD	$\dot{V}O_2$/HR ml/beat	R	pH	HCO₃⁻ meq/L	P_{O_2} ET	P_{O_2} a	P_{O_2} (A−a)	P_{CO_2} ET	P_{CO_2} a	P_{CO_2} (a−ET)	$\dot{V}E/\dot{V}CO_2$	$\dot{V}E/\dot{V}O_2$	V_D/V_T
	Rest	176/92								7.41	27		82			43				
	Rest		76	28	15.0	0.28	0.30	3.9	0.93			108			40			45	42	
	Rest		76	19	13.7	0.33	0.38	5.0	0.87			107			38			37	32	
	Rest		76	19	9.8	0.22	0.26	3.4	0.85			106			39			37	31	
	Rest	164/92	76	16	9.3	0.20	0.24	3.2	0.83	7.43	26	105	96	8	39	40	1	40	33	0.39
	Rest		80	22	12.3	0.29	0.36	4.5	0.81			103			40			36	29	
	Rest		80	22	11.4	0.25	0.32	4.0	0.78			103			40			38	30	
	Unloaded		87	30	11.2	0.17	0.20	2.3	0.85			104			41			51	43	
	Unloaded		87	17	15.7	0.54	0.79	9.1	0.68			79			49			26	18	
	Unloaded		86	19	11.8	0.42	0.63	7.3	0.67			79			49			24	16	
	Unloaded		89	18	11.6	0.42	0.59	6.6	0.71			88			47			24	17	
	Unloaded		82	25	13.1	0.40	0.55	6.7	0.73			93			46			27	20	
	Unloaded	185/92	82	25	15.1	0.47	0.62	7.6	0.76	7.40	27	92	85	10	47	44	−3	28	21	0.25
0.5	20		88	14	16.5	0.61	0.79	9.0	0.77			93			46			25	19	
1.0	20		89	14	14.9	0.54	0.69	7.8	0.78			93			47			25	20	
1.5	40		92	15	19.5	0.70	0.89	9.7	0.79			93			46			26	20	
2.0	40	194/89	95	16	20.7	0.73	0.92	9.7	0.79	7.40	27	94	84	12	46	45	−1	26	21	0.26
2.5	60		98	22	20.5	0.74	0.94	9.6	0.79			88			48			25	20	
3.0	60		102	17	25.1	0.92	1.16	11.4	0.79			95			45			26	20	
3.5	80		103	19	29.5	1.05	1.30	12.6	0.81			96			45			27	21	
4.0	80	203/89	107	20	30.0	1.10	1.31	12.2	0.84	7.40	26	98	85	16	46	43	−3	26	22	0.21
4.5	100		111	21	32.6	1.19	1.39	12.5	0.86			97			46			26	22	
5.0	100		115	22	37.4	1.38	1.54	13.4	0.90			100			46			26	23	
5.5	120	209/89	116	28	36.6	1.34	1.52	13.1	0.88	7.38	26	96	82	18	49	45	−4	26	23	0.23
6.0	120		127	26	47.2	1.74	1.87	14.7	0.93			93			51			26	24	
6.5	140		130	27	38.1	1.51	1.59	12.2	0.95			94			53			24	23	
7.0	140	215/92	140	29	43.6	1.65	1.61	11.5	1.02	7.35	26	96	81	22	54	48	−6	25	26	0.26
7.5	160		142	27	55.5	2.13	1.94	13.7	1.10			105			47			25	27	
	Recovery		132	29	49.0	1.80	1.58	12.0	1.14			105			49	38	−4	26	29	
	Recovery		121	27	46.8	1.56	1.14	9.4	1.37			111			47			29	39	
	Recovery		113	24	35.4	1.09	0.70	6.2	1.56			121			40			31	48	
	Recovery	209/92	109	29	23.7	0.71	0.48	4.4	1.48	7.37	22	118	115	7	42			30	44	0.22

Case 9 Exceptionally Fit Man with Mild Lung Disease

Clinical Findings

This 59-year-old shipyard worker had no complaints or history of heart or lung disease. He had sustained a gunshot wound to the right chest at age 24 that was not surgically treated. He had been exposed to asbestos 20 years previously and had smoked one pack of cigarettes daily for 12 years until 20 years ago. He cycled approximately 50 miles a week. Physical, roentgenographic, and ECG examinations were normal except for evidence of focal, old granulomatous disease and an old rib fracture.

Exercise Findings

The patient performed exercise on a cycle ergometer. He pedaled at 60 rpm without added load for 3 minutes. The work rate was then increased 20 W per minute to his symptom-limited maximum. Arterial blood was sampled every second minute, and intraarterial blood pressure was recorded from a percutaneously placed brachial artery catheter. He stopped exercise because of general exhaustion. Exercise ECGs were normal.

Interpretation

Comments

The results of this patient's respiratory function studies are within normal limits (Table 10.9.1). The resting ECG is normal. When starting to breathe on the mouthpiece, the patient hyperventilates to a pH of 7.52, Pa_{CO_2} of 27 mm Hg, and Pa_{O_2} of 120. The respiratory alkalosis at rest, while breathing on the mouthpiece, is acute, developing in anticipation of exercise. It disappears after exercise starts. The extraordinarily large increase in Pa_{O_2} when starting to breathe on the mouthpiece at rest is probably due to (a) hypoxemia off the mouthpiece due to microatelectasis associated with obesity (a common problem in overweight subjects); and (b) the large increase in Pa_{O_2}, which accompanies acute hyperventilation, and a high R.

Analysis

Referring to flowchart 1, this patient's peak $\dot{V}_{O_2}$ and anaerobic threshold are above predicted (Table 10.9.2). Because he cycled regularly to maintain his fitness, he performed exceedingly well. Referring to flowchart 2, the ECG and O_2 pulse (high because of fitness) at maximal exercise are normal, but the blood gases are abnormal (branch point 2.1). V_D/V_T and $P(a - _{ET})_{CO_2}$ are normal, but $P(_A - a)_{O_2}$ at maximum exercise is increased and suggests the presence of mild lung disease (branch point 2.3).

Conclusion

This exceptionally fit man of 59 years has features of mild lung disease.

TABLE 10.9.1. Selected Respiratory Function Data

Measurement	Predicted	Measured
Age, yr		59
Sex		Male
Height, cm		175
Weight, kg	78	93
Hematocrit, %		46
VC, L	4.21	4.34
IC, L	2.79	3.57
TLC, L	6.36	5.86
FEV_1, L	3.58	3.57
FEV_1/ VC, %	80	82
MVV, L/min	137	152
$D_L{CO}$, ml/mm Hg/min	28.2	29.5

TABLE 10.9.2. Selected Exercise Data

Measurement	Predicted	Measured
Peak $\dot{V}_{O_2}$, L/min	2.32	3.40
Maximum HR, beats/min	161	195
Maximum O_2 pulse, ml/beat	14.4	17.4
$\Delta\dot{V}_{O_2}/\Delta$WR, ml/min/W	10.3	12.7
AT, L/min	>1.02	1.4
Blood pressure, mmHg (rest, max)		125/75, 200/88
Maximum $\dot{V}_E$, L/min		174
Exercise breathing reserve, L/min	>15	−22
Pa_{O_2}, mmHg (rest, max ex)		120, 71
$P(_A - a)_{O_2}$, mmHg (rest, max ex)		5, 49
$P(a - _{ET})_{CO_2}$, mmHg (rest, max ex)		−4, −13
V_D/V_T (rest, heavy ex)		0.17, 0.02
HCO_3^-, mEq/L (rest, 2-min recov)		25, 10

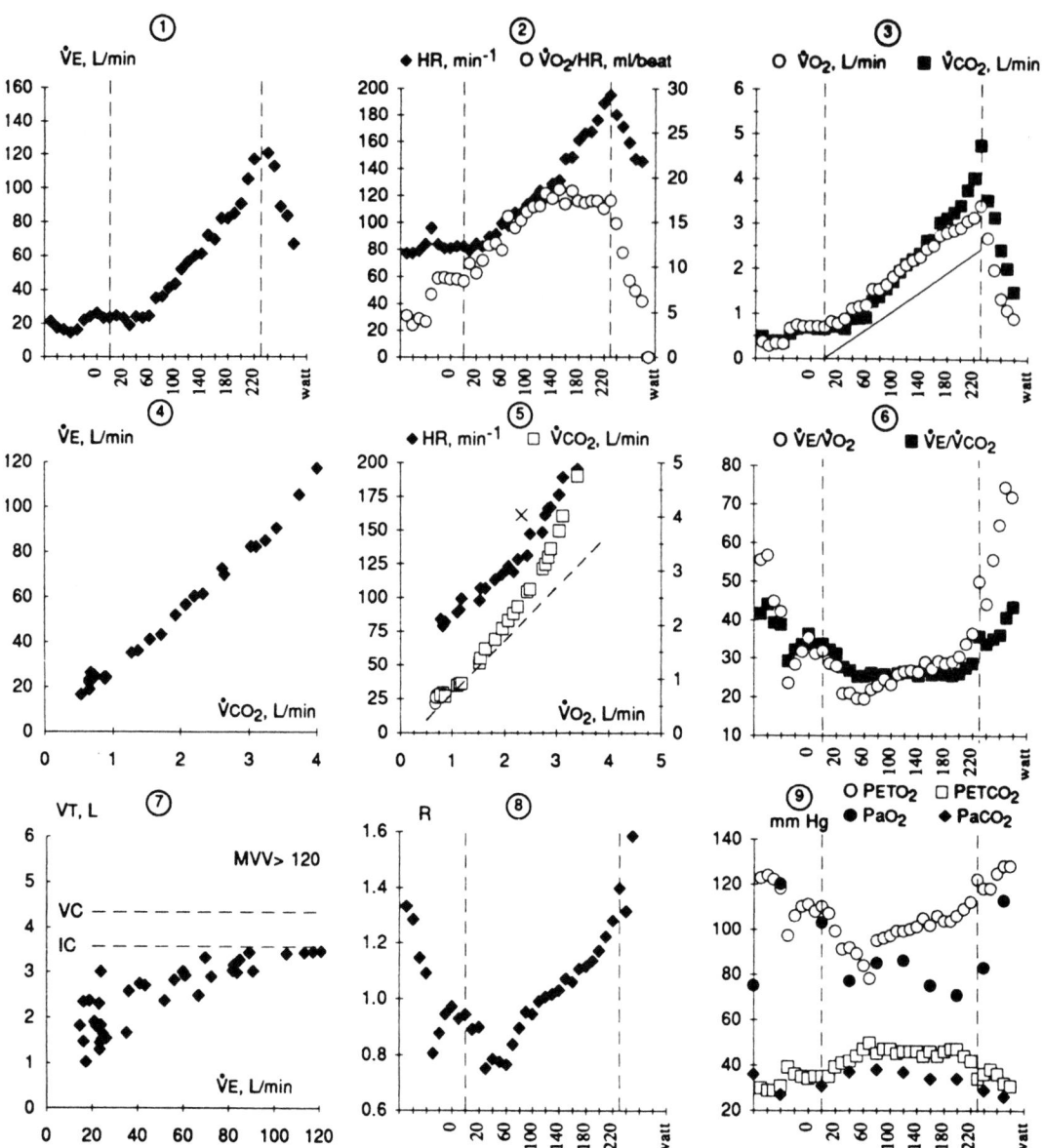

FIGURE 10.9.1. **1:** Vertical dashed lines in panels 1 to 3 and 6, 8, and 9 indicate the beginning and the end of the increasing work period. **2:** Unloaded cycling is performed for 3 minutes before the left vertical dashed line. **3:** In panel 3, the diagonal line shows the increase of $\dot{V}O_2$ at a slope of 10 ml/min/W. **4:** In panel 5, the diagonal dashed line has a slope of 1; the x in the upper right is the predicted maximum heart rate and $\dot{V}O_2$ for the subject.

TABLE 10.9.3.   Air Breathing

Time min	Work rate watts	BP mmHg	HR min⁻¹	f min⁻¹	$\dot{V}_E$ L/min BTPS	$\dot{V}_{CO_2}$ L/min STPD	$\dot{V}_{O_2}$ L/min STPD	$\dot{V}_{O_2}$/HR ml/beat	R	pH	HCO₃⁻ meq/L	Po₂, mmHg ET	a	(A−a)	Pco₂, mmHg ET	a	(a−ET)	$\dot{V}_E/\dot{V}_{CO_2}$	$\dot{V}_E/\dot{V}_{O_2}$	V_D/V_T
	Rest	125/75								7.45	25	75			36					
	Rest		77	11	20.9	0.48	0.36	4.7	1.33			123			30			42	55	
	Rest		77	17	17.3	0.36	0.28	3.6	1.29			124			29			44	57	
	Rest		79	11	16.2	0.39	0.34	4.3	1.15			122			29			39	45	
	Rest	119/75	84	8	14.6	0.36	0.33	3.9	1.09	7.52	22	118	120	5	31	27	−4	39	42	0.17
	Unloaded		96	7	16.4	0.54	0.67	7.0	0.81			97			39			29	24	
	Unloaded		84	12	21.9	0.65	0.74	8.8	0.88			106			36			32	28	
	Unloaded		81	13	23.9	0.68	0.72	8.9	0.94			110			35			34	32	
	Unloaded		81	17	26.2	0.68	0.70	8.6	0.97			111			34			36	35	
	Unloaded		82	10	23.0	0.66	0.71	8.7	0.93			108			35			34	31	
	Unloaded	156/81	82	16	23.3	0.65	0.69	8.4	0.94	7.47	22	110	103	14	35	31	−4	34	32	0.17
0.5	20		79	15	24.7	0.73	0.82	10.4	0.89			107			35			32	29	
1.0	20		84	18	23.3	0.70	0.78	9.3	0.90			99			39			31	28	
1.5	40		82	8	18.9	0.66	0.88	10.7	0.75			91			41			28	21	
2.0	40	163/81	89	8	24.0	0.87	1.11	12.5	0.78	7.43	24	92	77	28	42	37	−5	27	21	0.13
2.5	60		91	13	23.5	0.89	1.15	12.6	0.77			89			44			25	19	
3.0	60		99	16	24.2	0.90	1.18	11.9	0.76			84			47			25	19	
3.5	80		98	21	35.2	1.28	1.53	15.6	0.84			78			50			26	22	
4.0	80	175/81	107	14	36.1	1.38	1.54	14.4	0.90	7.41	24	95	85	24	45	38	−7	25	23	0.10
4.5	100		107	15	41.1	1.55	1.63	15.2	0.95			96			47			26	24	
5.0	100		113	16	43.4	1.72	1.82	16.1	0.95			97			47			24	23	
5.5	120		117	22	52.0	1.93	1.95	16.7	0.99			99			45			26	26	
6.0	120		123	20	56.5	2.08	2.07	16.8	1.00	7.37	21	99	86	27	46	37	−9	26	26	0.11
6.5	140		119	20	60.0	2.20	2.17	18.2	1.01			100			46			27	27	
7.0	140		128	21	61.2	2.33	2.26	17.7	1.03			101			46			26	26	
7.5	160		131	25	72.5	2.61	2.44	18.6	1.07			105			44			27	29	
8.0	160	200/88	147	21	69.8	2.65	2.50	17.0	1.06	7.35	18	102	75	43	46	34	−12	26	27	0.01
8.5	180		148	27	82.1	3.03	2.74	18.5	1.11			106			44			26	29	
9.0	180		161	26	82.2	3.11	2.79	17.3	1.11			104			46			26	29	
9.5	200		166	26	85.0	3.24	2.85	17.2	1.14			104			47			26	29	
10.0	200		167	30	90.6	3.40	2.90	17.4	1.17	7.29	16	106	71	49	47	34	−13	26	30	0.02
10.5	220		176	31	105.5	3.74	3.06	17.4	1.22			109			44			28	34	
11.0	220		189	34	117.3	4.01	3.13	16.6	1.28			112			42			29	37	
11.5	240		195	55	174.5	4.75	3.40	17.4	1.40			122			34			36	50	
	Recovery	200/88	180	35	121.1	3.52	2.68	14.9	1.31	7.26	13	118	83	43	36	29	−7	34	44	0.11
	Recovery		171	33	113.3	3.15	1.99	11.6	1.58			118			38			35	56	
	Recovery		159	26	89.2	2.42	1.35	8.5	1.79			125			36			36	64	
	Recovery	163/75	147	28	83.7	2.01	1.09	7.4	1.84	7.20	10	128	113	20	32	26	−6	40	75	0.17
	Recovery		145	27	67.1	1.50	0.90	6.2	1.67			128			31			43	72	
	Recovery																			

Case 10 Normal Subject: Cycle and Treadmill Studies

Clinical Findings

This 37-year-old hospital employee was asymptomatic and volunteered for an exercise study. He did not exercise regularly or smoke. Physical examination, chest roentgenograms, and resting ECG were normal.

Exercise Findings

On two separate days, 1 month apart, the subject exercised to maximum tolerance using an incremental protocol, first on the cycle and second on the treadmill. He stopped on both occasions because of calf fatigue. There were no arrhythmias or abnormalities in the ECG.

Interpretation

Comments

The results of this subject's resting respiratory function studies are normal (Table 10.10.1). The resting ECG is normal. This study is presented to contrast the results when the same subject performed on the cycle and on the treadmill.

Analysis

Referring to flowchart 1, the peak $\dot{V}O_2$ and the anaerobic threshold are normal for both cycle and treadmill exercise (Table 10.10.2). Referring to flowchart 2, the ECG and O_2 pulse are normal at maximum work rate (branch point 2.1). The subject is not obese (branch point 2.2). The peak $\dot{V}O_2$ is about 10% higher on the treadmill than on the cycle.

Conclusion

This subject shows normal exercise performance.

TABLE 10.10.1.   Selected Respiratory Function Data

Measurement	Predicted	Measured
Age, yr		37
Sex		Male
Height, cm		161
Weight, kg	66	53
Hematocrit, %		45
VC, L	3.56	3.21
IC, L	2.37	2.51
TLC, L	4.90	5.01
FEV_1, L	2.87	2.64
FEV_1/VC, %	81	82
MVV, L/min	132	107
$D_L CO$, ml/mm Hg/min	23.1	22.3

TABLE 10.10.2.   Selected Exercise Data

Measurement	Predicted		Measured	
	Cycle	Treadmill	Cycle	Treadmill
Peak $\dot{V}O_2$, L/min	2.21	2.45	1.87	2.07
Maximum HR, beats/min	183	183	173	183
Maximum O_2 pulse, ml/beat	12.1	13.4	10.8	11.3
$\Delta \dot{V}O_2/\Delta WR$, ml/min/W	10.3		8.4	
AT, L/min	>0.93	>1.03	1.1	1.15
Maximum $\dot{V}E$, L/min			76	85
Exercise breathing reserve, L/min	>15	>15	31	22

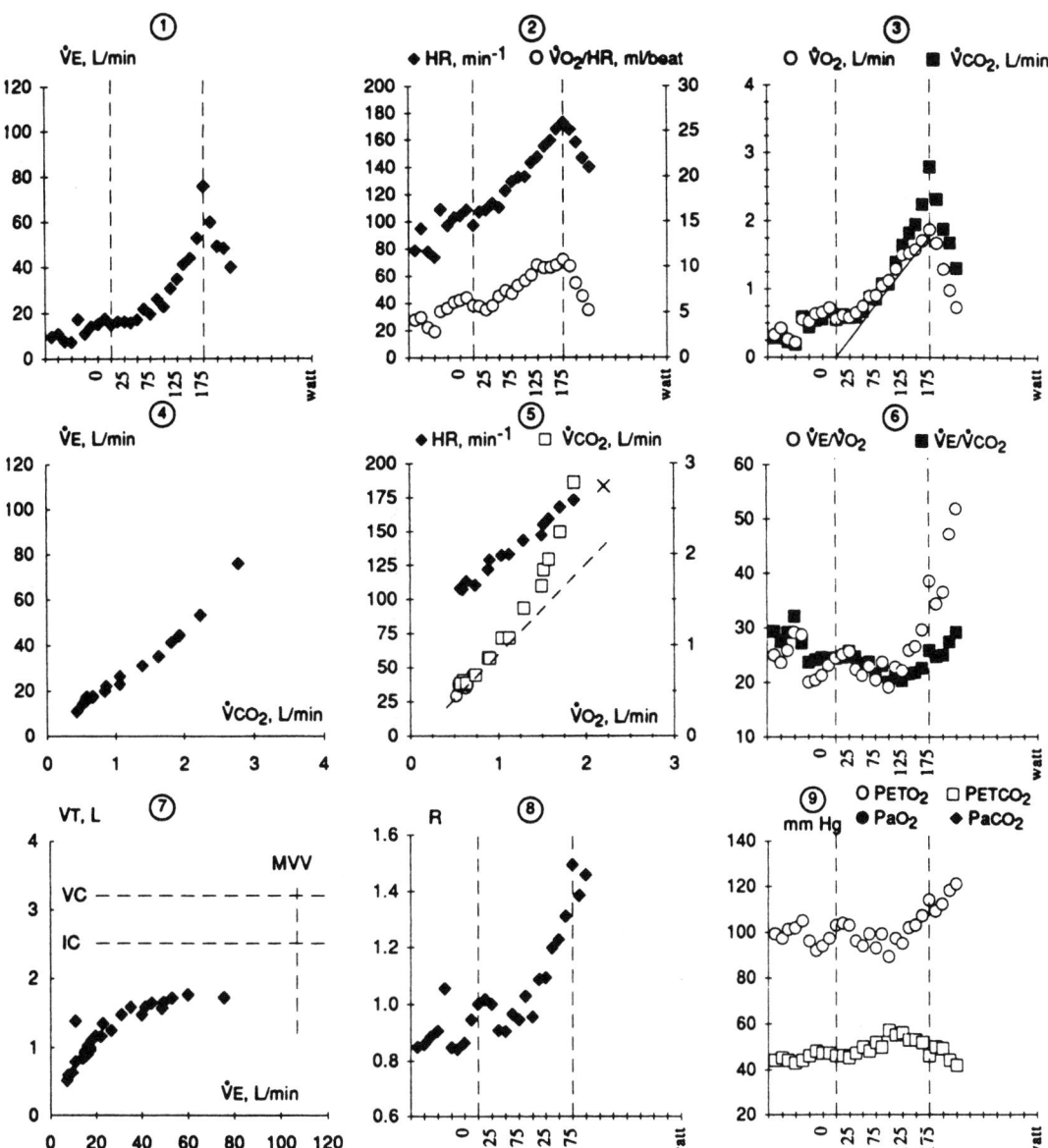

FIGURE 10.10.1.   Cycle ergometry. **1:** Vertical dashed lines in panels 1 to 3 and 6, 8, and 9 indicate the beginning and the end of the increasing work period. **2:** Unloaded cycling is performed for 3 minutes before the left vertical dashed line. **3:** In panel 3, the diagonal line shows the increase of $\dot{V}O_2$ at a slope of 10 ml/min/W. **4:** In panel 5, the diagonal dashed line has a slope of 1; the *x* in the upper right is the predicted maximum heart rate and $\dot{V}O_2$ for the subject.

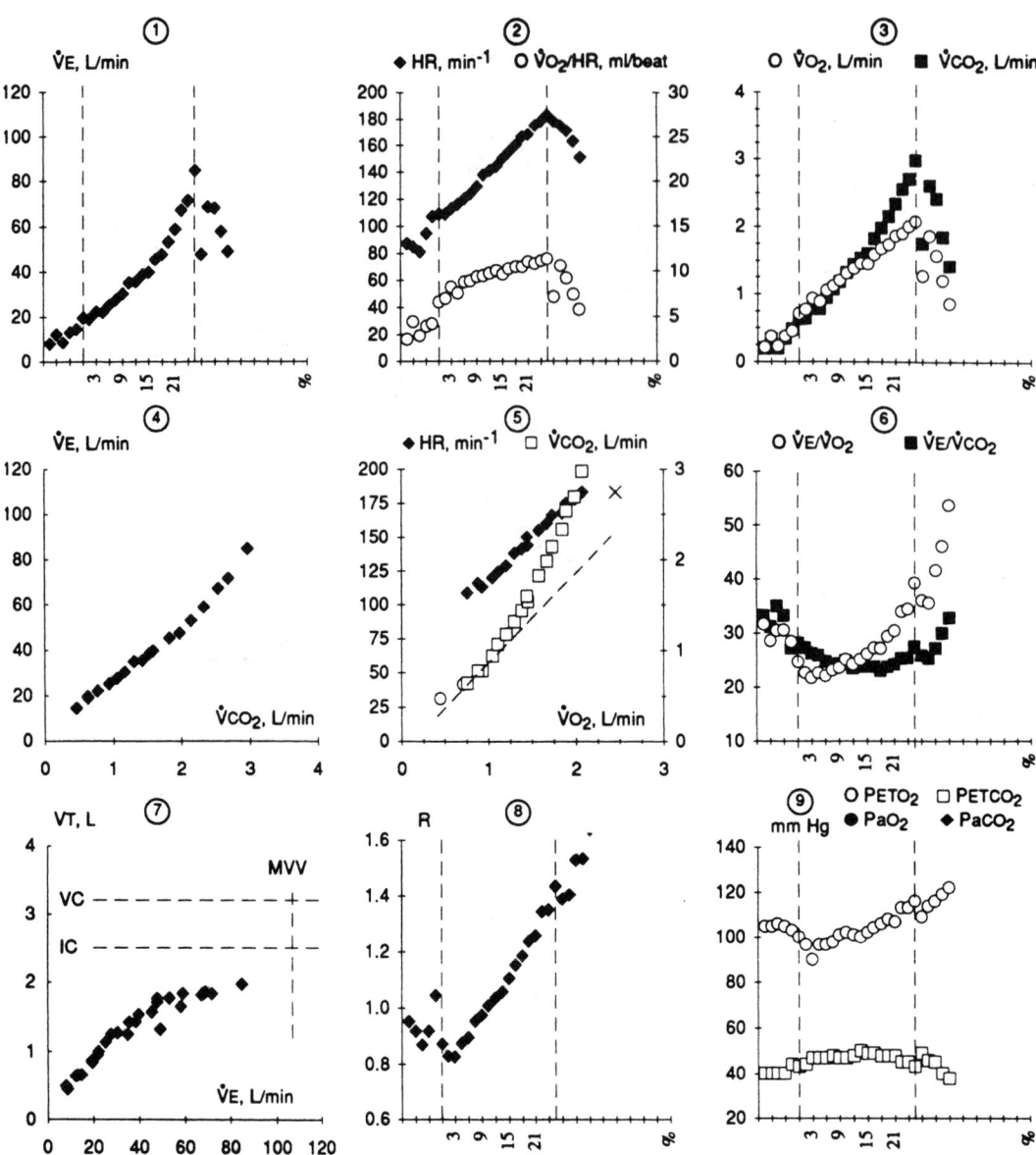

FIGURE 10.10.2.   Treadmill ergometry. **1:** Vertical dashed lines in panels 1 to 3 and 6, 8, and 9 indicate the beginning and the end of the increasing work period. **2:** Zero-grade walking is performed for 1 minute before the left vertical dashed line. **3:** In panel 5, the diagonal dashed line has a slope of 1; the x in the upper right is the predicted maximum heart rate and $\dot{V}O_2$ for the subject.

TABLE 10.10.3.   Cycle Ergometry

Time min	Work rate watts	BP mmHg	HR min⁻¹	f min⁻¹	$\dot{V}_E$ L/min BTPS	$\dot{V}_{CO_2}$ L/min STPD	$\dot{V}_{O_2}$ L/min STPD	$\dot{V}_{O_2}$/HR ml/beat	R	pH	HCO₃⁻ meq/L	P_{O_2}, mmHg ET	a	(A − a)	P_{CO_2}, mmHg ET	a	(a − ET)	$\dot{V}_E/\dot{V}_{CO_2}$	$\dot{V}_E/\dot{V}_{O_2}$	V_D/V_T
	Rest		79	15	9.5	0.28	0.33	4.2	0.85			99			44			29	25	
	Rest		95	14	11.1	0.36	0.42	4.4	0.86			97			45			28	24	
	Rest		78	13	7.8	0.23	0.26	3.3	0.88			101			44			29	26	
	Rest		74	14	7.3	0.19	0.21	2.8	0.90			102			43			32	29	
	Unloaded		109	18	17.3	0.58	0.55	5.0	1.05			105			44			27	29	
	Unloaded		97	8	11.1	0.44	0.52	5.4	0.85			96			46			24	20	
	Unloaded		103	17	14.3	0.53	0.63	6.1	0.84			92			48			24	20	
	Unloaded		104	16	15.1	0.56	0.65	6.3	0.86			94			47			25	21	
	Unloaded		108	16	17.7	0.67	0.71	6.6	0.94			97			47			24	23	
	Unloaded		97	16	14.8	0.55	0.55	5.7	1.00			103			46			24	24	
0.5	25		107	16	16.4	0.61	0.60	5.6	1.02			104			46			25	25	
1.0	25		108	18	16.2	0.57	0.57	5.3	1.00			103			45			26	26	
1.5	50		113	18	15.8	0.58	0.64	5.7	0.91			96			47			25	22	
2.0	50		110	17	17.1	0.67	0.74	6.7	0.91			94			50			23	21	
2.5	75		122	19	22.0	0.86	0.89	7.3	0.97			99			48			24	23	
3.0	75		129	17	19.8	0.85	0.90	7.0	0.94			93			52			22	20	
3.5	100		132	21	26.4	1.07	1.04	7.9	1.03			99			50			23	24	
4.0	100		133	17	22.9	1.07	1.12	8.4	0.96			89			57			20	19	
4.5	125		143	21	31.1	1.40	1.29	9.0	1.09			97			55			21	23	
5.0	125		147	22	35.1	1.64	1.50	10.2	1.09			95			56			20	22	
5.5	150		155	26	41.1	1.82	1.52	9.8	1.20			102			53			22	26	
6.0	150		159	27	44.4	1.94	1.58	9.9	1.23			103			53			22	27	
6.5	175		168	31	53.2	2.24	1.71	10.2	1.31			107			53			23	30	
7.0	175		173	44	75.8	2.79	1.87	10.8	1.49			114			46			26	29	
	Recovery		167	34	60.1	2.31	1.67	10.0	1.38			109			50			25	34	
	Recovery		158	30	49.5	1.88	1.29	8.2	1.46			112			49			25	36	
	Recovery		146	31	48.8	1.68	0.98	6.7	1.71			118			44			27	47	
	Recovery		140	27	40.1	1.30	0.73	5.2	1.78			121			42			29	52	

TABLE 10.10.4.   Treadmill Ergometry

Time min	Treadmill grade, %	BP mmHg	HR min⁻¹	f min⁻¹	$\dot{V}_E$ L/min BTPS	$\dot{V}_{CO_2}$ L/min STPD	$\dot{V}_{O_2}$ L/min STPD	$\dot{V}_{O_2}$/HR ml/beat	R	pH	HCO₃⁻ meq/L	P_{O_2}, mmHg ET	a	(A − a)	P_{CO_2}, mmHg ET	a	(a − ET)	$\dot{V}_E/\dot{V}_{CO_2}$	$\dot{V}_E/\dot{V}_{O_2}$	V_D/V_T
	Rest		87	16	8.0	0.20	0.21	2.4	0.95			105			40			33	32	
	Rest		85	19	12.2	0.34	0.37	4.4	0.92			105			40			31	29	
	Rest		81	19	8.6	0.20	0.23	2.8	0.87			106			40			35	30	
	Rest		95	20	13.0	0.34	0.37	3.9	0.92			105			40			33	31	
	0		107	22	14.6	0.47	0.45	4.2	1.04			103			44			27	28	
	0		109	23	19.4	0.62	0.71	6.5	0.87			100			43			28	25	
0.5	3		109	22	19.1	0.63	0.76	7.0	0.83			97			44			27	23	
1.0	3		113	22	22.1	0.77	0.93	8.2	0.83			90			47			26	22	
1.5	6		116	23	21.9	0.77	0.88	7.6	0.88			97			47			26	23	
2.0	6		120	22	25.1	0.94	1.05	8.8	0.90			97			47			25	22	
2.5	9		124	22	27.5	1.06	1.11	9.0	0.95			98			48			24	23	
3.0	9		129	24	30.4	1.17	1.20	9.3	0.98			101			47			24	24	
3.5	12		138	28	35.0	1.31	1.30	9.4	1.01			102			47			25	25	
4.0	12		141	25	35.6	1.43	1.38	9.8	1.04			101			48			23	24	
4.5	15		144	27	38.6	1.53	1.45	10.1	1.06			100			50			24	25	
5.0	15		150	26	39.8	1.59	1.44	9.6	1.10			102			49			24	26	
5.5	18		155	29	45.6	1.82	1.58	10.2	1.15			104			49			24	27	
6.0	18		160	27	47.8	1.98	1.67	10.4	1.19			106			48			23	27	
6.5	21		166	30	53.3	2.14	1.73	10.4	1.24			108			48			24	29	
7.0	21		168	32	59.0	2.33	1.85	11.0	1.26			107			48			24	30	
7.5	24		175	37	67.3	2.54	1.89	10.8	1.34			113			45			25	34	
8.0	24		178	39	71.7	2.69	1.99	11.2	1.35			113			45			25	34	
8.5	27		183	43	84.9	2.97	2.07	11.3	1.43			116			43			27	39	
	Recovery		178	28	47.8	1.75	1.26	7.1	1.39			109			49			26	36	
	Recovery		175	37	68.8	2.60	1.85	10.6	1.41			114			46			25	35	
	Recovery		171	37	68.3	2.40	1.57	9.2	1.53			116			45			27	42	
	Recovery		163	35	58.1	1.84	1.20	7.4	1.53			119			40			30	46	
	Recovery		151	37	49.2	1.41	0.86	5.7	1.64			122			38			33	54	

Case 11 Normal Subject: Before and After β-Adrenergic Blockade

Clinical Findings

This 23-year-old asthmatic student voluntarily participated in a double-blind study evaluating the effect of a β-adrenergic blocker, pindolol, on exercise-induced asthma. He had had hay fever and asthma since childhood but was otherwise in excellent health. He was taking no medications. Physical examination, chest roentgenograms, ECG, and hemogram were normal.

Exercise Findings

Two similar cycle exercise studies were performed a week apart. After baseline spirometry, 0.4 mg of pindolol or placebo was given over a 20-minute period through a venous catheter. After repeat spirometry, the subject pedaled without added resistance at 60 rpm for 3 minutes and at 60 W for an additional 3 minutes. Thereafter, the work rate was increased 20 W every minute. On each occasion the subject stopped because of fatigue. ECG pattern remained normal. Repeat spirometry in duplicate or triplicate, performed 2, 7, 12, 17, 22, and 27 minutes after exercise, did not reveal exercise-induced bronchospasm.

Interpretation

Comments

This study is presented to demonstrate the effect of β-adrenergic blockade on exercise. The lowest work rate after unloaded cycling is 60 W, followed by 1-minute increments of 20 W. This uneven increase in the work rate increment causes the upward distortion in the $\dot{V}O_2$–work rate slope (panel 3, Figs. 10.11.1 and 10.11.2). Results of respiratory function testing are normal at the time of study (Table 10.11.1).

Analysis

Referring to flowchart 1, the maximum aerobic capacity and *AT* are within normal limits on both pre-

and post-β-adrenergic blockade exercise tests (Table 10.11.2). See flowchart 2. The ECG and O_2 pulse at maximum work rate are normal (branch point 2.1). The large reduction in maximum HR, with slight reduction in peak $\dot{V}O_2$ and increase in maximum O_2 pulse, is typical of the effect of β-adrenergic blockade. The chronotropic effect of the β-blockade increases the time for ventricular filling and results in a larger O_2 pulse at the same work rate.

Conclusion

This study is normal, with demonstration of heart rate slowing and the slight decrease in peak $\dot{V}O_2$ following β-adrenergic blockade.

TABLE 10.11.1.   Selected Respiratory Function Data

Measurement	Predicted	Measured
Age, yr		23
Sex		Male
Height, cm		170
Weight, kg	68	64
Hematocrit, %		45
VC, L	4.79	4.86
IC, L	3.21	3.40
TLC, L	6.46	6.72
FEV$_1$, L	4.04	3.58
FEV$_1$/VC, %	84	74
MVV, L/min	175	142
D$_L$CO, ml/mm Hg/min	33.2	32.5

TABLE 10.11.2.   Selected Exercise Data

Measurement	Predicted	Placebo	Pindolol
Peak $\dot{V}O_2$, L/min	2.90	2.57	2.39
Maximum HR, beats/min	197	189	156
Maximum O_2 pulse, ml/beat	14.7	13.6	15.3
$\Delta\dot{V}O_2$/ΔWR, ml/min/W	10.3	10.5	9.7
AT, L/min	>1.16	1.5	1.4
Maximum $\dot{V}E$, L/min		94	85
Exercise breathing reserve, L/min	>15	48	57

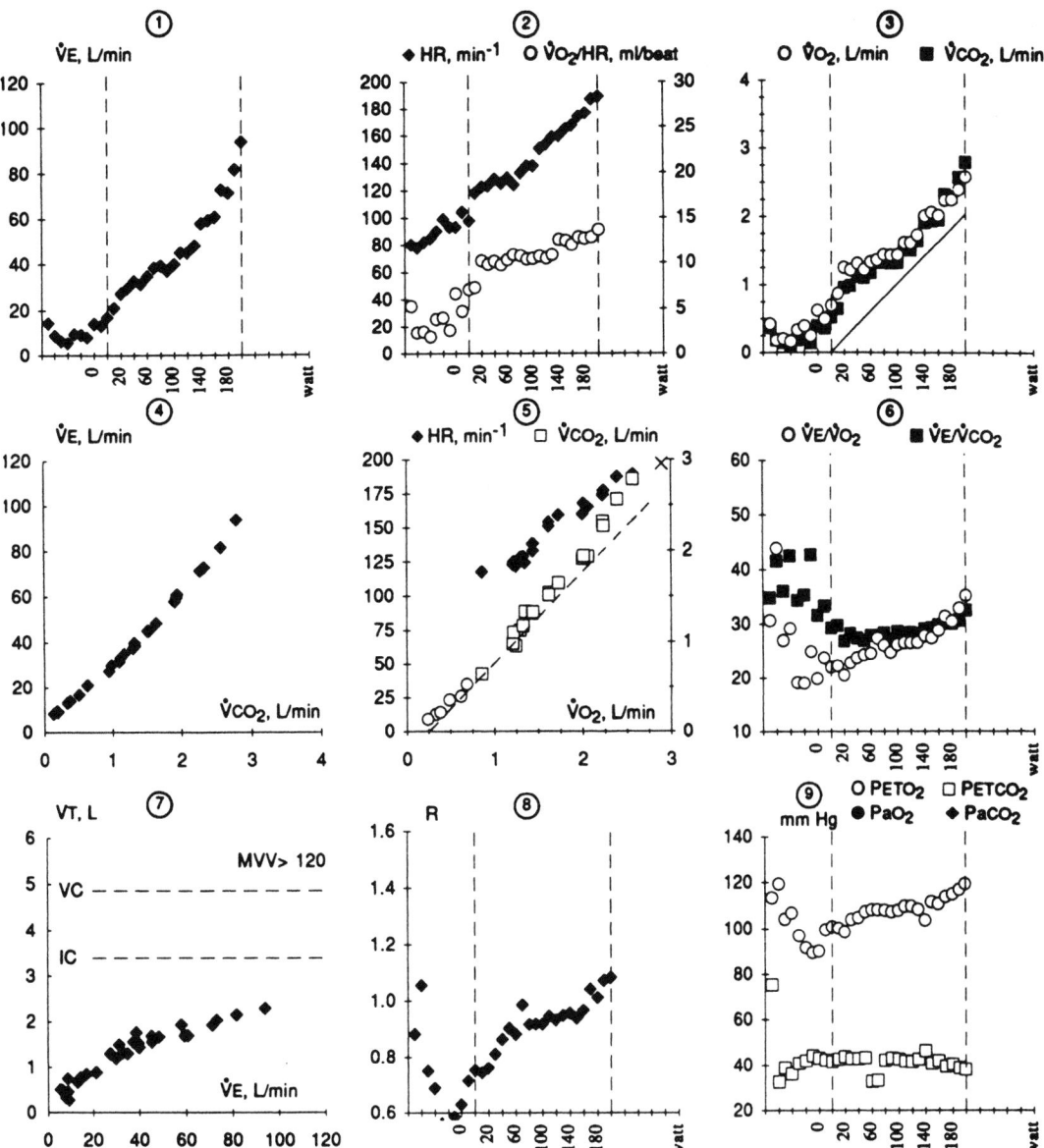

FIGURE 10.11.1.   Before β-adrenergic blockade. **1:** Vertical dashed lines in panels 1 to 3 and 6, 8, and 9 indicate the beginning and the end of the increasing work period. **2:** Unloaded cycling is performed for 3 minutes before the left vertical dashed line. **3:** In panel 3, the diagonal line shows the increase of $\dot{V}O_2$ at a slope of 10 ml/min/W. **4:** In panel 5, the diagonal dashed line has a slope of 1; the x in the upper right is the predicted maximum heart rate and $\dot{V}O_2$ for the subject.

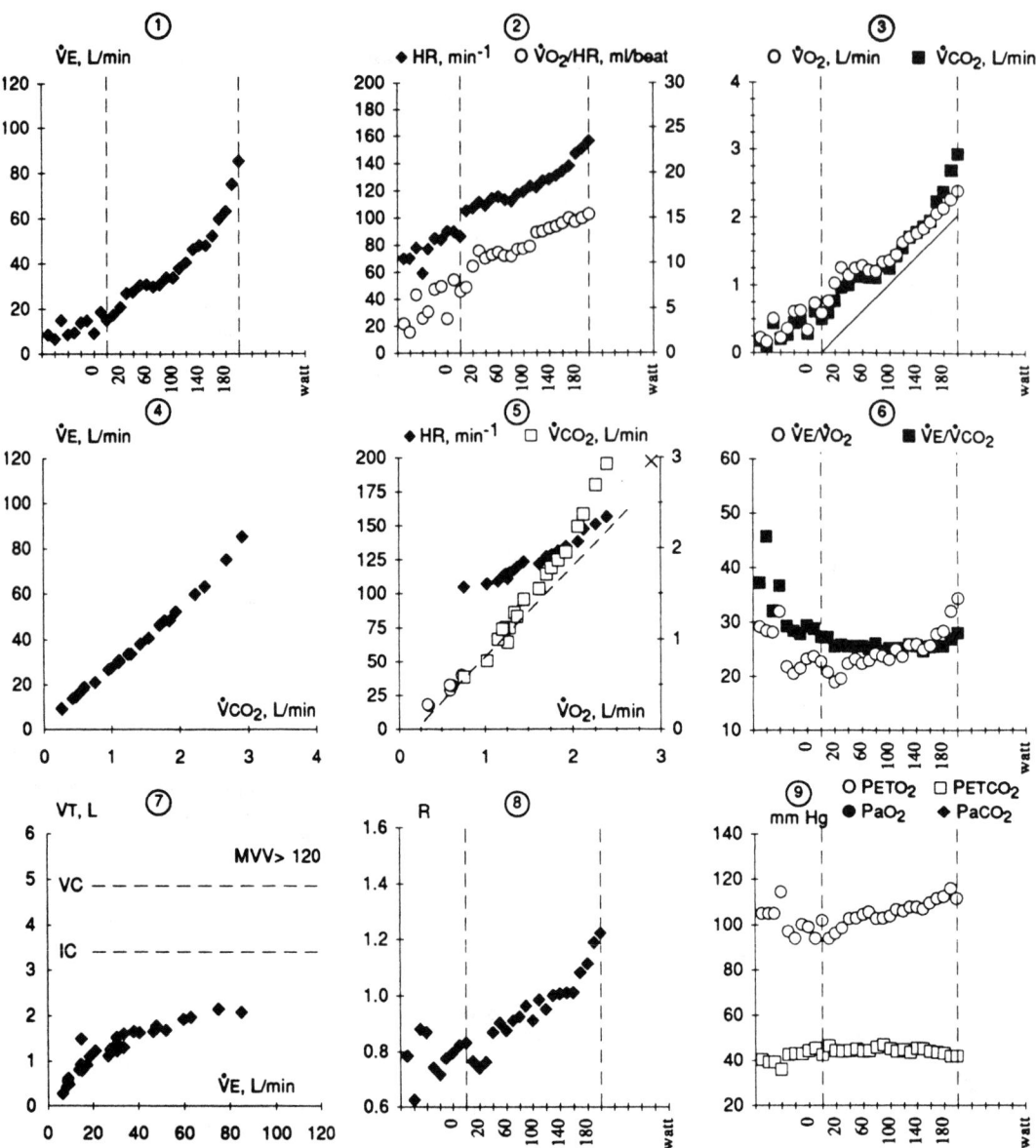

FIGURE 10.11.2.   After β-adrenergic blockade. **1:** Vertical dashed lines in panels 1 to 3 and 6, 8, and 9 indicate the beginning and the end of the increasing work period. **2:** Unloaded cycling is performed for 3 minutes before the left vertical dashed line. **3:** In panel 3, the diagonal line shows the increase of $\dot{V}O_2$ at a slope of 10 ml/min/W. **4:** In panel 5, the diagonal dashed line has a slope of 1; the x in the upper right is the predicted maximum heart rate and $\dot{V}O_2$ for the subject.

TABLE 10.11.3.   Pre-β-adrenergic Blockade

Time min	Work rate watts	BP mmHg	HR min⁻¹	f min⁻¹	$\dot{V}_E$ L/min BTPS	$\dot{V}_{CO_2}$ L/min STPD	$\dot{V}_{O_2}$ L/min STPD	$\dfrac{\dot{V}_{O_2}}{HR}$ ml/beat	R	pH	HCO₃⁻ meq/L	P_{O_2}, mmHg ET	a	(A − a)	P_{CO_2}, mmHg ET	a	(a − ET)	$\dfrac{\dot{V}_E}{\dot{V}_{CO_2}}$	$\dfrac{\dot{V}_E}{\dot{V}_{O_2}}$	$\dfrac{V_D}{V_T}$
	Rest		80	19	14.5	0.37	0.42	5.3	0.88			113			75			35	31	
	Rest		78	12	8.9	0.19	0.18	2.3	1.06			119			32			41	44	
	Rest		82	13	6.5	0.15	0.20	2.4	0.75			104			39			36	27	
	Rest		85	11	5.6	0.11	0.16	1.9	0.69			107			36			42	29	
	Unloaded		90	34	9.4	0.19	0.34	3.8	0.56			97			41			34	19	
	Unloaded		99	20	9.1	0.21	0.39	3.9	0.54			92			42			35	19	
	Unloaded		93	25	8.1	0.14	0.24	2.6	0.58			90			44			43	25	
	Unloaded		93	20	14.0	0.39	0.62	6.7	0.63			90			43			32	20	
	Unloaded		104	20	13.3	0.35	0.49	4.7	0.71			99			42			33	24	
	Unloaded		98	20	16.9	0.52	0.69	7.0	0.75			101			41			29	22	
0.5	20		118	24	21.1	0.64	0.86	7.3	0.74			100			42			30	22	
1.0	20		122	21	27.3	0.95	1.25	10.2	0.76			99			44			27	20	
1.5	40		123	25	29.8	0.98	1.21	9.8	0.81			104			43			28	23	
2.0	40		128	25	32.9	1.12	1.30	10.2	0.86			105			43			27	24	
2.5	60		125	21	31.4	1.10	1.22	9.8	0.90			107			43			27	24	
3.0	60		129	27	34.9	1.17	1.33	10.3	0.88			108			33			28	25	
3.5	80		124	22	38.7	1.33	1.35	10.9	0.99			108			33			28	27	
4.0	80		133	26	39.7	1.32	1.44	10.8	0.92			108			42			28	26	
4.5	100		138	24	37.5	1.31	1.43	10.4	0.92			107			43			27	25	
5.0	100		138	28	40.1	1.32	1.44	10.4	0.92			108			42			29	26	
5.5	120		151	27	45.3	1.53	1.62	10.7	0.94			110			42			28	27	
6.0	120		154	29	45.4	1.51	1.62	10.5	0.93			110			41			28	27	
6.5	140		159	29	48.5	1.64	1.73	10.9	0.95			108			42			28	27	
7.0	140		160	30	58.0	1.91	2.00	12.5	0.96			104			46			29	28	
7.5	160		165	35	59.4	1.93	2.06	12.5	0.94			112			41			29	27	
8.0	160		168	36	61.0	1.94	2.01	12.0	0.97			111			42			30	29	
8.5	180		174	36	72.9	2.32	2.23	12.8	1.04			114			39			30	31	
9.0	180		177	37	71.3	2.27	2.24	12.7	1.01			115			40			30	30	
9.5	200		187	38	81.7	2.56	2.39	12.8	1.07			117			39			31	33	
10.0	200		189	41	93.8	2.78	2.57	13.6	1.08			119			38			32	35	

TABLE 10.11.4. Post-β-adrenergic Blockade

Time min	Work rate watts	BP mmHg	HR min⁻¹	f min⁻¹	$\dot{V}_E$ L/min BTPS	$\dot{V}_{CO_2}$ L/min STPD	$\dot{V}_{O_2}$ L/min STPD	$\dfrac{\dot{V}_{O_2}}{HR}$ ml/beat	R	pH	HCO_3^- meq/L	P_{O_2}, mmHg ET	a	(A − a)	P_{CO_2}, mmHg ET	a	(a − ET)	$\dfrac{\dot{V}_E}{\dot{V}_{CO_2}}$	$\dfrac{\dot{V}_E}{\dot{V}_{O_2}}$	$\dfrac{V_D}{V_T}$
	Rest		70	20	8.4	0.18	0.23	3.3	0.78			105			40			37	29	
	Rest		70	24	6.6	0.10	0.16	2.3	0.63			105			39			46	29	
	Rest		78	10	14.9	0.44	0.50	6.4	0.88			105			39			32	28	
	Rest		59	16	8.7	0.20	0.23	3.9	0.87			114			36			37	32	
	Unloaded		77	20	9.3	0.26	0.35	4.5	0.74			97			42			29	22	
	Unloaded		85	17	13.7	0.43	0.60	7.1	0.72			94			43			29	20	
	Unloaded		84	16	14.7	0.48	0.62	7.4	0.77			100			43			28	22	
	Unloaded		90	15	9.2	0.27	0.34	3.8	0.79			99			44			29	23	
	Unloaded		90	17	18.7	0.60	0.73	8.1	0.82			94			46			29	24	
	Unloaded		86	19	15.0	0.49	0.59	6.9	0.83			102			42			27	23	
0.5	20		105	19	17.4	0.58	0.76	7.2	0.76			94			47			27	21	
1.0	20		107	17	20.9	0.76	1.03	9.6	0.74			96			44			26	19	
1.5	40		111	24	26.8	0.96	1.26	11.4	0.76			99			44			26	20	
2.0	40		109	22	27.5	1.00	1.15	10.6	0.87			103			45			26	22	
2.5	60		114	20	30.4	1.12	1.24	10.9	0.90			103			45			26	23	
3.0	60		115	25	30.7	1.12	1.28	11.1	0.88			104			44			26	22	
3.5	80		113	23	29.9	1.11	1.22	10.8	0.91			106			44			25	23	
4.0	80		112	22	30.7	1.11	1.20	10.7	0.93			103			46			26	24	
4.5	100		117	21	33.6	1.29	1.34	11.5	0.96			103			47			25	24	
5.0	100		119	26	33.7	1.25	1.37	11.5	0.91			104			45			25	23	
5.5	120		123	23	38.0	1.43	1.45	11.8	0.99			107			44			25	25	
6.0	120		122	25	40.6	1.55	1.63	13.4	0.95			106			45			25	24	
6.5	140		127	28	46.5	1.71	1.71	13.5	1.00			108			44			26	26	
7.0	140		128	28	48.2	1.78	1.77	13.8	1.01			108			46			26	26	
7.5	160		131	27	48.1	1.86	1.84	14.0	1.01			107			45			25	25	
8.0	160		134	31	52.2	1.95	1.93	14.4	1.01			110			44			25	26	
8.5	180		138	31	59.8	2.23	2.06	14.9	1.08			111			44			26	28	
9.0	180		147	32	63.1	2.37	2.13	14.5	1.11			112			43			25	28	
9.5	200		151	35	75.1	2.69	2.26	15.0	1.19			116			42			27	32	
10.1	200		156	41	85.2	2.92	2.39	15.3	1.22			111			42			28	34	

Case 12 Normal Subject: Immediate Effects of Cigarette Smoking

Clinical Findings

This 27-year-old subject was one of several men who volunteered for a study to investigate the effect of recent cigarette smoking on cardiovascular and respiratory function during exercise. The subject was apparently in excellent general health, but had smoked cigarettes for 10 years. Physical examination, chest roentgenogram, and ECG were normal.

Exercise Findings

Two similar exercise studies were performed 6 days apart on a cycle ergometer. In the 5 hours before the first study, the subject smoked 15 medium-tar cigarettes. In the second study, the subject was under observation for 5 hours without smoking. He breathed oxygen for the first 3 of those 5 hours to reduce the carboxyhemoglobin in his blood. On both occasions he pedaled without added load at 60 rpm for 3 minutes. The work rate was then increased 25 W every minute to his symptom-limited maximum. On both occasions, the subject stopped exercise because of fatigue. ECG remained normal. Carboxyhemoglobin levels were 6.1% at the start of the first study and 1.5% at the start of the second study.

Interpretation

Comments

This study is presented because it illustrates the small but significant effects of short-term cigarette smoking on the peak $\dot{V}O_2$ and the anaerobic threshold. It also illustrates the reproducibility of the cardiac and gas exchange responses to exercise performed on different days, and the effects of obesity.

Results of resting respiratory function studies are normal (Table 10.12.1). The resting ECG is normal.

TABLE 10.12.1.   Selected Respiratory Function Data

Measurement	Predicted	With Prior Smoking	Without Smoking
Age, yr		27	
Sex		Male	
Height, cm		168	
Weight, kg	69	83	
Hematocrit, %		47	47
VC, L	4.65	4.18	4.20
IC, L	3.10	3.43	3.43
TLC, L	6.19	6.26	6.68
FEV_1, L	3.79	3.57	3.55
FEV_1/VC, %	81	85	85
MVV, L/min	168	149	163
$D_L CO$, ml/mm Hg/min	31.2	34.7	37.4

TABLE 10.12.2.   Selected Exercise Data

Measurement	Predicted	With Prior Smoking	Without Prior Smoking
Peak $\dot{V}O_2$, L/min	2.99	2.55	2.73
Maximum HR, beats/min	193	178	182
Maximum O_2 pulse, ml/beat	15.5	14.3	15.0
$\Delta\dot{V}O_2/\Delta WR$, ml/min/W	10.3	9.0	9.9
AT, L/min	>1.23	1.1	1.25
Blood pressure, mmHg (rest, max)		138/84, 183/110	132/84, 186/105
Maximum $\dot{V}E$, L/min		110	121
Exercise breathing reserve, L/min	>15	39	42
PaO_2, mmHg (rest, max ex)		102, 103	109, 106
$P(A - a)O_2$, mmHg (rest, max ex)		5, 19	−1, 16
$P(a - ET)CO_2$, mmHg (rest, max ex)		−1, −3	−2, −3
VD/VT (rest, heavy ex)		0.37, 0.18	0.27, 0.20
HCO_3^-, mEq/L (rest, 2-min recov)		25, 14	26, 15

TABLE 10.12.3. With Prior Smoking

Time min	Work rate watts	BP mmHg	HR min⁻¹	f min⁻¹	$\dot{V}_E$ L/min BTPS	$\dot{V}_{CO_2}$ L/min STPD	$\dot{V}_{O_2}$ L/min STPD	$\dot{V}_{O_2}$/HR ml/beat	R	pH	HCO₃⁻ meq/L	PO₂, mmHg ET	a	(A − a)	PCO₂, mmHg ET	a	(a − ET)	$\dot{V}_E$/$\dot{V}_{CO_2}$	$\dot{V}_E$/$\dot{V}_{O_2}$	VD/VT
	Rest	138/84								7.42	24		98			38				
	Rest		76	26	12.1	0.24	0.31	4.1	0.77			100			41			41	32	
	Rest		77	27	13.4	0.27	0.31	4.0	0.87			106			39			41	36	
	Rest		76	27	11.1	0.21	0.27	3.6	0.78			97			42			42	33	
	Rest	138/84	77	25	13.2	0.28	0.32	4.2	0.88	7.42	25	107	102	5	40	39	−1	40	35	0.37
	Rest		76	25	12.4	0.26	0.30	3.9	0.87			105			40			40	34	
	Rest		75	25	11.7	0.23	0.26	3.5	0.88			104			41			42	37	
	Unloaded		99	19	15.8	0.50	0.51	5.2	0.98			104			43			28	28	
	Unloaded		101	20	17.1	0.56	0.65	6.4	0.86			97			43			28	24	
	Unloaded		103	21	19.2	0.69	0.89	8.6	0.78			93			46			25	20	
	Unloaded		103	21	23.6	0.87	0.96	9.3	0.91			97			45			25	23	
	Unloaded		102	24	21.8	0.76	0.84	8.2	0.90			100			45			26	24	
	Unloaded	156/96	105	23	23.8	0.85	0.92	8.8	0.92	7.39	24	102	98	8	45	41	−4	26	24	0.17
0.5	25		107	22	22.5	0.81	0.89	8.3	0.91			99			45			25	23	
1.0	25		109	21	24.0	0.90	0.99	9.1	0.91			100			44			25	22	
1.5	50		113	25	27.0	0.97	1.03	9.1	0.94			99			46			26	24	
2.0	50	165/93	115	23	32.1	1.16	1.17	10.2	0.99	7.38	24	101	95	13	45	42	−3	26	26	0.20
2.5	75		123	25	31.6	1.20	1.24	10.1	0.97			100			46			25	24	
3.0	75		124	25	35.4	1.36	1.33	10.7	1.02			103			46			24	25	
3.5	100		129	27	36.8	1.42	1.38	10.7	1.03			102			47			24	25	
4.0	100	177/96	135	26	43.4	1.68	1.53	11.3	1.10	7.36	24	102	94	16	47	43	−4	25	27	0.17
4.5	125		145	29	43.0	1.70	1.61	11.1	1.06			103			47			24	25	
5.0	125		150	30	50.8	2.01	1.88	12.5	1.07			103			48			24	26	
5.5	150		154	33	57.5	2.21	1.99	12.9	1.11			105			47			25	27	
6.0	150	177/99	162	36	66.6	2.47	2.09	12.9	1.18	7.33	22	107	95	18	46	42	−4	26	30	0.19
6.5	175		171	36	70.4	2.66	2.24	13.1	1.19			108			46			25	30	
7.0	175		172	43	84.8	2.95	2.34	13.6	1.26			112			43			28	35	
7.5	200		176	51	101.2	3.27	2.51	14.3	1.30			115			41			30	39	
8.0	200		178	62	110.6	3.36	2.55	14.3	1.32	7.32	17	119	103	19	37	34	−3	31	41	0.18
	Recovery		176	45	95.2	2.99	2.18	12.4	1.37			119			39			31	42	
	Recovery		164	43	81.4	2.46	1.49	9.1	1.65			123			37			32	52	
	Recovery		160	43	70.6	1.93	1.15	7.2	1.68			125			36			35	58	
	Recovery	165/84	153	35	53.3	1.46	0.98	6.4	1.49	7.27	14	123	112	14	35	32	−3	34	51	0.21

Analysis

Referring to flowchart 1, the peak $\dot{V}_{O_2}$ is reduced with prior smoking as compared with the non-smoking study and is borderline normal. However, it was clearly normal without prior smoking (Table 10.12.2). The anaerobic threshold is reduced after smoking but is normal without prior smoking (Table 10.12.2). Referring to flowchart 2, the subject is 20% overweight (branch point 2.2). This obese subject's $\dot{V}_{O_2}$ during unloaded cycling is approximately 0.95 L/min (Table 10.12.3 and panel 3 of Figs. 10.12.1 and 10.12.2).

Indices other than peak $\dot{V}_{O_2}$ and AT that might reflect the effect of the increased carboxyhemoglobin during exercise are the O_2 pulse and $\Delta\dot{V}_{O_2}/\Delta WR$. These are both reduced after cigarette smok-

ing (Table 10.12.2). Although the indices of ventilation–perfusion matching are normal at maximum exercise in this and most normal subjects, they tend to become abnormal immediately after smoking (1).

Conclusion

Cigarette smoking and obesity have affected exercise performance in an otherwise normal subject.

Reference

1. Hirsch GL, Sue DY, Wasserman K, et al. Immediate effects of cigarette smoking on cardiorespiratory responses to exercise. *J Appl Physiol* 1985;58:1975–1981.

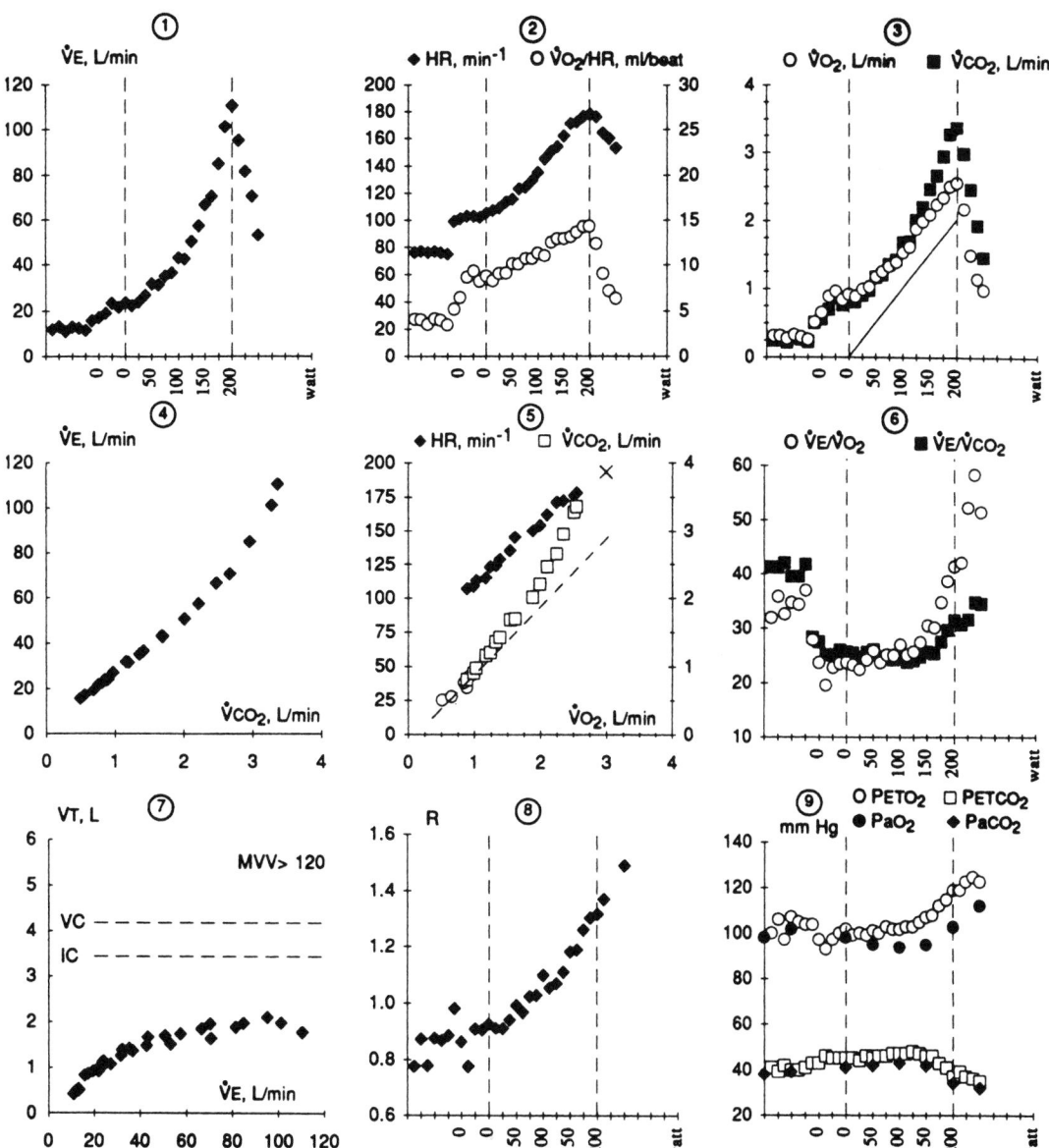

FIGURE 10.12.1.   With prior smoking. **1:** Vertical dashed lines in panels 1 to 3 and 6, 8, and 9 indicate the beginning and the end of the increasing work period. **2:** Unloaded cycling is performed for 3 minutes before the left vertical dashed line. **3:** In panel 3, the diagonal line shows the increase of $\dot{V}O_2$ at a slope of 10 ml/min/W. **4:** In panel 5, the diagonal dashed line has a slope of 1; the *x* in the upper right is the predicted maximum heart rate and $\dot{V}O_2$ for the subject.

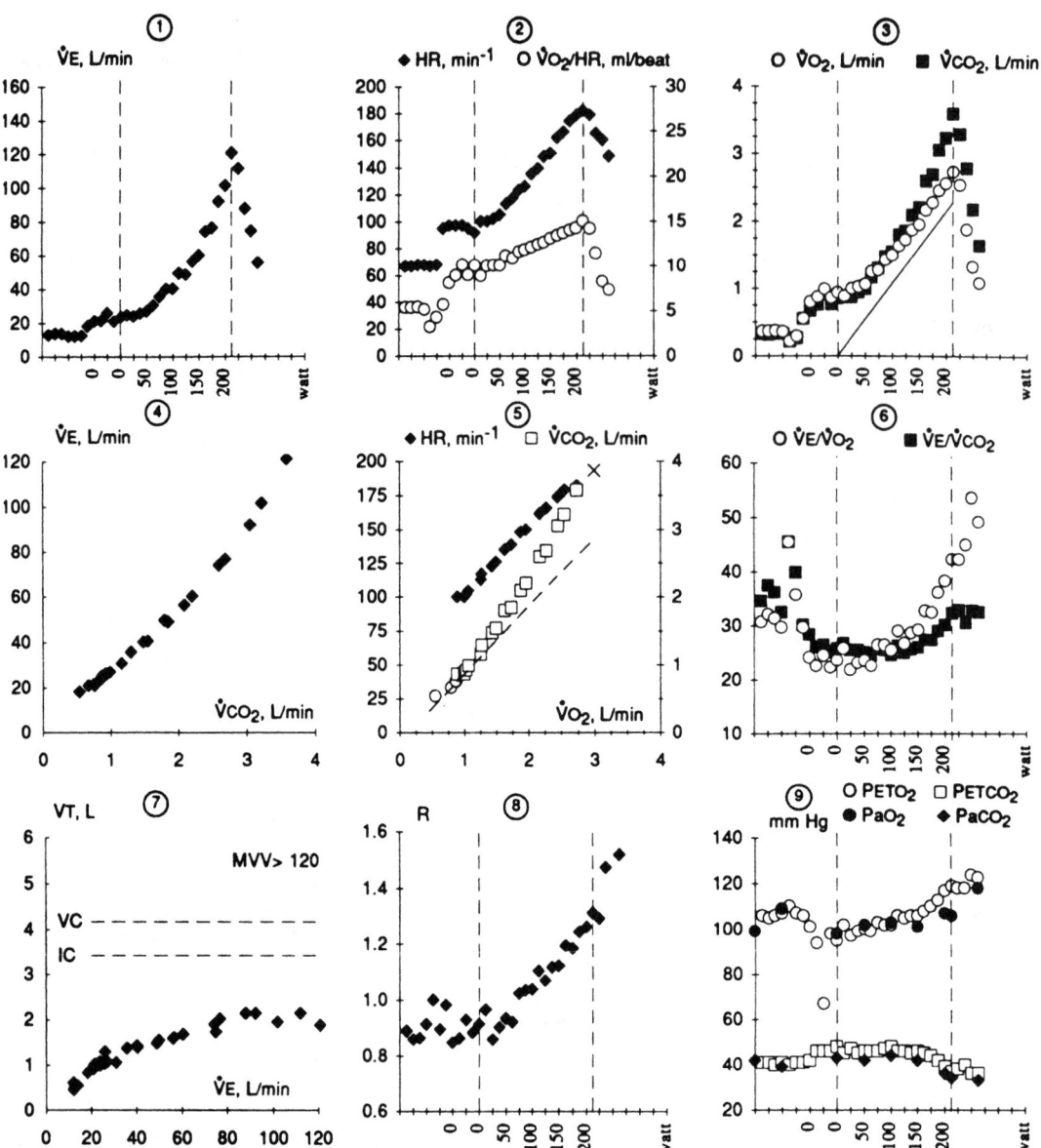

FIGURE 10.12.2.   Without prior smoking. **1:** Vertical dashed lines in panels 1 to 3 and 6, 8, and 9 indicate the beginning and the end of the increasing work period. **2:** Unloaded cycling is performed for 3 minutes before the left vertical dashed line. **3:** In panel 3, the diagonal line shows the increase of $\dot{V}O_2$ at a slope of 10 ml/min/W. **4:** In panel 5, the diagonal dashed line has a slope of 1; the x in the upper right is the predicted maximum heart rate and $\dot{V}O_2$ for the subject.

TABLE 10.12.4.   Without Prior Smoking

Time min	Work rate watts	BP mmHg	HR min⁻¹	f min⁻¹	$\dot{V}_E$ L/min BTPS	$\dot{V}_{CO_2}$ L/min STPD	$\dot{V}_{O_2}$ L/min STPD	$\dot{V}_{O_2}$/HR ml/beat	R	pH	HCO_3^- meq/L	P_{O_2} ET	P_{O_2} a	P_{O_2} (A−a)	P_{CO_2} ET	P_{CO_2} a	P_{CO_2} (a−ET)	$\dot{V}_E/\dot{V}_{CO_2}$	$\dot{V}_E/\dot{V}_{O_2}$	V_D/V_T
	Rest	129/84								7.40	26	99			42					
	Rest		67	24	13.1	0.32	0.36	5.4	0.89			106			41			35	31	
	Rest		67	26	13.8	0.31	0.36	5.4	0.86			105			41			37	32	
	Rest		68	26	13.8	0.32	0.37	5.4	0.86			106			40			36	31	
	Rest	132/84	68	20	12.1	0.32	0.35	5.1	0.91	7.43	25	107	109	−1	41	39	−2	33	30	0.27
	Rest		67	27	12.3	0.22	0.22	3.3	1.00			110			40			45	45	
	Rest		68	25	12.5	0.26	0.29	4.3	0.90			107			41			40	36	
	Unloaded		95	22	18.2	0.54	0.55	5.8	0.98			106			41			30	30	
	Unloaded		97	23	21.0	0.67	0.79	8.1	0.85			101			42			28	24	
	Unloaded		97	21	21.4	0.75	0.87	9.0	0.86			94			46			26	23	
	Unloaded		97	20	26.0	0.92	0.99	10.2	0.93			67			46			26	25	
	Unloaded		95	21		0.76	0.86	9.1	0.88			98			46			25	22	
	Unloaded	141/87	92	22	23.8	0.85	0.93	10.1	0.91	7.39	26	95	98	6	48	43	−5	26	24	0.20
0.5	25		100	24	25.0	0.86	0.89	8.9	0.97			102			45			27	26	
1.0	25		100	24	24.0	0.86	1.00	10.0	0.86			97			47			26	22	
1.5	50		102	25	25.9	0.93	1.03	10.1	0.90			99			45			26	23	
2.0	50	153/90	105	25	27.0	0.99	1.06	10.1	0.93	7.39	25	100	102	4	46	42	−4	25	23	0.17
2.5	75		113	29	30.9	1.16	1.26	11.2	0.92			99			46			25	23	
3.0	75		117	26	35.8	1.30	1.27	10.9	1.02			103			46			26	26	
3.5	100		123	28	40.3	1.48	1.43	11.6	1.03			102			47			26	27	
4.0	100	168/93	126	29	40.6	1.55	1.49	11.8	1.04	7.37	25	102	103	4	48	44	−4	25	26	0.19
4.5	125		135	32	50.0	1.80	1.63	12.1	1.10			106			46			26	29	
5.0	125		139	33	49.0	1.85	1.73	12.4	1.07			105			46			25	27	
5.5	150		148	35	56.6	2.09	1.87	12.6	1.12			106			45			26	29	
6.0	150	177/99	150	36	60.4	2.20	1.96	13.1	1.12	7.36	23	106	101	11	46	42	−4	26	29	0.20
6.5	175		162	39	74.3	2.59	2.17	13.4	1.19			108			45			27	33	
7.0	175		166	38	76.8	2.69	2.27	13.7	1.19			110			44			27	32	
7.5	200		174	43	92.2	3.05	2.45	14.1	1.24			113			42			29	36	
8.0	200	186/105	179	52	101.8	3.22	2.55	14.2	1.26	7.35	20	117	107	13	39	36	−3	30	38	0.20
8.5	225		182	64	121.0	3.58	2.73	15.0	1.31	7.32	17	119	106	16	37	34	−3	32	42	0.20
	Recovery		179	52	111.9	3.28	2.54	14.2	1.29			118			38			33	42	
	Recovery		165	41	88.0	2.77	1.88	11.4	1.47			118			40			31	45	
	Recovery		160	43	74.9	2.18	1.33	8.3	1.64			124			36			33	54	
	Recovery	162/90	148	35	56.1	1.64	1.08	7.3	1.52	7.26	15	123	118	8	36	33	−3	32	49	0.18

Case 13 Cardiologic Misdiagnoses in a Man at Ages 65 and 72

Clinical Findings

At age 65, this self-employed male executive had cardiopulmonary exercise testing to evaluate dyspnea that had occurred while he was hiking with a group of young men at an altitude of 10,000 ft (3 km). He had been an avid hiker but had noted a decreased ability to hike at high altitudes in the last 3 to 4 years. He was referred by his private physician to a cardiologist, who peformed an extensive cardiologic workup, including treadmill exercise tests (without gas exchange measurements), gated cardiac wall motion studies, echocardiogram, and a coronary angiogram. The results of these were negative. He was told that he probably had heart failure secondary to a cardiomyopathy and was prescribed an angiotensin-converting enzyme inhibitor. The patient believed that the drug did not help him but caused untoward side effects. The results of the cardiopulmonary exercise tests done at Harbor-UCLA reported here show that this man did not have heart failure and, in fact, had above-normal parameters of aerobic function, indicating good cardiac function.

Seven years later, he still liked to hike, but he no longer did it at high altitude. Because he experienced exercise fatigue and found that he was not able to maintain the pace of his female companion, he went to a cardiologist, who gave him an extensive cardiologic workup that included an exercise study without gas exchange measurements. During the exercise test, he developed ST-segment depression in the left precordial leads that became more marked as exercise progressed, and had a run of three premature ventricular contractions (PVCs) at a heart rate of 150, his maximum. The cardiologist concluded that the patient had "excellent exercise tolerance" and discounted the ECG changes as a "false positive ECG response" based on normal echocardiographic studies. The pulmonary artery systolic pressure was estimated to be 70 to 75 mm Hg during exercise. Because of the pulmonary hypertension, the patient was referred to a pulmonologist. $\dot{V}/\dot{Q}$ scans were read as showing a low probability of pulmonary embolus. This patient was referred by the pulmonologist to Harbor-UCLA for evaluation because of fatigue with exercise and a diagnosis of pulmonary hypertension, based on the interpretation of echocardiographic studies, which the pulmonologist felt could not be attributed to lung disease.

TABLE 10.13.1.   Selected Respiratory Function Data, Age 65

Measurement	Predicted	Measured
Age, yr		65
Sex		Male
Height, cm		183
Weight, kg	83	83
Hematocrit, %		44
VC, L	4.60	4.70
IC, L	3.06	3.70
FEV$_1$, L	3.45	3.47
FEV$_1$/VC, %	75	74
MVV, L/min	142	129
D$_L$CO, ml/mm Hg/min	28.0	28.6

TABLE 10.13.2.   Selected Exercise Data, Age 65

Measurement	Predicted (Room air)	Measured	
		Air	15% O$_2$
Peak $\dot{V}$O$_2$, L/min	2.21	2.69	2.19
Maximum HR, beats/min	155	175	172
Maximum O$_2$ pulse, ml/beat	14.3	15.9	12.9
$\Delta\dot{V}$O$_2$/ΔWR, ml/min/W	10.3	10.3	7.8
AT, L/min	>0.99	1.9	1.2
Blood pressure, mmHg (rest, max ex)		132/72, 210/90	114/66, 198/96
Maximum $\dot{V}$E, L/min		115	108
Exercise breathing reserves, L/min	>15	14	21
PaO$_2$, mmHg (rest, max ex)		113, 106	77, 52
P(A − a)O$_2$ mmHg (rest, max ex)		−1, 16	0, 27
P(a − ET)CO$_2$, mmHg (rest, max ex)		1, −3	2, 0
VD/VT (rest, max ex)		0.25, 0.21	0.36, 0.19
HCO$_3^-$, mEq/L (rest, 2-min recovery)		21, 15	21, 17

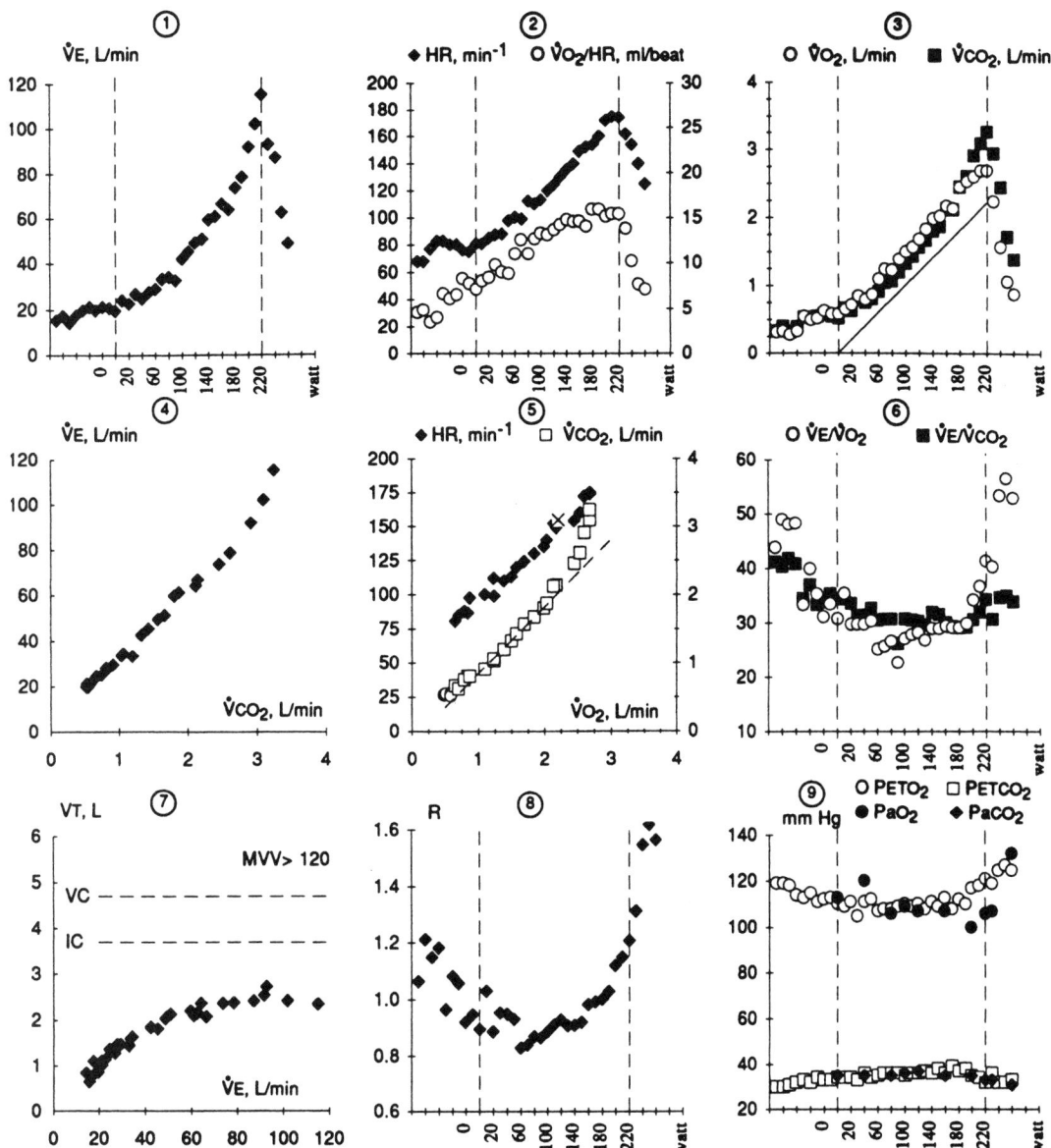

FIGURE 10.13.1.   Room air, age 65. **1:** Vertical dashed lines in panels 1 to 3 and 6, 8, and 9 indicate the beginning and the end of the increasing work period. **2:** Unloaded cycling is performed for 3 minutes before the left vertical dashed line. **3:** In panel 3, the diagonal line shows the increase of $\dot{V}O_2$ at a slope of 10 ml/min/W. **4:** In panel 5, the diagonal dashed line has a slope of 1; the x in the upper right is the predicted maximum heart rate and $\dot{V}O_2$ for the subject.

Exercise Findings

Age 65

The patient performed exercise on a cycle ergometer while he breathed room air and a second time breathing 15% O_2 (equivalent to an 8,000-ft altitude). On both occasions, he pedaled at 60 rpm without an added load for 3 minutes. The work rate was then increased 20 W per minute to tolerance. Arterial blood was sampled every second minute, and intraarterial pressure was recorded from a per-

cutaneously placed brachial artery catheter. The patient stopped exercise because of fatigue and shortness of breath on both occasions. No ECG abnormalities were noted at rest or during exercise.

Age 72

The air-breathing exercise study was repeated using the same protocol as that used in the initial evaluation at age 65, including arterial blood sampling and pressure measurements. The ST segment

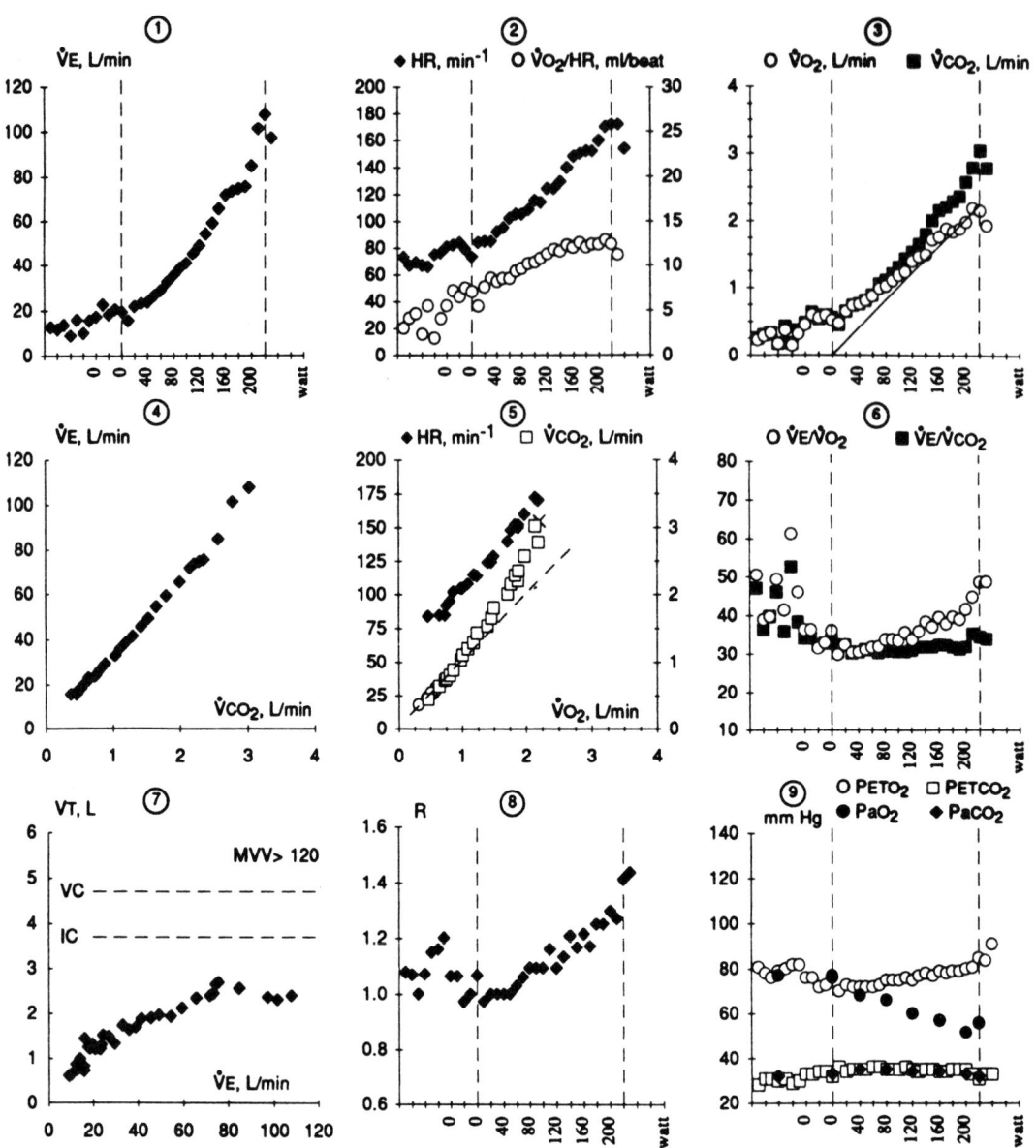

FIGURE 10.13.2.   Fifteen percent oxygen, age 65. **1:** Vertical dashed lines in panels 1 to 3 and 6, 8, and 9 indicate the beginning and the end of the increasing work period. **2:** Unloaded cycling is performed for 3 minutes before the left vertical dashed line. **3:** In panel 3, the diagonal line shows the increase of $\dot{V}O_2$ at a slope of 10 ml/min/W. **4:** In panel 5, the diagonal dashed line has a slope of 1; the x in the upper right is the predicted maximum heart rate and $\dot{V}O_2$ for the subject.

was depressed in aVF by 1.5 mm at a heart rate of 125. At a heart rate of 137, the ST segment was depressed by 2 mm in lead III, aVF, and V_5, with smaller depression in V_4 and V_6. He had no ectopic beats or chest pain.

Interpretation

Comments

Resting respiratory function studies were normal.

Analysis

Age 65. Referring to flowchart 1, peak $\dot{V}O_2$ and the anaerobic threshold are both normal, well above predicted values for sedentary men. Proceeding to flowchart 2 through branch points 2.1 and 2.2, it is apparent that the patient is an exceptionally fit man. The low breathing reserve is compatible with good motivation. While the patient was breathing 15% O_2, peak $\dot{V}O_2$ and the anaerobic threshold decreased. $\Delta\dot{V}O_2/\Delta WR$ and exercise tolerance de-

TABLE 10.13.3.   Room Air, Age 65

Time min	Work rate watts	BP mmHg	HR min⁻¹	f min⁻¹	$\dot{V}_E$ L/min BTPS	$\dot{V}_{CO_2}$ L/min STPD	$\dot{V}_{O_2}$ L/min STPD	$\dot{V}_{O_2}$/HR ml/beat	R	pH	HCO₃⁻ meq/L	P_{O_2}, mmHg ET	a	(A − a)	P_{CO_2}, mmHg ET	a	(a − ET)	$\dot{V}_E$/$\dot{V}_{CO_2}$	$\dot{V}_E$/$\dot{V}_{O_2}$	VD/VT
	Rest		68	24	15.6	0.33	0.31	4.6	1.06			119			30			41	44	
	Rest		68	16	17.5	0.40	0.33	4.9	1.21			119			30			40	49	
	Rest		77	17	14.4	0.31	0.27	3.5	1.15			118			31			42	48	
	Rest		83	22	17.8	0.39	0.33	4.0	1.18			114			32			41	48	
	Unloaded		83	19	19.9	0.53	0.55	6.6	0.96			113			33			35	33	
	Unloaded		80	21	21.3	0.53	0.49	6.1	1.08			115			32			37	40	
	Unloaded		80	19	19.9	0.55	0.52	6.5	1.06			111			34			33	35	
	Unloaded		76	19	21.2	0.58	0.63	8.3	0.92			112			33			34	31	
	Unloaded		75	19	21.0	0.55	0.58	7.7	0.95			113			33			35	33	
	Unloaded	135/72	81	23	19.8	0.52	0.58	7.2	0.90	7.40	21	110	113	−1	34	35	1	34	31	0.25
0.5	20		81	18	24.5	0.67	0.65	8.0	1.03			109			34			34	35	
1.0	20		85	20	22.8	0.63	0.71	8.4	0.89			111			34			33	30	
1.5	40		87	21	27.1	0.81	0.85	9.8	0.95			105			33			31	30	
2.0	40	144/75	88	19	25.1	0.75	0.79	9.0	0.95	7.40	21	111	120	−6	36	35	−1	31	30	0.20
2.5	60		98	19	28.0	0.81	0.87	8.9	0.93			112			34			33	30	
3.0	60		100	20	29.4	0.91	1.10	11.0	0.83			107			35			30	25	
3.5	80		99	21	33.7	1.04	1.24	12.5	0.84			108			36			31	26	
4.0	80	144/75	112	21	34.5	1.07	1.23	11.0	0.87	7.40	21	108	106	5	36	35	−1	31	27	0.18
4.5	100		110	23	33.3	1.20	1.39	12.6	0.86			109			36			26	23	
5.0	100	162/84	113	23	42.6	1.33	1.50	13.3	0.89	7.40	22	110	109	1	35	36	1	31	27	0.21
5.5	120		120	25	45.6	1.43	1.57	13.1	0.91			109			36			30	28	
6.0	120	168/84	124	24	49.6	1.57	1.69	13.6	0.93	7.40	23	110	107	4	36	37	1	30	28	0.22
6.5	140		130	24	51.2	1.67	1.84	14.2	0.91			108			37			29	27	
7.0	140		135	27	59.8	1.81	1.99	14.7	0.91			111			36			32	29	
7.5	160		140	29	61.2	1.87	2.03	14.5	0.92			109			38			31	29	
8.0	160	174/84	149	32	66.7	2.14	2.18	14.6	0.98	7.40	21	113	107	7	36	35	−1	30	29	0.17
8.5	180		152	27	64.3	2.12	2.14	14.1	0.99			108			39			29	29	
9.0	180		154	31	73.7	2.45	2.45	15.9	1.00			112			37			29	29	
9.5	200		160	33	78.7	2.61	2.54	15.9	1.03			110			38			29	30	
10.0	200	207/84	172	36	91.8	2.91	2.60	15.1	1.12	7.40	21	117	100	18	35	35	0	30	34	0.19
10.5	220		175	42	102.1	3.09	2.69	15.4	1.15			118			34			32	37	
11.0	220	210/90	174	49	115.3	3.25	2.69	15.5	1.21	7.40	20	121	106	15	32	33	1	34	41	0.23
	Recovery		162	34	92.9	2.94	2.24	13.8	1.31	7.30	16	119	107	16	36	33	−3	31	40	0.14
	Recovery		154	36	87.3	2.44	1.58	10.3	1.54			125			32			35	53	
	Recovery		140	29	62.8	1.73	1.07	7.6	1.62			127			32			35	56	
	Recovery		125	24	49.1	1.39	0.89	7.1	1.56	7.30	15	125	132	−4	33	31	−2	34	53	0.17

creased somewhat; these decreases are expected because all of these measurements are O_2 transport dependent.

Age 72. The patient's predicted peak $\dot{V}_{O_2}$ had decreased by 0.2 L/min, but his actual peak $\dot{V}_{O_2}$ had decreased by 0.7 L/min. Referring to flowchart 1, his peak $\dot{V}_{O_2}$ is still within normal limits (branch point 1.1). Referring to flowchart 2, his ECG is abnormal (branch point 2.1). His VD/VT, P(A − a)O_2, and P(a − ET)CO_2 are normal (branch point 2.3), indicating that the patient probably has early cardiovascular disease but does not have functionally significant lung or pulmonary vascular disease.

Because there were important changes in O_2 transport—such as decreasing slope of the $\dot{V}_{O_2}$–work rate relation, O_2 pulse becoming constant at a lower than predicted value, and steepening of the heart rate response to increasing $\dot{V}_{O_2}$ (panel 5 of Fig. 10.13.3) above the heart rate at which the ST segments begin to decrease—it should be concluded that the ECG changes reflected functionally important myocardial ischemia. This patient probably developed significant myocardial ischemia with exercise at a $\dot{V}_{O_2}$ of about 1.4 L/min and a heart rate of about 110 beats per minute (heart rate at which the heart rate–$\dot{V}_{O_2}$ relation starts to become more steep and O_2 pulse becomes constant). Because C(a − $\bar{v}$)O_2 increases with increasing $\dot{V}_{O_2}$, the constant O_2 pulse could be interpreted as indicating that the stroke volume starts to decrease above the work rate at which the O_2 pulse becomes constant. The decreasing stroke volume is the likely cause of the nonlinear steepening of the heart rate–$\dot{V}_{O_2}$ relation (Fig.

TABLE 10.13.4.   15% Oxygen, Age 65

Time min	Work rate watts	BP mmHg	HR min⁻¹	f min⁻¹	V̇E L/min BTPS	V̇CO₂ L/min STPD	V̇O₂ L/min STPD	V̇O₂/HR ml/beat	R	pH	HCO₃⁻ meq/L	PO₂, mmHg ET	a	(A − a)	PCO₂, mmHg ET	a	(a − ET)	V̇E/V̇CO₂	V̇E/V̇O₂	VD/VT
	Rest		73	17	12.7	0.24	0.22	3.0	1.08			81			28			47	51	
	Rest		67	14	12.1	0.30	0.28	4.2	1.07			78			31			36	39	
	Rest		69	14	13.9	0.32	0.32	4.6	1.00			76			31			40	40	
	Rest	114/56	67	15	9.1	0.17	0.16	2.4	1.07	7.44	21	79	77	0	30	32	2	46	49	0.36
	Rest		66	11	16.0	0.42	0.37	5.5	1.15			80			31			36	41	
	Rest		75	16	10.3	0.17	0.15	2.0	1.16			82			29			53	61	
	Unloaded		76	19	15.8	0.37	0.31	4.0	1.20			82			30			38	46	
	Unloaded		81	14	17.5	0.48	0.45	5.6	1.07			76			33			34	36	
	Unloaded		82	19	23.1	0.63	0.59	7.2	1.07			76			33			34	36	
	Unloaded		84	15	18.4	0.53	0.54	6.5	0.97			72			34			32	31	
	Unloaded		79	17	20.8	0.59	0.59	7.5	1.00			73			34			33	33	
	Unloaded	132/36	73	15	19.8	0.55	0.51	7.1	1.07	7.39	20	77	76	0	32	33	1	34	36	0.21
0.5	20		84	22	15.7	0.45	0.46	5.5	0.97			70			36			31	30	
1.0	20		85	18	22.2	0.64	0.64	7.5	1.00			73			34			32	32	
1.5	40		85	18	23.6	0.73	0.73	8.6	1.00			72			35			30	30	
2.0	40	114/60	92	16	24.2	0.75	0.75	8.1	1.00	7.41	22	72	68	4	35	35	0	30	30	0.18
2.5	60		95	18	26.8	0.81	0.81	8.5	1.00			72			35			31	31	
3.0	60		102	22	29.4	0.89	0.86	8.5	1.03			72			36			31	32	
3.5	80		105	19	33.0	1.04	0.98	9.3	1.06			73			36			30	32	
4.0	80	144/66	105	22	36.0	1.11	1.01	9.7	1.10	7.42	22	75	66	9	35	35	0	31	34	0.19
4.5	100		108	23	38.9	1.20	1.10	10.1	1.10			75			35			31	34	
5.0	100		115	22	41.5	1.30	1.19	10.3	1.10			75			35			30	33	
5.5	120		114	24	45.7	1.43	1.23	10.8	1.16			76			36			31	36	
6.0	120	144/66	124	25	49.2	1.53	1.40	11.3	1.10	7.42	22	75	60	15	35	34	−1	31	34	0.17
6.5	140		124	28	54.5	1.65	1.45	11.7	1.14			77			34			32	36	
7.0	140		129	28	59.4	1.80	1.49	11.5	1.21			78			35			32	38	
7.5	160		140	28	65.7	2.00	1.71	12.2	1.17			77			35			32	37	
8.0	160	174/73	148	30	72.0	2.15	1.77	11.9	1.22	7.41	21	79	57	21	34	34	0	32	39	0.21
8.5	180		150	30	73.6	2.21	1.88	12.5	1.17			78			34			32	38	
9.0	180		152	28	74.6	2.29	1.83	12.0	1.25			79			35			32	39	
9.5	200		152	28	75.6	2.36	1.88	12.4	1.25			79			35			31	39	
10.0	200	195/84	160	33	84.8	2.57	1.98	12.4	1.30	7.38	19	80	52	28	35	33	−2	32	41	0.17
10.5	220		170	44	101.6	2.78	2.19	12.9	1.27			81			33			35	45	
11.0	220	198/96	172	45	107.9	3.03	2.15	12.5	1.41	7.33	17	85	56	27	31	32	1	34	49	0.21
	Recovery		172	41	97.3	2.77	1.93	11.2	1.44			84			33			34	49	
	Recovery		154									91			33					

10.13.3, panel 5) as peak V̇O₂ is approached. The heart rate–V̇O₂ plot at age 72 contrasts with the same plot at age 65.

Conclusion

Age 65. This man had excellent cardiovascular function with no evidence to support the diagnosis of cardiomyopathy. His symptoms were most likely due to the decrease in cardiovascular function associated with aging while he tried to continue his physical feats of earlier years.

Age 72. This man's aerobic function decreased considerably more rapidly than predicted despite his maintenance of an exercise schedule. At this time, he has physiologic and ECG evidence of myocardial ischemia during exercise above a V̇O₂ of 1.4 L/min and heart rate of 110 beats per minute. He did not have significant pulmonary vascular dis-

ease, as evidenced by the blood gas and VD/VT data during exercise and the normal V̇E/V̇CO₂ at the AT.

Two different cardiologists misdiagnosed this patient because they did not have the benefit of exercise gas exchange measurements. At age 65, the patient was given the diagnosis of heart failure and accordingly treated, when he in fact had better than normal cardiac function as evidenced by his ability to transport more than the predicted amount of O₂ to the tissues. At age 72, he was told that he had "excellent exercise tolerance" and also that he had pulmonary vascular disease (not compatible conclusions), and that he did not have myocardial ischemia. The cardiopulmonary exercise test showed that his overall cardiovascular function was average for sedentary men of his age and size, that he had myocardial ischemia at submaximal exercise, both electrocardiographically and functionally, and that he did not have significant pulmonary vascular disease.

TABLE 10.13.5. Selected Respiratory Function Data, Age 72

Measurement	Predicted	Measured
Age, yr		72
Sex		Male
Height, cm		184
Weight, kg	83	84
Hematocrit, %		47
VC, L	4.61	4.39
IC, L	3.08	3.82
FEV_1, L	3.29	2.94
FEV_1 VC, %	75	68
MVV, L/min	134	130
D_LCO, ml/mm Hg/min	27.0	19.2

TABLE 10.13.6. Selected Exercise Data, Age 72

Measurement	Predicted	Measured
Peak $\dot{V}O_2$, L/min	2.02	1.99
Maximum HR, beats/min	148	152
Maximum O_2 pulse, ml/beat	13.6	13.1
$\Delta\dot{V}O_2/\Delta WR$, ml/min/W	10.3	8.6
AT, L/min	>0.95	1.4
Blood pressure, mmHg (rest, max)		110/60, 200/75
Maximum $\dot{V}E$, L/min		85
Exercise breathing reserve, L/min	>15	46
PaO_2, mmHg (rest, max ex)		102, 105
$P(A - a)O_2$, mmHg (rest, max ex)		15, 21
$P(a - ET)CO_2$, mmHg (rest, max ex)		5, −2
VD/VT (rest, heavy ex)		0.53, 0.18
HCO_3^-, mEq/L (rest, 2-min recov)		24, 20

TABLE 10.13.7. Room Air, Age 72

Time min	Work rate watts	BP mmHg	HR min⁻¹	f min⁻¹	$\dot{V}E$ L/min BTPS	$\dot{V}CO_2$ L/min STPD	$\dot{V}O_2$ L/min STPD	$\dot{V}O_2$/HR ml/beat	R	pH	HCO_3^- meq/L	PO_2 ET	PO_2 a	PO_2 (A−a)	PCO_2 ET	PCO_2 a	PCO_2 (a−ET)	$\dot{V}E/\dot{V}CO_2$	$\dot{V}E/\dot{V}O_2$	VD/VT
	Rest																			
	Rest		65	24	15.9	0.26	0.21	3.3	1.20			139			29			55	67	
	Rest		65	24	12.9	0.23	0.22	3.4	1.03			134			32			48	50	
	Rest	110/60	65	18	10.6	0.20	0.21	3.3	0.93	7.42	24	130	102	9	33	37	4	46	43	0.43
	Rest		63	21	17.1	0.37	0.39	6.2	0.96			131			33			42	40	
	Rest		72	26	19.3	0.39	0.37	5.2	1.04			136			31			45	46	
	Rest		67	23	18.4	0.35	0.32	4.8	1.08			136			30			48	52	
	Unloaded		75	24	22.0	0.49	0.49	6.5	1.00			132			31			41	41	
	Unloaded		77	17	21.1	0.53	0.51	6.6	1.04			133			33			38	39	
	Unloaded		70	17	24.2	0.58	0.55	7.8	1.06			132			32			39	42	
	Unloaded		69	18	17.3	0.41	0.41	5.9	1.01			133			33			39	39	
	Unloaded		68	21	21.8	0.50	0.46	6.8	1.08			132			31			41	44	
	Unloaded	130/65	66	19	16.2	0.34	0.34	5.2	0.99	7.40	22	135	103	11	33	36	3	44	43	0.41
0.5	7		65	25	19.4	0.40	0.40	6.2	1.00			133			32			43	44	
1.0	18		70	31	19.6	0.39	0.42	6.0	0.93			130			33			44	41	
1.5	29		75	22	21.7	0.54	0.60	8.0	0.90			127			34			37	33	
2.0	39	105/40	76	20	20.5	0.50	0.52	6.8	0.97	7.47	23	129	110	7	34	32	−2	38	37	0.27
2.5	50		77	19	22.5	0.59	0.68	8.8	0.87			125			35			36	31	
3.0	62	105/40	84	20	27.4	0.75	0.85	10.2	0.88	7.41	24	123	97	10	36	39	3	35	30	0.34
3.5	71		86	22	32.4	0.88	0.92	10.7	0.95			127			35			35	33	
4.0	80	120/50	89	23	33.7	0.97	1.07	12.0	0.90	7.42	24	123	103	7	37	37	0	33	30	0.28
4.5	90		99	26	43.9	1.18	1.18	11.9	1.01			129			34			36	36	
5.0	100	115/40	94	23	45.7	1.29	1.31	13.9	0.98	7.41	24	127	99	12	36	39	3	34	34	0.34
5.5	109		101	23	45.5	1.35	1.41	13.9	0.96			125			37			33	31	
6.0	120	135/50	108	25	50.0	1.46	1.47	13.6	0.99	7.43	24	126	107	6	36	37	1	33	33	0.28
6.5	129		111	27	53.9	1.60	1.57	14.1	1.02			127			36			32	33	
7.0	141	145/55	114	25	55.8	1.70	1.65	14.4	1.03	7.42	23	126	106	9	37	36	−1	32	33	0.23
7.5	149		118	24	54.7	1.71	1.63	13.8	1.04			126			38			31	32	
8.0	162	150/55	123	27	61.7	1.91	1.81	14.7	1.05	7.40	22	126	106	9	38	36	−2	31	33	0.23
8.5	169		130	30	71.3	2.10	1.84	14.2	1.14			130			36			33	38	
9.0	177	175/65	136	32	71.2	2.14	1.89	13.9	1.14	7.40	21	129	103	15	37	35	−2	32	36	0.22
9.5	192		143	32	79.1	2.34	1.95	13.7	1.20			132			36			33	39	
10.0	201	180/65	150	32	81.1	2.34	1.94	12.9	1.21	7.40	21	132	100	21	35	34	−1	34	41	0.24
	Recovery		154	29	74.5	2.31	1.95	12.7	1.18	7.39	20	129	105	15	39	34	−5	31	37	0.18
	Recovery		138	29	74.7	2.13	1.47	10.7	1.44			136			36			34	49	
	Recovery		121	30	61.2	1.62	0.97	8.0	1.67			141			34			36	61	
	Recovery		108	32	47.3	1.17	0.70	6.5	1.66			142			32			38	64	
	Recovery		101	27	44.1	1.07	0.67	6.6	1.60			142			31			40	63	

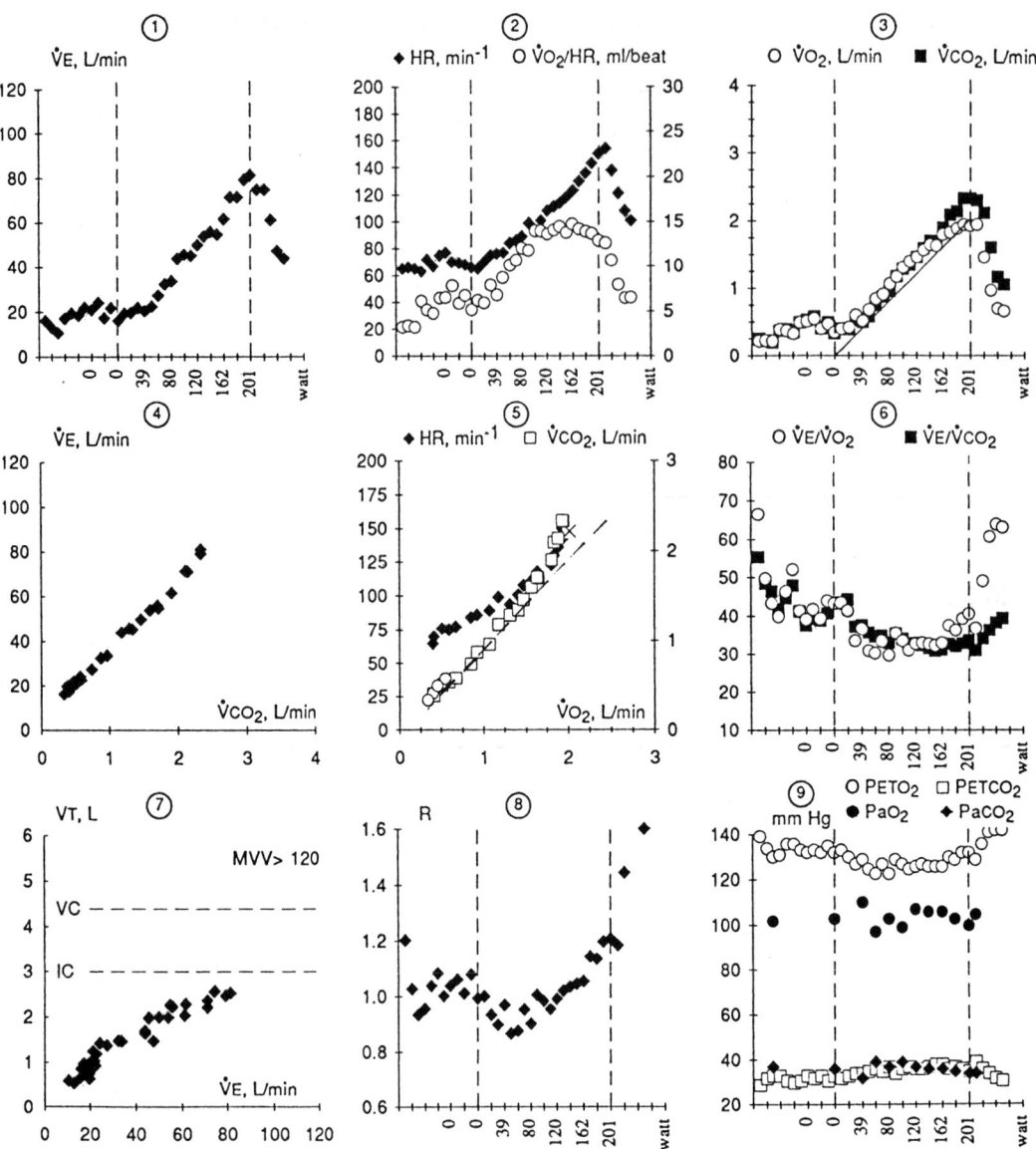

FIGURE 10.13.3.   Room air, age 72. **1:** Vertical dashed lines in panels 1 to 3 and 6, 8, and 9 indicate the beginning and the end of the increasing work period. **2:** Unloaded cycling is performed for 3 minutes before the left vertical dashed line. **3:** In panel 3, the diagonal line shows the increase of $\dot{V}O_2$ at a slope of 10 ml/min/W. **4:** In panel 5, the diagonal dashed line has a slope of 1; the x in the upper right is the predicted maximum heart rate and $\dot{V}O_2$ for the subject.

Case 14 Obesity, Hypertension, and Cigarette Smoking

Clinical Findings

This 53-year-old former mechanic had retired because of medical disability 3 years previously with symptoms of vertigo, nausea, and ataxia and a diagnosis of vestibular neuronitis. He had no other complaints except for some shortness of breath when bicycling uphill. He had 30 years of cigarette smoking and claimed to be smoking one-half a pack per day. Hypertension, diagnosed 14 years ago, was being treated with methyldopa. Chest roentgenograms were normal except for symmetric pleural thickening considered to represent extrapleural fat.

Exercise Findings

The patient performed exercise on a cycle ergometer. He pedaled at 60 rpm without added load for 3 minutes. The work rate was then increased 15 W per minute to his symptom-limited maximum. Arterial blood was sampled every second minute, and intraarterial blood pressure was recorded from a percutaneously placed brachial artery catheter. Resting and exercise ECGs were normal. Resting carboxyhemoglobin was 7.4%. The patient stopped exercise complaining of leg fatigue.

Interpretation

Comments

Results of this patient's resting respiratory function studies are normal except for a low ratio of expiratory reserve volume (ERV) to inspiratory capacity (IC) consistent with obesity (Table 10.14.1). The resting ECG is normal. The patient is 30 kg overweight (Table 10.14.1); his resting carboxyhemoglobin of 7.4% suggests recent cigarette smoking.

Analysis

Referring to flowchart 1, peak $\dot{V}O_2$ and anaerobic threshold are within normal limits (Table 10.14.2). See flowchart 2. The ECG, arterial blood gases, and

O_2 pulse at peak $\dot{V}O_2$ are normal (branch point 2.1). The patient is 30 kg overweight (branch point 2.2). Supporting the diagnosis of obesity as the cause of this patient's shortness of breath are his high oxygen cost for unloaded cycling ($\dot{V}O_2 = 0.9$ L/min), and low breathing reserve at the maximum work rate (Table 10.14.2).

Conclusion

Obesity has contributed to dyspnea in an otherwise normal, cigarette-smoking, hypertensive patient.

TABLE 10.14.1.   Selected Respiratory Function Data

Measurement	Predicted	Measured
Age, yr		53
Sex		Male
Height, cm		171
Weight, kg	74	104
Hematocrit, %		51
VC, L	4.15	4.00
IC, L	2.77	3.64
TLC, L	6.15	5.69
FEV$_1$, L	3.28	3.25
FEV$_1$ VC, %	79	81
MVV, L/min	140	126
D$_L$CO, ml/mm Hg/min	28.8	29.8

TABLE 10.14.2.   Selected Exercise Data

Measurement	Predicted	Measured
Peak $\dot{V}O_2$, L/min	2.48	2.45
Maximum HR, beats/min	167	168
Maximum O$_2$ pulse, ml/beat	14.9	15.6
$\Delta\dot{V}O_2/\Delta$WR, ml/min/W	10.3	10.4
AT, L/min	>1.07	1.45
Blood pressure, mmHg (rest, max)		160/90, 274/137
Maximum $\dot{V}E$, L/min		116
Exercise breathing reserve, L/min	>15	10
PaO$_2$, mmHg (rest, max ex)		81, 85
P(A − a)O$_2$, mmHg (rest, max ex)		26, 37
P(a − ET)CO$_2$, mmHg (rest, max ex)		1, −7
VD/VT (rest, heavy ex)		0.31, 0.23
HCO$_3^-$, mEq/L (rest, 2-min recov)		24, 14

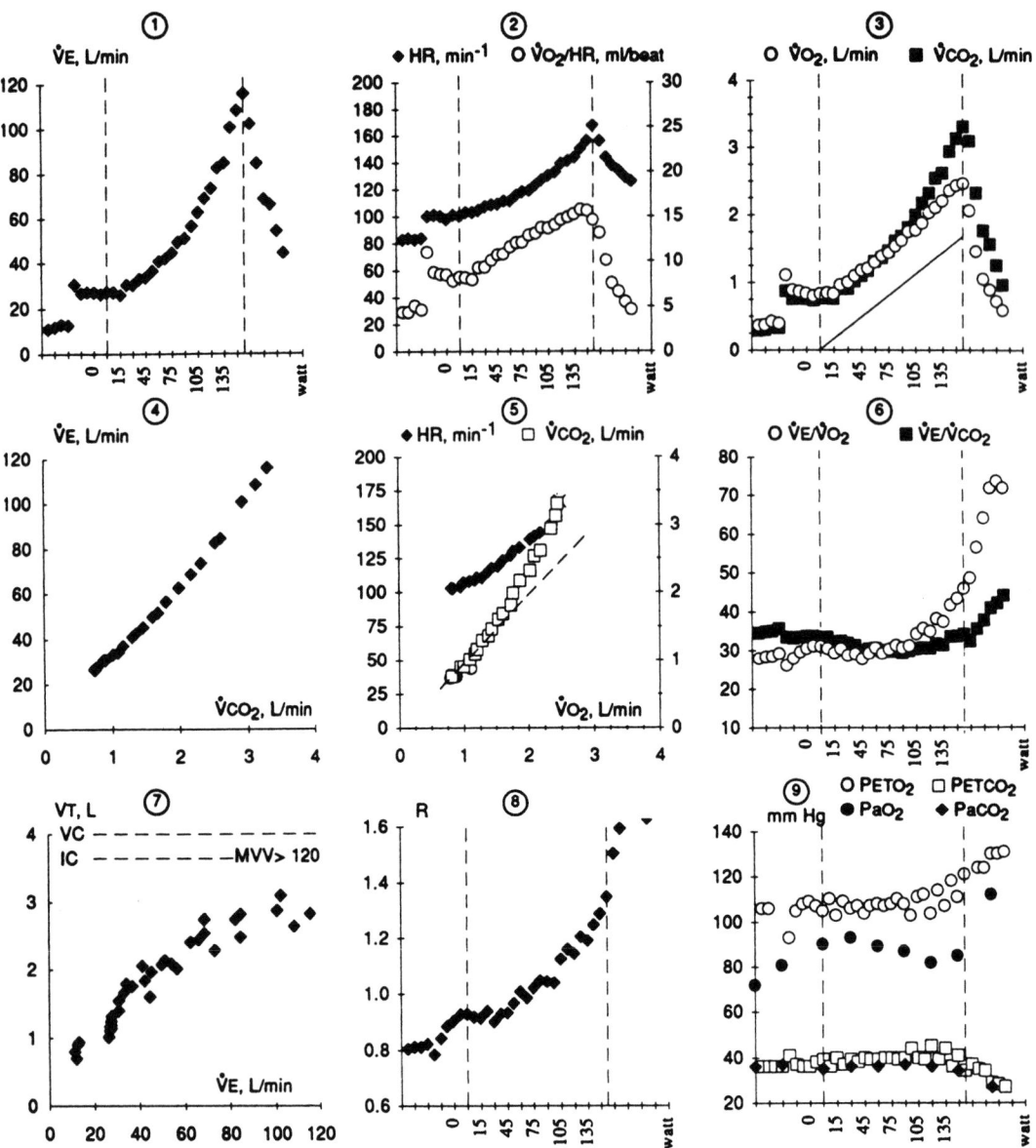

FIGURE 10.14.1.   **1:** Vertical dashed lines in panels 1 to 3 and 6, 8, and 9 indicate the beginning and the end of the increasing work period. **2:** Unloaded cycling is performed for 3 minutes before the left vertical dashed line. **3:** In panel 3, the diagonal line shows the increase of $\dot{V}O_2$ at a slope of 10 ml/min/W. **4:** In panel 5, the diagonal dashed line has a slope of 1; the x in the upper right is the predicted maximum heart rate and $\dot{V}O_2$ for the subject.

TABLE 10.14.3.

Time min	Work rate watts	BP mmHg	HR min⁻¹	f min⁻¹	$\dot{V}_E$ L/min BTPS	$\dot{V}_{CO_2}$ L/min STPD	$\dot{V}_{O_2}$ L/min STPD	$\dot{V}_{O_2}$/HR ml/beat	R	pH	HCO_3^- meq/L	P_{O_2} ET	P_{O_2} a	P_{O_2} (A−a)	P_{CO_2} ET	P_{CO_2} a	P_{CO_2} (a−ET)	$\dot{V}_E/\dot{V}_{CO_2}$	$\dot{V}_E/\dot{V}_{O_2}$	V_D/V_T
	Rest	160/100								7.44	24		72			36				
	Rest		83	14	11.2	0.29	0.36	4.3	0.81			106			36			35	28	
	Rest		84	17	11.9	0.30	0.37	4.4	0.81			106			36			35	28	
	Rest		83	14	13.1	0.34	0.42	5.1	0.81			167			36			35	28	
	Rest	160/90	84	14	12.6	0.32	0.39	4.6	0.82	7.43	24	168	81	26	36	37	1	36	29	0.2
	Unloaded		100	20	30.8	0.87	1.11	11.1	0.78			93			41			33	26	
	Unloaded		101	23	26.9	0.75	0.89	8.8	0.84			105			37			33	28	
	Unloaded		100	22	27.3	0.76	0.86	8.6	0.88			108			36			33	30	
	Unloaded		98	23	27.3	0.75	0.83	8.5	0.90			109			36			34	31	
	Unloaded		101	24	26.6	0.73	0.79	7.8	0.92			107			38			34	31	
	Unloaded	200/110	100	24	27.4	0.76	0.82	8.2	0.93	7.43	23	105	90	23	39	35	−4	33	31	0.2
0.5	15		103	21	27.5	0.77	0.84	8.2	0.92			110			36			33	31	
1.0	15		103	26	26.3	0.75	0.82	8.0	0.91			103			40			32	29	
1.5	30		104	20	30.8	0.90	0.96	9.2	0.94			109			37			32	30	
2.0	30	200/110	107	22	30.6	0.90	1.00	9.3	0.90	7.43	23	106	93	18	39	36	−3	32	29	0.2
2.5	45		108	20	33.3	1.01	1.09	10.1	0.93			107			38			31	29	
3.0	45		109	19	34.0	1.09	1.17	10.7	0.93			104			40			30	28	
3.5	60		111	21	36.9	1.16	1.20	10.8	0.97			107			39			30	29	
4.0	60		111	20	41.2	1.30	1.29	11.6	1.01	7.42	23	108	89	25	39	36	−3	30	31	0.2
4.5	75		115	23	42.4	1.36	1.38	12.0	0.99			107			40			30	29	
5.0	75		118	23	45.2	1.46	1.43	12.1	1.02			108			40			30	30	
5.5	90		119	24	49.9	1.60	1.53	12.9	1.05			110			39			30	31	
6.0	90	215/106	123	24	51.4	1.68	1.61	13.1	1.04	7.39	22	108	87	27	40	37	−3	29	31	0.2
6.5	105		127	28	56.6	1.81	1.74	13.7	1.04			103			44			30	31	
7.0	105		130	26	62.6	1.99	1.77	13.6	1.12			111			40			30	34	
7.5	120		133	27	68.8	2.17	1.87	14.1	1.16			112			39			31	36	
8.0	120		139	32	73.3	2.32	2.03	14.6	1.14	7.38	21	104	82	36	45	36	−9	30	35	0.2
8.5	135		141	30	82.4	2.53	2.10	14.9	1.20			114			39			32	38	
9.0	135		144	34	84.5	2.61	2.19	15.2	1.19			107			44			31	37	
9.5	150		150	35	100.8	2.93	2.35	15.7	1.25			118			36			33	42	
10.0	150	274/137	156	41	108.4	3.13	2.43	15.6	1.29	7.37	19	111	85	37	41	34	−7	34	43	0.2
10.5	165		168	41	115.8	3.30	2.45	14.6	1.35			121			34			34	46	
	Recovery		156	33	102.3	3.08	2.05	13.1	1.50			1			37			32	49	
	Recovery		144	30	84.5	2.31	1.45	10.1	1.59			124			35			35	57	
	Recovery		138	25	68.7	1.76	1.04	7.5	1.69			124			34			38	64	
	Recovery	210/100	134	27	66.1	1.56	0.89	6.6	1.75	7.32	14	130	112	20	29	27	−2	41	72	0.2
	Recovery		129	26	54.4	1.24	0.71	5.5	1.75			130			28			42	74	
	Recovery		126	28	44.7	0.96	0.59	4.7	1.63			131			27			44	72	

Case 15 Extreme Obesity

Clinical Findings

This 45-year-old man was referred for an exercise study to evaluate his capacity for work as a security guard. Because of his obesity, his employer believed that he was unable to perform his duties, which could include running up stairs and chasing after thieves. The evaluee denied any exercise limitation and is not taking any medications. He does not smoke or drink alcoholic beverages. Resting ECG was normal.

Exercise Findings

The patient performed exercise on a treadmill because this was believed to best simulate the tasks he might be called on to perform. He walked on the level at 3 miles per hour (4.8 km per hour) for 3 minutes, after which the grade was increased 2 degrees per minute to tolerance. Heart rate and rhythm were continuously monitored. Blood pressure was measured by sphygmomanometry, and oxygen saturation by ear oximetry. Multiple-lead ECGs were taken during rest, exercise, and recovery. The patient appeared to give an excellent effort and stopped exercise because of fatigue; he denied chest pain or dyspnea during or after the study. No ectopy or abnormal ECG changes occurred during or after exercise.

Interpretation

Comments

Resting lung studies are typical of extreme obesity.

Analysis

Referring to flowchart 1, peak $\dot{V}O_2$ and the anaerobic threshold are high normal as predicted from height (Table 10.15.1). Through branch point 1.1 in this flowchart and branch points 2.1 and 2.2 in flowchart 2, the diagnosis of obesity is confirmed. The breathing reserve is low at maximal exercise. The metabolic cost ($\dot{V}O_2$) of walking at zero grade at

3 miles per hour is seen to be 2.5 L/min, which is much higher than would be seen in an individual of normal weight. The anaerobic threshold is reached at a grade of 6% to 8%, and peak $\dot{V}O_2$ is reached at a 16% grade. These are roughly the tasks that would correspond to the anaerobic threshold and peak $\dot{V}O_2$ in a subject of normal weight (albeit at a much lower $\dot{V}O_2$ cost).

Conclusion

Except for systolic hypertension, no evidence of cardiopulmonary disease was found. There is a fit thin person hiding in this obese man! Despite his fitness, obesity has added a significant burden to his ability to perform an exercise task as well as a normal-weight person of equal fitness.

TABLE 10.15.1.   Selected Respiratory Function Data

Measurement	Predicted	Measured
Age, yr		45
Sex		Male
Height, cm		168
Weight, kg	72	157
Hematocrit, %		47
VC, L	4.11	3.67
IC, L	2.74	3.63
FEV$_1$, L	3.31	3.19
FEV$_1$/VC, %	81	87
MVV, L/min	132	140

TABLE 10.15.2.   Selected Exercise Data

Measurement	Predicted	Measured
Peak $\dot{V}O_2$, L/min	3.28	4.14
Maximum HR, beats/min	175	191
Maximum O$_2$ pulse, ml/beat	18.7	21.8
AT, L/min	>1.39	3.25
Blood pressure, mmHg (rest, max)		160/90, 225/100
Maximum $\dot{V}E$, L/min		128
Exercise breathing reserve, L/min	>15	12

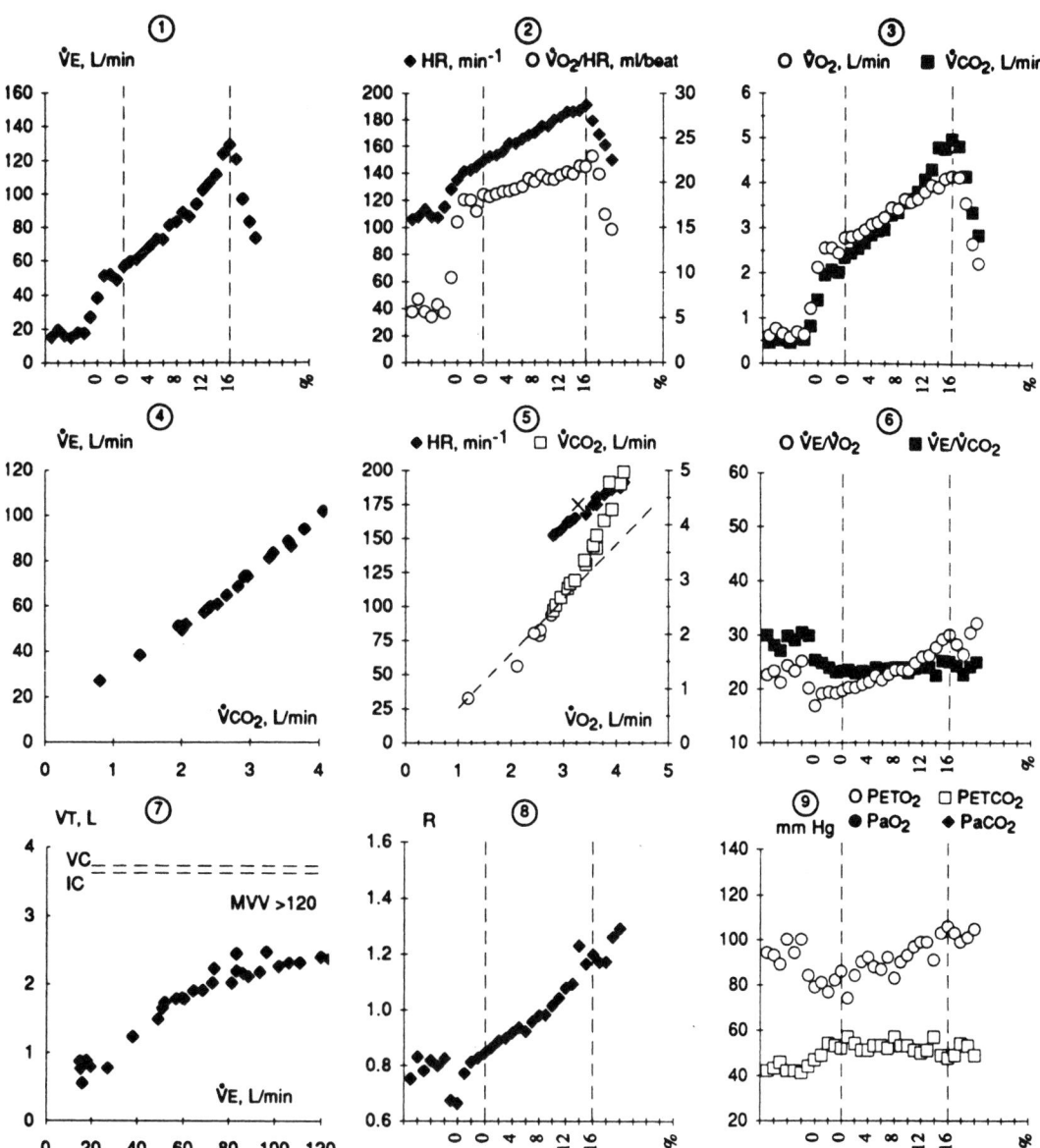

FIGURE 10.15.1.   **1:** Vertical dashed lines in panels 1 to 3 and 6, 8, and 9 indicate the beginning and the end of the increasing work period. **2:** Zero-grade walking is performed for 3 minutes before the left vertical dashed line. **3:** In panel 5, the diagonal dashed line has a slope of 1; the x in the upper right is the predicted maximum heart rate and $\dot{V}O_2$ for the subject.

TABLE 10.15.3. Air Breathing

Time min	Treadmill grade, %	BP mmHg	HR min⁻¹	f min⁻¹	$\dot{V}_E$ L/min BTPS	$\dot{V}_{CO_2}$ L/min STPD	$\dot{V}_{O_2}$ L/min STPD	$\dfrac{\dot{V}_{O_2}}{HR}$ ml/beat	R	pH	HCO_3^- meq/L	P_{O_2}, mmHg ET	a	(A − a)	P_{CO_2}, mmHg ET	a	(a − ET)	$\dfrac{\dot{V}_E}{\dot{V}_{CO_2}}$	$\dfrac{\dot{V}_E}{\dot{V}_{O_2}}$	$\dfrac{V_D}{V_T}$
	Rest	160/90																		
	Rest		106	20	15.2	0.45	0.60	5.7	0.75			94			42			30	23	
	Rest		108	25	19.8	0.63	0.76	7.0	0.83			93			43			28	23	
	Rest		113	29	16.0	0.50	0.64	5.7	0.78			89			46			27	21	
	Rest	150/100	108	17	14.8	0.45	0.55	5.1	0.82			100			42			30	24	
	Rest		107	20	17.7	0.55	0.69	6.4	0.80			94			42			29	23	
	Rest		115	20	17.5	0.52	0.63	5.5	0.83			100			41			30	25	
0.5	0		128	35	27.1	0.81	1.20	9.4	0.68			84			44			30	20	
1.0	0		135	31	38.1	1.40	2.11	15.6	0.66			79			47			25	17	
1.5	0		141	31	51.1	1.96	2.54	18.0	0.77			81			49			25	19	
2.0	0		142	30	52.0	2.07	2.55	18.0	0.81			77			54			24	19	
2.5	0		145	33	49.2	2.01	2.43	16.8	0.83			82			53			23	19	
3.0	0	210/100	149	32	57.0	2.34	2.77	18.6	0.84			86			52			23	20	
3.5	2		152	33	59.5	2.42	2.80	18.4	0.86			74			57			23	20	
4.0	2		153	34	60.6	2.53	2.85	18.6	0.89			84			54			23	20	
4.5	4		156	34	64.6	2.66	2.96	19.0	0.90			90			51			23	21	
5.0	4	210/90	162	36	68.6	2.83	3.08	19.0	0.92			92			51			23	21	
5.5	6		162	36	72.7	2.92	3.12	19.3	0.94			88			53			24	22	
6.0	6		165	36	72.8	2.97	3.22	19.5	0.92			87			53			23	22	
6.5	8		168	40	81.1	3.28	3.43	20.4	0.96			92			52			24	23	
7.0	8	210/90	170	38	83.4	3.34	3.41	20.1	0.98			83			57			24	24	
7.5	10		175	42	88.7	3.56	3.63	20.7	0.98			90			53			24	23	
8.0	10		175	40	86.3	3.61	3.56	20.3	1.01			93			53			23	23	
8.5	12		180	43	93.6	3.79	3.64	20.2	1.04			97			51			24	25	
9.0	12	220/90	182	45	101.8	4.07	3.78	20.8	1.08			99			50			24	26	
9.5	14		186	46	106.3	4.28	3.92	21.1	1.09			99			51			24	26	
10.0	14		186	48	111.0	4.77	3.88	20.9	1.23			91			57			22	28	
10.5	16		187	52	123.5	4.75	4.08	21.8	1.16			103			49			25	29	
11.0	16	225/100	191	53	128.4	4.96	4.14	21.7	1.20			106			48			25	30	
	Recovery		179	50	120.1	4.80	4.10	22.9	1.17			103			49			24	28	
	Recovery	200/80	169	39	96.4	4.13	3.53	20.9	1.17			99			54			23	26	
	Recovery		161	34	83.2	3.34	2.65	16.5	1.26			101			53			24	30	
	Recovery	180/80	150	33	73.6	2.85	2.21	14.7	1.29			105			49			25	32	

Case 16 Coronary Artery Disease

Clinical Findings

This 58-year-old man had been exposed to asbestos, sandblasting, and 35 years of cigarettes. On questioning, he admitted to a grinding chest pain, originating in the midback and radiating around the left chest into the substernal area. The pain, brought on when walking on cold days and relieved in a few minutes by rest, had not previously been treated or diagnosed. He denied shortness of breath. A physical examination revealed no evidence of peripheral vascular disease, heart murmurs, or abnormal heart sounds. The resting 12-lead ECG was within normal limits.

Exercise Findings

The patient performed exercise on a cycle ergometer. He pedaled at 60 rpm without added load for 3 minutes. The work rate was then increased 20 W per minute to his symptom-limited maximum. Arterial blood was sampled every second minute, and intraarterial blood pressure was recorded from a percutaneously placed brachial artery catheter. The patient stopped exercise because of interscapular pain and right anterior chest pain. The ECG showed a 2-mm ST-segment depression in leads II, III, aVF, and V_3 through V_6 during exercise but returned to normal after 9 minutes of recovery. The chest pain resolved within 1 minute of cessation of exercise.

Interpretation

Comments

Resting respiratory function is normal (Table 10.16.1).

Analysis

In flowchart 1, the peak $\dot{V}O_2$ is reduced, whereas the anaerobic threshold is normal (Table 10.16.2), which directs us through branch points 1.1, 1.2, and 1.3 to flowchart 3. The breathing reserve (branch point 3.1) is high and the ECG (branch point 3.3) is abnormal, directing us to a diagnosis of myocardial ischemia. The patient's chest pain and low $\Delta\dot{V}O_2/\Delta WR$ are confirmatory; even more significant is the

plateau in $\dot{V}O_2$ and O_2 pulse that occurs concurrently with the onset of abnormal ST-segment changes. The rise in O_2 pulse after heavy exercise ceased is evidence for recovery of stroke volume from ischemia-induced left ventricular dysfunction. None of these abnormalities would have been evident if exercise had been terminated at a heart rate below 140 beats per minute.

Conclusion

Myocardial ischemia secondary to coronary artery disease.

TABLE 10.16.1.   Selected Respiratory Function Data

Measurement	Predicted	Measured
Age, yr		58
Sex		Male
Height, cm		173
Weight, kg	76	82
Hematocrit, %		41
VC, L	4.09	4.04
IC, L	2.73	3.39
TLC, L	6.20	5.93
FEV_1, L	3.21	3.43
FEV_1/VC, %	79	85
MVV, L/min	135	155
D_LCO, ml/mm Hg/min	25.5	25.9

TABLE 10.16.2.   Selected Exercise Data

Measurement	Predicted	Measured
Peak $\dot{V}O_2$, L/min	2.25	1.47
Maximum HR, beats/min	162	146
Maximum O_2 pulse, ml/beat	13.9	10.3
$\Delta\dot{V}O_2/\Delta WR$, ml/min/W	10.3	7.2
AT, L/min	>0.99	1.0
Blood pressure, mmHg (rest, max)		174/81, 222/99
Maximum $\dot{V}E$, L/min		75
Exercise breathing reserve, L/min	>15	80
PaO_2, mmHg (rest, max ex)		87, 115
$P(A-a)O_2$, mmHg (rest, max ex)		18, 10
$P(a-ET)CO_2$, mmHg (rest, max ex)		−3, −6
VD/VT (rest, heavy ex)		0.21, 0.12
HCO_3^-, mEq/L (rest, 2-min recov)		22, 16

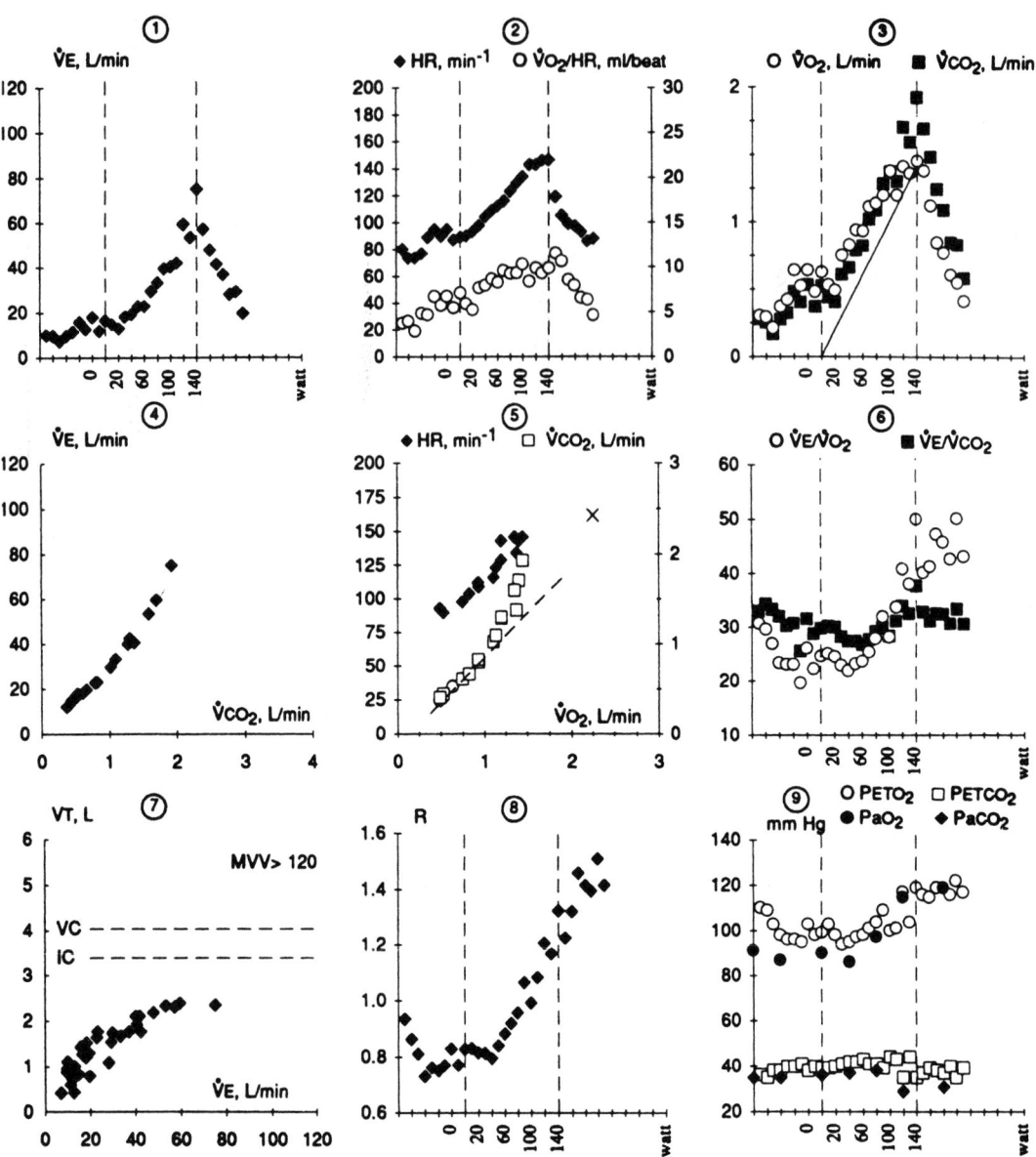

FIGURE 10.16.1.   **1:** Vertical dashed lines in panels 1 to 3 and 6, 8, and 9 indicate the beginning and the end of the increasing work period. **2:** Unloaded cycling is performed for 3 minutes before the left vertical dashed line. **3:** In panel 3, the diagonal line shows the increase of $\dot{V}_{O_2}$ at a slope of 10 ml/min/W. **4:** In panel 5, the diagonal dashed line has a slope of 1; the x in the upper right is the predicted maximum heart rate and $\dot{V}_{O_2}$ for the subject.

TABLE 10.16.3.   Air Breathing

Time min	Work rate watts	BP mmHg	HR min⁻¹	f min⁻¹	$\dot{V}_E$ L/min BTPS	$\dot{V}_{CO_2}$ L/min STPD	$\dot{V}_{O_2}$ L/min STPD	$\dfrac{\dot{V}_{O_2}}{HR}$ ml/beat	R	pH	HCO_3^- meq/L	P_{O_2}, mmHg ET	P_{O_2}, mmHg a	P_{O_2}, mmHg (A − a)	P_{CO_2}, mmHg ET	P_{CO_2}, mmHg a	P_{CO_2}, mmHg (a − ET)	$\dot{V}_E$ $\dot{V}_{CO_2}$	$\dot{V}_E$ $\dot{V}_{O_2}$	V_D V_T
	Rest									7.42	22		91			35				
	Rest		80	9	10.0	0.28	0.30	3.8	0.93			110			36			33	31	
	Rest		74	11	9.5	0.25	0.29	3.9	0.86			109			35			34	30	
	Rest		74	17	7.1	0.17	0.21	2.8	0.81			103			38			33	27	
	Rest		77	10	9.5	0.27	0.37	4.8	0.73	7.41	22	98	87	18	38	35	−3	32	23	0.21
	Rest		89	19	11.3	0.32	0.42	4.7	0.76			96			40			30	23	
	Rest		95	11	15.7	0.48	0.64	6.7	0.75			96			40			31	23	
	Unloaded		90	30	12.8	0.40	0.52	5.8	0.77			95			41			26	20	
	Unloaded		95	15	18.0	0.53	0.64	6.7	0.83			103			38			32	26	
	Unloaded		87	17	12.1	0.37	0.48	5.5	0.77			98			40			29	22	
	Unloaded	174/81	89	13	16.6	0.52	0.63	7.1	0.83	7.41	22	99	90	18	39	36	−3	30	25	0.18
0.5	20		90	18	14.8	0.44	0.53	5.9	0.83			103			39			30	25	
1.0	20		93	13	13.1	0.40	0.49	5.3	0.82			98			40			30	24	
1.5	40		98	12	18.2	0.61	0.75	7.7	0.81			94			41			28	23	
2.0	40	192/84	104	15	19.4	0.66	0.83	8.0	0.80	7.40	23	95	86	19	42	37	−5	27	22	0.14
2.5	60		109	14	22.9	0.79	0.94	8.6	0.84			97			42			27	23	
3.0	60		112	13	23.0	0.82	0.93	8.3	0.88			98			43			27	24	
3.5	80		116	17	29.6	1.02	1.11	9.6	0.92			101			41			28	25	
4.0	80	204/90	123	20	33.4	1.09	1.14	9.3	0.96	7.39	23	104	97	14	41	38	−3	29	28	0.21
4.5	100		129	19	39.9	1.28	1.20	9.3	1.07			109			39			30	32	
5.0	100		134	21	40.5	1.37	1.38	10.3	0.99			100			44			28	28	
5.5	120		143	24	42.4	1.30	1.20	8.4	1.08			101			43			31	34	
6.0	120	222/99	143	25	59.6	1.70	1.41	9.9	1.21	7.42	18	117	115	10	35	29	−6	34	41	0.12
6.5	140		146	23	53.6	1.59	1.36	9.3	1.17			104			44			32	38	
7.0	140		146	32	75.1	1.92	1.45	9.9	1.32			119			35			38	50	
	Recovery	210/72	119	25	57.4	1.69	1.38	11.6	1.22			116			37			33	40	
	Recovery		105	22	48.0	1.48	1.12	10.7	1.32			115			39			31	41	
	Recovery		99	20	41.9	1.24	0.85	8.6	1.46			119			38			32	47	
	Recovery		97	21	37.0	1.09	0.77	7.9	1.42	7.34	16	119	119	7	37	31	−6	32	46	0.13
	Recovery		93	26	28.2	0.85	0.61	6.6	1.39			116			40			31	43	
	Recovery		86	19	29.2	0.83	0.55	6.4	1.51			122			35			33	50	
	Recovery		88	25	19.8	0.58	0.41	4.7	1.41			117			39			30	43	

Case 17 Coronary Artery Disease

Clinical Findings

This 61-year-old retired shipyard worker complained of breathing difficulties that he could not quantify or describe well. He denied shortness of breath but stated that he stopped using stairs because of a "peculiar feeling in his chest." He also complained of a stabbing substernal and right flank pain not associated with exertion or stress and of neck pain associated with movement of the head attributed to degenerative cervical spine arthritis. He had never smoked cigarettes. Examination revealed psoriasis and normal blood pressure, heart sounds, and peripheral pulses. He had bilateral pleural plaques on chest roentgenograms. He also had ECG findings suggestive of left ventricular hypertrophy.

Exercise Findings

The patient performed exercise on a cycle ergometer. He pedaled at 60 rpm without added load for 3 minutes. The work rate was then increased 20 W per minute to his symptom-limited maximum. Arterial blood was sampled every second minute, and intraarterial blood pressure was recorded from a percutaneously placed brachial artery catheter. The patient stopped exercise because of shortness of breath and tired thighs. He denied chest pain. The ECG developed slight ST-segment depression in leads II, III, aVF, V_5, and V_6 at 120 W of exercise (HR 150) that gradually became more prominent, with a maximum ST depression of 5 mm at the cessation of exercise (180 W). A rare, unifocal, premature ventricular contraction was noted. The ECG returned to baseline after 14 minutes of recovery.

Interpretation

Comments

Resting respiratory function (Table 10.17.1) and ECG are normal.

Analysis

Referring to flowchart 1, the peak $\dot{V}O_2$ and anaerobic threshold are normal (Table 10.17.2), which directs us through branch point 1.1 to flowchart 2. The ECG is abnormal and the O_2 pulse is reduced, reaching a plateau for the last 5 minutes of incremental exercise (panel 2, Fig. 10.17.1) (branch point 2.1). The indices of ventilation–perfusion matching are normal (branch point 2.3). The low O_2 pulse, steep heart rate–$\dot{V}O_2$ relationship and reduced $\Delta\dot{V}O_2/\Delta WR$ indicate that the ST-segment changes are functionally significant, that is, consistent with coronary artery disease.

Conclusion

Silent myocardial ischemia.

TABLE 10.17.1. Selected Respiratory Function Data

Measurement	Predicted	Measured
Age, yr		61
Sex		Male
Height, cm		176
Weight, kg	78	70
Hematocrit, %		39
VC, L	4.23	3.95
IC, L	2.82	2.60
TLC, L	6.47	6.01
FEV_1, L	3.32	3.25
FEV_1/VC, %	78	82
MVV, L/min	137	121
D_LCO, ml/mm Hg/min	25.5	33.3

TABLE 10.17.2. Selected Exercise Data

Measurement	Predicted	Measured
Peak $\dot{V}O_2$, L/min	2.08	1.90
Maximum HR, beats/min	159	180
Maximum O_2 pulse, ml/beat	13.1	10.6
$\Delta\dot{V}O_2/\Delta WR$, ml/min/W	10.3	7.5
AT, L/min	>0.91	1.1
Blood pressure, mmHg (rest, max)		144/75, 246/108
Maximum $\dot{V}E$, L/min		86
Exercise breathing reserve, L/min	>15	35
PaO_2, mmHg (rest, max ex)		87, 103
$P(A - a)O_2$, mmHg (rest, max ex)		5, 15
$P(a - ET)CO_2$, mmHg (rest, max ex)		2, −1
VD/VT (rest, heavy ex)		0.48, 0.24
HCO_3^-, mEq/L (rest, 2-min recov)		26, 20

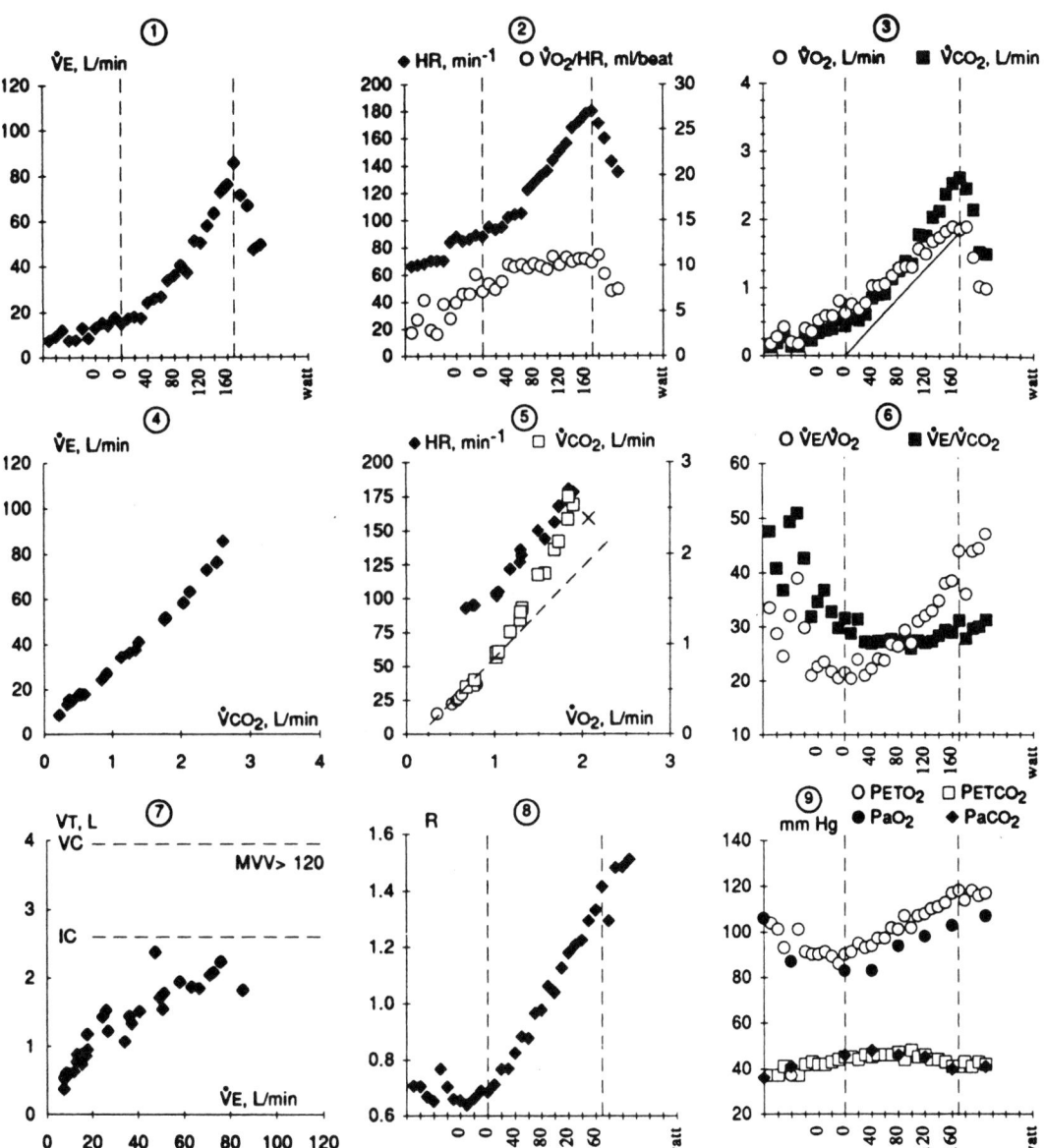

FIGURE 10.17.1.   **1:** Vertical dashed lines in panels 1 to 3 and 6, 8, and 9 indicate the beginning and the end of the increasing work period. **2:** Unloaded cycling is performed for 3 minutes before the left vertical dashed line. **3:** In panel 3, the diagonal line shows the increase of $\dot{V}O_2$ at a slope of 10 ml/min/W. **4:** In panel 5, the diagonal dashed line has a slope of 1; the x in the upper right is the predicted maximum heart rate and $\dot{V}O_2$ for the subject.

TABLE 10.17.3.

Time min	Work rate watts	BP mmHg	HR min⁻¹	f min⁻¹	$\dot{V}_E$ L/min BTPS	$\dot{V}_{CO_2}$ L/min STPD	$\dot{V}_{O_2}$ L/min STPD	$\dot{V}_{O_2}$/HR ml/beat	R	pH	HCO₃⁻ meq/L	P_{O_2}, mmHg ET	a	(A − a)	P_{CO_2}, mmHg ET	a	(a − ET)	$\dot{V}_E$/$\dot{V}_{CO_2}$	$\dot{V}_E$/$\dot{V}_{O_2}$	V_D/V_T
	Rest	144/75								7.48	26		106			36				
	Rest		66	20	7.4	0.12	0.17	2.6	0.71			104			37			48	34	
	Rest		67	16	9.1	0.19	0.27	4.0	0.70			101			37			41	29	
	Rest		68	19	11.9	0.28	0.42	6.2	0.67			93			41			37	24	
	Rest	150/75	70	14	7.6	0.13	0.20	2.9	0.65	7.44	27	37	87	5	39	41	2	49	32	0.48
	Rest		70	15	7.9	0.13	0.17	2.4	0.76			101			37			51	39	
	Rest		70	15	13.2	0.28	0.40	5.7	0.70			91			42			43	30	
	Unloaded		84	14	8.5	0.23	0.35	4.2	0.66			90			43			32	21	
	Unloaded		88	17	13.2	0.34	0.52	5.9	0.65			90			42			35	23	
	Unloaded		85	21	15.4	0.37	0.58	6.8	0.64			91			42			37	23	
	Unloaded		86	17	14.2	0.39	0.59	6.9	0.66			89			43			33	22	
	Unloaded		89	15	17.7	0.55	0.80	9.0	0.69			86			44			30	21	
	Unloaded	171/78	88	17	15.0	0.43	0.63	7.2	0.68	7.41	29	90	83	4	45	46	1	32	22	0.37
0.5	20		95	20	17.2	0.54	0.76	8.0	0.71			91			45			29	20	
1.0	20		93	19	17.9	0.52	0.68	7.3	0.76			95			44			31	24	
1.5	40		95	15	17.6	0.60	0.78	8.2	0.77			93			46			27	21	
2.0	40	192/78	102	17	24.3	0.85	1.03	10.1	0.83	7.40	29	94	83	11	45	48	3	27	22	0.31
2.5	60		104	17	26.0	0.90	1.02	9.8	0.88			97			46			27	24	
3.0	60		105	22	26.9	0.92	1.05	10.0	0.88			97			46			27	24	
3.5	80		122	32	34.2	1.14	1.18	9.7	0.97			102			46			28	27	
4.0	80	216/87	127	25	36.1	1.26	1.29	10.2	0.98	7.40	28	101	94	9	47	46	−1	27	26	0.29
4.5	100		132	27	40.8	1.39	1.31	9.9	1.06			107			44			28	29	
5.0	100		136	28	37.4	1.35	1.30	9.6	1.04			102			48			26	27	
5.5	120		144	29	51.4	1.78	1.58	11.0	1.13			107			45			27	31	
6.0	120	231/96	150	33	50.8	1.77	1.50	10.0	1.18	7.39	27	108	98	12	46	45	−1	27	32	0.28
6.5	140		156	30	58.1	2.04	1.69	10.8	1.21			110			44			27	33	
7.0	140		168	34	63.3	2.13	1.74	10.4	1.22			111			44			28	35	
7.5	160		172	35	72.8	2.38	1.84	10.7	1.29			113			43			29	38	
8.0	160	234/99	178	34	76.0	2.53	1.90	10.7	1.33	7.39	24	117	103	15	41	40	−1	29	38	0.24
8.5	180	246/108	180	47	85.5	2.62	1.85	10.3	1.42			118			41			31	44	
	Recovery		171	35	71.3	2.46	1.90	11.1	1.29			114			43			28	36	
	Recovery		160	36	66.6	2.15	1.45	9.1	1.48			118			41			30	44	
	Recovery		143	20	47.5	1.53	1.03	7.2	1.49			116			43			30	44	
	Recovery	192/78	135	29	49.6	1.51	1.00	7.4	1.51	7.30	20	117	107	13	42	41	−1	31	47	0.31

Case 18 Small Vessel Coronary Artery Disease

Clinical Findings

This 47-year-old asymptomatic man was referred for cardiopulmonary exercise testing because of a strong family history of coronary artery disease and the finding of coronary artery calcification on an ultrafast computed tomographic (CT) cardiac scan. Physical examination, chest roentgenograms, and resting ECGs were normal.

Exercise Findings

The patient performed exercise on a cycle ergometer. He pedaled at 60 rpm without an added load for 3 minutes. The work rate was then increased 25 W per minute to tolerance. Heart rate and rhythm were continuously monitored; 12-lead ECGs were obtained during rest, exercise, and recovery. Blood pressure was measured with a sphygmomanometer, and oxygen saturation with an ear oximeter. The patient appeared to give an excellent effort and stopped exercise because of leg fatigue. He denied chest pain during or after the study. The ECGs showed progressive downsloping ST-segment depression in leads II, III, aVF, and V_3 to V_6 after 150 W of exercise, which reached approximately 3 mm in leads II and V_4 at the cessation of exercise. These changes resolved by 5 minutes of recovery. No ectopy was present.

Interpretation

Comments

Spirometry was normal (Table 10.18.1).

Analysis

Referring to flowchart 1, peak $\dot{V}O_2$ is reduced, but the anaerobic threshold is within normal limits (Table 10.18.2). Proceeding next to flowchart 3, the high breathing reserve (branch point 3.1) and abnormal ECG that developed during exercise (branch point 3.3) lead us to the diagnosis of myocardial ischemia. The low O_2 pulse and the failure of $\dot{V}O_2$

and the O_2 pulse to rise appropriately for the last 2.5 minutes of exercise indicate that an O_2 delivery problem developed at that time. The constant O_2 pulse indicates that the product of the arterial–mixed venous O_2 content difference and stroke volume reached its maximum value prematurely. The constant value might reflect a decreasing stroke volume while arteriovenous difference is increasing.

Conclusion

The combination of O_2 delivery abnormalities (which imply a failure of cardiac output to increase appropriately for the work rate) and ECG findings consistent with myocardial ischemia suggests that the patient had functionally important coronary artery disease. Follow-up coronary angiograms showed diffuse distal coronary artery disease.

TABLE 10.18.1. Selected Respiratory Function Data

Measurement	Predicted	Measured
Age, yr		47
Sex		Male
Height, cm		175
Weight, kg	78	64
Hematocrit, %		42
VC, L	4.78	5.04
IC, L	3.19	3.70
FEV$_1$, L	3.91	4.03
FEV$_1$/VC, %	81	80
MVV, L/min	153	180

TABLE 10.18.2. Selected Exercise Data

Measurement	Predicted	Measured
Peak $\dot{V}O_2$, L/min	2.35	1.68
Maximum HR, beats/min	173	181
Maximum O_2 pulse, ml/beat	13.6	10.4
$\Delta\dot{V}O_2/\Delta$WR, ml/min/W	10.3	6.4
AT, L/min	>1.01	1.3
Blood pressure, mmHg (rest, max)		125/82, 160/90
Maximum $\dot{V}E$, L/min		78
Exercise breathing reserve, L/min	>15	102
O_2 saturation, oximeter (rest, max)		99, 95

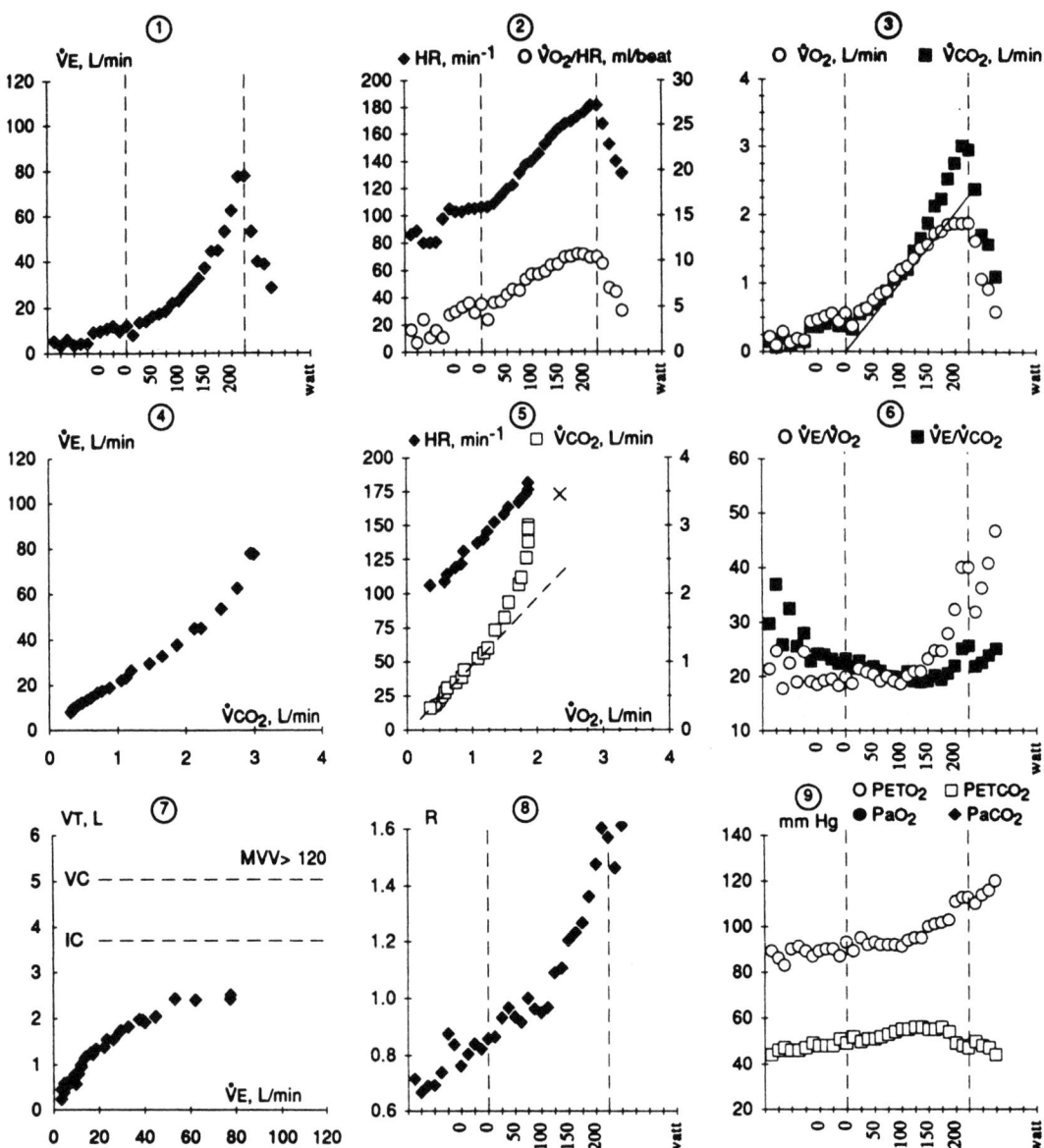

FIGURE 10.18.1. **1:** Vertical dashed lines in panels 1 to 3 and 6, 8, and 9 indicate the beginning and the end of the increasing work period. **2:** Unloaded cycling is performed for 3 minutes before the left vertical dashed line. **3:** In panel 3, the diagonal line shows the increase of $\dot{V}O_2$ at a slope of 10 ml/min/W. **4:** In panel 5, the diagonal dashed line has a slope of 1; the x in the upper right is the predicted maximum heart rate and $\dot{V}O_2$ for the subject.

TABLE 10.18.3.   Air Breathing

Time min	Work rate watts	BP mmHg	HR min⁻¹	f min⁻¹	$\dot{V}_E$ L/min BTPS	$\dot{V}_{CO_2}$ L/min STPD	$\dot{V}_{O_2}$ L/min STPD	$\dfrac{\dot{V}_{O_2}}{HR}$ ml/beat	R	pH	HCO_3^- meq/L	P_{O_2}, mmHg ET	a	(A − a)	P_{CO_2}, mmHg ET	a	(a − ET)	$\dfrac{\dot{V}_E}{\dot{V}_{CO_2}}$	$\dfrac{\dot{V}_E}{\dot{V}_{O_2}}$	$\dfrac{V_D}{V_T}$
	Rest	125/82																		
	Rest		86	11	5.4	0.15	0.21	2.4	0.71			89			44			30	21	
	Rest		89	14	3.4	0.06	0.09	1.0	0.67			86			46			37	25	
	Rest		80	10	6.0	0.20	0.29	3.6	0.69			83			47			26	18	
	Rest	110/60	80	8	3.6	0.09	0.13	1.6	0.69			90			46			32	22	
	Rest		81	12	4.6	0.14	0.19	2.3	0.74			91			46			26	19	
	Rest		98	8	4.6	0.14	0.16	1.6	0.88			89			47			28	25	
	Unloaded		105	12	9.2	0.36	0.43	4.1	0.84			87			49			23	19	
	Unloaded		103	12	9.5	0.35	0.46	4.5	0.76			89			48			24	18	
	Unloaded		103	14	11.0	0.41	0.51	5.0	0.80			90			48			24	19	
	Unloaded		105	12	11.9	0.47	0.56	5.3	0.84			90			48			23	19	
	Unloaded		105	17	9.7	0.37	0.45	4.3	0.82			87			51			22	18	
	Unloaded	120/82	106	13	12.2	0.48	0.56	5.3	0.86			93			49			23	20	
0.5	25		106	13	8.0	0.32	0.37	3.5	0.86			89			52			22	19	
1.0	20		109	12	13.6	0.55	0.59	5.4	0.93			95			50			23	21	
1.5	50		114	12	14.1	0.61	0.63	5.5	0.97			92			51			21	21	
2.0	50	130/90	119	13	16.3	0.70	0.75	6.3	0.93			93			51			22	20	
2.5	75		122	14	17.3	0.77	0.84	6.9	0.92			92			52			21	19	
3.0	75		131	14	18.7	0.88	0.88	6.7	1.00			92			53			20	20	
3.5	100		137	16	22.2	1.05	1.09	8.0	0.96			92			54			20	19	
4.0	100	130/90	140	15	23.3	1.13	1.19	8.5	0.95			91			55			19	19	
4.5	125		145	17	26.3	1.20	1.24	8.6	0.97			94			55			21	20	
5.0	125		152	17	29.5	1.47	1.35	8.9	1.09			95			56			19	21	
5.5	150		158	18	32.8	1.66	1.50	9.5	1.11			95			56			19	21	
6.0	150	145/90	163	19	37.7	1.88	1.56	9.6	1.21			100			55			19	23	
6.5	175		167	22	44.8	2.13	1.73	10.4	1.23			101			55			20	25	
7.0	175		169	22	45.1	2.23	1.76	10.4	1.27			102			56			19	25	
7.5	200		173	22	53.4	2.52	1.85	10.7	1.36			103			54			20	28	
8.0	200	160/90	176	26	62.5	2.76	1.87	10.6	1.48			111			49			22	32	
8.5	225		181	32	77.5	3.00	1.87	10.3	1.60			113			48			25	40	
9.0	225		181	31	77.8	2.95	1.88	10.4	1.57			113			47			25	40	
	Recovery		167	22	53.4	2.37	1.62	9.7	1.46			110			50			22	32	
	Recovery		152	21	40.2	1.71	1.06	7.0	1.61			114			48			22	36	
	Recovery		140	20	39.1	1.57	0.92	6.6	1.71			116			47			24	41	
	Recovery	160/75	131	17	28.9	1.10	0.59	4.5	1.86			120			44			25	47	

Case 19 Coronary Artery Disease Developed Over a Three-Year Interval

Clinical Findings

This 57-year-old male asbestos worker was evaluated at a 3-year interval. At the time of his first evaluation he had a several-year history of diabetes mellitus treated with insulin injections, hypertension treated with hydrochlorothiazide, obesity, arthritis of the hip, and moderate exertional dyspnea. He had never smoked tobacco. Examination at that time revealed moderate obesity and minimal pleural thickening on his chest roentgenograms. The respiratory function and exercise study data of that evaluation are shown in Tables 10.19.1 to 10.19.3 and Figure 10.19.1. When evaluated 3 years later (Tables 10.19.4 to 10.19.6 and Figure 10.19.2), he had developed left-sided "gas" pains at the left sternal border associated with exercise, which were being treated with cimetidine.

Exercise Findings

On both occasions, the patient performed exercise on a cycle ergometer. He pedaled at 60 rpm without an added load for 2 or 3 minutes. The work rate was then increased 20 W per minute to tolerance. On the first occasion, arterial blood was sampled every second minute and intraarterial pressure was recorded from a percutaneously placed brachial artery catheter. The patient was well motivated and cooperative and stopped exercise because of thigh pain, without chest or abdominal pain. No ECG abnormalities were noted at rest, but during high work levels, 1- to 2-mm J-point depression with upsloping ST segments was seen in a few leads.

On the second exercise test, the patient stopped exercise because of calf fatigue and an inability to maintain his cycling frequency. During the last 1 to 2 minutes of exercise, he noted left parasternal nonradiating "gas" pain that subsided within 3 minutes of recovery. He denied shortness of breath. The resting ECG was entirely normal. However, at 120 W, 1.5 mm of ST-segment depression was seen in leads II, III, aVF, V_3, and V_4; at 140 W, 2.5- to 3-mm ST-segment depression was seen in the same leads, plus V_5 and V_6. The ECG returned to normal by 3 minutes after exercise.

Interpretation

Comments

Resting respiratory function studies and arterial blood gases and pH were normal at both evaluations.

TABLE 10.19.1.   Selected Respiratory Function Data: First Study

Measurement	Predicted	Measured
Age, yr		57
Sex		Male
Height, cm		171
Weight, kg	74	96
Hematocrit, %		46
VC, L	3.99	4.25
IC, L	2.66	3.37
TLC, L	6.03	6.00
FEV_1, L	3.14	3.52
FEV_1/VC, %	79	83
MVV, L/min	134	135
$D_L CO$, ml/mm Hg/min	26.4	36.4

TABLE 10.19.2.   Selected Exercise Data: First Study

Measurement	Predicted	Measured
Peak $\dot{V}O_2$, L/min	2.32	2.20
Maximum HR, beats/min	163	148
Maximum O_2 pulse, ml/beat	14.2	14.9
$\Delta \dot{V}O_2 / \Delta WR$, ml/min/W	10.3	10.3
AT, L/min	>1.02	1.2
Blood pressure, mmHg (rest, max ex)		156/94, 250/113
Maximum $\dot{V}E$, L/min		143
Exercise breathing reserves, L/min	>15	−8
PaO_2, mmHg (rest, max ex)		100, 129
$P(A − a)O_2$, mmHg (rest, max ex)		10, 3
$P(a − ET)CO_2$, mmHg (rest, max ex)		−4, −2
VD/VT (rest, max ex)		0.16, 0.19
HCO_3^-, mEq/L (rest, 2-min recovery)		24, 15

TABLE 10.19.3.   First Study

Time min	Work rate watts	BP mmHg	HR min⁻¹	f min⁻¹	$\dot{V}E$ L/min BTPS	$\dot{V}CO_2$ L/min STPD	$\dot{V}O_2$ L/min STPD	$\dot{V}O_2$/HR ml/beat	R	pH	HCO₃⁻ meq/L	PO₂ mmHg ET	a	(A−a)	PCO₂ mmHg ET	a	(a−ET)	$\dot{V}E/\dot{V}CO_2$	$\dot{V}E/\dot{V}O_2$	VD/VT
	Rest	156/94								7.37	24		84			43				
	Rest		80	10	11.9	0.36	0.40	5.0	0.90			109			36			31	28	
	Rest		85	11	10.0	0.32	0.39	4.6	0.82			103			39			28	23	
	Rest		87	7	9.4	0.30	0.36	4.1	0.83			104			39			29	24	
	Rest	175/100	84	7	10.1	0.32	0.38	4.5	0.84	7.40	21	105	100	10	39	35	−4	30	25	0.16
	Unloaded		97	21	21.8	0.65	0.85	8.8	0.76			94			43			31	24	
	Unloaded		96	18	17.4	0.55	0.74	7.7	0.74			99			40			29	21	
	Unloaded		100	22	23.7	0.77	1.01	10.1	0.76			99			40			28	22	
	Unloaded	206/113	98	21	20.8	0.63	0.71	7.2	0.89	7.41	19	105	103	13	40	31	−9	30	27	0.07
0.5	20		101	21	28.3	0.91	1.01	10.0	0.90			104			39			29	26	
1.0	20		101	20	29.2	0.92	1.02	10.1	0.90			106			39			30	27	
1.5	40		102	16	29.4	0.96	1.07	10.5	0.90			104			40			29	26	
2.0	40	219/106	108	20	26.3	0.89	1.04	9.6	0.86	7.39	21	103	100	9	40	36	−4	28	24	0.12
2.5	60		111	21	30.3	1.01	1.14	10.3	0.89			104			41			28	25	
3.0	60		115	22	35.2	1.17	1.22	10.6	0.96			107			40			28	27	
3.5	80		117	25	40.7	1.36	1.36	11.6	1.00			110			39			28	28	
4.0	80	238/106	129	26	45.7	1.50	1.41	10.9	1.06	7.39	21	112	103	13	39	36	−3	29	31	0.16
4.5	100		123	28	50.9	1.65	1.53	12.4	1.08			114			38			29	32	
5.0	100		125	29	51.9	1.70	1.56	12.5	1.09			114			38			29	32	
5.5	120		127	32	67.8	2.02	1.68	13.2	1.20			119			35			32	39	
6.0	120	250/113	131	39	80.3	2.24	1.84	14.0	1.22	7.41	19	122	114	9	32	31	−1	34	42	0.18
6.5	140		131	41	91.5	2.42	1.99	15.2	1.22			120			34			36	44	
7.0	140		141	55	121.3	2.79	2.15	15.2	1.30			128			27			42	54	
7.5	160	235/110	148	59	142.8	2.95	2.20	14.9	1.34	7.42	15	130	129	3	25	23	−2	47	63	0.19
	Recovery		131	39	80.8	2.04	1.73	13.2	1.18			124			30			38	45	
	Recovery		119	33	50.4	1.18	0.98	8.2	1.20			127			27			40	49	

Analysis

Referring to flowchart 1, in the first study all findings were normal with the exception of a negative breathing reserve, which we interpret as indicating the patient's sensitive ventilatory response to the exercise-induced metabolic acidosis with precise pH regulation. To maintain this normal pH, he lowered his $PaCO_2$ from 35 to 23 mm Hg over a 3.5-minute period. He had no evidence of pulmonary or cardiovascular dysfunction.

In the second study, 3 years later, the peak $\dot{V}O_2$ was reduced while the anaerobic threshold, although lower than that of the earlier study, remained normal (Table 10.19.5). Referring to flowchart 3, the breathing reserve was normal (branch point 3.1). The ECG during the second exercise study was clearly abnormal, leading to the diagnosis of myocardial ischemia. The low $\Delta\dot{V}O_2/\Delta WR$ and flat O_2 pulse during the period of increasing work rate are supportive of this diagnosis.

Conclusion

This patient, with several risk factors for coronary artery disease, had an initially normal cardiovascular response to incremental exercise. Three years later, his O_2 flow became clearly abnormal during incremental exercise. At about the same time, he developed ECG abnormalities and chest pain. The ECG changes, symptoms, and the gas exchange abnormalities establish the diagnosis of myocardial ischemia.

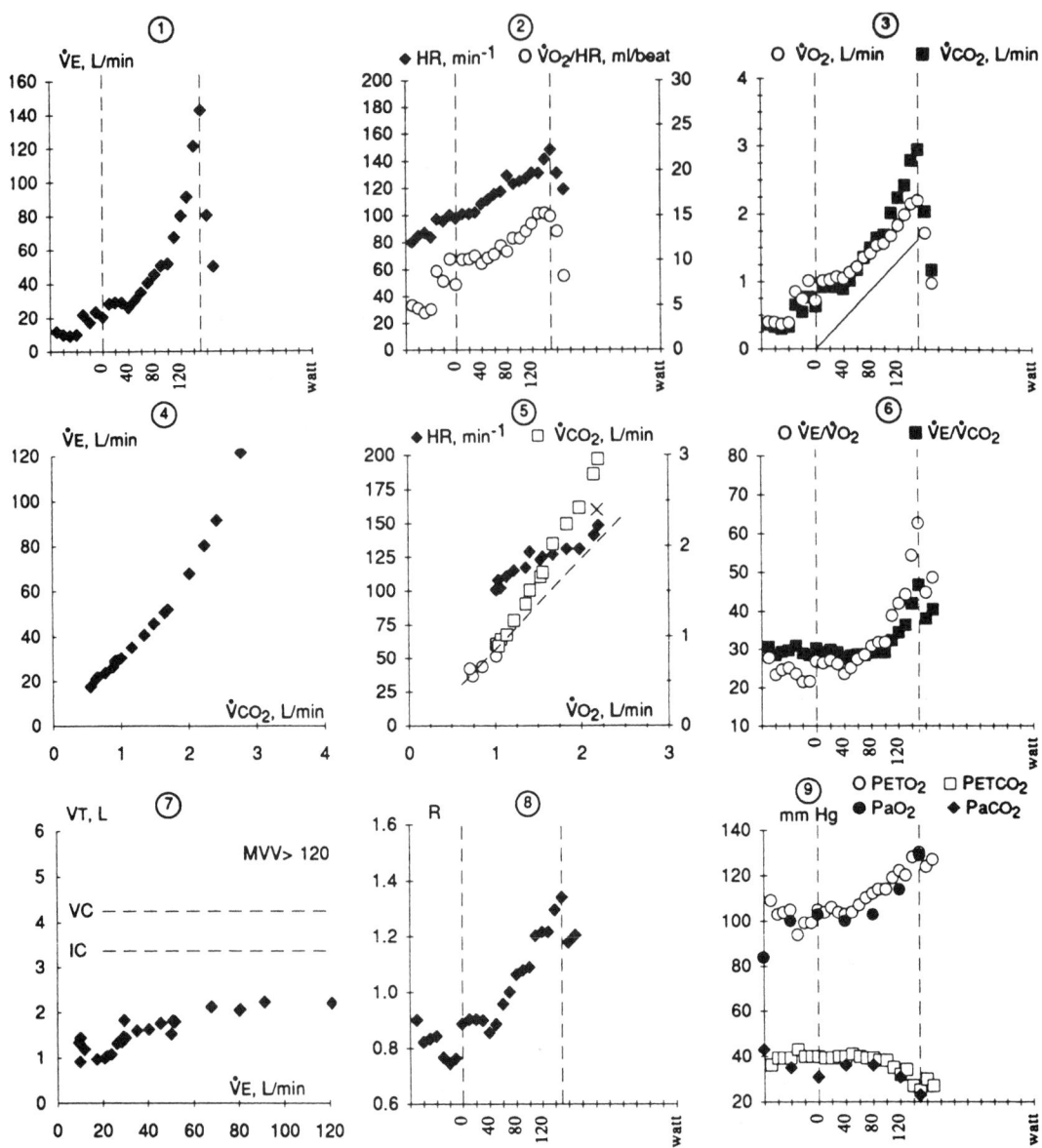

FIGURE 10.19.1.   First study. **1:** Vertical dashed lines in panels 1 to 3 and 6, 8, and 9 indicate the beginning and the end of the increasing work period. **2:** Unloaded cycling is performed for 3 minutes before the left vertical dashed line. **3:** In panel 3, the diagonal line shows the increase of $\dot{V}O_2$ at a slope of 10 ml/min/W. **4:** In panel 5, the diagonal dashed line has a slope of 1; the x in the upper right is the predicted maximum heart rate and $\dot{V}O_2$ for the subject.

TABLE 10.19.4.   Selected Respiratory Function Data: Second Study

Measurement	Predicted	Measured
Age, yr		60
Sex		Male
Height, cm		171
Weight, kg	74	87
VC, L	3.92	4.38
IC, L	2.61	2.53
TLC, L	6.11	5.87
FEV_1, L	3.06	3.59
FEV_1/VC, %	78	81
MVV, L/min	132	158
D_LCO, ml/mm Hg/min	26.4	31.8

TABLE 10.19.5.   Selected Exercise Data: Second Study

Measurement	Predicted	Measured
Peak $\dot{V}O_2$, L/min	2.19	1.63
Maximum HR, beats/min	160	118
Maximum O_2 pulse, ml/beat	13.7	14.2
$\Delta\dot{V}O_2/\Delta WR$, ml/min/W	10.3	6.8
AT, L/min	>0.96	1.05
Blood pressure, mmHg (rest, max ex)		140/80, 210/100
Maximum $\dot{V}E$, L/min		79
Exercise breathing reserve, L/min	>15	79

TABLE 10.19.6.   Second Study

Time min	Work rate watts	BP mmHg	HR min^{-1}	f min^{-1}	$\dot{V}E$ L/min BTPS	$\dot{V}CO_2$ L/min STPD	$\dot{V}O_2$ L/min STPD	$\dot{V}O_2$/HR ml/beat	R	pH	HCO_3^- meq/L	PO_2, mmHg ET	PO_2 a	PO_2 (A − a)	PCO_2, mmHg ET	PCO_2 a	PCO_2 (a − ET)	$\dot{V}E/\dot{V}CO_2$	$\dot{V}E/\dot{V}O_2$	V_D/V_T
	Rest	140/80																		
	Rest		59	12	9.1	0.25	0.31	5.3	0.81			102			39			32	26	
	Rest	140/90	57	12	9.6	0.25	0.29	5.1	0.86			106			37			34	30	
	Rest		54	13	6.2	0.13	0.15	2.8	0.87			104			38			39	34	
	Rest	140/90	55	15	7.7	0.16	0.22	4.0	0.73			99			39			40	39	
	Rest		57	13	10.5	0.28	0.37	6.5	0.76			99			39			34	25	
	Rest		57	19	10.8	0.27	0.34	6.0	0.79			101			39			34	27	
	Unloaded		70	18	16.8	0.56	0.70	10.0	0.80			100			41			27	22	
	Unloaded		70	13	16.7	0.52	0.58	8.3	0.90			108			38			30	27	
	Unloaded		70	14	17.0	0.56	0.66	9.4	0.85			104			39			28	24	
	Unloaded		72	19	21.3	0.65	0.69	9.6	0.94			109			38			30	29	
	Unloaded		72	19	19.8	0.63	0.73	10.1	0.86			103			40			29	25	
	Unloaded	145/90	76	16	21.2	0.68	0.80	10.5	0.85			100			41			29	25	
0.5	20		76	13	18.0	0.59	0.66	8.7	0.89			106			39			29	26	
1.0	20		76	15	19.9	0.66	0.76	10.0	0.87			103			40			28	25	
1.5	40		76	16	21.8	0.74	0.87	11.4	0.85			102			41			28	23	
2.0	40	180/90	83	19	28.2	0.92	0.98	11.8	0.94			104			41			29	27	
2.5	60		85	17	27.1	0.95	1.06	12.5	0.90			102			42			27	24	
3.0	60		88	20	36.8	1.23	1.23	14.0	1.00			102			42			29	29	
3.5	80		93	24	37.4	1.25	1.18	12.7	1.06			109			41			28	30	
4.0	80	195/85	100	23	42.1	1.38	1.26	12.6	1.10			113			38			29	32	
4.5	100		102	25	48.4	1.53	1.36	13.3	1.13			114			38			30	34	
5.0	100		105	29	57.6	1.72	1.42	13.5	1.21			118			35			32	39	
5.5	120		103	34	68.8	1.92	1.50	14.6	1.28			121			33			34	44	
6.0	120	210/100	113	49	79.3	2.02	1.54	13.6	1.31			121			33			37	49	
6.5	140		118	40	78.0	2.06	1.58	13.4	1.30			119			34			36	47	
7.0	140		115	42	76.5	2.16	1.63	14.2	1.33			119			33			34	45	
	Recovery		98	27	66.8	1.89	1.35	13.8	1.40			120			34			34	48	
	Recovery	210/90	97	27	61.9	1.71	1.23	12.7	1.39			123			32			35	48	
	Recovery		91	23	45.5	1.27	0.94	10.3	1.35			122			33			34	46	
	Recovery	180/90	91	23	41.9	1.16	0.88	9.7	1.32			122			33			34	45	

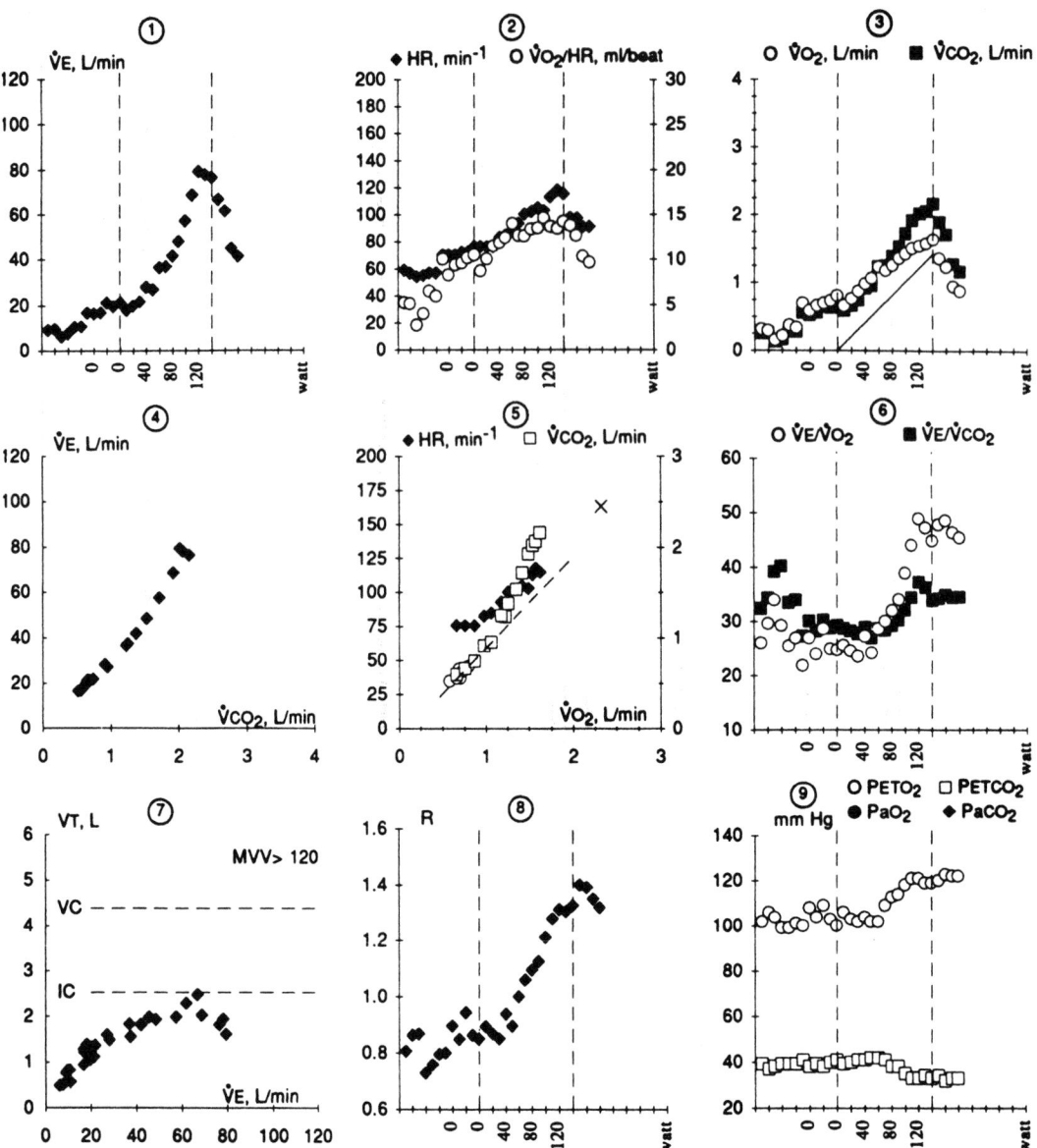

FIGURE 10.19.2.   Second study. **1:** Vertical dashed lines in panels 1 to 3 and 6, 8, and 9 indicate the beginning and the end of the increasing work period. **2:** Unloaded cycling is performed for 3 minutes before the left vertical dashed line. **3:** In panel 3, the diagonal line shows the increase of $\dot{V}O_2$ at a slope of 10 ml/min/W. **4:** In panel 5, the diagonal dashed line has a slope of 1; the x in the upper right is the predicted maximum heart rate and $\dot{V}O_2$ for the subject.

Case 20 Myocardial Ischemia with Mild Interstitial and Obstructive Airway Disease

Clinical Findings

This 54-year-old man was referred by a government agency for cardiopulmonary exercise testing because of his work exposure to asbestos of 15 years. He no longer smoked but had a 30-year history of cigarette smoking. He denied dyspnea, cough, chest pain, weight change, or ankle edema. He got little exercise and felt numbness in his legs after 20 minutes of walking. He had borderline hypertension and an elevated serum cholesterol level. There were crackles at the left lung base, and a chest roentgenogram showed linear scarring in that area. Heart sounds and the resting ECGs were normal.

Exercise Findings

The patient performed exercise on a cycle ergometer. He pedaled at 60 rpm without an added load for 3 minutes. The work rate was then increased 15 W per minute to tolerance. Heart rate and rhythm were continuously monitored; 12-lead ECGs were obtained during rest, exercise, and recovery. Blood pressure was measured with a sphygmomanometer, and arterial oxygen saturation was estimated with an ear oximeter. The patient appeared to give a good effort and stopped exercise because of leg fatigue; he denied chest pain or dyspnea during or after the study. Significant ST-segment depression in leads II, III, aVF, and V_3 to V_6 was noted beginning at the 120-W work rate, with a maximum of 2.5 mm depression at end of exercise. The ST-segment abnormalities resolved after 9 minutes of recovery. No ectopy was present. Saturation as estimated by oximetry remained normal.

Interpretation

Comments

Resting studies showed a mild obstructive ventilatory defect (Table 10.20.1).

Analysis

Referring to flowchart 1, peak $\dot{V}O_2$ is mildly decreased, but the anaerobic threshold is normal (Table 10.20.2). Proceeding next to flowchart 3, the high breathing reserve (branch point 3.1) and ab-

normal exercise ECG (branch point 3.3) lead to the diagnosis of myocardial ischemia, although the patient had no chest pain or distress. The $\Delta\dot{V}O_2/\Delta WR$ is within normal limits, but the plateau in the O_2 pulse for the last 4 minutes of exercise suggests the inability to further increase stroke volume and the arteriovenous O_2 difference or that stroke volume is decreasing as arteriovenous O_2 difference is increasing. This is coincident with the onset of abnormal ECG findings and is further supported by a slowing of $\dot{V}O_2$ increase as work rate is increased.

Conclusion

The patient has evidence of myocardial ischemia associated with concurrent evidence of myocardial dysfunction. This is most likely due to coronary artery disease. The normal ventilatory equivalents indicate essentially normal ventilation–perfusion matching despite the mild obstructive and interstitial lung disease. The patient was referred to his private internist for further diagnostic and therapeutic evaluation of his cardiac disease.

TABLE 10.20.1. Selected Respiratory Function Data

Measurement	Predicted	Measured
Age, yr		54
Sex		Male
Height, cm		191
Weight, kg	90	98
Hematocrit, %		47
VC, L	5.36	4.79
IC, L	3.58	3.78
FEV$_1$, L	4.25	3.05
FEV$_1$/VC, %	79	64
MVV, L/min	164	126
D$_L$CO, ml/mm Hg/min	29.5	27.7

TABLE 10.20.2. Selected Exercise Data

Measurement	Predicted	Measured
Peak $\dot{V}O_2$, L/min	2.81	2.09
Maximum HR, beats/min	166	142
Maximum O$_2$ pulse, ml/beat	16.9	14.8
$\Delta\dot{V}O_2/\Delta WR$, ml/min/W	10.3	8.9
AT, L/min	>1.21	1.4
Blood pressure, mmHg (rest, max)		154/90, 198/78
Maximum $\dot{V}E$, L/min		72
Exercise breathing reserve, L/min	>15	54

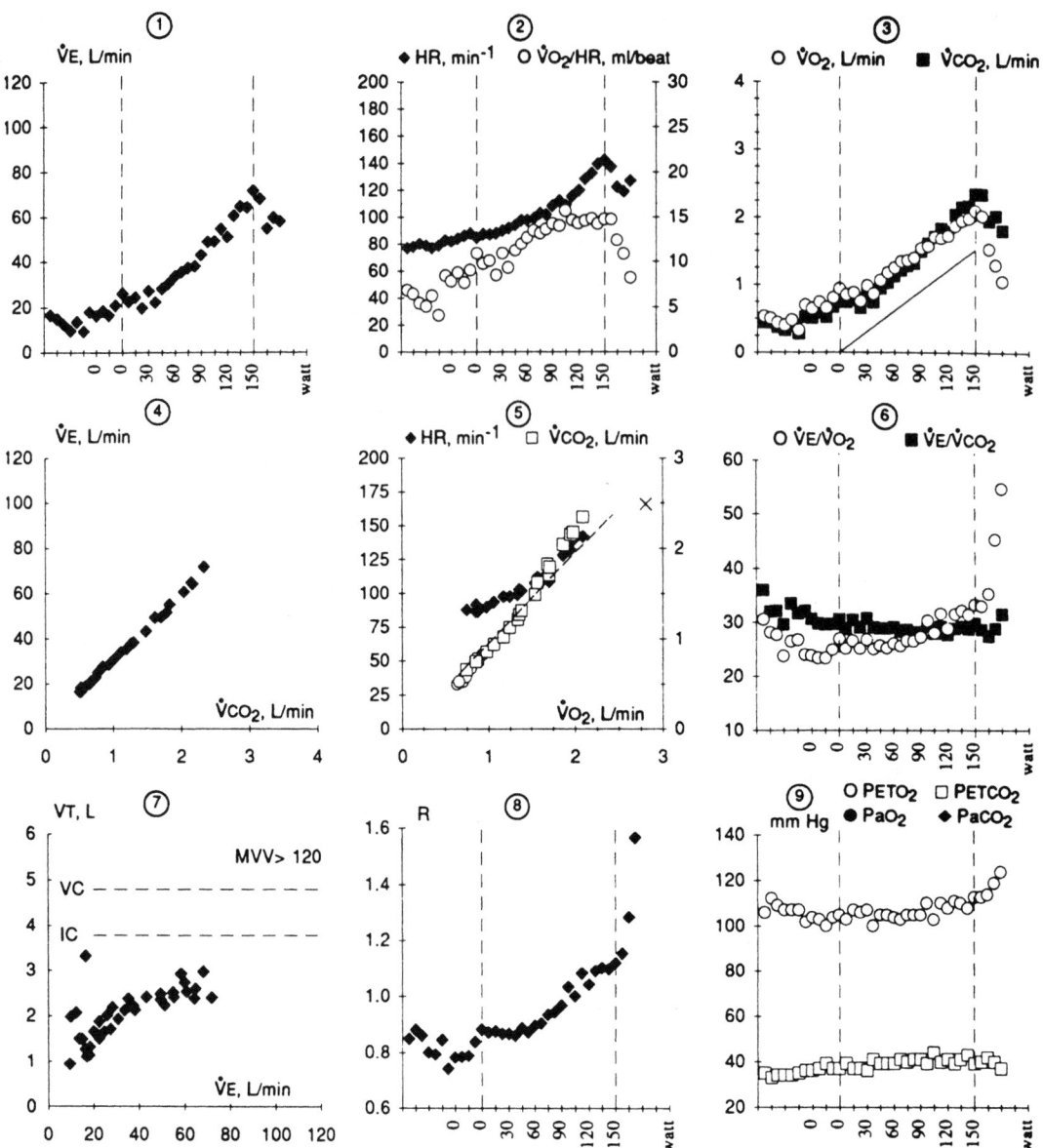

FIGURE 10.20.1.   **1:** Vertical dashed lines in panels 1 to 3 and 6, 8, and 9 indicate the beginning and the end of the increasing work period. **2:** Unloaded cycling is performed for 3 minutes before the left vertical dashed line. **3:** In panel 3, the diagonal line shows the increase of $\dot{V}O_2$ at a slope of 10 ml/min/W. **4:** In panel 5, the diagonal dashed line has a slope of 1; the *x* in the upper right is the predicted maximum heart rate and $\dot{V}O_2$ for the subject.

TABLE 10.20.3.   Air Breathing

Time min	Work rate watts	BP mmHg	HR min⁻¹	f min⁻¹	V̇E L/min BTPS	V̇CO₂ L/min STPD	V̇O₂ L/min STPD	V̇O₂/HR ml/beat	R	pH	HCO₃⁻ meq/L	PO₂ mmHg ET	a	(A−a)	PCO₂ mmHg ET	a	(a−ET)	V̇E/V̇CO₂	V̇E/V̇O₂	VD/VT
	Rest	154/90																		
	Rest		77	5	16.6	0.45	0.53	6.9	0.85			106			35			36	31	
	Rest		78	10	14.9	0.44	0.50	6.4	0.88			112			33			32	28	
	Rest		80	6	12.4	0.37	0.43	5.4	0.86			109			34			32	28	
	Rest	150/96	79	5	9.9	0.32	0.40	5.1	0.80			107			34			30	24	
	Rest		77	9	13.5	0.38	0.48	6.2	0.79			107			34			34	27	
	Rest		79	10	9.4	0.27	0.32	4.1	0.84			107			35			32	27	
	Unloaded		83	16	18.1	0.52	0.70	8.4	0.74			102			36			32	24	
	Unloaded		82	13	16.4	0.50	0.64	7.8	0.78			104			36			31	24	
	Unloaded		84	14	18.5	0.58	0.74	8.8	0.78			103			37			30	23	
	Unloaded		86	15	16.7	0.52	0.66	7.7	0.79			100			39			30	23	
	Unloaded		88	13	21.0	0.67	0.80	9.1	0.84			104			37			30	25	
	Unloaded	148/88	85	13	26.1	0.82	0.93	10.9	0.88			105			37			30	27	
0.5	15		87	15	22.6	0.74	0.85	9.8	0.87			103			39			29	25	
1.0	15		87	15	24.7	0.77	0.88	10.1	0.88			107			37			30	27	
1.5	30		88	12	19.9	0.65	0.75	8.5	0.87			106			37			29	25	
2.0	30	152/90	90	16	27.5	0.85	0.98	10.9	0.87			107			36			31	27	
2.5	45		92	12	22.5	0.74	0.86	9.3	0.86			100			41			29	25	
3.0	45		94	13	28.3	0.94	1.06	11.3	0.89			105			39			29	26	
3.5	60		98	16	30.9	1.02	1.17	11.9	0.87			105			39			29	25	
4.0	60	148/84	98	16	33.9	1.12	1.25	12.8	0.90			104			39			29	26	
4.5	75		99	15	35.6	1.21	1.34	13.5	0.90			103			41			28	26	
5.0	75		103	17	37.7	1.27	1.36	13.2	0.93			105			40			29	27	
5.5	90		102	18	38.3	1.31	1.39	13.6	0.94			105			41			28	26	
6.0	90	178/86	108	18	43.4	1.49	1.54	14.3	0.97			105			41			28	27	
6.5	105		112	21	49.4	1.62	1.57	14.0	1.03			110			39			29	30	
7.0	105		109	20	49.6	1.71	1.71	15.7	1.00			103			44			28	28	
7.5	120		115	22	55.1	1.83	1.69	14.7	1.08			110			40			29	31	
8.0	120	170/88	120	23	51.4	1.79	1.72	14.3	1.04			108			41			28	29	
8.5	135		128	24	60.8	2.04	1.87	14.6	1.09			111			39			29	31	
9.0	135		132	25	64.8	2.15	1.95	14.8	1.10			110			41			29	32	
9.5	150		139	27	64.4	2.17	1.98	14.2	1.10			108			43			29	31	
10.0	150	198/78	142	30	71.9	2.34	2.09	14.7	1.12			113			39			30	33	
	Recovery		137	23	68.4	2.33	2.02	14.7	1.15			113			40			29	33	
	Recovery		122	23	55.4	1.95	1.52	12.5	1.28			114			42			27	35	
	Recovery		119	22	60.1	2.02	1.29	10.8	1.57			119			40			29	45	
	Recovery		127	20	58.5	1.81	1.04	8.2	1.74			124			37			31	55	

Case 21 Silent Myocardial Ischemia, Systemic Hypertension, and Mild Interstitial Lung Disease

Clinical Findings

This 65-year-old man was referred for evaluation. He had retired from work in the shipyard 5 years previously. He had noted slight dyspnea on exertion beginning 6 years prior to evaluation but could still climb two flights of stairs without shortness of breath. He had smoked half a pack of cigarettes a day between the ages of 24 and 40. He denied cough, sputum production, or wheezing. He had recently become short of breath on a fishing trip at high altitude. At age 25, he was discharged from the Army because of a "cardiac murmur," but this was not noted on later examinations. There was no history of rheumatic fever or congestive heart failure. He took no medications. Physical examination was normal except for bilateral arcus senilis. Chest roentgenograms revealed bilateral pleural plaques and possible bibasilar interstitial disease.

Exercise Findings

The patient performed exercise on a cycle ergometer. He pedaled at 60 rpm without added load for 3 minutes. The work rate was then increased 20 W per minute. Blood was sampled every second minute, and intraarterial blood pressure was recorded from a percutaneously placed brachial artery catheter. Resting ECG showed deep Q waves in leads II, III, and aVF compatible with an old inferior infarction. During exercise, occasional single premature ventricular contractions were noted. At 120 W the ST segments were depressed 2 mm in V_4 through V_6; they were depressed 4 mm before exercise was stopped at 160 W. The ST segments became isoelectric within 5 minutes of recovery. The patient experienced leg fatigue but denied any chest pain or discomfort.

Interpretation

Comments

Results of the resting respiratory function studies are within normal limits (Table 10.21.1). The resting ECG is abnormal and suggests that the patient had an inferior wall myocardial infarction in the past.

Analysis

Referring to flowchart 1, the peak $\dot{V}O_2$ is reduced, but the anaerobic threshold is within normal limits (Table 10.21.2). Proceeding to flowchart 3, the breathing reserve is high (branch point 3.1). The ECG became abnormal as the maximum work rate was approached (branch point 3.3). Although the patient did not experience chest pain, the diagnosis of myocardial ischemia is supported by the marked change in slope in $\dot{V}O_2$ in response to increasing work rate (panel 3, Fig. 10.21.1) and a reduced $\Delta\dot{V}O_2/\Delta WR$. The very marked increase in R starting at 80 W (Table 10.21.3 and panel 8, Fig. 10.21.1) reflects the development of a significant metabolic acidosis as the anaerobic threshold is exceeded. The steepening heart rate response with increasing oxygen uptake (panel 5, Fig. 10.21.1) and the failure

TABLE 10.21.1. Selected Respiratory Function Data

Measurement	Predicted	Measured
Age, yr		65
Sex		Male
Height, cm		174
Weight, kg	77	65
Hematocrit, %		45
VC, L	3.97	3.58
IC, L	2.64	2.24
TLC, L	6.21	6.68
FEV_1, L	3.09	2.60
FEV_1/VC, %	78	73
MVV, L/min	128	117
D_LCO, ml/mm Hg/min	25.6	21.7

TABLE 10.21.2. Selected Exercise Data

Measurement	Predicted	Measured
Peak $\dot{V}O_2$, L/min	1.88	1.41
Maximum HR, beats/min	155	176
Maximum O_2 pulse, ml/beat	12.1	8.0
$\Delta\dot{V}O_2/\Delta WR$, ml/min/W	10.3	7.3
AT, L/min	>0.84	1.05
Blood pressure, mmHg (rest, max)		189/108, 234/126
Maximum $\dot{V}E$, L/min		74
Exercise breathing reserve, L/min	>15	43
PaO_2, mmHg (rest, max ex)		93, 89
$P(A-a)O_2$, mmHg (rest, max ex)		15, 35
$P(a-ET)CO_2$, mmHg (rest, max ex)		3, 1
VD/VT (rest, heavy ex)		0.32, 0.37

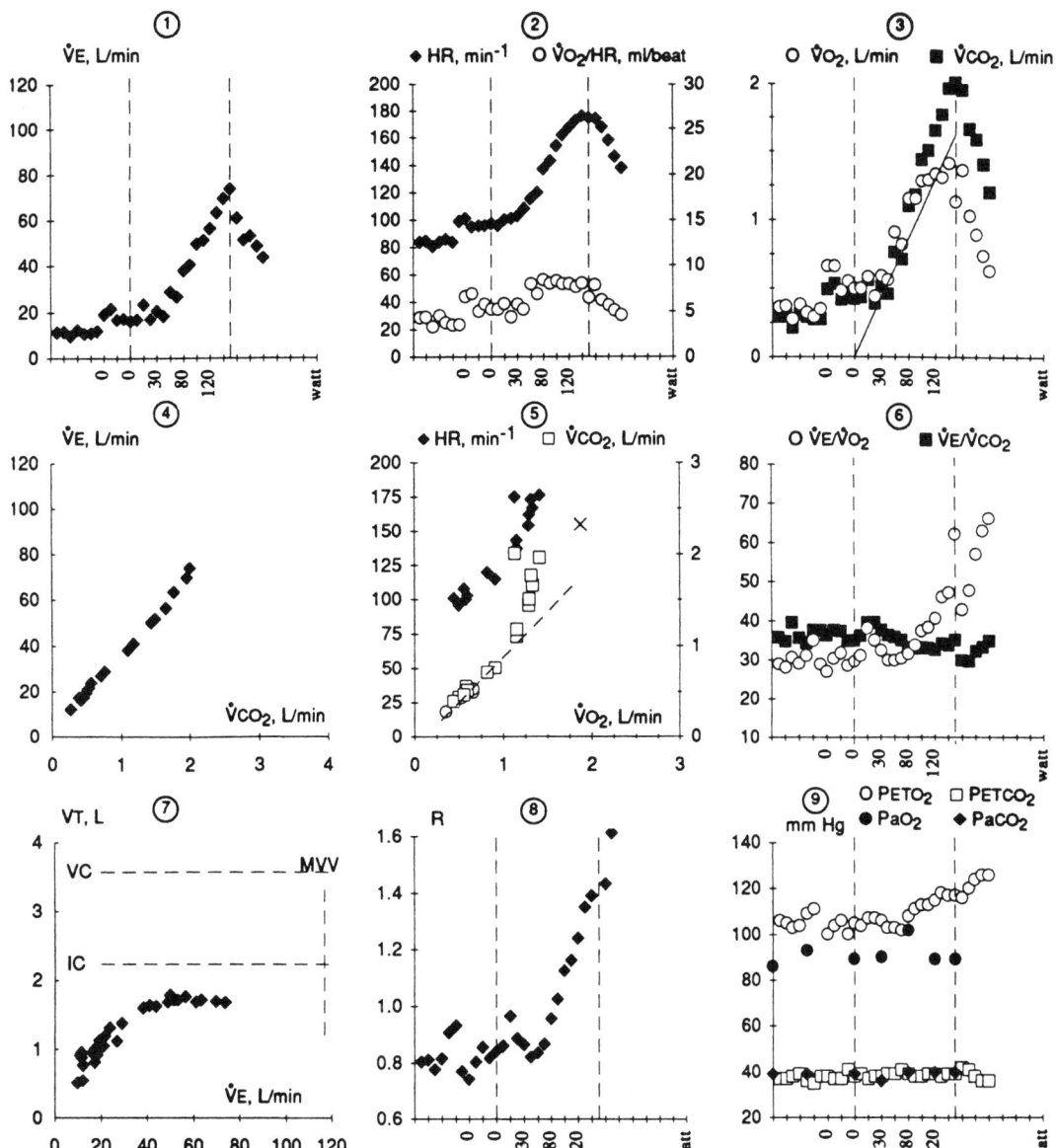

FIGURE 10.21.1.   **1:** Vertical dashed lines in panels 1 to 3 and 6, 8, and 9 indicate the beginning and the end of the increasing work period. **2:** Unloaded cycling is performed for 3 minutes before the left vertical dashed line. **3:** In panel 3, the diagonal line shows the increase of $\dot{V}O_2$ at a slope of 10 ml/min/W. **4:** In panel 5, the diagonal dashed line has a slope of 1; the x in the upper right is the predicted maximum heart rate and $\dot{V}O_2$ for the subject.

of O_2 pulse to increase at a low work rate (panel 2, Fig. 10.21.1) reflect a low stroke volume and a maximal $C(a - \bar{v})O_2$ being reached at a relatively low work rate.

This patient has significant systemic hypertension. We cannot therefore exclude the possibility that the myocardial ischemia and impaired cardiac function demonstrated here are due, in part, to abnormally increased myocardial work and coronary artery disease.

There is evidence of ventilation–perfusion mismatching [high V_D/V_T and positive $P(a - ET)CO_2$]. These abnormal findings might be due to the abnormalities that develop in the lungs in response to chronic heart failure (due to an ischemic cardiomyopathy), as described in Chapter 5. The normal resting respiratory function suggests that the decrease in perfusion of ventilated lung reflected by these blood gas abnormalities is unlikely to be due to primary lung disease.

TABLE 10.21.3. Air Breathing

Time min	Work rate watts	BP mmHg	HR min⁻¹	f min⁻¹	V̇E L/min BTPS	V̇CO₂ L/min STPD	V̇O₂ L/min STPD	V̇O₂/HR ml/beat	R	pH	HCO₃⁻ meq/L	PO₂ mmHg ET	a	(A−a)	PCO₂ mmHg ET	a	(a−ET)	V̇E/V̇CO₂	V̇E/V̇O₂	VD/VT
	Rest	189/108								7.44	26		86			39				
	Rest		84	12	11.4	0.29	0.36	4.3	0.81			106			37			36	29	
	Rest		85	13	11.5	0.30	0.37	4.4	0.81			105			37			35	28	
	Rest		81	19	9.9	0.21	0.27	3.3	0.78			103			38			39	31	
	Rest		84	16	12.4	0.31	0.38	4.5	0.82			104			39			36	29	
	Rest	192/114	86	12	11.0	0.29	0.32	3.7	0.91	7.44	26	109	93	15	36	39	3	34	31	0.32
	Rest		84	12	11.2	0.27	0.29	3.5	0.93			111			35			38	35	
	Unloaded		99	22	12.0	0.27	0.35	3.5	0.77			193			38			38	29	
	Unloaded		101	17	19.2	0.49	0.66	6.5	0.74			100			38			36	27	
	Unloaded		95	18	21.5	0.53	0.66	6.9	0.80			104			37			38	30	
	Unloaded		96	18	16.8	0.41	0.48	5.0	0.85			106			37			37	32	
	Unloaded		96	19	17.3	0.45	0.55	5.7	0.82			100			41			35	29	
	Unloaded	213/120	97	17	16.2	0.42	0.50	5.2	0.84	7.43	25	105	89	16	38	39	1	35	30	0.34
0.5	20		96	17	17.0	0.43	0.50	5.2	0.86			104			39			36	31	
1.0	20		100	18	23.6	0.56	0.58	5.8	0.97			107			37			39	38	
1.5	30		101	21	17.2	0.39	0.44	4.4	0.89			107			38			40	35	
2.0	30	210/114	103	20	20.9	0.51	0.59	5.7	0.86	7.50	28	106	90	20	38	36	−2	38	33	0.33
2.5	60		108	20	18.4	0.46	0.56	5.2	0.82			103			39			36	30	
3.0	60		115	21	29.0	0.76	0.91	7.9	0.84			103			39			36	30	
3.5	80		120	24	26.9	0.71	0.82	6.8	0.87			102			41			35	30	
4.0	80	219/117	137	24	38.3	1.10	1.15	8.4	0.96	7.36	22	108	102	7	39	40	1	33	32	0.33
4.5	100		143	25	41.0	1.18	1.15	8.0	1.03			111			38			33	34	
5.0	100		154	28	50.1	1.44	1.28	8.3	1.13			113			38			33	37	
5.5	120		162	30	51.8	1.50	1.29	8.0	1.16			113			39			33	38	
6.0	120	234/126	167	32	56.6	1.65	1.33	8.0	1.24	7.35	22	115	89	27	39	40	1	33	41	0.32
6.5	140		173	37	63.5	1.77	1.31	7.6	1.35			118			38			34	46	
7.0	140		176	41	69.8	1.96	1.41	8.0	1.39			117			39			34	47	
7.5	160	234/126	175	44	73.9	2.00	1.13	6.5	1.77	7.35	22	117	89	35	39	40	1	35	62	0.37
	Recovery		174	36	61.1	1.95	1.36	7.8	1.43			116			42			30	43	
	Recovery		168	30	51.6	1.66	1.03	6.1	1.61			120			41			30	48	
	Recovery		158	31	53.3	1.58	0.89	5.6	1.78			124			38			32	57	
	Recovery	220/120	146	29	49.0	1.40	0.74	5.1	1.89			126			36			33	63	
	Recovery		138	27	44.0	1.20	0.63	4.6	1.90			126			36			35	66	

Conclusion

Myocardial ischemia with reduced exercise performance secondary to coronary artery disease and systemic hypertension.

Case 22 Ischemic Cardiomyopathy

Clinical Findings

This 65-year-old man had sustained an acute myocardial infarction 6 years ago. Since then he had required one to two nitroglycerin tablets per day and propranolol for "stable angina." He had had 30 years of asbestos exposure in the shipyards and had smoked for 23 years. He could walk 2 to 3 miles before becoming dyspneic and admitted to a scantily productive morning cough. Resting ECG was normal. An exercise study was performed to evaluate the relative contributions of his pulmonary and cardiac illnesses.

Exercise Findings

The patient performed exercise on a cycle ergometer. He pedaled at 60 rpm without added load for 3 minutes. The work rate was then increased 10 W per minute. Arterial blood was sampled every second minute, and intraarterial blood pressure was recorded from a percutaneously placed brachial artery catheter. The incremental cycle exercise test was terminated at 70 W because of moderate substernal chest pain; the development of 3 mm of ST-segment depression in leads II, III, and aVF; and occasional premature ventricular beats. These abnormalities resolved promptly after termination of exercise.

Interpretation

Comments

The resting respiratory function studies indicate that the patient has mild airflow obstruction (Table 10.22.1). The resting ECG is normal.

Analysis

Referring to flowchart 1, the peak $\dot{V}_{O_2}$ is reduced and the anaerobic threshold is normal (Table 10.22.2). See flowchart 3. The breathing reserve is high (branch point 3.1), while the exercise ECG (branch point 3.3) was clearly abnormal. The chest pain, low

$\Delta\dot{V}_{O_2}/\Delta WR$, and low O_2 pulse that fails to rise during exercise all support the primary diagnosis of myocardial ischemia. The breathing reserve is high. Indices of ventilation–perfusion matching are borderline abnormal. In contrast, the cardiovascular response to exercise is abnormal.

Conclusion

Reduced exercise performance secondary to ischemic cardiomyopathy with mild airflow obstruction.

TABLE 10.22.1.   Selected Respiratory Function Data

Measurement	Predicted	Measured
Age, yr		65
Sex		Male
Height, cm		167
Weight, kg	71	55
Hematocrit, %		41
VC, L	3.54	3.42
IC, L	2.36	1.81
TLC, L	5.57	6.16
FEV_1, L	2.75	2.33
FEV_1/VC, %	78	68
MVV, L/min	120	101
$D_L CO$, ml/mm Hg/min	22.6	26.4

TABLE 10.22.2.   Selected Exercise Data

Measurement	Predicted	Measured
Peak $\dot{V}_{O_2}$, L/min	1.68	1.01
Maximum HR, beats/min	155	152
Maximum O_2 pulse, ml/beat	10.8	7.3
$\Delta\dot{V}_{O_2}/\Delta WR$, ml/min/W	10.3	5.7
AT, L/min	>0.74	0.9
Blood pressure, mmHg (rest, max)		165/87, 159/84
Maximum $\dot{V}E$, L/min		39
Exercise breathing reserve, L/min	>15	62
Pa_{O_2}, mmHg (rest, max ex)		94, 95
$P(A - a)_{O_2}$, mmHg (rest, max ex)		13, 18
$P(a - ET)_{CO_2}$, mmHg (rest, max ex)		4, 2
V_D/V_T (rest, heavy ex)		0.40, 0.29
HCO_3^-, mEq/L (rest, 2-min recov)		27, 23

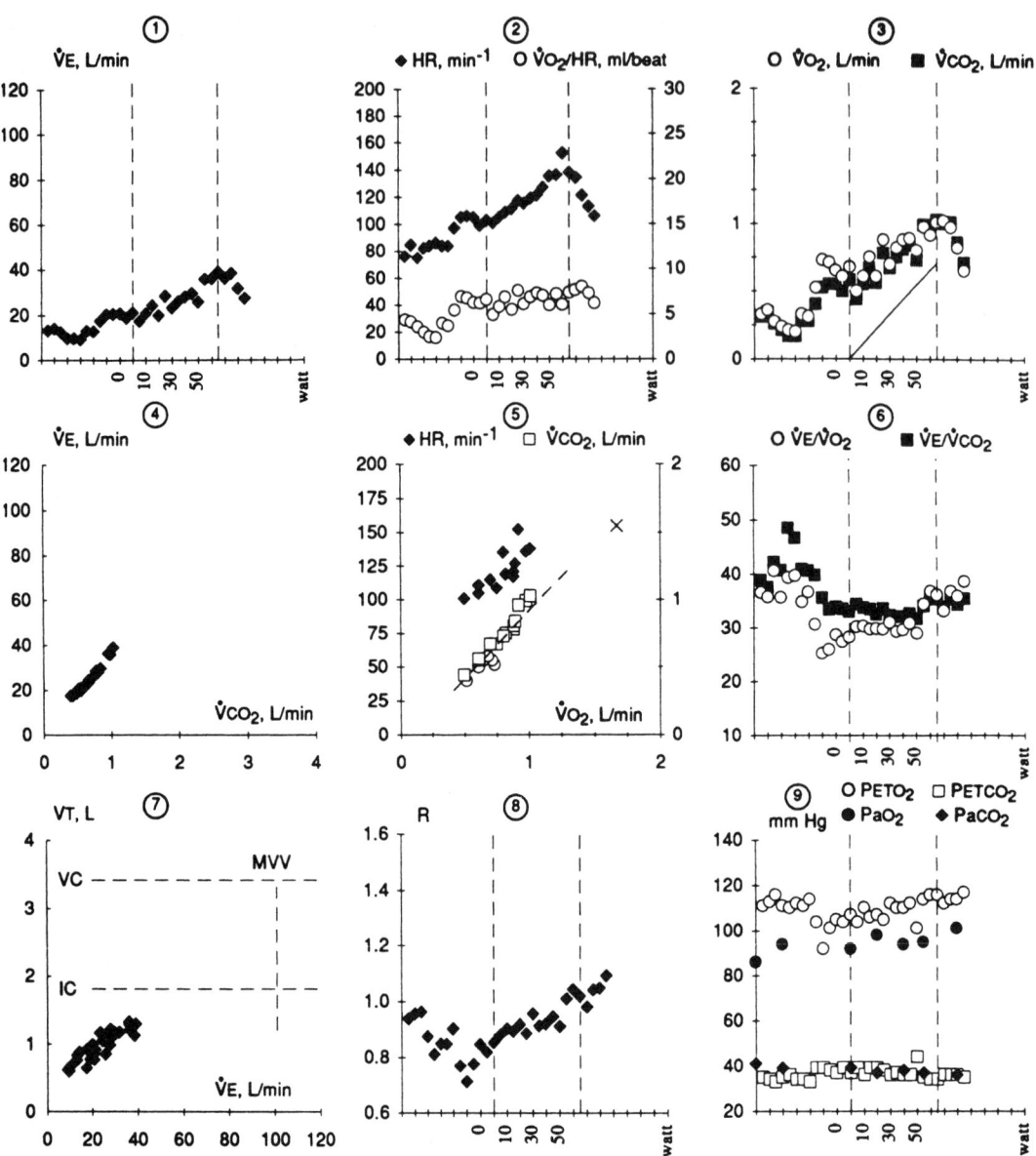

FIGURE 10.22.1. **1:** Vertical dashed lines in panels 1 to 3 and 6, 8, and 9 indicate the beginning and the end of the increasing work period. **2:** Unloaded cycling is performed for 3 minutes before the left vertical dashed line. **3:** In panel 3, the diagonal line shows the increase of $\dot{V}O_2$ at a slope of 10 ml/min/W. **4:** In panel 5, the diagonal dashed line has a slope of 1; the x in the upper right is the predicted maximum heart rate and $\dot{V}O_2$ for the subject.

TABLE 10.22.3. Air Breathing

Time min	Work rate watts	BP mmHg	HR min⁻¹	f min⁻¹	V̇E L/min BTPS	V̇CO₂ L/min STPD	V̇O₂ L/min STPD	V̇O₂/HR ml/beat	R	pH	HCO₃⁻ meq/L	PO₂ mmHg ET	a	(A−a)	PCO₂ mmHg ET	a	(a−ET)	V̇E/V̇CO₂	V̇E/V̇O₂	VD/VT
	Rest	165/87								7.43	27		86			41				
	Rest		76	16	13.4	0.31	0.33	4.3	0.94			111			35			39	36	
	Rest		85	16	14.1	0.34	0.36	4.2	0.96			113			34			37	36	
	Rest		75	17	12.4	0.26	0.27	3.6	0.96			116			33			42	41	
	Rest		82	15	9.8	0.21	0.24	2.9	0.88	7.44	26	111	94	13	35	39	4	41	36	0.40
	Rest	156/84	84	16	9.6	0.17	0.21	2.5	0.81			110			36			48	39	
	Rest		86	15	9.2	0.17	0.20	2.3	0.85			112			34			47	40	
	Rest		84	17	12.9	0.28	0.33	3.9	0.85			111			34			41	35	
	Rest		84	17	12.8	0.28	0.31	3.7	0.90			114			33			41	37	
	Unloaded		97	19	17.5	0.40	0.52	5.4	0.77			104			39			40	31	
	Unloaded		105	22	20.3	0.52	0.73	7.0	0.71			92			39			35	25	
	Unloaded		106	24	20.4	0.55	0.71	6.7	0.77			101			38			33	26	
	Unloaded		105	23	20.6	0.55	0.65	6.2	0.85			105			37			34	29	
	Unloaded		99	24	18.8	0.50	0.61	6.2	0.82			104			39			34	27	
	Unloaded	162/84	103	23	21.1	0.58	0.68	6.6	0.85	7.44	26	107	92	14	37	39	2	33	28	0.30
0.5	10		101	27	17.4	0.44	0.50	5.0	0.88			104			39			34	30	
1.0	10		105	27	20.8	0.55	0.61	5.8	0.90			110			36			34	30	
1.5	20		109	23	24.3	0.67	0.75	6.9	0.89			106			39			33	30	
2.0	20	165/87	111	20	19.9	0.56	0.61	5.5	0.92	7.45	25	107	98	12	39	37	−2	33	30	0.26
2.5	30		117	26	28.4	0.78	0.88	7.5	0.89			105			38			34	30	
3.0	30		115	20	23.3	0.67	0.70	6.1	0.96			112			36			32	31	
3.5	40		119	23	26.0	0.75	0.82	6.9	0.91			110			37			32	29	
4.0	40	156/84	121	23	27.9	0.81	0.88	7.3	0.92	7.44	25	110	94	15	36	38	2	32	29	0.27
4.5	50		127	25	29.5	0.84	0.89	7.0	0.94			112			36			33	31	
5.0	50		135	30	25.7	0.73	0.80	5.9	0.91			101			44			32	29	
5.5	60	162/84	136	27	35.9	0.99	0.98	7.2	1.01	7.44	25	114	5	18	35	37	2	34	34	0.29
6.0	60		152	28	36.2	0.96	0.92	6.1	1.04			116			34			35	37	
6.5	70	159/84	138	30	38.9	1.03	1.01	7.3	1.02			116			34			35	36	
	Recovery		134	30	36.3	1.00	1.02	7.6	0.98			112			36			34	33	0.28
	Recovery		121	34	38.5	1.01	0.97	8.0	1.04			114			36			35	37	
	Recovery	162/84	113	27	31.7	0.86	0.82	7.3	1.05	7.43	23	114	101	14	36	36	0	34	36	
	Recovery		106	28	27.5	0.71	0.65	6.1	1.09			117			35			35	39	

Case 23 Cardiomyopathy

Clinical Findings

This 41-year-old former brickworker, woodworker, sandblaster, and security guard had been placed on disability for a back injury 9 years ago. Hypertension had been diagnosed 6 years ago. He had started complaining of dyspnea and a productive cough 3 years ago. He had been diagnosed as having "probable pulmonary asbestosis" and "asthmatic bronchitis" 2 years ago. He denied smoking but had had repeated hospitalizations for alcoholism. He was being treated with propranolol, hydrochlorothiazide, oxtriphylline, and potassium supplementation. Auscultation of the heart and lungs were normal, as were posteroanterior, lateral, and oblique chest roentgenograms.

Exercise Findings

The patient performed exercise on a cycle ergometer. He pedaled at 60 rpm without added load for 3 minutes. The work rate was then increased 20 W per minute to his symptom-limited maximum. Arterial blood was sampled every second minute, and intraarterial blood pressure was recorded from a percutaneously placed brachial artery catheter. Resting ECG was normal. He stopped exercise with complaints of shortness of breath, a feeling that he was "going to faint," and leg "tiredness." One premature ventricular contraction occurred during exercise, but exercise and recovery ECGs were otherwise normal.

Interpretation

Comments

Resting pulmonary function (Table 10.23.1) and ECG are normal.

Analysis

Referring to flowchart 1, the peak $\dot{V}O_2$ and anaerobic threshold are reduced (Table 10.23.2). See flowchart 4. The breathing reserve is normal (branch point 4.1), and the ventilatory equivalent at the anaerobic threshold (branch point 4.3) and the indices of ventilation–perfusion matching are normal. These findings indicate that this patient does not have an abnormal pulmonary circulation, but does have a nonpulmonary O_2 flow problem. Because the hematocrit is normal (branch point 4.4), this is most likely due to cardiovascular disease. The exercise ECG is essentially normal throughout exercise. His $\Delta\dot{V}O_2/\Delta WR$ is low, and he has a low but rising O_2 pulse at maximum work rate (panel 2, Fig. 10.23.1). The patient's blood pressure response to exercise and heart rate reserve are normal (Table 10.23.2), and the patient did not have leg pain with exercise, making peripheral arterial disease unlikely. Because propranolol, one of this patient's medications, ordinarily gives a high O_2 pulse during exercise, the finding of a low O_2 pulse at maxi-

TABLE 10.23.1.   Selected Respiratory Function Data

Measurement	Predicted	Measured
Age, yr		41
Sex		Male
Height, cm		170
Weight, kg	74	78
Hematocrit, %		44
VC, L	3.95	4.00
IC, L	2.63	3.30
TLC, L	5.58	5.28
FEV_1, L	3.16	3.43
FEV_1/VC, %	80	86
MVV, L/min	137	118
D_LCO, ml/mm Hg/min	25.8	24.7

TABLE 10.23.2.   Selected Exercise Data

Measurement	Predicted	Measured
Peak $\dot{V}O_2$, L/min	2.64	1.75
Maximum HR, beats/min	179	150
Maximum O_2 pulse, ml/beat	14.7	11.7
$\Delta\dot{V}O_2/\Delta WR$, ml/min/W	10.3	8.3
AT, L/min	>1.11	0.85
Blood pressure, mmHg (rest, max)		132/87, 204/108
Maximum $\dot{V}E$, L/min		78
Exercise breathing reserve, L/min	>15	40
PaO_2, mmHg (rest, max ex)		87, 117
$P(A - a)O_2$, mmHg (rest, max ex)		4, 3
$P(a - ET)CO_2$, mmHg (rest, max ex)		2, −2
VD/VT (rest, heavy ex)		0.36, 0.23
HCO_3^-, mEq/L (rest, 2-min recov)		27, 18

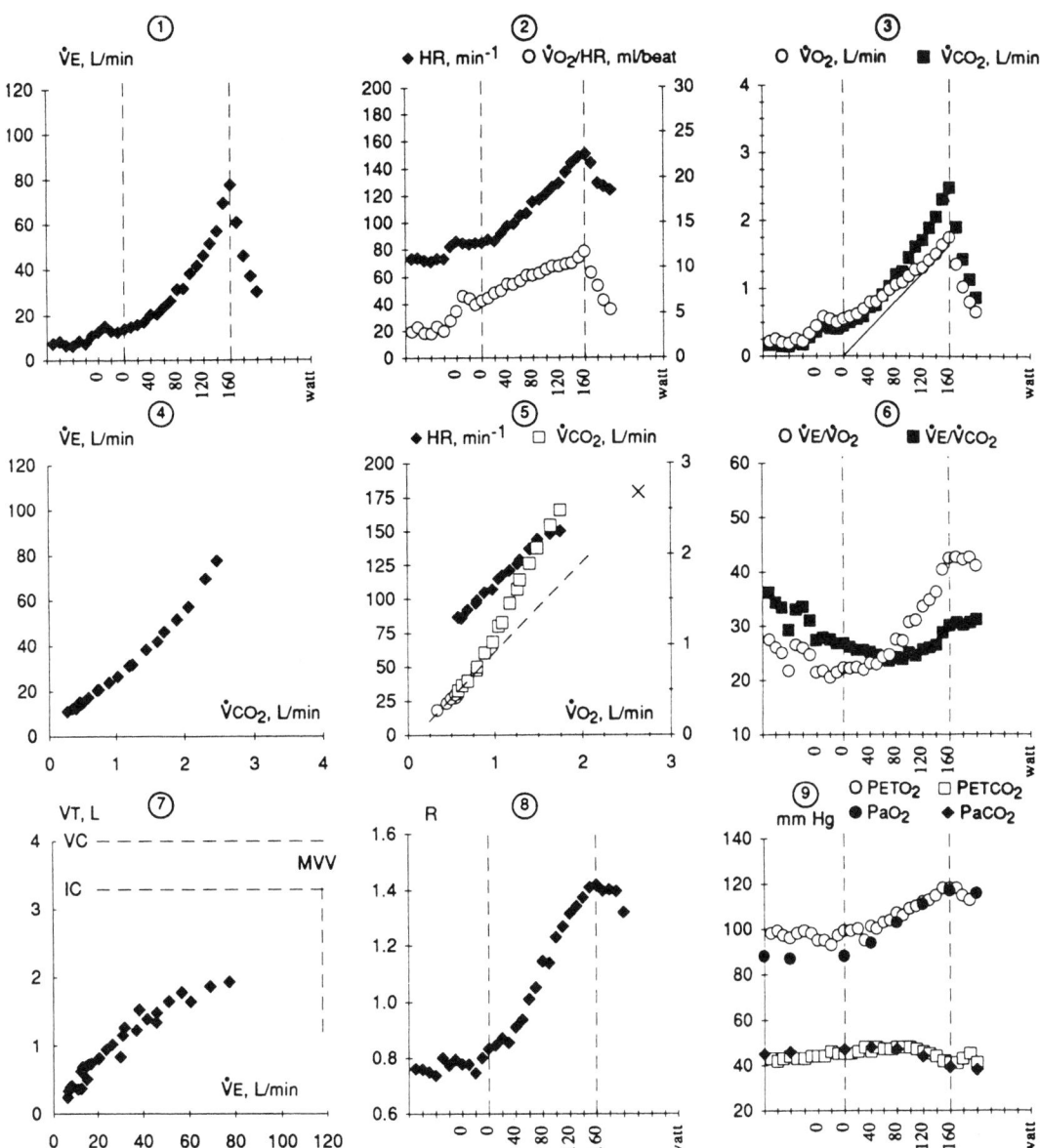

FIGURE 10.23.1. **1:** Vertical dashed lines in panels 1 to 3 and 6, 8, and 9 indicate the beginning and the end of the increasing work period. **2:** Unloaded cycling is performed for 3 minutes before the left vertical dashed line. **3:** In panel 3, the diagonal line shows the increase of $\dot{V}O_2$ at a slope of 10 mL/min/W. **4:** In panel 5, the diagonal dashed line has a slope of 1; the x in the upper right is the predicted maximum heart rate and $\dot{V}O_2$ for the subject.

mum exercise supports the diagnosis of primary heart disease. (Pulmonary vascular disease has already been ruled out.)

Conclusion

This patient is a 41-year-old chronic alcoholic with cardiovascular limitation. Pulmonary vascular, pe-

ripheral arterial, and coronary artery disease were shown to be unlikely causes of the limitation. Two-dimensional echocardiography with exercise supported the diagnosis of cardiomyopathy.

TABLE 10.23.3. Air Breathing

Time min	Work rate watts	BP mmHg	HR min⁻¹	f min⁻¹	V̇E L/min BTPS	V̇CO₂ L/min STPD	V̇O₂ L/min STPD	V̇O₂/HR ml/beat	R	pH	HCO₃⁻ meq/L	PO₂, mmHg ET	a	(A−a)	PCO₂, mmHg ET	a	(a−ET)	V̇E/V̇CO₂	V̇E/V̇O₂	VD/VT
	Rest	132/87								7.39	27		88			45				
	Rest		73	19	7.4	0.16	0.21	2.9	0.76			98			43			36	28	
	Rest		74	21	8.3	0.19	0.25	3.4	0.76			99			42			34	26	
	Rest		72	20	6.7	0.15	0.20	2.8	0.75			97			43			33	25	
	Rest	126/84	71	17	6.4	0.14	0.19	2.7	0.74	7.39	27	96	87	4	44	46	2	35	26	0.36
	Rest		73	21	8.4	0.20	0.25	3.4	0.80			98			43			33	26	
	Rest		73	20	7.4	0.17	0.22	3.0	0.77			99			43			34	26	
	Unloaded		82	31	11.0	0.27	0.34	4.1	0.79			98			44			31	25	
	Unloaded		86	34	12.5	0.35	0.45	5.2	0.78			95			44			27	21	
	Unloaded		85	30	15.1	0.45	0.58	6.8	0.78			95			44			28	22	
	Unloaded		84	19	12.9	0.41	0.55	6.5	0.75			93			46			28	21	
	Unloaded		85	20	12.4	0.40	0.50	5.9	0.80			97			45			27	21	
	Unloaded	138/84	85	21	13.8	0.45	0.54	6.4	0.83	7.37	27	99	88	8	45	47	2	27	22	0.27
0.5	20		87	21	14.6	0.49	0.58	6.7	0.84			99			45			26	22	
1.0	20		86	22	15.7	0.54	0.62	7.2	0.87			100			46			26	22	
1.5	40		92	23	17.0	0.59	0.69	7.5	0.86			95			48			26	22	
2.0	40	147/90	97	25	20.3	0.72	0.79	8.1	0.91	7.38	28	101	94	4	46	48	2	25	23	0.26
2.5	60		99	25	20.5	0.75	0.80	8.1	0.94			100			48			25	23	
3.0	60		105	25	23.6	0.90	0.89	8.5	1.01			103			47			24	24	
3.5	80		107	26	26.4	1.03	0.98	9.2	1.05			104			47			23	25	
4.0	80	159/90	115	27	31.2	1.20	1.05	9.1	1.14	7.36	26	107	103	5	48	47	−1	24	28	0.22
4.5	100		117	25	31.7	1.24	1.09	9.3	1.14			106			48			24	27	
5.0	100		121	25	38.3	1.45	1.18	9.8	1.23			109			48			25	31	
5.5	120		126	30	41.9	1.61	1.27	10.1	1.27			110			47			24	31	
6.0	120	192/105	129	31	46.2	1.71	1.30	10.1	1.32	7.35	24	112	111	3	46	44	−2	25	34	0.22
6.5	140		137	31	51.5	1.89	1.41	10.3	1.34			113			45			26	35	
7.0	140		144	32	57.0	2.06	1.50	10.4	1.37			115			44			26	36	
7.5	160		148	37	69.3	2.31	1.64	11.1	1.41			118			42			29	40	
8.0	160	204/108	150	40	77.6	2.48	1.75	11.7	1.42	7.34	21	118	117	3	41	39	−2	30	42	0.25
	Recovery		144	37	61.0	1.90	1.36	9.4	1.40			118			41			30	43	
	Recovery		129	34	45.8	1.43	1.02	7.9	1.40			115			43			30	42	
	Recovery		127	30	37.0	1.13	0.81	6.4	1.40			113			45			30	43	
	Recovery	150/78	124	36	30.1	0.87	0.66	5.3	1.32	7.28	18	116	116	3	41	38	−3	31	41	0.24

Case 24 Cardiomyopathy, Hypertrophic Type

Clinical Findings

This 65-year-old female real estate broker was referred for evaluation of exertional dyspnea of 1 year's duration. She noted dyspnea without chest pain when walking half a block on the level or climbing less than one flight of stairs. She denied asthma but had smoked cigarettes until 6 years previously. She had been treated 2 decades ago for hyperthyroidism. Workup elsewhere revealed mild airway obstruction, hypertension, and normal thyroid status. Cardiac catheterization showed 40% stenosis of one coronary artery. Echocardiogram was interpreted as normal, and a wall motion study showed a left ventricular ejection fraction of 72%, decreasing slightly during exercise. Medications were clonidine, triamterene, and hydrochlorothiazide. Examination was normal except for systemic hypertension, mild obesity, and a variable systolic murmur at the third left interspace near the sternum. Resting ECG showed left ventricular hypertrophy.

Exercise Findings

The patient performed cycle ergometer exercise on two occasions. During the first study, the murmur was loud, her O_2 pulse decreased as exercise progressed, and she was more hypertensive and became symptomatic with minimal exercise. Two weeks later she returned for the second study (Fig. 10.24.1) shortly after taking clonidine. She had less hypertension and a barely audible systolic murmur.

She pedaled at 60 rpm without added load for 3 minutes. The work rate was then increased 10 W per minute to her symptom-limited maximum. Arterial blood was sampled every second minute, and intraarterial blood pressure was recorded from a percutaneously placed brachial artery catheter. The patient stopped exercise because of overall fatigue and shortness of breath. Less than 1 mm of downsloping ST-segment depression developed in leads I, aVL, and V_6, while an increasing number of atrial and ventricular premature contractions developed near the end of exercise. A recording of brachial artery pressure is shown in Figure 10.24.2.

Interpretation

Comments

The results of the resting respiratory function studies are compatible with mild airflow obstruction

TABLE 10.24.1.   Selected Respiratory Function Data

Measurement	Predicted	Measured
Age, yr		65
Sex		Female
Height, cm		164
Weight, kg	64	69
Hematocrit, %		40
VC, L	2.86	2.78
IC, L	1.91	2.30
TLC, L	4.93	5.45
FEV_1, L	2.26	1.88
FEV_1/VC, %	79	67
MVV, L/min	85	67
D_LCO, ml/mm Hg/min	21.0	19.3

TABLE 10.24.2.   Selected Exercise Data

Measurement	Predicted	First Study	Second Study
Peak $\dot{V}O_2$, L/min	1.28	0.88	1.15
Maximum HR, beats/min	155	142	148
Maximum O_2 pulse, ml/beat	8.3	5.8	7.8
$\Delta\dot{V}O_2/\Delta WR$, ml/min/W	10.3		6.3
AT, L/min	>0.63	Indeterminate	1.0
Blood pressure, mmHg (rest, max)		168/80, 243/102	159/69, 240/79
Maximum $\dot{V}E$, L/min		54	65
Exercise breathing reserve, L/min	>15	13	2
PaO_2, mmHg (rest, max ex)			84, 109
$P(A - a)O_2$, mmHg (rest, max ex)			20, 16
$P(a - ET)CO_2$, mmHg (rest, max ex)			5, 2
VD/VT (rest, heavy ex)			0.35, 0.32
HCO_3, mEq/L (rest, 2-min recov)			26, 22

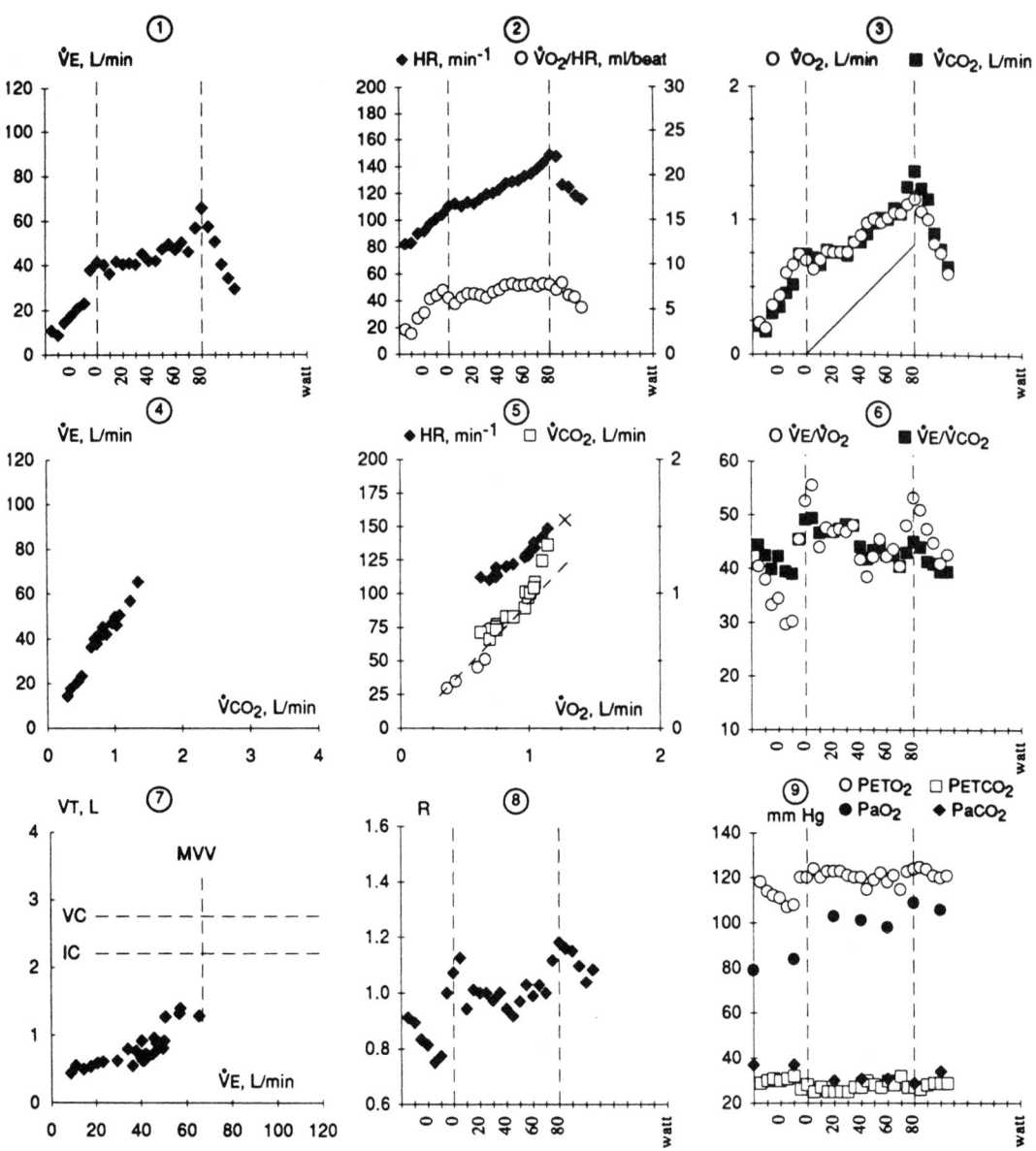

FIGURE 10.24.1.   Second study **1:** Vertical dashed lines in panels 1 to 3 and 6, 8, and 9 indicate the beginning and the end of the increasing work period. **2:** Unloaded cycling is performed for 3 minutes before the left vertical dashed line. **3:** In panel 3, the diagonal line shows the increase of $\dot{V}O_2$ at a slope of 10 ml/min/W. **4:** In panel 5, the diagonal dashed line has a slope of 1; the x in the upper right is the predicted maximum heart rate and $\dot{V}O_2$ for the subject.

Analysis

Referring to flowchart 1, in the first study the peak $\dot{V}O_2$ is reduced and the anaerobic threshold is indeterminate. In the second study, the peak $\dot{V}O_2$ and anaerobic threshold are normal (Table 10.24.2). If we use flowchart 2, because of the abnormal blood gases, we go to the right sides of branch points 2.1

(Table 10.24.1). A resting ECG is normal except for left ventricular hypertrophy. Her left ventricular ejection fraction at rest is 72%.

and 2.3 and arrive at the diagnoses of lung or pulmonary vascular disease. In view of the findings of the anaerobic threshold, we should refer to flowchart 5. Addressing the question of branch point 5.1, VD/VT and $P(a - ET)CO_2$ are mildly abnormal, but $P(A - a)O_2$ is normal (Tables 10.24.2, 10.24.3). Taking the abnormal branch of branch point 5.1, we address the question of the breathing reserve (branch point 5.3). In this patient, it is borderline in the first study and reduced in the second study, primarily because of hyperventilation that she developed during exercise. Because of the normal heart

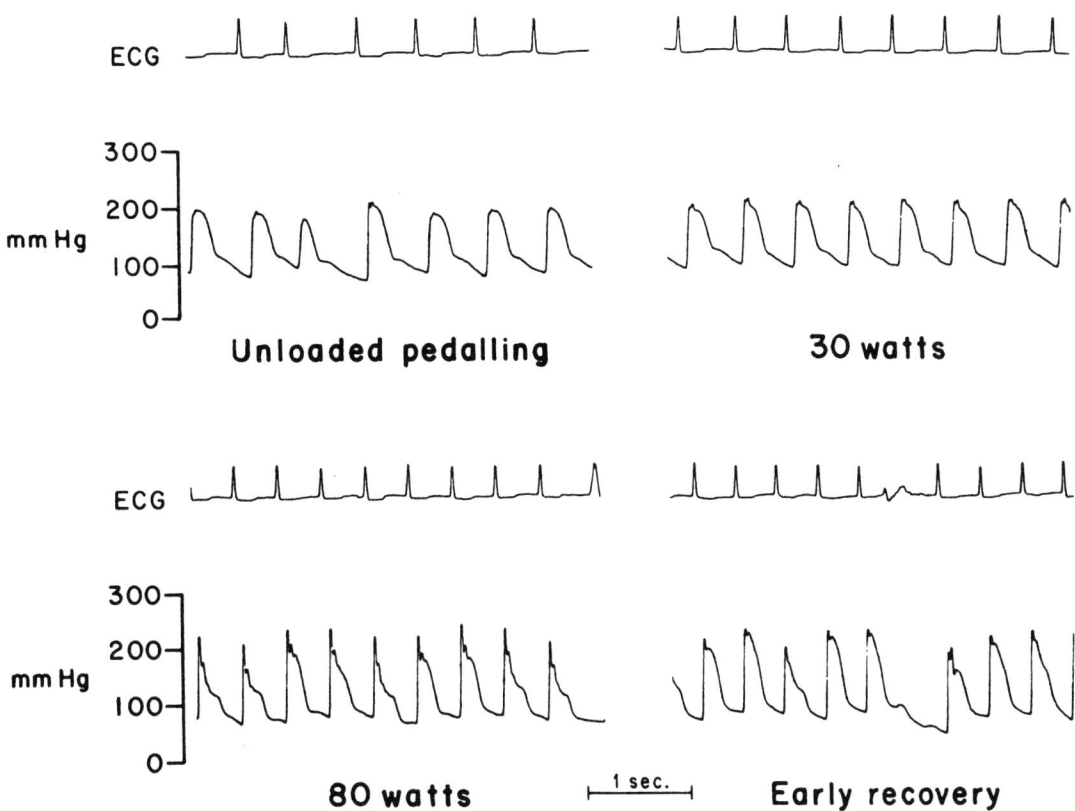

FIGURE 10.24.2.   Four tracings of ECG **(upper)** and brachial artery blood pressure **(lower)** during and immediately after cycle ergometer exercise: **(1)** unloaded pedaling, **(2)** 30 W, **(3)** 80W, and **(4)** early recovery. Each tracing is 4 seconds in duration. Note premature contractions at unloaded pedaling and early recovery and their effect on the contour of the following pulse.

rate reserve and the absence of respiratory acidosis at maximal exercise, we must examine the other side of branch point 5.1.

In this study the prominent disorders are a low $\Delta\dot{V}O_2/\Delta WR$ and a low O_2 pulse that does not increase with increasing work rate (Table 10.24.2 and panel 2 of Fig. 10.24.1). Therefore, it seems more likely that this patient has a cardiovascular defect. Taking the left sides of branch points 5.1, 5.2, and 5.4, we should conclude that the cause of this patient's exercise limitation is myocardial ischemia or a heart disease that prevents the normal increase in cardiac output with work rate increase. Supporting this diagnosis are the observations that the $\dot{V}O_2$ does not rise normally in response to increasing work rate (panel 3, Fig. 10.24.1), the O_2 pulse is flat (panel 2, Fig. 10.24.1), and the heart rate becomes steeper with increasing $\dot{V}O_2$ (panel 5, Fig. 10.24.1). During her more symptomatic test (not shown here), not only was her limitation greater, but her

O_2 pulse actually decreased with increasing work rate.

The directly recorded arterial pressures are unusual and provide a clue to her cardiac diagnosis. The upstrokes in arterial pressure during systole are steep and abruptly stop increasing. Thus, the pressure wave takes on a spike-and-dome pattern. This pattern becomes more prominent with increasing work rate and remains so during early recovery (Fig. 10.24.2), which is characteristic of idiopathic hypertrophic cardiomyopathy. Premature ventricular contractions in recovery were followed by heart beats with a reduced, rather than increased, systolic and pulse pressure, a finding also characteristic of this disorder.

Conclusion

Reduced exercise tolerance secondary to hypertrophic cardiomyopathy.

TABLE 10.24.3. Second Study

Time min	Work rate watts	BP mmHg	HR min⁻¹	f min⁻¹	$\dot{V}_E$ L/min BTPS	$\dot{V}_{CO_2}$ L/min STPD	$\dot{V}_{O_2}$ L/min STPD	$\dot{V}_{O_2}$/HR ml/beat	R	pH	HCO_3^- meq/L	P_{O_2} ET	P_{O_2} a	P_{O_2} (A−a)	P_{CO_2} ET	P_{CO_2} a	P_{CO_2} (a−ET)	$\dot{V}_E/\dot{V}_{CO_2}$	$\dot{V}_E/\dot{V}_{O_2}$	V_D/V_T
	Rest	159/69								7.46	26		79			37				
	Rest		82	20	11.0	0.21	0.23	2.8	0.91			118			29			44	40	
	Rest		83	20	8.9	0.17	0.19	2.3	0.89			114			30			42	38	
	Unloaded		90	29	14.4	0.30	0.36	4.0	0.83			112			31			40	33	
	Unloaded		92	33	17.6	0.35	0.43	4.7	0.81			111			30			42	34	
	Unloaded		97	35	20.7	0.45	0.60	6.2	0.75			107			31			39	30	
	Unloaded	184/75	101	38	23.1	0.51	0.66	6.5	0.77	7.47	26	108	84	20	32	37	5	39	30	0.35
	Unloaded		104	49	37.8	0.74	0.74	7.1	1.00			120			26			45	45	
	Unloaded		110	58	41.2	0.74	0.69	6.3	1.07			120			28			49	53	
0.5	10		112	60	40.1	0.71	0.63	5.6	1.13			124			25			49	56	
1.0	10		110	66	36.3	0.66	0.70	6.4	0.94			120			27			47	44	
1.5	20		113	66	41.7	0.77	0.76	6.7	1.01			123			25			47	47	
2.0	20	201/90	112	63	40.4	0.75	0.75	6.7	1.00	7.52	24	123	103	17	25	30	5	47	47	0.33
2.5	30		115	65	40.9	0.75	0.75	6.5	1.00			123			25			47	47	
3.0	30		119	62	40.4	0.73	0.75	6.3	0.97			121			25			48	47	
3.5	40		120	63	45.1	0.83	0.83	6.9	1.00			120			27			48	48	
4.0	40	193/73	122	64	42.0	0.83	0.88	7.2	0.94	7.51	24	120	101	17	27	31	4	44	42	0.32
4.5	50		127	58	42.1	0.89	0.97	7.6	0.92			115			30			42	38	
5.0	50		128	60	47.1	0.97	1.00	7.8	0.97			119			28			43	42	
5.5	60		129	61	49.7	1.01	0.98	7.6	1.03			122			27			44	45	
6.0	60	220/73	132	53	47.0	1.00	1.01	7.7	0.99	7.49	23	118	98	21	30	31	1	42	42	0.31
6.5	60		134	55	50.4	1.08	1.05	7.8	1.03			121			28			42	44	
7.0	70		138	48	46.0	1.04	1.04	7.5	1.00			115			32			40	40	
7.5	80		142	43	56.8	1.24	1.11	7.8	1.12			123			27			43	48	
8.0	80	240/79	148	51	65.5	1.36	1.15	7.8	1.18	7.49	22	124	109	16	27	29	2	45	53	0.32
	Recovery		147	41	57.4	1.23	1.06	7.2	1.16			125			26			44	51	
	Recovery		126	40	50.8	1.15	1.00	7.9	1.15			124			28			41	47	
	Recovery		124	44	40.4	0.90	0.82	6.6	1.10			121			29			41	45	
	Recovery	261/92	118	43	34.3	0.78	0.75	6.4	1.04	7.42	22	120	106	11	29	34	5	39	41	0.32
	Recovery		115	47	29.5	0.65	0.60	5.2	1.08			121			29			39	43	

Case 25 Chronic Heart Failure: Before and After Therapy

Clinical Findings

This 64-year-old retired man had recurrent episodic shortness of breath for 11 years, initially diagnosed as "asthma," and hypertension. He had recently been hospitalized repeatedly for congestive heart failure without evidence of prior myocardial infarction or valvular heart disease. He had been a cigarette smoker and was being treated with digoxin, furosemide, hydralazine, potassium chloride, prednisone, ranitidine, occasional albuterol, and diazepam. Examination revealed a heavy-set man without peripheral edema or abnormal physical findings on examination of the chest. Chest roentgenograms showed cardiomegaly and Kerley B lines; resting ECG showed left atrial enlargement and probable left ventricular hypertrophy. Exercise studies were performed after stabilization and every several weeks during 3 months of a drug study. The patient had progressive improvement; the first and final exercise tests of this period are presented.

Exercise Findings

On both occasions, the patient performed exercise on a cycle ergometer. He pedaled at 60 rpm without an added load for 3 minutes. The work rate was then increased in a ramp fashion 10 W per minute to tolerance. Blood pressure was measured with a sphygmomanometer. On both occasions, the patient was well motivated and cooperative and stopped exercise because of generalized fatigue. The patient had no chest pain, arrhythmia, or abnormal ST-T wave changes.

Interpretation

Comments

Initial resting respiratory function studies showed respiratory restriction and mild airway obstruction with some response to inhaled albuterol (Table 10.25.1). The resting respiratory function tests were not repeated 3 months later.

Analysis

Referring to flowchart 1 (first study), the patient has a reduced peak $\dot{V}O_2$ and anaerobic threshold (Table 10.25.2 and Fig. 10.25.1), which leads us to flowchart 4. Referring to flowchart 4, the breathing reserve is high (branch point 4.1), and the $\dot{V}E/\dot{V}CO_2$ at the anaerobic threshold is also high (branch point 4.3), suggesting an abnormal pulmonary circulation. Because the vital capacity is low (branch point

TABLE 10.25.1.   Selected Respiratory Function Data

Measurement	Predicted	Measured
Age, yr		64
Sex		Male
Height, cm		170
Weight, kg	73	82
VC, L	3.65	2.70 (2.80*)
IC, L	2.43	1.92
TLC, L	5.95	4.33
FEV$_1$, L	2.92	2.01 (2.30*)
FEV$_1$/VC, %	80	74
MVV, L/min	117	80 (92*)
D$_L$CO, ml/mm Hg/min	23.4	22
Hematocrit		44

*After 4 breaths of aerosolized albuterol.

TABLE 10.25.2.   Selected Exercise Data

Measurement	Predicted	First Study	Final Study
Peak $\dot{V}O_2$, L/min	2.03	0.91	1.34
Maximum HR, beats/min	156	131	160
Maximum O$_2$ pulse, ml/beat	13.0	7.0	9.0
$\Delta\dot{V}O_2$/ΔWR, ml/min/W	10.3	8.0	9.2
AT, L/min	>0.89	0.6	1.0
Blood pressure, mmHg (rest, max ex)		112/95, 139/88	139/88, 204/104
Maximum $\dot{V}E$, L/min		44	55
Exercise breathing reserve, L/min	>15	36	25

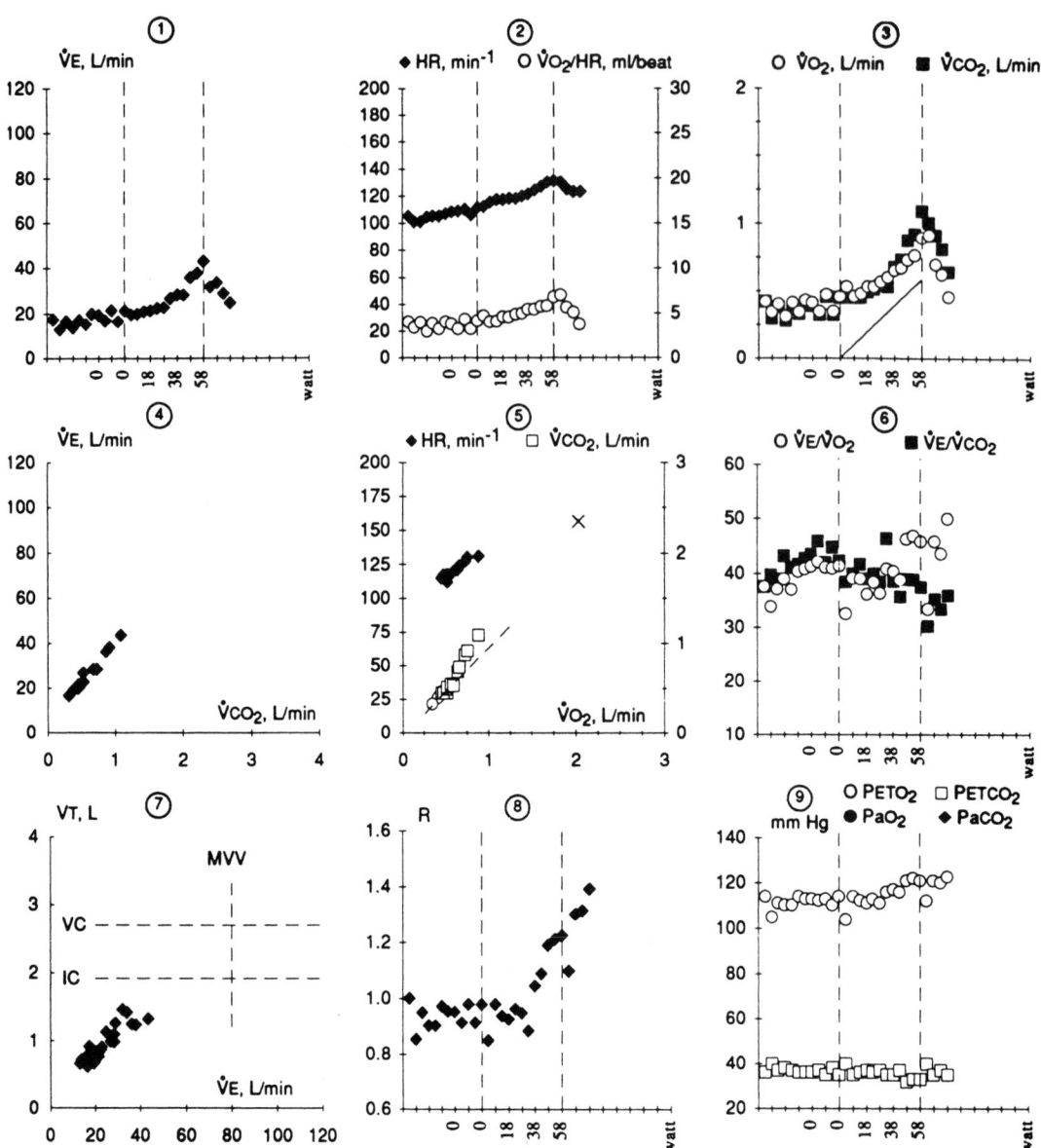

FIGURE 10.25.1.   First study. **1:** Vertical dashed lines in panels 1 to 3 and 6, 8, and 9 indicate the beginning and the end of the increasing work period. **2:** Unloaded cycling is performed for 3 minutes before the left vertical dashed line. **3:** In panel 3, the diagonal line shows the increase of $\dot{V}O_2$ at a slope of 10 ml/min/W. **4:** In panel 5, the diagonal dashed line has a slope of 1; the x in the upper right is the predicted maximum heart rate and $\dot{V}O_2$ for the subject.

4.5), we are directed to consider moderate to severe left ventricular failure. The patient has physiologic features of this problem, including low O_2 pulse and low $\Delta\dot{V}O_2/\Delta$WR. The reduced and slowly increasing O_2 pulse during exercise and the increase when exercise stopped are consistent with left ventricular dysfunction.

Three months after treatment that included afterload reduction, the maximum work rate, peak $\dot{V}O_2$, maximum O_2 pulse, anaerobic threshold, and $\Delta\dot{V}O_2/\Delta$WR findings are considerably improved (Table 10.25.4 and Fig. 10.25.2).

Conclusion

This study is presented to show the findings of severe left ventricular dysfunction, as may be seen with cardiomyopathy of any cause, and the improvement in the functional abnormalities with effective therapy.

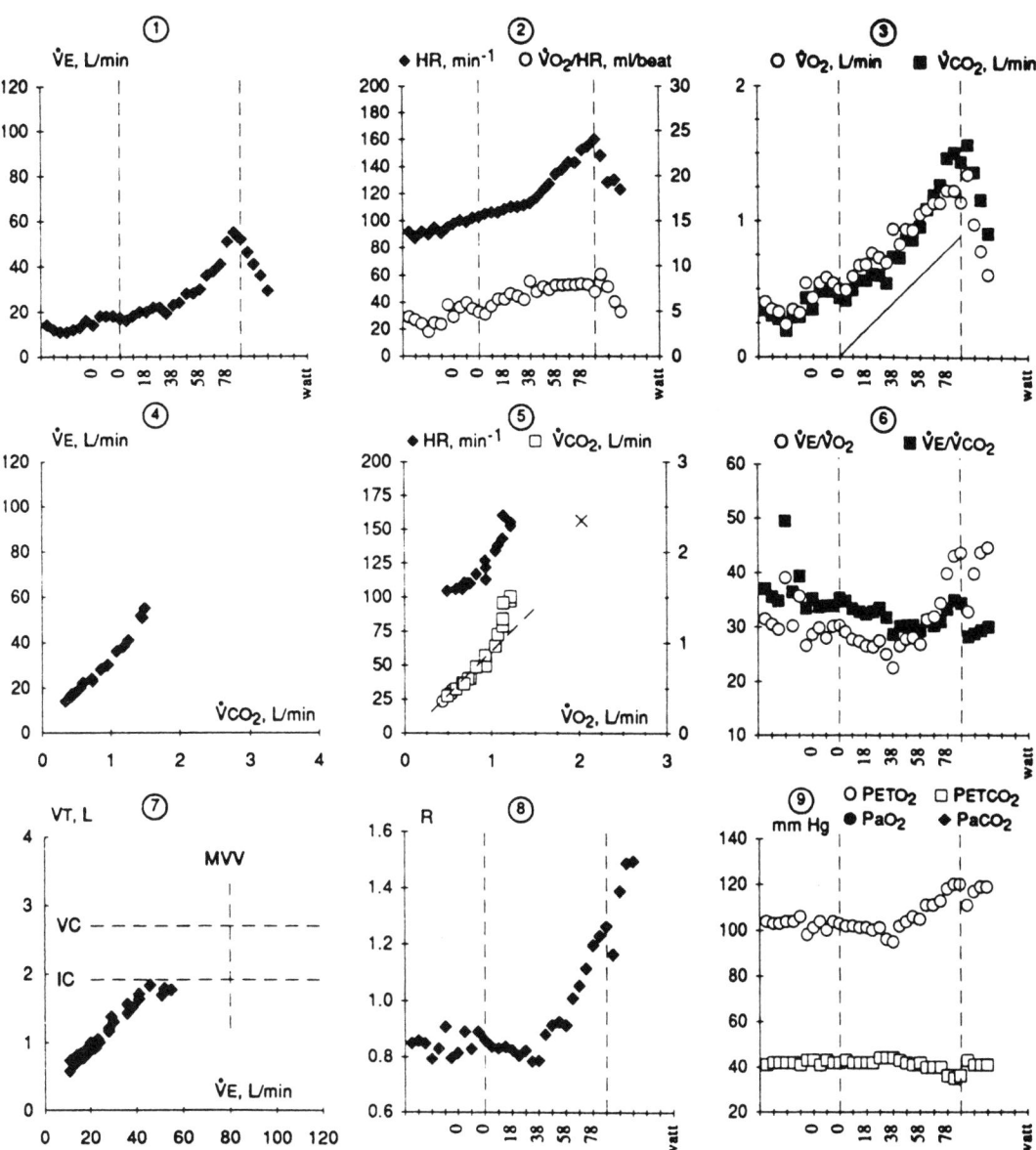

FIGURE 10.25.2.   Final study. **1:** Vertical dashed lines in panels 1 to 3 and 6, 8, and 9 indicate the beginning and the end of the increasing work period. **2:** Unloaded cycling is performed for 3 minutes before the left vertical dashed line. **3:** In panel 3, the diagonal line shows the increase of $\dot{V}_{O_2}$ at a slope of 10 ml /min/W. **4:** In panel 5, the diagonal dashed line has a slope of 1; the x in the upper right is the predicted maximum heart rate and $\dot{V}_{O_2}$ for the subject.

TABLE 10.25.3. First Study

Time min	Work rate watts	BP mmHg	HR min⁻¹	f min⁻¹	$\dot{V}_E$ L/min BTPS	$\dot{V}_{CO_2}$ L/min STPD	$\dot{V}_{O_2}$ L/min STPD	$\dot{V}_{O_2}$/HR ml/beat	R	pH	HCO₃⁻ meq/L	PO₂, mmHg ET	a	(A − a)	PCO₂, mmHg ET	a	(a − ET)	$\dot{V}_E$/$\dot{V}_{CO_2}$	$\dot{V}_E$/$\dot{V}_{O_2}$	VD/VT
	Rest	112/95	105	19	17.4	0.42	0.42	4.0	1.00			114			36			38	38	
	Rest		101	20	13.2	0.29	0.34	3.4	0.85			105			40			40	34	
	Rest		101	21	16.6	0.38	0.40	4.0	0.95			111			37			39	37	
	Rest		104	19	13.7	0.28	0.31	3.0	0.90			110			38			43	39	
	Rest		105	24	17.2	0.37	0.41	3.9	0.90			110			37			41	37	
	Rest		105	22	15.6	0.33	0.34	3.2	0.97			114			36			42	40	
	Unloaded		107	28	19.9	0.41	0.43	4.0	0.95			113			36			43	41	
	Unloaded		108	29	19.4	0.39	0.41	3.8	0.95			113			36			43	41	
	Unloaded		109	26	16.9	0.32	0.35	3.2	0.91			112			37			46	42	
	Unloaded		110	26	21.5	0.46	0.47	4.3	0.98			113			35			42	41	
	Unloaded		106	27	16.6	0.32	0.35	3.3	0.91			110			38			45	41	
	Unloaded		111	28	21.4	0.45	0.46	4.1	0.98			114			35			42	41	
0.5	3		112	29	19.7	0.45	0.53	4.7	0.85			104			40			38	33	
1.0	8		115	24	20.0	0.45	0.46	4.0	0.98			114			35			40	39	
1.5	13		117	28	21.1	0.45	0.48	4.1	0.94			112			36			42	39	
2.0	18		117	25	21.2	0.49	0.53	4.5	0.92			111			37			39	36	
2.5	23		118	26	22.5	0.51	0.53	4.5	0.96			113			36			40	38	
3.0	28		118	25	22.8	0.54	0.57	4.8	0.95			111			37			38	36	
3.5	33		120	27	26.8	0.53	0.60	5.0	0.88			116			35			46	41	
4.0	38		121	26	28.4	0.68	0.65	5.4	1.05			117			35			39	40	
4.5	43		124	29	28.4	0.73	0.67	5.4	1.09			116			37			36	39	
5.0	48		127	29	36.2	0.87	0.73	5.7	1.19			121			32			39	46	
5.5	53		130	31	38.2	0.92	0.76	5.8	1.21			122			33			39	47	
6.0	58	139/88	131	33	43.5	1.09	0.89	6.8	1.22			121			33			37	46	
	Recovery		130	22	32.1	1.00	0.91	7.0	1.10			112			40			30	33	
	Recovery		125	24	34.0	0.91	0.70	5.6	1.30			121			35			35	46	
	Recovery		123	23	29.0	0.81	0.62	5.0	1.31			120			37			33	44	
	Recovery		123	22	24.8	0.64	0.46	3.7	1.39			123			35			36	50	

TABLE 10.25.4. Final Study

Time min	Work rate watts	BP mmHg	HR min⁻¹	f min⁻¹	V̇E L/min BTPS	V̇CO₂ L/min STPD	V̇O₂ L/min STPD	V̇O₂/HR ml/beat	R	pH	HCO₃⁻ meq/L	PO₂, mmHg ET	a	(A−a)	PCO₂, mmHg ET	a	(a−ET)	V̇E/V̇CO₂	V̇E/V̇O₂	VD/VT
	Rest	139/88	92	17	14.0	0.34	0.40	4.3	0.85			104			41			37	31	
	Rest		87	16	12.0	0.30	0.35	4.0	0.86			103			42			35	30	
	Rest		92	15	11.0	0.28	0.33	3.6	0.85			103			42			35	29	
	Rest		90	19	11.0	0.19	0.24	2.7	0.79			104			42			49	39	
	Rest		95	17	12.0	0.29	0.35	3.7	0.83			104			42			36	30	
	Rest		91	19	13.0	0.29	0.32	3.5	0.91			106			41			39	36	
	Unloaded		95	19	16.0	0.43	0.54	5.7	0.80			98			43			33	27	
	Unloaded		98	20	14.0	0.35	0.43	4.4	0.81			101			43			35	29	
	Unloaded		100	22	18.0	0.48	0.54	5.4	0.89			104			41			34	30	
	Unloaded		99	21	18.0	0.48	0.58	5.9	0.83			100			43			34	28	
	Unloaded		102	21	18.0	0.48	0.54	5.3	0.89			104			42			34	30	
	Unloaded		103	22	17.0	0.43	0.50	4.9	0.86			103			42			35	30	
0.5	3		105	21	16.0	0.41	0.49	4.7	0.84			102			43			35	29	
1.0	8		106	20	18.0	0.49	0.59	5.6	0.83			102			42			33	28	
1.5	13		106	20	20.0	0.56	0.67	6.3	0.84			101			42			33	27	
2.0	18		108	23	20.0	0.56	0.68	6.3	0.82			101			42			32	27	
2.5	23		110	24	22.0	0.61	0.76	6.9	0.80			100			42			33	26	
3.0	28		110	23	22.0	0.60	0.73	6.6	0.82			101			44			33	27	
3.5	33		111	22	19.0	0.54	0.69	6.2	0.78			96			44			32	25	
4.0	38		113	22	23.0	0.74	0.94	8.3	0.79			95			44			29	22	
4.5	43		117	24	24.0	0.73	0.83	7.1	0.88			102			43			30	26	
5.0	48		122	24	28.0	0.86	0.94	7.7	0.91			104			42			30	28	
5.5	53		127	23	28.0	0.86	0.93	7.3	0.92			106			41			30	28	
6.0	58		134	23	30.0	0.96	1.05	7.8	0.91			105			42			29	27	
6.5	63		138	25	36.0	1.09	1.08	7.8	1.01			111			40			31	31	
7.0	68		143	25	38.0	1.19	1.13	7.9	1.05			111			40			30	32	
7.5	73		143	25	41.0	1.26	1.13	7.9	1.12			113			40			31	34	
8.0	78		152	30	51.0	1.46	1.22	8.0	1.20			118			36			33	40	
8.5	83		155	31	55.0	1.50	1.22	7.9	1.23			120			35			35	43	
9.0	88	204/104	160	29	52.0	1.44	1.14	7.1	1.26			120			36			34	43	
	Recovery		148	25	46.0	1.56	1.34	9.1	1.16			111			43			28	33	
	Recovery		128	24	41.0	1.36	0.98	7.7	1.39			117			41			29	40	
	Recovery		130	23	36.0	1.16	0.78	6.0	1.49			119			41			29	44	
	Recovery		123	21	29.0	0.91	0.61	5.0	1.49			119			41			30	45	

Case 26 Cardiomyopathy with Oscillatory Function

Clinical Findings

This 57-year-old housewife reported to the clinic because she started to experience shortness of breath, exercise limitation, and easy fatigability starting about 6 months previously. She had two-pillow orthopnea and paroxysmal nocturnal dyspnea. She did not experience chest pain with activity. She had 2+ pitting pretibial edema, but no hepatomegaly or jugular venous distention. An echocardiogram interpretation reported a 15% ejection fraction. She was started on treatment with lisinopril, digoxin, warfarin (Coumadin), atorvastatin (Lipitor), furosemide (Lasix) as needed, and conjugated estrogens (Premarin), and referred to the cardiopulmonary exercise lab for quantification of the severity of her heart failure. At the time of referral, she was symptomatically improved on therapy, and pretibial edema was trace. Chest roentgenograms were normal except for mild left ventricular enlargement. Resting ECG revealed sinus rhythm and left bundle branch block with rare premature ventricular contractions.

Exercise Findings

The patient was studied during exercise on a cycle ergometer (Fig. 10.26.1). After 3 minutes of rest, she pedaled at 60 rpm without added load for 3 minutes. The work rate was then increased in a ramp pattern at 10 W per minute to her symptom-limited maximum. Arm blood pressure was measured with a sphygmomanometer. Arterial oxyhemoglobin saturation was measured with a pulse oximeter on the finger. The patient stopped exercise on her own volition because of leg fatigue. During unloaded cycling, premature ventricular contractions occurred at about one per minute, but did not recur at higher work rates. The ST pattern did not change with exercise. At rest and during early exercise, an oscillatory breathing pattern with a period of about 1 minute was observed (Fig. 10.26.2).

Interpretation

Comments

This patient has an idiopathic cardiomyopathy with symptoms compatible with New York Heart Associ-

ation classes II to III. Respiratory function shows mild airway obstruction and mild reduction in diffusing capacity (Table 10.26.1). An oscillatory pattern in $\dot{V}O_2$, $\dot{V}CO_2$, and $\dot{V}E$ is seen at rest and at exercise intensities below the anaerobic threshold, as found in some patients with left ventricular failure (Fig. 10.26.2).

Analysis

Referring to flowchart 1, the peak $\dot{V}O_2$ and anaerobic threshold are reduced (Table 10.26.2). Go to flowchart 4. The breathing reserve is normal

TABLE 10.26.1.   Selected Respiratory Function Data

Measurement	Predicted	Measured
Age, yr		57
Sex		Female
Height, cm		168
Weight, kg		59.1
Hematocrit, %		38.5
VC, L	3.27	3.17
IC, L	2.18	1.98
ERV, L	1.09	1.19
FEV_1, L	2.64	2.17
FEV_1/VC, %	81	69
MVV, L/min	97	86
D_LCO, ml/mm Hg/min	22.7	17.8

TABLE 10.26.2.   Selected Exercise Data

Measurement	Predicted	Measured
Peak $\dot{V}O_2$, L/min	1.35	0.83
Maximum HR, beats/min	163	134
Maximum O_2 pulse, ml/beat	8.3	6.2
$\Delta\dot{V}O_2/\Delta WR$, ml/min/W	10.3	6.9
AT, L/min	>0.70	0.53
Blood pressure, mmHg (rest, max)		102/66, 120/85
Maximum $\dot{V}E$, L/min		43
Exercise breathing reserve, L/min	>15	43
$\dot{V}E/\dot{V}CO_2$ @AT	<33	39
$PETCO_2$ @AT	>40	33
$\dot{V}E$ vs $\dot{V}CO_2$	<32	38
SaO_2 rest, ex − pulse oximeter (%)	>95	98, 98

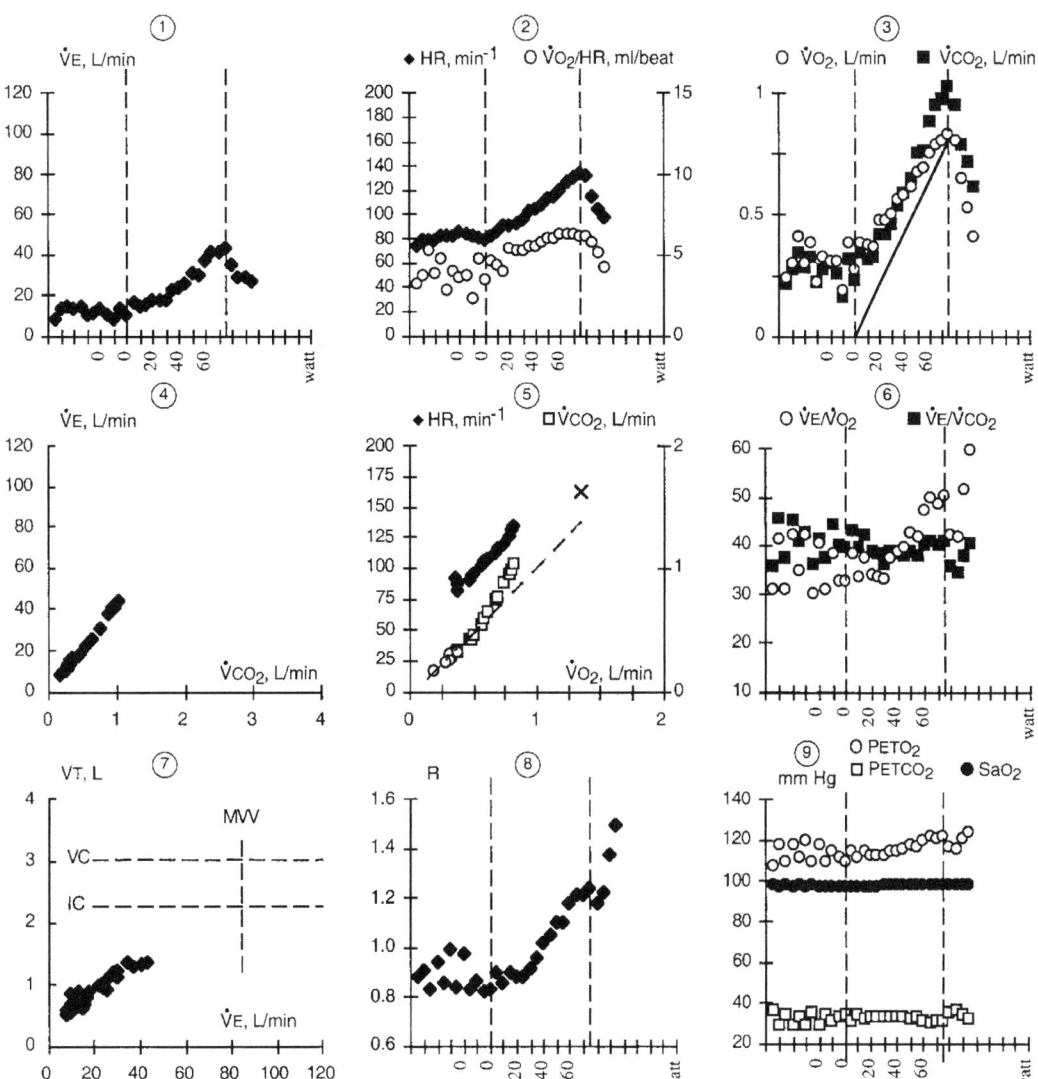

FIGURE 10.26.1. **1:** Vertical dashed lines in panels 1 to 3 and 6, 8, and 9 indicate the beginning and the end of the increasing work period. **2:** Unloaded cycling is performed for 3 minutes before the left vertical dashed line. **3:** In panel 3, the diagonal line shows the increase of $\dot{V}O_2$ at a slope of 10 mL/min/W. **4:** In panel 5, the diagonal dashed line has a slope of 1; the x in the upper right is the predicted maximum heart rate and $\dot{V}O_2$ for the subject.

(branch point 4.1), whereas the ventilatory equivalent for CO_2 at the AT is high (branch point 4.3), probably due to the increased VD/VT (1). The rightward direction takes us to the diagnostic box labeled "abnormal pulmonary circulation" (branch point 4.5). It is now necessary to distinguish between high $\dot{V}A/\dot{Q}$ mismatch due to primary pulmonary vascular disease (left branch) and high $\dot{V}A/\dot{Q}$ mismatch due to relative stasis of pulmonary blood flow caused by left ventricular failure (right branch). At branch point 4.5, the arterial oxyhemoglobin saturation is normal throughout exercise, which is characteristic of the slow pulmonary blood flow (long transit time) of moderate to severe left

ventricular function (right branch) as opposed to the shortened transit time associated with exercise arterial hypoxemia of primary pulmonary vascular disease (left branch).

Because the points in the nine-panel plots are at 30-second intervals, the gas exchange appears to be extra noisy, without pattern. But at the time of testing, using a moving average, a systematic oscillatory pattern in gas exchange is evident, accounting for the noisy gas exchange signals at rest and low levels of exercise seen in the nine-panel graphical display. This oscillatory breathing pattern at rest and low levels of exercise is characteristically found in patients with left ventricular failure, and might

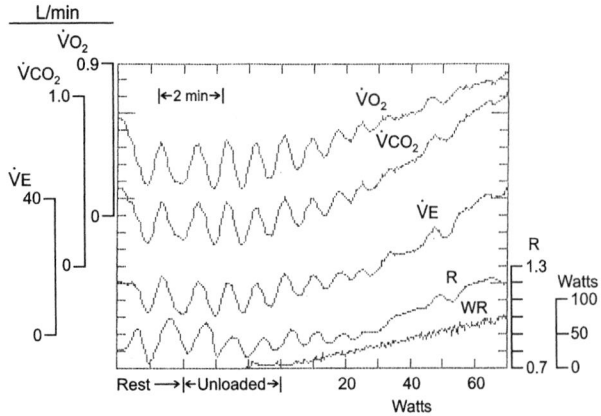

FIGURE 10.26.2. $\dot{V}O_2$, $\dot{V}CO_2$, $\dot{V}E$, R, and work rate (WR), from top to bottom. The oscillations have a period of 1 minute from peak to peak and are greatest at rest and mild to moderate exercise. To obtain an essentially noise-free graph of these variables, which are plotted separated vertically in this figure, the moving interval (MI) type of filtering method is used. For numerical calculation, the breath-by-breath data points are first translated into equal time intervals (0.1 sec) by interpolation. For each data point, the data in the averaging width are fitted by a fifth-order polynomial, and the center point of the MI is given by the center point of the polynomial. This method gives a superior fitting for data with rapid changes of slope. The variables have a wavy shape similar to a sinusoid, and the time delays from $\dot{V}O_2$ are measured by the time between their peaks. The oscillation width for this subject is 1.0 minute, and time delay from $\dot{V}O_2$ is 0.05 minute for $\dot{V}CO_2$, 0.1 minute for $\dot{V}E$, and 0.34 minute for R. The oscillations and time delays of respiratory variables are compatible with oscillatory pulmonary blood flow followed by ventilatory changes. See the analysis in the case section "Interpretation" for further discussion of mechanism.

be an awake form of Cheyne-Stokes respiration. The periodic (oscillatory) gas exchange pattern is analyzed in greater detail in the search for a mechanism (Fig. 10.26.2). The oscillations have a period of 1 minute from peak to peak and are greatest at rest and during mild to moderate exercise.

The $\dot{V}O_2$ is the leading oscillation, followed in the order of time lag by $\dot{V}CO_2$, $\dot{V}E$, and R. To obtain essentially noise-free graphs of these variables, which are plotted separated vertically in Figure 10.26.2, a moving interval (MI) type of filtering method is used.

The mechanism for the oscillation in pulmonary blood flow is thought to be oscillating vasomotor tone that causes blood pressure to increase and decrease with a period of 1 minute, combined with a heart that is failing and functioning on the flat or descending limb of the Frank–Starling curve. The oscillations in arterial pressure are known as Traube–Hering waves and have a period ranging from 0.75 to 1.5 minutes. These oscillating arterial pressures do not affect cardiac output (and therefore pulmonary blood flow) in normal individuals because forward output normally depends on venous return (ascending limb of the Frank–Starling curve). With left ventricular failure, however, the cardiac output is less dependent on cardiac preload (Starling's law of the heart) and more dependent on afterload (systemic arterial pressure). Thus, cardiac output (pulmonary blood flow) and $\dot{V}O_2$ will oscillate as vasomotor tone oscillates in the systemic arterial bed in patients with heart failure. $\dot{V}E$ will oscillate secondary to the pulmonary blood flow oscillation because arterial $PaCO_2$, PaO_2, and H^+ oscillate as a result of transient pulmonary blood flow–alveolar ventilation mismatch.

It is thought that the increased production of catecholamines that occurs with heavy exercise obliterates the changing vasomotor tone stimulus from the central nervous system. This oscillatory gas exchange pattern is characteristic of some patients with more severe forms of left ventricular failure (2).

Conclusion

This patient is presented to illustrate the oscillatory pattern in $\dot{V}O_2$ and other abnormalities that frequently occur in patients with left ventricular failure.

References

1. Wasserman K, Zhang Y-Y, Gitt A, et al. Lung function and exercise gas exchange in chronic heart failure. *Circulation* 1997;96:2221–2227.
2. Ben-Dov I, Sietsema KE, Casaburi R, et al. Evidence that circulatory oscillations accompany ventilatory oscillations during exercise in patients with heart failure. *Am Rev Respir Dis* 1992;145:776–781.

TABLE 10.26.3. Air Breathing

Time min	Work rate watts	BP mmHg	HR min⁻¹	f min⁻¹	$\dot{V}_E$ L/min BTPS	$\dot{V}_{CO_2}$ L/min STPD	$\dot{V}_{O_2}$ L/min STPD	$\frac{\dot{V}_{O_2}}{HR}$ ml/beat	R	pH	HCO_3^- meq/L	P_{O_2}, mmHg ET	a	(A − a)	P_{CO_2}, mmHg ET	a	(a − ET)	$\frac{\dot{V}_E}{\dot{V}_{CO_2}}$	$\frac{\dot{V}_E}{\dot{V}_{O_2}}$	$\frac{V_D}{V_T}$
	Rest		74	14	8.1	0.21	0.24	3.2	0.87			107			36			36	31	
	Rest		79	21	13.2	0.27	0.30	3.7	0.91			118			29			45	41	
	Rest		79	19	13.7	0.34	0.41	5.2	0.83			109			34			38	31	
	Rest	102/66	78	20	13.5	0.28	0.30	3.8	0.94			118			29			45	42	
	Rest		81	20	14.4	0.33	0.38	4.7	0.85			111			33			41	35	
	Rest		81	15	10.2	0.22	0.22	2.8	0.99			120			29			43	42	
	Unloaded		82	15	10.5	0.27	0.32	4.0	0.84			109			35			36	30	
	Unloaded		85	15	13.0	0.30	0.31	3.6	0.97			118			29			41	40	
	Unloaded		83	12	10.0	0.25	0.31	3.7	0.83			109			34			37	31	
	Unloaded		82	16	7.8	0.16	0.18	2.2	0.86			115			31			44	38	
	Unloaded		80	19	13.4	0.31	0.38	4.8	0.82			111			33			40	33	
	Unloaded		79	19	9.9	0.23	0.28	3.5	0.83			109			34			39	33	
0.5	5		82	24	15.8	0.34	0.38	4.6	0.90			115			31			43	38	
1.0	10		86	21	13.6	0.32	0.38	4.4	0.85			111			34			39	33	
1.5	15		91	25	14.9	0.33	0.36	4.0	0.89			115			32			42	38	
2.0	20		90	22	17.3	0.42	0.48	5.3	0.88			112			33			39	34	
2.5	25		93	21	17.2	0.42	0.48	5.2	0.88			112			33			38	34	
3.0	30		95	20	17.6	0.46	0.50	5.3	0.91			112			33			36	33	
3.5	35		102	23	22.2	0.54	0.57	5.5	0.96			114			33			39	37	
4.0	40		105	25	23.6	0.59	0.58	5.5	1.02			115			33			38	39	
4.5	45		107	24	25.6	0.65	0.62	5.8	1.05			116			33			38	40	
5.0	50		112	25	30.2	0.75	0.68	6.1	1.10			118			32			39	43	
5.5	55		115	27	30.0	0.76	0.69	6.0	1.10			117			33			38	41	
6.0	60		119	29	37.0	0.89	0.75	6.3	1.18			120			31			40	47	
6.5	65		126	31	40.5	0.95	0.79	6.2	1.21			122			30			41	50	
7.0	70	120/85	130	31	40.7	0.98	0.81	6.2	1.21			121			31			40	48	
7.5	75		134	32	43.4	1.03	0.83	6.2	1.24			122			31			41	50	
	Recovery		131	26	35.1	0.95	0.80	6.1	1.18			117			35			36	42	
	Recovery		114	24	28.2	0.79	0.65	5.7	1.22			116			36			34	42	
	Recovery		104	25	28.4	0.72	0.53	5.1	1.37			121			34			38	52	
	Recovery	127/75	97	29	26.1	0.61	0.41	4.2	1.49			124			32			40	60	

Case 27 Mitral Insufficiency

Clinical Findings

This 43-year-old female electronics assembler had rheumatic fever at age 10. In the last 6 months she developed increasing dyspnea and orthopnea, with intermittent atrial fibrillation and pleural effusion, requiring repeated hospitalizations. There was no evidence of mitral stenosis or coronary artery disease on catheterization, angiography, or echocardiography. At the time of exercise study, she had a sinus rhythm, findings of mitral regurgitation with left atrial and left ventricular enlargement, but no pleural effusion or dependent edema. Her medications were digoxin, furosemide, and potassium chloride.

Exercise Findings

The patient performed exercise on a cycle ergometer. She pedaled at 60 rpm without added load for 3 minutes. The work rate was then increased 5 W per minute to her symptom-limited maximum. She stopped cycling because of general fatigue. There were no ST-segment changes or arrhythmia.

Interpretation

Comments

Respiratory function at rest is compatible with a restrictive defect, but the diffusing capacity ($D_{L}CO$) is normal (Table 10.27.1).

Analysis

Referring to flowchart 1, the peak $\dot{V}O_2$ and anaerobic threshold are low (Table 10.27.2). See flowchart 4. The breathing reserve is high (branch point 4.1). The ventilatory equivalent for CO_2 is slightly elevated at the anaerobic threshold (branch point 4.3). Therefore, we are led to consider an abnormal pulmonary circulation. The vital capacity is reduced (branch point 4.5), leading us to the diagnosis of left ventricular failure, undoubtedly due to the valvular heart disease. The striking findings are the low and flat O_2 pulse throughout exercise (panel 2, Fig. 10.27.1) and steep heart rate–$\dot{V}O_2$ relationship (panel 5, Fig. 10.27.1), low heart rate reserve,

and low $\Delta\dot{V}O_2/\Delta WR$, all findings confirming the diagnosis of heart disease. The low and unchanging O_2 pulse suggests that the patient's effective stroke volume is very low and the arterial–mixed venous O_2 difference is maximized at a low work rate. Note that if the $\dot{V}E/\dot{V}CO_2$ at the AT were normal (branch point 4.3), we would have been led to the same diagnosis of heart disease through branch point 4.6. The difference reflects on the extent to which the pulmonary circulation has been affected by the left-sided heart failure.

Conclusion

Valvular heart disease, as suggested by the patient's history, has caused marked exercise intolerance because of an inadequate cardiac output response to exercise (heart failure).

TABLE 10.27.1.   Selected Respiratory Function Data

Measurement	Predicted	Measured
Age, yr		43
Sex		Female
Height, cm		160
Weight, kg	61	56
Hematocrit, %		40
VC, L	2.88	2.03
IC, L	1.92	1.49
TLC, L	4.33	3.32
FEV_1, L	2.36	1.81
FEV_1/VC, %	82	89
MVV, L/min	90	90
$D_{L}CO$, ml/mm Hg/min	21.7	23.5

TABLE 10.27.2.   Selected Exercise Data

Measurement	Predicted	Measured
Peak $\dot{V}O_2$, L/min	1.57	0.79
Maximum HR, beats/min	177	186
Maximum O_2 pulse, ml/beat	8.9	4.2
$\Delta\dot{V}O_2/\Delta WR$, ml/min/W	10.3	5.6
AT, L/min	>0.74	0.65
Maximum $\dot{V}E$, L/min		31
Exercise breathing reserve, L/min	>15	59

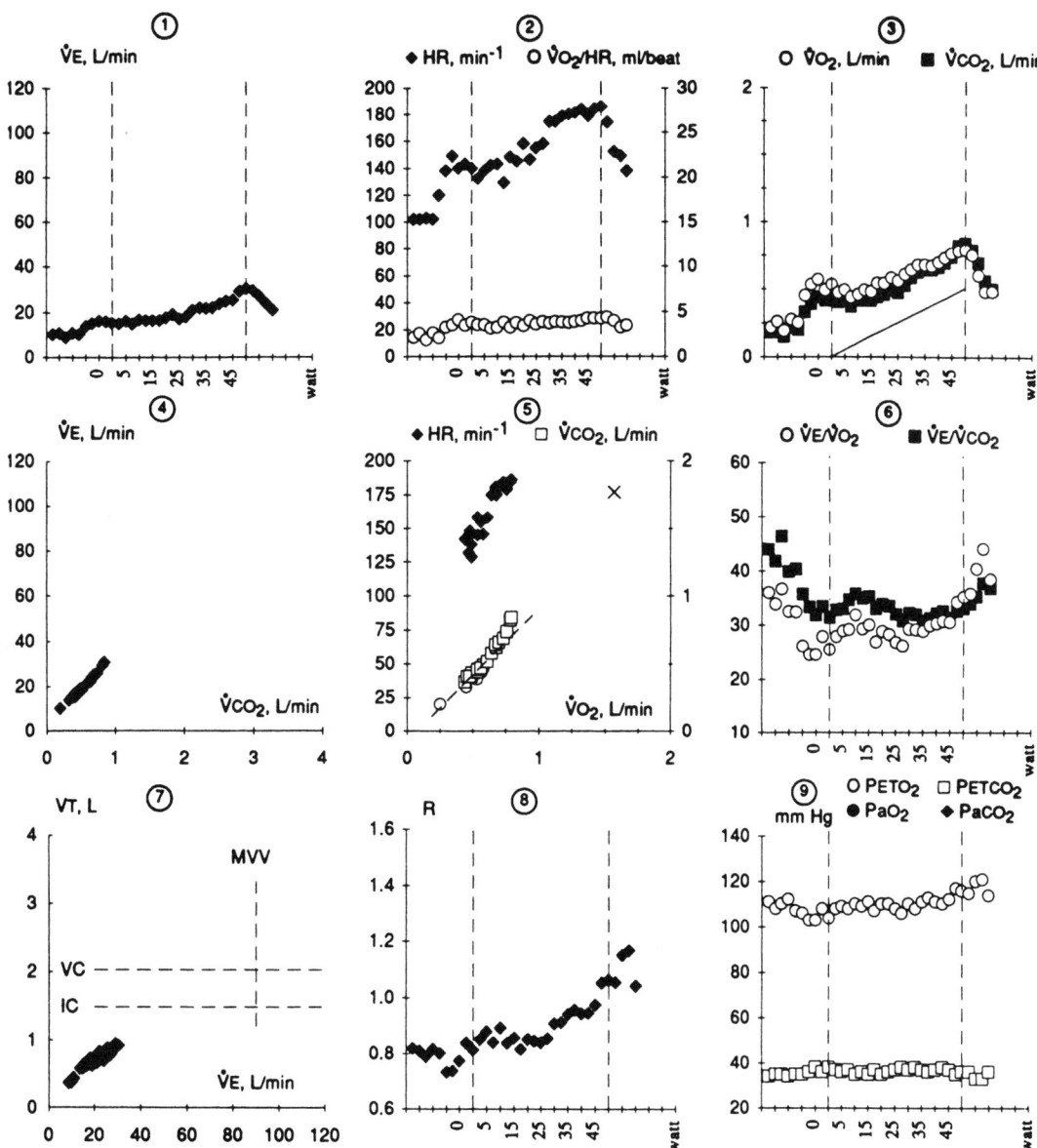

FIGURE 10.27.1.   **1:** Vertical dashed lines in panels 1 to 3 and 6, 8, and 9 indicate the beginning and the end of the increasing work period. **2:** Unloaded cycling is performed for 3 minutes before the left vertical dashed line. **3:** In panel 3, the diagonal line shows the increase of $\dot{V}O_2$ at a slope of 10 ml/min/W. **4:** In panel 5, the diagonal dashed line has a slope of 1; the *x* in the upper right is the predicted maximum heart rate and $\dot{V}O_2$ for the subject.

TABLE 10.27.3. Air Breathing

Time min	Work rate watts	BP mmHg	HR min⁻¹	f min⁻¹	$\dot{V}_E$ L/min BTPS	$\dot{V}_{CO_2}$ L/min STPD	$\dot{V}_{O_2}$ L/min STPD	$\dfrac{\dot{V}_{O_2}}{HR}$ ml/beat	R	pH	HCO₃⁻ meq/L	Po₂, mmHg ET	a	(A − a)	Pco₂, mmHg ET	a	(a − ET)	$\dfrac{\dot{V}_E}{\dot{V}_{CO_2}}$	$\dfrac{\dot{V}_E}{\dot{V}_{O_2}}$	VD VT
	Rest		102	27	10.2	0.18	0.22	2.2	0.82			111			34			44	36	
	Rest		102	26	11.0	0.21	0.26	2.5	0.81			108			35			42	34	
	Rest		103	24	9.0	0.15	0.19	1.8	0.79			110			35			46	37	
	Rest		102	25	10.9	0.22	0.27	2.6	0.81			112			34			40	33	
	Unloaded		120	25	10.2	0.20	0.25	2.1	0.80			107			35			40	32	
	Unloaded		138	24	13.8	0.33	0.45	3.3	0.73			106			35			36	26	
	Unloaded		149	25	15.1	0.39	0.53	3.6	0.74			103			36			33	24	
	Unloaded		140	26	16.2	0.44	0.57	4.1	0.77			103			38			32	25	
	Unloaded		143	26	15.9	0.41	0.49	3.4	0.84			108			36			33	28	
	Unloaded		140	24	15.5	0.43	0.53	3.8	0.81			104			38			31	25	
0.5	5		132	25	15.2	0.40	0.47	3.6	0.85			108			37			33	28	
1.0	5		138	26	16.4	0.43	0.49	3.6	0.88			109			36			33	29	
1.5	10		142	26	15.0	0.37	0.44	3.1	0.84			108			37			35	29	
2.0	10		143	27	16.9	0.41	0.46	3.2	0.89			110			35			36	32	
2.5	15		129	27	16.6	0.41	0.49	3.8	0.84			109			36			35	29	
3.0	15		148	26	16.6	0.41	0.48	3.2	0.85			111			35			35	30	
3.5	20		145	26	16.7	0.44	0.54	3.7	0.81			107			37			33	27	
4.0	20		158	27	17.8	0.46	0.54	3.4	0.85			110			35			34	29	
4.5	25		146	31	19.0	0.49	0.58	4.0	0.84			110			36			33	28	
5.0	25		155	25	17.1	0.47	0.56	3.6	0.84			108			37			32	27	
5.5	30		158	25	18.1	0.52	0.61	3.9	0.85			106			38			31	26	
6.0	30		175	28	21.0	0.58	0.64	3.7	0.91			110			37			32	29	
6.5	35		175	29	22.2	0.62	0.68	3.9	0.91			108			38			32	29	
7.0	35		179	27	21.9	0.64	0.68	3.8	0.94			111			37			31	29	
7.5	40		180	28	22.3	0.64	0.67	3.7	0.96			113			36			31	30	
8.0	40		181	30	23.7	0.66	0.70	3.9	0.94			111			37			32	30	
8.5	45		184	30	24.9	0.69	0.73	4.0	0.95			110			38			32	31	
9.0	45		179	29	25.6	0.74	0.76	4.2	0.97			112			37			31	30	
9.5	50		184	31	29.2	0.82	0.78	4.2	1.05			117			35			32	34	
10.0	50		186	33	30.5	0.84	0.79	4.2	1.06			116			36			33	35	
	Recovery		174	33	29.6	0.79	0.75	4.3	1.05			115			36			34	36	
	Recovery		152	35	27.2	0.69	0.60	3.9	1.15			120			33			35	40	
	Recovery		149	35	24.1	0.56	0.48	3.2	1.17			121			33			38	44	
	Recovery		138	32	21.1	0.50	0.48	3.5	1.04			114			36			37	38	

Case 28 Mitral Stenosis: Before and After β-Adrenergic Blockade

Clinical Findings

This 57-year-old former receptionist had had rheumatic fever at age 16. She had had orthopnea during pregnancy at age 24. She was otherwise well except for gradually increasing dyspnea of 6 years' duration and exertional dull substernal aching radiating to the jaw and left arm of 3 months' duration. Examination revealed a grade 2 presystolic murmur and an opening snap. The mitral valve area was mildly decreased and the left atrium was moderately dilated. Coronary arteriography was normal. The second exercise study was performed 17 months after the first while the patient was receiving propranolol three times daily. At that time she complained of increasing dyspnea, even at rest, associated with lightheadedness, sweating, numbness of the fingers, and perioral tingling.

Exercise Findings

On both occasions the patient exercised on a cycle ergometer to her symptom-limited maximum. She pedaled at 60 rpm without added load for 3 minutes. During the first test the work rate was increased 10 W per minute; during the second test (17 months later), it was increased 5 W per minute. Arterial blood was sampled every second minute, and intraarterial blood pressure was recorded from a percutaneously placed brachial artery catheter. Resting ECGs showed left atrial enlargement and

sinus rhythm; there were no abnormal ST-segment changes, nor arrhythmia during exercise. She stopped exercise in both studies complaining of leg fatigue, not dyspnea or chest pain.

Interpretation

Comments

Resting pulmonary function is normal on both occasions of study (Table 10.28.1). The ECG is normal except for evidence of left atrial enlargement. This case is presented because it illustrates the abnormalities of mitral stenosis and changes in O_2 pulse with propranolol. Moreover, it is presented because the development of respiratory alkalosis during exercise is unusual.

TABLE 10.28.1.   Selected Respiratory Function Data

Measurement	Predicted	Before Blockade	After Blockade
Age, yr		57	59
Sex		Female	
Height, cm		166	
Weight, kg	65	67	
Hematocrit, %		40	
Vc, L	3.10	3.16	2.73
IC, L	2.07	2.26	2.19
TLC, L	5.15	5.01	4.62
FEV$_1$, L	2.48	2.58	2.26
FEV$_1$/Vc, %	80	82	83
MVV, L/min	93	96	81
D$_L$CO, ml/mmHg/min	21.9	20.3	18.7

TABLE 10.28.2.   Selected Exercise Data

Measurement	Predicted	Before Blockade	After Blockade
Peak V̇O$_2$, L/min	1.42	0.74	0.91
Maximum HR, beats/min	162	120	108
Maximum O$_2$ pulse, ml/beat	8.7	6.2	8.4
ΔV̇O$_2$/ΔWR, ml/min/W	10.3	Indeterminate	7.4
AT, L/min	>0.70	Indeterminate	Indeterminate
Blood pressure, mmHg (rest, max)		128/62, 164/83	153/72, 168/78
Maximum V̇E, L/min		43	47
Exercise breathing reserve, L/min	>15	53	34
PaO$_2$, mmHg (rest, max ex)		97, 125	87, 122
P(A − a)O$_2$, mmHg (rest, max ex)		10, 2	11, 5
P(a − ET)CO$_2$, mmHg (rest, max ex)		0, −1	3, −1
VD/VT (rest, heavy ex)		0.26, 0.25	0.28, 0.19
HCO$_3^-$, mEq/L (rest, 2-min recov)		24, 18	24, 18

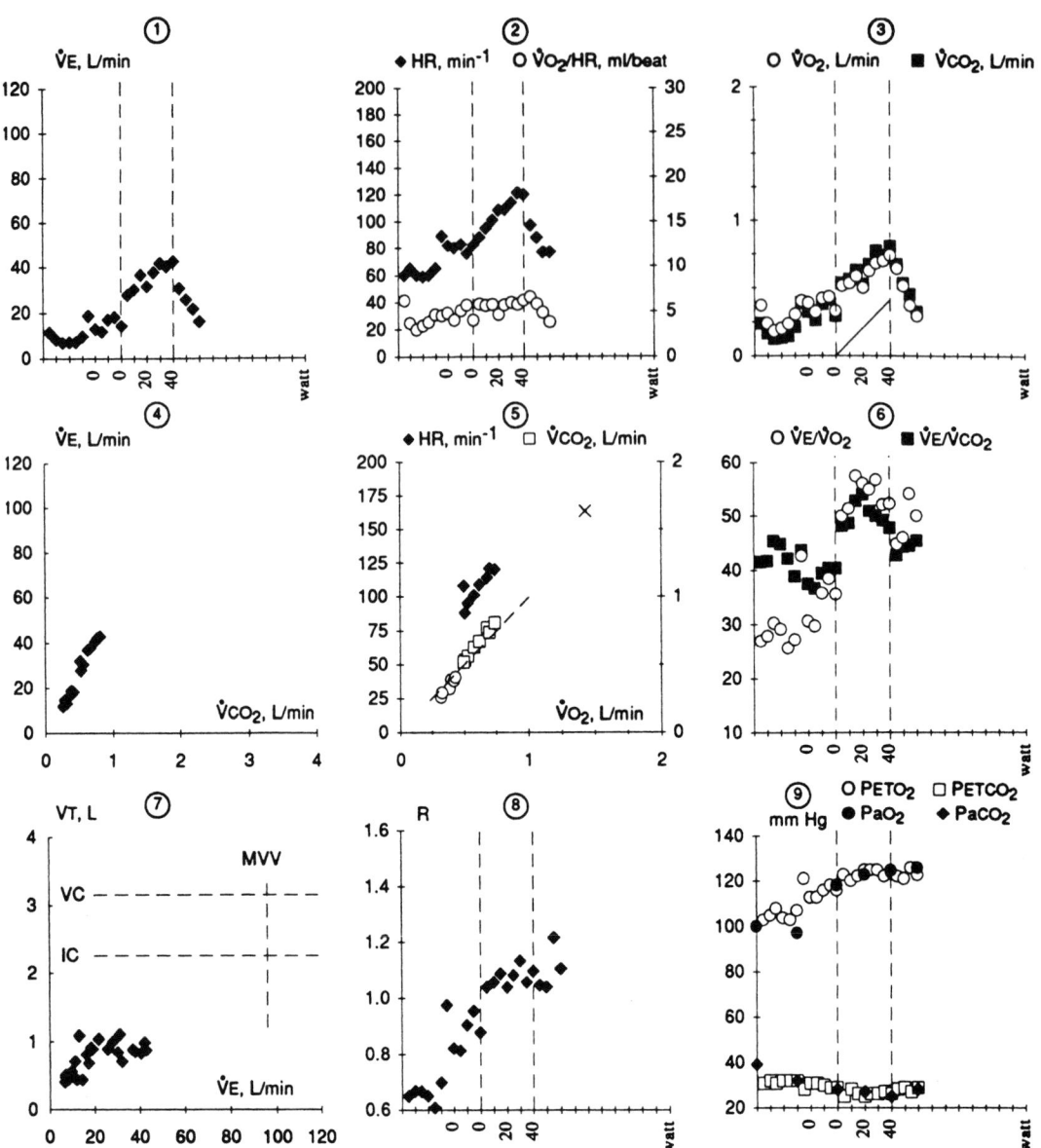

FIGURE 10.28.1.   Before β-adrenergic blockade. **1:** Vertical dashed lines in panels 1 to 3 and 6, 8, and 9 indicate the beginning and the end of the increasing work period. **2:** Unloaded cycling is performed for 3 minutes before the left vertical dashed line. **3:** In panel 3, the diagonal line shows the increase of $\dot{V}_{O_2}$ at a slope of 10 ml/min/W. **4:** In panel 5, the diagonal dashed line has a slope of 1; the x in the upper right is the predicted maximum heart rate and $\dot{V}_{O_2}$ for the subject.

Analysis

During exercise, the peak $\dot{V}_{O_2}$ is decreased and the anaerobic threshold is indeterminate (Table 10. 28.2). See flowchart 5. The indices of distribution of ventilation relative to perfusion are normal at maximum exercise, making lung disease and pulmonary vascular disease unlikely diagnoses (branch point 5.1). The heart rate reserve was high before β-adrenergic blockade, leading us to branch point 5.5. We only had enough data to calculate $\Delta\dot{V}_{O_2}/\Delta WR$

after β-adrenergic blockade; it was low, taking us to branch point 5.8. The arterial pressure response to exercise was not high, leading us to the diagnosis of left ventricular failure. Consistent with heart disease as the primary diagnosis is the low O_2 pulse that fails to rise as the work rate increases.

Commonly, an anticipatory respiratory alkalosis occurs at rest, but disappears with the start of exercise. Respiratory alkalosis in response to exercise, as observed in this patient on both study occasions, is unusual and probably abnormal.

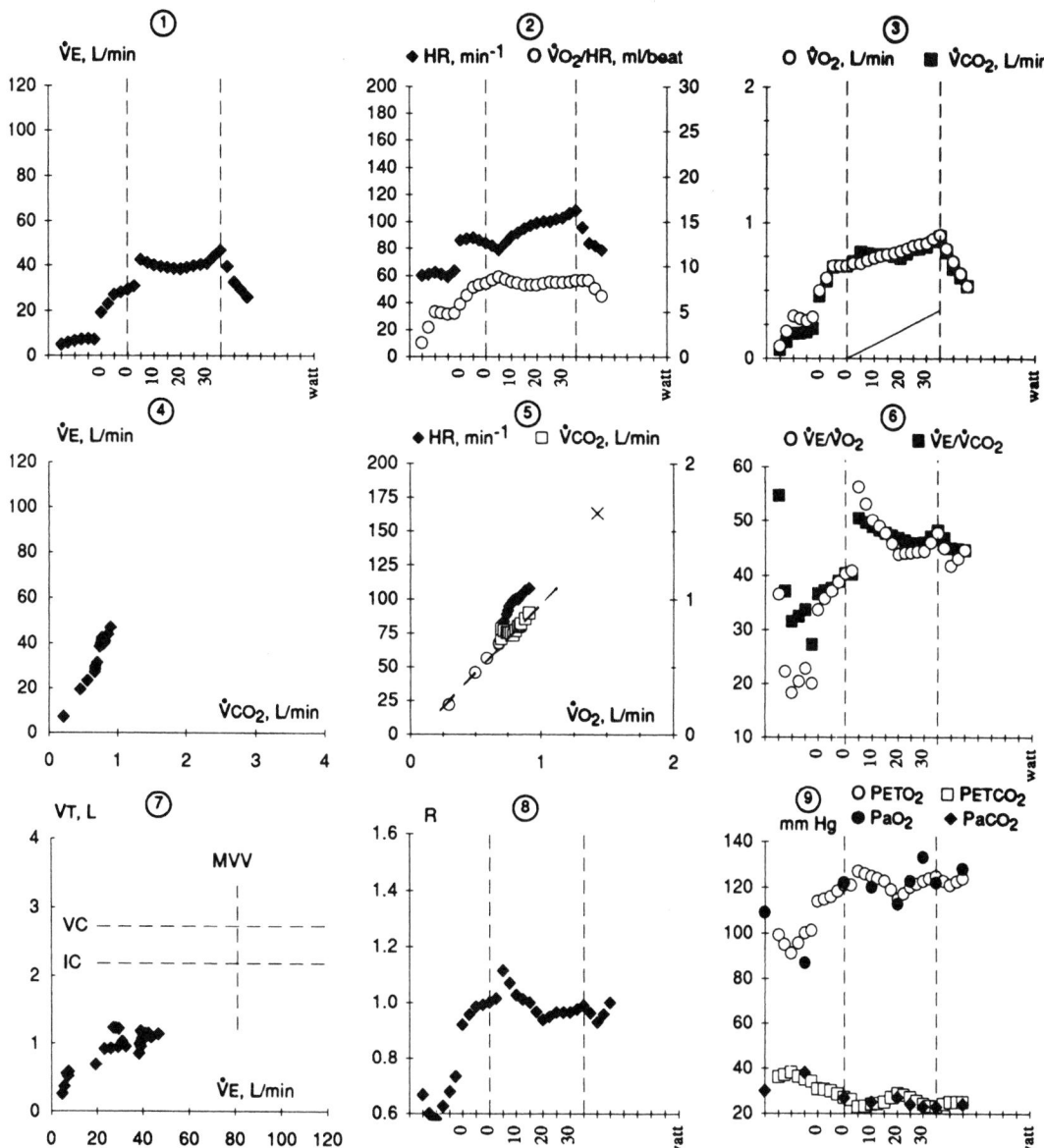

FIGURE 10.28.2.   After β-adrenergic blockade. **1:** Vertical dashed lines in panels 1 to 3 and 6, 8, and 9 indicate the beginning and the end of the increasing work period. **2:** Unloaded cycling is performed for 3 minutes before the left vertical dashed line. **3:** In panel 3, the diagonal line shows the increase of $\dot{V}_{O_2}$ at a slope of 10 ml/min/W. **4:** In panel 5, the diagonal dashed line has a slope of 1; the *x* in the upper right is the predicted maximum heart rate and $\dot{V}_{O_2}$ for the subject.

In the postpropranolol study (Fig. 10.28.2), after an initial elevation, $\dot{V}_E$ remains relatively unchanged (panel 1, Fig. 10.28.2) while R remains high (panel 8, Fig. 10.28.2) and Pa_{CO_2} falls further as work rate is increased (panel 9, Fig. 10.28.2 and Table 10.28.4). The further hyperventilation of the arterial blood (decrease in Pa_{CO_2}) without an increase in $\dot{V}_E$ probably results from an inordinately small pulmonary blood flow increase in response to increasing work rate. This also accounts for the

shallow $\dot{V}_{O_2}$ response as work rate is increased (panel 3, Fig. 10.28.2) and the low, flat O_2 pulse response (panel 2, Fig. 10.28.2).

Conclusion

Response to exercise reflecting left-sided heart failure due to mitral stenosis, with and without β-adrenergic blockade. A rare occurrence of exercise-induced respiratory alkalosis is presented.

TABLE 10.28.3. Pre-β-adrenergic Blockade

Time min	Work rate watts	BP mmHg	HR min⁻¹	f min⁻¹	$\dot{V}_E$ L/min BTPS	$\dot{V}_{CO_2}$ L/min STPD	$\dot{V}_{O_2}$ L/min STPD	$\dot{V}_{O_2}$/HR ml/beat	R	pH	HCO_3^- meq/L	P_{O_2} ET	a	(A−a)	P_{CO_2} ET	a	(a−ET)	$\dot{V}_E/\dot{V}_{CO_2}$	$\dot{V}_E/\dot{V}_{O_2}$	V_D/V_T
	Rest	128/62								7.40	24		100			39				
	Rest		60	16	11.3	0.24	0.37	6.2	0.65			103			31			41	27	
	Rest		65	18	8.2	0.16	0.24	3.7	0.67			105			32			42	28	
	Rest		60	17	6.9	0.12	0.18	3.0	0.67			108			31			45	30	
	Rest		59	15	7.1	0.13	0.20	3.4	0.65			104			32			45	29	
	Rest		60	14	7.1	0.14	0.23	3.8	0.61			103			32			42	26	
	Rest	140/77	65	17	9.6	0.21	0.30	4.6	0.70	7.43	21	107	97	10	32	32	0	39	27	0.26
	Unloaded		89	21	18.8	0.39	0.40	4.5	0.98			121			28			44	43	
	Unloaded		82	12	13.0	0.32	0.39	4.8	0.82			113			31			37	31	
	Unloaded		80	27	11.8	0.26	0.32	4.0	0.81			113			31			37	30	
	Unloaded		83	25	17.1	0.38	0.42	5.1	0.90			116			30			39	36	
	Unloaded		76	20	18.2	0.41	0.43	5.7	0.95			118			29			40	38	
	Unloaded	146/80	82	33	14.5	0.29	0.33	4.0	0.88	7.47	20	116	118	1	29	28	−1	40	35	0.19
0.5	10		88	28	27.9	0.53	0.51	5.8	1.04			123			25			48	50	
1.0	10		95	36	30.3	0.56	0.53	5.6	1.06			120			28			49	51	
1.5	20		101	42	36.9	0.63	0.58	5.7	1.09			122			26			53	57	
2.0	20	152/80	108	45	31.9	0.52	0.50	4.6	1.04	7.50	21	125	123	1	25	27	2	54	56	0.36
2.5	30		109	44	37.8	0.67	0.62	5.7	1.08			125			26			51	55	
3.0	30		114	43	42.2	0.77	0.68	6.0	1.13			125			26			50	57	
3.5	40		121	49	40.6	0.74	0.70	5.8	1.06			122			27			49	52	
4.0	40	164/83	120	49	42.9	0.81	0.74	6.2	1.09	7.49	19	124	125	2	26	25	−1	48	52	0.25
	Recovery		97	28	31.0	0.67	0.64	6.6	1.05			122			28			43	45	
	Recovery		88	29	25.9	0.53	0.51	5.8	1.04			121			29			44	46	
	Recovery		77	21	21.8	0.45	0.37	4.8	1.22			126			27			44	54	
	Recovery	149/71	77	20	16.2	0.32	0.29	3.8	1.10	7.42	18	123	126	−2	29	28	−1	45	50	0.29

TABLE 10.28.4. Post-β-adrenergic Blockade

Time min	Work rate watts	BP mmHg	HR min⁻¹	f min⁻¹	$\dot{V}_E$ L/min BTPS	$\dot{V}_{CO_2}$ L/min STPD	$\dot{V}_{O_2}$ L/min STPD	$\dot{V}_{O_2}$/HR ml/beat	R	pH	HCO_3^- meq/L	P_{O_2} ET	a	(A−a)	P_{CO_2} ET	a	(a−ET)	$\dot{V}_E/\dot{V}_{CO_2}$	$\dot{V}_E/\dot{V}_{O_2}$	V_D/V_T
	Rest	153/72								7.48	22		109			30				
	Rest																			
	Rest		60	19	4.9	0.06	0.09	1.5	0.67			99			36			55	37	
	Rest		61	16	5.8	0.12	0.20	3.3	0.60			95			37			37	22	
	Rest		62	12	6.7	0.18	0.31	5.0	0.58			91			38			32	18	
	Rest		61	13	7.1	0.19	0.30	4.8	0.63			96			37			32	20	
	Rest	159/72	59	13	7.5	0.19	0.28	4.7	0.68	7.41	24	100	87	11	35	38	3	34	23	0.28
	Unloaded		63	14	7.2	0.22	0.30	4.8	0.73			101			34			27	20	
	Unloaded		86	28	19.2	0.46	0.50	5.8	0.92			114			31			37	34	
	Unloaded		87	25	23.2	0.57	0.59	6.8	0.96			115			31			37	36	
	Unloaded		88	22	27.1	0.67	0.68	7.7	0.99			116			30			38	37	
	Unloaded		86	23	28.3	0.68	0.68	7.9	0.99			119			29			39	39	
	Unloaded	162/78	84	24	29.4	0.68	0.68	8.1	1.00	7.50	21	121	122	1	27	27	0	40	40	0.19
0.5	5		82	30	31.1	0.71	0.70	8.5	1.01			121			26			40	41	
1.0	5		79	37	42.5	0.78	0.70	8.9	1.11			127			23			50	56	
1.5	10		84	36	41.3	0.77	0.72	8.6	1.07			126			24			50	53	
2.0	10	168/78	89	35	40.1	0.76	0.74	8.3	1.03	7.52	20	125	120	6	24	25	1	49	50	0.27
2.5	15		92	34	39.6	0.76	0.75	8.2	1.01			124			25			48	49	
3.0	15		95	33	39.1	0.76	0.76	8.0	1.00			123			25			48	48	
3.5	20		97	39	38.8	0.75	0.78	8.0	0.97			119			27			47	46	
4.0	20	171/81	99	45	38.4	0.74	0.79	8.0	0.94	7.49	20	115	113	9	29	27	−2	47	44	0.28
4.5	25		100	41	39.1	0.77	0.81	8.1	0.95			118			28			46	44	
5.0	25	168/78	100	37	39.8	0.80	0.83	8.3	0.96	7.51	19	120	123	2	27	24	−3	46	44	0.20
5.5	30		102	38	40.4	0.81	0.84	8.2	0.96			122			26			46	44	
6.0	30	168/78	103	38	40.9	0.82	0.85	8.3	0.96	7.51	18	123	133	−7	24	23	−1	46	44	0.17
6.5	35		106	40	43.9	0.86	0.88	8.3	0.98			124			24			47	46	
7.0	35	168/78	108	41	46.8	0.90	0.91	8.4	0.99	7.50	18	125	122	5	23	23	0	48	48	0.20
	Recovery		96	38	39.7	0.78	0.81	8.4	0.96			123			24			47	45	
	Recovery		84	34	32.5	0.66	0.71	8.5	0.93			121			25			45	42	
	Recovery		82	31	29.3	0.60	0.62	7.6	0.96			123			25			45	43	
	Recovery	156/72	79	28	26.0	0.53	0.53	6.7	1.00	7.49	18	124	128	−2	25	24	−1	45	45	0.18

Case 29 Congenital Heart Disease

Clinical Findings

This 18-year-old woman was referred to evaluate exercise dyspnea. She had a known history of dextrocardia and had had a pulmonic valve replacement as a child. Pulmonary hypertension and pulmonic valve insufficiency were recently diagnosed. She had experienced dyspnea from climbing less than one flight of stairs. She had smoked cigarettes for 1 year. Examination revealed normal breath sounds and a grade 2 diastolic murmur over the upper sternum.

Exercise Findings

Exercise studies with the patient breathing room air and 100% O_2 were performed on a cycle ergometer during the same morning, with an intermediate rest period. On both occasions, arterial blood was sampled every second minute and intraarterial pressure was recorded from a percutaneously placed brachial artery catheter. The patient pedaled at 60 rpm without an added load for 3 minutes. The work rate was then increased in a ramp of 7 W per minute to tolerance. The patient was cooperative, appeared to give good effort, and stopped exercise on both occasions because of dyspnea. Resting and repeated ECGs during exercise (taken with reversed limb and right chest leads) did not reveal arrhythmias or evidence of myocardial ischemia. Ar-

terial saturation by ear oximetry fell from 97% at rest to 87% at maximal exercise, but direct arterial blood gas measurements did not support this change.

Interpretation

Comments

This is a patient with known congenital heart disease, previously surgically repaired, with recent deterioration and mild restrictive lung disease. The arterial oxyhemoglobin saturation did not fall during the brief exercise period when directly measured, but ear oximetry saturation declined 10% during the same time.

TABLE 10.29.1.   Selected Respiratory Function Data

Measurement	Predicted	Measured
Age, yr		18
Sex		Female
Height, cm		160
Weight, kg	61	49
Hematocrit, %		39
VC, L	3.38	2.20
IC, L	2.25	1.61
TLC, L	4.81	3.62
FEV_1, L	2.97	1.91
FEV_1/VC, %	88	87
MVV, L/min		
Direct	118	58
Indirect	119	76
D_LCO, ml/mm Hg/min	25.1	12.6

TABLE 10.29.2.   Selected Exercise Data

Measurement	Predicted	Room Air	Oxygen
Peak $\dot{V}O_2$, L/min	1.93	0.76	
Maximum HR, beats/min	202	111	113
Maximum O_2 pulse, ml/beat	9.6	6.8	
$\Delta\dot{V}O_2/\Delta$WR, ml/min/W	10.3	6.3	
AT, L/min	>0.87	<0.65	
Work rate, max, W		<35	35
Blood pressure, mmHg (rest, max ex)		96/60, 126/66	102/60, 114/66
Maximum $\dot{V}E$, L/min		47	38
Exercise breathing reserve, L/min			
Using direct MVV	>15	11	20
Using indirect MVV	>15	19	38
O_2 saturation, oximeter (rest, max ex)		97, 87	
PaO_2, mmHg (rest, max ex)		75, 81	479, 532
P(A − a)O_2, mmHg (rest, max ex)		40, 42	203, 150
P(a − ET)CO_2 mmHg (rest, max ex)		5, 6	3, 4
VD/VT (rest, max ex)		0.31, 0.37	0.35, 0.35
HCO_3^-, mEq/L (rest, recovery)		20, 19	21, 20

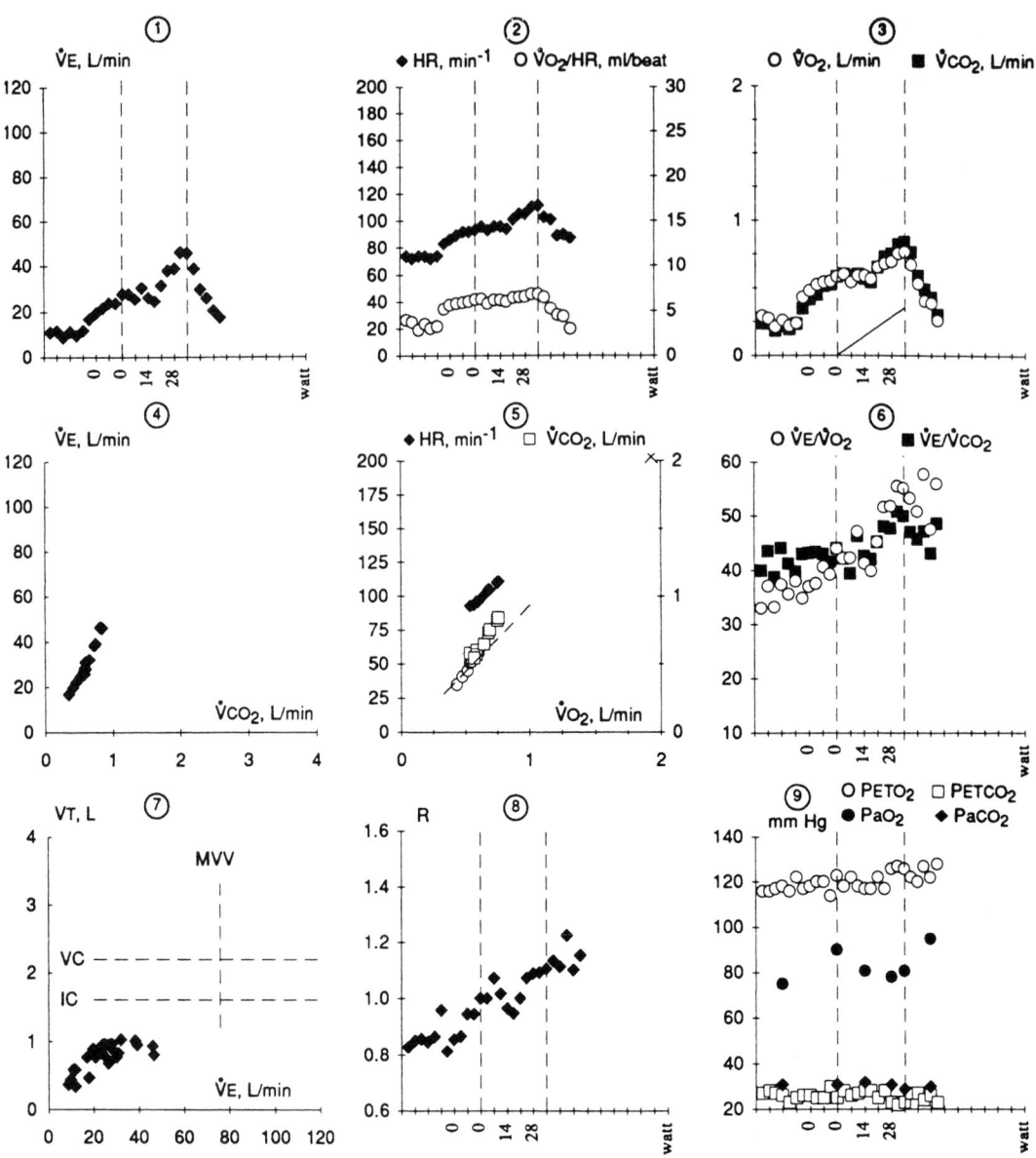

FIGURE 10.29.1.   Air breathing. 1: Vertical dashed lines in panels 1 to 3 and 6, 8, and 9 indicate the beginning and the end of the increasing work period. 2: Unloaded cycling is performed for 3 minutes before the left vertical dashed line. 3: In panel 3, the diagonal line shows the increase of $\dot{V}O_2$ at a slope of 10 ml/min/W. 4: In panel 5, the diagonal dashed line has a slope of 1; the x in the upper right is the predicted maximum heart rate and $\dot{V}O_2$ for the subject.

Analysis

Referring to flowchart 1, in the room air study the peak $\dot{V}O_2$ was reduced while the anaerobic threshold was also low (Table 10.29.2). This directs us to flowchart 4. Using the indirect MVV measurement, the breathing reserve is normal (branch point 4.1). This leads us to branch point 4.3, in which we address the $\dot{V}E/\dot{V}CO_2$ at the AT, which is elevated. This leads us to a diagnosis of abnormal pulmonary circulation, taking us to branch point 4.5. The vital capacity is reduced, leading us to the diagnosis of moderate to severe left-sided heart failure. However, the differential feature between left ventricular failure disorder and pulmonary vascular disease based on the reduced vital capacity might be incorrect because her prior surgery, rather than moderate severe heart failure, might have accounted for the reduction. Addressing the diagnosis through flowchart 5, the V_D/V_T, $P(A - a)O_2$, and $P(a - ET)CO_2$ are abnormal (branch point 5.1), whereas the breathing reserve is normal (branch point 5.3). Evidence of a reduced cardiac output response and of a reduced $\Delta\dot{V}O_2/\Delta WR$ is indicative of a circulatory limitation.

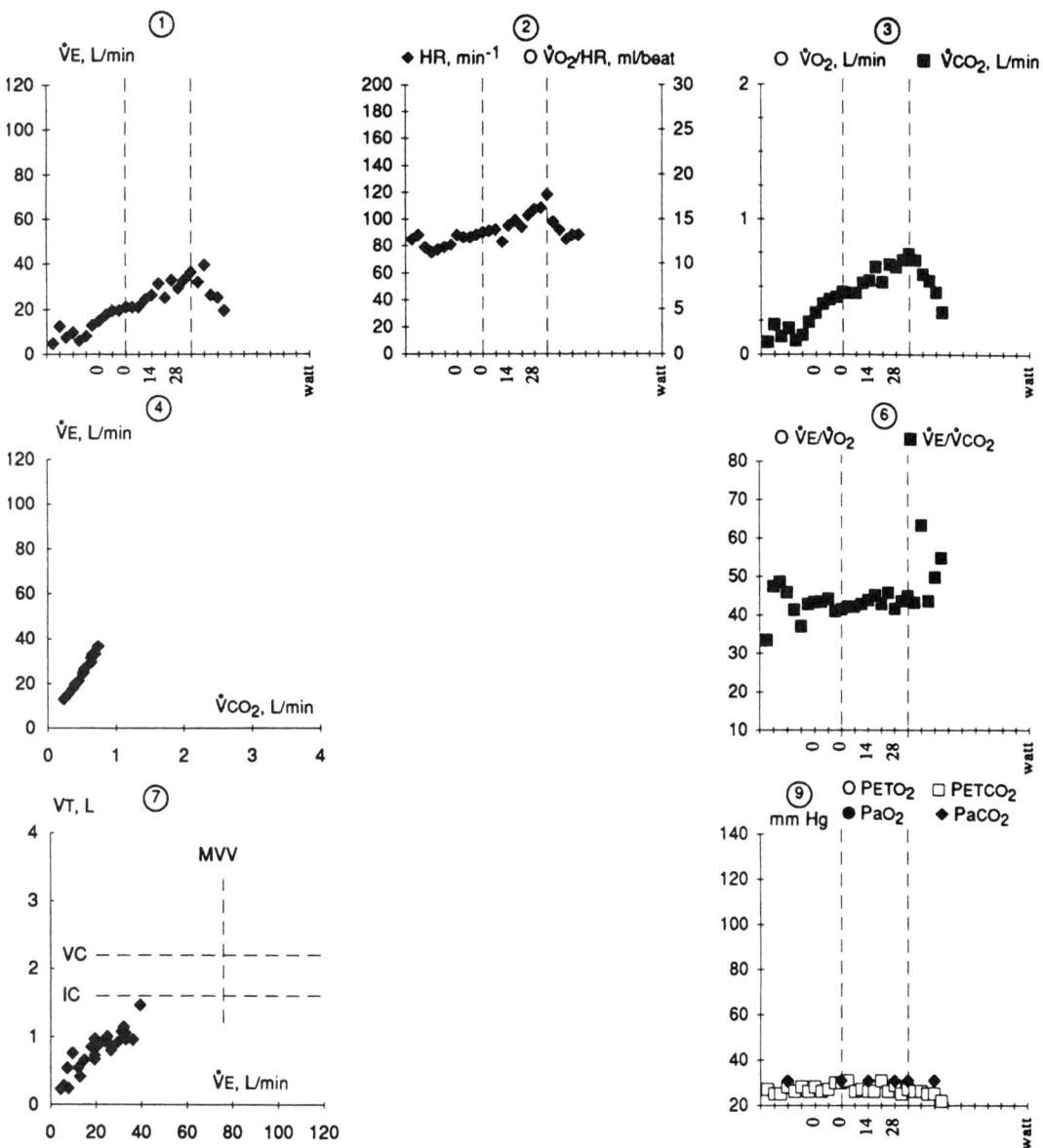

FIGURE 10.29.2.   Oxygen breathing. **1:** Vertical dashed lines in panels 1 to 3 and 6 and 9 indicate the beginning and the end of the increasing work period. **2:** Unloaded cycling is performed for 3 minutes before the left vertical dashed line.

O_2 breathing provided no benefit to the patient with respect to work capacity or the ventilatory response. Neither the breathing frequency nor the V_T/IC is abnormally high on either test. The high heart rate reserve suggests chronotropic insufficiency. The high PaO_2 during O_2 breathing excludes a significant right-to-left shunt. The tight control of pH and the failure to recruit new pulmonary blood vessels during exercise, reflected in the increase in ventilatory equivalent for CO_2 during exercise (i.e., decrease in gas exchange efficiency, panel 6), might account for this patient's dyspnea.

Conclusion

This patient demonstrates a severe cardiovascular limitation to exercise, secondary to congenital heart disease, that is subjectively experienced as dyspnea. For some reason, the patient regulates her $PaCO_2$ at a low level (has a low set point), thereby requiring a high ventilation to eliminate the metabolic CO_2 of exercise (see the high $\dot{V}_E/\dot{V}CO_2$ at the anaerobic threshold in panel 6 of Fig. 10.29.1). This high ventilatory requirement is likely the main factor stimulating dyspnea and limiting exercise tolerance.

TABLE 10.29.3. Air Breathing

Time min	Work rate watts	BP mmHg	HR min⁻¹	f min⁻¹	$\dot{V}_E$ L/min BTPS	$\dot{V}_{CO_2}$ L/min STPD	$\dot{V}_{O_2}$ L/min STPD	$\dot{V}_{O_2}$/HR ml/beat	R	pH	HCO_3^- meq/L	P_{O_2}, mmHg ET	a	(A − a)	P_{CO_2}, mmHg ET	a	(a − ET)	$\dot{V}_E$/$\dot{V}_{CO_2}$	$\dot{V}_E$/$\dot{V}_{O_2}$	V_D/V_T
	Rest		74	19	11.2	0.24	0.29	3.9	0.83			116			27			40	33	
	Rest		72	20	11.7	0.23	0.27	3.8	0.85			116			28			43	37	
	Rest		74	24	9.0	0.18	0.21	2.8	0.86			117			27			39	33	
	Rest	96/60	74	20	11.4	0.22	0.26	3.5	0.85	7.43	20	118	75	40	26	31	5	44	37	0.31
	Rest		72	22	9.7	0.19	0.22	3.1	0.86			116			23			41	36	
	Rest		74	35	12.1	0.23	0.24	3.2	0.96			122			25			40	38	
	Unloaded		83	22	16.9	0.35	0.43	5.2	0.81			117			26			43	35	
	Unloaded		86	22	19.6	0.41	0.48	5.6	0.85			118			26			43	37	
	Unloaded		89	27	21.8	0.45	0.52	5.8	0.87			120			25			43	38	
	Unloaded		92	25	24.0	0.51	0.54	5.9	0.94			120			25			43	41	
	Unloaded		92	29	24.0	0.52	0.55	6.0	0.95			114			30			41	39	
	Unloaded	102/66	93	29	28.0	0.58	0.58	6.2	1.00	7.46	22	123	90	29	25	31	6	44	44	0.34
0.5	4		96	31	27.9	0.60	0.60	6.3	1.00			118			28			42	42	
1.0	7		93	34	25.7	0.58	0.54	5.8	1.07			122			26			39	42	
1.5	11		96	37	30.9	0.60	0.59	6.1	1.02			118			27			46	47	
2.0	14	114/66	96	28	26.7	0.57	0.59	6.1	0.97	7.43	21	117	81	36	28	32	4	43	41	0.34
2.5	18		94	26	24.9	0.54	0.57	6.1	0.95			117			28			42	40	
3.0	21		101	31	32.0	0.65	0.65	6.4	1.00			122			25			45	45	
3.5	25		105	38	38.3	0.73	0.68	6.5	1.07			117			28			48	52	
4.0	28	126/66	105	41	39.2	0.75	0.69	6.6	1.09	7.43	20	126	78	43	23	31	8	48	52	0.38
4.5	32		110	57	46.5	0.82	0.75	6.8	1.09			127			22			51	56	
5.0	35		111	49	46.1	0.84	0.76	6.8	1.11	7.45	20	126	81	42	23	29	6	50	55	0.37
	Recovery		103	41	39.2	0.76	0.67	6.5	1.13			122			27			47	53	
	Recovery		101	39	30.2	0.59	0.53	5.2	1.11			120			27			46	51	
	Recovery		89	39	26.4	0.49	0.40	4.5	1.23			127			24			47	58	
	Recovery	108/60	90	27	20.8	0.43	0.39	4.3	1.10	7.41	19	122	95	27	26	30	4	43	47	0.29
	Recovery		87	38	17.8	0.30	0.26	3.0	1.15			128			23			49	56	

As is not uncommonly seen in patients with cardiovascular limitation to exercise, the ear oximeter values were falsely decreased at maximal exercise, probably because of inadequate cardiac output and reduced perfusion of the ear lobe (1).

Reference

1. Hansen JE, Casaburi R. Validity of ear oximetry in clinical exercise testing. *Chest* 1987;91:333–337.

TABLE 10.29.4.   Oxygen Breathing

Time min	Work rate watts	BP mmHg	HR min⁻¹	f min⁻¹	$\dot{V}_E$ L/min BTPS	$\dot{V}_{CO_2}$ L/min STPD	$\dot{V}_{O_2}$ L/min STPD	$\dfrac{\dot{V}_{O_2}}{HR}$ ml/beat	R	pH	HCO₃⁻ meq/L	P_{O_2}, mmHg ET	a	(A−a)	P_{CO_2}, mmHg ET	a	(a−ET)	$\dfrac{\dot{V}_E}{\dot{V}_{CO_2}}$	$\dfrac{\dot{V}_E}{\dot{V}_{O_2}}$	$\dfrac{V_D}{V_T}$
	Rest		85	20	4.7	0.09									27			33		
	Rest		88	23	12.4	0.22									25			47		
	Rest		79	14	7.5	0.13									25			49		
	Rest	102/60	75	13	9.8	0.19				7.45	21		479	203	28	31	3	46		0.35
	Rest		77	22	6.0	0.10									26			41		
	Rest		79	33	8.0	0.14									28			37		
	Unloaded		81	31	12.9	0.24									26			43		
	Unloaded		88	23	14.9	0.30									28			43		
	Unloaded		86	21	17.8	0.37									26			43		
	Unloaded		86	20	19.4	0.40									27			44		
	Unloaded		88	27	19.5	0.42									30			41		
	Unloaded	114/66	90	23	21.0	0.46				7.42	20		533	149	30	31	1	41		0.30
0.5	4		91	24	21.0	0.45									31			42		
1.0	7		92	24	21.0	0.45									26			42		
1.5	11		83	26	24.4	0.52									27			43		
2.0	14	120/72	95	33	26.4	0.54				7.44	21		536	146	26	31	5	44		0.32
2.5	18		99	29	31.3	0.64									26			45		
3.0	21		94	28	25.1	0.53									31			43		
3.5	25		103	31	32.8	0.66									26			46		
4.0	28	114/72	107	32	29.4	0.64				7.42	20		534	148	29	31	2	42		0.30
4.5	32		108	34	33.0	0.69									25			44		
5.0	35	114/66	118	38	36.4	0.74				7.43	20		532	150	27	31	4	45		0.35
	Recovery		98	28	32.1	0.69									26			43		
	Recovery		92	27	39.6	0.59									26			63		
	Recovery		85	30	26.1	0.54									25			44		
	Recovery	90/48	88	25	25.0	0.46				7.42	20		543	139	25	31	6	50		0.40
	Recovery		88	29	19.4	0.31									22			55		

Case 30 Peripheral Arterial Disease

Clinical Findings

This 65-year-old cigarette-smoking man was evaluated as part of a research study looking for coronary artery calcification. He had been overweight and a known diabetic for approximately 6 years. He had continued to lead an active life, but had been limited in his speed of walking for approximately 5 years, with pain in his thighs and calves, especially on the right side. He had had some cough and sputum production for a decade. He denied chest pain, shortness of breath, wheezing, edema, or skin problems. Pulses could not be palpated in the legs except for a faint right femoral artery pulse. The patient had no edema; skin warmth and color were good. The coronary arteries were free of calcification.

Exercise Findings

The patient performed exercise on a cycle ergometer. He pedaled at 60 rpm without an added load for 3 minutes. The work rate was then increased 15 W per minute to tolerance. Heart rate and rhythm were continuously monitored; 12-lead ECGs were obtained during rest, exercise, and recovery. Blood pressure was measured with a sphygmomanometer every minute. The patient appeared to give an excellent effort and stopped exercise because of bilateral thigh and calf pain. He denied chest pain or discomfort during or after the study. The ECGs showed occasional premature ventricular contractions both at rest and during exercise, but were otherwise normal. No abnormal ST segments or T waves were noted before, during, or after exercise.

Interpretation

Comments

The patient has mild, asymptomatic airways obstruction, diabetes mellitus, obesity, and clinical evidence of peripheral arterial disease without heart disease.

Analysis

Referring to flowchart 1, peak $\dot{V}O_2$ and the anaerobic threshold are reduced (Table 10.30.2). Proceeding next to flowchart 4, the high breathing reserve (branch point 4.1) and normal $\dot{V}E/\dot{V}CO_2$ at the anaerobic threshold (branch point 4.3) lead us to a diagnosis of "O_2 flow problem of nonpulmonary origin." The normal hematocrit (branch point 4.4) indicates a cardiovascular disorder with a low nonchanging O_2 pulse (branch point 4.6). The findings of exercise-induced systemic hypertension, leg pain, low $\Delta\dot{V}O_2/\Delta WR$ and $\Delta\dot{V}CO_2/\Delta WR$ and high heart rate reserve all support the diagnosis of peripheral arterial disease. The absence of ECG changes indicative of myocardial ischemia suggests that the coronary vessels are relatively uninvolved.

TABLE 10.30.1. Selected Respiratory Function Data

Measurement	Predicted	Measured
Age, yr		65
Sex		Male
Height, cm		170
Weight, kg	74	88
Hematocrit, %		42
VC, L	3.43	3.65
IC, L	2.44	3.20
FEV$_1$, L	2.74	2.48
FEV$_1$/VC, %	79	68
MVV, L/min	110	92

TABLE 10.30.2. Selected Exercise Data

Measurement	Predicted	Measured
Peak $\dot{V}O_2$, L/min	2.04	1.06
Maximum HR, beats/min	155	135
Maximum O_2 pulse, ml/beat	13.2	7.9
$\Delta\dot{V}O_2/\Delta WR$, ml/min/W	10.3	6.9
AT, L/min	>0.95	0.8
Blood pressure, mmHg (rest, max)		164/88, 278/110
Maximum $\dot{V}E$, L/min		33
Exercise breathing reserve, L/min	>15	59

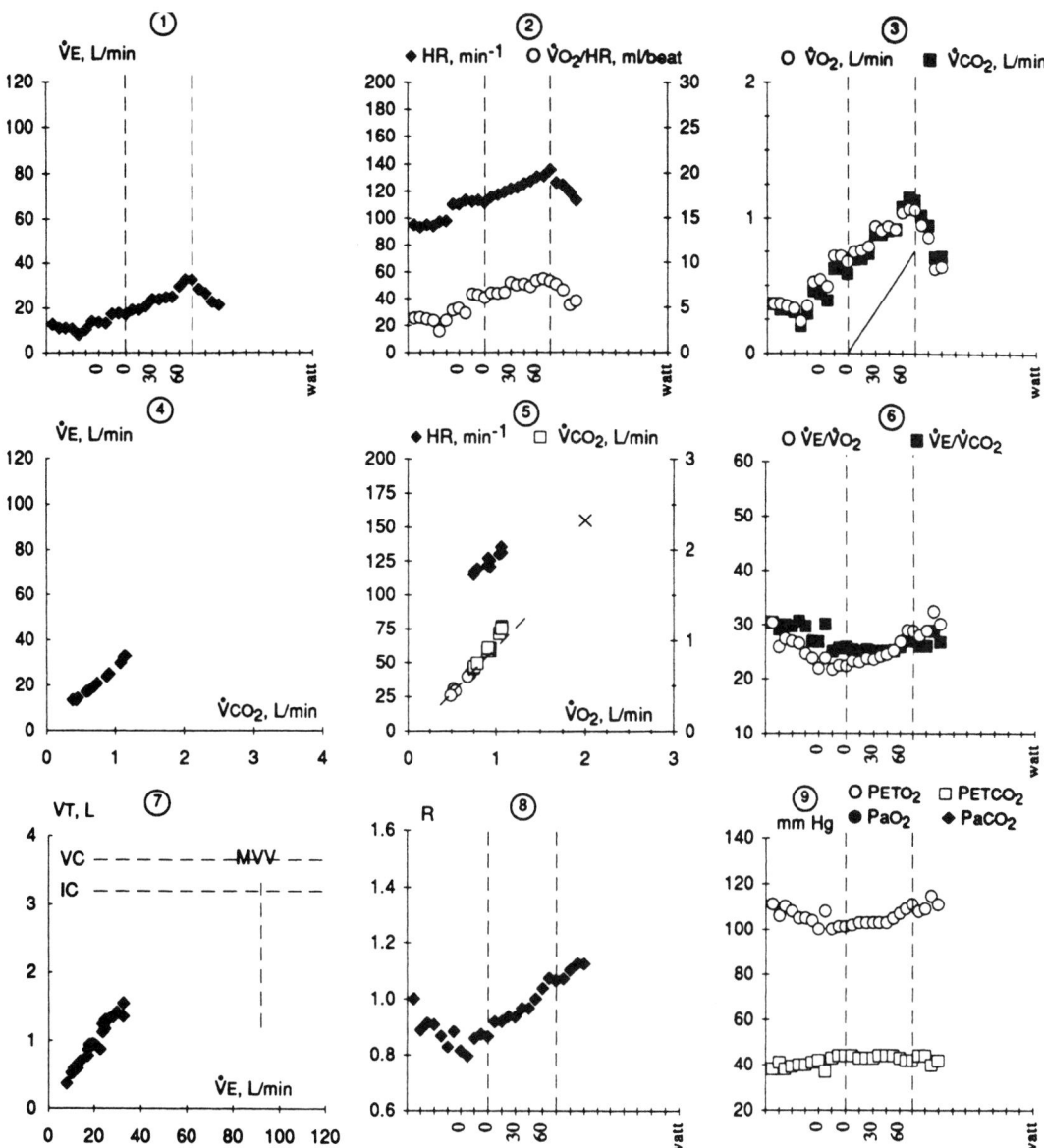

FIGURE 10.30.1.   **1:** Vertical dashed lines in panels 1 to 3 and 6, 8, and 9 indicate the beginning and the end of the increasing work period. **2:** Unloaded cycling is performed for 3 minutes before the left vertical dashed line. **3:** In panel 3, the diagonal line shows the increase of $\dot{V}O_2$ at a slope of 10 ml/min/W. **4:** In panel 5, the diagonal dashed line has a slope of 1; the x in the upper right is the predicted maximum heart rate and $\dot{V}O_2$ for the subject.

Conclusion

The exercise-induced hypertension is especially typical of peripheral arterial disease. In addition, the increase in $\dot{V}CO_2$ with work rate is reduced similar to the $\dot{V}O_2$–work rate relationship, in contrast to the findings in primary heart disease or disease of the pulmonary circulation. Perhaps this is because the leg blood flow contributes in a relatively small way to the total systemic circulation, and the reduction in $\dot{V}O_2$ results in a reduction in aerobic CO_2 production. Although many patients with peripheral arterial disease are limited by associated coronary artery disease, this does not seem to be true for this man.

TABLE 10.30.3. Air Breathing

Time min	Work rate watts	BP mmHg	HR min⁻¹	f min⁻¹	$\dot{V}_E$ L/min BTPS	$\dot{V}_{CO_2}$ L/min STPD	$\dot{V}_{O_2}$ L/min STPD	$\dfrac{\dot{V}_{O_2}}{HR}$ ml/beat	R	pH	HCO_3^- meq/L	P_{O_2}, mmHg ET	a	(A − a)	P_{CO_2}, mmHg ET	a	(a − ET)	$\dfrac{\dot{V}_E}{\dot{V}_{CO_2}}$	$\dfrac{\dot{V}_E}{\dot{V}_{O_2}}$	$\dfrac{V_D}{V_T}$
	Rest	164/88										111								
	Rest		95	22	12.8	0.36	0.36	3.8	1.00			106			38			30	30	
	Rest	188/80	93	21	11.1	0.32	0.36	3.9	0.89			110			41			29	26	
	Rest		95	19	11.2	0.32	0.35	3.7	0.91			108			38			30	27	
	Rest	218/80	94	20	10.6	0.30	0.33	3.5	0.91			105			39			30	27	
	Rest		97	22	8.0	0.20	0.23	2.4	0.87			105			40			31	27	
	Rest	198/82	98	20	10.3	0.29	0.35	3.6	0.83						40			30	25	
	Unloaded		110	20	14.1	0.46	0.52	4.7	0.88			104			41			27	24	
	Unloaded	214/100	110	20	13.5	0.44	0.54	4.9	0.81			100			42			27	22	
	Unloaded		113	20	13.4	0.39	0.49	4.3	0.80			108			37			30	24	
	Unloaded	238/96	112	20	17.3	0.62	0.72	6.4	0.86			100			43			25	22	
	Unloaded		113	19	17.8	0.63	0.72	6.4	0.88			101			44			26	22	
	Unloaded	254/90	111	22	17.1	0.59	0.68	6.1	0.87			101			44			26	22	
0.5	7.5		115	20	19.2	0.69	0.75	6.5	0.92			102			44			25	23	
1.0	15	255/100	117	20	19.2	0.70	0.76	6.5	0.92			103			43			25	23	
1.5	22.5		119	22	20.6	0.74	0.79	6.6	0.94			103			43			25	24	
2.0	30	245/114	121	19	23.7	0.88	0.94	7.8	0.94			103			43			25	23	
2.5	37.5		122	21	23.7	0.88	0.91	7.5	0.97			103			44			25	24	
3.0	45	252/110	125	21	24.7	0.91	0.94	7.5	0.97			103			44			25	24	
3.5	52.5		127	19	24.8	0.92	0.92	7.2	1.00			105			44			25	25	
4.0	60	256/114	130	21	29.7	1.08	1.04	8.0	1.04			107			43			26	27	
4.5	67.5		131	21	32.7	1.15	1.07	8.2	1.07			109			42			27	29	
5.0	75	278/110	135	24	32.6	1.13	1.06	7.9	1.07			111			42			27	29	
	Recovery		126	21	28.4	1.02	0.95	7.5	1.07			108			44			26	26	
	Recovery	268/90	124	20	26.5	0.95	0.86	6.9	1.10			109			44			26	29	
	Recovery		119	26	22.6	0.71	0.63	5.3	1.13			115			40			29	32	
	Recovery	241/86	113	23	21.2	0.72	0.64	5.7	1.13			111			42			27	30	

Case 31 Peripheral Arterial Disease with Pulmonary Vascular and Obstructive Airway Disease

Clinical Findings

This 69-year-old retired shipyard worker had been a heavy cigarette smoker until 5 years before examination. For more than a decade he had noted excessive shortness of breath on climbing one flight of stairs. For the last several years his activity had been limited by cramps in the calves after walking approximately 100 yards; they were relieved by rest. He took no medication. Examination revealed a left cataract and reduced arterial pulsations in the legs, but no rales, wheezing, or edema. Chest roentgenographic studies showed pleural thickening on the right, an elevated left leaf of the diaphragm, and normal heart size.

Exercise Findings

The patient performed exercise on a cycle ergometer. He pedaled at 60 rpm without added load for 3 minutes. The work rate was then increased 10 W per minute to his symptom-limited maximum. Blood was sampled every second minute, and intraarterial blood pressure was recorded from a percutaneously placed brachial artery catheter. The patient stopped exercise because of pain in both calves. He developed frequent premature ventricular contractions and hypertension during exercise that resolved during recovery. Resting, exercise, and recovery ECG tracings were otherwise normal.

Interpretation

Comments

Resting respiratory function studies show the patient to have moderate airflow obstruction (Table 10.31.1). The resting electrocardiogram is normal.

Analysis

Referring to flowchart 1, the peak $\dot{V}O_2$ is reduced, and the anaerobic threshold was not measurable (Table 10.31.2). The latter is not unexpected for peripheral arterial disease because of the difficulty for muscle lactic acidosis to be reflected systemically,

as discussed in Case 30. Therefore, we consider the anaerobic threshold to be indeterminate and use flowchart 5. Although the maximum work rate performed is quite low, the maximum exercise VD/VT is high, and $P(a - ET)CO_2$ and $P(A - a)O_2$ are at the borderline of abnormality (branch point 5.1). The breathing reserve is high (branch point 5.3). This suggests that the disease process is either that of pulmonary vascular or left ventricular failure. However, neither diagnosis fits very well with the measurements shown in the two supporting boxes. The failure to develop a systemic metabolic acidosis, the high heart rate reserve, and the systemic hypertension are particularly incompatible with either diagnosis and suggest that this patient has a mixed disorder, with neither of the two choices derived by

TABLE 10.31.1.   Selected Respiratory Function Data

Measurement	Predicted	Measured
Age, yr		69
Sex		Male
Height, cm		165
Weight, kg	70	76
Hematocrit, %		40
VC, L	3.68	3.25
IC, L	2.45	2.69
TLC, L	6.11	6.05
FEV_1, L	2.87	1.92
FEV_1/VC, %	78	59
MVV, L/min	113	87
D_LCO, ml/mm Hg/min	21.8	17.5

TABLE 10.31.2.   Selected Exercise Data

Measurement	Predicted	Measured
Peak $\dot{V}O_2$, L/min	1.78	0.83
Maximum HR, beats/min	151	115
Maximum O_2 pulse, ml/beat	11.8	7.2
$\Delta\dot{V}O_2/\Delta WR$, ml/min/W	10.3	5.2
AT, L/min	>0.80	not reached
Blood pressure, mmHg (rest, max)		198/84, 264/120
Maximum $\dot{V}E$, L/min		30
Exercise breathing reserve, L/min	>15	57
PaO_2, mmHg (rest, max ex)		87, 80
$P(A - a)O_2$, mmHg (rest, max ex)		11, 28
$P(a - ET)CO_2$, mmHg (rest, max ex)		5, 1
VD/VT (rest, heavy ex)		0.47, 0.38
HCO_3^-, mEq/L (rest, 2-min recov)		24, 23

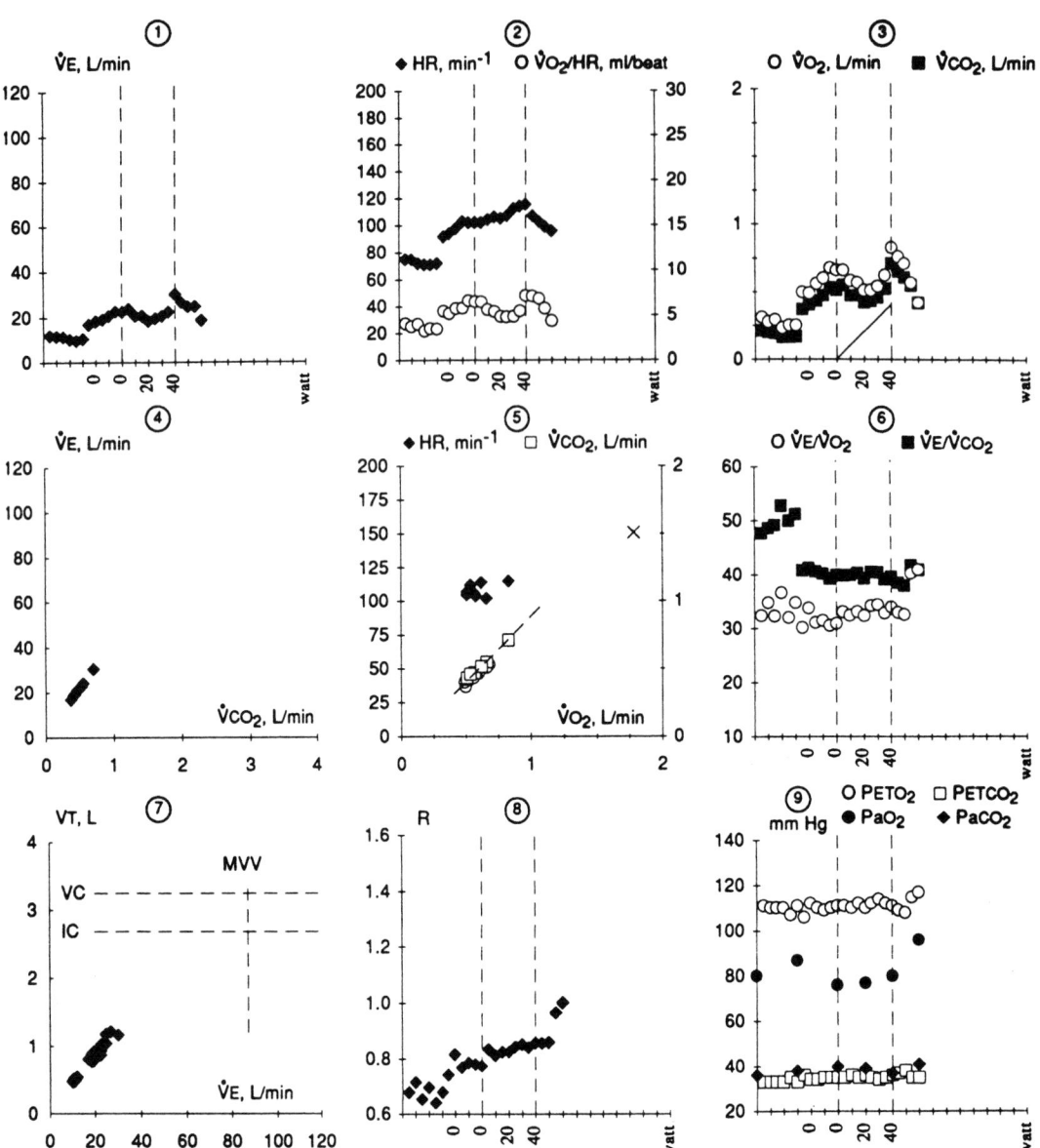

FIGURE 10.31.1. **1:** Vertical dashed lines in panels 1 to 3 and 6, 8, and 9 indicate the beginning and the end of the increasing work period. **2:** Unloaded cycling is performed for 3 minutes before the left vertical dashed line. **3:** In panel 3, the diagonal line shows the increase of $\dot{V}O_2$ at a slope of 10 ml/min/W. **4:** In panel 5, the diagonal dashed line has a slope of 1; the x in the upper right is the predicted maximum heart rate and $\dot{V}O_2$ for the subject.

the flowchart being the dominant limiting disorder. Returning to branch point 5.1 and taking the normal branch for arterial blood gases, we continue through branch points 5.2, high HRR, and 5.5, low $\Delta\dot{V}O_2/\Delta WR$, and finally reach branch point 5.8. The patient has systemic hypertension, reduced arterial pulses in the legs, and lower extremity pain with exercise, suggesting that peripheral arterial disease is the diagnosis that is limiting exercise performance. Supporting this is the failure to develop a systemic metabolic acidosis. ($\dot{V}O_2$ and $\dot{V}CO_2$ could increase only slightly above that required for unloaded cycling.)

Conclusion

Both peripheral arterial and lung disease are present, with the former being the primary limiting disorder. The exercise-induced arrhythmia also suggests the presence of myocardial ischemia, perhaps from the high cardiac afterload induced by systemic hypertension. The poor perfusion of the exercising muscles probably prevented the cellular metabolic acidosis from being reflected in the arterial blood. Note that although this patient has moderate airflow obstruction, it does not appear to be an important factor in his exercise limitation.

TABLE 10.31.3. Air Breathing

Time min	Work rate watts	BP mmHg	HR min⁻¹	f min⁻¹	$\dot{V}_E$ L/min BTPS	$\dot{V}_{CO_2}$ L/min STPD	$\dot{V}_{O_2}$ L/min STPD	$\dfrac{\dot{V}_{O_2}}{HR}$ ml/beat	R	pH	HCO₃⁻ meq/L	P_{O_2}, mmHg ET	a	(A − a)	P_{CO_2}, mmHg ET	a	(a − ET)	$\dfrac{\dot{V}_E}{\dot{V}_{CO_2}}$	$\dfrac{\dot{V}_E}{\dot{V}_{O_2}}$	$\dfrac{V_D}{V_T}$
	Rest	210/84								7.43	23		80			36				
	Rest		75	22	11.9	0.21	0.31	4.1	0.68			111			33			48	32	
	Rest		75	22	11.6	0.20	0.28	3.7	0.71			110			33			49	35	
	Rest		72	23	11.3	0.19	0.29	4.0	0.66			110			33			49	32	
	Rest		71	22	10.3	0.16	0.23	3.2	0.70			110			33			53	37	
	Rest		71	20	9.7	0.16	0.25	3.5	0.64			107			33			50	32	
	Rest	198/84	72	20	10.4	0.17	0.25	3.5	0.68	7.41	24	111	87	11	33	38	5	51	35	0.47
	Unloaded		92	21	16.9	0.37	0.50	5.4	0.74			106			36			41	30	
	Unloaded		94	21	18.3	0.40	0.49	5.2	0.82			112			34			41	34	
	Unloaded		98	21	19.2	0.43	0.56	5.7	0.77			110			34			41	31	
	Unloaded		103	22	20.7	0.47	0.60	5.8	0.78			109			35			40	31	
	Unloaded		102	22	22.6	0.53	0.68	6.7	0.78			110			35			39	30	
	Unloaded	246/93	102	24	22.4	0.51	0.66	6.5	0.77	7.40	24	111	76	25	35	40	5	40	31	0.42
0.5	10		102	23	23.8	0.55	0.66	6.5	0.83			111			35			40	3	
1.0	10		104	23	20.7	0.47	0.58	5.6	0.81			110			36			40	32	
1.5	20		106	24	20.9	0.47	0.57	5.4	0.82			112			35			40	33	
2.0	20	252/114	105	24	18.5	0.42	0.51	4.9	0.82	7.40	24	110	77	27	36	39	3	39	32	0.39
2.5	30		107	25	19.5	0.43	0.51	4.8	0.84			112			35			40	34	
3.0	40		112	25	20.7	0.46	0.54	4.8	0.85			114			34			40	34	
3.5	40		114	26	22.5	0.52	0.62	5.4	0.84			112			35			39	33	
4.0	40	264/120	115	26	30.3	0.71	0.83	7.2	0.86	7.40	23	111	80	28	36	37	1	40	34	0.38
	Recovery		107	22	26.8	0.65	0.76	7.1	0.86			109			37			38	33	
	Recovery		103	21	24.8	0.61	0.71	6.9	0.86			108			38			38	32	
	Recovery		99	24	24.9	0.55	0.57	5.8	0.96			115			35			42	40	
	Recovery	210/96	96	21	18.9	0.42	0.42	4.4	1.00	7.37	23	117	96	13	35	41	6	41	41	0.44

Case 32 Heart Failure–Dominant Mixed Cardiovascular Disease in an Anemic Smoker

Clinical Findings

This 54-year-old male bartender was referred for preoperative study to evaluate his exercise capacity. He occasionally had calf pain at rest and always after walking one block. He had smoked at least 60 pack-years but denied cardiac or respiratory symptoms. The left iliac and superficial femoral arteries were demonstrated to be obstructed on angiography. He was moderately anemic (hematocrit = 34), with occult blood in the stool.

Exercise Findings

The patient performed exercise on a cycle ergometer. He pedaled at 60 rpm without added load for 3 minutes. The work rate was then increased 15 W per minute to his symptom-limited maximum. Blood was sampled every second minute, and intraarterial blood pressure was recorded from a percutaneously placed brachial artery catheter. Resting and exercise ECGs were normal. He stopped exercise because of severe leg pain, which was more prominent on the left. Carboxyhemoglobin was 5.6% in his resting arterial blood.

Interpretation

Comments

The resting respiratory function is normal, including the diffusing capacity (Table 10.32.1).

Analysis

Referring to flowchart 1, peak $\dot{V}O_2$ and anaerobic threshold are reduced during exercise testing (Table 10.32.2). See flowchart 4 for further analysis. The breathing reserve is high (branch point 4.1). This patient has a combination of abnormalities that fit the major diagnoses leading from both branches of branch point 4.3. Mildly elevated values of VD/VT and $P(a − ET)CO_2$, and normal $P(A − a)O_2$ and PaO_2 at maximal exercise suggest the reduced perfusion to ventilated lung seen in moderate to severe heart failure (right branch of branch point 4.5). The abnormality in VD/VT with normal $P(A − a)O_2$, low $\Delta\dot{V}O_2/\Delta WR$, and low and flat O_2 pulse are the abnormalities seen with moderate to severe left-sided heart failure. The patient's anemia and carboxyhe-

moglobinemia may contribute to the abnormality in peripheral oxygenation. The steep heart rate versus $\dot{V}O_2$ relation and low O_2 pulse noted with increasing work rate are consistent with either a cardiac abnormality or anemia, or a combination of both disorders.

Conclusion

Although the patient has ischemic peripheral arterial disease, as documented by angiography and reflected by his leg pain in response to exercise, the flat O_2 pulse pattern as work rate is increased, the manifestation of a systemic lactic acidosis, and the steep heart rate response to exercise suggest that heart failure with anemia and carboxyhemoglobinemia are dominant factors in the patient's pathophysiology.

TABLE 10.32.1. Selected Respiratory Function Data

Measurement	Predicted	Measured
Age, yr		59
Sex		Male
Height, cm		168
Weight, kg	72	60
Hematocrit, %		34
VC, L	3.94	3.84
IC, L	2.63	3.64
TLC, L	5.86	7.16
FEV$_1$, L	3.12	3.07
FEV$_1$/VC, %	79	80
MVV, L/min	136	110
D$_L$CO, ml/mm Hg/min	23.0	22.9

TABLE 10.32.2. Selected Exercise Data

Measurement	Predicted	Measured
Peak $\dot{V}O_2$, L/min	1.90	0.82
Maximum HR, beats/min	161	141
Maximum O_2 pulse, ml/beat	11.8	5.8
$\Delta\dot{V}O_2/\Delta WR$, ml/min/W	10.3	6.2
AT, L/min	>0.84	0.7
Blood pressure, mmHg (rest, max)		168/72, 255/114
Maximum $\dot{V}E$, L/min		60
Exercise breathing reserve, L/min	>15	50
PaO$_2$, mmHg (rest, max ex)		94, 117
P(A − a)O$_2$, mmHg (rest, max ex)		20, 11
P(a − ET)CO$_2$, mmHg (rest, max ex)		3, 2
VD/VT (rest, heavy ex)		0.45, 0.38
HCO$_3^-$, mEq/L (rest, 2-min recov)		20, 16

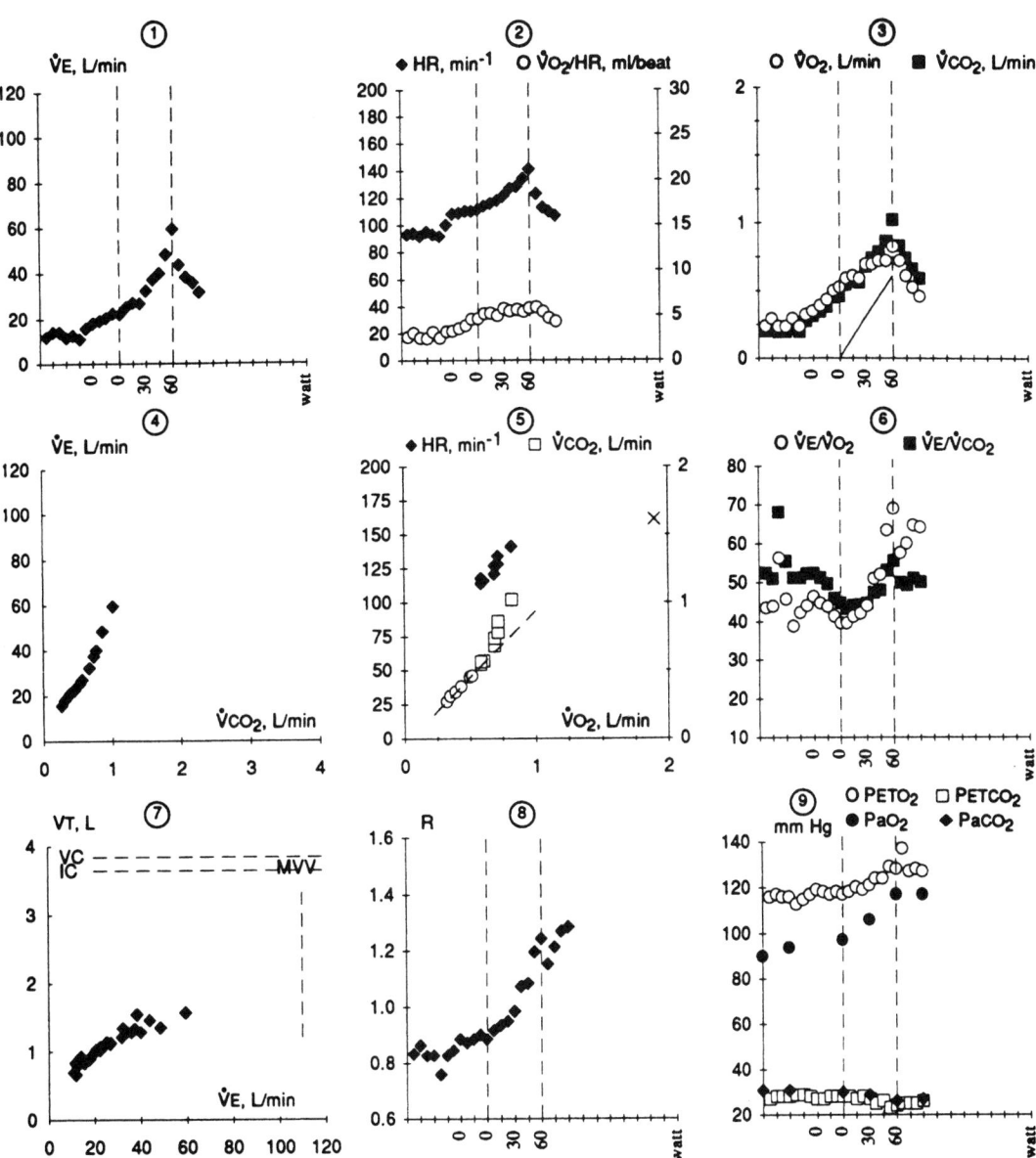

FIGURE 10.32.1. **1:** Vertical dashed lines in panels 1 to 3 and 6, 8, and 9 indicate the beginning and the end of the increasing work period. **2:** Unloaded cycling is performed for 3 minutes before the left vertical dashed line. **3:** In panel 3, the diagonal line shows the increase of $\dot{V}O_2$ at a slope of 10 ml/min/W. **4:** In panel 5, the diagonal dashed line has a slope of 1; the x in the upper right is the predicted maximum heart rate and $\dot{V}O_2$ for the subject.

TABLE 10.32.3.   Air Breathing

Time min	Work rate watts	BP mmHg	HR min⁻¹	f min⁻¹	$\dot{V}_E$ L/min BTPS	$\dot{V}_{CO_2}$ L/min STPD	$\dot{V}_{O_2}$ L/min STPD	$\dfrac{\dot{V}_{O_2}}{HR}$ ml/beat	R	pH	HCO₃⁻ meq/L	PO₂, mmHg ET	a	(A−a)	PCO₂, mmHg ET	a	(a−ET)	$\dfrac{\dot{V}_E}{\dot{V}_{CO_2}}$	$\dfrac{\dot{V}_E}{\dot{V}_{O_2}}$	$\dfrac{V_D}{V_T}$
	Rest	168/72								7.43	20		90			31				
	Rest		93	18	12.0	0.20	0.24	2.6	0.83			116			27			52	44	
	Rest		94	15	14.0	0.25	0.29	3.1	0.86			117			28			51	44	
	Rest		92	16	14.3	0.19	0.23	2.5	0.83			116			28			68	56	
	Rest	168/72	95	14	11.7	0.19	0.23	2.4	0.83	7.42	20	116	94	20	28	31	3	55	46	0.45
	Rest		93	16	12.6	0.22	0.29	3.1	0.76			113			29			51	39	
	Rest		92	16	11.1	0.19	0.23	2.5	0.83			115			29			51	42	
	Unloaded		100	19	15.7	0.27	0.32	3.2	0.84			117			28			52	44	
	Unloaded		108	20	17.9	0.31	0.35	3.2	0.89			119			27			52	46	
	Unloaded		109	20	19.1	0.34	0.39	3.6	0.87			118			27			51	45	
	Unloaded		110	20	20.5	0.38	0.43	3.9	0.88			117			28			49	44	
	Unloaded		110	22	22.5	0.45	0.50	4.5	0.90			118			28			46	41	
	Unloaded	231/93	111	21	22.3	0.46	0.52	4.7	0.88	7.43	20	117	97	20	28	30	2	45	39	0.33
0.5	15		114	22	25.2	0.54	0.59	5.2	0.92			118			28			43	40	
1.0	15		116	24	27.1	0.57	0.61	5.3	0.93			120			27			44	41	
1.5	30		118	24	26.8	0.56	0.59	5.0	0.95			119			28			44	42	
2.0	30	245/102	121	24	32.3	0.68	0.69	5.7	0.99	7.43	19	121	106	15	27	29	2	45	44	0.31
2.5	45		127	28	37.4	0.74	0.69	5.4	1.07			124			25			47	51	
3.0	45		128	31	40.1	0.78	0.72	5.6	1.08			124			26			48	52	
3.5	60		134	36	48.6	0.86	0.72	5.4	1.19			129			23			53	63	
4.0	60	255/114	141	38	59.7	1.02	0.82	5.8	1.24	7.44	17	128	117	11	24	26	2	55	69	0.38
	Recovery		123	30	43.9	0.83	0.72	5.9	1.15			137			25			50	57	
	Recovery		113	25	38.6	0.74	0.61	5.4	1.21			127			25			49	60	
	Recovery		110	28	35.9	0.66	0.52	4.7	1.27			128			25			51	64	
	Recovery	258/102	107	26	31.7	0.59	0.46	4.3	1.28	7.39	16	127	117	11	26	27	1	50	64	0.34

Case 33 Hypertensive Cardiovascular Disease and Carboxyhemoglobinemia

Clinical Findings

This 46-year-old current shipyard worker was referred for evaluation of shortness of breath. He complained of chronic cough and sputum production of 8 to 10 years' duration. He dated the shortness of breath to a hospitalization for a leg fracture 6 years before. He had previously abused alcohol and smoked. Physical examination revealed a smooth liver edge 5 cm below the right costal margin without other evidence of liver disease. There were no physical signs of cardiovascular or pulmonary disease. Chest roentgenogram showed small bilateral pleural plaques. ECG showed a left anterior hemiblock.

Exercise Findings

The patient performed exercise on a cycle ergometer. He pedaled at 60 rpm without added load for 3 minutes. The work rate was then increased 20 W per minute to his symptom-limited maximum. Arterial blood was sampled every second minute, and intraarterial blood pressure was recorded from a percutaneously placed brachial artery catheter. He stopped exercise complaining of shortness of breath and exhaustion. Carboxyhemoglobin level was 7.5% at the start of exercise, suggesting that the patient had recently smoked. There was no chest pain or abnormal ECG changes.

Interpretation

Comments

Respiratory function at rest is normal (Table 10. 33.1). Resting ECG is consistent with a left anterior hemiblock.

Analysis

Referring to flowchart 1, the peak $\dot{V}O_2$ and anaerobic threshold are reduced during exercise (Table 10.33.2). Proceeding to flowchart 4, the breathing reserve is high (Table 10.33.2) (branch point 4.1). The ventilatory equivalent for CO_2 at the anaerobic threshold is normal (Fig. 10.33.1), and the indices of distribution of ventilation relative to perfusion are normal (branch point 4.3), supporting the diagnosis of an O_2 flow problem of nonpulmonary origin. The hematocrit is normal (branch point 4.4). The maximum O_2 pulse is reduced but increasing

(branch point 4.6), supporting a diagnosis of peripheral arterial pathophysiology. Confirmatory findings are a high heart rate reserve, hypertension, and a shallow $\Delta\dot{V}O_2/\Delta WR$. The patient did not experience chest pain, and his ECG remained normal throughout the exercise test.

Conclusion

The patient evidently has exercise intolerance secondary to cardiovascular disease. This is possibly secondary to combined peripheral arterial disease due to essential hypertension and failure of the heart to respond adequately to the increased afterload; however, the reduced O_2 capacity of the blood and shift to the left of the oxyhemoglobin dissociation curve, caused by the elevated carboxyhemoglobin concentration, may also contribute to the patient's circulatory dysfunction.

TABLE 10.33.1.   Selected Respiratory Function Data

Measurement	Predicted	Measured
Age, yr		46
Sex		Male
Height, cm		161
Weight, kg	67	70
Hematocrit, %		43
VC, L	3.32	3.23
IC, L	2.22	2.24
TLC, L	4.77	4.77
FEV$_1$, L	2.65	2.62
FEV$_1$/VC, %	80	81
MVV, L/min	122	104
D$_L$CO, ml/mm Hg/min	22.3	22.1

TABLE 10.33.2.   Selected Exercise Data

Measurement	Predicted	Measured
Peak $\dot{V}O_2$, L/min	2.26	1.17
Maximum HR, beats/min	174	149
Maximum O$_2$ pulse, ml/beat	13.0	8.1
$\Delta\dot{V}O_2/\Delta WR$, ml/min/W	10.3	7.6
AT, L/min	>0.97	0.9
Blood pressure, mmHg (rest, max)		168/108, 228/126
Maximum $\dot{V}E$, L/min		45
Exercise breathing reserve, L/min	>15	59
PaO$_2$, mmHg (rest, max ex)		93, 101
P(A − a)O$_2$, mmHg (rest, max ex)		12, 21
P(a − ET)CO$_2$, mmHg (rest, max ex)		0, −2
VD/VT (rest, heavy ex)		0.25, 0.19
HCO$_3^-$, mEq/L (rest, 2-min recov)		23, 18

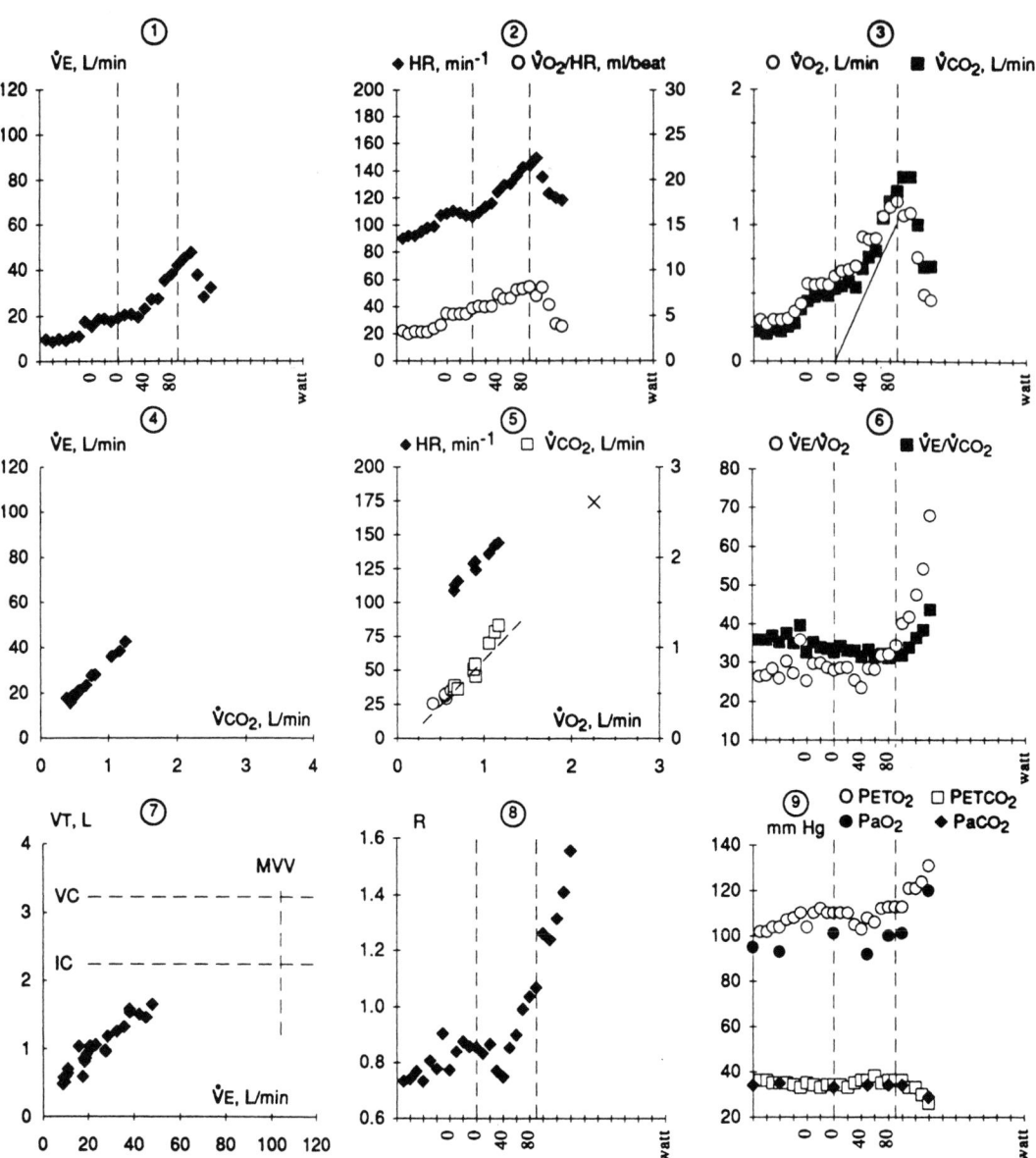

FIGURE 10.33.1.   **1:** Vertical dashed lines in panels 1 to 3 and 6, 8, and 9 indicate the beginning and the end of the increasing work period. **2:** Unloaded cycling is performed for 3 minutes before the left vertical dashed line. **3:** In panel 3, the diagonal line shows the increase of $\dot{V}O_2$ at a slope of 10 ml/min/W. **4:** In panel 5, the diagonal dashed line has a slope of 1; the x in the upper right is the predicted maximum heart rate and $\dot{V}O_2$ for the subject.

TABLE 10.33.3.   Air Breathing

Time min	Work rate watts	BP mmHg	HR min⁻¹	f min⁻¹	$\dot{V}_E$ L/min BTPS	$\dot{V}_{CO_2}$ L/min STPD	$\dot{V}_{O_2}$ L/min STPD	$\dot{V}_{O_2}$/HR ml/beat	R	pH	HCO_3^- meq/L	P_{O_2} ET	P_{O_2} a	P_{O_2} (A−a)	P_{CO_2} ET	P_{CO_2} a	P_{CO_2} (a−ET)	$\dot{V}_E/\dot{V}_{CO_2}$	$\dot{V}_E/\dot{V}_{O_2}$	V_D/V_T
	Rest	168/108								7.44	23		95			34				
	Rest		90	19	9.5	0.22	0.30	3.3	0.73			102			36			36	26	
	Rest		92	18	8.7	0.20	0.27	2.9	0.74			102			36			36	27	
	Rest		92	17	9.9	0.23	0.30	3.3	0.77			104			35			37	28	
	Rest	168/108	95	16	9.1	0.22	0.30	3.2	0.73	7.41	22	104	93	12	35	35	0	35	26	0.25
	Rest		98	17	10.8	0.25	0.31	3.2	0.81			107			35			37	30	
	Rest		99	16	11.1	0.28	0.36	3.6	0.78			108			34			35	27	
	Unloaded		107	30	17.6	0.38	0.42	3.9	0.90			110			33			40	36	
	Unloaded		108	15	15.6	0.44	0.57	5.3	0.77			104			35			33	25	
	Unloaded		110	23	18.5	0.47	0.56	5.1	0.84			110			34			35	30	
	Unloaded		109	22	18.8	0.50	0.57	5.2	0.88			112			33			34	30	
	Unloaded		107	21	17.8	0.48	0.56	5.2	0.86			110			34			33	29	
	Unloaded	186/111	106	21	19.1	0.53	0.62	5.8	0.85	7.45	23	110	101	12	34	33	−1	33	28	0.18
0.5	20		109	21	20.5	0.55	0.66	6.1	0.83			110			34			34	28	
1.0	20		113	20	20.8	0.58	0.67	5.9	0.87			110			33			33	29	
1.5	40		116	21	19.5	0.54	0.70	6.0	0.77			105			35			33	25	
2.0	40		124	22	23.2	0.68	0.91	7.3	0.75			103			36			31	23	
2.5	60	204/120	129	28	27.5	0.76	0.89	6.9	0.85	7.43	22	108	92	19	36	34	−2	33	28	0.21
3.0	60		130	29	27.8	0.81	0.90	6.9	0.90			106			38			31	28	
3.5	80		136	27	35.8	1.05	1.06	7.8	0.99			112			35			32	32	
4.0	80	225/123	142	25	38.3	1.17	1.13	8.0	1.04	7.41	21	113	100	17	36	34	−2	31	32	0.17
4.5	100		144	28	42.4	1.25	1.17	8.1	1.07			113			36			32	34	
	Recovery	228/126	149	31	45.3	1.35	1.07	7.2	1.26	7.40	21	113	101	21	36	34	−2	32	40	0.19
	Recovery		135	29	47.9	1.35	1.09	8.1	1.24			121			33			34	42	
	Recovery		123	24	38.1	1.00	0.76	6.2	1.32			121			33			36	47	
	Recovery		120	24	28.5	0.69	0.49	4.1	1.41			124			30			38	54	
	Recovery	183/111	118	26	32.7	0.70	0.45	3.8	1.56	7.41	18	131	120	9	26	29	3	44	68	0.30

Case 34 Patent Ductus Arteriosus

Clinical Findings

This 25-year-old man recently developed exertional dyspnea. He was found to have a patent ductus arteriosus. Cardiac angiography demonstrated normal coronary arteries, a left ventricular ejection fraction of 56%, a large flow from the aorta through the patent ductus to the pulmonary artery, and normal pulmonary artery pressures at rest. The surgeon desired a preoperative cycle ergometer study with a pulmonary artery catheter in place to assess pulmonary artery pressures during exercise. The patient was sent to the exercise laboratory with a right radial artery catheter and pulmonary artery catheter placed via the right subclavian vein. Resting 12-lead ECGs showed left atrial enlargement and left ventricular hypertrophy.

Exercise Findings

The patient performed exercise on a cycle ergometer. He pedaled at 60 rpm without an added load for 3 minutes. The work rate was then increased 15 W per minute to tolerance. Intraarterial pressures were recorded continuously, except when blood was simultaneously sampled every 2 minutes from the systemic and pulmonary arterial catheters. The patient stopped exercise because of calf and thigh fatigue. The patient had no chest pain and no further ECG abnormalities.

Interpretation

Comments

Resting respiratory function studies were normal, with a high-normal DLCO suggestive of an increase in pulmonary capillary blood volume (Table 10.34.1). For the level of $\dot{V}O_2$, the left ventricular output at rest and exercise, as calculated from the Fick equation, was considerably elevated. The exercise systemic blood pressure was high, but the pulmonary artery pressure was normal. The breathing reserve was high, and gas exchange measures were normal.

Analysis

Referring to flowchart 1, peak $\dot{V}O_2$ and the anaerobic threshold are decreased (Table 10.34.2). Proceeding to flowchart 4, the high breathing reserve (branch point 4.1), normal $\dot{V}E/\dot{V}CO_2$ (branch point 4.3), normal hematocrit (branch point 4.4), and low,

unchanging O_2 pulse (branch point 4.6) lead to the diagnosis of heart disease. The ECG does not show evidence of myocardial ischemia, but the low $\Delta\dot{V}O_2/\Delta WR$ and steep HR versus $\dot{V}O_2$ response confirm the presence of cardiovascular dysfunction.

Conclusion

The patient's large left-to-right shunt through the patent ductus arteriosus requires an increased left ventricular output to support the peripheral O_2 requirements. Thus, although the left ventricular output is high, the recirculation of part of it through the lungs deprives the peripheral tissues of the O_2 they need. Thus, the pathophysiology is similar to left ventricular failure, with a low anaerobic threshold and peak $\dot{V}O_2$. In addition, the noninvasively

TABLE 10.34.1.   Selected Respiratory Function Data

Measurement	Predicted	Measured
Age, yr		25
Sex		Male
Height, cm		170
Weight, kg	74	56
Hemoglobin, g/100 ml		14.6
VC, L	4.39	4.27
IC, L	2.93	2.42
TLC, L	5.81	6.62
FEV$_1$, L	3.57	3.62
FEV$_1$/VC, %	81	85
MVV, L/min	156	158
DLCO, ml/mm Hg/min	29.6	35.6

TABLE 10.34.2.   Selected Exercise Data

Measurement	Predicted	Measured
Peak $\dot{V}O_2$, L/min	2.68	1.68
Maximum HR, beats/min	195	166
Maximum O_2 pulse, ml/beat	13.7	10.1
$\Delta\dot{V}O_2/\Delta WR$, ml/min/W	10.3	8.2
AT, L/min	>1.09	1.0
Systemic blood pressure, mmHg (rest, max)		154/70, 228/105
Pulmonary artery pressure, mmHg (rest, max)		20/10, 30/15
Maximum $\dot{V}E$, L/min		54
Exercise breathing reserve, L/min	>15	104
PaO$_2$, mmHg (rest, max ex)		103, 95
P(A − a)O$_2$, mmHg (rest, max ex)		6, 17
P(a − ET)CO$_2$, mmHg (rest, max ex)		0, −3
VD/VT (rest, max ex)		0.39, 0.20
HCO$_3^-$, mEq/L (rest, 2-min recov)		25, 18

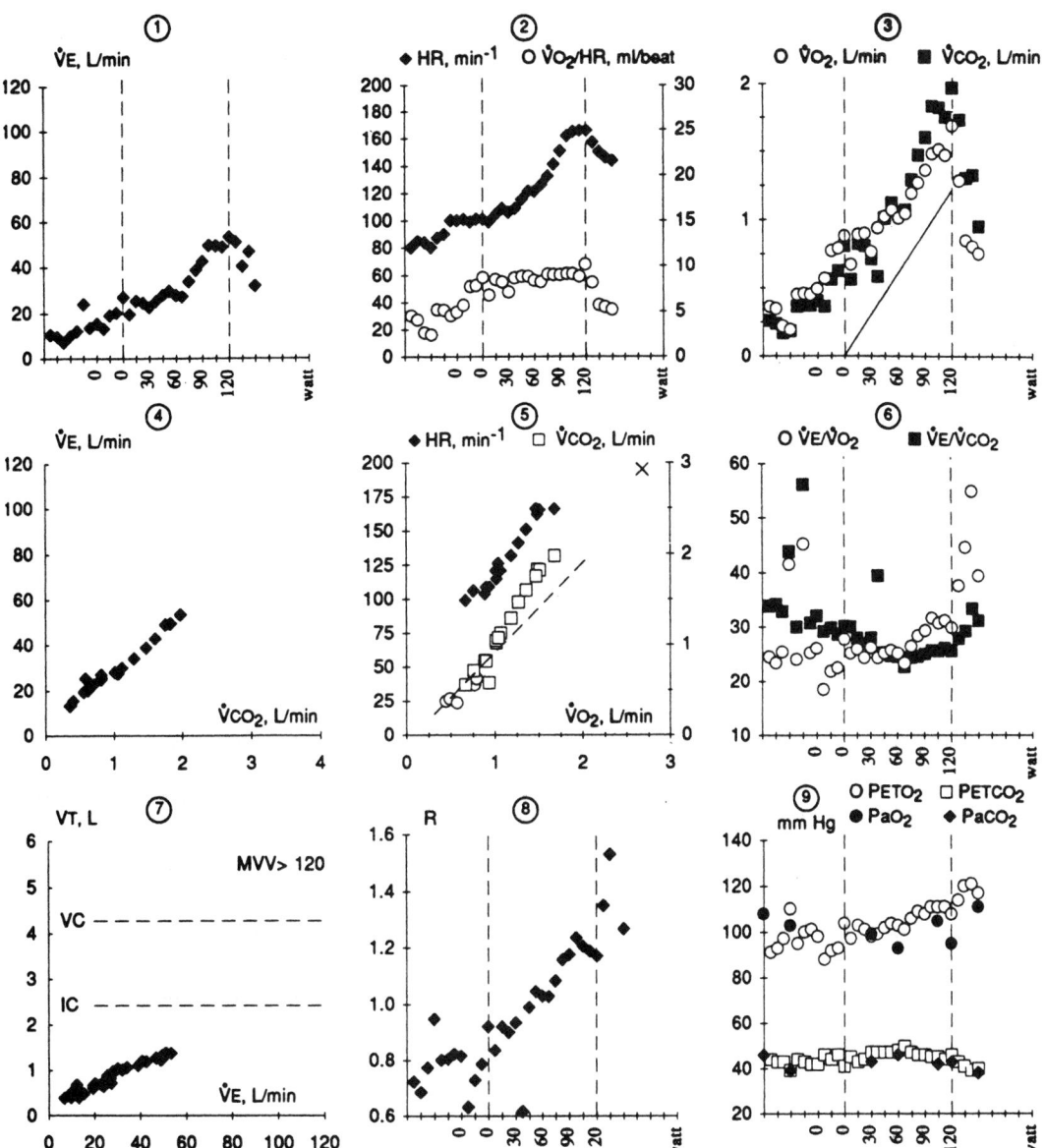

FIGURE 10.34.1.   **1:** Vertical dashed lines in panels 1 to 3 and 6, 8, and 9 indicate the beginning and the end of the increasing work period. **2:** Unloaded cycling is performed for 3 minutes before the left vertical dashed line. **3:** In panel 3, the diagonal line shows the increase of $\dot{V}O_2$ at a slope of 10 ml/min/W. **4:** In panel 5, the diagonal dashed line has a slope of 1; the x in the upper right is the predicted maximum heart rate and $\dot{V}O_2$ for the subject.

measured low and relatively unchanging O_2 pulse throughout incremental exercise indicates that the patient reached a maximum product of stroke volume and arterial–mixed venous O_2 difference early in the exercise study. Presumably, these abnormalities would be corrected by removing the pulmonary steal of systemic blood flow by closing the ductus. Following surgical correction of the patent ductus arteriosus, the patient's dyspnea and exercise tolerance improved considerably.

TABLE 10.34.3.   Air Breathing

Time min	Work rate watts	BP mmHg	HR min⁻¹	f min⁻¹	$\dot{V}_E$ L/min BTPS	$\dot{V}_{CO_2}$ L/min STPD	$\dot{V}_{O_2}$ L/min STPD	$\dot{V}_{O_2}/HR$ ml/beat	R	pH	HCO_3^- meq/L	P_{O_2}, mmHg ET	a	(A−a)	P_{CO_2}, mmHg ET	a	(a−ET)	$\dot{V}_E/\dot{V}_{CO_2}$	$\dot{V}_E/\dot{V}_{O_2}$	V_D/V_T
	Rest	154/69								7.32	23	108			46					
	Rest		80	20	10.5	0.26	0.36	4.5	0.72			91			44			34	24	
	Rest		85	19	9.8	0.24	0.35	4.1	0.69			93			43			34	23	
	Rest		84	18	7.1	0.17	0.22	2.6	0.77			97			43			33	25	
	Rest		80	25	10.0	0.18	0.19	2.4	0.95	7.42	25	110	103	6	39	39	0	44	41	0.39
	Rest	180/87	87	18	12.3	0.36	0.45	5.2	0.80			95			44			30	24	
	Rest		90	37	23.9	0.37	0.46	5.1	0.80			100			43			56	45	
	Unloaded		100	25	13.5	0.37	0.45	4.5	0.82			101			42			31	25	
	Unloaded		100	32	15.5	0.40	0.49	4.9	0.82			98			42			32	26	
	Unloaded		101	33	13.3	0.36	0.57	5.6	0.63			88			46			29	18	
	Unloaded		99	29	19.2	0.56	0.77	7.8	0.73			92			44			30	22	
	Unloaded		101	29	20.2	0.62	0.79	7.8	0.78			93			46			29	22	
	Unloaded		101	33	27.1	0.81	0.88	8.7	0.92			104			41			30	28	
0.5	15		99	32	19.5	0.56	0.67	6.8	0.84			97			45			30	25	
1.0	15		104	29	25.4	0.82	0.89	8.6	0.92			103			43			28	26	
1.5	30		109	33	24.7	0.81	0.90	8.3	0.90			101			44			27	24	
2.0	30	222/102	106	33	22.7	0.71	0.76	7.2	0.93	7.39	26	98	99	6	47	43	−4	28	26	0.25
2.5	45		109	30	25.4	0.58	0.94	8.6	0.62			99			47			39	24	
3.0	45		115	29	28.0	1.01	1.02	8.9	0.99			102			47			25	25	
3.5	60		121	29	30.0	1.12	1.07	8.8	1.05			104			47			25	26	
4.0	60	231/96	121	30	27.9	1.04	1.01	8.3	1.03	7.35	25	103	93	12	48	46	−2	24	25	0.21
4.5	75		126	38	27.4	1.07	1.04	8.3	1.03			101			50			23	23	
5.0	75		132	32	34.1	1.29	1.19	9.0	1.08			106			47			24	26	
5.5	90		141	35	38.9	1.47	1.27	9.0	1.16			109			46			24	28	
6.0	90		151	36	42.8	1.60	1.36	9.0	1.18			108			46			25	29	
6.5	105		162	37	49.8	1.83	1.48	9.1	1.24			111			45			25	32	
7.0	105	246/108	165	40	49.6	1.82	1.51	9.2	1.21	7.34	22	111	105	9	45	42	−3	25	31	0.18
7.5	120		166	40	49.0	1.75	1.47	8.9	1.19			111			44			26	31	
8.0	120	228/105	166	39	53.5	1.97	1.68	10.1	1.17	7.30	21	108	95	17	46	43	−3	25	30	0.20
	Recovery		157	37	51.1	1.73	1.28	8.2	1.35			114			43			28	37	
	Recovery		150	34	40.8	1.30	0.85	5.7	1.53			120			41			29	45	
	Recovery		146	37	47.0	1.32	0.80	5.5	1.65			121			39			33	55	
	Recovery	171/90	144	32	32.2	0.95	0.75	5.2	1.27	7.29	18	117	111	7	40	38	−2	31	39	0.25

Case 35 Vasoregulatory Asthenia

Clinical Findings

This 31-year-old woman was referred for exercise testing because of insidious and progressive fatigability of 10 months' duration. She had formerly been active as a homemaker, had worked frequent 12-hour shifts as a nurse in the intensive care unit, and had done 2 to 3 hours of vigorous exercise daily. At this time, she recognized dyspnea on walking two blocks and often experienced rapid, forceful palpitations with exertion or emotion. Her sleep requirements had increased markedly and she had gained 17 pounds. She frequently woke from sleep diaphoretic and with palpitations, but did not snore. She had had hypertension only during her two pregnancies. She did not smoke or use drugs. Workup elsewhere revealed a normal physical examination, chest roentgenograms, ECG, spirometry, echocardiograms, ejection fraction, resting blood gases, and thyroid function. Exercise studies elsewhere, including cardiac catheterization, showed tachycardia, normal ear oximetry, normal right- and left-sided arterial pressures, and a high mixed venous P_{O_2} during exercise. Examination here revealed a healthy-looking, animated woman with resting tachycardia and normal peripheral pulses. The oxyhemoglobin dissociation curve was normal, as assessed by measuring the P_{50}.

Exercise Findings

The patient performed exercise on a cycle ergometer. She pedaled at 60 rpm without an added load for 3 minutes. The work rate was then increased 15 W per minute to tolerance. Heart rate and rhythm were continuously monitored; 12-lead ECGs were obtained during rest, exercise, and recovery. Blood pressure was measured with a sphygmomanometer, and oxygen saturation with an ear oximeter. The patient appeared to give an excellent effort and stopped exercise because of generalized and thigh fatigue. She denied chest pain during or after the study. No arrhythmias or ischemic changes were noted on ECGs.

Interpretation

Comments

Resting respiratory function studies were better than average (Table 10.35.1).

Analysis

Referring to flowchart 1, the peak $\dot{V}_{O_2}$ is normal for a sedentary person (which this patient is not), but the anaerobic threshold is low (Table 10.35.2). We are directed through branch points 1.1, 1.2, and 1.3 to flowchart 4. The breathing reserve was high (branch point 4.1). The $\dot{V}_E/\dot{V}_{CO_2}$ at the anaerobic threshold is borderline elevated, but the P_{ETCO_2} is reduced, suggesting hyperventilation. If we take the normal branch for $\dot{V}_E/\dot{V}_{CO_2}$ at the AT, we go to the diagnosis labeled "O_2 flow problem of nonpulmonary origin." We are moderately confident that the patient does not have appreciable widening of the $P(A - a)_{O_2}$ because of the normal ear oximetry. The hematocrit is normal (branch point 4.4). The O_2 pulse is not low and nonchanging (branch point 4.6), leading us to the diagnosis of peripheral arterial disease. This diagnosis does not fit the patient well, considering her resting tachycardia, negative heart rate reserve, absence of hypertension, and good peripheral pulses.

TABLE 10.35.1.   Selected Respiratory Function Data

Measurement	Predicted	Measured
Age, yr		31
Sex		Female
Height, cm		167
Weight, kg	66	63
Hematocrit, %		40
VC, L	3.75	4.81
IC, L	2.50	3.34
TLC, L	5.51	6.64
FEV$_1$, L	3.08	4.27
FEV$_1$/VC, %	82	89
MVV, L/min	116	146
D$_L$CO, ml/mm Hg/min	27.1	28.8

TABLE 10.35.2.   Selected Exercise Data

Measurement	Predicted	Measured
Peak $\dot{V}_{O_2}$, L/min	1.88	1.73
Maximum HR, beats/min	189	195
Maximum O_2 pulse, ml/beat	10.1	8.9
$\Delta\dot{V}_{O_2}/\Delta$WR, ml/min/W	10.3	10.3
AT, L/min	>0.86	0.8
Blood pressure, mmHg (rest, max)		155/90, 155/90
Maximum $\dot{V}_E$, L/min		67
Exercise breathing reserve, L/min	>15	79
O_2 saturation, oximeter (rest, max)		99, 100

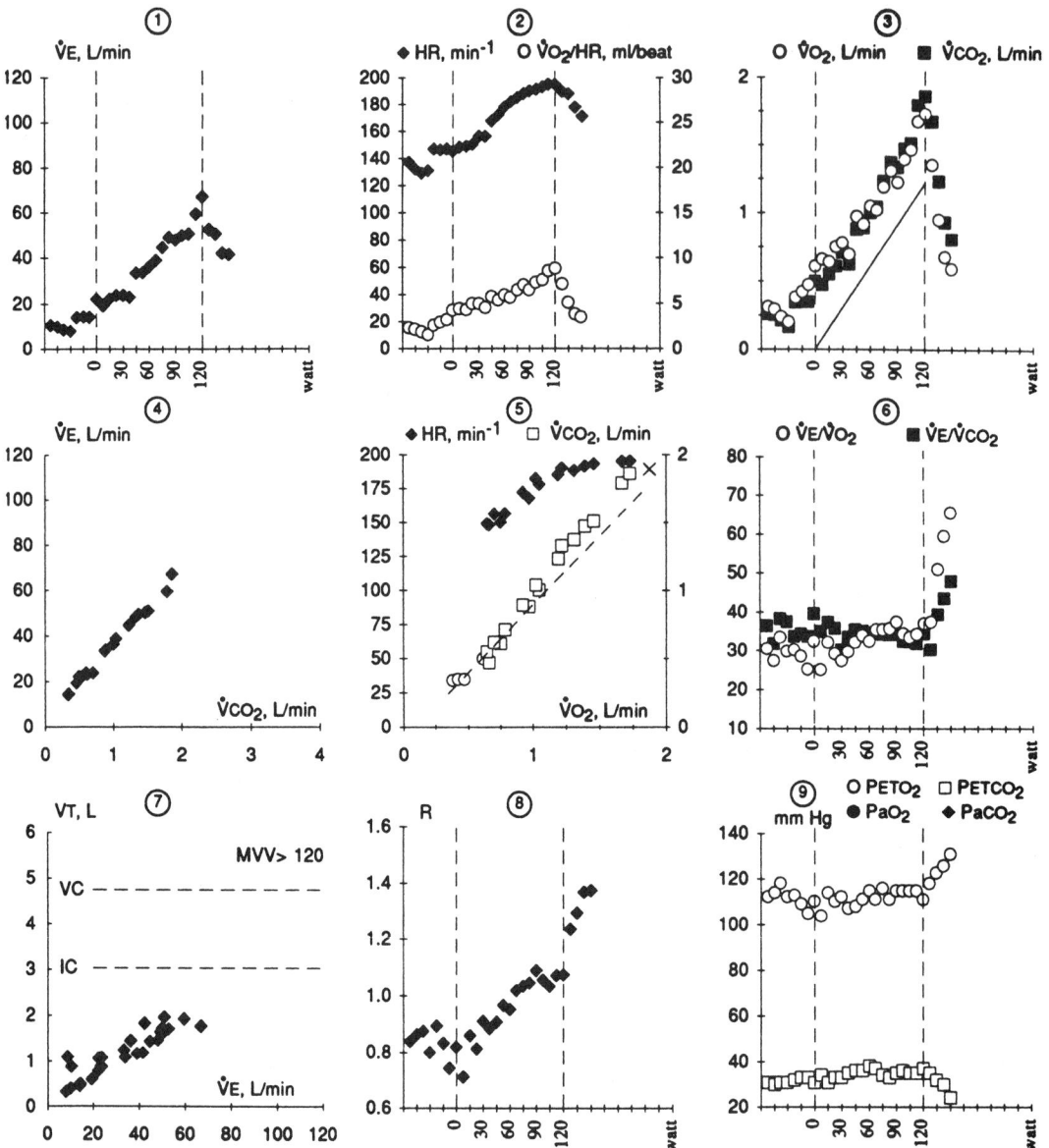

FIGURE 10.35.1.   **1:** Vertical dashed lines in panels 1 to 3 and 6, 8, and 9 indicate the beginning and the end of the increasing work period. **2:** Unloaded cycling is performed for 3 minutes before the left vertical dashed line. **3:** In panel 3, the diagonal line shows the increase of $\dot{V}O_2$ at a slope of 10 ml/min/W. **4:** In panel 5, the diagonal dashed line has a slope of 1; the *x* in the upper right is the predicted maximum heart rate and $\dot{V}O_2$ for the subject.

Exploring further, she does not fit the diagnosis of anemia or heart disease, but she does have a steep HR versus $\dot{V}O_2$ relationship and a low heart rate reserve. Knowing from prior studies that she did not have a low mixed venous P_{O_2} during heavy exercise, we can presume that the exercising muscles have difficulty extracting oxygen from their capillaries. These findings fit the diagnosis of vasoregulatory asthenia (1–3), which appears to be characterized by an inability to vasodilate the exercising muscle vascular beds and to vasoconstrict nonexercising organs. This may represent a specific defect in the autonomic nervous system.

Conclusion

The patient's findings were consistent with vasoregulatory asthenia, but follow-up evaluation was recommended. The patient was placed on a physical training program with some objective and subjective improvement in exercise tolerance, but there was no improvement with β-adrenergic blockade.

TABLE 10.35.3.   Air Breathing

Time min	Work rate watts	BP mmHg	HR min⁻¹	f min⁻¹	$\dot{V}_E$ L/min BTPS	$\dot{V}_{CO_2}$ L/min STPD	$\dot{V}_{O_2}$ L/min STPD	$\dot{V}_{O_2}$/HR ml/beat	R	pH	HCO₃⁻ meq/L	P_{O_2}, mmHg ET	a	(A – a)	P_{CO_2}, mmHg ET	a	(a – ET)	$\dot{V}_E/\dot{V}_{CO_2}$	$\dot{V}_E/\dot{V}_{O_2}$	V_D/V_T
	Rest	115/90	137	12	10.5	0.26	0.31	2.3	0.84			112			31			36	31	
	Rest		132	25	10.1	0.25	0.29	2.2	0.86			114			30			32	28	
	Rest		129	8	8.7	0.21	0.24	1.9	0.88			118			31			38	33	
	Rest		131	25	8.1	0.16	0.20	1.5	0.80			112			31			37	30	
	Unloaded		147	31	14.1	0.34	0.38	2.6	0.89			113			32			34	30	
	Unloaded		146	29	14.5	0.35	0.42	2.9	0.83			109			33			34	29	
	Unloaded		147	28	14.2	0.35	0.47	3.2	0.74			105			33			34	25	
	Unloaded	140/95	145	28	22.1	0.50	0.61	4.2	0.82			110			31			39	32	
0.5	15		148	32	19.2	0.47	0.66	4.5	0.71			104			34			35	25	
1.0	15		149	21	22.3	0.55	0.64	4.3	0.86			114			31			37	32	
1.5	30		150	22	23.7	0.61	0.75	5.0	0.81			110			33			36	29	
2.0	30		156	27	23.7	0.71	0.78	5.0	0.91			112			33			30	27	
2.5	45		156	26	23.0	0.62	0.70	4.5	0.89			107			35			34	30	
3.0	45		166	27	33.4	0.88	0.97	5.8	0.91			108			36			35	32	
3.5	60		172	31	33.8	0.89	0.92	5.3	0.97			111			36			35	34	
4.0	60	155/90	178	25	36.3	1.00	1.05	5.9	0.95			115			38			34	33	
4.5	75		182	33	38.9	1.04	1.02	5.6	1.02			111			37			35	35	
5.0	75		185	31	44.7	1.23	1.19	6.4	1.03			116			34			34	35	
5.5	90		188	30	49.2	1.37	1.31	7.0	1.05			111			33			34	36	
6.0	90		190	33	48.2	1.33	1.22	6.4	1.09			115			35			34	37	
6.5	105		191	29	50.1	1.47	1.39	7.3	1.06			115			36			32	34	
7.0	105		193	26	51.0	1.51	1.46	7.6	1.03			115			35			32	33	
7.5	120		195	31	59.7	1.79	1.67	8.6	1.07			115			35			32	34	
8.0	120		195	38	67.1	1.86	1.73	8.9	1.08			111			37			34	37	
	Recovery		190	31	53.0	1.67	1.35	7.1	1.24			118			35			30	37	
	Recovery		188	31	50.9	1.23	0.95	5.1	1.29			123			32			39	51	
	Recovery		178	23	42.3	0.93	0.68	3.8	1.37			126			30			43	59	
	Recovery	125/60	171	35	41.6	0.81	0.59	3.5	1.37			131			24			48	65	

Because the pathophysiologic mechanisms underlying vasoregulatory asthenia are unclear, a subsequent exercise test was performed in which serial venous blood samples were drawn. Blood lactate levels were markedly increased during exercise (reaching a peak of 8.2 mEq/L), ruling out McArdle's syndrome (4) as the cause of her exercise intolerance. Other muscle disorders (e.g., electron transport chain defects) were not excluded, however (5,6). This disorder may be due to autonomic dysfunction of the peripheral circulation (1–3).

References

1. Holmgren A, Jonsson B, Levander M, et al. Low physical work capacity in suspected heart cases due to inadequate adjustment of peripheral blood flow (vasoregulatory asthenia). *Acta Med Scand* 1957;158:413–436.
2. Holmgren A, Jonsson B, Levander M, et al. Physical training of patients with vasoregulatory asthenia. *Acta Med Scand* 1957;158:437–446.
3. Gillum RF, Teichholz LE, Herman MV, et al. The idiopathic hyperkinetic heart syndrome: clinical course and long-term prognosis. *Am Heart J* 1981;102:728–734.
4. McArdle B. Myopathy due to a defect in muscle glycogen breakdown. *Clin Sci* 1951;10:13–18.
5. Carroll JE, Hagberg JH, Brooke MH, et al. Bicycle ergometry and gas exchange measurements in neuromuscular diseases. *Arch Neurol* 1979;36:457–461.
6. DiMauro S, Bonilla E, Zevina M, et al. Mitochondrial myopathies. *Ann Neurol* 1985;17:521–538.

Case 36 Mild Chronic Bronchitis with Normal Exercise Performance

Clinical Findings

This 55-year-old shipyard worker complained of dyspnea after walking up one flight of stairs or a few blocks on a level surface. He had had morning cough several months of each year and had noted occasional retrosternal pain unrelated to exertion or emotional upset. He had 35 pack-years of smoking until stopping 12 years ago. He exercised regularly. The physical examination was normal except for mild obesity. Chest roentgenographic studies showed bilateral pleural thickening in the midlung zones and old granulomatous disease in the right upper lobe. Resting ECG was normal.

Exercise Findings

The patient performed exercise on a cycle ergometer. He first pedaled at 60 rpm without added load for 3 minutes. The work rate was then increased 20 W per minute to his symptom-limited maximum. Arterial blood was sampled every second minute, and intraarterial blood pressure was recorded from a percutaneously placed brachial artery catheter. The patient stopped exercise because of "exhaustion." The ECG remained normal throughout exercise.

Interpretation

Comments

Resting respiratory function is compatible with mild airflow obstruction (Table 10.36.1). The resting ECG is normal.

Analysis

Referring to flowchart 1, the peak oxygen uptake and anaerobic threshold are normal (Table 10.36.2). Referring to flowchart 2, arterial blood gases and ECG at peak $\dot{V}_{CO_2}$ are normal (branch point 2.1).

The patient is about 14% overweight (branch point 2.2). This is not a serious obesity problem but does contribute to the additional metabolic cost of work. The patient also has mild airflow obstruction, causing a characteristic obstructive pattern at high exercise levels.

Conclusion

This study illustrates normal exercise performance in a mildly obese man with airflow obstruction.

TABLE 10.36.1. Selected Respiratory Function Data

Measurement	Predicted	Measured
Age, yr		54
Sex		Male
Height, cm		174
Weight, kg	77	88
Hematocrit, %		45
VC, L	4.28	3.59
IC, L	2.86	3.12
TLC, L	6.38	6.15
FEV_1, L	3.39	2.40
FEV_1/VC, %	79	67
MVV, L/min	142	112
$D_{L}CO$, ml/mm Hg/min	28.8	29.8

TABLE 10.36.2. Selected Exercise Data

Measurement	Predicted	Measured
Peak $\dot{V}_{O_2}$, L/min	2.42	2.66
Maximum HR, beats/min	166	169
Maximum O_2 pulse, ml/beat	14.6	15.7
$\Delta\dot{V}_{O_2}/\Delta WR$, ml/min/W	10.3	9.9
AT, L/min	>1.04	1.3
Blood pressure, mmHg (rest, max)		144/93, 225/117
Maximum $\dot{V}_E$, L/min		86
Exercise breathing reserve, L/min	>15	26
Pa_{O_2}, mmHg (rest, max ex)		81, 92
$P(A - a)_{O_2}$, mmHg (rest, max ex)		18, 21
$P(a - ET)_{CO_2}$, mmHg (rest, max ex)		5, −3
V_D/V_T (rest, heavy ex)		0.41, 0.23
HCO_3^-, mEq/L (rest, 2-min recov)		26, 16

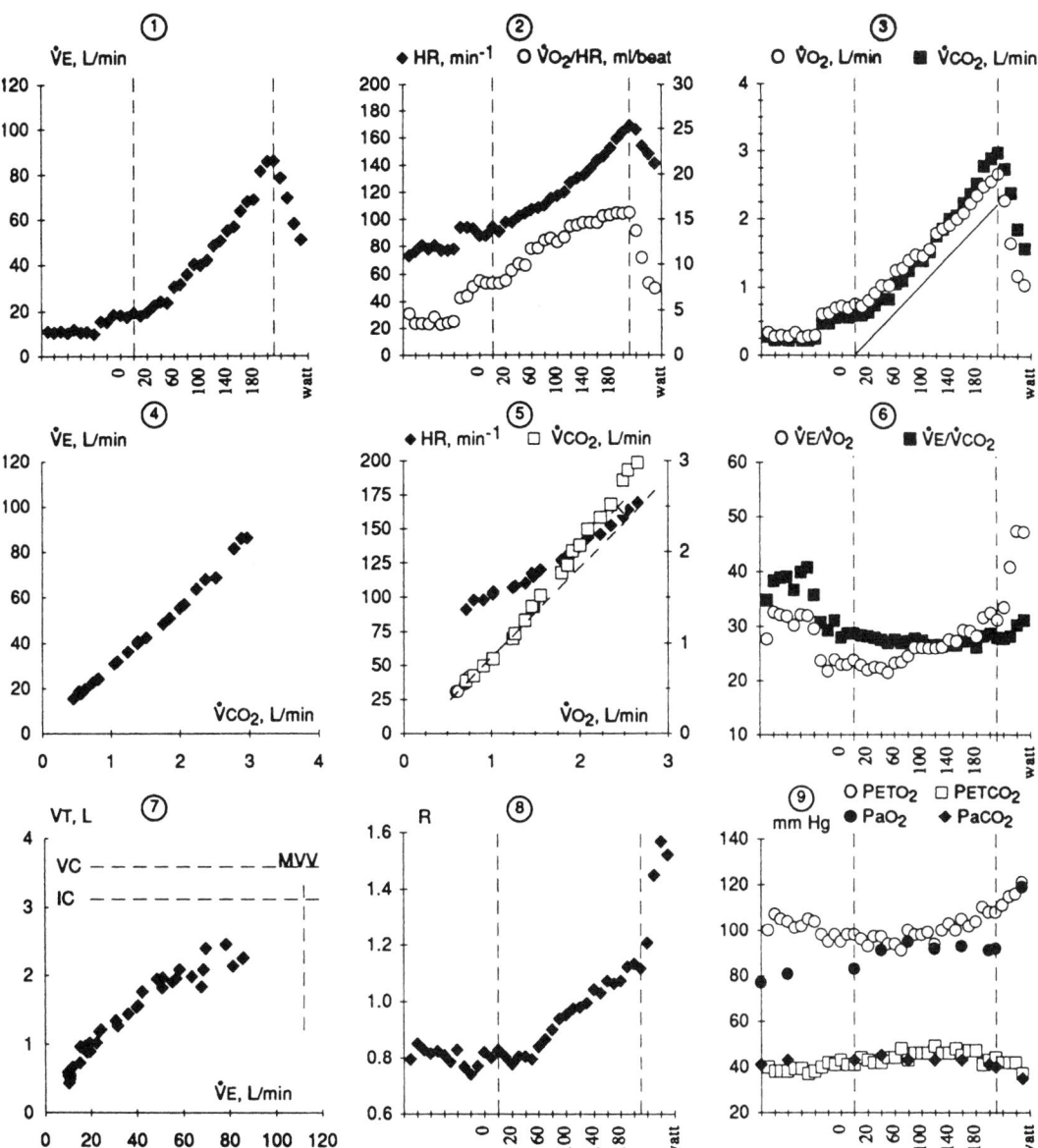

FIGURE 10.36.1.   **1:** Vertical dashed lines in panels 1 to 3 and 6, 8, and 9 indicate the beginning and the end of the increasing work period. **2:** Unloaded cycling is performed for 3 minutes before the left vertical dashed line. **3:** In panel 3, the diagonal line shows the increase of $\dot{V}_{O_2}$ at a slope of 10 ml/min/W. **4:** In panel 5, the diagonal dashed line has a slope of 1; the *x* in the upper right is the predicted maximum heart rate and $\dot{V}_{O_2}$ for the subject.

TABLE 10.36.3. Air Breathing

Time min	Work rate watts	BP mmHg	HR min⁻¹	f min⁻¹	$\dot{V}_E$ L/min BTPS	$\dot{V}_{CO_2}$ L/min STPD	$\dot{V}_{O_2}$ L/min STPD	$\dot{V}_{O_2}$/HR ml/beat	R	pH	HCO_3^- meq/L	P_{O_2}, mmHg ET	a	(A − a)	P_{CO_2}, mmHg ET	a	(a − ET)	$\dot{V}_E/\dot{V}_{CO_2}$	$\dot{V}_E/\dot{V}_{O_2}$	V_D/V_T
	Rest	141/93								7.42	26		77			41				
	Rest		73	20	11.1	0.27	0.34	4.7	0.79			100			40			35	28	
	Rest		76	20	10.5	0.23	0.27	3.6	0.85			107			38			38	33	
	Rest		81	21	11.1	0.24	0.29	3.6	0.83			105			38			39	32	
	Rest	144/90	78	19	10.2	0.22	0.27	3.5	0.81	7.40	26	104	81	18	38	43	5	39	32	0.41
	Rest		81	18	11.8	0.28	0.34	4.2	0.82			101			39			37	30	
	Rest		77	24	10.4	0.21	0.26	3.4	0.81			102			39			40	32	
	Rest		77	22	10.8	0.22	0.28	3.6	0.79			105			37			41	32	
	Rest		78	17	10.0	0.24	0.29	3.7	0.83			104			38			36	30	
	Unloaded		94	16	15.5	0.46	0.60	6.4	0.77			98			40			31	24	
	Unloaded		94	21	15.2	0.46	0.62	6.6	0.74			95			42			29	22	
	Unloaded		93	21	18.5	0.54	0.70	7.5	0.77			98			41			31	24	
	Unloaded		88	20	18.2	0.59	0.72	8.2	0.82			95			43			28	23	
	Unloaded		88	18	17.6	0.56	0.70	8.0	0.80			98			41			29	23	
	Unloaded	162/99	94	19	19.4	0.62	0.75	8.0	0.83	7.39	26	98	83	17	41	43	2	29	24	0.28
0.5	20		91	19	18.0	0.58	0.72	7.9	0.81			96			44			28	23	
1.0	20		98	22	19.6	0.63	0.81	8.3	0.78			93			43			28	22	
1.5	40		98	22	22.5	0.74	0.92	9.4	0.80			97			42			28	22	
2.0	40	174/96	102	20	24.3	0.82	1.02	10.0	0.80	7.37	26	97	91	5	42	45	3	28	22	0.28
2.5	60		104	20	23.8	0.82	1.03	9.9	0.80			94			44			27	21	
3.0	60		107	23	30.9	1.05	1.25	11.7	0.84			94			44			28	23	
3.5	80		108	25	31.8	1.10	1.27	11.8	0.87			91			48			27	23	
4.0	80	174/93	110	25	36.1	1.25	1.39	12.6	0.90	7.37	24	100	95	8	43	43	0	27	24	0.25
4.5	100		115	26	40.6	1.39	1.48	12.9	0.94			98			46			28	26	
5.0	100		117	26	40.1	1.39	1.46	12.5	0.95			98			46			27	26	
5.5	120		120	24	42.4	1.52	1.56	13.0	0.97			99			46			27	26	
6.0	120	204/99	127	25	48.7	1.76	1.80	14.2	0.98	7.36	24	94	92	14	49	43	−6	26	26	0.23
6.5	140		130	28	51.0	1.85	1.86	14.3	0.99			100			46			26	26	
7.0	140		132	29	55.4	2.00	1.92	14.5	1.04			103			46			26	28	
7.5	160		137	29	56.9	2.06	2.00	14.6	1.03			100			48			26	27	
8.0	160	210/105	143	32	63.7	2.24	2.09	14.6	1.07	7.35	23	105	93	16	45	43	−2	27	29	0.25
8.5	180		146	37	67.9	2.37	2.23	15.3	1.06			102			47			27	29	
9.0	180		152	33	68.8	2.52	2.35	15.5	1.07			104			47			26	28	
9.5	200		159	38	81.4	2.78	2.48	15.6	1.12			110			41			28	32	
10.0	200	228/114	164	38	85.7	2.89	2.55	15.5	1.13	7.33	21	108	91	22	43	41	−2	29	32	0.25
10.5	220	225/117	169	38	86.0	2.97	2.66	15.7	1.12	7.31	20	108	92	21	44	40	−4	28	31	0.22
	Recovery		166	32	78.5	2.74	2.27	13.7	1.21			111			42			28	33	
	Recovery		154	29	69.7	2.39	1.65	10.7	1.45			115			42			28	41	
	Recovery		148	28	58.3	1.85	1.18	8.0	1.57			116			42			30	47	
	Recovery	183/96	141	26	51.2	1.58	1.04	7.4	1.52	7.27	16	121	119	5	37	35	−2	31	47	0.20

Case 37 Chronic Bronchitis and Obesity

Clinical Findings

This 69-year-old former shipyard worker had first noted dyspnea on exertion 16 years earlier, later accompanied by cough, sputum production, and frequent wheezing. He had been receiving bronchodilators and antibiotics intermittently for 16 years. Physical examination revealed obesity, bilaterally decreased breath sounds, and some expiratory wheezes. There was no evidence of cardiovascular disease. Chest roentgenographic study revealed moderate pleural thickening bilaterally and scattered parenchymal calcifications compatible with inactive granulomatous disease. The heart was not enlarged. The ECG was compatible with left atrial enlargement and left ventricular hypertrophy. He admitted to a 15 pack-year history of cigarette smoking.

Exercise Findings

The patient performed exercise on a cycle ergometer. He pedaled at 60 rpm without added load for 3 minutes. The work rate was then increased 10 W per minute to his symptom-limited maximum. Arterial blood was sampled every second minute, and intraarterial blood pressure was recorded from a percutaneously placed brachial artery catheter. The patient stopped exercising complaining of shortness of breath and chest tightness. There were no ST-segment changes or arrhythmia.

Interpretation

Comments

Respiratory function studies indicate that this patient has a moderate obstructive defect (Table 10.37.1). The ECG is interpreted to demonstrate left ventricular hypertrophy and left atrial enlargement.

Analysis

Referring to flowchart 1, peak $\dot{V}O_2$ is low and anaerobic threshold is normal (Table 10.37.2). Proceeding to flowchart 3, the breathing reserve is low

(branch point 3.1), suggesting that lung disease accounts for this patient's reduced exercise performance. Supporting this is the finding that the indices of ventilation–perfusion matching [V_D/V_T, $P(A - a)O_2$, and $P(a - ET)CO_2$] are abnormal and the heart rate reserve is high.

The actual maximum work rate performed by the patient is quite low, despite a mildly reduced peak $\dot{V}O_2$, because the patient has an exceptionally high oxygen cost for unloaded cycling ($\dot{V}O_2 = 0.85$ L/ min). This is most likely due to his obesity (added metabolic cost of moving his lower extremities). The fall

TABLE 10.37.1.   Selected Respiratory Function Data

Measurement	Predicted	Measured
Age, yr		69
Sex		Male
Height, cm		166
Weight, kg	70	98
Hematocrit, %		45
VC, L	3.31	2.91 (2.15*)
IC, L	2.21	2.35 (1.89*)
TLC, L	5.38	7.32
FEV_1, L	2.55	1.47 (1.30*)
FEV_1/VC, %	77	51 (60*)
MVV, L/min	112	56 (44*)
D_LCO, ml/mm Hg/min	22.6	26.0

*On day of exercise study

TABLE 10.37.2.   Selected Exercise Data

Measurement	Predicted	Measured
Peak $\dot{V}O_2$, L/min	1.93	1.50
Maximum HR, beats/min	151	125
Maximum O_2 pulse, ml/beat	12.8	12.0
$\Delta\dot{V}O_2/\Delta WR$, ml/min/W	10.3	10.4
AT, L/min	>0.87	1.35
Blood pressure, mmHg (rest, max)		142/72, 234/99
Maximum $\dot{V}E$, L/min		55
Exercise breathing reserve, L/min	>15	1
PaO_2, mmHg (rest, max ex)		73, 92
$P(A - a)O_2$, mmHg (rest, max ex)		32, 17
$P(a - ET)CO_2$, mmHg (rest, max ex)		6, 1
V_D/V_T (rest, heavy ex)		0.40, 0.35
HCO_3^-, mEq/L (rest, 2-min recov)		26, 22

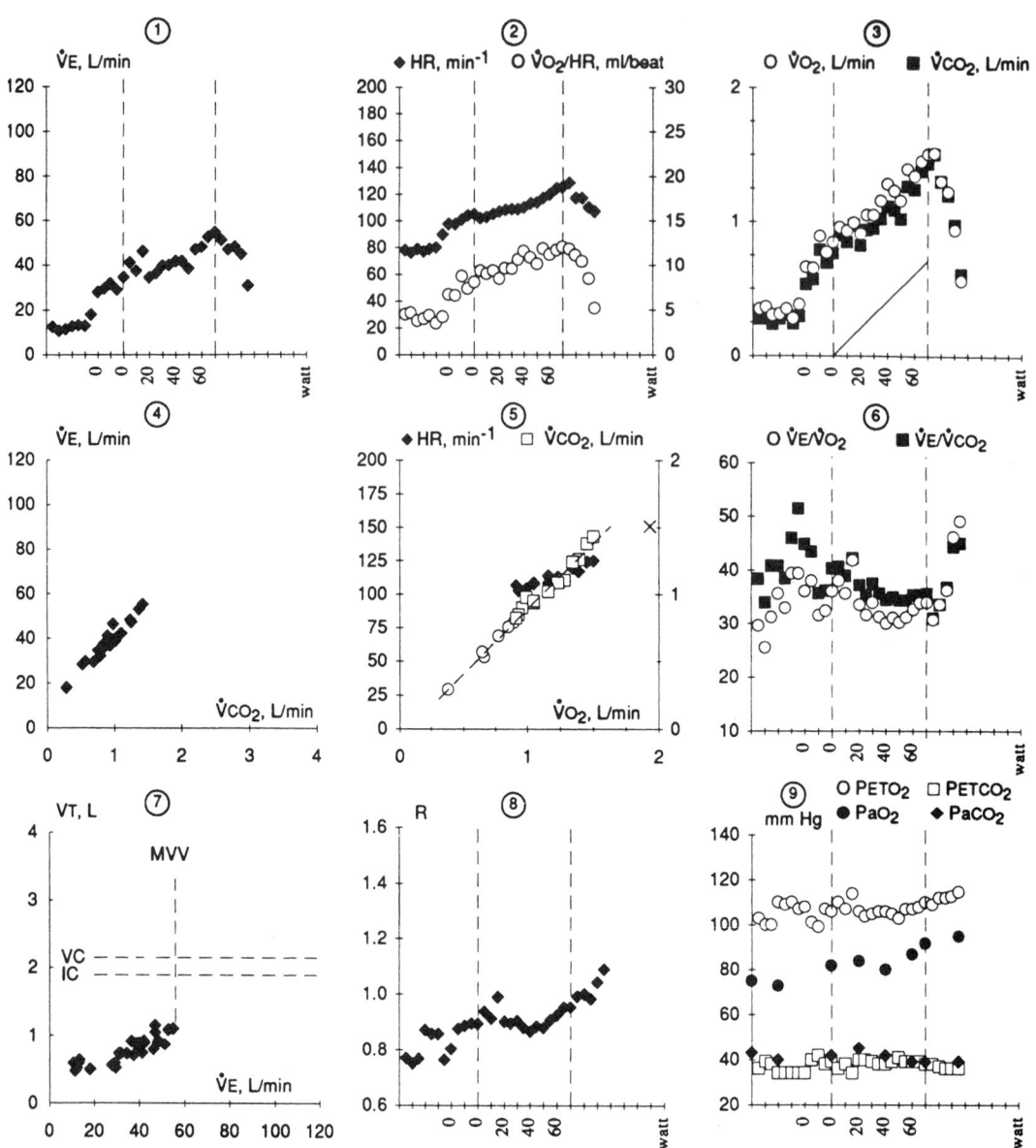

FIGURE 10.37.1.   **1:** Vertical dashed lines in panels 1 to 3 and 6, 8, and 9 indicate the beginning and the end of the increasing work period. **2:** Unloaded cycling is performed for 3 minutes before the left vertical dashed line. **3:** In panel 3, the diagonal line shows the increase of $\dot{V}O_2$ at a slope of 10 ml/min/W. **4:** In panel 5, the diagonal dashed line has a slope of 1; the x in the upper right is the predicted maximum heart rate and $\dot{V}O_2$ for the subject.

in $P(A - a)O_2$ and rise in PaO_2 when changing activity from rest to exercise suggest that the resting hypoxemia in this patient is attributable to obesity-related basilar microatelectasis at rest that disappears with the increased ventilation accompanying exercise.

The elevated dead space fraction of the tidal volume (VD/VT) and high metabolic cost of exercise caused by obesity, combined with mechanical limitation to breathing due to obstructive lung disease, are all potential contributors to exertional dyspnea.

Evidence against primary heart disease causing this patient's symptom is the absence of myocardial ischemia on the 12-lead ECG, the high heart rate reserve at maximum exercise, the normal anaerobic threshold, and the normal $\Delta\dot{V}O_2/\Delta WR$.

Conclusion

Exertional dyspnea is secondary to moderate obstructive lung disease and obesity in this patient.

TABLE 10.37.3.   Air Breathing

Time min	Work rate watts	BP mmHg	HR min⁻¹	f min⁻¹	$\dot{V}_E$ L/min BTPS	$\dot{V}_{CO_2}$ L/min STPD	$\dot{V}_{O_2}$ L/min STPD	$\dot{V}_{O_2}$/HR ml/beat	R	pH	HCO₃⁻ meq/L	ET	PO₂ a	(A−a)	ET	PCO₂ a	(a−ET)	$\dot{V}_E/\dot{V}_{CO_2}$	$\dot{V}_E/\dot{V}_{O_2}$	VD/VT
	Rest	142/72								7.40	26		75			43				
	Rest		78	24	12.4	0.27	0.35	4.5	0.77			103			36			38	30	
	Rest		76	18	10.7	0.27	0.36	4.7	0.75			100			39			34	25	
	Rest		79	24	11.4	0.23	0.30	3.8	0.77			100			38			41	31	
	Rest	156/81	77	21	12.8	0.27	0.31	4.0	0.87	7.42	25	110	73	32	34	40	6	41	36	0.41
	Rest		79	21	13.3	0.30	0.35	4.4	0.86			109			34			38	33	
	Rest		80	22	12.9	0.24	0.28	3.5	0.86			110			34			46	39	
	Unloaded		90	36	18.0	0.29	0.38	4.2	0.76			107			34			52	39	
	Unloaded		98	50	28.0	0.53	0.66	6.7	0.80			108			34			45	36	
	Unloaded		98	56	29.5	0.57	0.65	6.6	0.88			101			40			43	38	
	Unloaded		101	43	31.8	0.79	0.89	8.8	0.89			99			42			36	32	
	Unloaded		104	49	29.1	0.69	0.77	7.4	0.90			107			38			36	32	
	Unloaded	198/93	105	47	34.6	0.76	0.85	8.1	0.89	7.40	26	106	82	22	39	42	3	40	36	0.43
0.5	10		102	55	41.2	0.90	0.96	9.4	0.94			110			36			41	38	
1.0	10		103	53	37.6	0.85	0.93	9.0	0.91			107			38			39	36	
1.5	20		105	58	46.3	0.98	0.99	9.4	0.99			114			34			42	42	
2.0	20	204/87	107	47	34.5	0.82	0.91	8.5	0.90	7.37	26	106	84	17	40	45	5	37	34	0.43
2.5	30		108	40	36.6	0.94	1.05	9.7	0.90			104			40			35	32	
3.0	30		109	50	39.8	0.95	1.05	9.6	0.90			105			39			37	34	
3.5	40		109	45	40.1	1.02	1.16	10.6	0.88			106			38			36	31	
4.0	40	207/87	110	46	42.2	1.11	1.28	11.6	0.87	7.38	24	106	80	23	38	42	4	34	30	0.37
4.5	50		113	47	42.1	1.09	1.23	10.9	0.89			105			39			35	31	
5.0	50		114	44	38.7	1.02	1.16	10.2	0.88			103			41			34	30	
5.5	60		117	45	47.1	1.26	1.39	11.9	0.91			107			39			34	31	
6.0	60	219/90	120	54	48.3	1.24	1.34	11.2	0.93	7.38	23	107	87	22	39	39	0	35	33	0.34
6.5	70		124	49	53.0	1.38	1.45	11.7	0.95			108			39			35	34	
7.0	70	234/99	125	50	55.0	1.43	1.50	12.0	0.95	7.37	32	110	92	17	38	39	1	35	34	0.35
	Recovery		128	59	51.3	1.50	1.51	11.8	0.99			109			38			31	31	
	Recovery		117	41	47.1	1.30	1.30	11.1	1.00			112			37			34	34	
	Recovery		117	52	48.5	1.20	1.22	10.4	0.98			112			36			37	36	
	Recovery		110	51	45.1	0.98	0.94	8.5	1.04			113			36			42	43	
	Recovery	204/84	107	42	31.0	0.61	0.56	5.2	1.09	7.37	22	115	95	19	36	39	3	45	49	0.45

Case 38 Chronic Bronchitis, Cigarette Smoking, and Obesity

Clinical Findings

This 50-year-old shipyard worker was referred for evaluation. He had a 65 pack-year history of smoking and had complained of shortness of breath and frequent chest colds with cough and sputum production for the last 7 years. He had been told that he had borderline hypertension but took no medications for this or his pulmonary symptoms. Examination was normal except for obesity, blood pressure of 140/100, and expiratory wheezes on forced expiration. Chest roentgenograms showed focal pleural plaques.

Exercise Findings

The patient performed exercise on a cycle ergometer. He pedaled at 60 rpm without added load for 3 minutes. The work rate was then increased 20 W per minute to his symptom-limited maximum. Arterial blood was sampled every second minute, and intraarterial blood pressure was recorded from a percutaneously placed brachial artery catheter. Resting carboxyhemoglobin level was 9.4%. He stopped exercise complaining of shortness of breath. After exercise, while sitting quietly on the cycle, he became lightheaded and hypotensive. He was put in the supine position and his legs elevated; this provided immediate relief of his lightheadedness and return of his systemic blood pressure to preexercise levels. Resting, exercise, and recovery ECGs showed no abnormalities.

Interpretation

Comments

Resting respiratory function studies reveal mild airflow obstruction that improves following treatment with an aerosolized bronchodilator (Table 10.38.1). The patient is 36 kg overweight. His resting carboxyhemoglobin is 9.4% (normal < 2.0%). The patient's resting ECG is normal. This case is also presented because of the orthostasis that the patient developed when stopping exercise; this phenomenon is occasionally observed when heavy, upright exercise is abruptly terminated. To avoid this, we usually ask a patient who has exercised hard to continue very light exercise (unloaded cycling or slow walking) after completing the maximum work rate.

Analysis

Referring to flowchart 1, the peak $\dot{V}O_2$ and anaerobic threshold are reduced (Table 10.38.2), which directs us through branch points 1.1, 1.2, and 1.3 to flowchart 4. The breathing reserve is low (branch point 4.1), and the V_D/V_T is high (branch point 4.2). The diagnosis of lung disease with impaired peripheral oxygenation is reached. The patient does have a positive $P(a - _{ET})CO_2$ and obstructive airway disease and probably a significant component of pulmonary vascular dysfunction that contributes to the low AT. The resting oxyhemoglobin saturation is reduced because of carboxyhemoglobinemia and a low PaO_2. When due to obesity, the latter improves with the deeper breathing of exercise. The heart rate reserve is also high, consistent with ventilatory limitation to exercise. Both the obesity and

TABLE 10.38.1.   Selected Respiratory Function Data

Measurement	Predicted	Before Bronchodilator	After Bronchodilator
Age, yr		50	
Sex		Male	
Height, cm		174	
Weight, kg	77	113	
Hematocrit, %		45	
VC, L	4.40	3.95	4.36
IC, L	2.94	3.30	3.75
TLC, L	6.44	6.08	
FEV$_1$, L	3.49	2.53	2.96
FEV$_1$/VC, %	79	64	
MVV, L/min	147	96	101
D$_L$CO, ml/mm Hg/min	28.6	30.6	

TABLE 10.38.2.   Selected Exercise Data

Measurement	Predicted	Measured
Peak $\dot{V}O_2$, L/min	2.68	1.84
Maximum HR, beats/min	170	131
Maximum O$_2$ pulse, ml/beat	15.8	14.3
$\Delta\dot{V}O_2/\Delta$WR, ml/min/W	10.3	10.2
AT, L/min	>1.15	1.0
Blood pressure, mmHg (rest, max)		131/88, 206/106
Maximum $\dot{V}E$, L/min		93
Exercise breathing reserve, L/min	>15	3
PaO$_2$, mmHg (rest, max ex)		73, 97
P(A − a)O$_2$, mmHg (rest, max ex)		34, 23
P(a − $_{ET}$)CO$_2$, mmHg (rest, max ex)		7, 2
V$_D$/V$_T$ (rest, heavy ex)		0.41, 0.31

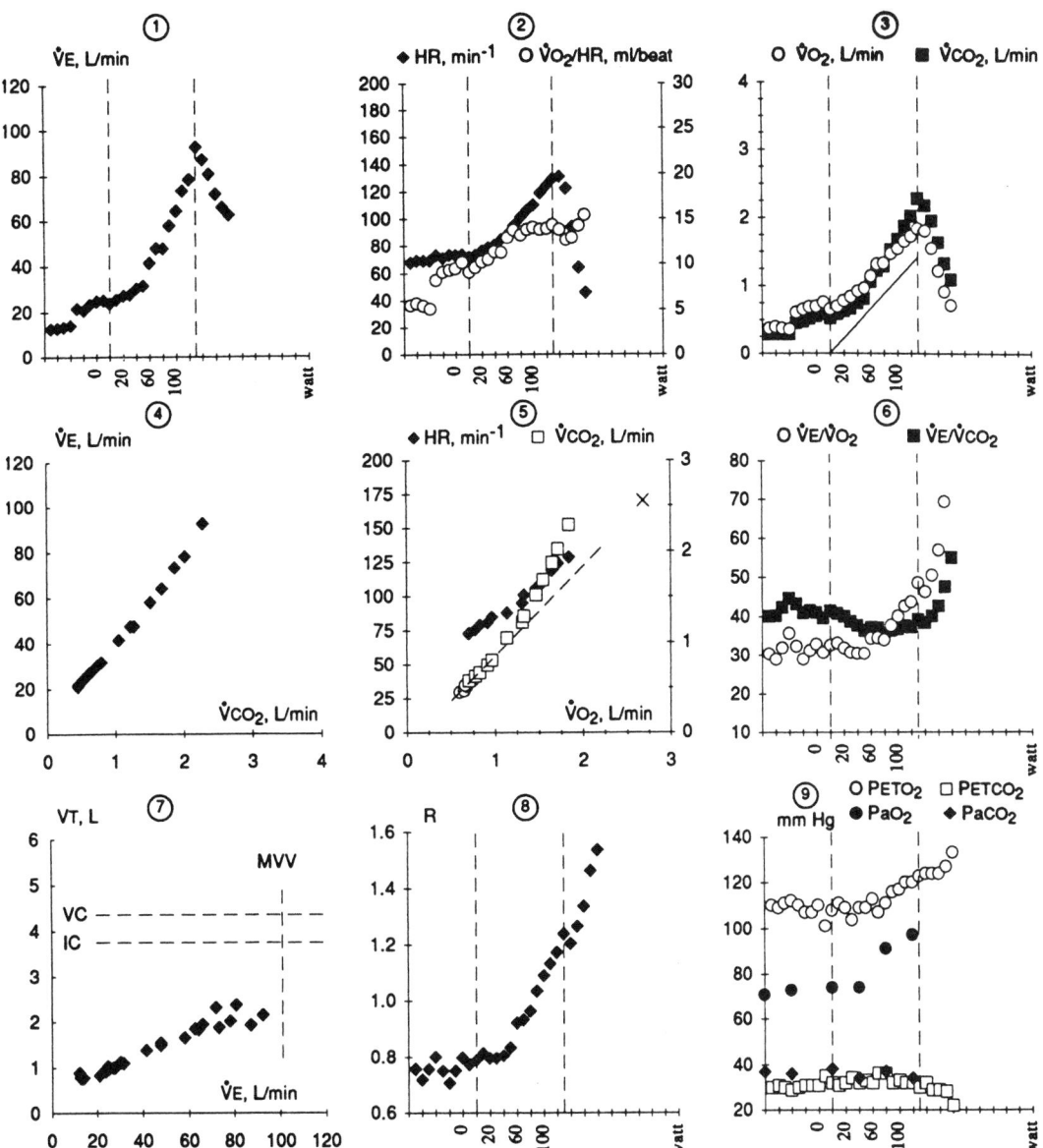

FIGURE 10.38.1.   **1:** Vertical dashed lines in panels 1 to 3 and 6, 8, and 9 indicate the beginning and the end of the increasing work period. **2:** Unloaded cycling is performed for 3 minutes before the left vertical dashed line. **3:** In panel 3, the diagonal line shows the increase of $\dot{V}O_2$ at a slope of 10 ml/min/W. **4:** In panel 5, the diagonal dashed line has a slope of 1; the x in the upper right is the predicted maximum heart rate and $\dot{V}O_2$ for the subject.

cigarette smoking add to the degree of dysfunction caused by the obstructive airway disease.

The development of a metabolic acidosis at a low $\dot{V}O_2$ (i.e., a low *AT*) also contributed to the exercise limitation, because it stimulated ventilation at all work rates above the *AT*, evidenced by the steep rise in $\dot{V}E/\dot{V}O_2$ in panel 6 of Figure 10.38.1. This response is in contrast to that seen in Cases 37, 40, and 42, where the $\dot{V}E/\dot{V}O_2$ does not rise as steeply toward the end of exercise and where a circulatory-induced metabolic acidosis did not contribute to a low breathing reserve and ventilatory limitation. Sedentary lifestyle and the carboxyhemoglobinemia from cigarette smoking contribute to the low *AT*. Thus, this patient has reversible elements to his illness.

Conclusion

Mild airflow obstruction, obesity, and cigarette smoking all contribute to ventilatory limitation to exercise in this patient.

TABLE 10.38.3.   Air Breathing

Time min	Work rate watts	BP mmHg	HR min⁻¹	f min⁻¹	V̇E L/min BTPS	V̇CO₂ L/min STPD	V̇O₂ L/min STPD	V̇O₂/HR ml/beat	R	pH	HCO₃⁻ meq/L	Po₂ ET	Po₂ a	Po₂ (A−a)	Pco₂ ET	Pco₂ a	Pco₂ (a−ET)	V̇E/V̇CO₂	V̇E/V̇O₂	VD/VT
	Rest	131/88								7.41	23		71			37				
	Rest		68	14	12.4	0.28	0.37	5.4	0.76			110			30			40	30	
	Rest		68	16	12.6	0.28	0.39	5.7	0.72			109			31			40	29	
	Rest		69	17	13.3	0.28	0.37	5.4	0.76			111			30			42	32	
	Rest	138/88	69	18	14.0	0.28	0.35	5.1	0.80	7.38	21	112	73	34	29	36	7	45	36	0.41
	Unloaded		73	25	21.5	0.45	0.60	8.2	0.75			110			30			43	32	
	Unloaded		71	25	20.9	0.46	0.65	9.2	0.71			107			31			41	29	
	Unloaded		73	25	23.3	0.51	0.68	9.3	0.75			107			31			42	31	
	Unloaded		73	24	24.6	0.55	0.69	9.5	0.80			110			31			41	33	
	Unloaded		74	26	25.2	0.58	0.75	10.1	0.77			101			35			40	31	
	Unloaded	150/88	72	26	23.7	0.51	0.66	9.2	0.79	7.39	23	108	74	30	32	38	6	41	33	0.41
0.5	20		73	26	25.4	0.57	0.70	9.6	0.81			111			31			41	33	
1.0	20		76	27	27.0	0.62	0.78	10.3	0.79			109			32			40	32	
1.5	40		79	28	27.8	0.66	0.83	10.5	0.80			104			34			39	31	
2.0	40	156/88	81	27	30.2	0.74	0.92	11.4	0.80	7.42	22	109	74	35	32	34	2	38	30	0.30
2.5	60		85	29	31.6	0.80	0.96	11.3	0.83			109			33			36	30	
3.0	60		88	29	41.5	1.05	1.14	13.0	0.92			113			32			37	34	
3.5	80		95	32	47.8	1.22	1.31	13.8	0.93			107			36			37	34	
4.0	80	169/94	101	31	47.8	1.28	1.33	13.2	0.96	7.36	21	111	91	21	36	37	1	35	34	0.32
4.5	100		106	35	58.1	1.52	1.47	13.9	1.03			116			32			36	38	
5.0	100		110	35	64.4	1.68	1.54	14.0	1.09			117			33			37	40	
5.5	120		119	39	73.3	1.87	1.65	13.9	1.13			120			32			37	42	
6.0	120	200/100	124	39	78.3	2.02	1.72	13.9	1.17	7.35	18	120	97	23	32	34	2	37	44	0.30
6.5	140		129	43	92.6	2.28	1.84	14.3	1.24			123			30			39	48	
	Recovery		131	45	87.3	2.18	1.81	13.8	1.20			124			32			38	46	
	Recovery	131/72	122	34	80.9	1.96	1.55	12.7	1.26			124			29			40	50	
	Recovery	113/63	94	31	71.9	1.63	1.22	13.0	1.34			124			29			42	57	
	Recovery	88/44	64	34	66.1	1.33	0.91	14.2	1.46			127			28			48	69	
	Recovery	75/31	46	34	62.7	1.09	0.71	15.4	1.54			133			22			55	84	

Case 39 Emphysema with Mild Airway Obstruction

Clinical Findings

This 50-year-old male long-term smoker was referred for cardiopulmonary exercise testing for evaluation of his exertional dyspnea. He became symptomatic after walking one block. He had mild obstructive lung disease of long duration consistent with emphysema. His only current medication was a frequently used inhaled β-agonist. The study was done to determine whether his exercise limitation was due to his lung disease.

Exercise Findings

The patient performed exercise on a cycle ergometer. He pedaled at 60 rpm without an added load for 3 minutes. The work rate was then increased 15 W per minute to tolerance. Heart rate and rhythm were continuously monitored; 12-lead ECGs were obtained during rest, exercise, and recovery. Blood pressure was measured with a sphygmomanometer, and oxygen saturation with an ear oximeter. The patient appeared to give an excellent effort and stopped exercise because of shortness of breath. He denied chest pain during or after the study. Resting, exercise, and recovery ECGs were not remarkable except for occasional multifocal premature ventricular contractions during exercise and recovery.

Interpretation

Comments

Resting respiratory function studies showed mild obstruction, an insignificant bronchodilator response to inhaled β-agonist, and a moderately reduced D_LCO (Table 10.39.1).

Analysis

Referring to flowchart 1, peak $\dot{V}_{O_2}$ and the anaerobic threshold are low (Table 10.39.2). Going next to flowchart 4, the breathing reserve (branch point 4.1) is very low, consistent with exercise limitation from lung disease. Although blood gases are not available, the very high ventilatory equivalents, without a high R to support acute hyperventilation, indicate increased dead space ventilation (branch

point 4.2). The high $\dot{V}_E/\dot{V}_{CO_2}$ at the *AT* indicates that the patient requires an inordinately high ventilatory response to exercise. The patient became hypoxic during exercise. The high heart rate reserve is also consistent with ventilation limiting exercise. The low $\Delta\dot{V}_{O_2}/\Delta WR$ might be due to pulmonary vascular disease secondary to the patient's obstructive lung disease or to reduced venous return during exercise resulting from high intrapleural pressure consequent to air trapping and hyperinflation.

Conclusion

This patient has mild to moderate obstructive lung disease with ventilatory limitation to exercise due to the increased ventilatory requirements secondary to ventilation–perfusion mismatching and low *AT*.

TABLE 10.39.1.   Selected Respiratory Function Data

Measurement	Predicted	Measured
Age, yr		50
Sex		Male
Height, cm		168
Weight, kg	72	66
Hematocrit, %		46
VC, L	4.06	4.10
IC, L	2.71	3.30
TLC, L	5.92	7.07
FEV_1, L	3.22	2.57
FEV_1/VC, %	79	63
MVV, L/min	141	91
D_LCO, ml/mm Hg/min	25.4	14.7

TABLE 10.39.2.   Selected Exercise Data

Measurement	Predicted	Measured
Peak $\dot{V}_{O_2}$, L/min	2.22	1.39
Maximum HR, beats/min	170	126
Maximum O_2 pulse, ml/beat	13.1	11.0
$\Delta\dot{V}_{O_2}/\Delta WR$, ml/min/W	10.3	7.3
AT, L/min	>0.95	0.9
Blood pressure, mmHg (rest, max)		120/80, 160/100
Maximum $\dot{V}_E$, L/min		89
Exercise breathing reserve, L/min	>15	2
O_2 saturation (oximeter) (rest, max)		93, 88

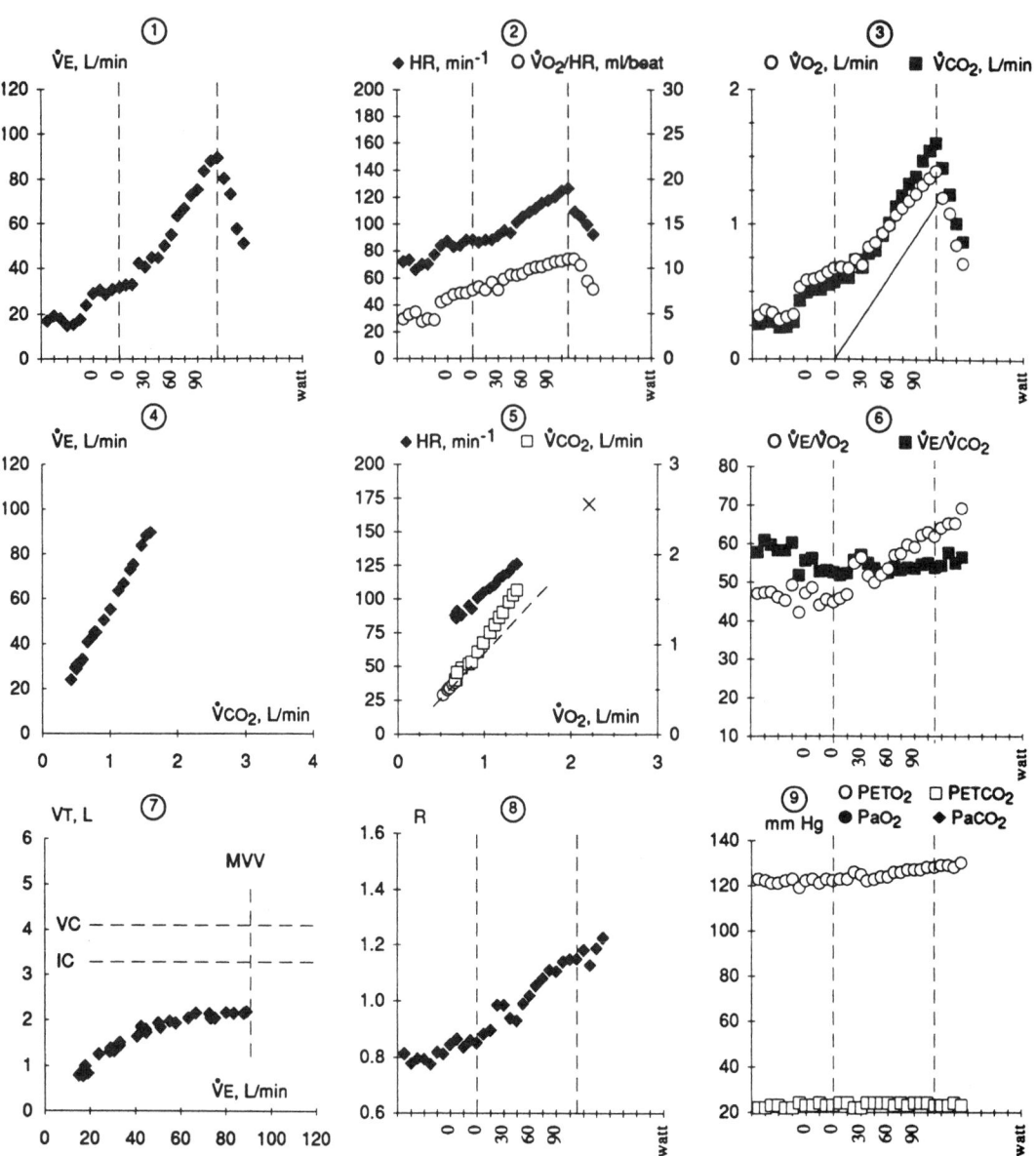

FIGURE 10.39.1.   **1:** Vertical dashed lines in panels 1 to 3 and 6, 8, and 9 indicate the beginning and the end of the increasing work period.
2: Unloaded cycling is performed for 3 minutes before the left vertical dashed line. **3:** In panel 3, the diagonal line shows the increase of $\dot{V}_{O_2}$ at a slope of 10 ml/min/W. **4:** In panel 5, the diagonal dashed line has a slope of 1; the x in the upper right is the predicted maximum heart rate and $\dot{V}_{O_2}$ for the subject.

TABLE 10.39.3.   Air Breathing

Time min	Work rate watts	BP mmHg	HR min⁻¹	f min⁻¹	V̇E L/min BTPS	V̇CO₂ L/min STPD	V̇O₂ L/min STPD	V̇O₂/HR ml/beat	R	pH	HCO₃⁻ meq/L	PO₂ ET	PO₂ a	PO₂ (A−a)	PCO₂ ET	PCO₂ a	PCO₂ (a−ET)	V̇E/V̇CO₂	V̇E/V̇O₂	VD/VT
	Rest	120/80																		
	Rest		72	22	16.9	0.26	0.32	4.4	0.81			123			22			58	47	
	Rest		73	23	19.0	0.28	0.36	4.9	0.78			122			22			61	47	
	Rest		66	21	17.9	0.27	0.34	5.2	0.79			121			23			60	47	
	Rest	120/80	70	19	15.0	0.23	0.29	4.1	0.79			121			23			58	46	
	Rest		70	19	15.6	0.24	0.31	4.4	0.77			122			22			58	45	
	Rest		77	18	17.8	0.27	0.33	4.3	0.82			123			22			60	49	
	Unloaded		84	19	23.9	0.43	0.53	6.3	0.81			119			24			52	42	
	Unloaded		87	21	29.1	0.49	0.58	6.7	0.84			122			23			56	47	
	Unloaded		83	23	30.6	0.51	0.59	7.1	0.86			123			23			56	49	
	Unloaded		84	22	28.8	0.51	0.61	7.3	0.84			121			24			53	44	
	Unloaded		88	23	31.1	0.55	0.64	7.3	0.86			123			23			53	46	
	Unloaded	140/90	88	22	31.9	0.57	0.67	7.6	0.85			122			23			53	25	
0.5	8		86	23	33.0	0.60	0.68	7.9	0.88			123			24			52	46	
1.0	15		88	22	33.2	0.60	0.67	7.6	0.90			123			24			52	47	
1.5	23		88	23	42.5	0.73	0.74	8.4	0.99			126			22			56	55	
2.0	30	140/90	91	25	40.9	0.68	0.69	7.6	0.99			125			22			57	56	
2.5	38		95	26	45.0	0.78	0.83	8.7	0.94			122			24			55	52	
3.0	45		93	25	44.9	0.80	0.86	9.2	0.93			123			24			53	50	
3.5	53		101	26	50.3	0.92	0.93	9.2	0.99			124			24			52	52	
4.0	60	150/92	105	28	55.3	1.01	1.02	9.4	1.02			124			24			52	53	
4.5	68		108	31	63.5	1.13	1.07	9.9	1.06			126			23			54	57	
5.0	75		111	31	66.8	1.21	1.12	10.1	1.08			126			24			53	57	
5.5	83		115	34	72.7	1.30	1.17	10.2	1.11			127			23			54	60	
6.0	90	160/100	117	37	75.2	1.35	1.22	10.4	1.11			127			24			53	59	
6.5	98		120	39	83.5	1.47	1.29	10.8	1.14			127			24			55	62	
7.0	105		124	41	87.9	1.54	1.34	10.8	1.15			128			24			55	63	
7.5	113		126	41	89.3	1.60	1.39	11.0	1.15			128			23			54	62	
	Recovery		109	37	80.1	1.42	1.20	11.0	1.18			129			23			54	64	
	Recovery	140/90	105	36	73.4	1.22	1.08	10.3	1.13			129			23			58	65	
	Recovery		99	30	57.9	1.01	0.85	8.6	1.19			128			24			55	65	
	Recovery	140/80	92	28	51.5	0.87	0.71	7.7	1.23			130			23			56	69	

Case 40 Severe Emphysema

Clinical Findings

This 65-year-old man had a long history of asbestos exposure and heavy cigarette smoking. He was being treated with aminophylline, inhaled bronchodilators, and home oxygen therapy. He was also receiving chlorothiazide for treatment of hypertension. He had stopped smoking 12 years previously. Resting ECG suggested left atrial enlargement. The question was raised with respect to the role of the patient's circulatory disease in his ventilatory impairment.

Exercise Findings

The patient performed exercise on a cycle ergometer. He pedaled at 60 rpm without added load for 3 minutes. The work rate was then increased 10 W per minute to his symptom-limited maximum. Blood was sampled every second minute, and intraarterial blood pressure was recorded from a brachial artery catheter. There were no abnormal ST-segment changes at rest or during exercise. He stopped exercise complaining of shortness of breath.

Interpretation

Comments

This patient clearly has evidence of very severe obstructive lung disease (Table 10.40.1). His resting ECG suggests left atrial enlargement.

Analysis

Referring to flowchart 1, the peak $\dot{V}O_2$ is reduced, while the anaerobic threshold is not reached but is above the lower limits of normal (Table 10.40.2), which directs us through branch points 1.1, 1.2, and 1.3 to flowchart 3. The breathing reserve is low (branch point 3.1), and there is confirmatory evidence for ventilation–perfusion mismatching [increased VD/VT, $P(A - a)O_2$, and $P(a - ET)CO_2$]. Although there is no breathing reserve at maximal exercise, there is a large heart rate reserve. The maximal ventilatory frequency is less than 50 (branch point 3.2), which is typical of obstructive lung disease. The mild respiratory acidosis during exercise is consistent with a diagnosis of ventilatory limitation.

Conclusion

The patient, although having ECG evidence of left atrial enlargement and significant systemic hypertension during exercise, clearly is limited by his obstructive lung disease and not by cardiac dysfunction. The presence of a high heart rate reserve and the absence of a ventilatory reserve, along with the development of a mild respiratory acidosis at this patient's maximum $\dot{V}O_2$, support the conclusion that he has ventilatory limitation. Circulatory limitation was not severe enough to cause a metabolic acidosis over the low range of work rates the patient was able to tolerate (only 1 mEq/L decrease in HCO_3^-). The patient's ventilation was inadequate to reduce $PETCO_2$ and $PaCO_2$ during exercise.

TABLE 10.40.1.   Selected Respiratory Function Data

Measurement	Predicted	Measured
Age, yr		65
Sex		Male
Height, cm		170
Weight, kg	74	99
Hematocrit, %		53
VC, L	3.72	2.17
IC, L	2.48	1.31
TLC, L	5.85	8.22
FEV$_1$, L	2.89	0.56
FEV$_1$/VC, %	78	26
MVV, L/min	123	31
D$_L$CO, ml/mm Hg/min	25.1	13.2

TABLE 10.40.2.   Selected Exercise Data

Measurement	Predicted	Measured
Peak $\dot{V}O_2$, L/min	2.11	0.90
Maximum HR, beats/min	155	129
Maximum O$_2$ pulse, ml/beat	13.6	7.0
$\Delta\dot{V}O_2/\Delta WR$, ml/min/W	10.3	8.9
AT, L/min	>0.93	not reached
Blood pressure, mmHg (rest, max)		175/94, 256/138
Maximum $\dot{V}E$, L/min		28
Exercise breathing reserve, L/min	>15	3
PaO$_2$, mmHg (rest, max ex)		56, 46
P(A − a)O$_2$, mmHg (rest, max ex)		39, 48
P(a − ET)CO$_2$, mmHg (rest, max ex)		4, 6
VD/VT (rest, heavy ex)		0.40, 0.41
HCO$_3^-$, mEq/L (rest, 2-min recov)		28, 27

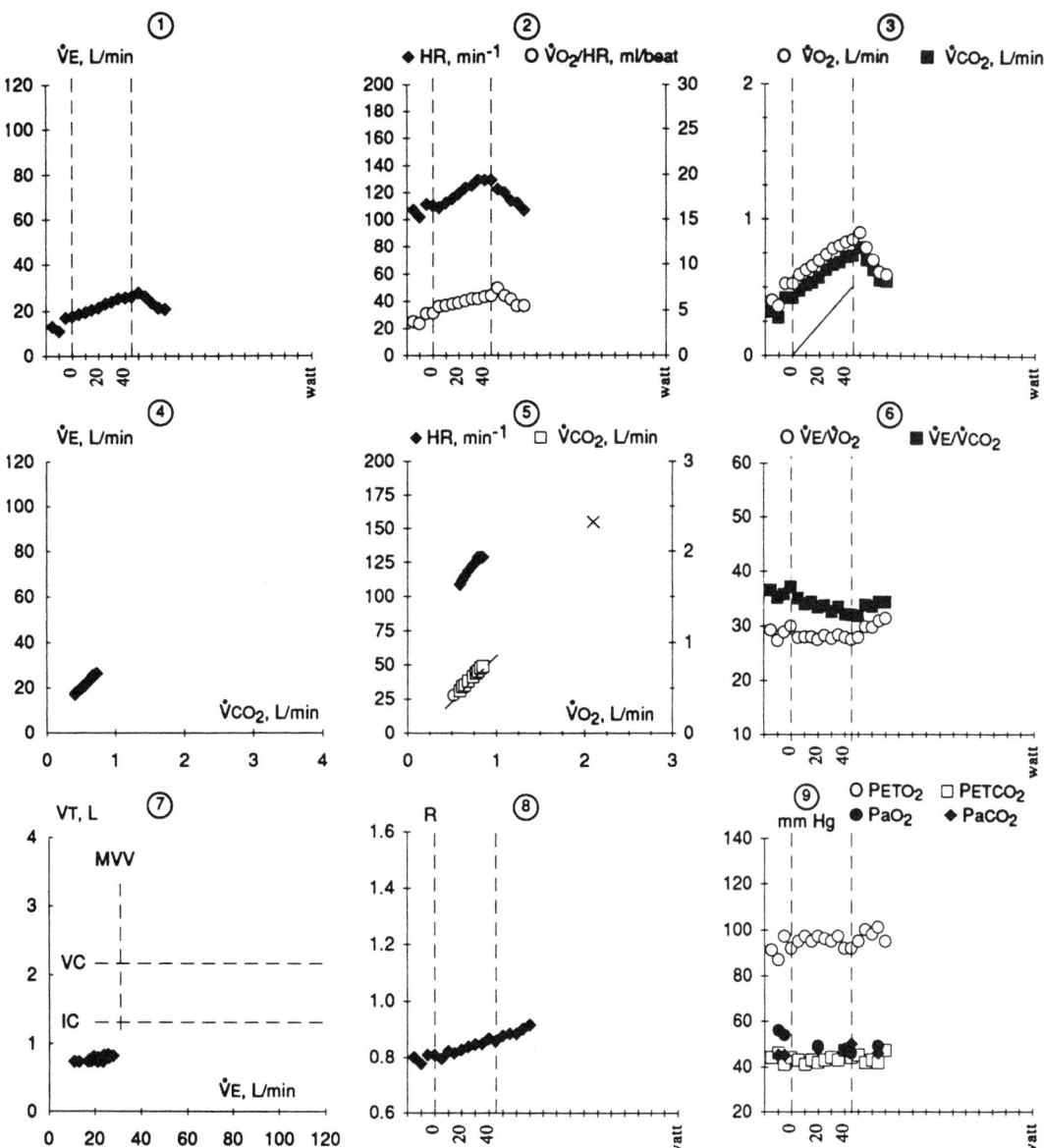

FIGURE 10.40.1.   **1:** Vertical dashed lines in panels 1 to 3 and 6, 8, and 9 indicate the beginning and the end of the increasing work period. **2:** Unloaded cycling is performed for 3 minutes before the left vertical dashed line. **3:** In panel 3, the diagonal line shows the increase of $\dot{V}_{O_2}$ at a slope of 10 ml/min/W. **4:** In panel 5, the diagonal dashed line has a slope of 1; the x in the upper right is the predicted maximum heart rate and $\dot{V}_{O_2}$ for the subject.

TABLE 10.40.3.   Air Breathing

Time min	Work rate watts	BP mmHg	HR min⁻¹	f min⁻¹	$\dot{V}_E$ L/min BTPS	$\dot{V}_{CO_2}$ L/min STPD	$\dot{V}_{O_2}$ L/min STPD	$\dfrac{\dot{V}_{O_2}}{HR}$ ml/beat	R	pH	HCO_3^- meq/L	P_{O_2}, mmHg ET	a	(A − a)	P_{CO_2}, mmHg ET	a	(a − ET)	$\dfrac{\dot{V}_E}{\dot{V}_{CO_2}}$	$\dfrac{\dot{V}_E}{\dot{V}_{O_2}}$	$\dfrac{V_D}{V_T}$
	Rest	175/94																		
	Rest		107	18	13.2	0.32	0.40	3.7	0.80			91			44			36	29	
	Rest	175/94	102	15	11.1	0.28	0.36	3.5	0.78	7.41	28	87	56	39	46	45		35	27	0.40
	Unloaded	194/100	111	23	17.0	0.42	0.52	4.7	0.81	7.41	28	97	54	43	41	45	4	36	29	0.41
	Unloaded		110	23	17.5	0.42	0.52	4.7	0.81			92			44			37	30	
0.5	10		109	25	18.6	0.47	0.59	5.4	0.80			95			43			35	28	
1.0	10		112	24	19.4	0.51	0.62	5.5	0.82			97			41			34	28	
1.5	20		115	27	20.5	0.53	0.65	5.7	0.82			95			43			34	28	
2.0	20	225/113	119	27	21.3	0.57	0.69	5.8	0.83	7.40	29	97	49	45	42	48	6	33	28	0.41
2.5	30		123	30	23.4	0.62	0.74	6.0	0.84			96			43			34	28	
3.0	30		125	29	24.0	0.66	0.78	6.2	0.85			95			44			33	28	
3.5	40		129	32	25.4	0.68	0.80	6.2	0.85			97			43			33	28	
4.0	40	250/131	129	31	25.8	0.72	0.83	6.4	0.87	7.37	27	92	47	49	47	48	1	32	28	0.40
4.5	50	256/138	129	33	26.2	0.73	0.85	6.6	0.86	7.37	28	92	46	48	44	50	6	32	28	0.41
	Recovery		122	34	28.0	0.79	0.90	7.4	0.88			95			45			32	28	
	Recovery		120	32	26.3	0.70	0.79	6.6	0.89			100			42			34	30	
	Recovery		114	32	23.5	0.62	0.70	6.1	0.89			98			43			34	30	
	Recovery	194/94	112	29	21.3	0.55	0.61	5.4	0.90	7.38	27	101	49	51	42	46	4	34	31	0.40
	Recovery		107	27	20.8	0.54	0.59	5.5	0.92			95			47			34	31	

Case 41 Emphysema with Pulmonary Vascular Disease

Clinical Findings

This 61-year-old man with bullous emphysema and right middle lobe scarring on chest roentgenogram was referred for evaluation regarding the need for oxygen supplementation. The patient had a 35 pack-year history of cigarette smoking. He had not sought medical care until 4 months previously, when he was hospitalized for pneumonia, severe dyspnea, and hemoptysis. Bronchoscopy, transbronchial biopsy, cytology, and mycobacterial studies were negative. Resting ECG showed poor R-wave progression.

Exercise Findings

The patient performed exercise on a cycle ergometer. He pedaled at 60 rpm without an added load for 3 minutes. The work rate was then increased 10 W per minute to tolerance. Arterial blood was sampled every second minute, and intraarterial pressure was recorded from a percutaneously placed brachial artery catheter. The patient stopped exercise because of leg fatigue. The patient had no chest pain or further ECG abnormalities.

Interpretation

Comments

Resting studies showed a moderate obstructive ventilatory defect, increased total lung capacity, and low D$_L$CO (Table 10.41.1). The ECG showed poor R-wave progression.

Analysis

Referring to flowchart 1, peak $\dot{V}O_2$ and anaerobic threshold are decreased (Table 10.41.2). Proceeding next to flowchart 4, the low breathing reserve (branch point 4.1) and high VD/VT (branch point 4.2) are consistent with lung disease with impaired peripheral oxygenation. The high VT/IC and low breathing reserve support ventilatory limitation, although ventilatory drive is increased because of the low work rate metabolic acidosis and the high VD/VT. Although the patient stated that he stopped exercise because of leg fatigue, his low breathing reserve indicated that he also had ventilatory limitation. The abnormal gas exchange [high ventila-

tory equivalents, high VD/VT, and positive P(a − ET) CO$_2$] with exercise is consistent with the presence of underperfusion of ventilated lung, which in turn is consistent with pulmonary vascular disease, presumably secondary to obstructive lung disease. The severity of the metabolic acidosis (decrease in HCO$_3^-$ from 22 to 13 mEq/L) is consistent with the low anaerobic threshold and suggests poor O$_2$ flow to the exercising muscle, most likely because the patient's pulmonary vascular disease limited his ability to increase cardiac output.

Conclusion

This patient has physiologic evidence of pulmonary vascular disease, secondary to obvious obstructive lung disease. The mild degree of hypoxemia does not qualify for O$_2$ supplementation under current

TABLE 10.41.1.   Selected Respiratory Function Data

Measurement	Predicted	Measured
Age, yr		61
Sex		Male
Height, cm		173
Weight, kg	76	63
Hematocrit, %		45
VC, L	4.00	4.37
IC, L	2.67	2.62
TLC, L	6.15	9.11
FEV$_1$, L	3.13	2.11
FEV$_1$/VC, %	78	48
MVV, L/min	131	87
D$_L$CO, ml/mm Hg/min	26.0	8.4

TABLE 10.41.2.   Selected Exercise Data

Measurement	Predicted	Measured
Peak $\dot{V}O_2$, L/min	1.95	1.25
Maximum HR, beats/min	159	149
Maximum O$_2$ pulse, ml/beat	12.3	8.4
$\Delta\dot{V}O_2/\Delta$WR, ml/min/W	10.3	8.5
AT, L/min	>0.86	0.7
Blood pressure, mmHg (rest, max)		127/75, 190/96
Maximum $\dot{V}E$, L/min		85
Exercise breathing reserve, L/min	>15	2
Pao$_2$, mmHg (rest, max ex)		83, 72
P(A − a)o$_2$, mmHg (rest, max ex)		32, 52
P(a − ET)co$_2$, mmHg (rest, max ex)		4, 8
VD/VT (rest, max ex)		0.28, 0.41
HCO$_3^-$, mEq/L (rest, 2-min recov)		22, 13

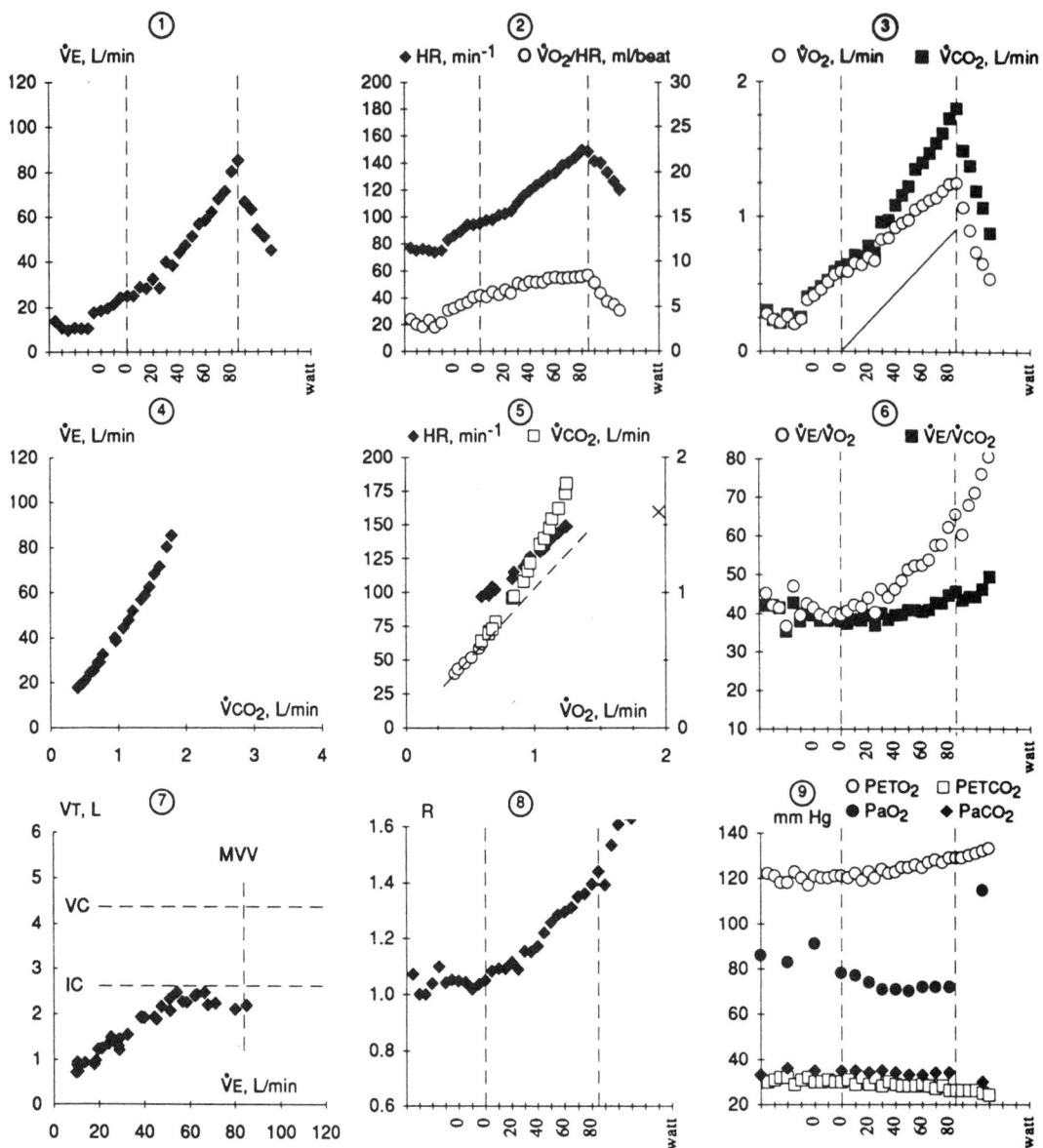

FIGURE 10.41.1. **1:** Vertical dashed lines in panels 1 to 3 and 6, 8, and 9 indicate the beginning and the end of the increasing work period. **2:** Unloaded cycling is performed for 3 minutes before the left vertical dashed line. **3:** In panel 3, the diagonal line shows the increase of $\dot{V}O_2$ at a slope of 10 ml/min/W. **4:** In panel 5, the diagonal dashed line has a slope of 1; the x in the upper right is the predicted maximum heart rate and $\dot{V}O_2$ for the subject.

federal funding guidelines, but dyspnea may well be less with O_2 supplementation. This is an example of lung disease causing secondary cardiovascular disease, which in turn results in a high ventilatory requirement as compensation for the exercise-induced lactic acidosis. This makes the patient more exercise limited than predicted from his moderate defect in spirometry.

TABLE 10.41.3.   Air Breathing

Time min	Work rate watts	BP mmHg	HR min⁻¹	f min⁻¹	$\dot{V}_E$ L/min BTPS	$\dot{V}_{CO_2}$ L/min STPD	$\dot{V}_{O_2}$ L/min STPD	$\dfrac{\dot{V}_{O_2}}{HR}$ ml/beat	R	pH	HCO_3^- meq/L	P_{O_2}, mmHg ET	a	(A − a)	P_{CO_2}, mmHg ET	a	(a − ET)	$\dfrac{\dot{V}_E}{\dot{V}_{CO_2}}$	$\dfrac{\dot{V}_E}{\dot{V}_{O_2}}$	$\dfrac{V_D}{V_T}$
	Rest	129/75								7.44	22		86			33				
	Rest		77	15	13.9	0.30	0.28	3.6	1.07			122			30			42	45	
	Rest		75	13	10.8	0.23	0.23	3.1	1.00			121			31			42	42	
	Rest		76	14	9.9	0.21	0.21	2.8	1.00			118			32			41	41	
	Rest	129/75	75	15	10.8	0.27	0.26	3.5	1.04	7.41	22	118	83	32	32	36	4	35	37	0.28
	Rest		74	12	10.4	0.22	0.20	2.7	1.10			123			29			43	47	
	Rest		75	11	10.4	0.25	0.24	3.2	1.04			120			31			38	39	
	Unloaded		83	20	17.8	0.40	0.38	4.6	1.05			117			32			40	42	
	Unloaded	138/41	86	19	18.6	0.43	0.41	4.8	1.05	7.41	22	121	91	25	30	35	5	40	41	0.34
	Unloaded		89	16	19.6	0.48	0.46	5.2	1.04			120			30			38	40	
	Unloaded		94	17	21.2	0.52	0.51	5.4	1.02			120			31			38	39	
	Unloaded		94	18	24.4	0.59	0.57	6.1	1.04			121			30			39	40	
	Unloaded	168/90	95	18	25.0	0.62	0.59	6.2	1.05	7.40	21	121	78	38	30	35	5	38	40	0.33
0.5	10		97	17	25.3	0.64	0.59	6.1	1.08			120			31			37	40	
1.0	10	168/90	98	20	29.0	0.71	0.65	6.6	1.09	7.41	22	122	77	40	29	35	6	38	42	0.34
1.5	20		101	22	28.5	0.70	0.64	6.3	1.09			119			32			38	42	
2.0	20	174/90	102	21	32.5	0.78	0.70	6.9	1.11	7.40	21	123	74	45	29	34	5	39	44	0.34
2.5	30		104	24	28.9	0.73	0.67	6.4	1.09			120			32			37	40	
3.0	30	174/40	110	21	40.1	0.96	0.83	7.5	1.16	7.40	21	124	71	48	28	35	7	40	46	0.37
3.5	40		115	20	38.7	0.97	0.84	7.3	1.15			122			30			38	44	
4.0	40	180/90	119	23	44.4	1.08	0.92	7.7	1.17	7.39	20	123	71	49	29	34	5	39	46	0.34
4.5	50		123	22	47.7	1.16	0.95	7.7	1.22			125			28			40	48	
5.0	50	182/88	126	25	51.7	1.22	0.97	7.7	1.26	7.38	19	125	70	52	28	33	5	41	51	0.34
5.5	60		130	25	56.9	1.35	1.05	8.1	1.29			126			28			41	52	
6.0	60	189/93	132	26	58.7	1.40	1.08	8.2	1.30	7.36	18	125	72	51	29	33	4	40	52	0.34
6.5	70		138	26	62.3	1.47	1.12	8.1	1.31			127			28			41	54	
7.0	70	190/90	140	31	68.1	1.54	1.14	8.1	1.35	7.32	17	128	72	51	27	34	7	43	57	0.39
7.5	80		144	32	71.4	1.62	1.19	8.3	1.36			127			28			42	58	
8.0	80	190/96	149	38	80.2	1.73	1.24	8.3	1.40	7.32	17	129	72	52	26	34	8	44	62	0.41
8.5	90		148	39	85.2	1.80	1.25	8.4	1.44			129			26			45	66	
	Recovery		141	27	66.6	1.49	1.07	7.6	1.39			129			26			43	60	
	Recovery		140	26	63.3	1.38	0.90	6.4	1.53			130			26			44	68	
	Recovery		133	22	54.5	1.19	0.74	5.6	1.61			131			26			44	71	
	Recovery	174/87	126	22	51.3	1.07	0.65	5.2	1.65	7.26	13	132	115	14	25	30	5	46	76	0.36
	Recovery		120	24	45.5	0.88	0.54	4.5	1.63			133			24			49	80	

Case 42 Severe Emphysema and Bronchitis: Air and Oxygen Breathing Studies
Clinical Findings

This 62-year-old retired accountant had a long history of heavy cigarette smoking but had stopped 4 years previously. He had a chronic cough and shortness of breath. He had gradually increased his activity by physical training and rode his bicycle many miles daily. There was no history of heart failure. He took oral theophylline but no other medications. He participated in a study evaluating the effects of oxygen supplementation.

Exercise Findings

The patient performed exercise on a cycle ergometer. He pedaled at 60 rpm without added load for 3 minutes while breathing humidified compressed air. The work rate was then increased 10 W per minute to his symptom-limited maximum. Blood was sampled every second minute, and intraarterial blood pressure was recorded from a percutaneously placed brachial artery catheter. He stopped exercise complaining of shortness of breath. Following 30 minutes of rest, he was given humidified 100% O_2 to breathe while the exercise study was repeated. He again stopped exercise complaining of shortness of breath. The 12-lead ECG showed no ST-segment changes or arrhythmia. His maximum heart rate increased by 25 beats per minute, and maximum work rate increased by 40 W.

Interpretation
Comments

Resting respiratory function studies indicate that this patient has severe obstructive lung disease (Table 10.42.1); he also had significant systemic hypertension at rest.

Analysis

Referring to flowchart 1, peak $\dot{V}O_2$ is moderately severely reduced and the anaerobic threshold is not reached (Table 10.42.2). We could satisfactorily use flowchart 3, but we use flowchart 5 because it is more detailed. The indices of ventilation–perfusion mismatching [VD/VT, $P(a - ET)CO_2$, and $P(A - a)O_2$] are abnormal (branch point 5.1). The breathing re-

TABLE 10.42.1. Selected Respiratory Function Data

Measurement	Predicted	Measured
Age, yr		62
Sex		Male
Height, cm		173
Weight, kg	76	78
Hematocrit, %		51
VC, L	4.30	1.67
IC, L	2.87	1.22
TLC, L	6.87	8.30
FEV_1, L	3.40	0.54
FEV_1/VC, %	79	32
MVV, L/min	131	32
D_LCO, ml/mm Hg/min	30.9	18.5

TABLE 10.42.2. Selected Exercise Data

Measurement	Predicted	Room Air	100% O_2
Maximum WR, W		80	120
Peak $\dot{V}O_2$, L/min	2.11	0.96	
Maximum HR, beats/min	158	140	165
Maximum O_2 pulse, ml/beat	13.4	6.9	
$\Delta\dot{V}O_2/\Delta WR$, ml/min/W	10.3	8.3	
AT, L/min	>0.93	not reached	
Blood pressure, mmHg (rest, max)		169/106, 250/125	144/94, 234/119
Maximum $\dot{V}E$, L/min		32	40
Exercise breathing reserve, L/min	>15	0	−8
PaO_2, mmHg (rest, max ex)		78, 53	587, 583
$P(A - a)O_2$, mmHg (rest, max ex)		21, 51	77, 66
$P(a - ET)CO_2$, mmHg (rest, max ex)		6, 5	8, 3
VD/VT (rest, heavy ex)		0.42, 0.38	0.48, 0.37
HCO_3^-, mEq/L (rest, 2-min recov)		25, 24	27, 22

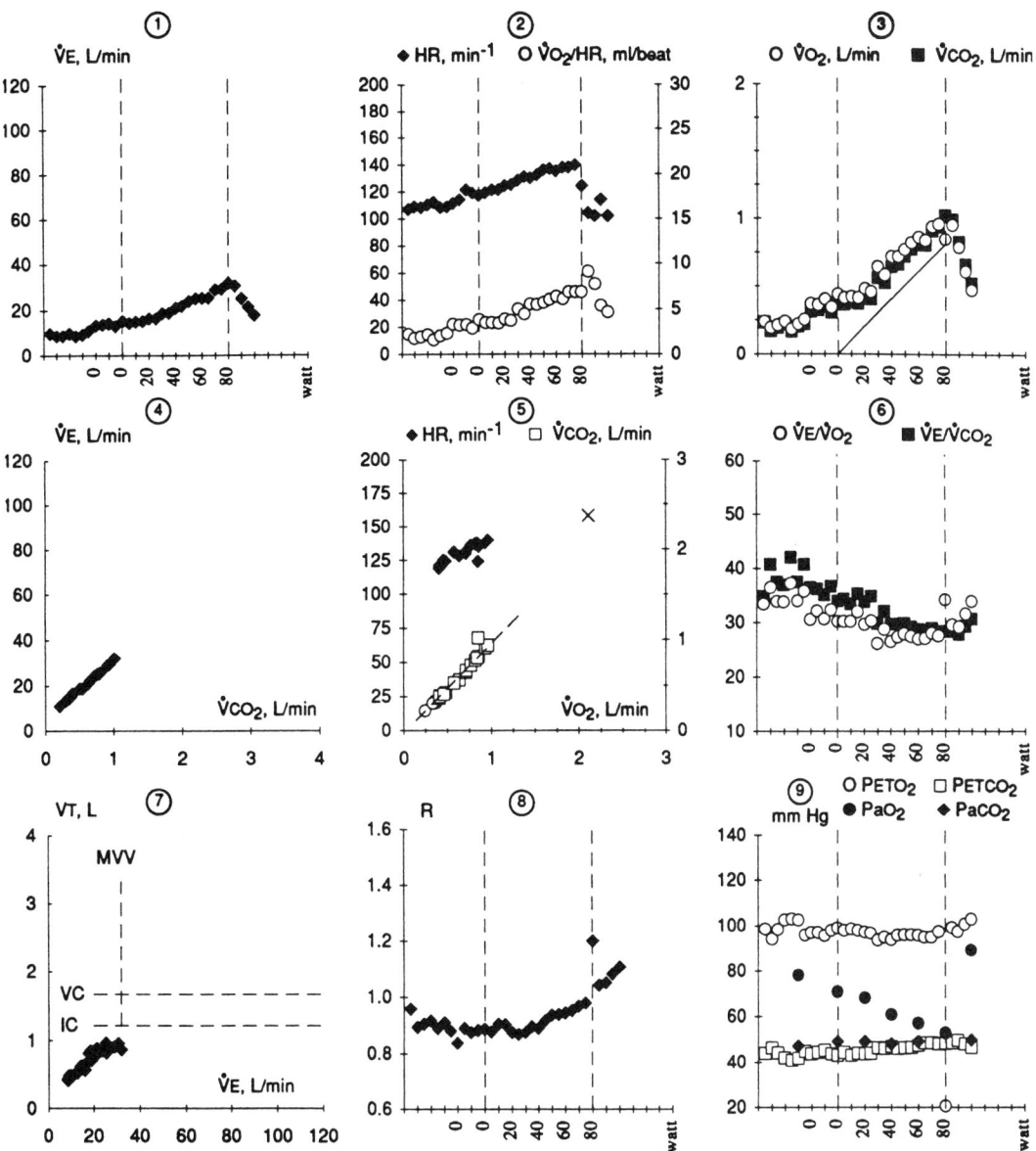

FIGURE 10.42.1   Air breathing. **1:** Vertical dashed lines in panels 1 to 3 and 6, 8, and 9 indicate the beginning and the end of the increasing work period. **2:** Unloaded cycling is performed for 3 minutes before the left vertical dashed line. **3:** In panel 3, the diagonal line shows the increase of $\dot{V}O_2$ at a slope of 10 ml/min/W. **4:** In panel 5, the diagonal dashed line has a slope of 1; the x in the upper right is the predicted maximum heart rate and $\dot{V}O_2$ for the subject.

serve is zero (branch point 5.3), indicating that the patient's exercise limitation is a result of lung disease. The breathing frequency (f) is less than 50 at the maximum work rate (branch point 5.7), consistent with the diagnosis of lung disease of the obstructive type. Other abnormal findings are an obstructive expiratory flow pattern (not shown), arterial oxygen tension and $P(A - a)O_2$ that are borderline at rest but abnormal with exercise, a high heart rate reserve, and a respiratory acidosis at the maximum $\dot{V}O_2$ (Table 10.42.3).

As a result of breathing 100% O_2, the patient was able to increase his maximal work rate by 40 W and the maximum heart rate by 25 beats per minute (i.e., from 140 during air breathing to 165 during 100% oxygen breathing). These results demonstrate that the high heart rate reserve seen during the air breathing test results from his ventilatory limitation. Moreover, the maximum exercise ventilation increases from 32 L/min while breathing air, the value of his resting MVV, to 40 L/min while breathing oxygen.

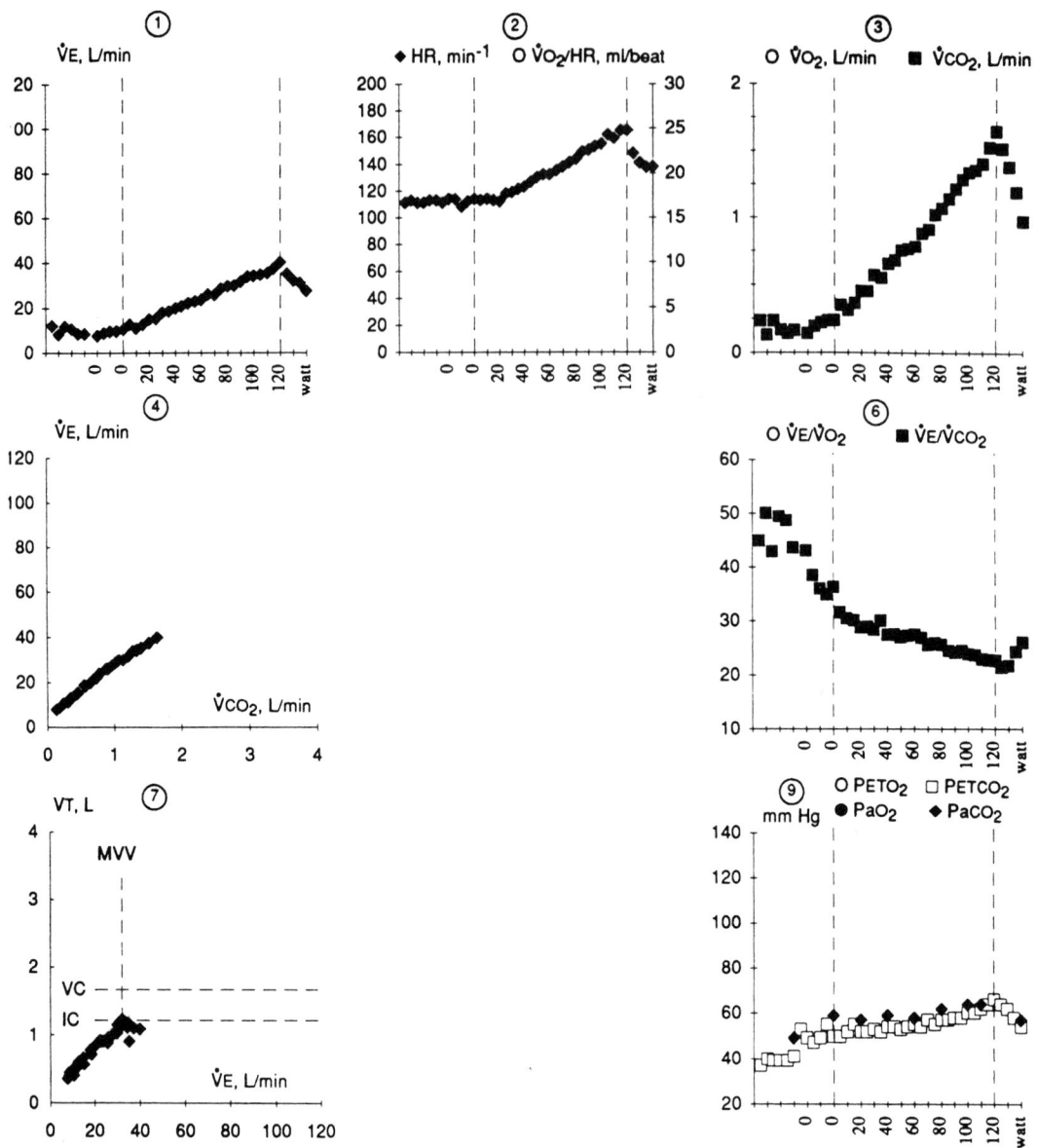

FIGURE 10.42.2.   Oxygen breathing 1: Vertical dashed lines in panels 1 to 3 and 6 and 9 indicate the beginning and the end of the increasing work period. 2: Unloaded cycling is performed for 3 minutes before the left vertical dashed line.

The increased work rate achieved during O_2 breathing is primarily the result of depression in the ventilatory response to exercise. Consequently, the patient develops more significant respiratory and metabolic acidoses as compared with the air breathing test (increase in $PaCO_2$ of 6 mm Hg above rest during air breathing, as compared with 15 mm Hg for oxygen breathing). PaO_2 remains above 580 mm Hg when breathing oxygen, indicating that no significant right-to-left shunt develops during exercise. Bicarbonate does not decrease in either study until 2 minutes after the exercise is terminated, because of the increase in $PaCO_2$ during exercise, which subsequently decreases in recovery.

Conclusion

Exercise performance is limited by severe obstructive lung disease. Oxygen breathing results in an increased work capacity, despite a normal resting PaO_2.

TABLE 10.42.3. Air Breathing

Time min	Work rate watts	BP mmHg	HR min⁻¹	f min⁻¹	$\dot{V}_E$ L/min BTPS	$\dot{V}_{CO_2}$ L/min STPD	$\dot{V}_{O_2}$ L/min STPD	$\dot{V}_{O_2}$/HR ml/beat	R	pH	HCO_3^- meq/L	P_{O_2}, mmHg ET	a	(A−a)	P_{CO_2}, mmHg ET	a	(a−ET)	$\dot{V}_E$/$\dot{V}_{CO_2}$	$\dot{V}_E$/$\dot{V}_{O_2}$	V_D/V_T
	Rest		107	20	9.7	0.23	0.24	2.2	0.96			99			44			35	33	
	Rest		109	21	8.7	0.17	0.19	1.7	0.89			94			46			41	36	
	Rest		108	20	8.8	0.19	0.21	1.9	0.90			98			44			37	34	
	Rest		110	20	9.8	0.22	0.24	2.2	0.92			102			42			37	34	
	Rest		112	20	8.4	0.16	0.18	1.6	0.89			103			41			42	37	
	Rest	169/106	108	19	9.1	0.20	0.22	2.0	0.91	7.35	25	102	78	21	42	47	6	37	34	0.42
	Unloaded		109	23	10.9	0.22	0.25	2.3	0.88			96			45			41	36	
	Unloaded		111	25	13.4	0.31	0.37	3.3	0.84			97			44			36	30	
	Unloaded		114	24	13.6	0.32	0.36	3.2	0.89			97			44			36	32	
	Unloaded		121	23	14.2	0.35	0.40	3.3	0.88			96			45			35	31	
	Unloaded		119	25	13.1	0.30	0.34	2.9	0.88			98			44			37	32	
	Unloaded	181/100	117	24	15.3	0.39	0.44	3.8	0.89	7.35	27	99	71	25	43	49	6	34	30	0.42
0.5	10		119	24	14.4	0.36	0.41	3.4	0.88			98			44			34	30	
1.0	10		121	25	14.8	0.38	0.42	3.5	0.90			99			43			33	30	
1.5	20		121	24	15.1	0.37	0.41	3.4	0.90			98			44			35	32	
2.0	20	187/106	124	25	16.3	0.42	0.48	3.9	0.88	7.35	27	97	68	27	44	49	6	34	30	0.42
2.5	30		125	29	16.4	0.40	0.46	3.7	0.87			97			44			35	30	
3.0	30		128	22	18.6	0.56	0.64	5.0	0.88	7.35	27	94			46			30	26	
3.5	40		131	27	18.9	0.52	0.58	4.4	0.90			95			46			32	29	
4.0	40	213/113	130	24	21.1	0.64	0.72	5.5	0.89	7.35	26	94	61	36	47	48	1	30	26	0.36
4.5	50		132	27	21.9	0.66	0.72	5.5	0.92			96			46			30	27	
5.0	50		136	28	23.9	0.72	0.77	5.7	0.94			96			46			30	28	
5.5	60		137	30	25.0	0.77	0.82	6.0	0.94			96			47			29	27	
6.0	60	225/119	135	28	25.6	0.81	0.86	6.4	0.94	7.35	27	96	57	42	48	49	1	29	27	0.35
6.5	70		138	31	25.4	0.80	0.84	6.1	0.95			95			49			28	27	
7.0	70		138	32	29.0	0.91	0.94	6.8	0.97			95			48			29	28	
7.5	80		140	32	29.2	0.94	0.96	6.9	0.98			98			48			28	28	
8.0	80	250/125	124	37	32.1	1.02	0.85	6.9	1.20	7.32	27	101	53	51	48	53	5	28	34	0.38
	Recovery		104	32	30.7	0.99	0.95	9.1	1.04			99			48			28	29	
	Recovery		102	26	25.2	0.83	0.79	7.7	1.05			98			50			28	29	
	Recovery		114	24	21.3	0.66	0.61	5.4	1.08			101			48			29	32	
	Recovery		102	22	17.8	0.52	0.47	4.6	1.11	7.30	24	103	89	15	47	50	3	31	34	0.39

TABLE 10.42.4. Oxygen Breathing

Time min	Work rate watts	BP mmHg	HR min⁻¹	f min⁻¹	V̇E L/min BTPS	V̇CO₂ L/min STPD	V̇O₂ L/min STPD	V̇O₂/HR ml/beat	R	pH	HCO₃⁻ meq/L	Po₂ ET	Po₂ a	Po₂ (A−a)	Pco₂ ET	Pco₂ a	Pco₂ (a−ET)	V̇E/V̇CO₂	V̇E/V̇O₂	VD/VT
	Rest		111	23	12.3	0.23									37			45		
	Rest		113	21	8.3	0.13									40			50		
	Rest		111	23	11.8	0.23									39			43		
	Rest		111	26	10.6	0.17									39			49		
	Rest		113	22	8.7	0.14									39			49		
	Rest	144/94	113	19	8.6	0.16				7.35	27		587	77	41	49	8	44		0.48
	Unloaded		111	11											53					
	Unloaded		114	22	7.9	0.14									49			43		
	Unloaded		114	20	9.0	0.19									47			38		
	Unloaded		108	20	9.6	0.22									49			36		
	Unloaded		112	22	9.9	0.23									55			35		
	Unloaded	181/106	114	21	10.5	0.24				7.29	28		587	67	50	59	9	36		0.50
0.5	10		113	21	12.8	0.35									50			31		
1.0	10		114	21	11.2	0.31									52			30		
1.5	20		113	21	12.6	0.36									55			30		
2.0	20	194/106	112	22	14.8	0.45				7.30	28		584	72	52	57	5	29		0.41
2.5	30		118	27	15.3	0.45									52			29		
3.0	30		119	23	18.1	0.57									53			28		
3.5	40		121	26	18.7	0.55									52			30		
4.0	40	200/106	123	24	19.9	0.65				7.29	28		580	74	54	59	5	27		0.42
4.5	50		127	24	20.8	0.68									54			28		
5.0	50		130	24	22.2	0.75									53			27		
5.5	60		132	25	22.8	0.76									54			27		
6.0	60	206/100	132	26	23.6	0.78				7.29	27		595	60	55	58	3	27		0.41
6.5	70		135	27	25.9	0.88									54			27		
7.0	70		138	29	25.8	0.91									57			26		
7.5	80		141	28	28.7	1.02									55			26		
8.0	80	213/106	144	29	29.8	1.07				7.27	28		601	50	57	62	5	26		0.42
8.5	90		149	26	30.0	1.14									57			24		
9.0	90		150	28	31.5	1.21									58			24		
9.5	100		153	30	33.8	1.28									58			24		
10.0	100	231/106	155	29	34.2	1.33				7.24	27		606	43	60	64	4	24		0.40
10.5	110		162	31	34.5	1.35									60			24		
11.0	110	234/119	159	39	35.4	1.40				7.23	26		583	66	62	64	2	23		0.37
11.5	120		165	34	37.3	1.52									64			23		
12.0	120		165	37	40.1	1.64									66			23		
	Recovery		148	30	35.0	1.51									64			21		
	Recovery		141	26	32.1	1.38									62			22		
	Recovery		138	26	31.1	1.19									58			24		
	Recovery	214/100	138	28	27.6	0.97				7.21	22		587	69	54	57	3	26		0.38

Case 43 Lung Cancer and Chronic Bronchitis: Preoperative Evaluation

Clinical Findings

This 62-year-old man with a long history of chronic obstructive pulmonary disease was referred for exercise testing to assess operative risk because of the finding of a malignant pulmonary nodule. The patient had quit smoking approximately 3 months earlier and was being treated aggressively with bronchodilator therapy, including oral corticosteroids. He had no known history of cardiovascular disease and stated he could walk 2 miles.

Exercise Findings

The patient performed exercise on a cycle ergometer. He pedaled at 60 rpm without an added load for 3 minutes. The work rate was then increased 10 W per minute to tolerance. Heart rate and rhythm were continuously monitored, and ECGs were repeatedly obtained. Blood pressure was measured with a sphygmomanometer, and arterial saturation was estimated with an ear oximeter. The patient gave an excellent effort and stopped exercise because of shortness of breath and leg fatigue. Resting and exercise ECGs and oximetry were normal.

Interpretation

Comments

Resting studies showed a moderately severe obstructive ventilatory defect (Table 10.43.1). The anaerobic threshold was low. During unloaded pedaling, the R rose over 1.0 and persisted thereafter, which was evidence of excess CO_2 production because of lactic acid buffering at a low $\dot{V}O_2$.

Analysis

The most distinctive abnormalities are the exercise tachycardia, low and early plateaus of the $\dot{V}O_2$ and the O_2 pulse, and the low $\Delta\dot{V}O_2/\Delta WR$. Peak $\dot{V}O_2$ and the anaerobic threshold are decreased (Table 10.43.2), leading us to flowchart 4. The breathing reserve is borderline low (branch point 4.1). We do not have arterial blood gas measurements to address the question of VD/VT (branch point 4.2), but the $\dot{V}E/\dot{V}CO_2$ at the anaerobic threshold is normal, suggesting that the VD/VT is within normal limits. The high ratio of tidal volume to inspiratory capacity and the borderline breathing reserve are com-

patible with obstructive lung disease. We know from panels 2, 3, 5, and 8 of the exercise test that the patient has a significant circulatory problem. Because of the normal VD/VT, the circulatory problem is not due to disease of the pulmonary circulation. Also, because of the large release of buffer CO_2 during exercise, the circulatory problem is not due to peripheral arterial disease. The steep heart rate response; low, flat O_2 pulse response to exercise; low plateau in $\dot{V}O_2$ at maximal work rate; low AT; and reduced $\Delta\dot{V}O_2/\Delta WR$ are all consistent with primary heart disease (such as left ventricular failure) limiting exercise performance.

Conclusion

The patient's $\dot{V}O_2$max of 18 ml/min/kg is associated with an intermediate risk for morbidity and mortality for lung resection. Values below 15 ml/min/kg indicate a higher risk. Unfortunately, the patient was found to have an enlarged axillary lymph node with metastatic malignant cells a few days later and was no longer a potential operative candidate.

TABLE 10.43.1.   Selected Respiratory Function Data

Measurement	Predicted	Measured
Age, yr		62
Sex		Male
Height, cm		170
Weight, kg	74	68
Hematocrit, %		49
VC, L	3.35	2.76
IC, L	2.23	2.07
TLC, L	5.20	5.46
FEV_1, L	2.62	1.28
FEV_1/VC, %	78	46
MVV, L/min	113	62
D_LCO, ml/mm Hg/min	22.9	20.2

TABLE 10.43.2.   Selected Exercise Data

Measurement	Predicted	Measured
Peak $\dot{V}O_2$, L/min	1.98	1.22
Maximum HR, beats/min	158	175
Maximum O_2 pulse, ml/beat	12.5	7.1
$\Delta\dot{V}O_2/\Delta WR$, ml/min/W	10.3	6.7
AT, L/min	>0.87	0.6
Blood pressure, mmHg (rest, max)		130/80, 220/110
Maximum $\dot{V}E$, L/min		48
Exercise breathing reserve, L/min	>15	14
O_2 saturation, oximeter (rest, max)		96, 96

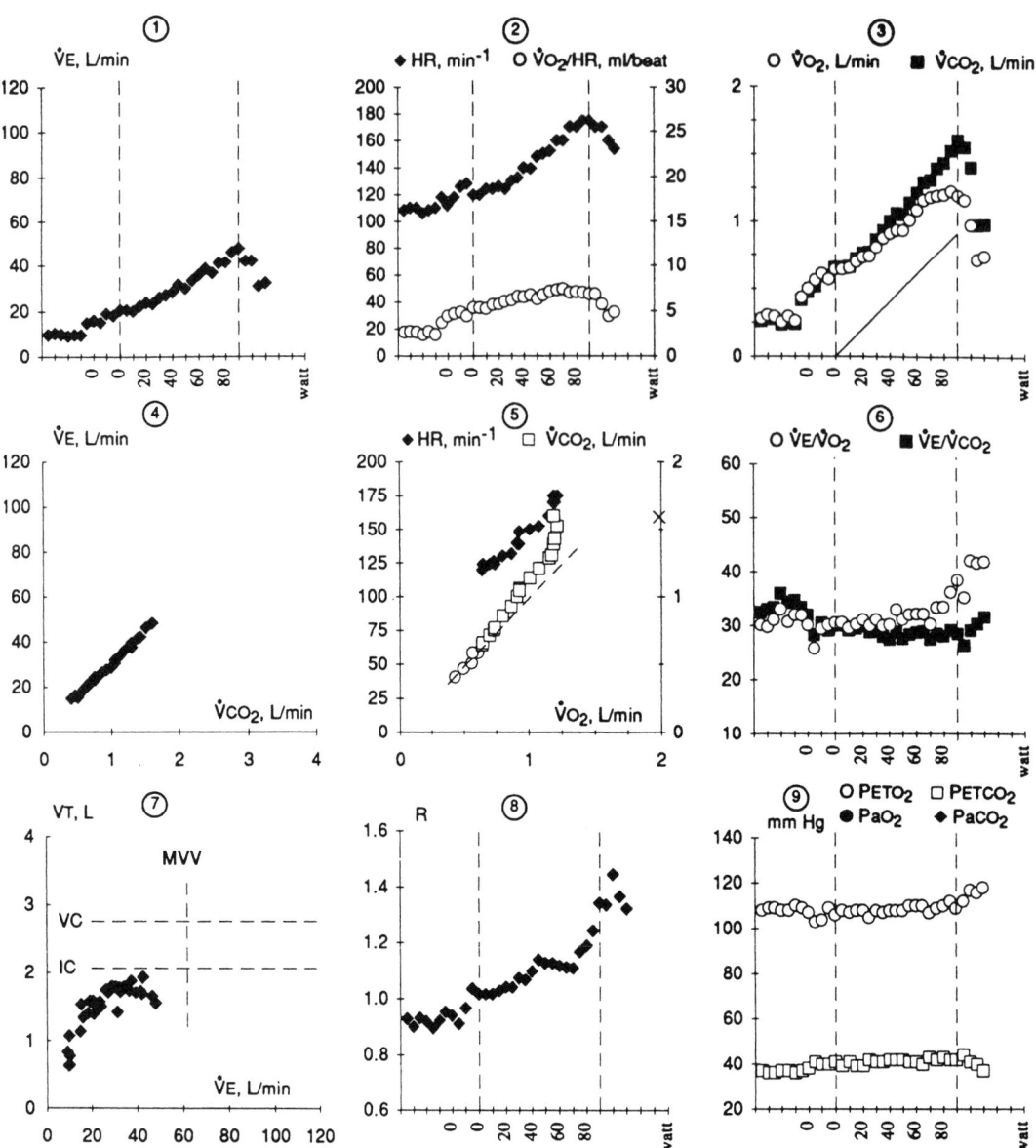

FIGURE 10.43.1.   **1:** Vertical dashed lines in panels 1 to 3 and 6, 8, and 9 indicate the beginning and the end of the increasing work period. **2:** Unloaded cycling is performed for 3 minutes before the left vertical dashed line. **3:** In panel 3, the diagonal line shows the increase of $\dot{V}O_2$ at a slope of 10 ml/min/W. **4:** In panel 5, the diagonal dashed line has a slope of 1; the x in the upper right is the predicted maximum heart rate and $\dot{V}O_2$ for the subject.

TABLE 10.43.3.   Air Breathing

Time min	Work rate watts	BP mmHg	HR min^{-1}	f min^{-1}	$\dot{V}_E$ L/min BTPS	$\dot{V}_{CO_2}$ L/min STPD	$\dot{V}_{O_2}$ L/min STPD	$\dfrac{\dot{V}_{O_2}}{HR}$ ml/beat	R	pH	HCO$_3^-$ meq/L	P_{O_2}, mmHg ET	a	(A − a)	P_{CO_2}, mmHg ET	a	(a − ET)	$\dfrac{\dot{V}_E}{\dot{V}_{CO_2}}$	$\dfrac{\dot{V}_E}{\dot{V}_{O_2}}$	$\dfrac{V_D}{V_T}$
	Rest	130/80																		
	Rest		108	15	9.7	0.26	0.28	2.6	0.93			108			37			32	30	
	Rest		110	16	10.3	0.27	0.30	2.7	0.90			109			36			33	30	
	Rest		110	13	10.1	0.27	0.29	2.6	0.93			109			36			33	31	
	Rest	130/80	106	11	9.2	0.23	0.25	2.4	0.92			108			37			36	33	
	Rest		108	9	9.7	0.26	0.29	2.7	0.90			108			37			34	31	
	Rest		110	15	9.6	0.24	0.26	2.4	0.92			110			36			35	32	
	Unloaded		118	13	14.8	0.41	0.43	3.6	0.95			109			37			33	32	
	Unloaded		112	12	16.1	0.47	0.50	4.5	0.94			107			38			32	30	
	Unloaded		118	10	15.3	0.51	0.56	4.7	0.91			103			41			28	26	
	Unloaded		126	12	19.0	0.59	0.61	4.8	0.97			104			40			30	29	
	Unloaded		128	13	18.3	0.59	0.57	4.5	1.04			109			40			29	30	
	Unloaded	140/80	120	13	20.6	0.65	0.64	5.3	1.02			106			41			30	30	
0.5	10		120												39			30	31	
1.0	10	159/90	124	15	20.9	0.65	0.64	5.3	1.02			108			41			29	30	
1.5	20		124	13	20.3	0.66	0.65	5.2	1.02			107			39			29	30	
2.0	20		126	15	22.5	0.72	0.70	5.6	1.03			108			39			30	31	
				16	24.1	0.76	0.73	5.8	1.04			108								
2.5	30		124	15	23.5	0.77	0.74	6.0	1.04			105			42			29	30	
3.0	30		130	15	26.2	0.86	0.80	6.2	1.08			108			41			29	31	
3.5	40		132	16	27.4	0.93	0.87	6.6	1.07			107			41			28	30	
4.0	40	150/90	140	16	28.8	1.00	0.91	6.5	1.10			108			42			27	30	
4.5	50		139	18	32.1	1.06	0.93	6.7	1.14			108			42			29	33	
5.0	50		148	17	30.4	1.05	0.93	6.3	1.13			108			42			28	31	
5.5	60		150	19	34.0	1.14	1.01	6.7	1.13			110			41			28	32	
6.0	60	200/100	152	21	36.5	1.21	1.08	7.1	112			110			41			29	32	
6.5	70		160	23	39.3	1.29	1.16	7.3	1.11			110			40			29	32	
7.0	70		160	20	37.5	1.31	1.18	7.4	1.11			107			43			27	30	
7.5	80		170	24	41.6	1.39	1.19	7.0	1.17			109			42			28	33	
8.0	80	200/100	170	25	42.2	1.43	1.20	7.1	1.19			110			43			28	33	
8.5	90		175	28	46.5	1.52	1.22	7.0	1.25			112			42			29	36	
9.0	90		175	31	48.2	1.60	1.19	6.8	1.34			109			42			28	38	
	Recovery		170	22	42.6	1.55	1.16	6.8	1.34			112			44			26	35	
	Recovery		170	22	42.5	1.40	0.97	5.7	1.44			117			41			29	42	
	Recovery		160	22	31.3	0.97	0.71	4.4	1.37			116			40			30	41	
	Recovery	220/110	154	19	32.6	0.98	0.74	4.8	1.32			118			37			32	42	

Case 44 Bullous Emphysema: Before and After Bullectomy

Clinical Findings

This 50-year-old computer technician had retired approximately 10 years prior to initial evaluation because of progressive dyspnea. He denied cough, sputum production, wheezing, or chest pain. There was no family history of lung disease. Chest roentgenographic studies showed large bullous lesions in the right middle and upper lung fields. Flow rates did not improve following four breaths of nebulized isoproterenol. Perfusion scan demonstrated no perfusion in the right middle and upper hemithorax or at the left apex. α_1-Antitrypsin levels were normal. One month after the first exercise test, the patient's right upper lobe and portions of the right middle lobe were resected. The resected lung showed bullous and centriacinar emphysema with patchy atelectasis; a small squamous cell scar carcinoma was found in the upper lobe. He continued to smoke heavily.

Exercise Findings

Preoperatively, the patient performed exercise on a cycle ergometer while breathing room air and, following a 90-minute rest, breathing 100% oxygen. Three months postoperatively, only an air breathing study was performed. On each occasion, he pedaled at 60 rpm on an unloaded cycle for 2, 3, or 4 minutes. The work rate was then increased 20 W every minute. Arterial blood was sampled every second minute, and intraarterial blood pressure was recorded from a percutaneous brachial artery

catheter. Resting ECGs were normal. Preoperatively, the patient stopped exercise because of dyspnea without an exercise-induced abnormality in the ECG. He stopped during the postoperative test because of dyspnea and pressurelike right-sided chest pain. There were multifocal, back-to-back, and salvos of premature ventricular contractions at the end of exercise and for 2 minutes of recovery without abnormal ST-segment changes.

Interpretation

Comments

Resting respiratory function studies show moderate obstructive lung disease with marked reduction in diffusing capacity ($D_{L}CO$). Following a bullectomy, the vital capacity increased, and the residual volume decreased with improvement in expiratory flow (Table 10.44.1). Although the diffusing capac-

TABLE 10.44.1.   Selected Respiratory Function Data

Measurement	Predicted	Preoperative	Postoperative
Age, yr		50	
Sex		Male	
Height, cm		170	
Weight, kg	74	71	
Hematocrit, %		46	
VC, L	3.89	3.01	3.57
IC, L	2.59	2.03	2.46
TLC, L	5.69	7.05	5.56
FEV$_1$, L	3.09	1.93	2.44
FEV$_1$/VC, %	79	64	68
MVV, L/min	131	90	110
D$_{L}$CO, ml/mm Hg/min	26.5	10.0	13.0

TABLE 10.44.2.   Selected Exercise Data

Measurement	Predicted	Preoperative	Postoperative
Peak V̇O$_2$, L/min	2.32	0.99	1.06
Maximum HR, beats/min	170	144	144
Maximum O$_2$ pulse, ml/beat	13.7	7.5	7.9
ΔV̇O$_2$/ΔWR, ml/min/W	10.3	5.1	5.8
AT, L/min	>1.00	0.6	0.75
Blood pressure, mmHg (rest, max)		144/90, 187/100	144/88, 238/94
Maximum V̇E, L/min		84	80
Exercise breathing reserve, L/min	>15	6	30
PaO$_2$, mmHg (rest, max ex)		67, 54	74, 74
P(A − a)O$_2$, mmHg (rest, max ex)		47, 72	34, 52
P(a − ET)CO$_2$, mmHg (rest, max ex)		4, 8	4, 3
VD/VT (rest, heavy ex)		0.39, 0.47	0.41, 0.40
HCO$_3^-$, mEq/L (rest, 2-min recov)		21, 14	21, 14

TABLE 10.44.3.   Pre-bullectomy Study

Time min	Work rate watts	BP mmHg	HR min⁻¹	f min⁻¹	V̇E L/min BTPS	V̇CO₂ L/min STPD	V̇O₂ L/min STPD	V̇O₂/HR ml/beat	R	pH	HCO₃⁻ meq/L	PO₂ ET	PO₂ a	PO₂ (A−a)	PCO₂ ET	PCO₂ a	PCO₂ (a−ET)	V̇E/V̇CO₂	V̇E/V̇O₂	VD/VT
	Rest									7.41	21		63			34				
	Rest		69	21	9.7	0.12	0.14	2.0	0.86			120			25			66	57	
	Rest		69	17	10.3	0.16	0.20	2.9	0.80			117			26			55	44	
	Rest		70	15	8.5	0.14	0.18	2.6	0.78			115			27			52	40	
	Rest		70	19	10.7	0.18	0.22	3.1	0.82			117			27			50	41	
	Rest		70	14	10.0	0.18	0.21	3.0	0.86			119			26			49	42	
	Rest	144/90	69	15	10.1	0.17	0.21	3.0	0.81	7.41	19	119	67	47	26	30	4	52	42	0.39
	Unloaded		76	31	29.2	0.45	0.49	6.4	0.92			124			23			59	54	
	Unloaded		80	32	30.5	0.48	0.52	6.5	0.92			125			23			58	53	
	Unloaded		80	32	31.4	0.50	0.52	6.5	0.96			125			23			57	55	
	Unloaded		84	29	28.3	0.47	0.50	6.0	0.94			124			24			55	52	
	Unloaded		88	33	29.8	0.46	0.48	5.5	0.96			124			24			59	56	
	Unloaded	156/90	87	28	28.9	0.48	0.51	5.9	0.94	7.41	18	125	62	58	24	29	5	55	52	0.42
0.5	20		91	32	32.6	0.53	0.57	6.3	0.93			125			24			56	52	
1.0	20		93	30	32.8	0.55	0.57	6.1	0.96			125			24			55	53	
1.5	40		93	32	35.0	0.57	0.59	6.3	0.97			124			24			57	55	
2.0	40	162/94	96	32	37.4	0.62	0.62	6.5	1.00	7.40	17	125	59	63	24	28	4	56	56	0.42
2.5	60		100	35	42.9	0.70	0.68	6.8	1.03			156			24			57	59	
3.0	60		104	40	50.8	0.80	0.76	7.3	1.05			156			24			59	62	
3.5	80		111	43	57.5	0.91	0.82	7.4	1.11			159			22			59	66	
4.0	80	181/96	116	45	62.7	1.00	0.87	7.5	1.15	7.40	18	159	51	72	22	30	8	59	68	0.48
4.5	100		120	58	77.3	1.13	0.95	7.9	1.19			131			20			64	76	
5.0	100		132	60	84.2	1.20	0.97	7.3	1.24			132			20			66	82	
5.5	120	187/100	144	57	78.6	1.19	0.99	6.9	1.20	7.39	17	133	54	72	20	28	8	62	75	0.47
	Recovery		138	55	76.5	1.23	1.01	7.3	1.22			132			21			58	71	
	Recovery		132	47	70.3	1.12	0.92	7.0	1.22			132			20			59	72	
	Recovery		120	44	66.2	1.08	0.83	6.9	1.30			133			20			58	75	
	Recovery	196/99	109	40	56.5	0.92	0.64	5.9	1.44	7.31	14	133	66	62	21	29	8	58	83	0.46

ity is slightly improved, it is still disproportionately reduced compared with the flow rate impairment. For example, postoperatively the MVV is 84% of predicted, whereas the diffusing capacity measurement is 50% of predicted. Exercise tolerance, surprisingly, is only slightly improved postoperatively.

Analysis

Referring to flowchart 1, the peak $\dot{V}O_2$ and anaerobic threshold are significantly reduced pre- and postoperatively (Table 10.44.2). See flowchart 4. Preoperatively the exercise breathing reserve is low, but postoperatively the breathing reserve is normal (branch point 4.1). Taking the low breathing reserve branch directed by the preoperative study, VD/VT is high, consistent with lung disease with impaired peripheral oxygenation (branch point 4.2). The confirmatory abnormalities noted in that diagnostic box are found in Table 10.44.3.

Postbullectomy, we must take the normal breathing reserve branch at branch point 4.1. The ventilatory equivalent for CO_2 at the AT is high and the indices of ventilation–perfusion mismatching are

abnormal, supporting the diagnosis of an abnormal pulmonary circulation (branch point 4.5). The vital capacity is normal, suggesting that the abnormality in the pulmonary circulation is due to pulmonary vascular disease. This is supported by a low resting DLCO. There is no abrupt reduction in PaO₂ postoperatively, as might be expected with a right-to-left shunt. This was confirmed by a repeat exercise test with the patient breathing 100% oxygen (not shown). Referring to the diagnostic box under abnormal pulmonary circulation, confirmatory observations are as follows: (a) a steep heart rate response to the increase in $\dot{V}O_2$, becoming steeper as the peak $\dot{V}O_2$ is approached (panel 5); (b) a low O_2 pulse with a flat contour as work rate is increased (panel 2); and (c) a decreasing $\Delta\dot{V}O_2/\Delta WR$ as work rate is increased (panel 3) for both the preoperative (Fig. 10.44.1) and postoperative (Fig. 19.44.2) studies. All these findings are consistent with an oxygen flow problem of the type seen with functionally important pulmonary vascular disease. Bullectomy did not improve the abnormalities in O_2 flow, although it improved the ventilatory mechanics. Despite improvement in respiratory mechanics, exercise per-

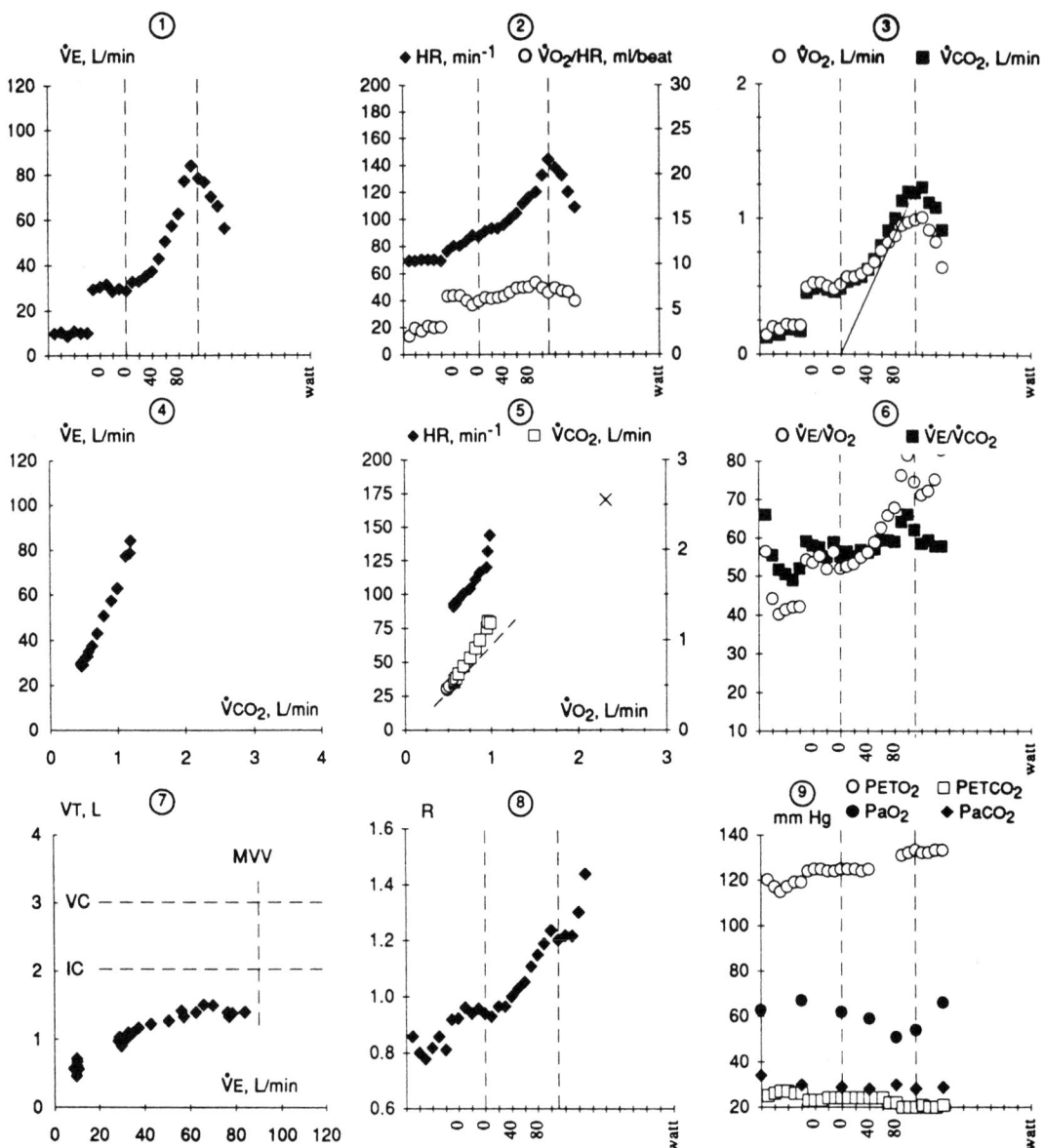

FIGURE 10.44.1.   Prebullectomy study. **1:** Vertical dashed lines in panels 1 to 3 and 6, 8, and 9 indicate the beginning and the end of the increasing work period. **2:** Unloaded cycling is performed for 3 minutes before the left vertical dashed line. **3:** In panel 3, the diagonal line shows the increase of $\dot{V}O_2$ at a slope of 10 ml/min/W. **4:** In panel 5, the diagonal dashed line has a slope of 1; the x in the upper right is the predicted maximum heart rate and $\dot{V}O_2$ for the subject.

formance did not significantly improve postoperatively. Pulmonary vascular disease was the predominant factor limiting exercise preoperatively. The ectopy noted during exercise after bullectomy might be secondary to the development of critically important pulmonary hypertension.

Conclusion

The patient has bullous emphysema. Pulmonary vascular occlusive disease limited exercise performance after bullectomy.

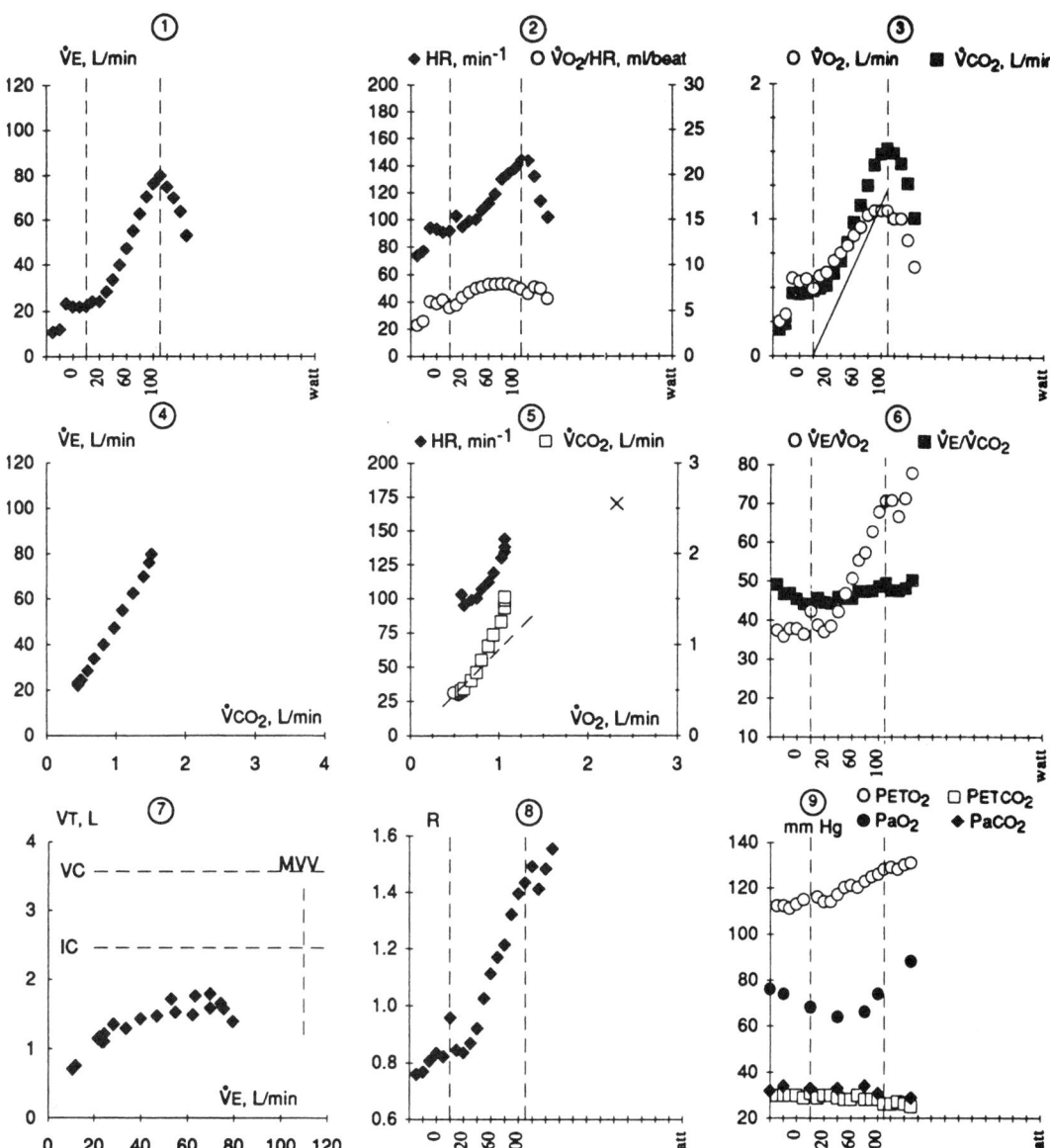

FIGURE 10.44.2.   Postbullectomy study. **1:** Vertical dashed lines in panels 1 to 3 and 6, 8, and 9 indicate the beginning and the end of the increasing work period. **2:** Unloaded cycling is performed for 3 minutes before the left vertical dashed line. **3:** In panel 3, the diagonal line shows the increase of $\dot{V}O_2$ at a slope of 10 ml/min/W. **4:** In panel 5, the diagonal dashed line has a slope of 1; the x in the upper right is the predicted maximum heart rate and $\dot{V}O_2$ for the subject.

TABLE 10.44.4. Post-bullectomy Study

Time min	Work rate watts	BP mmHg	HR min⁻¹	f min⁻¹	$\dot{V}_E$ L/min BTPS	$\dot{V}_{CO_2}$ L/min STPD	$\dot{V}_{O_2}$ L/min STPD	$\dot{V}_{O_2}$/HR ml/beat	R	pH	HCO_3^- meq/L	P_{O_2}, mmHg ET	a	(A−a)	P_{CO_2}, mmHg ET	a	(a−ET)	$\dot{V}_E/\dot{V}_{CO_2}$	$\dot{V}_E/\dot{V}_{O_2}$	V_D/V_T
	Rest	150/94								7.44	21		76			32				
	Rest		74	15	10.6	0.19	0.25	3.4	0.76			112			30			49	37	
	Rest	144/88	77	16	12.1	0.23	0.30	3.9	0.77	7.42	22	112	74	34	30	34		47	36	0.41
	Unloaded		94	21	23.3	0.46	0.57	6.1	0.81			111			30			47	38	
	Unloaded		93	19	22.0	0.45	0.54	5.8	0.83			113			30			45	38	
	Unloaded		91	19	21.9	0.46	0.56	6.2	0.82			115			29			44	36	
	Unloaded	163/38	92	19	22.2	0.47	0.49	5.3	0.96	7.42	21		68	48	31	33	2	44	42	0.37
0.5	20		103	22	24.2	0.49	0.58	5.6	0.84			116			29			46	39	
1.0	20		95	20	24.3	0.51	0.61	6.4	0.84			114			30			44	37	
1.5	40		99	21	28.3	0.60	0.69	7.0	0.87			114			30			44	38	
2.0	40	175/94	100	26	33.7	0.69	0.75	7.5	0.92	7.42	21	117	64	51	29	33	4	46	42	0.40
2.5	60		107	28	40.1	0.83	0.81	7.6	1.02			120			28			45	47	
3.0	60		112	32	47.2	0.98	0.88	7.9	1.11			121			28			45	51	
3.5	80		119	36	54.9	1.10	0.94	7.9	1.17			120			30			47	55	
4.0	80	225/94	130	42	62.4	1.25	1.03	7.9	1.21	7.39	20	123	66	55	28	34	6	47	57	0.43
4.5	100		134	44	69.9	1.40	1.06	7.9	1.32			125			28			47	62	
5.0	100	238/94	138	48	75.7	1.48	1.06	7.7	1.40	7.35	17	126	74	52	28	31	3	48	68	0.40
5.5	120		144	57	79.5	1.52	1.06	7.4	1.43			128			26			49	70	
	Recovery		144	45	74.5	1.49	1.00	6.9	1.49			129			26			47	71	
	Recovery		132	39	69.8	1.41	1.00	7.6	1.41			128			27			47	66	
	Recovery		114	36	63.5	1.26	0.85	7.5	1.48			130			26			48	71	
	Recovery	231/100	102	31	53.2	1.01	0.65	6.4	1.55	7.31	14	131	88	41	25	29	4	50	78	0.39

Case 45 Obstructive Airway Disease: Before and After Rehabilitation

Clinical Findings

This 69-year-old man with known chronic obstructive lung disease was evaluated before and after a pulmonary rehabilitation program of 2 months' duration, which featured (among other components) a program of cycle ergometer exercise. The patient exercised for 45 minutes per day, 3 days per week, on a stationery bicycle at exercise intensities approaching his maximum tolerance. Resting respiratory and exercise testing data for both evaluations are shown. The patient had recently stopped smoking, although he had a 51-year history of cigarette smoking. His medications included theophylline and inhaled α-agonist and anticholinergic agents.

Exercise Findings

The patient performed exercise on a cycle ergometer before and after a 2-month training period. He pedaled at 60 rpm without an added load for 3 minutes. The work rate was then increased 5 W per minute to tolerance. Heart rate and rhythm were continuously monitored; 12-lead ECGs were obtained during rest, exercise, and recovery. Every 2 minutes, blood pressure was measured by a sphygmomanometer, and a sample of blood was drawn from a venous catheter placed in the back of the hand. Blood samples were assayed for blood lactate concentration. The patient was well motivated and cooperative and stopped exercise on both occasions because of dyspnea. No ECG abnormalities were noted at rest or during exercise.

Interpretation

Comments

This case shows the effects of a training program on resting respiratory function, work capacity, and peak $\dot{V}O_2$. Resting studies show moderate obstructive lung disease, with severe loss of effective pulmonary capillary bed.

Analysis

Referring to flowchart 1, on the initial study the peak $\dot{V}O_2$ was low, whereas the anaerobic threshold was at the lower limits of normal (Table 10.45.2). Regardless of which flowchart is used, we would arrive at the diagnosis of obstructive lung disease for both studies. Using flowchart 3 for the first study, we would go through branch points 3.1 and 3.2 to reach that diagnosis. Using flowchart 4,

TABLE 10.45.1.   Selected Respiratory Function Data

Measurement	Predicted	Measured	
Age, yr		69	
Sex		Male	
Height, cm		170	
Weight, kg	60	74	
Hematocrit, %		40	
		Before	After*
VC, L	3.60	1.99	2.19
IC, L	2.40	1.50	1.65
FEV_1, L	2.78	0.99	1.11
FEV_1/VC, %	77	50	51
MVV, indirect, L/min	111	40	44
D_LCO, ml/mm Hg/min	22.4	10.6	12.7

*After training.

TABLE 10.45.2.   Selected Exercise Data

Measurement	Predicted	Before	After
Peak $\dot{V}O_2$, L/min	1.67	0.90	1.0
Maximum HR, beats/min	151	136	140
Work rate, max W		30	50
Maximum O_2 pulse, ml/beat	11.1	6.6	7.6
$\Delta\dot{V}O_2/\Delta WR$, ml/min/W	10.3		8.2
AT, L/min	>0.75	0.75	Indeterminate*
Maximum $\dot{V}E$, L/min		40	42
Exercise breathing reserve, L/min using indirect MVV	>15	0	2
Peak lactate, mEq/L		3.0	2.3

*Apparently, because of the small increase in lactate after training, a breakpoint in the V-slope plot (panel 5) is not observed.

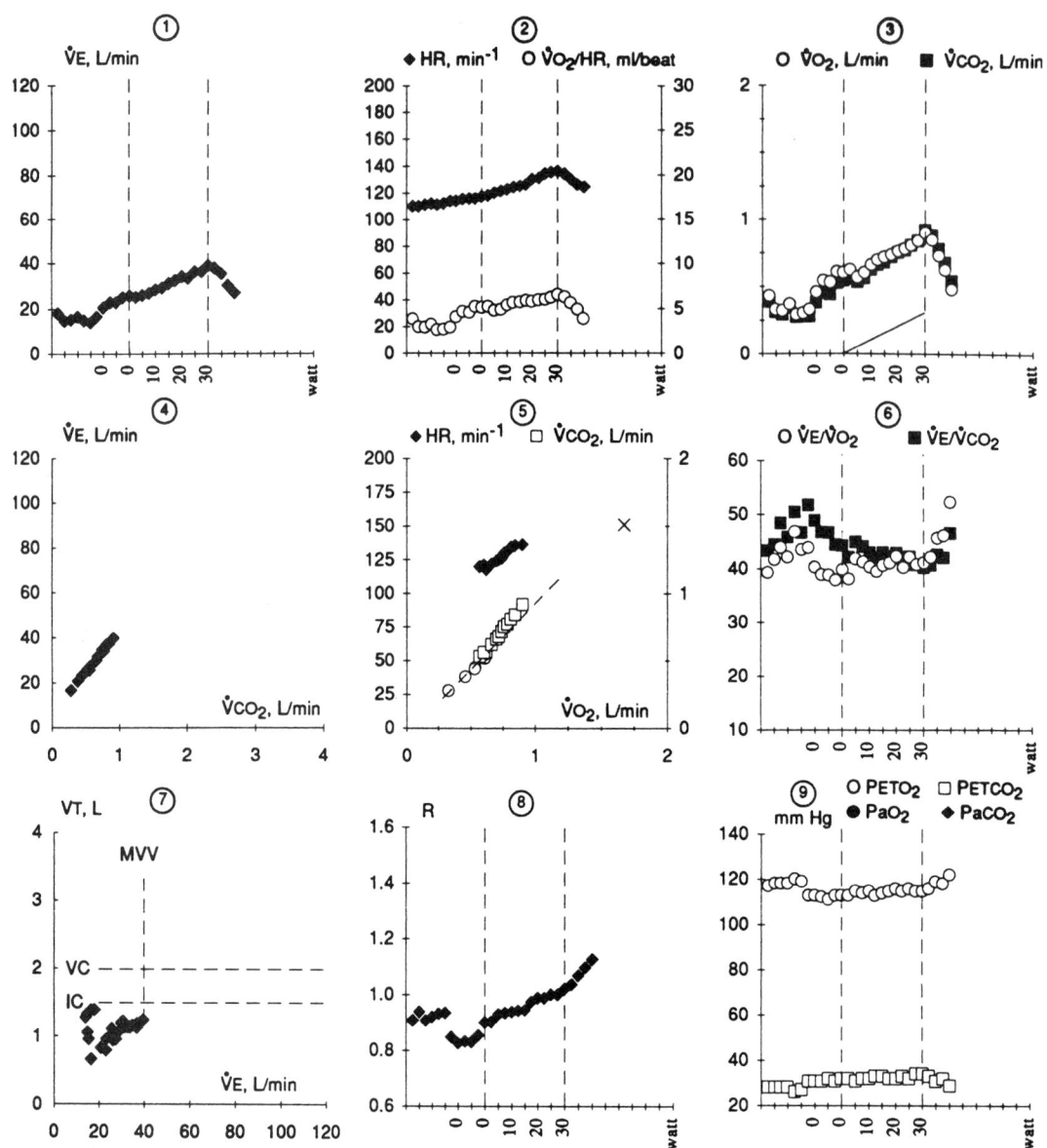

FIGURE 10.45.1.   Before training. **1:** Vertical dashed lines in panels 1 to 3 and 6, 8, and 9 indicate the beginning and the end of the increasing work period. **2:** Unloaded cycling is performed for 3 minutes before the left vertical dashed line. **3:** In panel 3, the diagonal line shows the increase of $\dot{V}O_2$ at a slope of 10 ml/min/W. **4:** In panel 5, the diagonal dashed line has a slope of 1; the x in the upper right is the predicted maximum heart rate and $\dot{V}O_2$ for the subject.

the low breathing reserve (branch point 4.1) and presumed high VD/VT because of the high $\dot{V}E/\dot{V}CO_2$ (branch point 4.2) lead us to the diagnosis of lung disease with impaired peripheral oxygenation. If we had used flowchart 5, we would have arrived at the diagnosis of obstructive lung disease through branch points 5.1, 5.3, and 5.7.

Conclusion

Comparing the studies performed before and after pulmonary rehabilitation, it is apparent that this patient's exercise tolerance has improved appreciably. This can be explained only in part by the small improvement in airways obstruction. Insight into

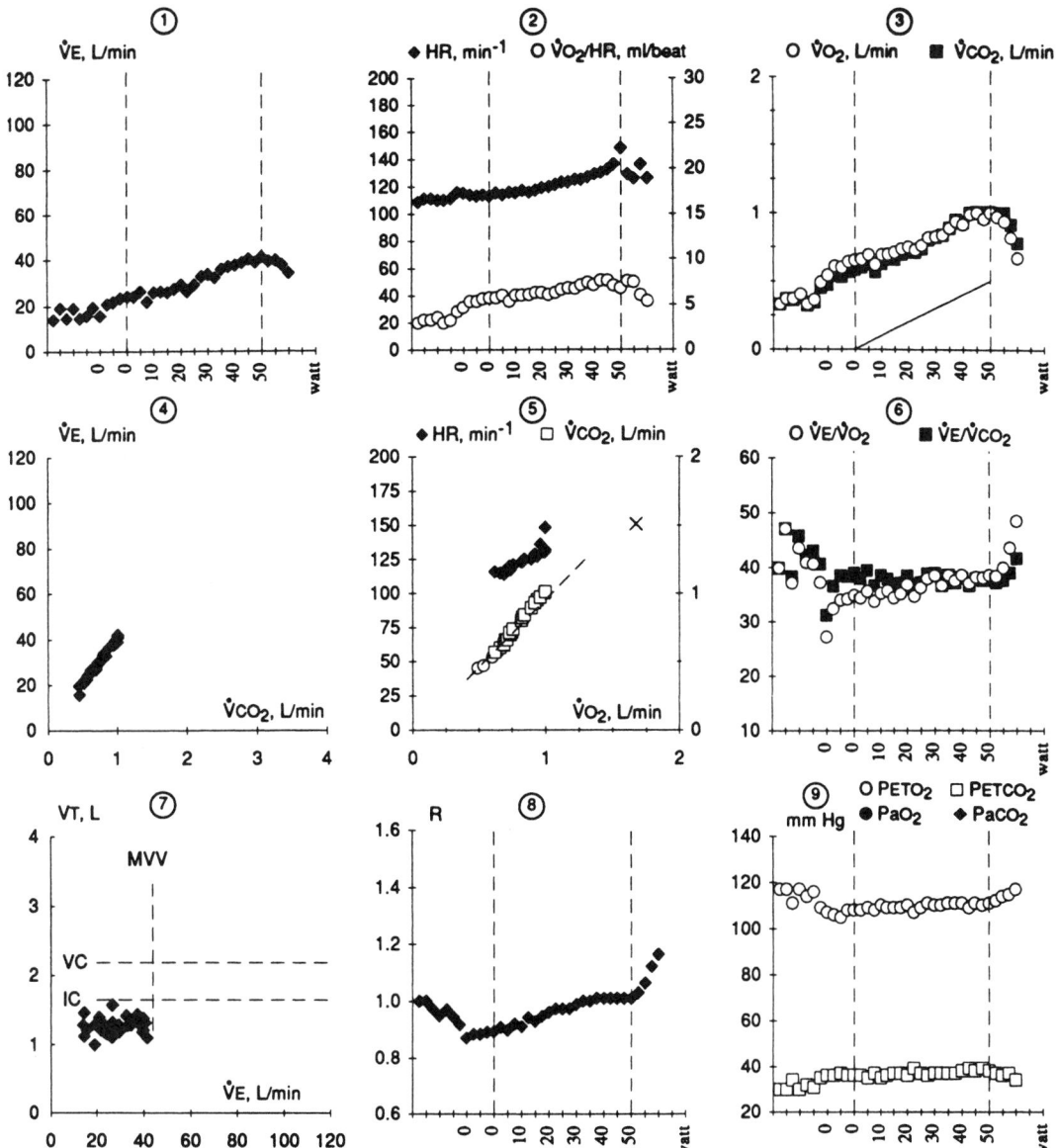

FIGURE 10.45.2.   After training. **1:** Vertical dashed lines in panels 1 to 3 and 6, 8, and 9 indicate the beginning and the end of the increasing work period. **2:** Unloaded cycling is performed for 3 minutes before the left vertical dashed line. **3:** In panel 3, the diagonal line shows the increase of $\dot{V}O_2$ at a slope of 10 ml/min/W. **4:** In panel 5, the diagonal dashed line has a slope of 1; the x in the upper right is the predicted maximum heart rate and $\dot{V}O_2$ for the subject.

the cause of the improvement can be gained by comparing the physiologic responses at identical work rates in the two studies (Table 10.45.5).

The reduction in lactate at a given work rate is characteristic of a physiologic training effect. This is also reflected in a lower $\dot{V}CO_2$ (less CO_2 release from

HCO_3^- buffering). The reduction in $\dot{V}E$ and the improved exercise tolerance are likely due to the reduced acid stimulus to breathing, reduced CO_2 production, and improved ventilation–perfusion relations (reduced V_D/V_T) reflected in a reduced ventilatory requirement for O_2 and CO_2.

TABLE 10.45.3. Before Training

Time min	Work rate watts	BP mmHg	HR min⁻¹	f min⁻¹	$\dot{V}_E$ L/min BTPS	$\dot{V}_{CO_2}$ L/min STPD	$\dot{V}_{O_2}$ L/min STPD	$\dfrac{\dot{V}_{O_2}}{HR}$ ml/beat	R	pH	HCO_3^- meq/L	Po₂, mmHg ET	a	(A − a)	Pco₂, mmHg ET	a	(a − ET)	$\dfrac{\dot{V}_E}{\dot{V}_{CO_2}}$	$\dfrac{\dot{V}_E}{\dot{V}_{O_2}}$	$\dfrac{V_D}{V_T}$
	Rest		110	13	18.0	0.39	0.43	3.9	0.91			117			28			43	39	
	Rest		110	11	14.7	0.31	0.33	3.0	0.94			118			28			44	42	
	Rest		111	16	15.4	0.29	0.32	2.9	0.91			118			28			48	44	
	Rest		112	12	16.6	0.34	0.37	3.3	0.92			118			28			46	42	
	Rest		111	14	14.8	0.27	0.29	2.6	0.93			120			26			50	47	
	Rest		112	11	14.0	0.28	0.30	2.7	0.93			119			27			47	44	
	Unloaded		114	25	16.6	0.28	0.33	2.9	0.85			113			31			52	44	
	Unloaded		114	25	20.7	0.38	0.46	4.0	0.83			113			31			49	40	
	Unloaded		115	24	23.1	0.45	0.54	4.7	0.83			112			31			47	39	
	Unloaded		116	29	23.0	0.44	0.53	4.6	0.83			111			32			47	39	
	Unloaded		116	25	25.2	0.52	0.61	5.3	0.85			113			31			44	38	
	Unloaded		117	25	26.0	0.54	0.60	5.1	0.90			113			32			44	40	
0.5	5		118	23	25.6	0.56	0.62	5.3	0.90			113			32			42	38	
1.0	5		120	28	26.2	0.53	0.57	4.8	0.93			115			31			45	42	
1.5	10		121	27	27.0	0.56	0.60	5.0	0.93			114			32			44	41	
2.0	10		122	27	28.9	0.62	0.66	5.4	0.94			115			32			43	40	
2.5	15		124	25	29.8	0.66	0.70	5.6	0.94			113			33			42	40	
3.0	15		125	28	31.6	0.68	0.72	5.8	0.94			114			33			43	41	
3.5	20		126	29	32.8	0.72	0.74	5.9	0.97			115			32			42	41	
4.0	20		130	30	34.7	0.75	0.76	5.8	0.99			116			32			43	42	
4.5	25		131	30	33.9	0.77	0.78	6.0	0.99			115			33			41	40	
5.0	25		134	33	36.9	0.81	0.81	6.0	1.00			116			32			42	42	
5.5	30		135	31	36.9	0.84	0.84	6.2	1.00			115			34			41	41	
6.0	30		136	32	39.7	0.92	0.90	6.6	1.02			115			34			40	41	
	Recovery		134	32	38.5	0.88	0.85	6.3	1.04			116			33			41	42	
	Recovery		130	31	35.9	0.78	0.73	5.6	1.07			119			31			43	46	
	Recovery		126	25	30.7	0.68	0.62	4.9	1.10			118			32			42	46	
	Recovery		124	29	27.6	0.54	0.48	3.9	1.13			122			29			47	52	

TABLE 10.45.4.   After Training

Time min	Work rate watts	BP mmHg	HR min⁻¹	f min⁻¹	V̇E L/min BTPS	V̇CO₂ L/min STPD	V̇O₂ L/min STPD	V̇O₂/HR ml/beat	R	pH	HCO₃⁻ meq/L	PO₂, mmHg ET	a	(A−a)	PCO₂, mmHg ET	a	(a−ET)	V̇E/V̇CO₂	V̇E/V̇O₂	VD/VT
	Rest		109	11	14.1	0.33	0.33	3.0	1.00			117			30			40	40	
	Rest		111	19	19.0	0.37	0.37	3.3	1.00			117			30			47	47	
	Rest		111	10	14.6	0.36	0.37	3.3	0.97			111			34			38	37	
	Rest		110	19	19.0	0.38	0.40	3.6	0.95			117			30			46	43	
	Rest		110	13	14.6	0.32	0.33	3.0	0.97			114			32			42	41	
	Rest		111	13	15.7	0.34	0.36	3.2	0.94			116			31			43	41	
	Unloaded		116	15	19.5	0.45	0.49	4.2	0.92			109			35			41	37	
	Unloaded		115	13	15.8	0.47	0.54	4.7	0.87			107			36			31	27	
	Unloaded		114	15	21.0	0.54	0.61	5.4	0.89			106			36			37	32	
	Unloaded		113	18	21.9	0.53	0.60	5.3	0.88			105			37			38	34	
	Unloaded		114	20	23.5	0.57	0.64	5.6	0.89			108			36			38	34	
	Unloaded		113	21	24.4	0.58	0.65	5.8	0.89			108			36			39	35	
0.5	5		115	20	24.4	0.60	0.66	5.7	0.91			108			36			38	34	
1.0	5		114	24	26.5	0.62	0.69	6.1	0.90			109			35			39	35	
1.5	10		116	17	22.3	0.57	0.62	5.3	0.92			108			37			37	34	
2.0	10		115	23	26.2	0.63	0.69	6.0	0.91			110			35			38	35	
2.5	15		117	20	26.6	0.66	0.70	6.0	0.94			109			36			38	36	
3.0	15		116	21	26.1	0.66	0.71	6.1	0.93			109			37			37	34	
3.5	20		117	22	27.8	0.70	0.74	6.3	0.95			109			37			37	35	
4.0	20		119	25	29.7	0.72	0.75	6.3	0.96			110			36			38	37	
4.5	25		120	17	26.7	0.71	0.73	6.1	0.97			107			39			36	35	
5.0	25		121	23	29.5	0.74	0.76	6.3	0.97			109			37			37	36	
5.5	30		123	26	33.2	0.80	0.82	6.7	0.98			111			36			39	38	
6.0	30		123	26	34.0	0.82	0.83	6.7	0.99			110			37			39	38	
6.5	35		125	23	32.6	0.84	0.84	6.7	1.00			110			37			36	36	
7.0	35		125	26	36.4	0.89	0.89	7.1	1.00			111			37			38	38	
7.5	40		127	26	37.4	0.95	0.94	7.4	1.01			111			37			37	37	
8.0	40		129	29	37.8	0.93	0.92	7.1	1.01			111			38			38	38	
8.5	45		130	29	39.0	1.00	0.99	7.6	1.01			109			39			37	37	
9.0	45		132	31	40.8	1.01	1.00	7.6	1.01			111			38			38	38	
9.5	50		136	33	39.3	0.97	0.96	7.1	1.01			110			39			38	38	
10.0	50		148	38	41.7	1.01	1.00	6.8	1.01			111			38			38	38	
	Recovery		129	33	39.9	1.00	0.97	7.5	1.03			112			37			37	38	
	Recovery		126	29	40.0	1.00	0.94	7.5	1.06			114			36			38	40	
	Recovery		136	29	38.2	0.92	0.82	6.0	1.12			115			37			39	44	
	Recovery		126	27	34.7	0.78	0.67	5.3	1.16			117			34			42	48	

TABLE 10.45.5.   Selected Comparisons

	Responses to 30 Watts	
	Before Rehabilitation	After Rehabilitation
V̇E, L/min	40	34
V̇O₂, L/min	0.9	0.83
V̇CO₂, L/min	0.92	0.82
Heart rate, beats/min	136	123
Lactate, mEq/L	3.0	1.7

Case 46 Early Asbestosis and Chronic Bronchitis

Clinical Findings

This 48-year-old shipyard worker denied having breathing difficulties and could climb three to four flights of stairs before noting shortness of breath. He had been treated for pneumonia 14 years earlier and for a pleural effusion 12 years ago. Two years previously, a benign "calcified mass" attached to a left lower rib had been removed. He had smoked a pack of cigarettes daily for 25 years and had a morning cough with small amounts of yellow sputum. No deformity, rhonchi, rales, or clubbing were noted on physical examination. Chest roentgenograms, including CT views, showed bilateral pleural plaques and marked coarse parenchymal scarring at both bases.

Exercise Findings

The patient performed exercise on a cycle ergometer. He pedaled at 60 rpm without added load for 3 minutes. The work rate was then increased 20 W per minute to his symptom-limited maximum. Arterial blood was sampled every second minute, and intraarterial blood pressure was recorded from a percutaneously placed brachial artery catheter. The patient stopped exercise because of chest discomfort. Resting and exercise ECGs were normal. Carboxyhemoglobin was 8.3%.

Interpretation

Comments

The results of the resting respiratory function studies indicate that this patient has mild, reversible airflow obstruction and a moderate reduction in diffusing capacity (Table 10.46.1). His resting and exercise ECGs are normal. The man is a cigarette smoker with a high carboxyhemoglobin level in his blood.

Analysis

Referring to flowchart 1, the peak $\dot{V}O_2$ and anaerobic threshold are at the lower limits of normal (Table 10.46.2). See flowchart 2. Even though these values are within the normal range and the ECG at the maximum work rate is normal, certain measurements become abnormal during exercise, indicating that the patient has ventilation–perfusion mismatching (branch point 2.3). These include mild arterial hypoxemia and a significant progressive increase in $P(A − a)O_2$ as work rate is increased.

Moreover, $P(a − ET)CO_2$ is increased at the peak $\dot{V}O_2$, and VD/VT is borderline normal.

Conclusion

This case shows ventilation–perfusion mismatching during exercise in an asymptomatic, 48-year-old man, with maximum exercise performance at the lower limit of normal. Putting this together with the history of a pleural effusion 12 years previously, pleural plaques, and pulmonary fibrosis evident on chest roentgenographic studies, the strong possibility exists that this patient is evidencing early features of pulmonary asbestosis. The persistent cigarette smoking (high level of blood carboxyhemoglobin) in this asbestos-exposed worker provides a major neoplastic threat. It also makes him a high-risk candidate for heart disease and emphysema.

TABLE 10.46.1.   Selected Respiratory Function Data

Measurement	Predicted	Measured
Age, yr		48
Sex		Male
Height, cm		180
Weight, kg	82	97
Hematocrit, %		49
VC, L	4.87	4.84 (5.04*)
IC, L	3.25	3.12
TLC, L	7.06	7.12
FEV$_1$, L	3.88	3.23 (3.59*)
FEV$_1$/VC, %	80	67
MVV, L/min	158	183
D$_L$CO, ml/mm Hg/min	31.8	20.0

*After 4 breaths of aerosolized isoproterenol

TABLE 10.46.2.   Selected Exercise Data

Measurement	Predicted	Measured
Peak $\dot{V}O_2$, L/min	2.77	2.37
Maximum HR, beats/min	172	149
Maximum O$_2$ pulse, ml/beat	16.1	15.9
$\Delta\dot{V}O_2$/ΔWR, ml/min/W	10.3	10.3
AT, L/min	>1.19	1.3
Blood pressure, mmHg (rest, max)		120/81, 213/84
Maximum $\dot{V}E$, L/min		98
Exercise breathing reserve, L/min	>15	85
PaO$_2$, mmHg (rest, max ex)		96, 72
P(A − a)O$_2$, mmHg (rest, max ex)		17, 47
P(a − ET)CO$_2$, mmHg (rest, max ex)		3, 1
VD/VT (rest, heavy ex)		0.41, 0.29
HCO$_3^-$, mEq/L (rest, 2-min recov)		25, 18

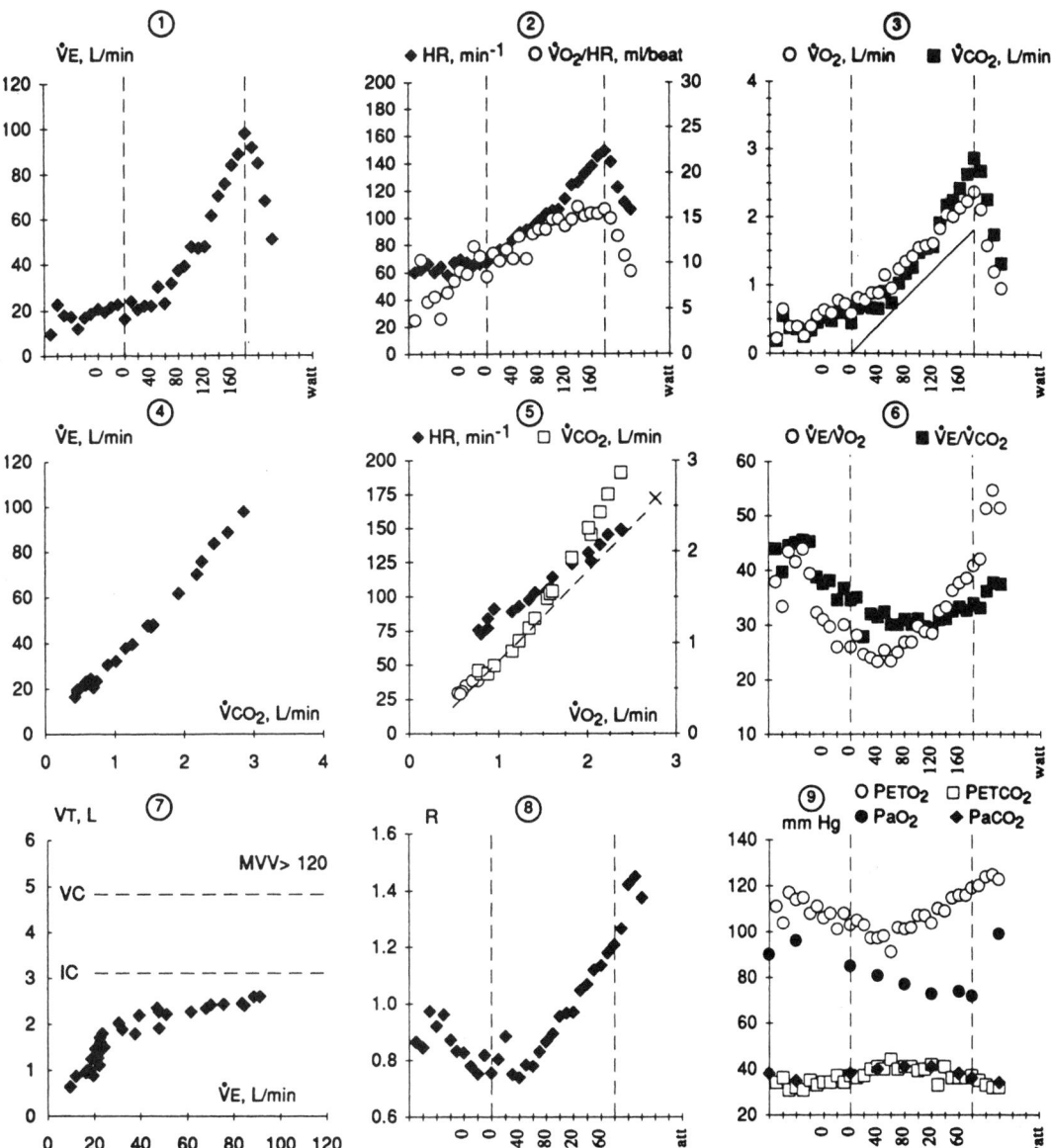

FIGURE 10.46.1.   **1:** Vertical dashed lines in panels 1 to 3 and 6, 8, and 9 indicate the beginning and the end of the increasing work period. **2:** Unloaded cycling is performed for 3 minutes before the left vertical dashed line. **3:** In panel 3, the diagonal line shows the increase of $\dot{V}O_2$ at a slope of 10 ml/min/W. **4:** In panel 5, the diagonal dashed line has a slope of 1; the x in the upper right is the predicted maximum heart rate and $\dot{V}O_2$ for the subject.

TABLE 10.46.3. Air Breathing

Time min	Work rate watts	BP mmHg	HR min⁻¹	f min⁻¹	$\dot{V}_E$ L/min BTPS	$\dot{V}_{CO_2}$ L/min STPD	$\dot{V}_{O_2}$ L/min STPD	$\dot{V}_{O_2}$/HR ml/beat	R	pH	HCO_3^- meq/L	P_{O_2}, mmHg ET	a	(A − a)	P_{CO_2}, mmHg ET	a	(a − ET)	$\dot{V}_E$/$\dot{V}_{CO_2}$	$\dot{V}_E$/$\dot{V}_{O_2}$	V_D/V_T
	Rest	120/81								7.43	25		90			38				
	Rest		60	15	9.6	0.19	0.22	3.7	0.86			111			34			44	38	
	Rest		62	14	22.6	0.54	0.64	10.3	0.84			104			36			40	33	
	Rest		66	18	18.0	0.37	0.38	5.8	0.97			117			31			45	43	
	Rest		66	18	18.0	0.37	0.38	5.8	0.97			117			31			45	43	
	Rest	120/78	60	18	17.3	0.35	0.38	6.3	0.92	7.45	24	114	96	17	32	35	3	45	42	0.41
	Rest		64	14	12.1	0.24	0.25	3.9	0.96			115			31			46	44	
	Rest		58	17	16.8	0.34	0.39	6.7	0.87			108			35			45	39	
	Unloaded		67	15	18.7	0.45	0.54	8.1	0.83			111			33			39	32	
	Unloaded		69	14	20.7	0.52	0.63	9.1	0.83			106			34			38	31	
	Unloaded		67	22	19.4	0.46	0.59	8.8	0.78			108			34			38	30	
	Unloaded		65	17	21.5	0.58	0.77	11.8	0.75			101			37			35	26	
	Unloaded		66	16	22.7	0.58	0.71	10.8	0.82			108			34			37	30	
	Unloaded	120/72	67	17	16.3	0.43	0.57	8.5	0.75	7.43	25	103	85	17	37	38	1	35	26	0.31
0.5	20		73	16	24.1	0.65	0.81	11.1	0.80			105			36			35	28	
1.0	20		76	14	20.4	0.69	0.78	10.3	0.88			103			37			28	25	
1.5	40		77	13	22.2	0.66	0.88	11.4	0.75			97			40			32	24	
2.0	40	129/72	84	20	22.1	0.65	0.88	10.5	0.74	7.42	25	97	81	18	41	40	−1	31	23	0.29
2.5	60		89	15	30.4	0.90	1.15	12.9	0.78			98			40			32	25	
3.0	60		91	13	23.3	0.74	0.95	10.4	0.78			91			44			30	23	
3.5	80		93	17	32.1	1.02	1.23	13.2	0.83			102			40			30	25	
4.0	80	150/75	98	21	37.7	1.16	1.34	13.7	0.87	7.39	24	101	77	27	41	41	0	31	27	0.30
4.5	100		103	18	39.4	1.26	1.41	13.7	0.89			102			41			30	27	
5.0	100		105	21	47.8	1.48	1.55	14.8	0.95			107			39			31	30	
5.5	120		106	20	47.2	1.53	1.58	14.9	0.97			107			40			30	29	
6.0	120	174/75	114	25	47.9	1.56	1.61	14.1	0.97	7.38	24	104	73	35	42	41	−1	29	28	0.27
6.5	140		124	27	61.6	1.92	1.83	14.8	1.05			110			33			31	32	
7.0	140		126	29	70.1	2.18	2.04	16.2	1.07			109			41			31	33	
7.5	160		132	31	75.6	2.25	2.01	15.2	1.12			115			36			32	36	
8.0	160	204/78	138	34	83.6	2.43	2.14	15.5	1.14	7.37	22	116	74	42	36	38	2	33	38	0.31
8.5	180		145	34	88.6	2.63	2.23	15.4	1.18			116			36			33	38	
9.0	180	213/84	149	10	97.6	2.86	2.37	15.9	1.21	7.36	20	119	72	47	37	36	−1	34	41	0.29
	Recovery		141	35	91.4	2.67	2.11	15.0	1.27			120			35			33	42	
	Recovery		122	35	84.5	2.26	1.59	13.0	1.42			124			33			36	51	
	Recovery		111	29	68.1	1.74	1.20	10.8	1.45			125			32			38	55	
	Recovery	213/72	106	23	51.2	1.32	0.96	9.1	1.38	7.33	18	123	99	24	32	34	2	37	51	0.31

Case 47 Mild Asbestosis

Clinical Findings

This 55-year-old male shipyard worker with a long history of asbestos exposure and former cigarette exposure complained of shortness of breath only after climbing three to four flights of stairs, and had a daily cough productive of scant, yellow-tinged sputum. He denied any other symptoms or illnesses. No rales were noted on examination. Chest roentgenogram revealed minimal, but definite, fibrosis, typical of asbestosis. Exercise testing was requested to ascertain whether physiologic abnormalities were associated with the asbestosis.

Exercise Findings

The patient performed exercise on a cycle ergometer. He pedaled at 60 rpm without an added load for 3 minutes. The work rate was then increased 10 W per minute to tolerance. Arterial blood was sampled every second minute, and intraarterial pressure was recorded from a percutaneously placed brachial artery catheter. The patient stopped exercise because of shortness of breath. The ECG showed nonspecific T-wave abnormalities and occasional premature ventricular contractions at rest and during exercise.

Interpretation

Comments

Resting pulmonary function studies showed a mild restrictive defect with parallel loss of pulmonary capillary bed (Table 10.47.1).

Analysis

Referring to flowchart 1, peak $\dot{V}O_2$ is decreased, but the anaerobic threshold is normal (Table 10.47.2). See flowchart 3. At branch point 3.1, the breathing reserve is borderline low. The V_D/V_T is borderline normal, but the $P(A - a)O_2$ and $P(a - ET)CO_2$ are normal. At branch point 3.2, the patient has a high breathing frequency, typical of restrictive lung disease. If we had used flowchart 2, we would have ar-

rived (through branch points 2.1 and 2.3) at the diagnosis of lung disease.

Conclusion

This patient with asbestosis shows mild abnormalities both at rest and with exercise. There is evidence of mild restrictive lung disease at rest. Exercise testing reveals a slightly low peak $\dot{V}O_2$. The high breathing frequency suggests ventilatory limitation; however, the disease at the time of testing has resulted in minimal physiologic impairments.

TABLE 10.47.1.   Selected Respiratory Function Data

Measurement	Predicted	Measured
Age, yr		55
Sex		Male
Height, cm		181
Weight, kg	82	84
Hematocrit, %		45
VC, L	4.24	3.50
IC, L	2.83	2.26
TLC, L	6.32	5.15
FEV$_1$, L	3.35	2.94
FEV$_1$/VC, %	79	84
MVV, L/min	135	107
D$_L$CO, ml/mm Hg/min	27.3	22.7

TABLE 10.47.2.   Selected Exercise Data

Measurement	Predicted	Measured
Peak $\dot{V}O_2$, L/min	2.50	2.03
Maximum HR, beats/min	165	154
Maximum O$_2$ pulse, ml/beat	15.1	13.2
$\Delta\dot{V}O_2/\Delta WR$, ml/min/W	10.3	8.7
AT, L/min	>1.08	1.3
Blood pressure, mmHg (rest, max)		156/90, 216/99
Maximum $\dot{V}E$, L/min		93
Exercise breathing reserve, L/min	>15	14
PaO$_2$, mmHg (rest, max ex)		88, 99
P(A − a)O$_2$, mmHg (rest, max ex)		14, 21
P(a − ET)CO$_2$, mmHg (rest, max ex)		3, −2
V$_D$/V$_T$ (rest, max ex)		0.37, 0.30
HCO$_3^-$, mEq/L (rest, 2-min recov)		25, 20

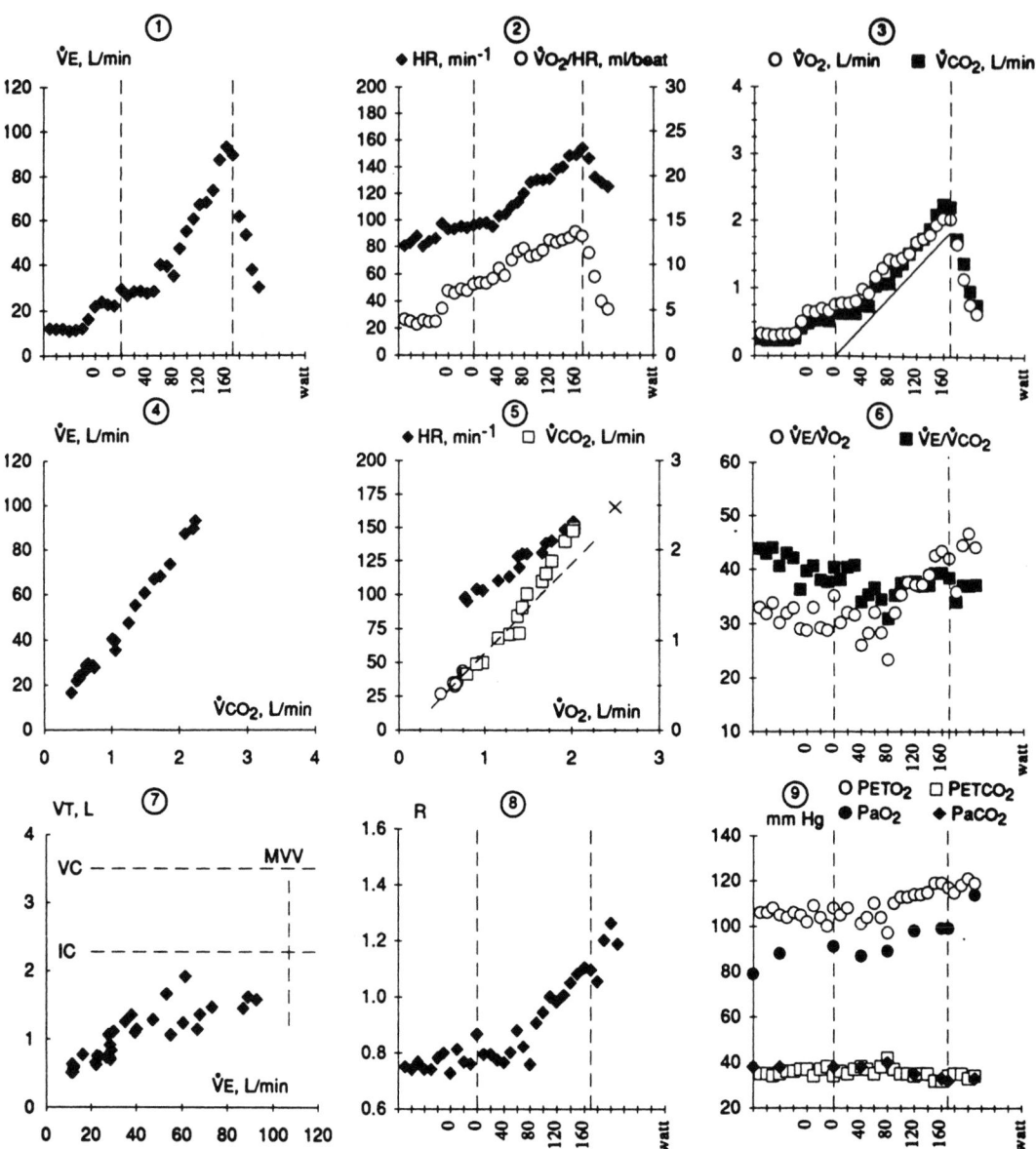

FIGURE 10.47.1.   **1:** Vertical dashed lines in panels 1 to 3 and 6, 8, and 9 indicate the beginning and the end of the increasing work period. **2:** Unloaded cycling is performed for 3 minutes before the left vertical dashed line. **3:** In panel 3, the diagonal line shows the increase of $\dot{V}O_2$ at a slope of 10 ml/min/W. **4:** In panel 5, the diagonal dashed line has a slope of 1; the *x* in the upper right is the predicted maximum heart rate and $\dot{V}O_2$ for the subject.

TABLE 10.47.3.   Air Breathing

Time min	Work rate watts	BP mmHg	HR min⁻¹	f min⁻¹	V̇E L/min BTPS	V̇CO2 L/min STPD	V̇O2 L/min STPD	V̇O2/HR ml/beat	R	pH	HCO3⁻ meq/L	PO2 ET	PO2 a	PO2 (A−a)	PCO2 ET	PCO2 a	PCO2 (a−ET)	V̇E/V̇CO2	V̇E/V̇O2	VD/VT
	Rest	156/90								7.43	25		79			38				
	Rest		81	21	12.3	0.24	0.32	4.0	0.75			106			35			44	33	
	Rest		83	23	11.8	0.23	0.31	3.7	0.74			106			35			43	32	
	Rest		88	21	11.9	0.23	0.30	3.4	0.77			108			34			44	34	
	Rest	162/96	80	22	11.2	0.23	0.31	3.9	0.74	7.42	24	105	88	14	35	38	3	41	30	0.37
	Rest		84	18	11.4	0.23	0.31	3.7	0.74			104			36			43	32	
	Rest		86	20	12.2	0.25	0.32	3.7	0.78			106			36			42	33	
	Unloaded		97	21	16.3	0.40	0.50	5.2	0.80			105			37			36	29	
	Unloaded		93	33	21.8	0.48	0.66	7.1	0.73			102			37			40	29	
	Unloaded		93	32	23.8	0.52	0.64	6.9	0.81			109			34			41	33	
	Unloaded		95	30	22.7	0.53	0.69	7.3	0.77			104			37			38	29	
	Unloaded		94	36	22.3	0.51	0.67	7.1	0.76			100			38			38	29	
	Unloaded	192/96	96	35	29.2	0.65	0.75	7.8	0.87	7.43	25	108	91	16	34	38	4	40	35	0.39
0.5	20		97	36	26.6	0.62	0.78	8.0	0.79			105			36			38	30	
1.0	20		98	39	28.3	0.62	0.78	8.0	0.79			108			35			40	32	
1.5	40		95	41	28.7	0.62	0.80	8.4	0.78			204			37			41	32	
2.0	40	192/90	103	26	27.7	0.75	0.98	9.5	0.77	7.43	25	101	87	16	38	38	0	34	26	0.31
2.5	60		104	31	28.3	0.73	0.91	8.8	0.80			104			37			35	28	
3.0	60		110	35	40.2	1.02	1.16	10.5	0.88			110			35			36	32	
3.5	80		113	36	39.6	1.06	1.29	11.4	0.82			104			38			34	28	
4.0	80	198/93	120	28	35.4	1.07	1.41	11.8	0.76	7.41	25	97	89	11	42	40	−2	31	23	0.28
4.5	100		128	37	47.4	1.26	1.39	10.9	0.91			110			37			35	32	
5.0	100		130	52	55.2	1.36	1.44	11.1	0.94			113			35			37	35	
5.5	120		130	49	60.6	1.50	1.50	11.5	1.00			113			35			38	38	
6.0	120	201/93	131	58	66.8	1.64	1.67	12.7	0.98	7.43	23	114	98	16	34	35	1	38	37	0.32
6.5	140		138	50	68.0	1.73	1.72	12.5	1.01			114			35			37	37	
7.0	140		140	50	73.4	1.87	1.78	12.7	1.05			115			35			37	39	
7.5	160		148	60	87.0	2.09	1.93	13.0	1.08			119			32			39	42	
8.0	160	198/99	149	59	92.9	2.24	2.03	13.6	1.10	7.43	22	119	99	20	32	33	1	39	43	0.32
8.5	180	216/99	154	55	89.3	2.21	2.02	13.1	1.09	7.42	20	117	99	21	34	32	−2	38	42	0.28
	Recovery		146	32	61.5	1.73	1.64	11.2	1.05			115			35			34	36	
	Recovery		132	32	53.4	1.37	1.14	8.6	1.20			118			35			37	44	
	Recovery		128	28	37.8	0.96	0.76	5.9	1.26			121			33			37	47	
	Recovery	189/93	125	27	30.1	0.75	0.63	5.0	1.19	7.39	20	119	114	7	34	33	−1	37	44	0.27

Case 48 Restrictive Lung Disease (Asbestosis)

Clinical Findings

This 67-year-old woman was referred for exercise testing. She had been exposed to asbestos for 3 years while working in a shipyard approximately 40 years earlier. She had never smoked. Three years prior to this evaluation, she noted fatigability, clubbing of fingernails, and shortness of breath. She was unable to climb a flight of stairs or walk rapidly on the level. A transbronchial lung biopsy at that time was reported as showing "fibrosis." Her symptoms improved markedly on 80 mg prednisone, but this medication was stopped after 1 year because of concern regarding its side effects. Five months prior to this evaluation she was started on oxygen therapy, but corticosteroids were not restarted. Examination revealed a thin woman with fine inspiratory rales in the lateral and inferior lung fields that did not clear with coughing. There was dramatic digital clubbing. Chest roentgenograms showed extensive pulmonary infiltrates, compatible with interstitial pulmonary fibrosis. There was also a small patch of pleural calcification on the left. Resting ECG was normal.

Exercise Findings

The patient performed exercise on a cycle ergometer. She pedaled at 60 rpm without added load for 3 minutes. The work rate was then increased 5 W per minute to her symptom-limited maximum. Arterial blood was sampled every second minute, and intraarterial blood pressure was recorded from a percutaneously placed brachial artery catheter. The patient stopped exercising because of dyspnea. She developed some premature atrial contractions during exercise, but the ECG otherwise was not remarkable.

Interpretation

Comments

Results of the respiratory function studies indicate that this patient has a moderately severe restrictive defect with a marked reduction in diffusing capacity (Table 10.48.1). The ECG is normal.

Analysis

Referring to flowchart 1, the peak $\dot{V}O_2$ is markedly reduced and the anaerobic threshold is indeterminate (Table 10.48.2). Referring to flowchart 5, VD/VT, $P(a - ET)CO_2$, and $P(A - a)O_2$ during exercise are markedly abnormal (branch point 5.1). The breathing reserve is low (branch point 5.3). The breathing frequency is high at rest and is maintained at a high level of approximately 50 breaths per minute through the incremental exercise period (branch point 5.7). The maximum ventilation achieved is approximately the patient's maximum ability to breathe. The foregoing findings lead to the diagnosis of restrictive lung disease. Supporting this diag-

TABLE 10.48.1.   Selected Respiratory Function Data

Measurement	Predicted	Measured
Age, yr		67
Sex		Female
Height, cm		163
Weight, kg	63	48
Hematocrit, %		38
VC, L	2.77	1.51
IC, L	1.85	0.70
TLC, L	4.82	2.65
FEV$_1$, L	2.19	1.24
FEV$_1$/VC, %	79	82
MVV, L/min	82	33
D$_L$CO, ml/mm Hg/min	22.3	6.4

TABLE 10.48.2.   Selected Exercise Data

Measurement	Predicted	Measured
Peak $\dot{V}O_2$, L/min	1.12	0.42
Maximum HR, beats/min	153	108
Maximum O$_2$ pulse, ml/beat	7.3	4.1
AT, L/min	>0.56	Indeterminate
Blood pressure, mmHg (rest, max)		122/74, 140/80
Maximum $\dot{V}E$, L/min		29
Exercise breathing reserve, L/min	>15	4
PaO$_2$, mmHg (rest, max ex)		58, 46
P(A − a)O$_2$, mmHg (rest, max ex)		41, 64
P(a − ET)CO$_2$, mmHg (rest, max ex)		8, 10
VD/VT (rest, heavy ex)		0.56, 0.55
HCO$_3^-$, mEq/L (rest, 2-min recov)		25, 24

TABLE 10.48.3.

Time min	Work rate watts	BP mmHg	HR min⁻¹	f min⁻¹	V̇E L/min BTPS	V̇CO₂ L/min STPD	V̇O₂ L/min STPD	V̇O₂/HR ml/beat	R	pH	HCO₃⁻ meq/L	PO₂ ET	PO₂ a	PO₂ (A−a)	PCO₂ ET	PCO₂ a	PCO₂ (a−ET)	V̇E/V̇CO₂	V̇E/V̇O₂	VD/VT
	Rest	122/74								7.44	25		48			37				
	Rest		86	38	14.3	0.14	0.19	2.2	0.74			111			32			79	58	
	Rest		89	36	15.2	0.18	0.23	2.6	0.78			113			32			67	53	
	Rest		87	37	13.4	0.12	0.16	1.8	0.75			110			32			85	64	
	Rest	119/71	90	36	15.0	0.17	0.22	2.4	0.77	7.40	25	109	58	41	33	41	8	70	54	0.56
	Rest		89	39	15.5	0.15	0.20	2.2	0.75			111			32			81	61	
	Rest		92	37	15.1	0.16	0.20	2.2	0.80			113			32			75	60	
	Unloaded		92	42	18.3	0.24	0.31	3.4	0.77			108			36			61	48	
	Unloaded		90	46	21.0	0.26	0.30	3.3	0.87			114			32			66	57	
	Unloaded		92	51	23.4	0.29	0.35	3.8	0.83			113			32			66	54	
	Unloaded		92	49	24.0	0.32	0.36	3.9	0.89			114			33			62	55	
	Unloaded	126/71	93	48	24.1	0.33	0.37	4.0	0.89	7.41	26	115	52	53	32	41	9	61	54	0.54
	Unloaded		95	50	24.3	0.30	0.33	3.5	0.91			117			31			67	61	
0.5	10		99	50	24.7	0.32	0.36	3.6	0.89			114			33			64	57	
1.0	10		97	51	25.0	0.32	0.36	3.7	0.89			114			33			65	57	
1.5	20		100	47	26.0	0.37	0.40	4.0	0.93			115			32			59	55	
2.0	20	137/74	105	47	25.8	0.37	0.40	3.8	0.93	7.41	25	116	49	58	32	40	8	59	55	0.54
2.5	30		104	49	28.6	0.43	0.46	4.4	0.93			118			31			57	53	
3.0	30		106	45	27.6	0.42	0.43	4.1	0.98			118			31			57	55	
3.5	40	140/80	108	45	29.1	0.44	0.42	3.9	1.05	7.39	24	120	46	64	31	41	10	57	60	0.55
	Recovery		101	39	24.8	0.41	0.40	4.0	1.03			116			34			52	54	
	Recovery		94	41	21.7	0.32	0.33	3.5	0.97			115			35			57	55	
	Recovery		92	40	20.8	0.30	0.30	3.3	1.00			115			34			58	58	
	Recovery	134/68	91	43	22.4	0.32	0.30	3.3	1.07	7.36	24	118	53	56	33	43	10	59	62	0.55
	Recovery		91	43	17.8	0.16	0.15	1.6	1.07			122			30			88	94	

nosis is the progressive decrease in PaO₂ and increase in P(A − a)O₂ at each work rate performed (Table 10.48.3 and panel 9, Fig. 10.48.1). An additional measurement consistent with restrictive lung disease is the high ratio of tidal volume to inspiratory capacity (panel 7, Fig. 10.48.1). An O₂ flow limitation is demonstrated by the small rise in V̇O₂ with increasing work rate and the failure of O₂ pulse to rise (panels 3 and 2, respectively, in Fig. 10.48.1) as work rate is increased.

Conclusion

Severe exercise intolerance with marked ventilation–perfusion mismatching in a patient with restrictive lung disease.

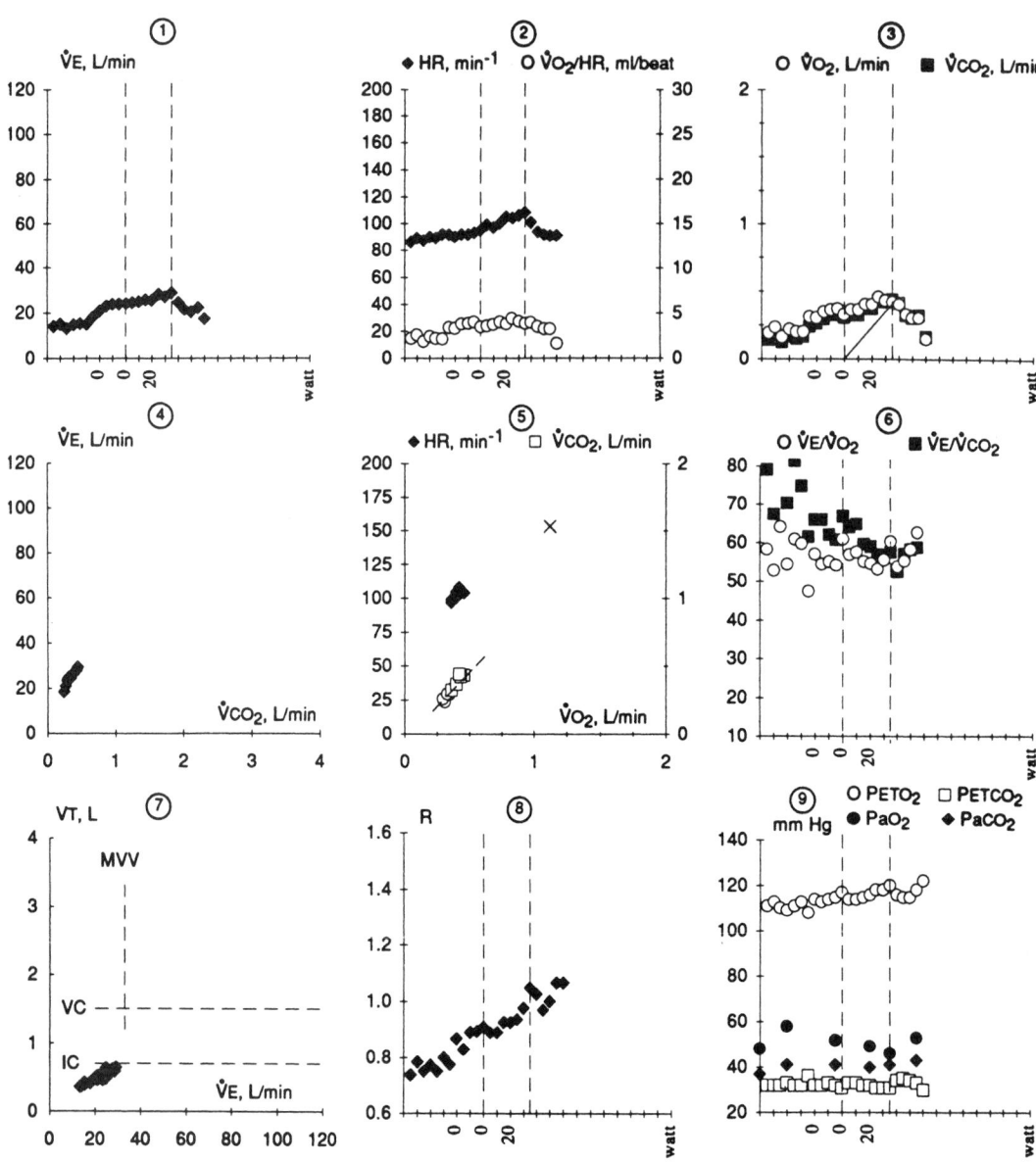

FIGURE 10.48.1.   **1:** Vertical dashed lines in panels 1 to 3 and 6, 8, and 9 indicate the beginning and the end of the increasing work period. **2:** Unloaded cycling is performed for 3 minutes before the left vertical dashed line. **3:** In panel 3, the diagonal line shows the increase of $\dot{V}_{O_2}$ at a slope of 10 ml/min/W. **4:** In panel 5, the diagonal dashed line has a slope of 1; the x in the upper right is the predicted maximum heart rate and $\dot{V}_{O_2}$ for the subject.

Case 49 Idiopathic Interstitial Lung Disease

Clinical Findings

This 45-year-old woman had developed dyspnea, diffuse pulmonary infiltrates, and hypoxemia 6 months previously and was treated with oral corticosteroids without lung biopsy or specific diagnosis. She was no longer receiving medication but still had dyspnea after walking three blocks. She had never smoked and had no known exposure to toxins, except that she worked in a pet shop and sprayed bleach on cages to clean them. She had no other significant illnesses. She was evaluated to determine the pathophysiology of her dyspnea.

Exercise Findings

The patient performed exercise on a cycle ergometer. She pedaled at 60 rpm without an added load for 3 minutes. The work rate was then increased 5 W per minute to her symptom-limited maximum. Arterial blood was sampled every second minute, and intraarterial blood pressure was recorded from a percutaneously placed brachial artery catheter. Resting and exercise ECGs were normal. The patient stopped exercise because of leg fatigue. By ear oximetry, the O_2 saturation was 96% at rest and 93% at peak exercise.

Interpretation

Comments

This case is presented to show the effects of severe pulmonary vascular disease accompanying interstitial lung disease. The resting respiratory studies show extremely severe DLCO reduction despite only mild to moderate restriction and normal resting PaO_2 (Table 10.49.1).

Analysis

Referring to flowchart 1, the patient has a low peak $\dot{V}O_2$ and anaerobic threshold (Table 10.49.2). In flowchart 4, the patient has a negligible breathing reserve (branch point 4.1) and a high VD/VT (branch point 4.2), leading to a tentative diagnosis of lung disease with impaired peripheral oxygenation. She has confirmatory findings of a high VT/IC ratio, low oximeter saturation, high breathing frequency, positive P(a − ET)CO_2, wide and increasing P(A − a)O_2, and a steep HR versus $\dot{V}O_2$ relationship. The $\Delta\dot{V}O_2$/

ΔWR is within normal limits, but the low and unchanging O_2 pulse is striking (panels 2 and 5 of Fig. 10.49.1). The decrease in O_2 saturation is small and gradual (branch point 4.5), making the development of a right-to-left shunt during exercise unlikely.

Conclusion

Although the patient has ventilatory limitation, she also has evidence of severe pulmonary vascular disease with decreased pulmonary blood flow (the steep heart rate response and the persistently low O_2 pulse). The pulmonary blood flow is so slow that there apparently is adequate time for near equilibration of pulmonary capillary PO_2 with alveolar gas even at peak exercise, the lowest exercise PaO_2 being 74.

TABLE 10.49.1. Selected Respiratory Function Data

Measurement	Predicted	Measured
Age, yr		45
Sex		Female
Height, cm		152
Weight, kg	56	51
Hematocrit, %		49
VC, L	2.92	1.81
IC, L	1.95	1.23
TLC, L	4.29	3.62
FEV_1, L	2.41	1.42
FEV_1/VC, %	83	78
MVV, L/min	92	56
D_LCO, ml/mm Hg/min	22.7	4.3

TABLE 10.49.2. Selected Exercise Data

Measurement	Predicted	Measured
Peak $\dot{V}O_2$, L/min	1.44	0.88
Maximum HR, beats/min	174	174
Maximum O_2 pulse, ml/beat	8.3	5.1
$\Delta\dot{V}O_2$/ΔWR, ml/min/W	10.3	8.7
AT, L/min	>0.69	0.65
Blood pressure, mmHg (rest, max)		150/90, 183/99
Maximum $\dot{V}E$, L/min		56
Exercise breathing reserve, L/min	>15	0
PaO_2, mmHg (rest, max ex)		93, 74
P(A − a)O_2, mmHg (rest, max ex)		24, 50
P(a − ET)CO_2, mmHg (rest, max ex)		1, 5
VD/VT (rest, max ex)		0.31, 0.38
HCO_3^-, mEq/L (rest, 2-min recov)		23, 17

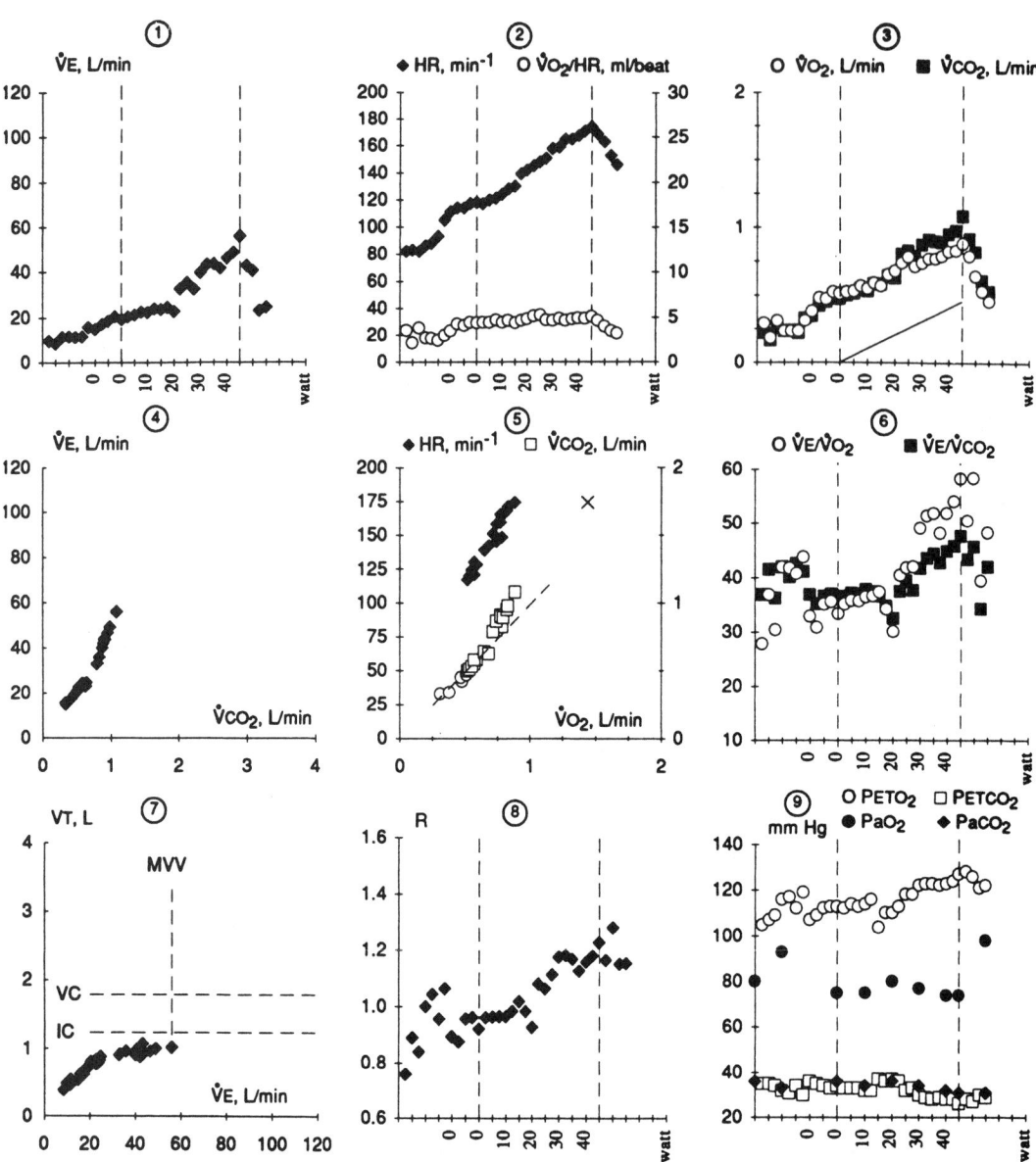

FIGURE 10.49.1.   **1:** Vertical dashed lines in panels 1 to 3 and 6, 8, and 9 indicate the beginning and the end of the increasing work period. **2:** Unloaded cycling is performed for 3 minutes before the left vertical dashed line. **3:** In panel 3, the diagonal line shows the increase of $\dot{V}_{O_2}$ at a slope of 10 ml/min/W. **4:** In panel 5, the diagonal dashed line has a slope of 1; the x in the upper right is the predicted maximum heart rate and $\dot{V}_{O_2}$ for the subject.

TABLE 10.49.3.   Air Breathing

Time min	Work rate watts	BP mmHg	HR min⁻¹	f min⁻¹	V̇E L/min BTPS	V̇CO₂ L/min STPD	V̇O₂ L/min STPD	V̇O₂/HR ml/beat	R	pH	HCO₃⁻ meq/L	PO₂, mmHg ET	a	(A − a)	PCO₂, mmHg ET	a	(a − ET)	V̇E/V̇CO₂	V̇E/V̇O₂	VD/VT
	Rest	150/84								7.42	23		80			36				
	Rest		82	20	9.8	0.22	0.29	3.5	0.76			105			35			37	28	
	Rest		83	22	8.5	0.16	0.18	2.2	0.89			107			35			41	37	
	Rest		82	22	11.3	0.26	0.31	3.8	0.84			109			34			36	30	
	Rest	150/90	86	23	11.6	0.23	0.23	2.7	1.00	7.45	23	116	93	24	32	33	1	42	42	0.31
	Rest		88	21	11.4	0.24	0.23	2.6	1.04			117			31			40	42	
	Rest		93	25	11.5	0.22	0.23	2.5	0.96			112			34			43	41	
	Unloaded		105	25	15.7	0.33	0.31	3.0	1.06			119			30			41	44	
	Unloaded		111	28	14.9	0.34	0.38	3.4	0.89			107			36			37	33	
	Unloaded		114	28	17.2	0.42	0.48	4.2	0.88			109			35			35	31	
	Unloaded		114	26	18.7	0.45	0.47	4.1	0.96			112			34			37	35	
	Unloaded		117	26	02.7	0.50	0.52	4.4	0.96			113			33			37	36	
	Unloaded	177/96	118	27	19.3	0.47	0.51	4.3	0.92	7.41	22	113	75	37	34	36	2	36	33	0.30
0.5	5		117	25	20.4	0.50	0.52	4.4	0.96			112			33			37	35	
1.0	5		120	27	21.3	0.51	0.53	4.4	0.96			114			33			37	36	
1.5	10		121	27	22.6	0.55	0.57	4.7	0.96			113			33			37	36	
2.0	10	177/96	124	29	22.5	0.53	0.55	4.4	0.96	7.41	21	114	75	40	32	34	2	38	36	0.29
2.5	15		128	29	24.1	0.58	0.59	4.6	0.98			116			32			37	37	
3.0	15		130	30	23.8	0.58	0.57	4.4	1.02			104			37			37	37	
3.5	20		139	28	24.6	0.64	0.65	4.7	0.98			110			36			35	34	
4.0	20	180/99	142	28	22.8	0.63	0.68	4.8	0.93	7.39	21	110	80	32	37	36	−1	32	30	0.23
4.5	25		145	36	33.0	0.80	0.74	5.1	1.08			113			36			37	40	
5.0	25		148	37	35.8	0.83	0.78	5.3	1.06			118			32			39	42	
5.5	30		151	36	32.8	0.79	0.71	4.7	1.11			118			33			38	42	
6.0	30	180/96	158	44	40.0	0.87	0.74	4.7	1.18	7.39	20	122	77	43	30	34	4	42	49	0.35
6.5	35		159	47	43.6	0.91	0.77	4.8	1.18			123			29			44	51	
7.0	35		165	46	43.8	0.90	0.77	4.7	1.17			123			28			44	52	
7.5	40		165	48	42.1	0.89	0.79	4.8	1.13			122			29			43	48	
8.0	40	180/96	168	48	46.6	0.95	0.82	4.9	1.16	7.39	19	123	74	47	28	32	4	45	52	0.36
8.5	45		171	49	49.0	0.98	0.83	4.9	1.18			124			28			46	54	
9.0	45	183/99	174	55	56.0	1.08	0.88	5.1	1.23	7.38	18	127	74	50	26	31	5	48	58	0.38
	Recovery		169	40	43.2	0.92	0.79	4.7	1.16			128			28			43	50	
	Recovery		163	41	40.9	0.82	0.64	3.9	1.28			126			27			46	58	
	Recovery		153	30	23.4	0.61	0.53	3.5	1.15			121			30			34	39	
	Recovery	165/90	146	28	24.6	0.53	0.46	3.2	1.15	7.35	17	122	98	24	29	31	2	42	48	0.30

Case 50 Mixed Connective Tissue Disease with Interstitial and Pulmonary Vascular Disease

Clinical Findings

This 38-year-old man with known connective tissue disease and restrictive lung disease of 3 years' duration was referred for evaluation to determine his level of disability. He had had a productive cough for 3 years and had been dyspneic for over 2 years. He had never smoked, but had been exposed to multiple chemical agents in a rubber factory. His current medications were prednisone, theophylline, and cimetidine.

Exercise Findings

The patient performed exercise on a cycle ergometer. He pedaled at 60 rpm without an added load for 3 minutes. The work rate was then increased 15 W per minute to his symptom-limited maximum. Arterial blood was sampled every second minute, and intraarterial blood pressure was recorded from a percutaneously passed brachial artery catheter. Resting ECG was normal except for occasional premature ectopic beats. The frequency of these increased during exercise to a maximum of 12 per minute. No ST-segment or T-wave abnormalities occurred. Exercise was stopped because the patient seemed unsteady and indicated that he was lightheaded. These symptoms cleared in a few minutes. He also indicated that he was out of breath, but did not identify this as the cause of stopping.

Interpretation

Comments

This patient shows the effect of severe interstitial lung disease on the cardiac output response to exercise, presumably because of increased pulmonary vascular resistance. The resting respiratory function studies show severe restriction with severe loss of available pulmonary capillary bed and mild hypoxemia (Table 10.50.1).

Analysis

Referring to flowchart 1, the patient has a low peak $\dot{V}O_2$ and an extremely low anaerobic threshold (Table 10.50.2). In flowchart 4, the patient has a low breathing reserve using the indirect MVV (branch point 4.1). At branch point 4.2 we are directed to a diagnosis of lung disease with impaired peripheral oxygenation by the finding of a high VD/VT. Confirmatory findings of ventilatory limitation to exercise are the high breathing frequency (64 breaths per minute) and high VT/IC. Especially impressive are the small increases in $\dot{V}O_2$ and O_2 pulse as compared with predicted, the arrhythmia, and the lightheadedness, all indicating difficulty in perfusion and/or oxygenation of the myocardium and brain as peak exercise is reached. [If we had decided that the breathing reserve were normal (branch point 4.1), we would also have been directed, through

TABLE 10.50.1.   Selected Respiratory Function Data

Measurement	Predicted	Measured
Age, yr		38
Sex		Male
Height, cm		188
Weight, kg	88	88
Hematocrit, %		43
VC, L	5.09	2.28
IC, L	3.39	1.36
TLC, L	7.14	3.43
FEV$_1$, L	4.09	1.99
FEV$_1$/VC, %	81	87
MVV, L/min		
Direct	163	107
Indirect	164	80
D$_L$CO, ml/mm Hg/min	32.7	10.7

TABLE 10.50.2.   Selected Exercise Data

Measurement	Predicted	Measured
Peak $\dot{V}O_2$, L/min	3.21	1.07
Maximum HR, beats/min	182	128
Maximum O_2 pulse, ml/beat	17.6	8.4
$\Delta\dot{V}O_2/\Delta WR$, ml/min/W	>10.3	7.3
AT, L/min	>1.35	<0.9
Blood pressure, mmHg (rest, max ex)		141/90, 222/102
Maximum $\dot{V}E$, L/min		76
Exercise breathing reserve, L/min		
Using direct MVV	>15	31
Using indirect MVV	>15	4
PaO_2, mmHg (rest, max ex)		79, 63
P(A − a)O_2, mmHg (rest, max ex)		16, 58
P(a − ET)CO_2, mmHg (rest, max ex)		5, 9
VD/VT (rest, max ex)		0.46, 0.48
HCO$_3^-$ mEq/L (rest, recov)		25, 20

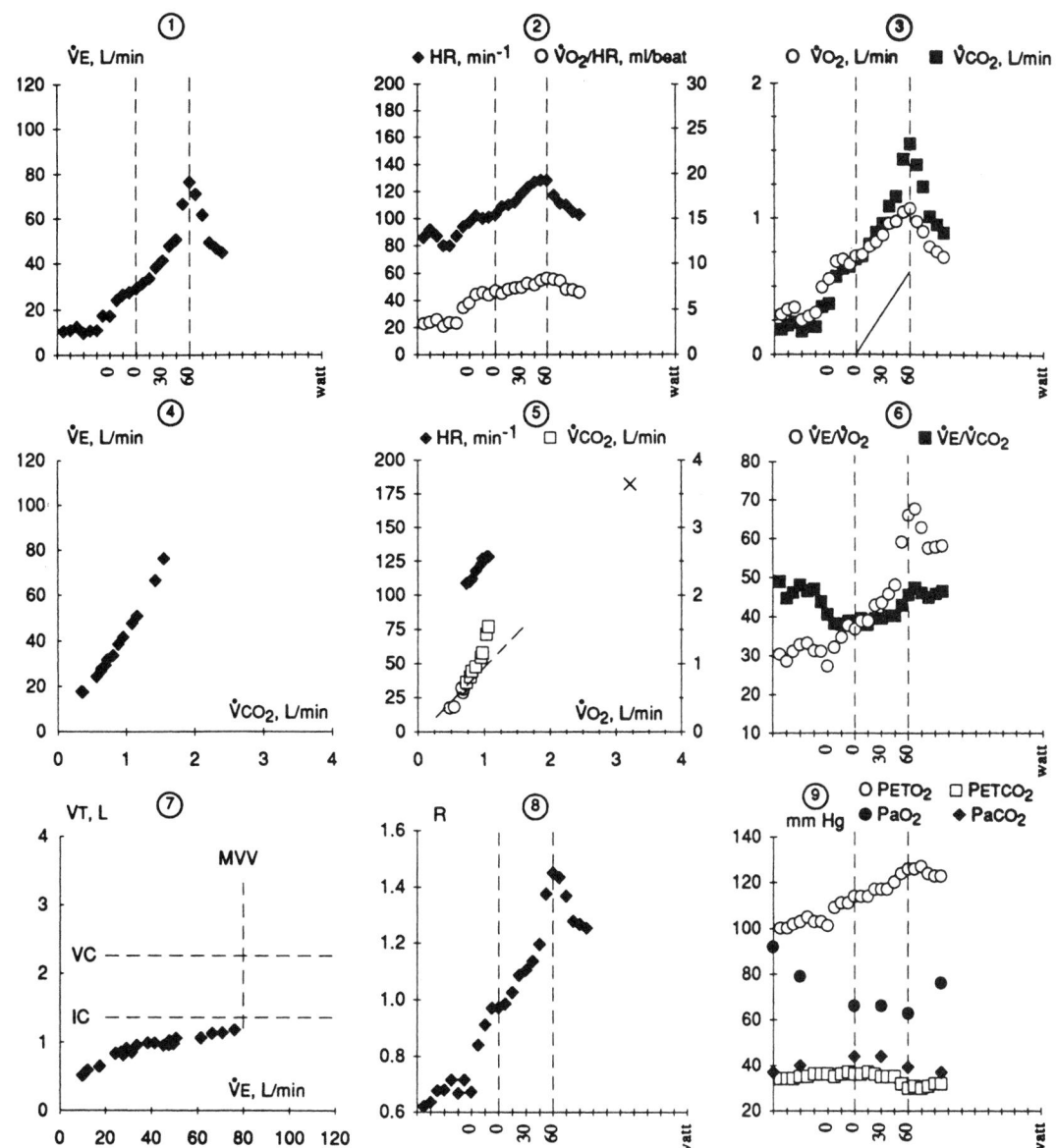

FIGURE 10.50.1.   **1:** Vertical dashed lines in panels 1 to 3 and 6, 8, and 9 indicate the beginning and the end of the increasing work period. **2:** Unloaded cycling is performed for 3 minutes before the left vertical dashed line. **3:** In panel 3, the diagonal line shows the increase of $\dot{V}O_2$ at a slope of 10 ml/min/W. **4:** In panel 5, the diagonal dashed line has a slope of 1; the x in the upper right is the predicted maximum heart rate and $\dot{V}O_2$ for the subject.

branch point 4.3 with high ventilatory equivalents, to a diagnosis of abnormal pulmonary circulation.]

Conclusion

This patient demonstrates significant gas exchange, ventilatory, and cardiovascular defects, all because of his severe interstitial lung disease. Although he has no evidence of intrinsic heart disease, he has severe impairment in his ability to increase cardiac output (pulmonary blood flow). The increased CO_2 production secondary to his metabolic acidosis and the high ventilatory requirement because of his increased V_D/V_T combine to create an unusually large ventilatory requirement in a patient with reduced ventilatory capacity.

TABLE 10.50.3. Air Breathing

Time min	Work rate watts	BP mmHg	HR min⁻¹	f min⁻¹	$\dot{V}_E$ L/min BTPS	$\dot{V}_{CO_2}$ L/min STPD	$\dot{V}_{O_2}$ L/min STPD	$\dfrac{\dot{V}_{O_2}}{HR}$ ml/beat	R	pH	HCO_3^- meq/L	P_{O_2}, mmHg ET	a	(A−a)	P_{CO_2}, mmHg ET	a	(a−ET)	$\dfrac{\dot{V}_E}{\dot{V}_{CO_2}}$	$\dfrac{\dot{V}_E}{\dot{V}_{O_2}}$	$\dfrac{V_D}{V_T}$
	Rest	141/90								7.45	25		92			37				
	Rest		86	20	10.5	0.18	0.29	3.4	0.62			100			34			49	30	
	Rest		92	20	11.1	0.21	0.33	3.6	0.64			100			34			45	28	
	Rest		87	21	12.4	0.23	0.34	3.9	0.68			102			34			46	31	
	Rest	156/96	80	19	9.8	0.17	0.25	3.1	0.68	7.41	25	103	79	16	35	40	5	48	33	0.46
	Rest		80	20	11.0	0.20	0.28	3.5	0.71			105			35			47	33	
	Rest		87	20	11.1	0.20	0.30	3.4	0.67			103			36			47	31	
	Unloaded		94	27	17.6	0.35	0.49	5.2	0.71			103			36			44	31	
	Unloaded		97	27	17.3	0.37	0.55	5.7	0.67			101			36			41	27	
	Unloaded		102	29	24.3	0.57	0.68	6.7	0.84			109			35			38	32	
	Unloaded		100	31	26.6	0.63	0.69	6.9	0.91			111			36			38	35	
	Unloaded		101	34	27.8	0.64	0.66	6.5	0.97			111			37			39	38	
	Unloaded	192/99	103	32	29.2	0.70	0.72	7.0	0.97	7.38	26	114	66	39	36	44	8	38	37	0.44
0.5	15		109	37	31.6	0.72	0.73	6.7	0.99			114			36			40	39	
1.0	15		110	35	33.7	0.81	0.79	7.2	1.03			114			37			38	39	
1.5	30		112	39	38.5	0.89	0.82	7.3	1.09			117			36			40	43	
2.0	30	204/102	118	42	41.5	0.96	0.87	7.4	1.10	7.38	26	117	66	43	35	44	9	40	44	0.46
2.5	45		123	47	47.8	1.09	0.96	7.8	1.14			117			35			40	46	
3.0	45		127	48	50.8	1.16	0.97	7.6	1.20			120			35			40	48	
3.5	60		128	59	66.5	1.43	1.04	8.1	1.38			124			32			43	59	
4.0	60	222/102	128	64	76.1	1.55	1.07	8.4	1.45	7.38	23	126	63	58	30	39	9	46	66	0.48
	Recovery		117	62	70.9	1.39	0.97	8.3	1.43			126			31			47	68	
	Recovery		111	58	61.5	1.23	0.90	8.1	1.37			127			30			46	63	
	Recovery		110	51	49.7	1.01	0.79	7.2	1.28			124			31			45	57	
	Recovery		105	49	47.5	0.95	0.75	7.1	1.27			123			32			46	58	
	Recovery	180/88	103	47	45.2	0.89	0.71	6.9	1.25	7.35	20	123	76	43	32	37	5	46	58	0.45

Case 51 Interstitial Lung Disease

Clinical Findings

This 20-year-old man with a history of exposure to crop dusting was found after extensive workup and open lung biopsy to have an interstitial pneumonitis with mica deposits. The patient noted severe dyspnea with walking one block or climbing two flights of stairs. He denied cough, wheezing, orthopnea, chest pain, syncope, peripheral edema, or cyanosis. He was being reevaluated following institution of daily prednisone.

Exercise Findings

The patient performed exercise on a cycle ergometer. He pedaled at 60 rpm without an added load for 3 minutes. The work rate was then increased 10 W per minute to tolerance. Arterial blood was sampled every second minute, and intraarterial pressure was recorded from a percutaneously placed brachial artery catheter. The patient was well motivated and cooperative and stopped exercise because of fatigue and shortness of breath. No ECG abnormalities occurred at rest or during exercise, but the patient developed a significant pulsus paradoxus (blood pressure variations with breathing).

Interpretation

Comments

Resting respiratory function studies showed severe restrictive lung disease (Table 10.51.1). Arterial blood gases revealed a chronic, compensated respiratory acidosis with mild hypoxemia.

Analysis

Referring to flowchart 1, peak $\dot{V}O_2$ and the anaerobic threshold are both markedly reduced (Table 10.51.2). Proceeding to flowchart 4 through branch points 4.1 and 4.2, we come to lung disease with impaired peripheral oxygenation. We are instructed to look at the pulmonary vascular disease box to confirm the diagnosis with other physiologic measurements. The high breathing frequency, high ratio of tidal volume to inspiratory capacity (panel 7 of

Fig. 10.51.1), and the low breathing reserve are all typical of severe restrictive lung disease. The elevated VD/VT and positive $P(a - ET)CO_2$ indicate inadequate perfusion of ventilated air spaces. The lack of severe hypoxemia is at first puzzling; the extremely low O_2 pulse and low anaerobic threshold tell us that stroke volume must be extremely low. On reflection, it seems likely that the right ventricle has not hypertrophied in response to the increased pulmonary vascular resistance caused by the underlying lung disease. Thus, the cardiac output is

TABLE 10.51.1.   Selected Respiratory Function Data

Measurement	Predicted	Measured
Age, yr		20
Sex		Male
Height, cm		160
Weight, kg	66	48
Hematocrit, %		51
VC, L	3.52	1.21
IC, L	2.37	0.74
FEV$_1$, L	2.99	1.21
FEV$_1$/VC, %	85	97
MVV, L/min	125	51

TABLE 10.51.2.   Selected Exercise Data

Measurement	Predicted	Measured
Peak $\dot{V}O_2$, L/min	2.46	0.74
Maximum HR, beats/min	200	182
Maximum O_2 pulse, ml/beat	12.3	4.1
$\Delta\dot{V}O_2/\Delta WR$, ml/min/W	10.3	4.2
AT, L/min	>0.98	<0.55
Blood pressure, mmHg (rest, max ex)		118/81, 165–126/102–63
Maximum $\dot{V}E$, L/min		47
Exercise breathing reserve, L/min	>15	4
PaO$_2$, mmHg (rest, max ex)		73, 85
P(A − a)O$_2$, mmHg (rest, max ex)		15, 36
P(a − ET)CO$_2$, mmHg (rest, max ex)		3, 4
VD/VT (rest, max ex)		0.37, 0.36
HCO$_3^-$, mEq/L (rest, 2-min recov)		28, 14

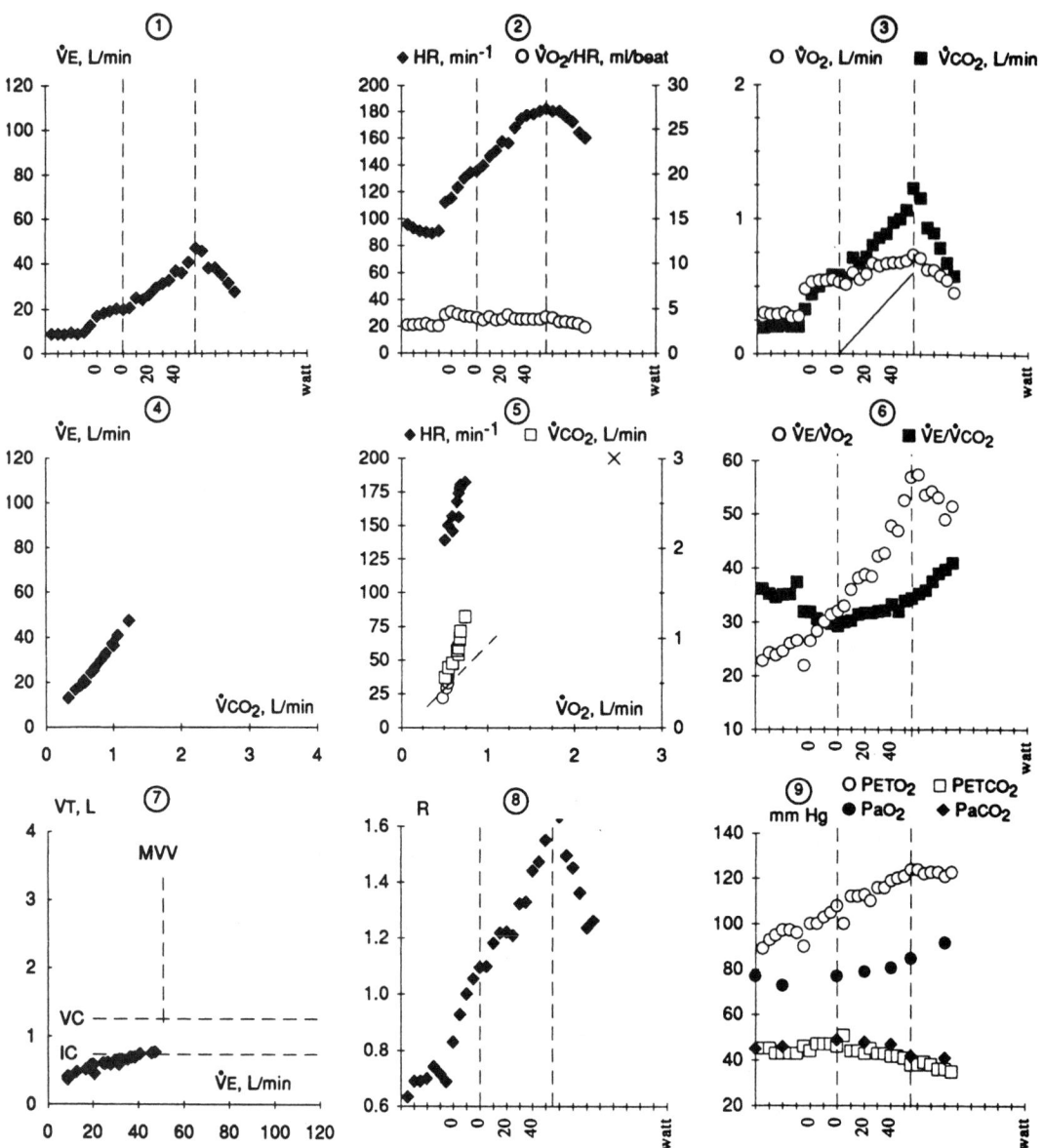

FIGURE 10.51.1.   **1:** Vertical dashed lines in panels 1 to 3 and 6, 8, and 9 indicate the beginning and the end of the increasing work period. **2:** Unloaded cycling is performed for 3 minutes before the left vertical dashed line. **3:** In panel 3, the diagonal line shows the increase of $\dot{V}_{O_2}$ at a slope of 10 mL/min/W. **4:** In panel 5, the diagonal dashed line has a slope of 1; the x in the upper right is the predicted maximum heart rate and $\dot{V}_{O_2}$ for the subject.

relatively fixed, as indicated by the failure of $\dot{V}_{O_2}$ to increase despite the increasing work rate. Because cardiac output does not increase, residence time in the pulmonary capillary remains unchanged. This allows the same equilibration time for the red cells to be exposed to the alveolar gas during exercise as at rest. The striking increase in $\dot{V}_{CO_2}$ is in contrast to $\dot{V}_{O_2}$. This is explained by the severe metabolic (lactic) acidosis that the patient develops as a result of the failure of cardiac output to increase in response to exercise (arterial HCO_3^- decreases 14 mEq/L in 8 minutes).

Conclusion

This is a young man with extremely severe restrictive lung disease and secondary pulmonary vascular disease with high dead space ventilation and extremely low stroke volume and cardiac output, but without significant hypoxemia.

TABLE 10.51.3. Air Breathing

Time min	Work rate watts	BP mmHg	HR min⁻¹	f min⁻¹	V̇E L/min BTPS	V̇CO₂ L/min STPD	V̇O₂ L/min STPD	V̇O₂/HR ml/beat	R	pH	HCO₃⁻ meq/L	PO₂ ET	PO₂ a	PO₂ (A−a)	PCO₂ ET	PCO₂ a	PCO₂ (a−ET)	V̇E/V̇CO₂	V̇E/V̇O₂	VD/VT
	Rest	96/68								7.40	27		77			45				
	Rest		96	24	8.9	0.19	0.30	3.1	0.63			89			45			36	23	
	Rest		93	23	9.0	0.20	0.29	3.1	0.69			93			45			35	24	
	Rest		91	21	8.7	0.20	0.29	3.2	0.69			95			43			35	24	
	Rest	118/81	90	23	9.3	0.21	0.30	3.3	0.70	7.40	28	97	73	15	43	46	3	35	24	0.37
	Rest		89	22	8.9	0.20	0.27	3.0	0.74			97			43			35	26	
	Rest		91	24	9.5	0.20	0.28	3.1	0.71			96			43			37	27	
	Unloaded		112	27	12.8	0.33	0.48	4.3	0.69			90			46			32	22	
	Unloaded		115	33	16.8	0.44	0.53	4.6	0.83			100			44			32	26	
	Unloaded		123	34	18.2	0.50	0.54	4.4	0.93			100			47			31	28	
	Unloaded		130	33	19.0	0.54	0.54	4.2	1.00			103			47			30	30	
	Unloaded		134	35	20.2	0.58	0.55	4.1	1.05			105			47			30	31	
	Unloaded	147/93	135	34	19.9	0.58	0.53	3.9	1.09	7.35	27	108	77	27	46	49	3	29	32	0.34
0.5	10		139	46	20.7	0.56	0.51	3.7	1.10			100			51			30	33	
1.0	10		146	42	25.1	0.71	0.60	4.1	1.18			112			44			30	36	
1.5	20		150	40	24.4	0.67	0.55	3.7	1.22			112			44			31	38	
2.0	20	156/96	157	43	26.5	0.72	0.59	3.8	1.22	7.33	25	113	79	30	43	48	5	32	39	0.37
2.5	30		156	46	29.6	0.81	0.67	4.3	1.21			110			45			32	38	
3.0	30		168	48	31.5	0.86	0.65	3.9	1.32			116			43			32	42	
3.5	40		174	50	32.9	0.89	0.67	3.9	1.33			116			43			32	43	
4.0	40	156/90	177	54	37.1	0.98	0.68	3.8	1.44	7.28	22	119	81	33	42	47	5	33	48	0.39
4.5	50		178	52	36.3	1.00	0.68	3.8	1.47			120			42			32	47	
5.0	50		180	55	40.9	1.07	0.69	3.8	1.55			121			41			34	53	
5.5	60	65–126/102–6	182	61	47.3	1.23	0.74	4.1	1.66	7.23	17	124	85	36	38	42	4	34	57	0.36
	Recovery		180	61	45.9	1.16	0.71	3.9	1.63			124			38			35	57	
	Recovery		180	55	38.4	0.94	0.63	3.5	1.49			122			39			36	54	
	Recovery		176	56	38.4	0.90	0.62	3.5	1.45			123			38			37	54	
	Recovery		172	54	35.4	0.79	0.58	3.4	1.36			123			36			39	53	
	Recovery	136/69	164	54	31.5	0.68	0.55	3.4	1.24	7.15	14	121	92	23	36	41	5	40	49	0.40
	Recovery		160	47	27.7	0.58	0.46	2.9	1.26			123			35			41	52	

Case 52 Sarcoidosis

Clinical Findings

This 39-year-old woman was referred for follow-up exercise testing with complaints of mild shortness of breath of 1 year's duration and diminished exercise tolerance of 18 months' duration. One year previously, following an episode of hepatitis of undetermined origin, she was found to have an enlarging right lower lung field cystic lesion. Noninvasive preoperative exercise testing at that time suggested cardiovascular limitation. During thoracic surgery, pulmonary artery pressure was normal. The resected lesion contained noncaseating granulomata compatible with sarcoidosis. No organisms were seen or cultured. The patient had never smoked cigarettes and took no medications. Her exercise test was repeated with an intraarterial catheter.

Exercise Findings

The patient performed exercise on a cycle ergometer. She pedaled at 60 rpm without an added load for 3 minutes. The work rate was then increased 15 W per minute to tolerance. Arterial blood was sampled every second minute, and intraarterial pressure was recorded from a percutaneously placed brachial artery catheter. The patient stopped exercise because of lightheadedness and shortness of breath. No ECG abnormalities occurred at rest or during exercise.

Interpretation

Comments

The resting respiratory function studies were similar to her pre–lung resection values and showed mild restrictive lung disease (Table 10.52.1). The resting blood gases reveal a mild compensated respiratory alkalosis or metabolic acidosis.

Analysis

Referring to flowchart 1, peak $\dot{V}O_2$ and the anaerobic threshold are both decreased (Table 10.52.2), sending us through branch point 1.3 to flowchart 4. The breathing reserve is high (branch point 4.1). The mildly elevated ventilatory equivalents can be accounted for by the low $PaCO_2$. The normal VD/VT, $P(a − ET)CO_2$, and $P(a − a)O_2$ (branch point 4.3) indicate uniform ventilation–perfusion ratios, and an O_2 flow problem of nonpulmonary origin. The he-

matocrit is normal (branch point 4.4). The maximum O_2 pulse is extremely low and increases minimally as work rate is increased. Thus, the choice is peripheral arterial disease or heart disease. Because the patient did not have symptoms of claudication and the CO_2 output from HCO_3^- buffering of lactic acid is high, the cause of the O_2 flow problem must be heart failure. The ECG was normal. These findings are compatible with a cardiomyopathy possibly secondary to sarcoidosis.

Conclusion

The patient exercised maximally and developed a significant lactic acidosis. Pulmonary disease does not explain her low peak $\dot{V}O_2$. The results are best explained by left-sided heart failure, presumably due to sarcoidosis that involves the myocardium.

TABLE 10.52.1.   Selected Respiratory Function Data

Measurement	Predicted	Measured
Age, yr		39
Sex		Female
Height, cm		162
Weight, kg	63	68
Hematocrit, %		41
VC, L	3.38	2.89
IC, L	2.25	1.80
TLC, L	5.84	4.34
FEV_1, L	2.75	2.40
FEV_1/VC, %	81	88
MVV, L/min	105	98
D_LCO, ml/mm Hg/min	24.2	17.9

TABLE 10.52.2.   Selected Exercise Data

Measurement	Predicted	Measured
Peak $\dot{V}O_2$, L/min	1.70	1.12
Maximum HR, beats/min	181	173
Maximum O_2 pulse, ml/beat	9.4	6.5
$\Delta \dot{V}O_2/\Delta WR$, ml/min/W	10.3	7.3
AT, L/min	>0.81	<0.65
Blood pressure, mmHg (rest, max)		146/88, 189/105
Maximum $\dot{V}E$, L/min		55
Exercise breathing reserve, L/min	>15	43
PaO_2, mmHg (rest, max ex)		104, 119
$P(A − a)O_2$, mmHg (rest, max ex)		7, 7
$P(a − ET)CO_2$, mmHg (rest, max ex)		0, −4
VD/VT (rest, max ex)		0.30, 0.19
HCO_3^-, mEq/L (rest, 2-min recov)		22, 13

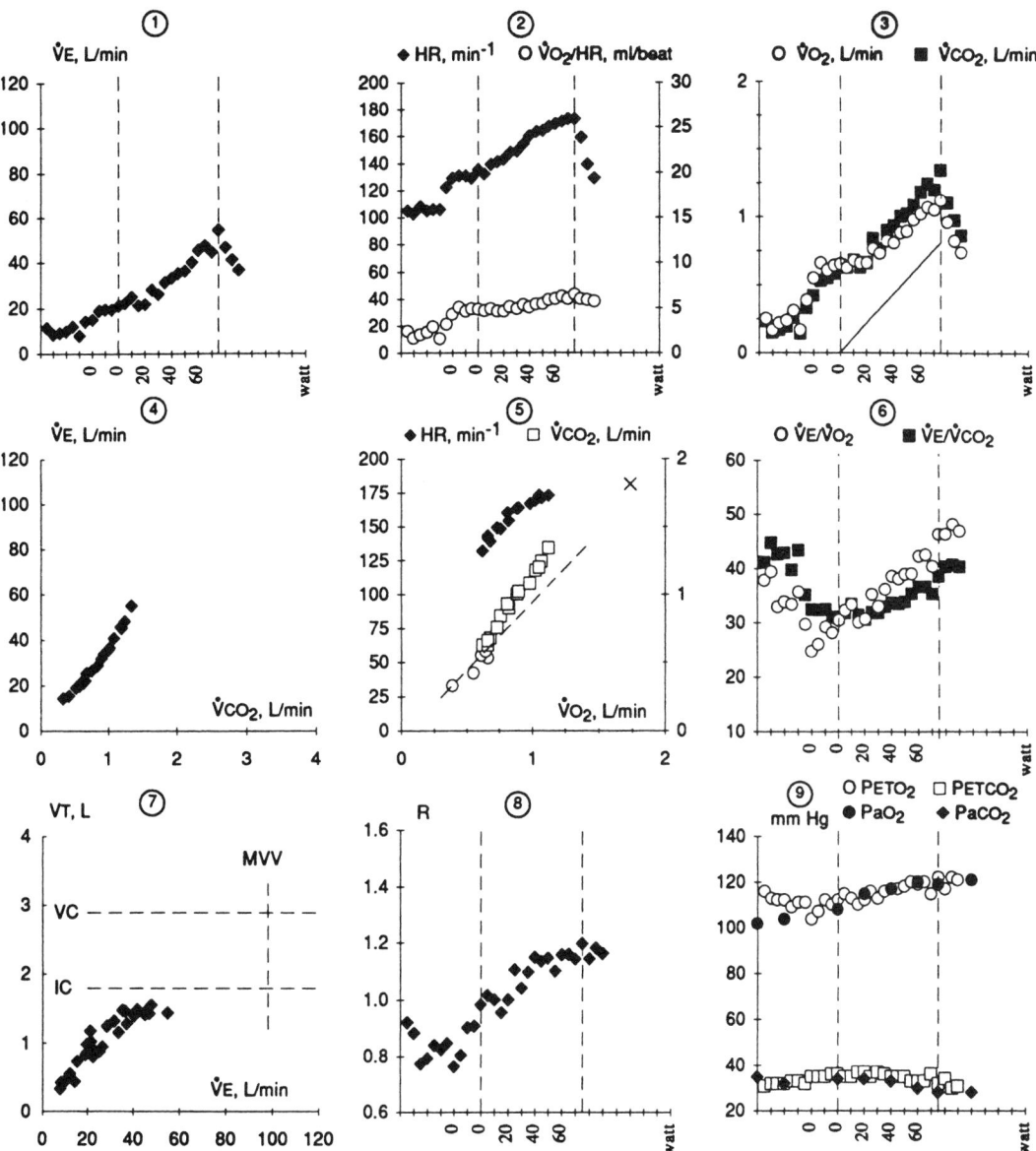

FIGURE 10.52.1.   **1:** Vertical dashed lines in panels 1 to 3 and 6, 8, and 9 indicate the beginning and the end of the increasing work period. **2:** Unloaded cycling is performed for 3 minutes before the left vertical dashed line. **3:** In panel 3, the diagonal line shows the increase of $\dot{V}O_2$ at a slope of 10 ml/min/W. **4:** In panel 5, the diagonal dashed line has a slope of 1; the x in the upper right is the predicted maximum heart rate and $\dot{V}O_2$ for the subject.

TABLE 10.52.3. Air Breathing

Time min	Work rate watts	BP mmHg	HR min⁻¹	f min⁻¹	$\dot{V}_E$ L/min BTPS	$\dot{V}_{CO_2}$ L/min STPD	$\dot{V}_{O_2}$ L/min STPD	$\dot{V}_{O_2}$/HR ml/beat	R	pH	HCO_3^- meq/L	P_{O_2}, mmHg ET	a	(A−a)	P_{CO_2}, mmHg ET	a	(a−ET)	$\dfrac{\dot{V}_E}{\dot{V}_{CO_2}}$	$\dfrac{\dot{V}_E}{\dot{V}_{O_2}}$	$\dfrac{V_D}{V_T}$
	Rest	156/90								7.41	22		102			35				
	Rest		105	23	11.4	0.23	0.25	2.4	0.92			116			31			41	38	
	Rest		103	20	8.4	0.15	0.17	1.7	0.88			113			32			45	39	
	Rest		108	23	9.2	0.17	0.22	2.0	0.77			112			32			43	33	
	Rest	146/88	105	23	10.1	0.19	0.24	2.3	0.79	7.43	21	112	104	7	32	32	0	43	34	0.30
	Rest		106	22	12.2	0.26	0.31	2.9	0.84			109			33			40	33	
	Rest		106	24	8.1	0.14	0.17	1.6	0.82			111			33			43	36	
	Unloaded		122	33	14.4	0.33	0.39	3.2	0.85			111			32			35	30	
	Unloaded		129	21	15.4	0.42	0.55	4.3	0.76			104			35			32	25	
	Unloaded		131	23	19.1	0.53	0.66	5.0	0.80			107			35			32	26	
	Unloaded		131	23	19.8	0.55	0.61	4.7	0.90			112			35			32	29	
	Unloaded		129	20	19.7	0.58	0.64	5.0	0.91			110			36			31	28	
	Unloaded	165/99	135	18	21.3	0.64	0.65	4.8	0.98	7.39	20	112	108	8	36	34	−2	31	30	0.17
0.5	10		132	28	22.4	0.63	0.62	4.7	1.02			115			35			32	32	
1.0	10		139	29	25.2	0.68	0.68	4.9	1.00			113			35			33	33	
1.5	20		141	21	21.6	0.63	0.66	4.7	0.95			110			37			31	30	
2.0	20	168/97	143	24	22.2	0.66	0.66	4.6	1.00	7.38	20	112	115	1	37	34	−3	31	31	0.15
2.5	30		148	23	28.7	0.84	0.76	5.1	1.11			116			35			32	35	
3.0	30		149	28	26.5	0.76	0.73	4.9	1.04			113			37			32	33	
3.5	40		154	24	31.7	0.90	0.82	5.3	1.10			116			36			33	36	
4.0	40	189/105	160	29	33.7	0.93	0.81	51	1.15	7.37	19	117	117	3	35	33	−2	34	39	0.21
4.5	50		163	24	35.6	1.00	0.88	5.4	1.14			117			35			34	38	
5.0	50		164	25	36.7	1.02	0.89	5.4	1.15			118			35			34	39	
5.5	60		167	29	40.7	1.08	0.98	5.9	1.10			120			33			35	39	
6.0	60	189/105	169	31	45.8	1.18	1.02	6.0	1.16	7.35	16	119	120	3	33	30	−3	37	42	0.20
6.5	70		171	31	48.1	1.24	1.07	6.3	1.16			120			33			37	42	
7.0	70		173	32	45.2	1.20	1.05	6.1	1.14			115			36			35	40	
7.5	80	189/105	173	38	55.0	1.34	1.12	6.5	1.20	7.32	14	122	119	7	32	28	−4	39	46	0.19
	Recovery		159	33	47.2	1.10	0.96	6.0	1.15			117			34			40	46	
	Recovery	118/60	139	28	41.8	0.97	0.82	5.9	1.18			122			30			41	48	
	Recovery		129	29	37.2	0.86	0.74	5.7	1.16			121			31			40	47	
										7.27	13		121			28				

Case 53 Severe Sarcoidosis: Air and Oxygen Breathing Studies

Clinical Findings

This 29-year-old man with a 6-year history of sarcoidosis was referred for evaluation of the pathophysiology of his worsening dyspnea. He was on continuous O_2 supplementation and beclomethasone dipropionate (Vanceril) inhaler, but he was not currently taking systemic corticosteroids. His weight was stable. He had smoked cigarettes for only 1 year.

Exercise Findings

The patient performed exercise on a cycle ergometer while he breathed room air. The test was repeated while he was breathing 100% O_2. On both occasions, he pedaled at 60 rpm without an added load for 3 minutes. The work rate was then increased 10 W per minute to tolerance. Arterial blood was sampled every second minute, and intraarterial pressure was recorded from a percutaneously placed brachial artery catheter. The patient stopped exercise because of shortness of breath while breathing room air and because of leg fatigue while breathing O_2. The resting ECG showed right axis deviation and inverted T waves anteriorly. The T waves became upright during exercise. No arrhythmias were noted.

Interpretation

Comments

Resting respiratory function studies showed mild to moderate restrictive and obstructive components in ventilatory mechanics, an extremely low DLCO, and severe arterial hypoxemia (Table 10.53.1).

Analysis

Referring to flowchart 1, both the peak $\dot{V}O_2$ and anaerobic threshold are severely reduced (Table 10.53.2). Proceeding to flowchart 4 through branch point 4.1, the breathing reserve is normal, but the high $\dot{V}E/\dot{V}CO_2$ at the *AT* (branch point 4.3) and high VD/VT (branch point 4.2) direct us to the boxes representing lung disease with impaired oxygenation

TABLE 10.53.1.   Selected Respiratory Function Data

Measurement	Predicted	Measured
Age, yr		29
Sex		Male
Height, cm		171
Weight, kg	73	58
Hematocrit, %		45
VC, L	4.28	3.11
IC, L	2.85	1.59
TLC, L	5.82	4.78
FEV$_1$, L	3.46	2.27
FEV$_1$/VC, %	81	73
MVV, L/min	138	91
D$_L$CO, ml/mm Hg/min	29.9	6.9

TABLE 10.53.2.   Selected Exercise Data

Measurement	Predicted	Measured	
		Air	100% O_2
Maximum work rate, W		40	70
Peak $\dot{V}O_2$, L/min	2.64	0.8	
Maximum HR, beats/min	191	149	150
Maximum O_2 pulse, ml/beat	13.6	5.7	
AT, L/min	>1.08	0.7	
Blood pressure, mmHg (rest, max ex)		114/72, 135/78	111/69, 141/87
Maximum $\dot{V}E$, L/min		64	70
Exercise breathing reserve, L/min	>15	27	21
PaO$_2$, mmHg (rest, max ex)		42, 35	585, 605
P(A − a)O$_2$, mmHg (rest, max ex)		52, 74	84, 57
P(a − ET)CO$_2$, mmHg (rest, max ex)		16, 22	19, 28
VD/VT (rest, max ex)		0.57, 0.67	0.63, 0.71
HCO$_3^-$, mEq/L (rest, 2-min recov)		27, 24	25, 24

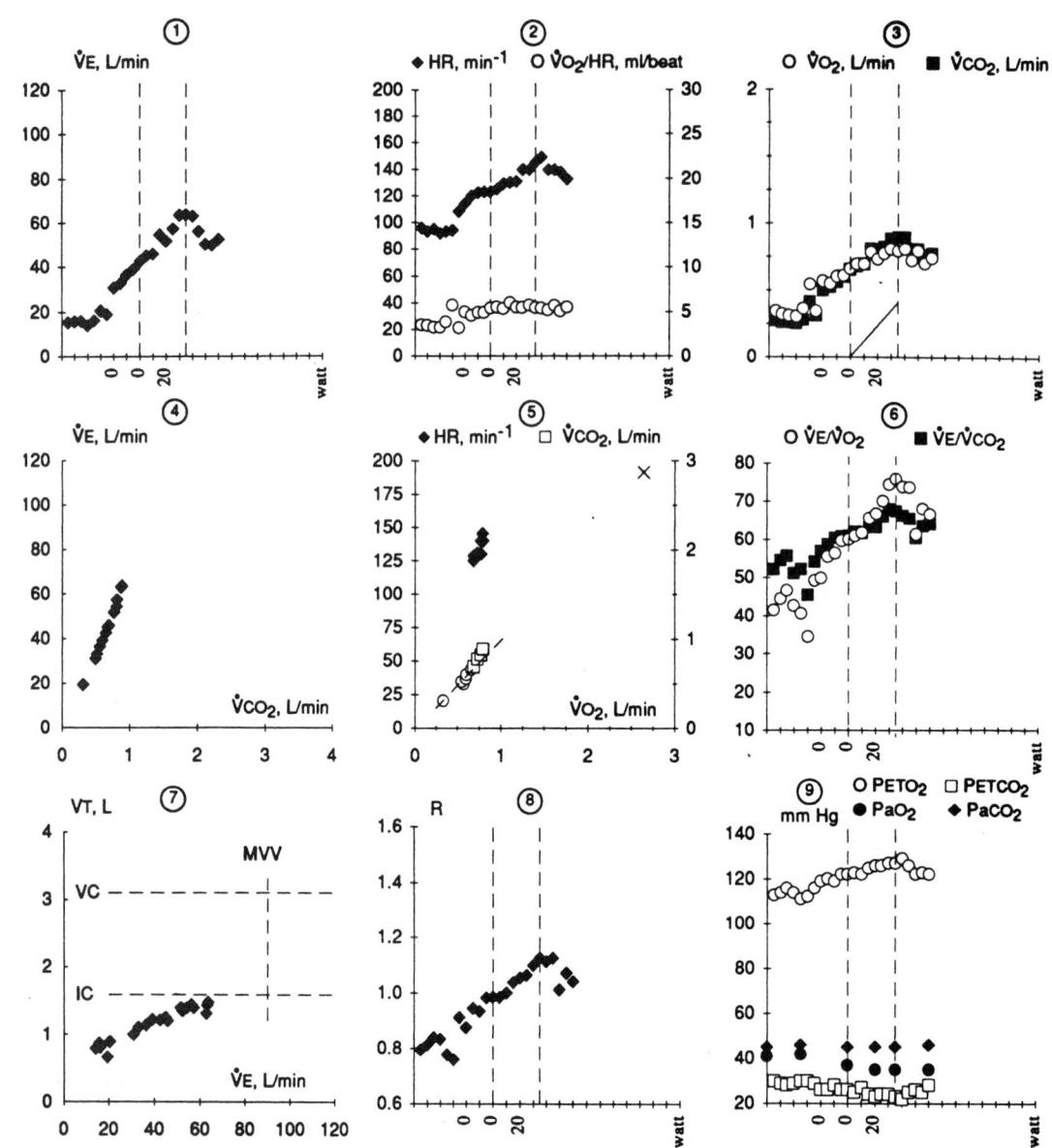

FIGURE 10.53.1.   Air breathing. **1:** Vertical dashed lines in panels 1 to 3 and 6, 8, and 9 indicate the beginning and the end of the increasing work period. **2:** Unloaded cycling is performed for 3 minutes before the left vertical dashed line. **3:** In panel 3, the diagonal line shows the increase of $\dot{V}O_2$ at a slope of 10 mL/min/W. **4:** In panel 5, the diagonal dashed line has a slope of 1; the x in the upper right is the predicted maximum heart rate and $\dot{V}O_2$ for the subject.

and abnormal pulmonary circulation. The findings support these diagnoses, with high dead space ventilation increasing the ventilatory requirements at rest and all work levels. With O_2 breathing, there is no evidence of a right-to-left shunt, but ventilatory drive is reduced and the patient is able to tolerate a considerably higher work rate.

Conclusion

This patient with sarcoidosis with some disturbance in ventilatory mechanics has severe gas ex-
change abnormality due to marked pulmonary vascular disease. He has severe hypoxemia at rest and during exercise without supplemental oxygen; his ability to perform work is increased with oxygen. From sequential exercise testing, it became evident that this man's pulmonary microcirculation was disappearing (increasing $\dot{V}D/\dot{V}T$ and $\dot{V}E/\dot{V}O_2$ and worsening hypoxemia) despite stable ventilatory mechanics. The patient was treated with unilateral lung transplantation.

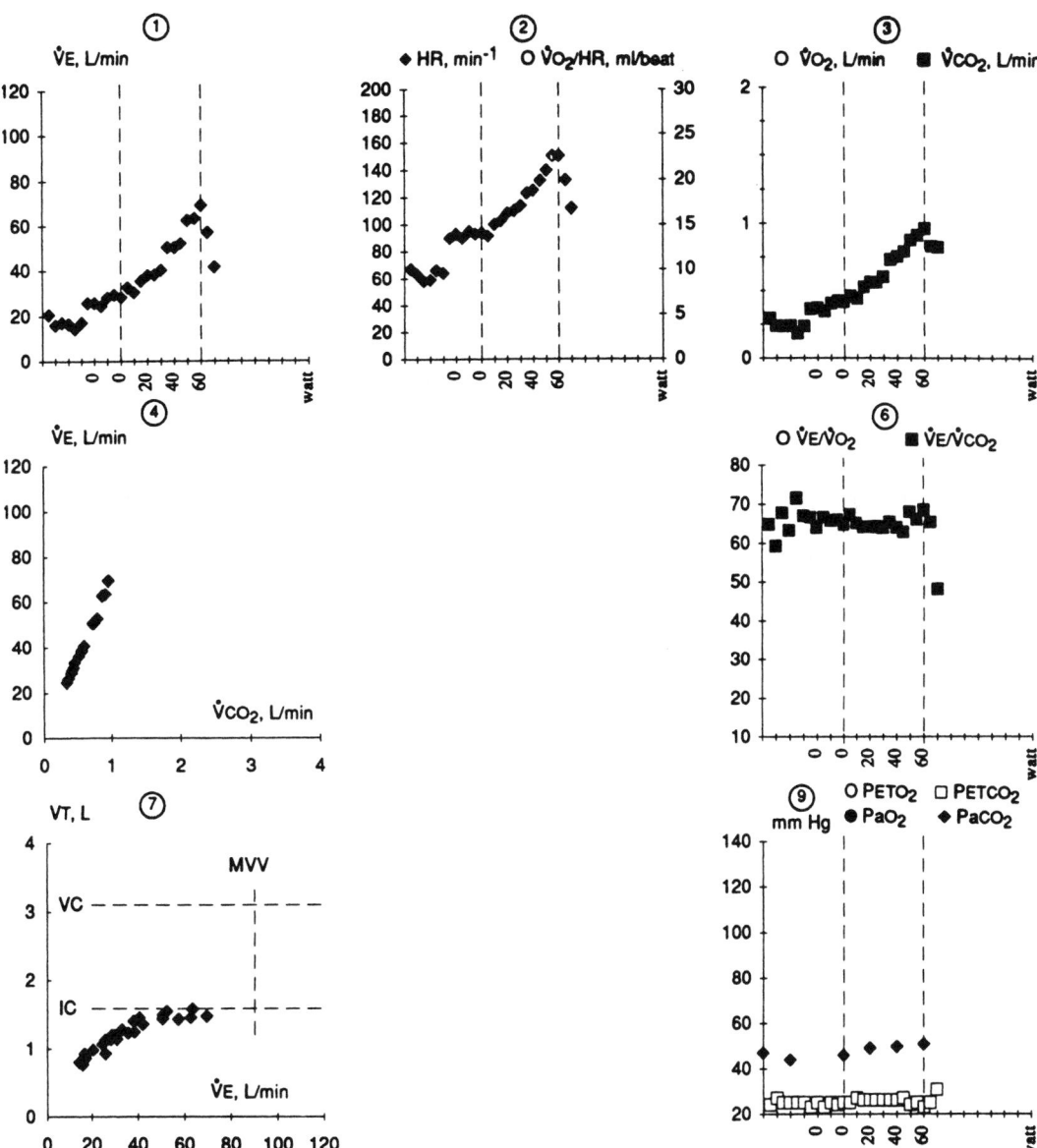

FIGURE 10.53.2.   Oxygen breathing. **1:** Vertical dashed lines in panels 1 to 3 and 6 and 9 indicate the beginning and the end of the increasing work period. **2:** Unloaded cycling is performed for 3 minutes before the left vertical dashed line.

TABLE 10.53.3.   Air Breathing

Time min	Work rate watts	BP mmHg	HR min⁻¹	f min⁻¹	$\dot{V}_E$ L/min BTPS	$\dot{V}_{CO_2}$ L/min STPD	$\dot{V}_{O_2}$ L/min STPD	$\dot{V}_{O_2}$ HR ml/beat	R	pH	HCO₃⁻ meq/L	P_{O_2}, mmHg			P_{CO_2}, mmHg			$\dfrac{\dot{V}_E}{\dot{V}_{CO_2}}$	$\dfrac{\dot{V}_E}{\dot{V}_{O_2}}$	$\dfrac{V_D}{V_T}$
												ET	a	(A − a)	ET	a	(a − ET)			
	Rest	111/66								7.39	27		41			45				
	Rest		96	18	15.6	0.27	0.34	3.5	0.79			113			30			52	41	
	Rest		93	19	15.8	0.26	0.32	3.4	0.81			114			29			55	44	
	Rest		95	19	16.1	0.26	0.31	3.3	0.84			116			28			56	47	
	Rest		92	18	14.3	0.25	0.30	3.3	0.83			114			29			51	43	
	Rest	114/72	93	20	16.3	0.28	0.36	3.9	0.78	7.38	27	111	42	52	30	46	16	52	41	0.57
	Rest		94	23	20.6	0.41	0.54	5.7	0.76			112			30			45	35	
	Unloaded		108	29	19.2	0.31	0.34	3.1	0.91			116			29			54	49	
	Unloaded		114	31	31.0	0.50	0.57	5.0	0.88			119			26			57	50	
	Unloaded		120	30	33.0	0.52	0.55	4.6	0.95			120			26			59	55	
	Unloaded		122	32	36.5	0.56	0.60	4.9	0.93			119			28			60	56	
	Unloaded		123	32	39.1	0.60	0.61	5.0	0.98			122			26			61	60	
	Unloaded	116/72	123	35	42.5	0.65	0.66	5.4	0.98	7.38	26	122	37	67	26	45	19	61	60	0.64
0.5	10		125	36	45.1	0.68	0.69	5.5	0.99			123			25			62	61	
1.0	10		129	38	45.8	0.69	0.69	5.3	1.00			122			27			62	62	
1.5	20		130	39	54.4	0.81	0.78	6.0	1.04			125			24			63	65	
2.0	20	129/78	131	37	51.7	0.77	0.73	5.6	1.05	7.37	26	126	35	72	23	45	22	63	67	0.65
2.5	30		140	41	57.4	0.82	0.77	5.5	1.06			126			24			66	70	
3.0	30		140	44	63.3	0.88	0.80	5.7	1.10			127			24			68	74	
3.5	40	135/78	145	43	63.6	0.89	0.79	5.4	1.13	7.35	24	127	35	74	23	45	22	67	76	0.67
	Recovery		149	48	63.0	0.89	0.80	5.4	1.11			129			22			66	74	
	Recovery		140	39	56.3	0.81	0.72	5.1	1.13			126			25			65	74	
	Recovery		140	36	50.5	0.80	0.79	5.6	1.01			122			26			59	60	
	Recovery		138	34	50.1	0.75	0.70	5.1	1.07			123			25			63	67	
	Recovery	114/69	133	39	52.5	0.77	0.74	5.6	1.04	7.33	24	122	35	70	28	46	18	64	66	0.66

TABLE 10.53.4.   Oxygen Breathing

Time min	Work rate watts	BP mmHg	HR min⁻¹	f min⁻¹	$\dot{V}_E$ L/min BTPS	$\dot{V}_{CO_2}$ L/min STPD	$\dot{V}_{O_2}$ L/min STPD	$\dot{V}_{O_2}$ HR ml/beat	R	pH	HCO₃⁻ meq/L	P_{O_2}, mmHg			P_{CO_2}, mmHg			$\dfrac{\dot{V}_E}{\dot{V}_{CO_2}}$	$\dfrac{\dot{V}_E}{\dot{V}_{O_2}}$	$\dfrac{V_D}{V_T}$
												ET	a	(A − a)	ET	a	(a − ET)			
	Rest									7.34	25		519			47				
	Rest		67	21	20.6	0.29									24			65		
	Rest		63	21	16.0	0.24									27			59		
	Rest		58	19	17.2	0.23									25			68		
	Rest	111/69	59	18	16.7	0.24				7.36	24		585	84	25	44	19	62		0.63
	Rest		66	18	14.4	0.18									25			72		
	Rest		64	20	17.1	0.23									25			67		
	Unloaded		90	23	25.9	0.36									23			67		
	Unloaded		93	28	26.0	0.37									25			64		
	Unloaded		90	23	24.6	0.34									23			67		
	Unloaded		95	25	28.4	0.40									25			66		
	Unloaded		93	25	29.8	0.42									24			66		
	Unloaded	116/75	94	24	28.6	0.41				7.35	25		615	52	25	46	21	65		0.66
0.5	10		92	26	33.1	0.46									25			67		
1.0	10		100	27	30.9	0.44									27			65		
1.5	20		103	29	35.8	0.52									26			64		
2.0	20	120/78	108	27	38.1	0.56				7.33	25		620	44	26	49	23	64		0.68
2.5	30		110	31	38.6	0.56									26			64		
3.0	30		114	28	40.6	0.60									26			64		
3.5	40		123	35	50.6	0.73									26			65		
4.0	40	132/81	125	34	50.8	0.75				7.31	25		612	51	26	50	24	64		0.69
4.5	50		132	34	52.5	0.79									27			63		
5.0	50		140	43	62.8	0.87									24			68		
5.5	60		150	40	63.5	0.91									25			66		
6.0	60	141/87	150	47	69.9	0.96				7.28	24		605	57	23	51	28	68		0.71
	Recovery		133	40	57.6	0.83									25			65		
	Recovery		112	31	42.1	0.82									31			48		

Case 54 Interstitial Pneumonitis: Before and After Corticosteroid Therapy

Clinical Findings

This 37-year-old housewife developed progressive shortness of breath. She was found to have a pattern of interstitial lung disease on chest roentgenographic studies and was referred for exercise testing.

Exercise Findings

The patient performed exercise on a cycle ergometer. She pedaled at 60 rpm without added load for 3 minutes. The work rate was then increased 15 W per minute to her symptom-limited maximum. Arterial blood was sampled every second minute, and intraarterial blood pressure was recorded from a percutaneously placed brachial artery catheter. Her resting and exercise ECGs were normal. In the initial study, she stopped exercise because of shortness of breath. After the first exercise test she was treated with prednisone. Her exercise test was repeated 6 months later, at which time she was taking 30 mg prednisone daily. She was asymptomatic at the time of the second test.

Interpretation

Comments

The resting respiratory function studies indicate that this patient had severe restrictive lung disease before therapy, which improved markedly after

therapy (Table 10.54.1). The resting ECG is normal. The after-treatment exercise test was performed 6 months after the first test.

Analysis

Referring to flowchart 1, the peak $\dot{V}O_2$ and the anaerobic threshold are abnormal (Table 10.54.2). Referring to flowchart 4, the patient's breathing reserve is low (branch point 4.1). VD/VT is high (branch point 4.2). This leads to the diagnosis of lung disease with an O_2 flow problem. Characteristically, this is a restrictive lung disease. Confirming restrictive lung disease as the major pathophysiologic disorder are a high VT/IC ratio (panel 7, Fig. 10.54.1), breathing frequency exceeding 50 breaths per minute at the patient's maximum work rate (Table 10.54.3), a $P(A − a)O_2$ that increases and a

TABLE 10.54.1.   Selected Respiratory Function Data

Measurement	Predicted	Before Treatment	After Treatment
Age, yr		37	
Sex		Female	
Height, cm		168	
Weight, kg	66	57	
Hematocrit, %		42	
VC, L	3.76	1.71	3.85
IC, L	2.50	1.31	2.25
FEV_1, L	3.08	1.52	3.10
FEV_1/VC, %	82	89	81
MVV, L/min	120	66	130
D_LCO, ml/mm Hg/min	28.5	16.2	

TABLE 10.54.2.   Selected Exercise Data

Measurement	Predicted	Before Treatment	After Treatment
Peak $\dot{V}O_2$, L/min	1.72	1.35	2.01
Maximum HR, beats/min	183	149	174
Maximum O_2 pulse, ml/beat	9.4	9.1	11.6
$\Delta\dot{V}O_2/\Delta WR$, ml/min/W	10.3	9.5	9.8
AT, L/min	>0.79	0.80	1.0
Blood pressure, mmHg (rest, max)		119/68, 190/81	125/75, 181/88
Maximum $\dot{V}E$, L/min		58	86
Exercise breathing reserve, L/min	>15	8	44
PaO_2, mmHg (rest, max ex)		65, 51	117, 98
$P(A − a)O_2$, mmHg (rest, max ex)		43, 65	−1, 26
$P(a − ET)CO_2$, mmHg (rest, max ex)		3, 3	−3, −2
VD/VT (rest, heavy ex)		0.40, 0.32	0.22, 0.15
HCO_3^-, mEq/L (rest, 2-min recov)		25, 21	24, 15

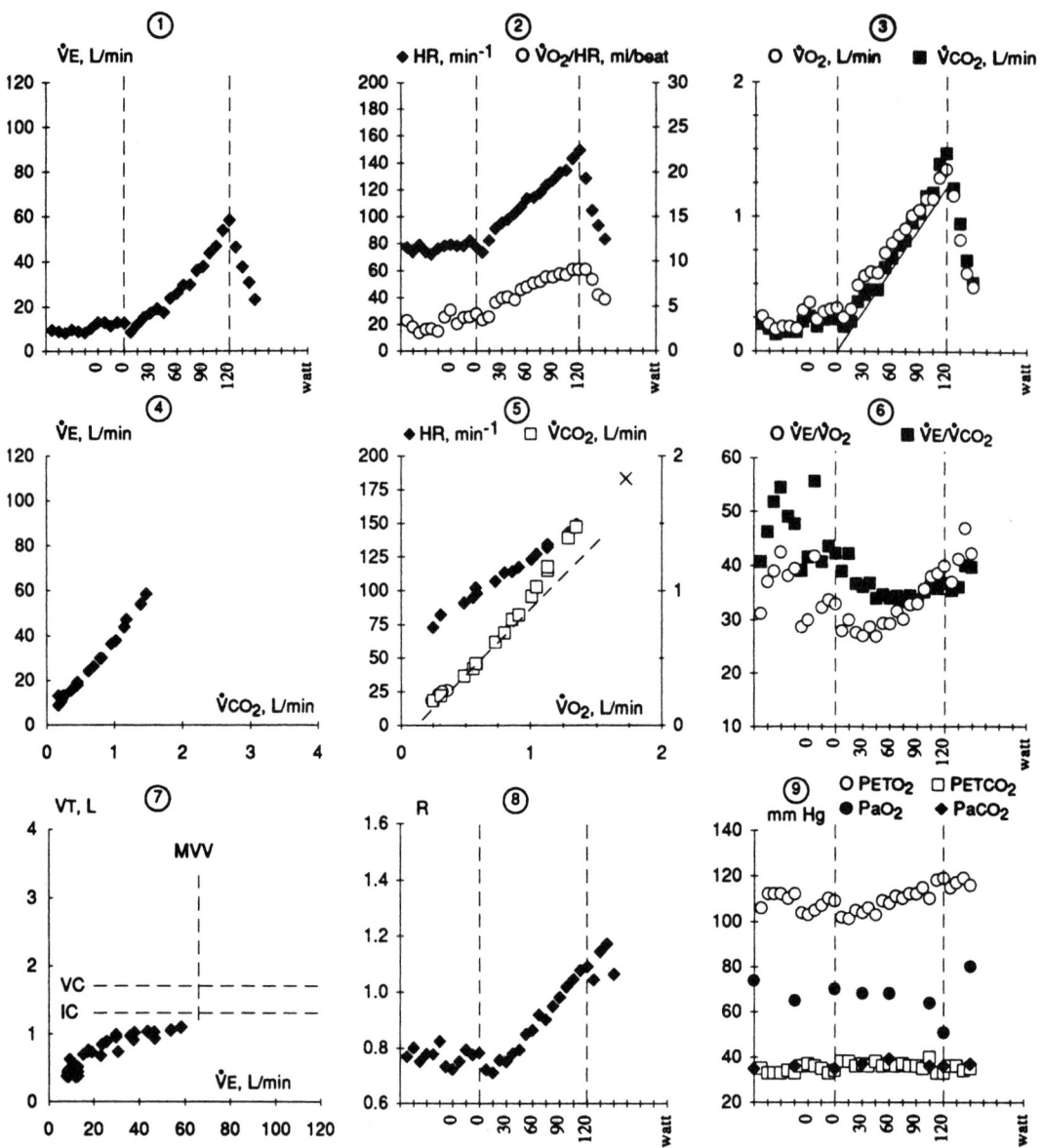

FIGURE 10.54.1.   Before treatment. **1:** Vertical dashed lines in panels 1 to 3 and 6, 8, and 9 indicate the beginning and the end of the increasing work period. **2:** Unloaded cycling is performed for 3 minutes before the left vertical dashed line. **3:** In panel 3, the diagonal line shows the increase of $\dot{V}O_2$ at a slope of 10 ml/min/W. **4:** In panel 5, the diagonal dashed line has a slope of 1; the x in the upper right is the predicted maximum heart rate and $\dot{V}O_2$ for the subject.

PaO_2 that decreases systematically with work rate, and increased values of $P(a - ET)CO_2$ and VD/VT (Table 10.54.3).

After treatment, the peak $\dot{V}O_2$ improved significantly and exceeded the predicted value. Arterial hypoxemia with exercise is no longer present, and $P(a - ET)CO_2$ and VD/VT are normal, suggesting that the ventilation–perfusion abnormality observed before treatment was corrected. Moreover, the re-

strictive breathing pattern observed during pretreatment exercise resolved after treatment (compare panels 7 of Figs. 10.54.1 and 10.54.2).

Conclusion

Reduced exercise capacity due to restrictive lung disease, reversed after 6 months of therapy.

TABLE 10.54.3.   Before Treatment

Time min	Work rate watts	BP mmHg	HR min⁻¹	f min⁻¹	$\dot{V}_E$ L/min BTPS	$\dot{V}_{CO_2}$ L/min STPD	$\dot{V}_{O_2}$ L/min STPD	$\dot{V}_{O_2}$/HR ml/beat	R	pH	HCO₃⁻ meq/L	PO₂, mmHg ET	a	(A−a)	PCO₂, mmHg ET	a	(a−ET)	$\dot{V}_E$/$\dot{V}_{CO_2}$	$\dot{V}_E$/$\dot{V}_{O_2}$	VD/VT
	Rest									7.47	25		74			35				
	Rest		77	15	9.4	0.20	0.26	3.4	0.77			106			35			41	31	
	Rest		74	19	9.0	0.16	0.20	2.7	0.80			112			33			46	37	
	Rest		79	21	8.0	0.12	0.16	2.0	0.75			112			33			52	39	
	Rest		74	22	9.5	0.14	0.18	2.4	0.78			112			33			55	42	
	Rest		72	24	8.9	0.14	0.18	2.5	0.78			110			34			49	38	
	Rest	119/68	76	19	8.3	0.14	0.17	2.2	0.82	7.45	25	112	65	43	33	36	3	48	39	0.40
	Unloaded		78	20	10.3	0.22	0.30	3.8	0.73			104			36			39	29	
	Unloaded		79	25	12.9	0.26	0.36	4.6	0.72			103			37			41	30	
	Unloaded		78	34	12.9	0.18	0.24	3.1	0.75			105			36			56	42	
	Unloaded		78	23	11.3	0.23	0.29	3.7	0.79			107			35			41	32	
	Unloaded		82	29	12.9	0.24	0.31	3.8	0.77			110			33			43	34	
	Unloaded	125/68	77	24	12.6	0.25	0.32	4.2	0.78	7.44	23	109	70	37	34	35	1	42	33	0.35
0.5	15		73	20	8.7	0.18	0.25	3.4	0.72			102			38			39	28	
1.0	15		82	32	12.0	0.22	0.31	3.8	0.71			101			38			42	30	
1.5	30		91	22	15.4	0.37	0.49	5.4	0.76			105			36			37	28	
2.0	30	131/68	95	23	17.1	0.42	0.56	5.9	0.75	7.44	25	104	68	35	37	37	0	36	27	0.31
2.5	45		98	26	19.1	0.46	0.59	6.0	0.78			106			36			37	29	
3.0	45		102	23	17.6	0.46	0.58	5.7	0.79			103			38			34	27	
3.5	60		107	28	23.8	0.62	0.73	6.8	0.85			109			36			35	29	
4.0	60	146/75	113	29	25.9	0.69	0.80	7.1	0.86	7.43	25	108	68	38	37	39	2	34	29	0.32
4.5	75		114	31	29.8	0.79	0.86	7.5	0.92			111			36			34	32	
5.0	75		117	30	29.9	0.82	0.91	7.8	0.90			110			37			33	30	
5.5	90		123	37	36.2	0.96	1.01	8.2	0.95			112			36			34	33	
6.0	90		127	37	37.8	1.03	1.05	8.3	0.98			112			36			34	33	
6.5	105		132	42	43.8	1.15	1.13	8.6	1.02			115			35			35	36	
7.0	105	190/78	134	50	47.0	1.18	1.13	8.4	1.04	7.42	23	110	64	51	40	36	−4	36	38	0.31
7.5	120		143	51	54.0	1.39	1.29	9.0	1.08			118			33			36	39	
8.0	120	190/81	149	53	58.4	1.47	1.35	9.1	1.09	7.41	22	119	51	65	33	36	3	37	40	0.32
	Recovery		128	45	46.6	1.21	1.16	9.1	1.04			115			36			35	37	
	Recovery		104	41	37.6	0.95	0.83	8.0	1.14			117			36			36	41	
	Recovery		93	41	30.7	0.68	0.58	6.2	1.17			119			34			40	47	
	Recovery	190/81	83	34	23.1	0.51	0.48	5.8	1.06	7.36	21	116	80	35	35	37	2	40	42	0.36

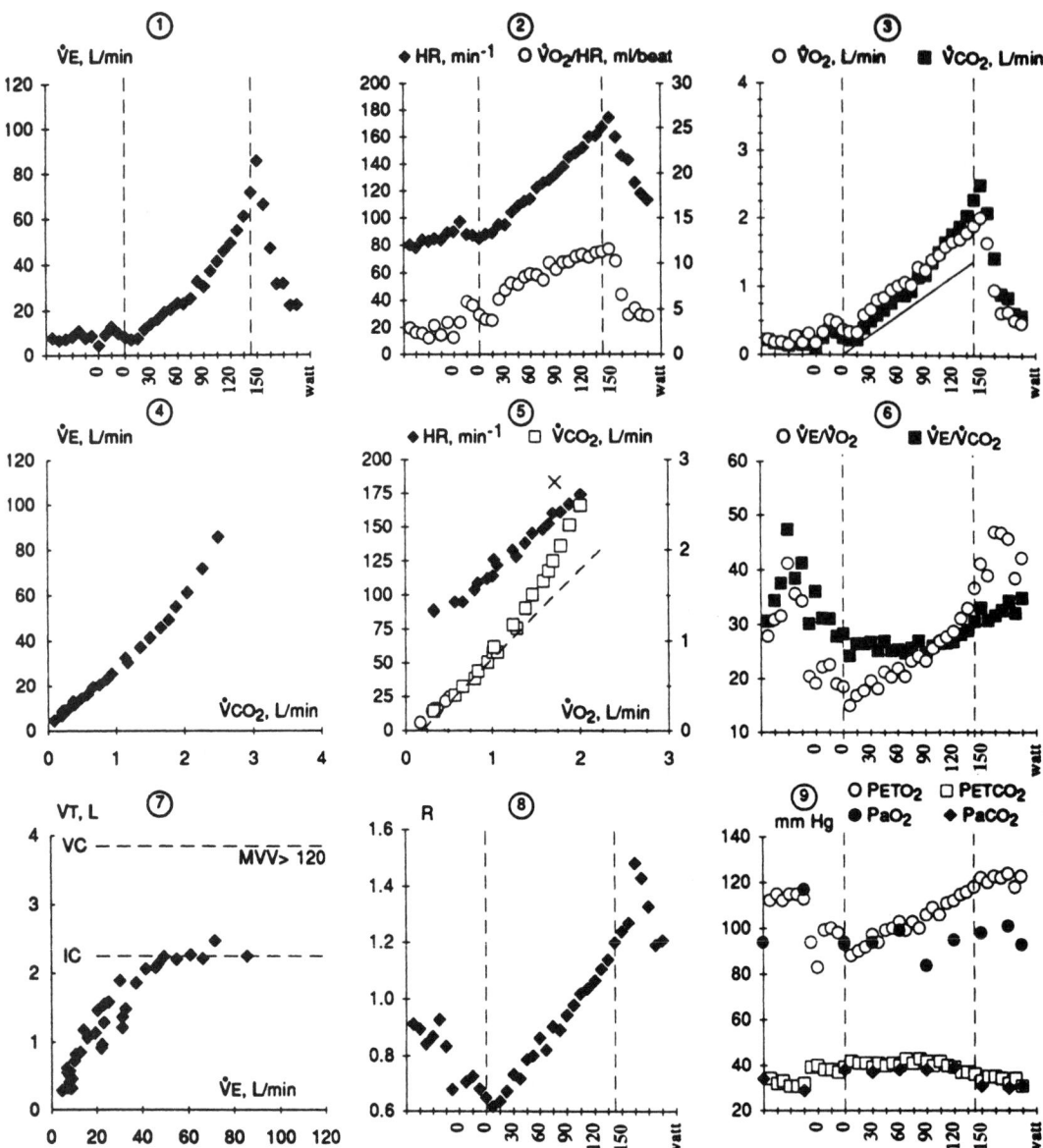

FIGURE 10.54.2.   After treatment. **1:** Vertical dashed lines in panels 1 to 3 and 6, 8, and 9 indicate the beginning and the end of the increasing work period. **2:** Unloaded cycling is performed for 3 minutes before the left vertical dashed line. **3:** In panel 3, the diagonal line shows the increase of $\dot{V}O_2$ at a slope of 10 ml/min/W. **4:** In panel 5, the diagonal dashed line has a slope of 1; the x in the upper right is the predicted maximum heart rate and $\dot{V}O_2$ for the subject.

TABLE 10.54.4.   After Treatment

Time min	Work rate watts	BP mmHg	HR min⁻¹	f min⁻¹	V̇E L/min BTPS	V̇CO₂ L/min STPD	V̇O₂ L/min STPD	V̇O₂/HR ml/beat	R	pH	HCO₃⁻ meq/L	PO₂ ET	PO₂ a	PO₂ (A−a)	PCO₂ ET	PCO₂ a	PCO₂ (a−ET)	V̇E/V̇CO₂	V̇E/V̇O₂	VD/VT
	Rest	125/75								7.45	23		94			34				
	Rest		80	15	7.7	0.21	0.23	2.9	0.91			112			34			31	28	
	Rest		78	11	6.8	0.17	0.19	2.4	0.89			115			32			35	31	
	Rest		84	13	7.1	0.16	0.19	2.3	0.84			112			33			37	32	
	Rest		83	24	8.2	0.13	0.15	1.8	0.87			115			31			47	41	
	Rest		85	13	10.7	0.25	0.27	3.2	0.98			115			31			38	36	
	Rest	119/75	84	19	7.8	0.15	0.18	2.1	0.83	7.50	22	113	117	−1	32	29	−3	41	34	0.22
	Unloaded		89	28	8.7	0.21	0.31	3.5	0.68			94			39			30	20	
	Unloaded		90	16	4.6	0.09	0.17	1.9	0.53			83			40			36	19	
	Unloaded		97	20	9.2	0.24	0.34	3.5	0.71			99			38			31	22	
	Unloaded		88	15	12.8	0.37	0.51	5.8	0.73			100			38			31	23	
	Unloaded		87	14	10.1	0.32	0.47	5.4	0.68			98			37			28	19	
	Unloaded	125/75	85	14	8.0	0.24	0.37	4.4	0.65	7.43	25	94	93	3	39	38	−1	28	18	0.17
0.5	15		88	21	6.9	0.21	0.34	3.9	0.62			88			42			24	15	
1.0	15		89	23	7.5	0.21	0.33	3.7	0.64			90			41			26	17	
1.5	30		95	14	11.5	0.39	0.58	6.1	0.67			92			41			26	18	
2.0	30	125/69	95	12	14.1	0.49	0.67	7.1	0.73	7.44	25	97	94	8	39	37	−2	27	20	0.12
2.5	45		104	15	15.9	0.58	0.81	7.8	0.72			94			41			25	18	
3.0	45		109	17	19.2	0.66	0.84	7.7	0.79			99			40			27	21	
3.5	60		112	14	20.4	0.76	0.95	8.5	0.80			100			41			25	20	
4.0	60	144/75	114	15	23.3	0.87	1.01	8.9	0.86	7.43	25	103	99	8	40	38	−2	25	22	0.10
4.5	75		122	18	23.1	0.87	1.06	8.7	0.82			99			43			25	20	
5.0	75		126	16	25.3	0.93	1.03	8.2	0.90			103			41			26	23	
5.5	90		128	22	32.6	1.14	1.28	10.0	0.89			100			43			27	24	
6.0	90	156/75	133	16	30.3	1.17	1.24	9.3	0.94	7.42	24	106	84	26	42	38	−4	25	23	0.08
6.5	105		138	20	37.2	1.36	1.39	10.1	0.98			109			40			26	26	
7.0	105		145	20	41.4	1.50	1.47	10.1	1.02			106			42			26	27	
7.5	120		148	22	45.8	1.65	1.59	10.7	1.04			111			40			27	28	
8.0	120	181/81	152	22	49.4	1.77	1.66	10.9	1.07	7.40	24	112	95	18	39	39	0	27	29	0.17
8.5	135		160	25	55.0	1.88	1.70	10.6	1.11			115			37			28	31	
9.0	135		161	27	61.2	2.04	1.79	11.1	1.14			116			37			29	33	
9.5	130		167	29	71.7	2.27	1.89	11.3	1.20			118			36			31	37	
10.0	130	181/88	174	38	85.6	2.49	2.01	11.6	1.24	7.40	19	122	98	26	33	31	−2	33	41	0.15
	Recovery		160	30	66.5	2.08	1.64	10.3	1.27			120			35			31	39	
	Recovery		146	22	46.9	1.42	0.96	6.6	148			123			35			32	47	
	Recovery		143	23	31.3	0.90	0.63	4.4	1.43			122			34			33	47	
	Recovery	181/81	126	26	31.4	0.85	0.64	5.1	1.33	7.36	17	124	101	25	32	30	−2	34	46	0.15
	Recovery		118	24	22.0	0.62	0.52	4.4	1.19			118			34			32	38	
	Recovery	175/75	113	23	22.2	0.58	0.48	4.2	1.21	7.36	17	123	93	30	31	31	0	35	42	0.18

Case 55 Interstitial Pulmonary Fibrosis: Air and Oxygen Breathing Studies

Clinical Findings

This 47-year-old man had developed dyspnea 12 years previously. A histologic diagnosis of pulmonary alveolar proteinosis was then made by open lung biopsy. Following whole-lung lavage, he became asymptomatic until 10 months prior to evaluation, when progressive dyspnea first became evident when he was skiing at high altitudes. Although previously active in sports, he was unable to walk more than 30 yards on flat ground at a normal pace. He coughed with exercise and sometimes produced clear sputum. He denied smoking, wheezing, or edema. The results of his examination were normal except for digital clubbing and infrequent fine inspiratory rales at the lung bases. Chest roentgenogram showed increased interstitial markings with honeycombing.

Exercise Findings

The patient performed exercise on a cycle ergometer breathing room air, and, after a 30-minute rest, breathing 100% oxygen. He pedaled at 60 rpm without added load for 3 minutes. The work rate was increased 15 W every minute to his symptom-limited maximum. Arterial blood was sampled every second minute, and intraarterial blood pressure was recorded from a percutaneously placed brachial artery catheter. When breathing room air, he stopped exercise because of fatigue and light-headedness. When breathing oxygen, he stopped because of leg pain and general fatigue. Resting and exercise ECGs were normal.

Interpretation

Comments

This case of severe interstitial lung disease is presented to illustrate two major findings: (a) the impaired peripheral oxygenation that may be caused by pulmonary fibrosis, and (b) the presence of a major increasing contribution of the carotid bodies to breathing, in association with arterial hypoxemia.

The results of the resting respiratory function studies indicate that this patient has a severe restric-

TABLE 10.55.1.   Selected Respiratory Function Data

Measurement	Predicted	Measured
Age, yr		47
Sex		Male
Height, cm		174
Weight, kg	77	85
Hematocrit, %		41
VC, L	4.49	2.20
IC, L	2.99	1.14
TLC, L	6.48	3.17
FEV_1, L	3.58	2.01
FEV_1/VC, %	80	91
MVV, L/min, direct	151	112
MVV, L/min, indirect	143	80
D_LCO, ml/mm Hg/min	30.7	13.9

TABLE 10.55.2.   Selected Exercise Data

Measurement	Predicted	Room Air	Oxygen
Peak $\dot{V}O_2$, L/min	2.60	1.23	
Maximum HR, beats/min	173	150	154
Maximum O_2 pulse, ml/beat	15.0	8.2	
$\Delta\dot{V}O_2/\Delta WR$, ml/min/W	10.3	8.6	
AT, L/min	>1.12	0.85	
Blood pressure, mmHg (rest, max)		120/75, 175/84*	138/87, 195/90*
Maximum $\dot{V}E$, L/min		72	56
Exercise breathing reserve, L/min	>15	8	32
PaO_2, mmHg (rest, max ex)		62, 37	568, 284
P(A − a)O_2, mmHg (rest, max ex)		30, 73	102, 365
P(a − ET)CO_2, mmHg (rest, max ex)		6, 10	4, 12
VD/VT (rest, heavy ex)		0.54, 0.54	0.51, 0.56
HCO_3^-, mEq/L (rest, 2-min recov)		23, 20	26, 22

*Systolic pulses paradoxus of 70 mmHg.

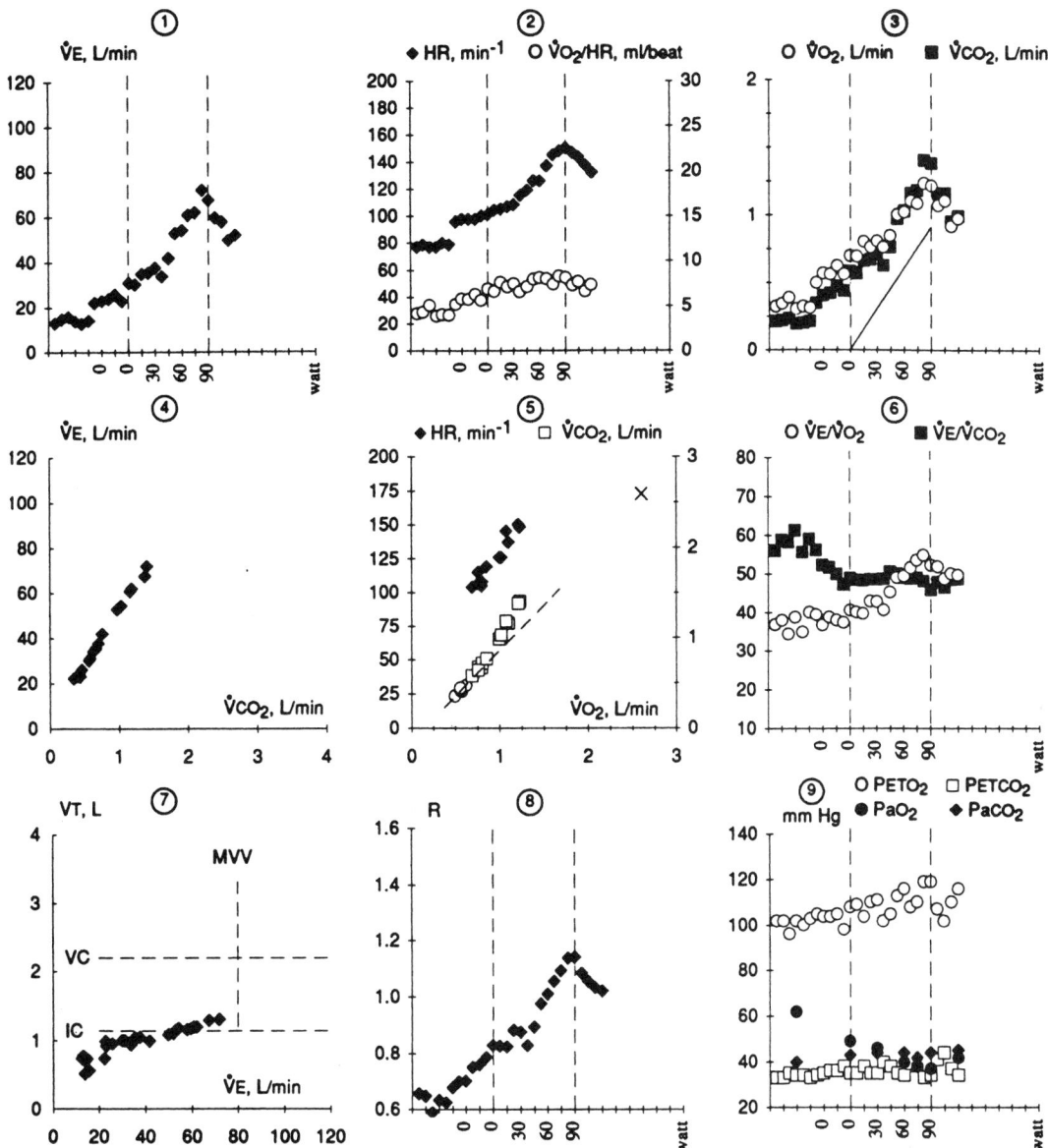

FIGURE 10.55.1. Air breathing. **1:** Vertical dashed lines in panels 1 to 3 and 6, 8, and 9 indicate the beginning and the end of the increasing work period. **2:** Unloaded cycling is performed for 3 minutes before the left vertical dashed line. **3:** In panel 3, the diagonal line shows the increase of $\dot{V}O_2$ at a slope of 10 ml/min/W. **4:** In panel 5, the diagonal dashed line has a slope of 1; the x in the upper right is the predicted maximum heart rate and $\dot{V}O_2$ for the subject.

tive disorder, with no evidence of airflow obstruction (Table 10.55.1). The resting ECG is normal.

Analysis

Referring to flowchart 1, the peak $\dot{V}O_2$ and anaerobic threshold are reduced (Table 10.55.2). Referring to flowchart 4, the breathing reserve is reduced (branch point 4.1). Following the low breathing reserve branch of branch point 4.1, we consider branch point 4.2 and the high VD/VT. From this, we conclude that this patient has restrictive lung dis-

ease with an O_2 flow problem. Findings confirming this diagnosis are as follows: (a) the high VT/IC ratio (panel 7, Fig. 10.55.1), (b) the low and progressively decreasing PaO_2 as work rate is increased (panel 9, Fig. 10.55.1), (c) a breathing frequency greater than 50 at the peak $\dot{V}O_2$ (Table 10.55.3), (d) an increased $P(a - ET)CO_2$ (panel 9, Fig. 10.55.1), (e) a steep heart rate response to the increasing oxygen uptake (panel 5, Fig. 10.55.1), (f) a low O_2 pulse with a flat contour as the work rate is increased (panel 2, Fig. 10.55.1), (g) a reduced $\Delta\dot{V}O_2/\Delta WR$ (Table 10.55.2 and panel 3, Fig. 10.55.1), and (h) $P(A - a)O_2$ in-

TABLE 10.55.3.   Air Breathing

Time min	Work rate watts	BP mmHg	HR min⁻¹	f min⁻¹	$\dot{V}_E$ L/min BTPS	$\dot{V}_{CO_2}$ L/min STPD	$\dot{V}_{O_2}$ L/min STPD	$\dot{V}_{O_2}$/HR ml/beat	R	pH	HCO$_3^-$ meq/L	PO$_2$, mmHg ET	a	(A − a)	PCO$_2$, mmHg ET	a	(a − ET)	$\dot{V}_E$/$\dot{V}_{CO_2}$	$\dot{V}_E$/$\dot{V}_{O_2}$	VD/VT
	Rest		77	17	13.2	0.21	0.32	4.2	0.66			102			33			56	37	
	Rest		79	20	14.6	0.22	0.34	4.3	0.65			102			33			59	38	
	Rest		77	28	15.8	0.23	0.39	5.1	0.59			96			35			58	34	
	Rest	120/75	77	27	13.9	0.19	0.30	3.9	0.63	7.37	23	102	62	30	34	40	6	61	39	0.54
	Rest		80	17	12.6	0.20	0.32	4.0	0.63			100			34			56	35	
	Rest		79	20	14.1	0.21	0.31	3.9	0.68			103			33			59	40	
	Unloaded		96	30	22.2	0.35	0.50	5.2	0.70			105			34			56	39	
	Unloaded		98	25	23.0	0.40	0.57	5.8	0.70			104			35			52	37	
	Unloaded		98	25	23.8	0.42	0.56	5.7	0.75			104			36			52	39	
	Unloaded		98	27	25.8	0.47	0.62	6.3	0.76			105			36			50	38	
	Unloaded		100	23	22.8	0.44	0.56	5.6	0.79			98			38			47	37	
	Unloaded	158/81	101	31	31.0	0.58	0.70	6.9	0.83	7.35	23	108	49	51	35	43	8	49	41	0.54
0.5	15		104	30	30.1	0.57	0.69	6.6	0.83			109			35			48	40	
1.0	15		105	35	34.8	0.66	0.80	7.6	0.83			104			38			48	40	
1.5	30		107	34	35.5	0.67	0.76	7.1	0.88			110			35			49	43	
2.0	30	159/75	108	36	37.6	0.71	0.81	7.5	0.88	7.34	23	111	46	55	35	44	9	49	43	0.55
2.5	45		115	36	33.8	0.63	0.76	6.6	0.83			102			40			49	40	
3.0	45		119	42	41.9	0.76	0.85	7.1	0.89			105			38			50	45	
3.5	60		126	46	52.8	0.98	1.00	7.9	0.98			113			35			50	49	
4.0	60	177/90	126	46	54.3	1.03	1.02	8.1	1.01	7.33	23	116	40	66	34	44	10	49	49	0.56
4.5	75		137	51	60.9	1.16	1.10	8.0	1.05			108			39			49	51	
5.0	75	186/90	145	52	62.1	1.18	1.08	7.4	1.09	7.33	22	110	38	73	38	42	4	49	53	0.54
5.5	90		148	55	72.0	1.40	1.23	8.3	1.14			119			33			48	55	
6.0	90	186/93	150	52	67.5	1.38	1.21	8.1	1.14	7.31	22	119	37	73	34	44	10	46	52	0.53
	Recovery		147	51	59.7	1.16	1.07	7.3	1.08			107			41			48	52	
	Recovery		144	50	57.9	1.16	1.10	7.6	1.05			102			44			46	49	
	Recovery		138	46	49.9	0.95	0.92	6.7	1.03			110			37			48	50	
	Recovery	174/90	132	47	52.1	0.99	0.97	7.3	1.02	7.27	20	116	42	64	34	45	11	49	50	0.56

creasing with increasing work rate (Table 10.55.3). Note that all these confirmatory findings are characteristic of restrictive lung disease.

O$_2$ breathing allows the patient to increase his maximum work rate from 90 to 135 W (Table 10.55.4 and Fig. 10.55.2). This was accomplished primarily by decreasing ventilatory drive. In contrast to regulating arterial PcO$_2$ around 40 as the patient did when breathing air, 100% O$_2$ breathing attenuated ventilatory drive (carotid body inhibition), causing PacO$_2$ to increase to 64 at the maximum work rate achieved. At each work rate during O$_2$ breathing, the breathing frequency (f) is decreased (compare Table 10.55.3 with Table 10.55.4). O$_2$ breathing allows the patient to breathe less and

to be less breathless. The breathing frequency is only 35 ($\dot{V}_E$ = 37.5) at 90 W when breathing O$_2$, as compared with 52 ($\dot{V}_E$ = 67.5) during air breathing at the same work rate. The heart rate is considerably more rapid during air breathing (150) than during O$_2$ breathing (132) at 90 W.

Conclusion

The patient has severe interstitial lung disease, with an important O$_2$ flow problem that was probably created by a combination of arterial hypoxemia and pulmonary vascular disease. O$_2$ breathing attenuates ventilatory drive and provides relief of dyspnea.

TABLE 10.55.4.   Oxygen Breathing

Time min	Work rate watts	BP mmHg	HR min⁻¹	f min⁻¹	V̇E L/min BTPS	V̇CO₂ L/min STPD	V̇O₂ L/min STPD	V̇O₂/HR ml/beat	R	pH	HCO₃⁻ meq/L	PO₂ ET	PO₂ a	PO₂ (A−a)	PCO₂ ET	PCO₂ a	PCO₂ (a−ET)	V̇E/V̇CO₂	V̇E/V̇O₂	VD/VT
	Rest	132/84								7.44	24	66			36					
	Rest		94	21	11.6	0.19									40			52		
	Rest		93	19	12.1	0.18									39			58		
	Rest		90	23	13.3	0.21									37			54		
	Rest	138/87	91	29	14.5	0.23				7.39	26	568	102		39	43	4	52		0.51
	Rest		92	23	14.5	0.22									38			57		
	Rest		96	25	14.0	0.18									36			66		
	Rest		96	22	17.8	0.30									37			53		
	Rest		89	30	16.7	0.24									37			59		
	Unloaded		102	28	19.8	0.33									37			53		
	Unloaded		100	26	20.1	0.34									39			53		
	Unloaded		100	25	18.9	0.33									39			51		
	Unloaded		100	21	15.7	0.31									45			45		
	Unloaded		104	22	16.4	0.37									45			39		
	Unloaded	192/108	114	24	17.2	0.42				7.33	26	540	122		46	51	5	36		0.47
0.5	15		122	22	16.9	0.49									48			31		
1.0	15		120	28	20.1	0.59									49			30		
1.5	15		120	35	39.6	0.79									39			46		
2.0	15		119	28	29.5	0.64									42			42		
2.5	30		116	37	32.2	0.64									47			45		
3.0	30	186/96	117	28	27.1	0.58				7.31	26	505	156		44	52	8	43		0.56
3.5	45		117	30	25.7	0.55									51			42		
4.0	45		120	32	32.0	0.74									44			40		
4.5	60		126	34	32.4	0.79									48			37		
5.0	60	192/99	128	29	33.5	0.83				7.28	25	467	191		48	55	7	37		0.54
5.5	75		131	32	34.6	0.85									47			38		
6.0	75		134	37	34.2	0.87									49			36		
6.5	90		136	33	36.5	0.94									51			36		
7.0	90	196/102	132	35	37.5	0.99				7.25	25	409	245		54	59	5	35		0.53
7.5	105		144	39	40.1	1.08									51			34		
8.0	105	207/102	145	37	41.3	1.10				7.23	25	350	302		54	51	7	35		0.55
8.5	120		145	40	47.0	1.31									52			33		
9.0	120		152	40	48.3	1.39									52			32		
9.5	135		153	45	54.7	1.54									53			33		
10.0	135	210/102	154	46	56.1	1.53				7.20	25	284	365		52	64	12	34		0.56
	Recovery		149	43	53.9	1.51									53			33		
	Recovery		144	43	51.7	1.38									52			35		
	Recovery		136	41	46.1	1.13									47			38		
	Recovery		133	39	44.1	1.03									47			40		
		192/102								7.22	22	475				55				

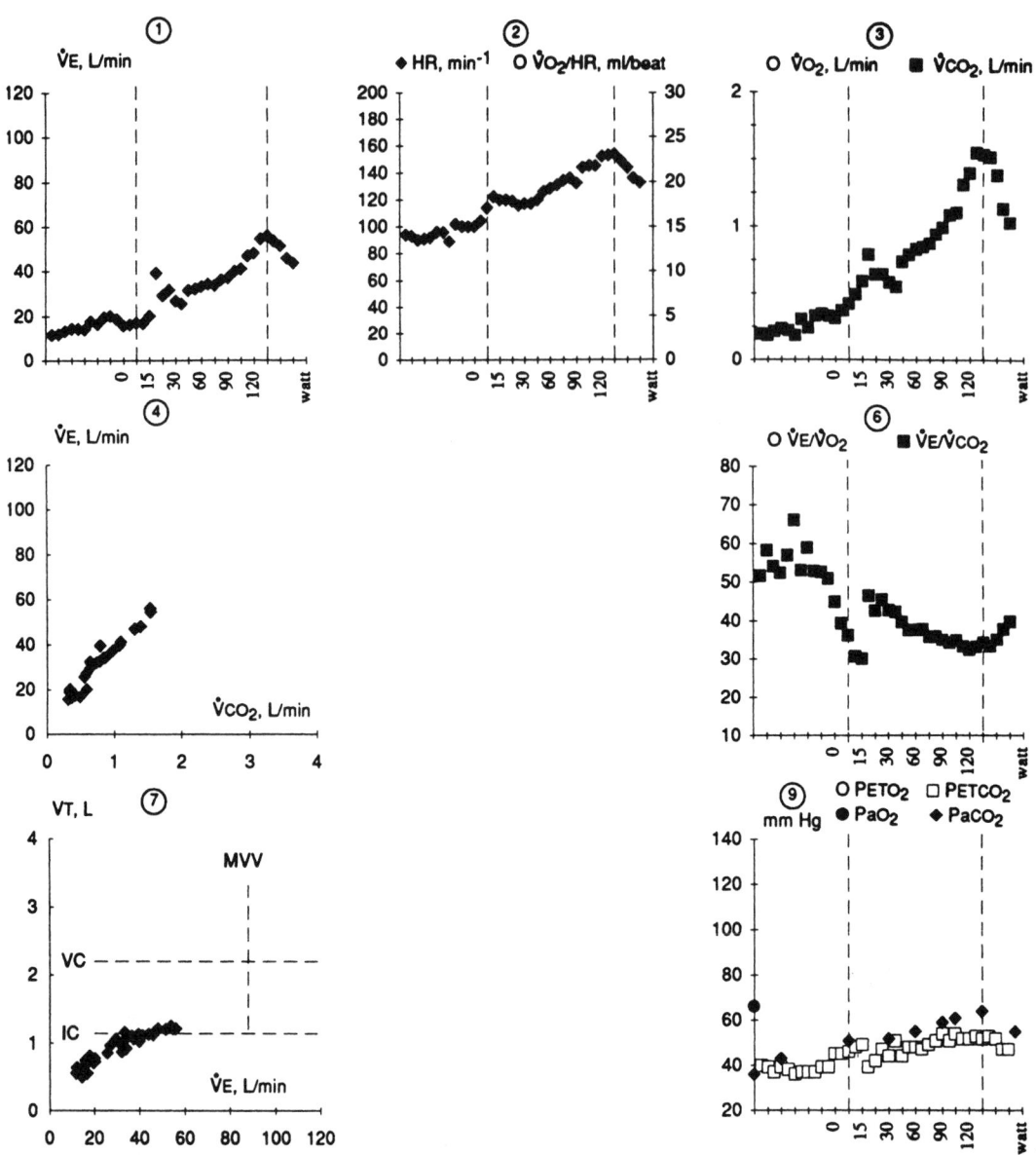

FIGURE 10.55.2.   Oxygen breathing. **1:** Vertical dashed lines in panels 1 to 3 and 6 and 9 indicate the beginning and the end of the increasing work period. **2:** Unloaded cycling is performed for 3 minutes before the left vertical dashed line.

Case 56 Pulmonary Alveolar Proteinosis: Air and Oxygen Breathing Studies

Clinical Findings

This 19-year-old man was hospitalized because of increasing shortness of breath, productive cough, and fatigue of 6 weeks' duration. He denied fever, sweats, chest pain, or exposure to infectious or toxic agents other than automobile paint fumes, tobacco, and occasional marijuana. He was thin, afebrile, tachycardic, and tachypneic with diffuse coarse rales bilaterally. Chest roentgenograms revealed a diffuse alveolar infiltrate, and blood gases showed hypoxemia and hypercapnia. An open lung biopsy showed pulmonary alveolar proteinosis. Exercise tests were performed while the patient was breathing room air and then 100% O_2 prior to bilateral lung lavage.

Exercise Findings

The patient performed exercise on a cycle ergometer twice in the same morning with a 40-minute rest period between tests. On both occasions, arterial blood was sampled every second minute, and intraarterial pressure was recorded from a percutaneously placed brachial artery catheter. He pedaled at 60 rpm without an added load for 3 minutes. The work rate was then increased 15 W per minute to tolerance. The patient was well motivated and co-

operative and stopped exercise on both occasions because of dyspnea and chest tightness. No ECG abnormalities were noted.

Interpretation

Comments

This case is presented to show the effects of O_2 breathing on work capacity in a patient with hypoxemia and restrictive lung disease and the differences between direct and indirect MVV measures in such patients. Resting respiratory function studies showed severe restrictive disease with low D_{LCO},

TABLE 10.56.1.   Selected Respiratory Function Data

Measurement	Predicted	Measured
Age, yr		19
Sex		Male
Height, cm		180
Weight, kg	82	68
Hematocrit, %		49
VC, L	4.46	2.46
IC, L	2.98	1.50
TLC, L	6.7	3.40
FEV$_1$, L	3.79	2.20
FEV$_1$/VC, %	85	89
MVV, L/min		
Direct	134	101
Indirect	152	88
D$_L$CO, ml/mm Hg/min	36.5	8.4

TABLE 10.56.2.   Selected Exercise Data

Measurement	Predicted	Room Air	Oxygen
Peak V̇O$_2$, L/min	3.26	1.42	
Maximum HR, beats/min	201	150	150
Maximum O$_2$ pulse, ml/beat	16.2	9.5	
ΔV̇O$_2$/ΔWR, ml/min/W	10.3	11.9	
AT, L/min	>1.31	1.4	
Work rate, max, W		75	120
Blood pressure, mmHg (rest, max ex)		120/57, 144/72	114/62, 132/72
Maximum V̇E, L/min		84	73
Exercise breathing reserve, L/min			
Using direct MVV	>15	17	28
Using indirect MVV	>15	4	15
PaO$_2$, mmHg (rest, max ex)		52, 38	306, 164
P(A − a)O$_2$, mmHg (rest, max ex)		57, 76	371. 506
P(a − ET)CO$_2$, mmHg (rest, max ex)		−1, 5	1, 5
VD/VT (rest, max ex)		0.42, 0.59	0.49, 0.48
HCO$_3^-$, mEq/L (rest, recov)		23, 21	23, 20

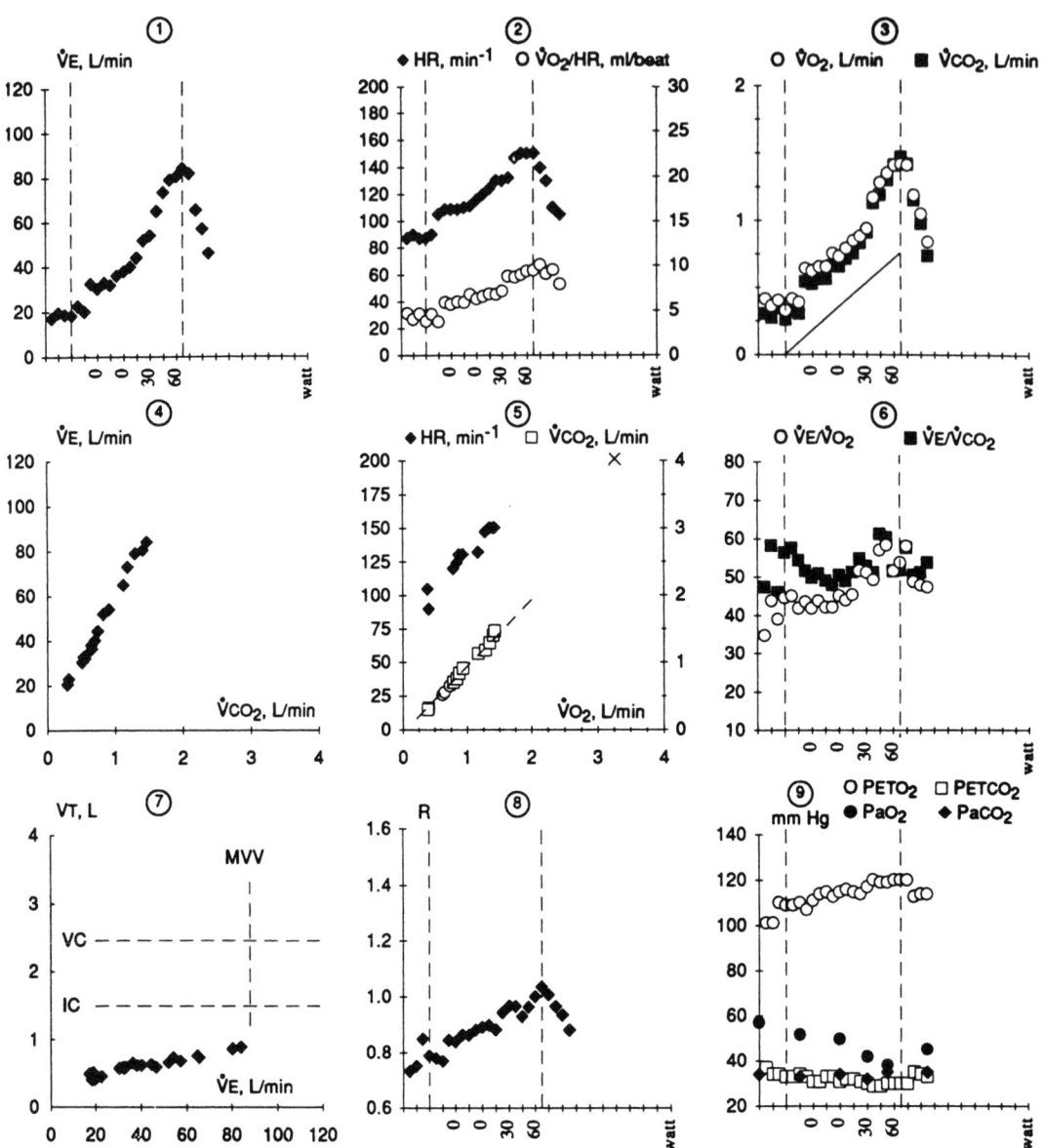

FIGURE 10.56.1.   Air breathing. **1:** Vertical dashed lines in panels 1 to 3 and 6, 8, and 9 indicate the beginning and the end of the increasing work period. **2:** Unloaded cycling is performed for 3 minutes before the left vertical dashed line. **3:** In panel 3, the diagonal line shows the increase of $\dot{V}O_2$ at a slope of 10 ml/min/W. **4:** In panel 5, the diagonal dashed line has a slope of 1; the x in the upper right is the predicted maximum heart rate and $\dot{V}O_2$ for the subject.

indicating loss of effective alveolar capillary bed, moderate hypoxemia, and mild hypocapnia (Table 10.56.1).

Analysis

Referring to flowchart 1, in the room air study the peak $\dot{V}O_2$ was low, but the anaerobic threshold was within normal limits (Table 10.56.2). This leads us to flowchart 3 and the category of lung disease through branch point 3.1 because of the borderline breathing reserve using the direct MVV. If we had used the indirect MVV, the breathing reserve would have been clearly low (abnormal). Confirmatory findings are high V_D/V_T, positive $P(a - ET)CO_2$, and wide $P(A - a)O_2$. Restrictive lung disease is further confirmed by the high breathing frequency of over 90 per minute (branch point 3.2). In the O_2 study, the patient exercised to a considerably higher work rate with a lower maximum $\dot{V}E$, confirming that the patient did indeed have ventilatory limitation during the room air study. The low O_2 pulse while the patient was breathing room air was predominantly due to the low arterial O_2 content (SaO_2 approxi-

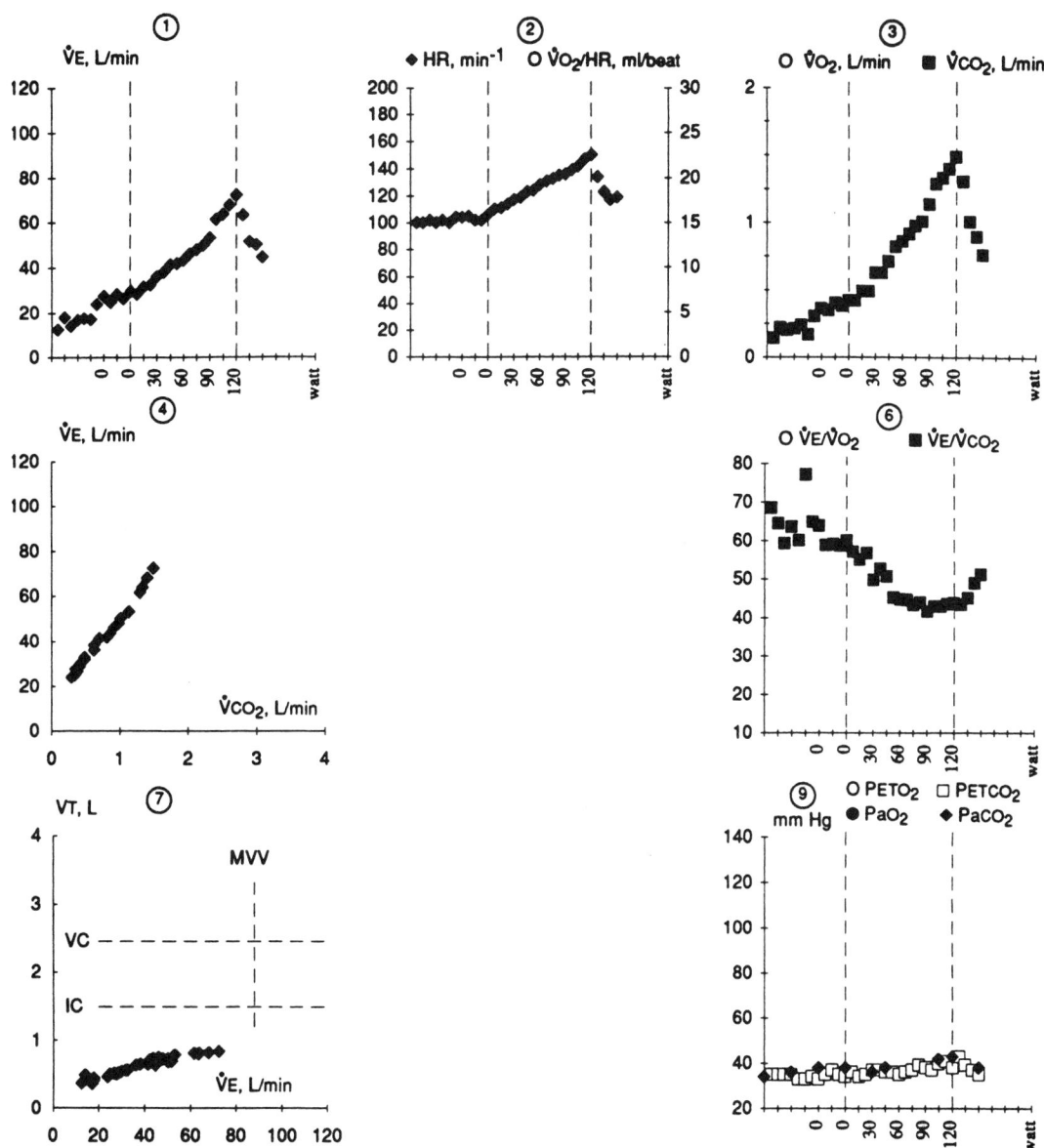

FIGURE 10.56.2.   Oxygen breathing. **1:** Vertical dashed lines in panels 1 to 3 and 6 and 9 indicate the beginning and the end of the increasing work period. **2:** Unloaded cycling is performed for 3 minutes before the left vertical dashed line.

mated 75% during late exercise). This contributed to a reduced arteriovenous O_2 content difference at maximal exercise. The patient developed a mild metabolic acidosis in both studies and some respiratory acidosis during O_2 breathing. The latter study demonstrates a large right-to-left shuntlike effect typical of this disorder (1).

Conclusion

This is a typical case of pulmonary alveolar proteinosis with restriction and severe gas exchange abnormalities. The patient was limited both by his ventilatory ability and by hypoxemia. Young patients with interstitial lung disease often develop strong ventilatory muscles that allow them to exercise at a higher rate than might otherwise be expected. The directly measured MVV, performed at a high breathing frequency, was 101 L/min, whereas the indirect MVV, calculated as 40 times the FEV_1, was 88 L/min. Bilateral lung lavage performed after this study was helpful in improving the patient's exercise tolerance.

Reference

1. Selecky PA, Wasserman K, Benfield JR, et al. The clinical and physiological effect of whole-lung lavage in pulmonary alveolar proteinosis: a ten-year experience. *Ann Thorac Surg* 1977;24:451–461.

TABLE 10.56.3. Air Breathing

Time min	Work rate watts	BP mmHg	HR min⁻¹	f min⁻¹	V̇E L/min BTPS	V̇CO₂ L/min STPD	V̇O₂ L/min STPD	V̇O₂/HR ml/beat	R	pH	HCO₃⁻ meq/L	Po₂ ET	Po₂ a	Po₂ (A−a)	Pco₂ ET	Pco₂ a	Pco₂ (a−ET)	V̇E/V̇CO₂	V̇E/V̇O₂	VD/VT
	Rest	102/57								7.45	23		57			34				
	Rest		87	35	17.2	0.30	0.41	4.7	0.73			101			37			47	35	
	Rest		90	48	19.8	0.27	0.36	4.0	0.75			101			34			58	44	
	Rest		87	37	18.8	0.34	0.40	4.6	0.85			110			34			46	39	
	Rest		87	45	18.5	0.26	0.33	3.8	0.79			109			33			56	44	
0.5			90	50	22.7	0.32	0.41	4.6	0.78			109			33			58	45	
1.0		99/60	105	47	20.3	0.30	0.39	3.7	0.77	7.45	23	110	52	57	34	33	−1	54	42	0.42
1.5	Unloaded		109	57	32.7	0.54	0.64	5.9	0.84			107			33			52	44	
2.0	Unloaded		109	53	30.4	0.52	0.62	5.7	0.84			111			31			50	42	
2.5	Unloaded		109	57	33.3	0.56	0.65	6.0	0.86			114			31			51	44	
3.0	Unloaded		110	55	32.1	0.56	0.65	5.9	0.86			115			33			49	42	
3.5	Unloaded		111	56	36.4	0.66	0.75	6.8	0.88			113			33			48	42	
4.0	Unloaded	123/69	116	62	38.1	0.65	0.73	6.3	0.89	7.45	23	115	50	63	31	34	3	51	45	0.43
4.5	15		120	65	40.2	0.71	.79	6.6	0.90			116			32			49	44	
5.0	15		124	70	44.4	0.75	0.85	6.9	0.88			115			32			51	45	
5.5	30		130	79	52.1	0.83	0.88	6.8	0.94			114			31			55	52	
6.0	30	126/72	130	73	54.2	0.91	0.94	7.2	0.97	7.46	22	117	42	75	30	32	2	53	51	0.43
6.5	45		132	85	64.9	1.13	1.17	8.9	0.97			120			29			51	49	
7.0	45		147	85	73.2	1.19	1.28	8.7	0.93			119			29			61	57	
7.5	60	144/72	150	93	78.8	1.30	1.35	9.0	0.96	7.43	23	119	38	76	30	35	5	60	58	0.59
8.0	60		150	93	80.4	1.41	1.41	9.4	1.00			120			30			51	51	
8.5	75		150	94	84.2	1.47	1.42	9.5	1.04			120			30			52	54	
	Recovery		140	92	81.8	1.42	1.41	10.1	1.01			120			30			57	58	
	Recovery		130	89	65.6	1.15	1.19	9.2	0.97			113			35			50	49	
	Recovery		110	84	57.3	0.98	1.05	9.5	0.93			114			34			51	48	
	Recovery	144/72	105	79	46.5	0.74	0.84	8.0	0.88	7.39	21	114	45	66	33	35	2	54	47	0.46

TABLE 10.56.4. Oxygen Breathing

Time min	Work rate watts	BP mmHg	HR min⁻¹	f min⁻¹	V̇E L/min BTPS	V̇CO₂ L/min STPD	V̇O₂ L/min STPD	V̇O₂/HR ml/beat	R	pH	HCO₃⁻ meq/L	Po₂ ET	Po₂ a	Po₂ (A−a)	Pco₂ ET	Pco₂ a	Pco₂ (a−ET)	V̇E/V̇CO₂	V̇E/V̇O₂	VD/VT
	Rest	114/62								7.44	23		359			34				
	Rest		100	34	12.5	0.14									35			69		
	Rest		100	44	17.9	0.22									35			69		
	Rest		102	29	14.3	0.20									35			59		
	Rest	99/63	100	43	17.0	0.21				7.41	22		306	371	35	36	1	64		0.49
	Rest		102	40	17.8	0.24									33			60		
	Rest		100	48	17.2	0.17									33			77		
	Unloaded		104	52	23.9	0.30									34			65		
	Unloaded	102/63	104	56	27.7	0.36				7.40	23		221	454	33	38	5	64		0.53
	Unloaded		105	50	24.8	0.35									35			59		
	Unloaded		102	55	28.3	0.40									37			59		
	Unloaded		102	51	26.6	0.38									35			59		
	Unloaded	102/69	106	56	29.9	0.42				7.40	23		227	448	34	38	4	60		0.52
0.5	15		110	54	28.6	0.42									36			57		
1.0	15		111	56	31.7	0.49									34			55		
1.5	30		114	58	32.7	0.49									35			57		
2.0	30	102/60	117	57	36.1	0.63				7.39	21		189	488	37	36	−1	50		0.45
2.5	45		119	59	38.2	0.63									37			53		
3.0	45	108/60	123	64	41.4	0.71				7.39	23		163	512	36	38	2	51		0.48
3.5	60		124	59	42.0	0.82									36			45		
4.0	60		128	60	43.5	0.86									35			45		
4.5	75		131	62	46.2	0.92									36			44		
5.0	75		133	66	48.0	0.98									37			43		
5.5	90		135	69	50.1	1.01									39			44		
6.0	90		136	68	53.3	1.14									38			42		
6.5	105		139	76	61.8	129									37			43		
7.0	105	126/66	142	79	63.9	1.33				7.34	22		157	514	40	42	2	43		0.47
7.5	120		147	83	68.1	1.40									41			44		
8.0	120	132/72	150	87	72.5	1.49				7.32	22		164	506	38	43	5	44		0.49
	Recovery		134	80	63.6	1.31									43			43		
	Recovery		123	75	51.8	1.01									39			45		
	Recovery		117	74	50.3	0.90									37			49		
	Recovery	117/60	119	70	44.8	0.76				7.33	20		185	490	35	38	3	51		0.48

Case 57 Alveolar Proteinosis: Before and After Whole-Lung Lavage

Clinical Findings

This 25-year-old graduate student was found to have alveolar proteinosis, proved by transbronchial lung biopsy, several years previously. He had had whole-lung lavage twice previously, at yearly intervals, with improvement on both occasions. Despite the dyspnea associated with this illness, he was very physically active, running an average of 70 miles per week. He returned because of increasing dyspnea. Examination revealed a thin, muscular man who was not cyanotic. Chest roentgenograms showed bilateral infiltrates typical of alveolar proteinosis.

Exercise Findings

The patient performed exercise on a cycle ergometer with similar protocols before and shortly after separate lavages of the right and left lungs. He pedaled at 60 rpm without added load for 3 minutes. The work rate was then increased 25 or 30 W per minute to his symptom-limited maximum. Arterial blood was sampled every second minute, and intraarterial blood pressure was recorded from a percutaneously placed brachial artery catheter. Resting 12-lead and exercise single-lead ECGs were normal. On both tests, the patient stopped exercise because of leg fatigue.

Interpretation

Comments

Respiratory function studies indicate moderately severe restrictive lung disease that improves after lung lavage (Table 10.57.1). The resting ECG is normal. The postlavage exercise study was done 7 days after completion of whole-lung lavage and 11 days after the prelavage study.

Analysis

Referring to flowchart 1, this patient's peak $\dot{V}O_2$ and anaerobic threshold are substantially greater than predicted because he is so exceptionally well trained. Nevertheless, the rate of rise in $\dot{V}O_2$ decreases above the anaerobic threshold before lavage (panel 3, Fig. 10.57.1). The peak $\dot{V}O_2$, even be-

fore lavage, is significantly above predicted (Table 10.57.2). Referring to flowchart 2, the O_2 pulse is supranormal, and the patient's ECG is normal at peak $\dot{V}O_2$. His blood gases, however, although normal at rest, become abnormal during exercise, with PaO_2 progressively decreasing and $P(A - a)O_2$ progressively increasing with work rate (Table 10.57.3) (branch point 2.1). The V_D/V_T is abnormal (branch point 2.3). At the maximum work rate performed, the patient has a marked tachypnea (Table 10.57.3). The tidal volume remains constant at the level of the inspiratory capacity from a relatively light work

TABLE 10.57.1.   Selected Respiratory Function Data

Measurement	Predicted	Pre-lavage	Post-lavage
Age, yr		25	
Sex		Male	
Height, cm		165	
Weight, kg	70	52	
Hematocrit, %		48	47
VC, L	4.46	2.06	2.98
IC, L	2.98	1.36	1.60
TLC, L	5.93	3.28	4.10
FEV$_1$, L	3.63	1.67	2.44
FEV$_1$/VC, %	81	81	82
MVV, L/min	163	97	121
D$_L$CO, ml/mm Hg/min	29.5	20.0	28.7

TABLE 10.57.2.   Selected Exercise Data

Measurement	Predicted	Pre-lavage	Post-lavage
Peak $\dot{V}O_2$, L/min	2.52	2.70	3.07
Maximum HR, beats/min	195	165	175
Maximum O$_2$ pulse, ml/beat	12.9	16.4	17.5
$\Delta\dot{V}O_2$/ΔWR, ml/min/W	10.3	9.2	9.1
AT, L/min	>1.02	2.1	2.1
Maximum $\dot{V}E$, L/min		125	133
Exercise breathing reserve L/min	>15	−28	−12
PaO$_2$, mmHg (rest, max ex)		82, 53	93, 64
P(A − a)O$_2$, mmHg (rest, max ex)		16, 64	12, 55
P(a − ET)CO$_2$, mmHg (rest, max ex)		−1, 6	−1, −5
VD/VT (rest, heavy ex)		0.20, 0.36	0.25, 0.21
HCO$_3^-$, mEq/L (rest, heavy ex)		26, 21	24, 15

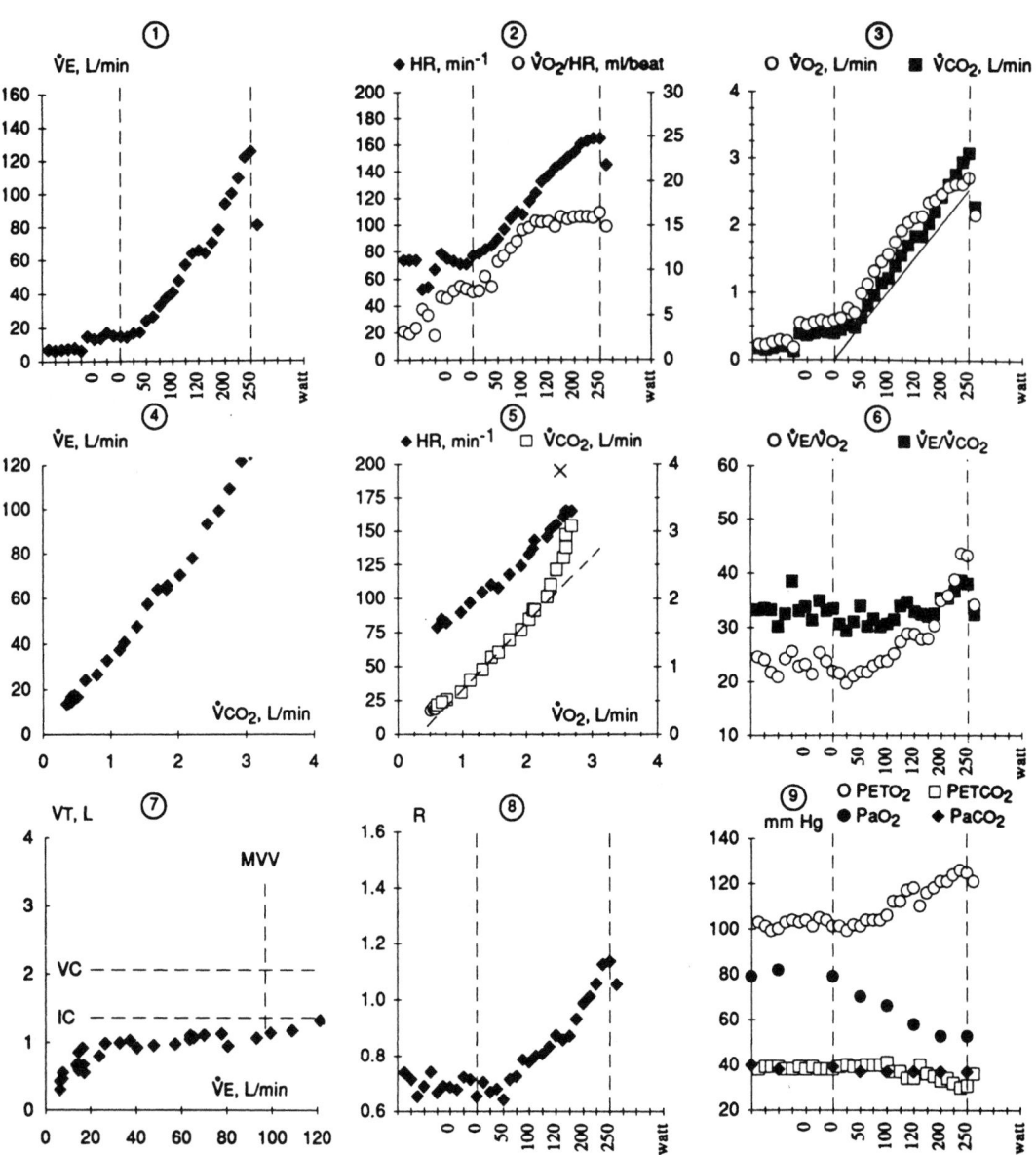

FIGURE 10.57.1.   Before whole-lung lavage. **1:** Vertical dashed lines in panels 1 to 3 and 6, 8, and 9 indicate the beginning and the end of the increasing work period. **2:** Unloaded cycling is performed for 3 minutes before the left vertical dashed line. **3:** In panel 3, the diagonal line shows the increase of $\dot{V}O_2$ at a slope of 10 ml/min/W. **4:** In panel 5, the diagonal dashed line has a slope of 1; the x in the upper right is the predicted maximum heart rate and $\dot{V}O_2$ for the subject.

rate to the maximum (panel 7, Fig. 10.57.1), with the increase in minute ventilation achieved almost solely by increasing breathing frequency. This exercise response is consistent with restrictive lung disease, despite a supranormal peak $\dot{V}O_2$.

Although the patient exceeds the predicted peak $\dot{V}O_2$ for sedentary males of his size, he clearly has physiologic abnormalities that limit his exercise performance, as evidenced by his improved exercise performance following bilateral whole-lung lavage (Table 10.57.2, and contrasting data in Tables 10.57.3 and 10.57.4). Because of the mechanical limitation to lung expansion imposed by the alveolar filling disorder, and perhaps some pulmonary fibrosis, the patient must increase minute ventilation during exercise primarily by increasing breathing rate. The minute ventilation at maximum exercise exceeds his MVV (negative breathing reserve), reflecting his high motivation and possibly some exercise bronchodilatation.

TABLE 10.57.3.   Pre-whole Lung Lavage

Time min	Work rate watts	BP mmHg	HR min⁻¹	f min⁻¹	V̇E L/min BTPS	V̇CO₂ L/min STPD	V̇O₂ L/min STPD	V̇O₂/HR ml/beat	R	pH	HCO₃⁻ meq/L	PO₂, mmHg			PCO₂, mmHg			V̇E/V̇CO₂	V̇E/V̇O₂	VD/VT
												ET	a	(A−a)	ET	a	(a−ET)			
	Rest									7.43	26		79			40				
	Rest		74	16	7.0	0.17	0.23	3.1	0.74			103			38			33	25	
	Rest		74	15	6.3	0.15	0.21	2.8	0.71			101			39			34	24	
	Rest		74	16	7.0	0.17	0.26	3.5	0.65			99			39			33	22	
	Rest		52	16	7.4	0.20	0.29	5.6	0.69	7.44	25	100	82	16	39	38	−1	30	21	0.20
	Rest		54	14	7.7	0.20	0.27	5.0	0.74			103			38			33	24	
	Rest		67	21	6.4	0.12	0.18	2.7	0.67			104			38			38	26	
	Unloaded		79	25	14.7	0.38	0.55	7.0	0.69			103			39			33	23	
	Unloaded		75	20	13.5	0.35	0.51	6.8	0.69			104			38			34	23	
	Unloaded		73	21	13.7	0.38	0.56	7.7	0.68			101			39			31	21	
	Unloaded		71	25	16.8	0.42	0.58	8.2	0.72			105			38			35	25	
	Unloaded		71	23	15.2	0.40	0.56	7.9	0.71			104			38			33	24	
	Unloaded		77	24	14.7	0.38	0.58	7.5	0.66	7.43	25	101	79	16	38	39	1	33	22	0.29
0.5	25		79	17	14.6	0.43	0.61	7.7	0.70			101			39			31	22	
1.0	25		82	18	16.5	0.51	0.76	9.3	0.67			99			40			29	20	
1.5	50		85	31	17.2	0.47	0.69	8.1	0.68			102			39			31	21	
2.0	50		90	30	23.9	0.63	0.98	10.9	0.64	7.43	24	101	70	27	39	37	−2	34	22	0.28
2.5	75		97	27	26.5	0.80	1.12	11.5	0.71			104			40			30	22	
3.0	75		105	33	32.8	0.95	1.31	12.5	0.73			104			40			32	23	
3.5	100		110	36	37.3	1.14	1.45	13.2	0.79			104			40			30	24	
4.0	100		108	44	40.7	1.21	1.56	14.4	0.78	7.44	25	106	66	39	41	37	−4	31	24	0.21
4.5	125		118	50	47.8	1.39	1.74	14.7	0.80			112			37			31	25	
5.0	125		124	59	57.4	1.55	1.92	15.5	0.81			112			37			34	27	
5.5	120		133	61	63.9	1.70	2.04	15.3	0.83			117			34			35	29	
6.0	120		137	61	65.6	1.84	2.11	15.4	0.87	7.43	24	118	58	51	34	37	3	33	29	0.27
6.5	175		143	58	64.1	1.83	2.13	14.9	0.86			110			40			32	28	
7.0	175		146	63	70.2	2.03	2.33	16.0	0.87			116			36			32	28	
7.5	200		151	69	77.8	2.21	2.37	15.7	0.93			118			35			33	30	
8.0	200		155	87	93.3	2.43	2.46	15.9	0.99	7.41	23	121	53	60	33	37	4	35	35	0.31
8.5	225		161	87	99.4	2.60	2.57	16.0	1.01			121			34			35	36	
9.0	225		163	93	108.9	2.76	2.61	16.0	1.06			124			32			37	39	
9.5	250		165	92	121.4	2.94	2.61	15.8	1.13			126			30			39	44	
10.0	250		165	96	124.9	3.07	2.70	16.4	1.14	7.36	21	125	53	64	31	37	6	38	43	0.36
	Recovery		145	85	80.6	2.27	2.15	14.8	1.06			121			36			32	34	

In the second study, the ventilatory pattern of restrictive disease persists but is more mild. The degree of arterial hypoxemia and the increase in $P(A - a)O_2$ are also considerably reduced following whole-lung lavage (compare Table 10.57.3 with Table 10.57.4), whereas the upper portion of the $\dot{V}CO_2$ versus $\dot{V}O_2$ plot is shallower and the O_2 pulse is increased at higher work rates (compare panels 5 and 2 of Figs. 10.57.1 and 10.57.2).

Conclusion

The patient has restrictive lung disease that improved following therapy.

TABLE 10.57.4. Post-whole Lung Lavage

Time min	Work rate watts	BP mmHg	HR min⁻¹	f min⁻¹	$\dot{V}_E$ L/min BTPS	$\dot{V}_{CO_2}$ L/min STPD	$\dot{V}_{O_2}$ L/min STPD	$\dot{V}_{O_2}$/HR ml/beat	R	pH	HCO_3^- meq/L	P_{O_2}, mmHg ET	a	(A − a)	P_{CO_2}, mmHg ET	a	(a − ET)	$\dot{V}_E/\dot{V}_{CO_2}$	$\dot{V}_E/\dot{V}_{O_2}$	V_D/V_T
	Rest									7.40	24		77			39				
	Rest		58	15	9.9	0.28	0.40	6.9	0.70			103			38			31	22	
	Rest		60	17	8.9	0.22	0.29	4.8	0.76			107			36			34	26	
	Rest		65	16	7.0	0.16	0.22	3.4	0.73	7.43	23	106	93	12	36	35	−1	35	26	0.24
	Rest		66	17	4.2	0.04	0.07	1.1	0.57			103			37			69	39	
	Rest		57	14	5.7	0.14	0.20	3.5	0.70			106			36			32	23	
	Rest		55	15	9.7	0.25	0.30	5.5	0.83			108			37			34	28	
	Unloaded		71	26	16.5	0.43	0.57	8.0	0.75			108			36			33	25	
	Unloaded		72	20	15.8	0.44	0.59	8.2	0.75			108			36			32	24	
	Unloaded		73	16	11.0	0.30	0.41	5.6	0.73			102			38			32	24	
	Unloaded		75	12	11.5	0.34	0.55	7.3	0.62			97			38			31	19	
	Unloaded		79	19	13.6	0.37	0.61	7.7	0.61			98			37			32	20	
	Unloaded		75	12	11.8	0.36	0.56	7.5	0.64	7.41	24	99	79	16	38	38	0	30	19	0.22
0.5	30		82	13	14.6	0.48	0.79	9.6	0.61			94			40			28	17	
1.0	30		85	21	16.5	0.50	0.85	10.0	0.59			94			40			29	17	
1.5	60		92	19	20.3	0.68	1.05	11.4	0.65			98			40			27	18	
2.0	60		92	24	20.8	0.64	0.95	10.3	0.67	7.41	23	99	79	20	40	37	−3	29	20	0.18
2.5	90		104	26	24.2	0.74	1.05	10.1	0.70			98			41			30	21	
3.0	90		107	27	29.8	0.97	1.30	12.1	0.75			103			40			28	21	
3.5	120		114	19	29.7	1.06	1.43	12.5	0.74			100			41			26	20	
4.0	120		117	31	40.0	1.30	1.59	13.6	0.82	7.40	23	104	75	31	41	37	−4	29	24	0.18
4.5	150		123	29	42.1	1.43	1.71	13.9	0.84			106			41			28	23	
5.0	150		127	31	43.7	1.48	1.74	13.7	0.85			106			41			28	24	
5.5	180		132	34	48.2	1.61	1.88	14.2	0.86			108			40			28	24	
6.0	180		140	41	56.8	1.81	2.05	14.6	0.88	7.40	23	109	71	38	40	37	−3	29	26	0.20
6.5	210		147	55	71.4	2.06	2.25	15.3	0.92			117			36			32	30	
7.0	210		152	58	75.8	2.18	2.36	15.5	0.92			115			37			33	30	
7.5	240		157	58	80.2	2.32	2.48	15.8	0.94			119			34			32	30	
8.0	240		158	57	81.3	2.36	2.56	16.2	0.92	7.40	21	109	65	49	40	34	−6	32	30	0.20
8.5	270		164	72	100.3	2.73	2.78	17.0	0.98			122			32			34	34	
9.0	270		168	75	113.0	3.04	2.96	17.6	1.03			124			32			35	36	
9.5	300		175	79	120.7	3.10	3.07	17.5	1.01	7.35	16	120	65	55	35	30	−5	37	37	0.21
10.0	300		176	96	132.8	3.17	3.06	17.4	1.04	7.30	15	125	64	55	31	32	1	39	41	0.29
	Recovery		157	84	102.9	2.80	2.50	15.9	1.12			118			40			34	38	
	Recovery		133	83	81.2	1.97	1.37	10.3	1.44			127			36			38	54	

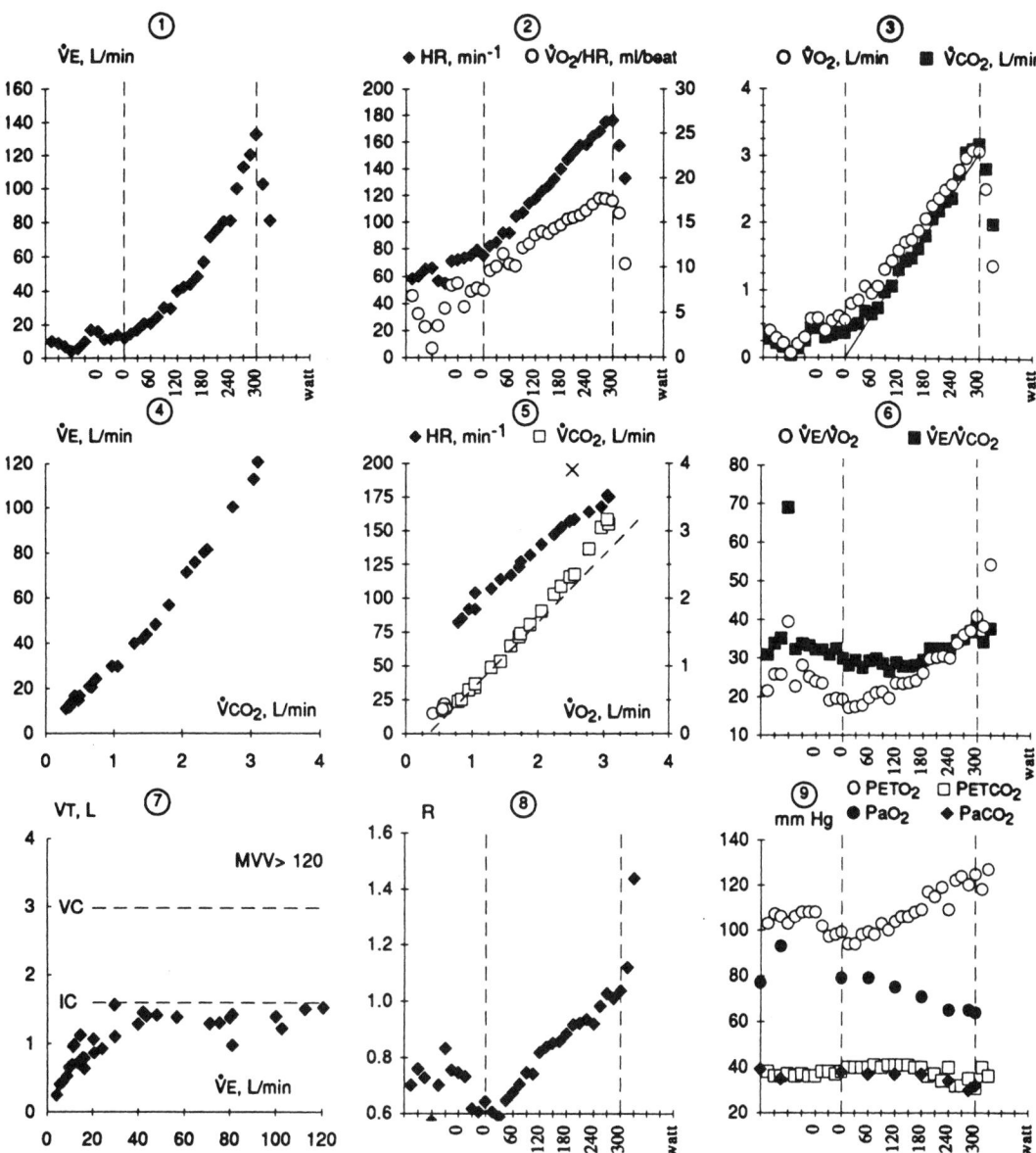

FIGURE 10.57.2.   After whole-lung lavage. **1:** Vertical dashed lines in panels 1 to 3 and 6, 8, and 9 indicate the beginning and the end of the in-creasing work period. **2:** Unloaded cycling is performed for 3 minutes before the left vertical dashed line. **3:** In panel 3, the diagonal line shows the increase of $\dot{V}O_2$ at a slope of 10 ml/min/W. **4:** In panel 5, the diagonal dashed line has a slope of 1; the x in the upper right is the predicted maximum heart rate and $\dot{V}O_2$ for the subject.

Case 58 Pulmonary Microlithiasis: Air and Oxygen Breathing Studies

Clinical Findings

This 63-year-old man had previously been diagnosed by lung biopsy as having pulmonary microlithiasis. He had never smoked. He had had slowly progressive dyspnea over 30 years until he was limited to walking a few steps. He occasionally had hemoptysis. He had been treated with corticosteroids and bronchodilators without apparent benefit. Exercise testing was requested to obtain optimal assessment of his cardiorespiratory function prior to possible therapeutic intervention. Resting ECG showed nonspecific ST-T wave changes.

Exercise Findings

Exercise tests recorded while the patient was breathing room air and then 100% O_2 were performed on the same day on a cycle ergometer, with an intermediate rest period. On both occasions, arterial blood was sampled every second minute, and intraarterial pressure was recorded from a percutaneously placed brachial artery catheter. The patient pedaled at 60 rpm without an added load for 3 minutes. The work rate was then increased 5 W per minute to tolerance. The patient was well motivated and cooperative and stopped exercise on both occasions because of dyspnea. No further ECG abnormalities were noted during or after exercise.

Interpretation

Comments

This case shows the effects of oxygen breathing on exercise capacity and blood gases in a patient severely disabled with interstitial lung disease. Resting respiratory function studies showed severe restrictive disease with low DLCO, severe hypoxemia, and moderate hypercapnia (Table 10.58.1).

Analysis

Referring to flowchart 1, the peak $\dot{V}O_2$ and the anaerobic threshold were reduced in the room air

TABLE 10.58.1.   Selected Respiratory Function Data

Measurement	Predicted	Measured
Age, yr		63
Sex		Male
Height, cm		164
Weight, kg	69	55
Hematocrit, %		51
VC, L	3.36	1.37
IC, L	2.24	0.73
TLC, L	5.28	2.70
FEV$_1$, L	2.61	1.31
FEV$_1$/VC, %	78	92
MVV, L/min		
Direct	117	62
Indirect	104	52
D$_L$CO, ml/mm Hg/min	23.9	6.0

TABLE 10.58.2.   Selected Exercise Data

Measurement	Predicted	Room air	Oxygen
Peak $\dot{V}O_2$, L/min	1.69	0.60	
Maximum HR, beats/min	151	110	138
Maximum O_2 pulse, ml/beat	11.2	5.6	
$\Delta\dot{V}O_2/\Delta WR$, ml/min/W	10.3	10.3	
AT, L/min	>0.75	<0.55	
Work rate, max, W		15	40
Blood pressure, mmHg (rest, max ex)		147/84, 186/87	135/81, 153/99
Maximum $\dot{V}E$, L/min		63	54
Exercise breathing reserve, L/min			
Using direct MVV	>15	−1	8
Using indirect MVV	>15	−11	−2
PaO_2, mmHg (rest, max ex)		40, 34	364, 344
P(A − a)O_2, mmHg (rest, max ex)		48, 88	292, 304
P(a − ET)CO_2, mmHg (rest, max ex)		16, 17	21, 22
VD/VT (rest, max ex)		0.65, 0.64	0.68, 0.71
HCO$_3^-$, mEq/L (rest, recov)		31, 27	29, 28

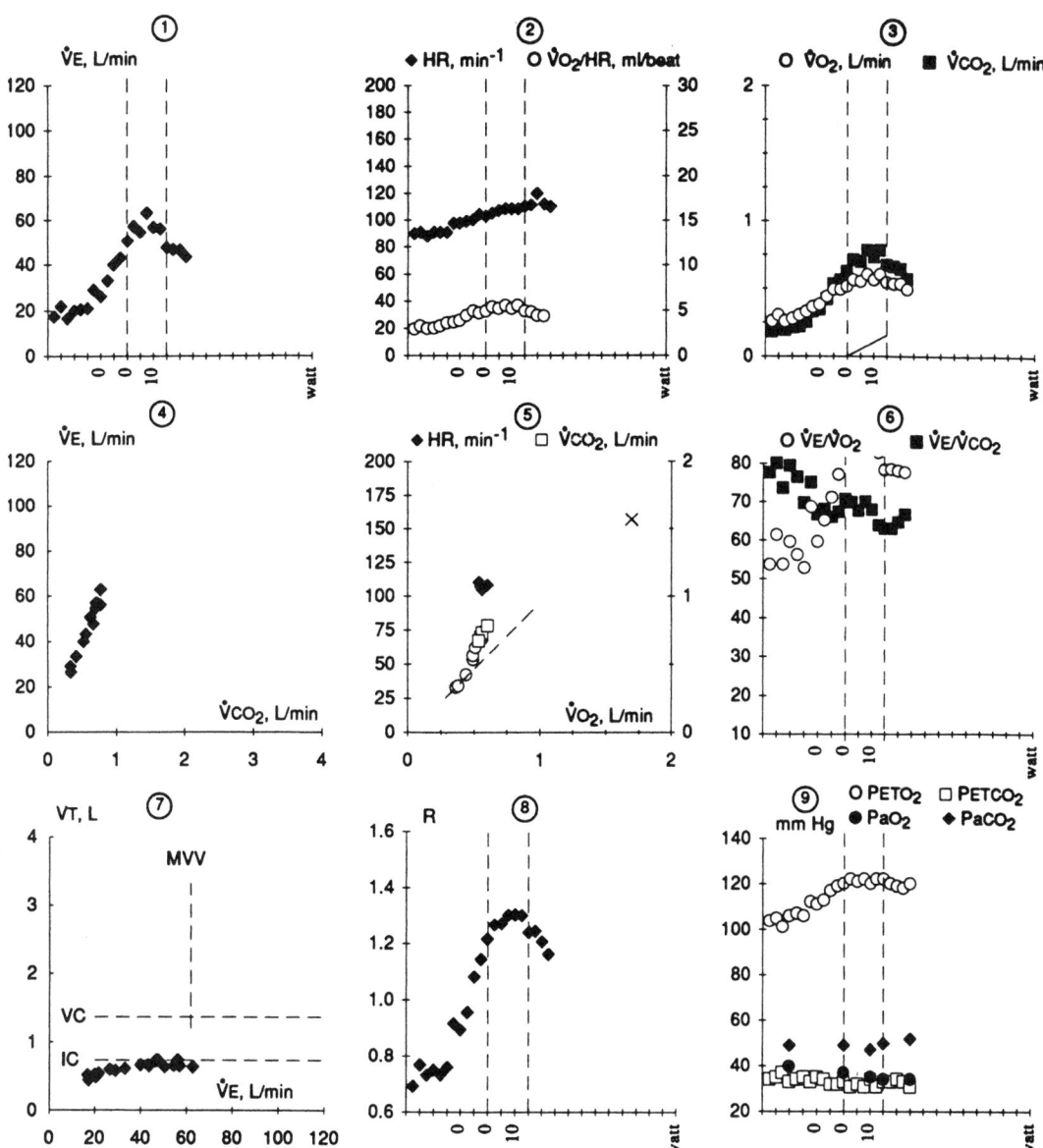

FIGURE 10.58.1.   Air breathing. **1:** Vertical dashed lines in panels 1 to 3 and 6, 8, and 9 indicate the beginning and the end of the increasing work period. **2:** Unloaded cycling is performed for 3 minutes before the left vertical dashed line. **3:** In panel 3, the diagonal line shows the increase of $\dot{V}O_2$ at a slope of 10 ml/min/W. **4:** In panel 5, the diagonal dashed line has a slope of 1; the x in the upper right is the predicted maximum heart rate and $\dot{V}O_2$ for the subject.

study (Table 10.58.2). This leads us through branch points 1.1, 1.2, and 1.3 to flowchart 4. We arrive at the diagnosis of lung disease with impaired peripheral oxygenation through branch point 4.1 (low breathing reserve) and branch point 4.2 (high V_D/V_T). The patient filled all the requirements in both this box and the "abnormal pulmonary circulation" box. With O_2 breathing, a large shunt was not found. The high breathing frequency, negative value for breathing reserve, and high ratio of tidal volume to inspiratory capacity all indicate severe ventila-

tory limitation. The gas exchange abnormalities [hypoxemia, positive $P(a - {\rm ET})CO_2$, and high V_D/V_T] were striking and reflect lung units with abnormally high and abnormally low ventilation–perfusion ratios. With O_2 breathing, exercise capacity was significantly increased as arterial O_2 saturation and content increased. As a consequence of carotid body suppression with O_2, the ventilatory response was decreased compared to air breathing, and a more severe respiratory acidosis developed. In addition, note the extremely low O_2 pulse while the

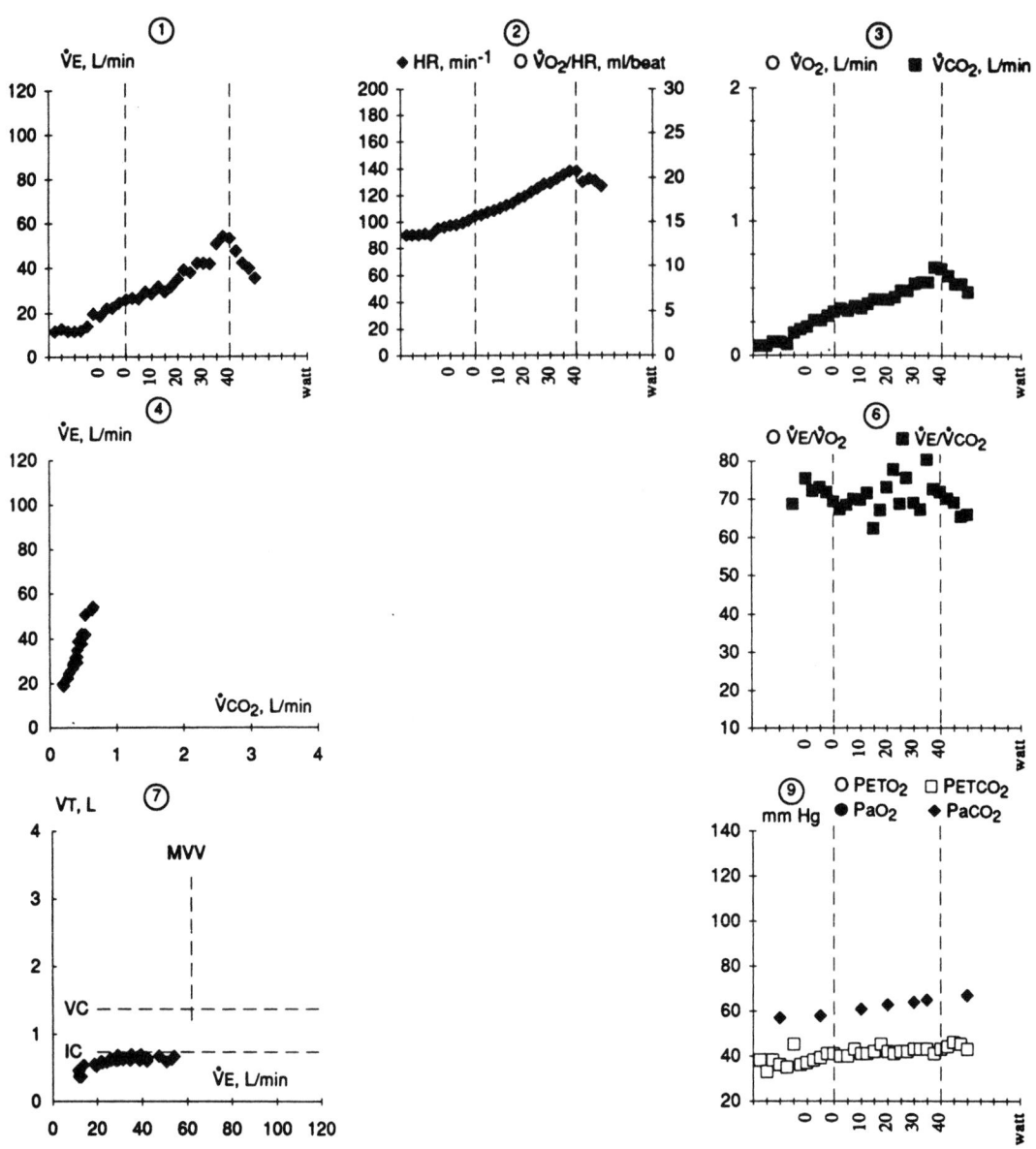

FIGURE 10.58.2.   Oxygen breathing. **1:** Vertical dashed lines in panels 1 to 3 and 6 and 9 indicate the beginning and the end of the increasing work period. **2:** Unloaded cycling is performed for 3 minutes before the left vertical dashed line.

patient was breathing air. Arterial O_2 capacity was 21.3 ml/100 ml, and air breathing O_2 content was approximately 15 ml/100 ml. Thus, a major part of the reduction in O_2 pulse is due to arterial hypoxemia, with some reduction likely due to a low stroke volume.

Conclusion

This patient demonstrates the gas exchange and ventilatory defects of severe interstitial lung disease and demonstrates the improvement in exercise tolerance from O_2 supplementation.

TABLE 10.58.3.   Air Breathing

Time min	Work rate watts	BP mmHg	HR min⁻¹	f min⁻¹	V̇E L/min BTPS	V̇CO₂ L/min STPD	V̇O₂ L/min STPD	V̇O₂/HR ml/beat	R	pH	HCO₃⁻ meq/L	PO₂ ET	PO₂ a	PO₂ (A−a)	PCO₂ ET	PCO₂ a	PCO₂ (a−ET)	V̇E/V̇CO₂	V̇E/V̇O₂	VD/VT
	Rest	147/84	90	39	17.3	0.18	0.26	2.9	0.69			104			34			78	54	
	Rest		91	40	21.8	0.23	0.30	3.3	0.77			105			35			80	61	
	Rest		88	32	16.7	0.19	0.26	3.0	0.73			101			37			74	54	
	Rest	147/84	91	38	19.9	0.21	0.28	3.1	0.75	7.41	31	106	40	48	33	49	16	79	60	0.65
	Rest		91	42	20.4	0.22	0.30	3.3	0.73			107			34			77	56	
	Rest		91	42	21.0	0.25	0.33	3.6	0.76			106			35			70	53	
	Unloaded		98	50	29.0	0.33	0.36	3.7	0.92			112			33			75	69	
	Unloaded		98	44	26.4	0.34	0.38	3.9	0.89			111			35			67	60	
	Unloaded		99	55	33.3	0.42	0.44	4.4	0.95			113			34			68	65	
	Unloaded		100	61	40.1	0.53	0.49	4.9	1.08			117			32			66	71	
	Unloaded		104	65	43.3	0.56	0.49	4.7	1.14			119			32			67	77	
	Unloaded	174/84	103	80	50.6	0.62	0.51	5.0	1.22	7.40	30	120	37	71	33	49	16	71	86	0.65
0.5	5		105	89	57.1	0.71	0.56	5.3	1.27			122			31			70	88	
1.0	5		107	84	54.5	0.70	0.55	5.1	1.27			121			32			68	86	
1.5	10		108	99	63.0	0.78	0.60	5.6	1.30			122			31			70	91	
2.0	10	186/90	108	83	56.7	0.73	0.56	5.2	1.30	7.39	28	120	35	77	34	47	13	68	89	0.64
2.5	15		108	77	56.2	0.78	0.60	5.6	1.30			122			31			64	83	
3.0	15	186/87	110	66	47.8	0.67	0.54	4.9	1.24	7.36	28	122	34	74	33	50	17	63	78	0.64
	Recovery		111	64	47.0	0.66	0.53	4.8	1.25			120			33			63	78	
	Recovery		120	65	46.8	0.64	0.53	4.4	1.21			119			34			64	78	
	Recovery		112	68	43.8	0.57	0.49	4.4	1.16			118			33			67	78	
	Recovery		110							7.33	27	120	34		31	52	21			

TABLE 10.58.4.   Oxygen Breathing

Time min	Work rate watts	BP mmHg	HR min⁻¹	f min⁻¹	V̇E L/min BTPS	V̇CO₂ L/min STPD	V̇O₂ L/min STPD	V̇O₂/HR ml/beat	R	pH	HCO₃⁻ meq/L	PO₂ ET	PO₂ a	PO₂ (A−a)	PCO₂ ET	PCO₂ a	PCO₂ (a−ET)	V̇E/V̇CO₂	V̇E/V̇O₂	VD/VT
	Rest	120/78	90	31	11.6	0.07									38			128		
	Rest		90	35	12.8	0.07									33			140		
	Rest		90	25	11.5	0.10									37			94		
	Rest	135/81	91	26	11.6	0.10				7.32	29		364	292	36	57	21	94		0.68
	Rest		90	31	12.1	0.08									35			118		
	Rest		95	26	13.9	0.17									45			69		
	Unloaded		96	37	19.6	0.19									36			87		
	Unloaded		97	34	18.7	0.21									37			75		
	Unloaded		98	37	21.9	0.26									38			72		
	Unloaded	147/90	99	39	22.3	0.26				7.32	29		437	218	39	58	19	73		0.68
	Unloaded		101	42	24.4	0.29									41			72		
	Unloaded		104	41	25.7	0.32									41			69		
0.5	5		105	43	26.5	0.34									40			67		
1.0	5		107	43	26.2	0.33									40			68		
1.5	10		108	48	29.3	0.36									43			70		
2.0	10	147/90	110	47	28.4	0.35				7.29	29		423	229	41	61	20	70		0.68
2.5	15		112	51	31.5	0.38									41			71		
3.0	15		114	43	29.2	0.41									42			62		
3.5	20		117	49	31.6	0.41									45			67		
4.0	20	141/84	119	57	34.8	0.41				7.28	29		387	263	42	63	21	73		0.70
4.5	25		122	64	38.9	0.43									41			78		
5.0	25		125	58	37.9	0.48									42			69		
5.5	30		128	70	42.2	0.48									42			76		
6.0	30	153/99	129	66	42.1	0.53				7.26	28		361	288	43	64	21	69		0.70
6.5	35		132	64	41.7	0.54									43			67		
7.0	35		135	86	50.7	0.54				7.25	28		344	304	43	65	22	80		0.71
7.5	40		138	81	54.1	0.65									41			73		
8.0	40		138	84	53.1	0.64									43			72		
	Recovery		130	70	47.3	0.59									44			70		
	Recovery		132	65	42.0	0.53									46			69		
	Recovery		131	57	39.4	0.53									45			65		
	Recovery	151/102	127	51	35.2	0.47				7.23	28		380	266	43	67	24	66		0.70

Case 59 Thromboembolic Pulmonary Vascular Disease

Clinical Findings

This 50-year-old shipyard worker had felt well until 1 year prior to evaluation, when he noted the insidious but progressive development of dyspnea and easy fatigability. Six months later, he experienced the abrupt onset of severe substernal chest pain and dyspnea, which resulted in hospitalization and treatment for a suspected myocardial infarction. Following discharge from the hospital, he had lost 25 to 30 pounds by watching his diet but remained somewhat dyspneic. There was no personal or family history of hypertension or diabetes mellitus. He had smoked three to four cigarettes daily until 2 years earlier. Physical examination was normal. Chest roentgenograms showed minimal pleural thickening bilaterally. Resting ECG showed normal QRS complexes and negative T waves in V_1 to V_3, suggesting right ventricular strain.

Exercise Findings

The patient performed exercise on a cycle ergometer. He pedaled at 60 rpm without added load for 3 minutes. The work rate was then increased 15 W per minute. Arterial blood was sampled every second minute, and intraarterial blood pressure was recorded from a percutaneously placed brachial artery catheter. At the 105-W work rate, the pedal came off the cycle ergometer. After 30 minutes rest, the study was restarted with an increase of 20 W every minute. The patient stopped exercise because of overall fatigue and exhaustion; he denied having chest pain or dyspnea. There was a 0.5-mm ST-segment depression in leads II, V_5, and V_6 that disappeared at 3 minutes of recovery.

Interpretation

Comments

This case is presented because it illustrates the use of exercise testing for detecting significant pulmonary vascular disease and correcting an erroneous diagnosis. The patient's physician assumed that symptoms of chest pain, dyspnea, and easy fatigability had been due to a myocardial infarction. That diagnosis could not be supported by myocardial enzyme concentrations or specific ECG changes. Radionuclide ventilation–perfusion scans, ordered because of the exercise study, confirmed the presence of many perfusion defects without ventilation defects, characteristic of pulmonary thromboembolic disease.

The results of the resting respiratory function studies indicate that this patient had normal lung mechanics. He had a significant reduction in diffusing capacity, however (Table 10.59.1). The ECG was suggestive of right ventricular strain.

Analysis

Referring to flowchart 1, the peak $\dot{V}O_2$ is reduced, and the anaerobic threshold is borderline low (Table 10.59.2). Referring to flowchart 4, the breathing reserve is normal, which directs us to branch point 4.3. $\dot{V}E/\dot{V}CO_2$ at the AT is abnormally high (panel 6, Fig. 10.59.1), leading us to the diagnosis of abnor-

TABLE 10.59.1.   Selected Respiratory Function Data

Measurement	Predicted	Measured
Age, yr		50
Sex		Male
Height, cm		185
Weight, kg	86	92
Hematocrit, %		46
VC, L	5.10	4.68
IC, L	3.40	2.94
TLC, L	7.45	5.94
FEV_1, L	4.06	3.62
FEV_1/VC, %	80	77
MVV, L/min	161	152
D_LCO, ml/mm Hg/min	32.3	21.2

TABLE 10.59.2.   Selected Exercise Data

Measurement	Predicted	Measured
Peak $\dot{V}O_2$, L/min	2.78	1.92
Maximum HR, beats/min	170	164
Maximum O_2 pulse, ml/beat	16.4	11.7
$\Delta\dot{V}O_2/\Delta WR$, ml/min/W	10.3	8.9
AT, L/min	>1.25	1.25
Blood pressure, mmHg (rest, max)		125/80, 161/92
Maximum $\dot{V}E$, L/min		104
Exercise breathing reserve, L/min	>15	48
PaO_2, mmHg (rest, max ex)		83, 56
$P(A - a)O_2$, mmHg (rest, max ex)		26, 63
$P(a - ET)CO_2$, mmHg (rest, max ex)		5, 9
VD/VT (rest, heavy ex)		0.40, 0.45
HCO_3^-, mEq/L (rest, 2-min recov)		22, 19

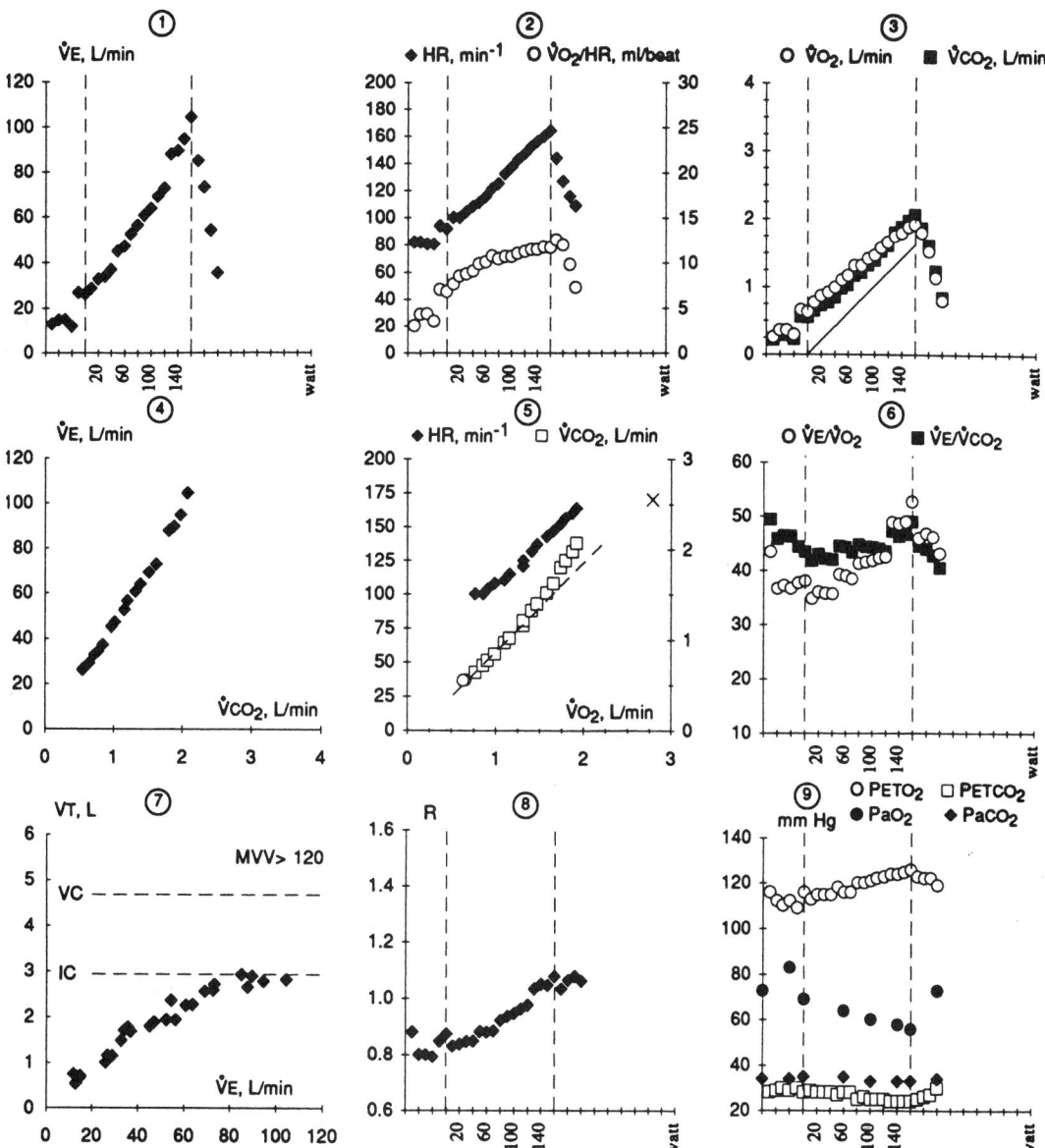

FIGURE 10.59.1.   **1:** Vertical dashed lines in panels 1 to 3 and 6, 8, and 9 indicate the beginning and the end of the increasing work period. **2:** Unloaded cycling is performed for 3 minutes before the left vertical dashed line. **3:** In panel 3, the diagonal line shows the increase of $\dot{V}O_2$ at a slope of 10 ml/min/W. **4:** In panel 5, the diagonal dashed line has a slope of 1; the x in the upper right is the predicted maximum heart rate and $\dot{V}O_2$ for the subject.

mal pulmonary circulation. The vital capacity is normal (branch point 4.5), differentiating the diagnosis of abnormal pulmonary circulatory physiology further to that of pulmonary vascular disease. We confirm this diagnosis with the abnormally high V_D/V_T, $P(A - a)O_2$, $P(a - ET)CO_2$, steep heart rate–$\dot{V}O_2$ relationship, and low, relatively nonchanging O_2 pulse. The patient was not tested with 100% O_2, but the lack of an abrupt decrease in PaO_2 during exercise

suggests that a right-to-left shunt through a potentially patent foramen ovale does not exist.

Conclusion

This patient had pulmonary vascular disease, previously unrecognized, probably of thromboembolic origin. The patient eventually died of thromboembolic disease.

TABLE 10.59.3. Air Breathing

Time min	Work rate watts	BP mmHg	HR min⁻¹	f min⁻¹	$\dot{V}_E$ L/min BTPS	$\dot{V}_{CO_2}$ L/min STPD	$\dot{V}_{O_2}$ L/min STPD	$\dot{V}_{O_2}$/HR ml/beat	R	pH	HCO₃⁻ meq/L	P_{O_2}, mmHg ET	a	(A−a)	P_{CO_2}, mmHg ET	a	(a−ET)	$\dfrac{\dot{V}_E}{\dot{V}_{CO_2}}$	$\dfrac{\dot{V}_E}{\dot{V}_{O_2}}$	$\dfrac{V_D}{V_T}$
	Rest	125/80								7.41	21		73			34				
	Rest		82	24	12.9	0.22	0.25	3.0	0.88			116			28			49	43	
	Rest		82	22	14.7	0.28	0.35	4.3	0.80			112			29			46	37	
	Rest		81	21	14.8	0.28	0.35	4.3	0.80			110			30			46	37	
	Rest	119/83	81	16	12.0	0.23	0.29	3.6	0.79	7.42	22	112	83	26	29	34	5	46	37	0.40
	Unloaded		94	23	26.8	0.56	0.66	7.0	0.85			109			30			44	38	
	Unloaded	140/86	92	26	26.1	0.55	0.63	6.8	0.87	7.42	22	116	69	42	28	35	7	43	38	0.40
0.5	20		100	25	28.9	0.64	0.77	7.7	0.83			113			29			42	35	
1.0	20		100	22	32.8	0.72	0.86	8.6	0.84			115			28			43	36	
1.5	40		104	20	34.2	0.77	0.91	8.8	0.85			115			28			42	36	
2.0	40		108	22	37.1	0.84	0.99	9.2	0.85			115			28			42	36	
2.5	60		111	25	45.2	0.97	1.10	9.9	0.88			118			27			44	39	
3.0	60	146/86	115	25	47.2	1.02	1.16	10.1	0.88	7.42	22	116	64	47	28	35	7	44	39	0.42
3.5	80		121	27	52.5	1.16	1.31	10.8	0.89			116			28			43	38	
4.0	80		125	29	56.5	1.21	1.31	10.5	0.92			120			25			45	41	
4.5	100		132	27	60.8	1.32	1.41	10.7	0.94			120			26			44	41	
5.0	100	155/89	137	28	63.9	1.39	1.47	10.7	0.95	7.43	22	121	60	55	25	33	8	44	42	0.39
5.5	120		143	27	69.1	1.52	1.58	11.0	0.96			122			25			44	42	
6.0	120		147	28	72.8	1.62	1.66	11.3	0.98			123			25			43	42	
6.5	140		152	33	87.8	1.80	1.74	11.4	1.03			124			24			47	49	
7.0	140	161/92	156	31	89.7	1.88	1.79	11.5	1.05	7.40	20	124	58	60	24	33	9	46	49	0.42
7.5	160		160	34	94.8	1.97	1.88	11.8	1.05			125			24			47	49	
8.0	160	155/86	164	37	104.5	2.07	1.92	11.7	1.08	7.40	20	126	56	63	24	33	9	49	53	0.45
	Recovery		144	29	85.2	1.86	1.80	12.5	1.03			123			25			44	46	
	Recovery		127	27	73.4	1.62	1.52	12.0	1.07			122			26			44	47	
	Recovery		116	23	54.5	1.23	1.14	9.8	1.08			122			27			43	46	
	Recovery	152/86	109	20	35.7	0.84	0.72	7.2	1.06	7.37	19	119	73	45	30	34	4	40	43	0.36

Case 60 Pulmonary Vasculitis: Air and Oxygen Breathing Studies

Clinical Findings

This 54-year-old executive had apparently been in good health until 11 years previously, when he had a documented acute myocardial infarction. Coronary arteriogram had been normal 1 year later. Five years ago he developed fatigue, jaundice, Raynaud's phenomenon, renal failure, and peripheral neuropathy with a histologic diagnosis of membranoproliferative glomerulonephritis secondary to vasculitis. Diffuse cerebritis with panhypopituitarism had followed; this had responded well to corticosteroids, cyclophosphamide, and endocrine replacement therapy. Three years ago, progressive exertional dyspnea had begun without cough, pleurisy, or wheezing. A pulmonary nodule had developed and was biopsied. Histologic examination showed an organizing exudate, hemorrhage, and severe arteriolar wall thickening. The patient never smoked or abused drugs or alcohol. Physical examination revealed acrocyanosis without clubbing, clear lungs, and normal heart sounds. Exercise testing was performed to evaluate the possible efficacy of supplemental oxygen.

Exercise Findings

The patient performed exercise tests on the cycle ergometer. On both occasions he pedaled at 60 rpm without added load for 3 minutes. The work rate was then increased 15 W every minute. The first test was done during air breathing, and the second was done while breathing 100% oxygen. Arterial blood was sampled every second minute, and intraarterial blood pressure was recorded from a percutaneously inserted brachial artery catheter.

During air breathing, the patient stopped because of leg fatigue and complained of shortness of breath. While breathing 100% O_2, the patient complained of leg fatigue only. Resting ECG showed a rightward axis, poor R-wave progression in the precordial leads, and T-wave inversion in V_4. There was no ectopy or abnormality of ST segments, although the T-wave inversion increased during exercise.

TABLE 10.60.1. Selected Respiratory Function Data

Measurement	Predicted	Measured
Age, yr		54
Sex		Male
Height, cm		170
Weight, kg	74	64
Hematocrit, %		38
VC, L	4.03	4.07
IC, L	2.68	3.16
FEV$_1$, L	3.18	3.38
FEV$_1$/VC, %	79	83
MVV, L/min	137	143
D$_L$CO, ml/mm Hg/min	26.5	8.0

TABLE 10.60.2. Selected Exercise Data

Measurement	Predicted	Room Air	Oxygen
Maximum work rate, W	160	90	90
Peak V̇O$_2$, L/min	2.11	0.96	
Maximum HR, beats/min	166	132	131
Maximum O$_2$ pulse, ml/beat	12.7	7.3	
ΔV̇O$_2$/ΔWR, ml/min/W	10.3	8.8	
AT, L/min	>0.91	<0.75	
Blood pressure, mmHg (rest, max)		129/69, 204/84	126/75, 201/87
Maximum V̇E, L/min		117	89
Exercise breathing reserve, L/min	>15	26	54
PaO$_2$, mmHg (rest, max ex)		114, 90	692, 678
P(A − a)O$_2$, mmHg (rest, max ex)		10, 41	−8, 4
P(a − ET)CO$_2$, mmHg (rest, max ex)		7, 9	10, 12
VD/VT (rest, heavy ex)		0.44, 0.52	0.52, 0.57
HCO$_3^-$, mEq/L (rest, 2-min recov)		18, 12	18, 15

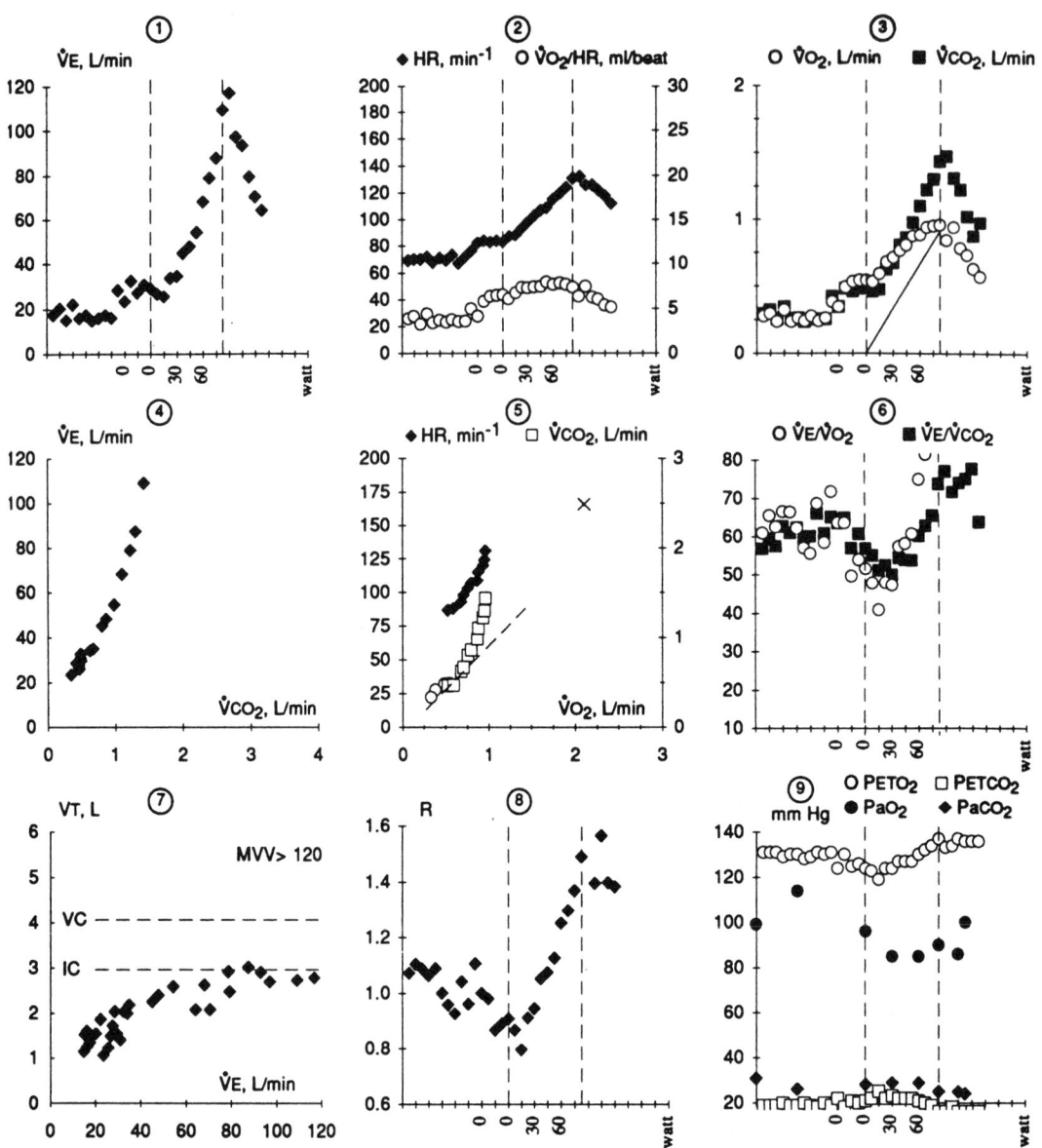

FIGURE 10.60.1.   Air breathing. **1:** Vertical dashed lines in panels 1 to 3 and 6, 8, and 9 indicate the beginning and the end of the increasing work period. **2:** Unloaded cycling is performed for 3 minutes before the left vertical dashed line. **3:** In panel 3, the diagonal line shows the increase of $\dot{V}O_2$ at a slope of 10 ml/min/W. **4:** In panel 5, the diagonal dashed line has a slope of 1; the x in the upper right is the predicted maximum heart rate and $\dot{V}O_2$ for the subject.

Interpretation

Comments

Except for the very low diffusing capacity, the results of this patient's respiratory function studies are normal (Table 10.60.1).

Analysis

Referring to flowchart 1, during air breathing the peak $\dot{V}O_2$ and the anaerobic threshold are significantly reduced (Table 10.60.2). See flowchart 4. The breathing reserve is normal (branch point 4.1). The $\dot{V}E/\dot{V}CO_2$ at the *AT* is significantly increased (Fig. 10.60.1, Table 10.60.3) (branch point 4.3), leading to the diagnosis of abnormal pulmonary circulation. The vital capacity is normal (branch point 4.5), leading to a diagnosis of pulmonary vascular disease as opposed to moderate to severe left ventricular failure. Confirmatory measurements are as follows: high VD/VT, $P(a - ET)CO_2$, and $P(A - a)O_2$ at the maximum work rate; steep heart rate–$\dot{V}O_2$ relationship; low, nonchanging O_2 pulse; and decreasing $\Delta\dot{V}O_2/\Delta WR$ with increasing work rate.

TABLE 10.60.3. Air Breathing

Time min	Work rate watts	BP mmHg	HR min⁻¹	f min⁻¹	$\dot{V}_E$ L/min BTPS	$\dot{V}_{CO_2}$ L/min STPD	$\dot{V}_{O_2}$ L/min STPD	$\dot{V}_{O_2}$/HR ml/beat	R	pH	HCO₃⁻ meq/L	PO₂, mmHg ET	a	(A−a)	PCO₂, mmHg ET	a	(a−ET)	$\dot{V}_E/\dot{V}_{CO_2}$	$\dot{V}_E/\dot{V}_{O_2}$	VD/VT
	Rest	129/69								7.38	18		99			31				
	Rest		69	12	17.5	0.29	0.27	3.9	1.07			131			19			57	61	
	Rest		70	13	20.1	0.32	0.29	4.1	1.10			131			19			59	66	
	Rest		70	10	15.2	0.25	0.23	3.3	1.09			131			19			57	62	
	Rest		72	12	22.3	0.34	0.32	4.4	1.06			129			20			63	67	
	Rest		68	10	16.1	0.25	0.23	3.4	1.09			130			19			61	66	
	Rest	126/69	71	13	17.3	0.26	0.26	3.7	1.00	7.44	17	130	114	10	19	26	7	62	62	0.44
	Rest		69	13	14.8	0.23	0.24	3.5	0.96			128			20			60	57	
	Rest		73	13	16.1	0.25	0.27	3.7	0.93			129			19			60	56	
	Rest		67	13	17.6	0.25	0.24	3.6	1.04			131			18			66	69	
	Rest		72	13	16.3	0.25	0.26	3.6	0.96			130			20			61	58	
	Unloaded		76	14	28.52	0.42	0.38	5.0	1.11			131			19			65	72	
	Unloaded		82	22	23.5	0.34	0.34	4.1	1.00			124			22			64	64	
	Unloaded		84	16	32.5	0.48	0.49	5.8	0.98			130			18			65	64	
	Unloaded		83	16	27.6	0.46	0.53	6.4	0.87			125			21			57	50	
	Unloaded		84	22	31.0	0.48	0.54	6.4	0.89			126			20			61	54	
	Unloaded	147/75	83	19	29.4	0.49	0.54	6.5	0.91	7.41	17	124	96	24	21	28	7	57	51	0.43
0.5	15		87	18	26.8	0.46	0.53	6.1	0.87			123			22			55	48	
1.0	15		88	21	25.8	0.47	0.59	6.7	0.80			119			25			51	41	
1.5	30		93	17	34.0	0.62	0.68	7.3	0.91			124			22			53	48	
2.0	30	156/78	98	16	34.9	0.67	0.71	7.2	0.94	7.39	17	124	85	35	23	29	6	50	47	0.39
2.5	45		103	20	45.2	0.80	0.76	7.4	1.05			127			22			54	57	
3.0	45		107	20	48.1	0.86	0.80	7.5	1.08			127			22			54	58	
3.5	60		109	21	54.5	0.98	0.87	8.0	1.13			127			22			54	61	
4.0	60	183/84	115	26	68.3	1.10	0.88	7.7	1.25	7.38	17	130	85	41	21	29	8	60	75	0.49
4.5	75		120	27	78.9	1.22	0.94	7.8	1.30			132			20			63	81	
5.0	75		124	29	87.6	1.30	0.95	7.7	1.37			134			19			65	90	
5.5	90	204/84	131	40	109.1	1.43	0.96	7.3	1.49	7.38	15	137	90	41	16	25	9	74	110	0.52
	Recovery		132	42	116.9	1.47	0.84	6.4	1.75			133			16			77	135	
	Recovery		126	36	97.1	1.31	0.94	7.5	1.39			134			18			72	100	
	Recovery	198/87	126	32	93.1	1.22	0.78	6.2	1.56	7.37	14	137	86	46	16	25	9	74	116	0.52
	Recovery	192/78	122	32	79.4	1.02	0.73	6.0	1.40	7.33	12	136	100	31	16	24	8	75	105	0.50
	Recovery		118	34	70.6	0.87	0.63	5.3	1.38			136			16			78	107	
	Recovery		112	31	64.4	0.97	0.57	5.1	1.70			136			16			64	108	

PaO₂ decreases during exercise but remains within the normal range (panel 9, Fig. 10.60.1). The high PaO₂ measured during exercise with the patient breathing 100% O₂ confirms the absence of the development of a right-to-left shunt (branch point 4.7). This might be contrasted with Case 61, a patient with pulmonary vascular disease in whom a right-to-left shunt through the foramen ovale did develop during exercise.

100% O₂ breathing had little effect on this patient's exercise performance. This suggests that this patient has little pulmonary vasodilatation in response to high O₂ breathing. Ventilation, however, is considerably reduced with O₂ breathing, demon-strating a suppression of ventilatory drive during exercise. Despite this reduction in ventilation and dyspnea, there was no improvement in exercise performance. This suggests that the patient is not ventilatory limited.

Resting arterial bicarbonate is low, demonstrating a compensated metabolic acidosis at rest. The metabolic acidosis worsens with exercise (Table 10.60.2).

Conclusion

Severe pulmonary vascular disease has limited this patient's exercise performance.

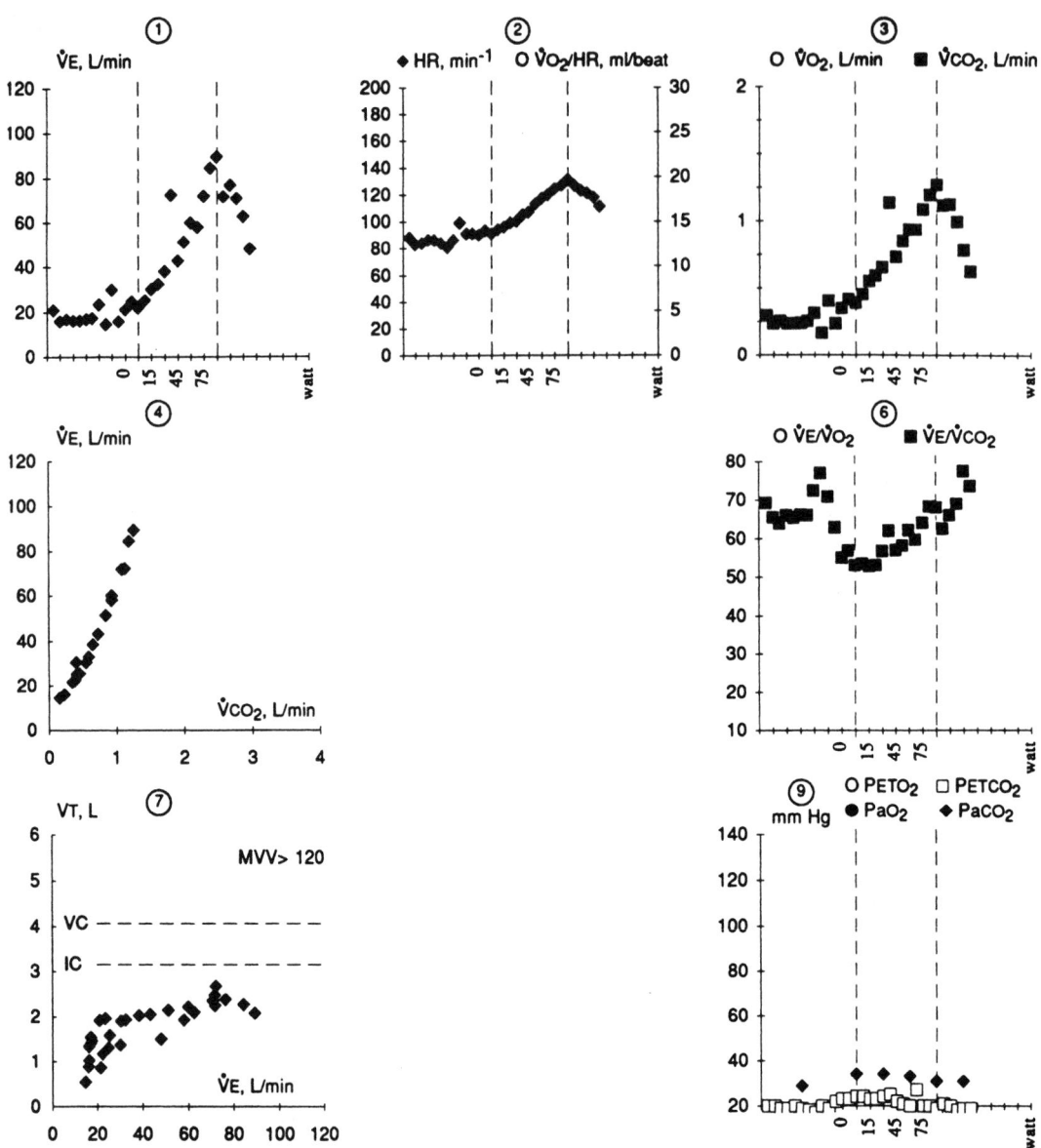

FIGURE 10.60.2.   Oxygen breathing. **1:** Vertical dashed lines in panels 1 to 3 and 6 and 9 indicate the beginning and the end of the increasing work period. **2:** Unloaded cycling is performed for 3 minutes before the left vertical dashed line.

TABLE 10.60.4.   Oxygen Breathing

Time min	Work rate watts	BP mmHg	HR min⁻¹	f min⁻¹	$\dot{V}_E$ L/min BTPS	$\dot{V}_{CO_2}$ L/min STPD	$\dot{V}_{O_2}$ L/min STPD	$\dfrac{\dot{V}_{O_2}}{HR}$ ml/beat	R	pH	HCO_3^- meq/L	P_{O_2}, mmHg ET	a	(A − a)	P_{CO_2}, mmHg ET	a	(a − ET)	$\dfrac{\dot{V}_E}{\dot{V}_{CO_2}}$	$\dfrac{\dot{V}_E}{\dot{V}_{O_2}}$	$\dfrac{V_D}{V_T}$
	Rest		88	11	21.0	0.29									20			69		
	Rest		83	12	16.1	0.23									20			66		
	Rest		84	11	16.9	0.25									19			64		
	Rest		86	12	16.2	0.23									19			66		
	Rest		86	16	16.4	0.23									20			65		
	Rest	120/72	84	12	16.9	0.24				7.40	18		692	−8	19	29	10	66		0.52
	Rest		81	12	17.5	0.25									18			66		
	Rest		86	12	23.5	0.31									17			73		
	Unloaded		99	27	14.6	0.16									20			77		
	Unloaded		91	22	30.2	0.40									19			71		
	Unloaded		91	18	16.0	0.23									22			63		
	Unloaded		90	25	21.4	0.35									23			55		
	Unloaded		93	19	24.9	0.41									23			57		
	Unloaded	132/72	91	19	22.3	0.39				7.36	19		678	1	24	34	10	53		0.48
0.5	15		94	16	25.4	0.45									24			53		
1.0	15		96	16	30.4	0.55									23			53		
1.5	30		99	17	32.7	0.59									23			53		
2.0	30	156/75	100	19	38.4	0.65				7.35	18		645	34	24	34	10	57		0.53
2.5	45		105	27	72.3	1.13									25			62		
3.0	45		107	21	43.3	0.73									22			57		
3.5	60		113	24	51.4	0.85									21			58		
4.0	60	189/81	117	27	60.1	0.93				7.35	18		683	−3	20	33	13	62		0.56
4.5	75		120	30	58.1	0.93									27			60		
5.0	75		124	32	72.0	1.08									20			64		
5.5	90		127	37	84.3	1.19									20			68		
6.0	90	201/87	131	43	89.4	1.26				7.34	16		678	4	19	31	12	68		0.57
	Recovery		127	29	71.7	1.11									21			62		
	Recovery		123	32	76.5	1.12									20			66		
	Recovery		121	30	70.8	0.99									18			69		
	Recovery	186/78	118	30	62.9	0.78				7.31	15		682	0	19	31	21	77		0.61
	Recovery		111	32	48.3	0.62									19			74		

Case 61 Pulmonary Hypertension with Patent Foramen Ovale

Clinical Findings

This 61-year-old woman had first noted mild exertional dyspnea 3 years prior to evaluation. Four months prior to evaluation she had "caught the flu" and soon thereafter developed recurring episodes of depression and confusion. Medical evaluation revealed hypoxemia. With oxygen therapy, her mental status returned to normal. She also admitted to squeezing substernal chest pain, usually associated with exercise, but this symptom was not prominent. There was no history of cigarette smoking, exposure to environmental toxins, pulmonary emboli, or thrombophlebitis. She was given alprazolam for her mental symptoms and propranolol for systemic hypertension. On referral, examination revealed mild obesity, hypertension, and a prominent S_4 heart sound. Chest roentgenogram showed enlarged pulmonary arteries. Resting ECG revealed right axis deviation, an R much greater than S in V_1, and negative T waves in leads V_1 to V_4.

Exercise Findings

The patient performed exercise on a cycle ergometer. She pedaled at 60 rpm without added load for 3 minutes. The work rate was then increased 5 W per minute to her symptom-limited maximum. Arterial blood was sampled every second minute, and intraarterial blood pressure was recorded from a percutaneously placed brachial artery catheter. She stopped exercise because of shortness of breath. There were no arrhythmias, ST-segment changes,

or T-wave changes with exercise. Following a rest period of 30 minutes, the exercise study was repeated while the patient was breathing 100% oxygen.

Interpretation

Comments

The results of this patient's resting respiratory function tests show mild airway obstruction (Table 10.61.1). The ECG is compatible with right ventricular hypertrophy. The exercise test was repeated with the subject breathing 100% oxygen to evaluate the possible development of a right-to-left shunt through a foramen ovale when exercise-induced right atrial pressure exceeds left atrial pressure—a possible cause of activity-induced hypoxemia, which might contribute to this patient's symptoms.

TABLE 10.61.1.   Selected Respiratory Function Data

Measurement	Predicted	Measured
Age, yr		61
Sex		Female
Height, cm		147
Weight, kg	53	61
Hematocrit, %		37
VC, L	2.33	2.31
IC, L	1.56	1.59
TLC, L	3.66	4.53
FEV_1, L	1.90	1.59
FEV_1/VC, %	81	69
MVV, L/min	73	59
D_LCO, ml/mm Hg/min	17.6	17.3

TABLE 10.61.2.   Selected Exercise Data

Measurement	Predicted	Room Air	Oxygen
Maximum work rate, W		20	25
Peak $\dot{V}O_2$, L/min	1.23	0.62	
Maximum HR, beats/min	159	87	85
Maximum O_2 pulse, ml/beat	7.8	7.1	
AT, L/min	>0.61	Indeterminate	
Blood pressure, mmHg (rest, max)		186/90, 204/90	172/84, 210/102
Maximum $\dot{V}E$, L/min		38	42
Exercise breathing reserve, L/min	>15	21	17
PaO_2, mmHg (rest, max ex)		71, 40	550, 70
$P(A - a)O_2$, mmHg (rest, max ex)		42, 79	138, 612
$P(a - ET)CO_2$, mmHg (rest, max ex)		5, 12	4, 9
VD/VT (rest, heavy ex)		0.31, 0.47	0.34, 0.47
HCO_3^-, mEq/L (rest, 2-min recov)		22, 20	22, 18

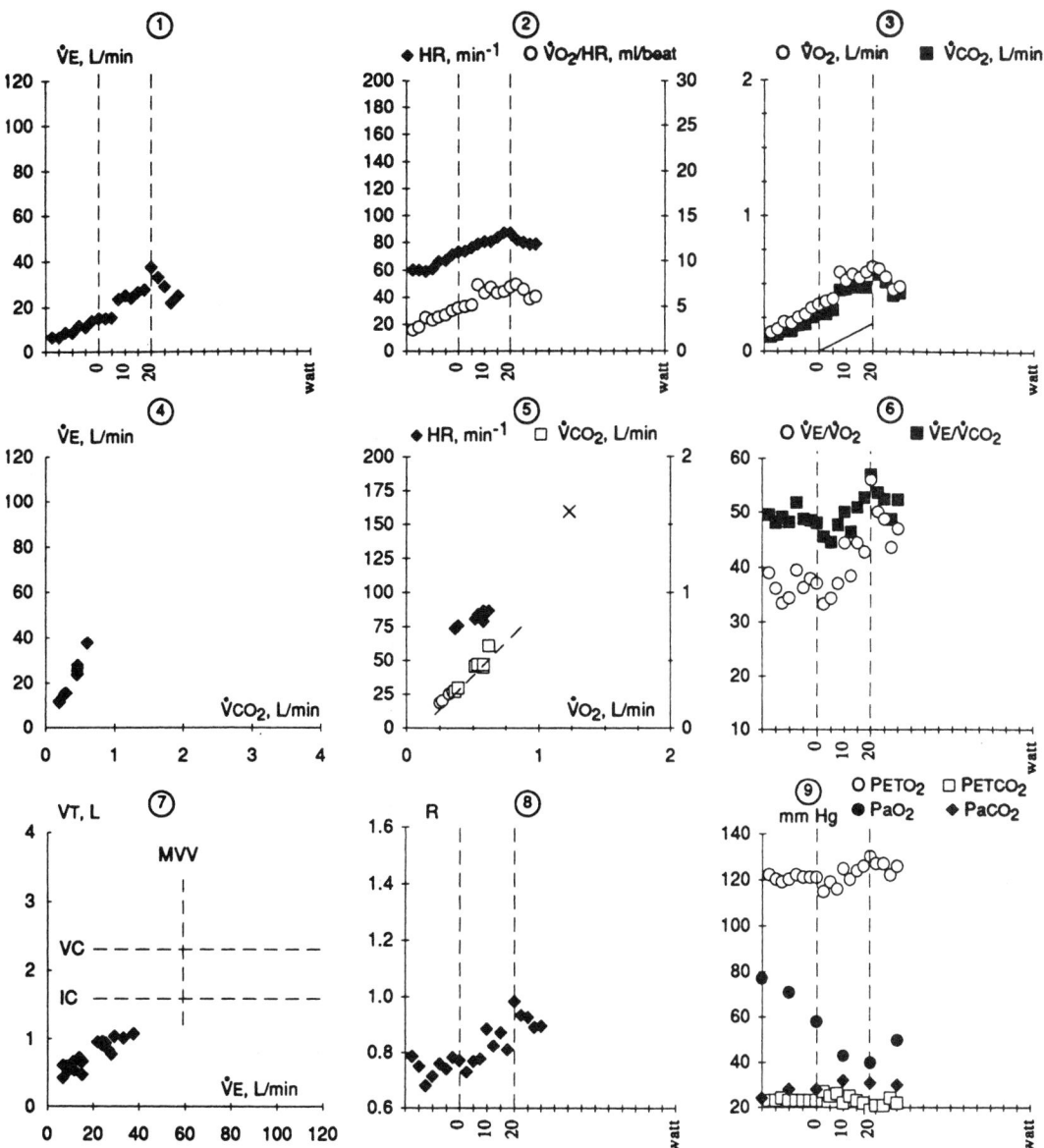

FIGURE 10.61.1.   Air breathing. **1:** Vertical dashed lines in panels 1 to 3 and 6, 8, and 9 indicate the beginning and the end of the increasing work period. **2:** Unloaded cycling is performed for 3 minutes before the left vertical dashed line. **3:** In panel 3, the diagonal line shows the increase of $\dot{V}O_2$ at a slope of 10 ml/min/W. **4:** In panel 5, the diagonal dashed line has a slope of 1; the x in the upper right is the predicted maximum heart rate and $\dot{V}O_2$ for the subject.

Analysis

Referring to flowchart 1, the peak oxygen uptake is reduced and the anaerobic threshold is indeterminate, but probably low (Table 10.61.2). Referring to flowchart 4, the breathing reserve is normal (branch point 4.1). The $\dot{V}E/\dot{V}CO_2$ during exercise is high (branch point 4.3), supporting the diagnosis of abnormal pulmonary circulation. The patient is hyperventilating, however, and the arterial PCO_2 must be taken into account so that true VD/VT is calculated. The latter is increased. Branch point 4.5 further distinguishes between abnormal pulmo-

nary circulation due to moderate to severe left ventricular failure and that due to pulmonary vascular disease, in that the vital capacity is normal. All confirmatory abnormalities are present, supporting the diagnosis of pulmonary vascular disease.

At the lowest work rate, PaO_2 abruptly decreases and continues to decrease as the work rate is increased. Moreover, $P(a - ET)CO_2$ continues to increase as work rate is increased, and the VD/VT become progressively more abnormal as work rate is increased (Tables 10.61.3 and 10.61.4). The changes in PaO_2, $PaCO_2$ and VD/VT suggest the development of a right-to-left shunt during exercise. Clearly, the

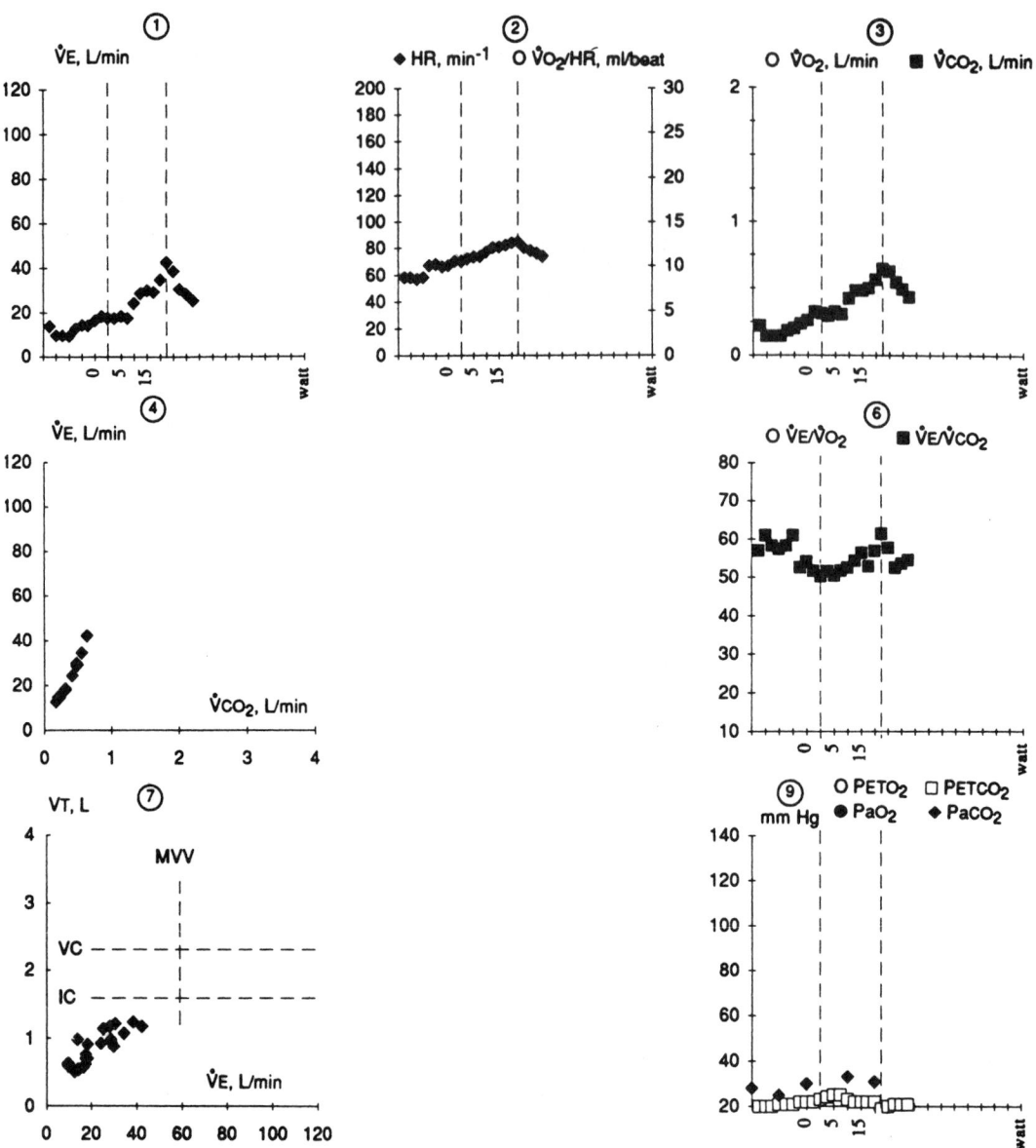

FIGURE 10.61.2.   Oxygen breathing. **1:** Vertical dashed lines in panels 1 to 3 and 6 and 9 indicate the beginning and the end of the increasing work period. **2:** Unloaded cycling is performed for 3 minutes before the left vertical dashed line.

patient is also oxygen flow limited in that $\dot{V}O_2$ and oxygen pulse fail to increase with increasing work rate (panels 3 and 2, respectively, Fig. 10.61.1).

To document that a right-to-left shunt develops with exercise, P_{AO_2} was measured at rest and during exercise while the patient was breathing 100% oxygen. At rest, P_{AO_2} is at the lower limits of normal (550 mm Hg); with mild exercise, it drops to 70 mm Hg. This can only be explained by the development of a right-to-left shunt with exercise (contrast with Case 60).

Subsequently, the patient had right heart catheterization. Pulmonary artery pressures were confirmed to be at systemic pressure levels; the cathe-

ter slipped easily through a foramen ovale into the left atrium.

Conclusion

After a diagnosis of pulmonary vascular occlusive disease with exercise-induced right-to-left shunt through a patent foramen ovale was made by the physicians who did the exercise studies, the patient had right heart catheterization. She was then diagnosed by the cardiologist who did the catheterization study as having "primary pulmonary hypertension with patent foramen ovale through which the catheter easily passed from right to left atrium."

TABLE 10.61.3. Air Breathing

Time min	Work rate watts	BP mmHg	HR min⁻¹	f min⁻¹	$\dot{V}_E$ L/min BTPS	$\dot{V}_{CO_2}$ L/min STPD	$\dot{V}_{O_2}$ L/min STPD	$\dot{V}_{O_2}$/HR ml/beat	R	pH	HCO_3^- meq/L	P_{O_2} ET	a	(A−a)	P_{CO_2} ET	a	(a−ET)	$\dot{V}_E/\dot{V}_{CO_2}$	$\dot{V}_E/\dot{V}_{O_2}$	V_D/V_T
	Rest	186/90								7.56	21		77			24				
	Rest		60	16	6.8	0.11	0.14	2.3	0.79			122			23			49	39	
	Rest		60	11	6.7	0.12	0.16	2.7	0.75			120			23			48	36	
	Rest		59	17	8.8	0.15	0.22	3.7	0.68			119			24			49	33	
	Rest	206/114	61	14	8.4	0.15	0.21	3.4	0.71	7.52	22	120	71	42	23	28	5	48	34	0.31
	Unloaded		66	22	11.7	0.19	0.25	3.8	0.76			122			23			52	39	
	Unloaded		67	17	11.2	0.20	0.27	4.0	0.74			121			23			49	36	
	Unloaded		71	19	13.7	0.25	0.32	4.5	0.78			121			23			48	38	
	Unloaded	191/94	73	23	14.9	0.27	0.35	4.8	0.77	7.50	21	121	58	57	23	28	5	48	37	0.31
0.5	5		74	32	15.0	0.27	0.37	5.0	0.73			115			27			45	33	
1.0	5		76	23	15.3	0.30	0.39	5.1	0.77			119			25			44	34	
1.5	10		79	26	23.6	0.45	0.58	7.3	0.78			116			26			48	37	
2.0	10	202/96	81	27	25.3	0.46	0.52	6.4	0.88	7.47	23	125	43	72	22	32	10	50	44	0.42
2.5	15		81	25	23.9	0.47	0.57	7.0	0.82			120			25			46	38	
3.0	15		84	32	26.6	0.47	0.54	6.4	0.87			124			23			51	44	
3.5	20		87	36	27.8	0.47	0.58	6.7	0.81			126			22			53	43	
4.0	20	204/90	87	35	37.7	0.61	0.62	7.1	0.98	7.45	21	130	40	79	19	31	12	57	56	0.47
	Recovery		82	33	33.3	0.57	0.61	7.4	0.93			127			21			54	50	
	Recovery		80	28	29.1	0.51	0.55	6.9	0.93			127			21			52	49	
	Recovery		79	23	21.9	0.41	0.46	5.8	0.89			122			24			49	43	
	Recovery	198/87	79	27	24.8	0.43	0.48	6.1	0.90	7.45	20	126	50	67	22	30	8	52	47	0.41

TABLE 10.61.4. Oxygen Breathing

Time min	Work rate watts	BP mmHg	HR min⁻¹	f min⁻¹	$\dot{V}_E$ L/min BTPS	$\dot{V}_{CO_2}$ L/min STPD	$\dot{V}_{O_2}$ L/min STPD	$\dot{V}_{O_2}$/HR ml/beat	R	pH	HCO_3^- meq/L	P_{O_2} ET	a	(A−a)	P_{CO_2} ET	a	(a−ET)	$\dot{V}_E/\dot{V}_{CO_2}$	$\dot{V}_E/\dot{V}_{O_2}$	V_D/V_T
	Rest	171/78								7.50	21		67			28				
	Rest		58	14	13.7	0.22									20			57		
	Rest		58	16	9.9	0.14									20			61		
	Rest		57	16	9.5	0.14									20			58		
	Rest	172/84	58	15	9.3	0.14				7.53	21		550	138	21	25	4	57		0.34
	Unloaded		67	25	12.6	0.18									21			58		
	Unloaded		68	27	14.5	0.20									21			61		
	Unloaded		66	26	14.3	0.23									22			53		
	Unloaded	180/87	67	29	16.5	0.26				7.48	22		386	297	22	30	8	54		0.40
	Unloaded		70	20	18.2	0.32									22			52		
	Unloaded		70	23	17.5	0.31									23			50		
0.5	5		72	28	17.3	0.29									24			51		
1.0	5		73	26	18.3	0.32									25			50		
1.5	10		74	25	17.6	0.30									25			52		
2.0	10	180/84	77	26	24.2	0.42				7.44	22		100	580	23	33	10	52		0.45
2.5	15		80	29	28.5	0.48									22			54		
3.0	15		81	34	29.9	0.48									22			56		
3.5	20		82	31	29.0	0.50									22			53		
4.0	20	210/102	84	32	34.5	0.56				7.45	21		70	612	22	31	9	57		0.47
4.5	25		85	36	42.3	0.64									19			61		
	Recovery		80	31	38.4	0.62									20			58		
	Recovery		78	25	30.5	0.54									21			53		
	Recovery		76	24	28.2	0.49									21			53		
	Recovery	198/92	74	22	25.2	0.43									21			54		

Case 62 Left Ventricular Failure with Accompanying Lung Function Changes

Clinical Findings

This 66-year-old shipyard worker stated that he was in excellent health. Two weeks prior to evaluation he experienced an episode of severe shortness of breath, awakening him from his sleep at a Colorado camp site at an altitude of 11,000 feet. He had driven there from Los Angeles in the previous 24 hours. He experienced no relief until he was driven down to an altitude of 7,000 feet. He had a 40 pack-year history of cigarette smoking with a nonproductive cough. He denied other symptoms. The physical examination was normal except for mild obesity. Chest roentgenograms revealed moderate nodular pleural plaques with evidence of minimal pulmonary fibrosis. Resting ECG showed left anterior superior hemiblock.

Exercise Findings

The patient performed exercise on a cycle ergometer. He pedaled at 60 rpm without added load for 3 minutes. The work rate was then increased 20 W per minute to his symptom-limited maximum. Arterial blood was sampled every second minute, and intraarterial blood pressure was recorded from a percutaneously placed brachial artery catheter. The patient stopped exercising because of leg fatigue and shortness of breath. Exercise ECG tracings were normal except for the appearance of infrequent premature ventricular contractions during the last two work rates.

Interpretation

Comments

Results of the resting respiratory function studies show the vital capacity to be at the low end of the normal range (Table 10.62.1). The resting ECG is abnormal, as noted previously in "Clinical Findings."

Analysis

Referring to flowchart 1, the peak $\dot{V}O_2$ is reduced and the anaerobic threshold is normal (Table 10.62.2). See flowchart 3. The breathing reserve is normal (branch point 3.1), and infrequent ventricular premature contractions appear during late exercise (branch point 3.3). This gives preference to the

diagnostic box labeled "myocardial ischemia," rather than "poor effort," especially because the reduced $\Delta\dot{V}O_2/\Delta WR$ strongly suggests a circulatory limitation. Because the low $\Delta\dot{V}O_2/\Delta WR$ is somewhat incompatible with a normal AT, perhaps this analysis should be performed using flowchart 4.

Because the breathing reserve is normal (branch point 4.1) and the $\dot{V}E/\dot{V}CO_2$ at the AT and the VD/VT are high (branch point 4.3), there is an abnormal pulmonary circulation. If we interpret the borderline reduced vital capacity as being low (branch point 4.5), this leads us to moderate to severe left ventricular failure. This is supported by the increase in $P(a - ET)CO_2$ while $P(A - a)O_2$ remains normal at the maximum work rate, a flattening of the O_2 pulse and $\dot{V}O_2$ as the maximum work rate is approached, and a reduced maximal O_2 pulse. The abnormalities in gas exchange at the lung are most

TABLE 10.62.1. Selected Respiratory Function Data

Measurement	Predicted	Measured
Age, yr		66
Sex		Male
Height, cm		178
Weight, kg	80	84
Hematocrit, %		41
VC, L	4.18	3.48
IC, L	2.79	2.96
TLC, L	6.56	5.95
FEV_1, L	3.26	2.76
FEV_1/VC, %	78	79
MVV, L/min	132	93
D_LCO, ml/mm Hg/min	25.6	22.7

TABLE 10.62.2. Selected Exercise Data

Measurement	Predicted	Measured
Peak $\dot{V}O_2$, L/min	2.12	1.58
Maximum HR, beats/min	154	141
Maximum O_2 pulse, ml/beat	13.7	11.6
$\Delta\dot{V}O_2/\Delta WR$, ml/min/W	10.3	7.7
AT, L/min	>0.95	1.1
Blood pressure, mmHg (rest, max)		167/86, 241/104
Maximum $\dot{V}E$, L/min		70
Exercise breathing reserve, L/min	>15	23
PaO_2, mmHg (rest, max ex)		87, 90
$P(A - a)O_2$, mmHg (rest, max ex)		19, 23
$P(a - ET)CO_2$, mmHg (rest, max ex)		−2, 3
VD/VT (rest, heavy ex)		0.38, 0.33
HCO_3^-, mEq/L (rest, 2-min recov)		24, 17

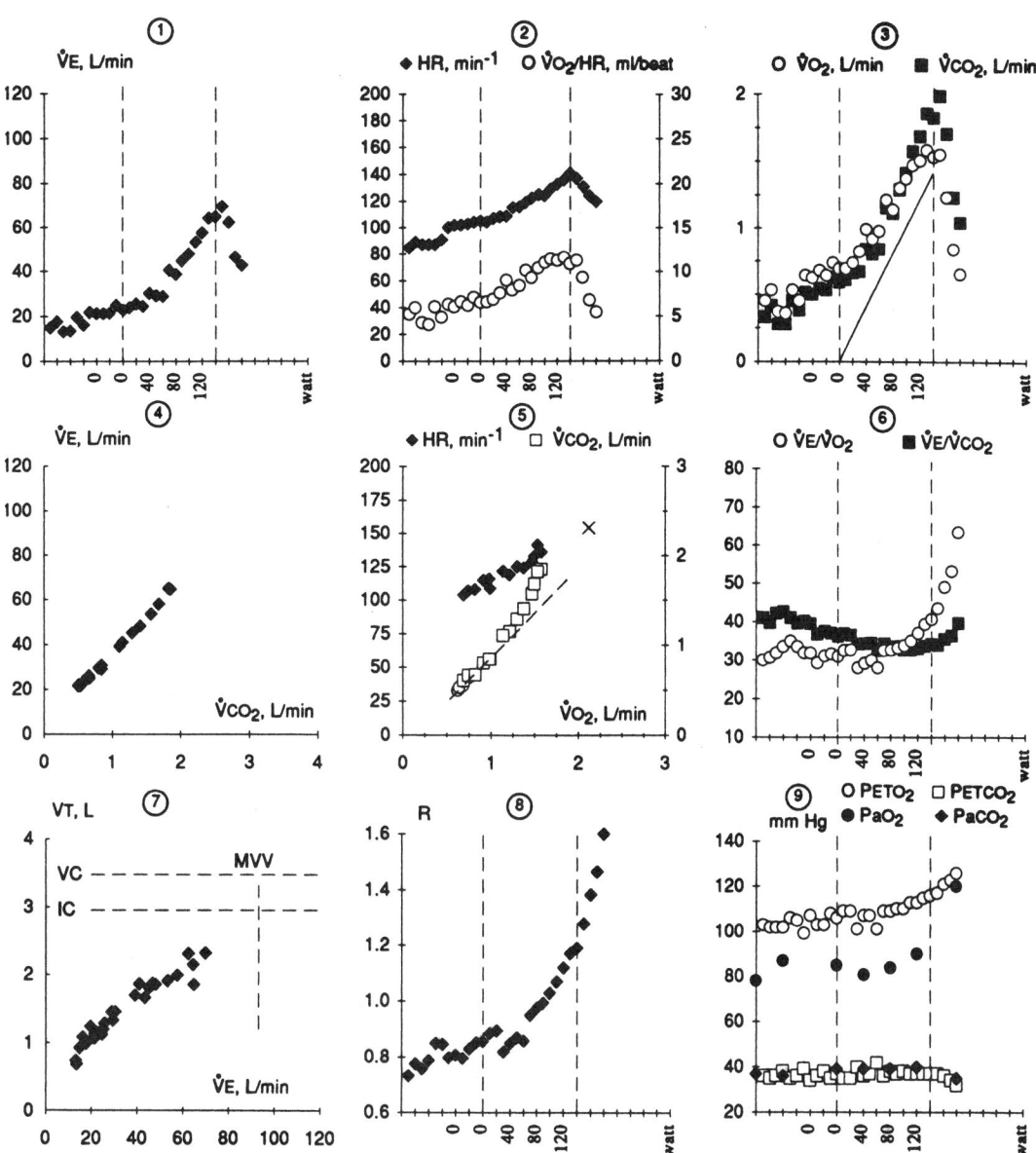

FIGURE 10.62.1.   **1:** Vertical dashed lines in panels 1 to 3 and 6, 8, and 9 indicate the beginning and the end of the increasing work period. **2:** Unloaded cycling is performed for 3 minutes before the left vertical dashed line. **3:** In panel 3, the diagonal line shows the increase of $\dot{V}_{O_2}$ at a slope of 10 ml/min/W. **4:** In panel 5, the diagonal dashed line has a slope of 1; the x in the upper right is the predicted maximum heart rate and $\dot{V}_{O_2}$ for the subject.

compatible with those found with left ventricular failure with disturbances in the pulmonary circulation, which commonly accompany this disorder when it is moderate to severe. The ECG changes are compatible with this diagnosis. Systemic arterial hypertension could be contributory to the cardiac failure or a response to it.

Conclusion

This patient has left ventricular failure with the abnormal changes in the pulmonary circulation that accompany this disease when it becomes moderate to severe, and systemic arterial hypertension.

TABLE 10.62.3.   Air Breathing

Time min	Work rate watts	BP mmHg	HR min⁻¹	f min⁻¹	$\dot{V}_E$ L/min BTPS	$\dot{V}_{CO_2}$ L/min STPD	$\dot{V}_{O_2}$ L/min STPD	$\dfrac{\dot{V}_{O_2}}{HR}$ ml/beat	R	pH	HCO₃⁻ meq/L	P_{O_2} ET	P_{O_2} a	P_{O_2} (A−a)	P_{CO_2} ET	P_{CO_2} a	P_{CO_2} (a−ET)	$\dfrac{\dot{V}_E}{\dot{V}_{CO_2}}$	$\dfrac{\dot{V}_E}{\dot{V}_{O_2}}$	$\dfrac{V_D}{V_T}$
	Rest	167/86								7.42	24		78			37				
	Rest		85	16	14.9	0.33	0.45	5.3	0.73			103			36			41	30	
	Rest		89	18	17.8	0.41	0.53	6.0	0.77			102			35			40	31	
	Rest		87	18	13.3	0.28	0.37	4.3	0.76			102			36			42	32	
	Rest	161/89	87	20	13.6	0.28	0.36	4.1	0.79	7.41	22	102	87	19	38	36	−2	43	33	0.38
	Rest		87	16	19.8	0.45	0.53	6.1	0.85			106			35			41	35	
	Rest		91	15	16.3	0.38	0.45	4.9	0.84			105			36			40	33	
	Unloaded		100	19	22.0	0.51	0.64	6.4	0.80			99			39			40	32	
	Unloaded		102	20	21.4	0.50	0.62	6.1	0.81			107			34			39	32	
	Unloaded		102	19	21.4	0.54	0.68	6.7	0.79			103			36			37	29	
	Unloaded		103	20	21.5	0.53	0.64	6.2	0.83			103			38			37	31	
	Unloaded		104	21	25.1	0.63	0.74	7.1	0.85			108			35			37	32	
	Unloaded	191/95	105	20	23.0	0.59	0.69	6.6	0.86	7.39	23	106	85	21	37	39	2	36	31	0.36
0.5	20		104	21	24.2	0.61	0.69	6.6	0.88			109			35			37	32	
1.0	20		107	20	25.8	0.66	0.74	6.9	0.89			109			35			37	33	
1.5	40		108	22	24.7	0.67	0.82	7.6	0.82			101			40			34	28	
2.0	40	194/92	109	21	30.5	0.84	0.99	9.1	0.85	7.39	23	107	81	24	36	39	3	34	29	0.33
2.5	60		115	22	29.4	0.80	0.92	8.0	0.87			107			37			34	30	
3.0	60		116	20	29.0	0.84	0.98	8.4	0.86			101			42			33	28	
3.5	80		119	22	41.1	1.15	1.21	10.2	0.95			109			36			34	32	
4.0	80	218/98	122	23	39.1	1.11	1.14	9.3	0.97	7.37	22	109	84	26	38	39	1	33	33	0.32
4.5	100		125	25	45.2	1.29	1.30	10.4	0.99			110			37			33	33	
5.0	100		124	26	48.3	1.41	1.37	11.0	1.03			110			38			33	34	
5.5	120		129	28	53.6	1.57	1.47	11.4	1.07			113			37			33	35	
6.0	120	239/98	133	29	57.8	1.68	1.50	11.3	1.12	7.34	21	113	90	23	37	40	3	33	37	0.33
6.5	140		136	30	64.5	1.85	1.58	11.6	1.17			115			37			33	39	
7.0	140	241/104	141	35	65.0	1.82	1.53	10.9	1.19			116			37			34	41	
	Recovery		137	30	69.7	1.98	1.55	11.3	1.28			117			37			34	43	
	Recovery		131	27	62.4	1.70	1.23	9.4	1.38			121			36			35	49	
	Recovery		124	25	46.8	1.23	0.84	6.8	1.46			123			34			36	53	
	Recovery	200/80	120	26	43.3	1.04	0.65	5.4	1.60	7.29	17	126	120	5	32	35	3	40	63	0.36

Case 63 Pulmonary Vascular Disease Secondary to Interstitial and Obstructive Lung Disease

Clinical Findings

This 70-year-old retired shipyard worker complained of shortness of breath after climbing a flight of stairs. He had a 50 pack-year smoking history but had stopped 3 months prior to the evaluation. He took triamterene, hydrochlorothiazide, and methyldopa for hypertension but denied any history of heart or lung disease. The physical examination was not remarkable. Resting ECG showed left axis deviation, left atrial enlargement, and left ventricular hypertrophy. Chest roentgenograms showed moderate pleural thickening with some calcification plus moderate interstitial fibrosis.

Exercise Findings

The patient performed exercise on a cycle ergometer. He pedaled at 60 rpm without added load for 3 minutes. The work rate was then increased 15 W per minute to his symptom-limited maximum. Arterial blood was sampled every second minute, and intraarterial blood pressure was recorded from a percutaneously placed brachial artery catheter. Except for an increase in rate, the ECG pattern remained unchanged during exercise. The patient stopped exercise because of shortness of breath and a dry mouth.

Interpretation

Comments

This case is presented because of its mixed pathophysiologic features. Despite the patient's denial of a history of lung disease, the results of his respiratory function studies indicate that he has mild to moderate obstructive as well as mild restrictive lung disease as evidenced by the reduced FEV_1/VC, total lung capacity, and vital capacity. Accompanying these changes is a marked reduction in diffusing capacity (Table 10.63.1). The resting ECG reflects changes associated with long-standing systemic hypertension, for which he is being treated.

Analysis

Referring to flowchart 1, the peak $\dot{V}O_2$ is reduced and the anaerobic threshold is borderline normal (Table 10.63.2). See flowchart 3. The breathing reserve is low (branch point 3.1), whereas the findings of a high VD/VT, $P(a - ET)CO_2$, and $P(A - a)O_2$ support the diagnosis of lung disease. There is no heart rate reserve, however. The high breathing frequency during most of the exercise period (branch point 3.2) is more typical of restrictive than obstructive lung disease, although the patient mani-

TABLE 10.63.1.   Selected Respiratory Function Data

Measurement	Predicted	Measured
Age, yr		70
Sex		Male
Height, cm		187
Weight, kg	87	76
Hematocrit, %		47
VC, L	4.69	3.64
IC, L	3.13	2.28
TLC, L	7.39	6.02
FEV_1, L	3.65	2.19
FEV_1/VC, %	78	60
MVV, L/min	140	90
D_LCO, ml/mm Hg/min	29.4	10.8

TABLE 10.63.2.   Selected Exercise Data

Measurement	Predicted	Measured
Peak $\dot{V}O_2$, L/min	2.01	1.32
Maximum HR, beats/min	150	152
Maximum O_2 pulse, ml/beat	13.4	8.7
$\Delta\dot{V}O_2/\Delta WR$, ml/min/W	10.3	7.4
AT, L/min	>0.91	0.95
Blood pressure, mmHg (rest, max)		176/86, 227/89
Maximum $\dot{V}E$, L/min		88
Exercise breathing reserve, L/min	>15	2
PaO_2, mmHg (rest, max ex)		54, 52
$P(A - a)O_2$, mmHg (rest, max ex)		43, 68
$P(a - ET)CO_2$, mmHg (rest, max ex)		6, 4
VD/VT (rest, heavy ex)		0.45, 0.48
HCO_3^-, mEq/L (rest, 2-min recov)		27, 19

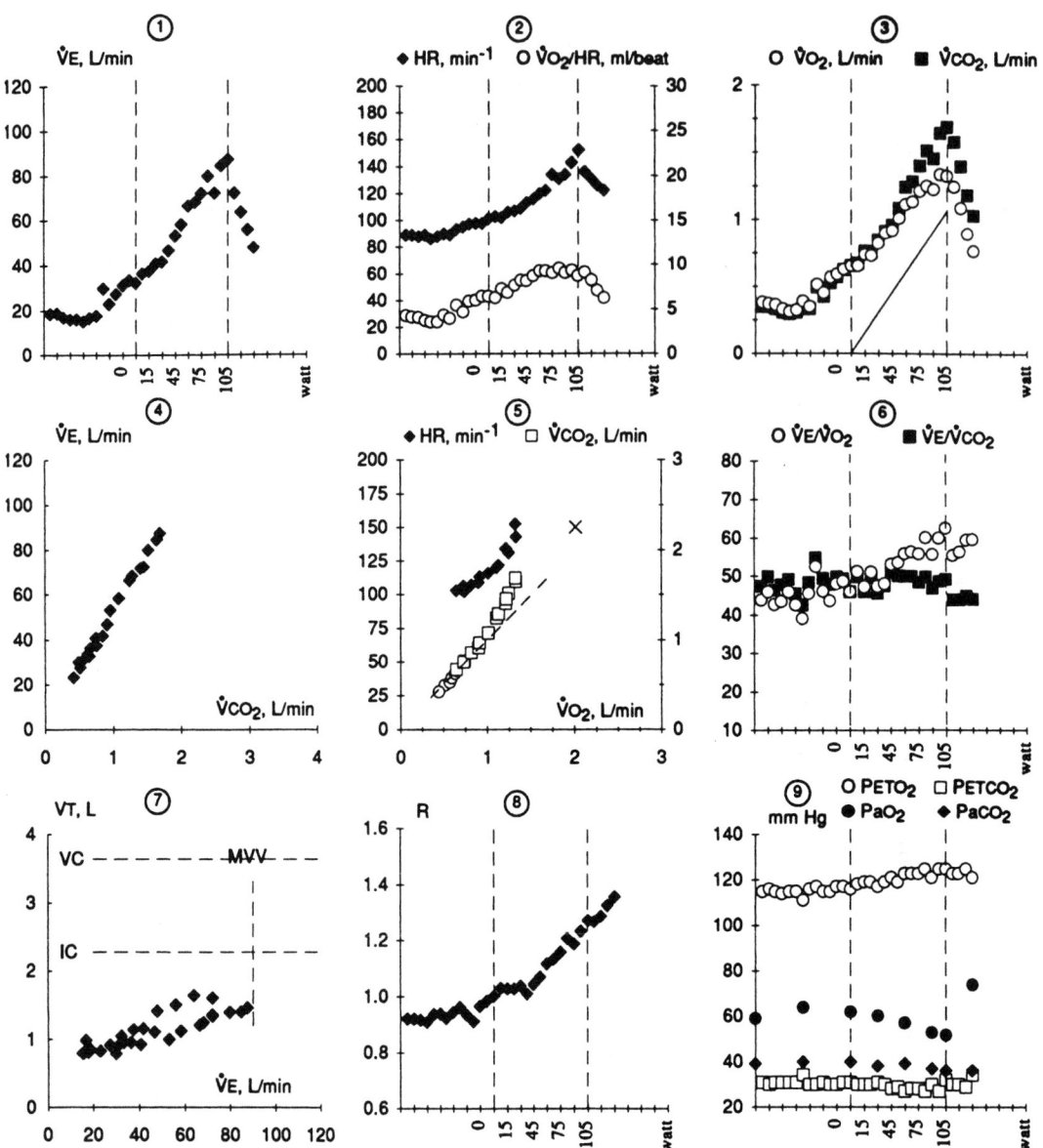

FIGURE 10.63.1.   **1:** Vertical dashed lines in panels 1 to 3 and 6, 8, and 9 indicate the beginning and the end of the increasing work period. **2:** Unloaded cycling is performed for 3 minutes before the left vertical dashed line. **3:** In panel 3, the diagonal line shows the increase of $\dot{V}O_2$ at a slope of 10 ml/min/W. **4:** In panel 5, the diagonal dashed line has a slope of 1; the x in the upper right is the predicted maximum heart rate and $\dot{V}O_2$ for the subject.

fests both disorders at rest. We must also consider the patient's other exercise findings. The plateau in $\dot{V}O_2$ and O_2 pulse at low values as well as the low $\Delta\dot{V}O_2/\Delta WR$, low heart rate reserve, and progressive hypoxemia are all characteristic of pulmonary vascular disease secondary to interstitial lung disease. See flowcharts 4 (abnormal pulmonary circulation) and 5 (pulmonary vascular disease) for details.

Conclusion

Pulmonary vascular disease with reduced exercise performance, probably secondary to an interstitial lung disease.

TABLE 10.63.3.   Air Breathing

Time min	Work rate watts	BP mmHg	HR min⁻¹	f min⁻¹	$\dot{V}_E$ L/min BTPS	$\dot{V}_{CO_2}$ L/min STPD	$\dot{V}_{O_2}$ L/min STPD	$\dfrac{\dot{V}_{O_2}}{HR}$ ml/beat	R	pH	HCO_3^- meq/L	P_{O_2}, mmHg ET	a	(A−a)	P_{CO_2}, mmHg ET	a	(a−ET)	$\dfrac{\dot{V}_E}{\dot{V}_{CO_2}}$	$\dfrac{\dot{V}_E}{\dot{V}_{O_2}}$	$\dfrac{V_D}{V_T}$
	Rest									7.45	27		59			39				
	Rest	176/86	89	22	18.5	0.35	0.38	4.3	0.92			115			31			48	44	
	Rest		89	22	18.8	0.34	0.37	4.2	0.92			116			30			50	46	
	Rest		88	20	17.0	0.33	0.36	4.1	0.92			115			31			46	43	
	Rest		89	20	16.0	0.30	0.33	3.7	0.91			114			31			48	43	
	Rest		86	20	15.9	0.29	0.31	3.6	0.94			115			31			49	46	
	Rest		88	19	15.2	0.30	0.32	3.6	0.94			115			31			45	42	
	Rest	185/89	90	17	16.7	0.36	0.39	4.3	0.92	7.43	26	111	64	43	34	40	6	42	39	0.45
	Rest		89	22	17.8	0.33	0.35	3.9	0.94			116			30			48	46	
	Unloaded		93	38	30.0	0.49	0.51	5.5	0.96			117			30			55	52	
	Unloaded		95	28	23.1	0.42	0.45	4.7	0.93			115			31			49	46	
	Unloaded		97	30	27.4	0.52	0.57	5.9	0.91			115			30			48	44	
	Unloaded		98	34	31.2	0.57	0.59	6.0	0.97			117			30			50	48	
	Unloaded		98	35	33.5	0.62	0.63	6.4	0.98			117			31			49	48	
	Unloaded	197/89	101	31	32.4	0.65	0.65	6.4	1.00	7.43	26	116	62	48	31	40	9	46	46	0.49
0.5	15		103	38	36.5	0.67	0.65	6.3	1.03			118			30			50	51	
1.0	15		102	33	37.6	0.76	0.74	7.3	1.03			119			30			46	47	
1.5	30		106	44	40.9	0.75	0.73	6.9	1.03			119			30			50	51	
2.0	30	206/86	107	36	41.8	0.85	0.82	7.7	1.04	7.42	24	117	60	53	31	38	7	46	47	0.46
2.5	45		109	42	46.8	0.91	0.90	8.3	1.01			119			30			48	48	
3.0	45		113	53	53.3	0.96	0.92	8.1	1.04			121			28			51	53	
3.5	60		116	52	58.4	1.08	1.01	8.7	1.07			119			29			50	53	
4.0	60	209/86	120	55	66.6	1.24	1.11	9.3	1.12	7.42	25	123	57	57	27	39	12	50	56	0.52
4.5	75		122	55	68.4	1.28	1.13	9.3	1.13			123			28			50	56	
5.0	75		134	53	72.1	1.40	1.21	9.0	1.16			123			28			48	56	
5.5	90		131	57	79.9	1.51	1.25	9.5	1.21			125			27			50	60	
6.0	90	221/92	134	54	72.4	1.45	1.22	9.1	1.19	7.40	23	121	53	65	30	37	7	47	56	0.47
6.5	105		143	60	84.7	1.64	1.33	9.3	1.23			125			27			49	60	
7.0	105	227/89	152	60	87.5	1.68	1.32	8.7	1.27	7.38	21	125	52	68	32	36	4	49	62	0.48
	Recovery		136	45	72.4	1.57	1.24	9.1	1.27			123			30			44	55	
	Recovery		131	39	64.1	1.39	1.08	8.2	1.29			123			30			44	56	
	Recovery		126	37	56.0	1.18	0.89	7.1	1.33			125			29			45	59	
	Recovery	233/98	122	34	48.1	1.03	0.76	6.2	1.36	7.34	19	121	74	47	34	36	2	44	59	0.43

Case 64 Pulmonary Arteriovenous Fistulae

Clinical Findings

This 26-year-old man with multiple pulmonary arteriovenous malformations and recurrent brain abscesses was referred for exercise testing to assess his pathophysiologic status before undergoing embolization therapy to his arteriovenous fistulae. He denied shortness of breath and, until recently, had worked as an aerobics instructor. The patient was well developed, muscular, and had no rales or murmurs on examination of the chest, but had marked finger clubbing and cyanosis. A recent study while the patient was at rest breathing oxygen showed a calculated right-to-left shunt of 53%.

Exercise Findings

The patient performed exercise on a cycle ergometer. He pedaled at 60 rpm without an added load for 3 minutes. The work rate was then increased continuously at a rate of 20 W per minute to tolerance. Blood was sampled every second minute, and intraarterial pressure was recorded from a percutaneously placed brachial artery catheter. Heart rate and rhythm were continuously monitored; 12-lead ECGs were obtained during rest, exercise, and recovery. The patient appeared to give an excellent effort and stopped exercise because of general and leg fatigue, without dyspnea or chest pain. No arrhythmias or ischemic changes were noted on ECGs.

Interpretation

Comments

Resting respiratory function studies showed restrictive lung disease with good ventilatory ability (Table 10.64.1). The patient was thin, cyanotic, and polycythemic. Resting arterial blood analysis showed hypoxemia and a chronic respiratory alkalosis.

Analysis

Referring to flowchart 1, the peak $\dot{V}O_2$ is low, but the anaerobic threshold is normal (Table 10.64.2). Also striking are the severe hypoxemia, low $P_{ET}CO_2$, and high V_D/V_T. We are directed through branch points 1.1, 1.2, and 1.3 to flowchart 3, which leads us

through branch points 3.1 and 3.3 to "poor effort or musculoskeletal disorder," which does not fit well with the patient's known findings. Using flowchart 4, the normal breathing reserve (branch point 4.1) and the high $\dot{V}E/\dot{V}CO_2$ at the AT (branch point 4.3) lead to the box labeled "abnormal pulmonary circulation pathophysiology," where the patient meets most of the criteria. If we had used flowchart 5, we would have arrived through branch points 5.1 and 5.3 at branch point 5.6, "pulmonary vascular disease." The sustained reduction in arterial oxyhemoglobin saturation during exercise suggests a large right-to-left shunt.

The finding of a lower than predicted O_2 pulse in the presence of polycythemia is of interest, espe-

TABLE 10.64.1.   Selected Respiratory Function Data

Measurement	Predicted	Measured
Age, yr		26
Sex		Male
Height, cm		189
Weight, kg	87	64
Hemoglobin, g/100 ml		21.8
VC, L	5.55	4.18
IC, L	3.70	2.94
FEV₁, L	4.50	3.95
FEV₁/VC, %	81	94
MVV, L/min		
Direct	183	169
Indirect	180	158

TABLE 10.64.2.   Selected Exercise Data

Measurement	Predicted	Measured
Peak $\dot{V}O_2$, L/min	3.12	2.19
Maximum HR, beats/min	194	160
Maximum O_2 pulse, ml/beat	16.1	13.7
Δ$\dot{V}O_2$/ΔWR, ml/min/W	10.3	9.9
AT, L/min	>1.28	1.5
Blood pressure, mmHg (rest, max)		144/84, 180/90
Maximum $\dot{V}E$, L/min		123
Exercise breathing reserve, L/min	>15	35
SaO₂, % (rest, max ex)		76, 64
PaO₂, mmHg (rest, max ex)		39, 39
P(A − a)O₂, mmHg (rest, max ex)		74, 76
P(a − ET)CO₂, mmHg (rest, max ex)		9, 15
VD/VT (rest, max ex)		0.42, 0.52
HCO₃⁻, mEq/L (rest, 2-min recov)		22, 16

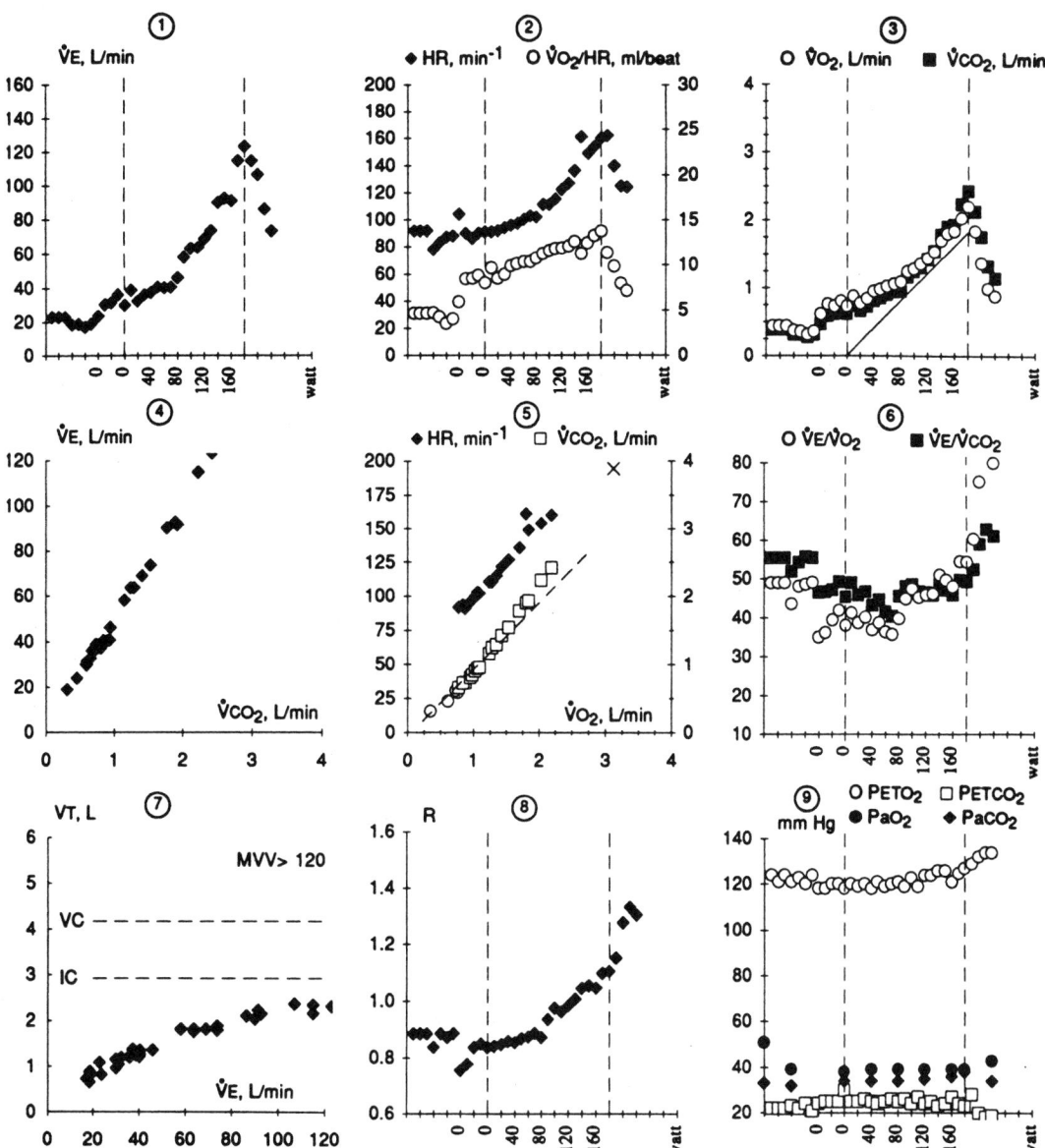

FIGURE 10.64.1.   **1:** Vertical dashed lines in panels 1 to 3 and 6, 8, and 9 indicate the beginning and the end of the increasing work period. **2:** Unloaded cycling is performed for 3 minutes before the left vertical dashed line. **3:** In panel 3, the diagonal line shows the increase of $\dot{V}O_2$ at a slope of 10 ml/min/W. **4:** In panel 5, the diagonal dashed line has a slope of 1; the x in the upper right is the predicted maximum heart rate and $\dot{V}O_2$ for the subject.

cially in view of the high oxyhemoglobin capacity of the blood (30.8 ml/100 ml versus the normal 21 ml/100 ml). Because of the low arterial oxyhemoglobin saturation, arterial content is only approximately 20 ml/100 ml. Likely, mixed venous oxyhemoglobin saturation is normal, resulting in a higher than normal oxyhemoglobin content (because of the polycythemia). Thus, there is no evidence of a reduced stroke volume or cardiac output. Much of the right ventricular output bypasses the aerated

alveoli. In order to compensate for the venous blood that bypasses the gas exchange vessels in the lungs, the blood that does go through the pulmonary capillaries must be exposed to alveoli with lower PCO_2 than that of the arterial blood. Because the $PaCO_2$ is about 35 mm Hg during exercise, the $PcCO_2$ and $PETCO_2$ values must be very low (panel 9, Fig. 10.64.1), and the VD/VT values are much increased (Table 10.64.3) despite probably no real parenchymal disease, because of the shunt.

TABLE 10.64.3. Air Breathing

Time min	Work rate watts	BP mmHg	HR min⁻¹	f min⁻¹	$\dot{V}_E$ L/min BTPS	$\dot{V}_{CO_2}$ L/min STPD	$\dot{V}_{O_2}$ L/min STPD	$\dot{V}_{O_2}$/HR ml/beat	R	pH	HCO_3^- meq/L	P_{O_2}, mmHg ET	a	(A − a)	P_{CO_2}, mmHg ET	a	(a − ET)	$\dot{V}_E/\dot{V}_{CO_2}$	$\dot{V}_E/\dot{V}_{O_2}$	V_D/V_T
	Rest									7.43	22		51			33				
	Rest		92	21	22.8	0.38	0.43	4.7	0.88			124			22			55	49	
	Rest		92	21	22.8	0.38	0.43	4.7	0.88			121			22			55	49	
	Rest		92	21	22.8	0.38	0.43	4.7	0.88			124			22			55	49	
	Rest		78	28	18.5	0.31	0.37	4.7	0.84	7.45	22	121	39	74	23	32	9	52	44	0.42
	Rest		83	21	18.6	0.31	0.35	4.2	0.89			123			22			54	48	
	Rest		87	23	17.0	0.27	0.31	3.6	0.87			120			24			56	49	
	Unloaded		88	23	19.1	0.31	0.35	4.0	0.89			124			21			55	49	
	Unloaded		104	29	23.8	0.46	0.61	5.9	0.75			118			24			46	35	
	Unloaded		90	31	30.1	0.59	0.76	8.4	0.78			118			25			47	36	
	Unloaded		86	30	31.3	0.61	0.73	8.5	0.84			120			25			47	39	
	Unloaded		90	30	36.0	0.68	0.80	8.9	0.85			120			25			49	42	
	Unloaded	144/84	91	26	26.9	0.61	0.73	8.0	0.84	7.43	22	118	38	73	30	34	4	45	38	0.41
0.5	10		91	31	38.8	0.74	0.88	9.7	0.84			120			25			49	41	
1.0	20		92	27	32.4	0.66	0.78	8.5	0.85			119			25			46	39	
1.5	30		94	29	36.1	0.72	0.84	8.9	0.86			120			26			47	40	
2.0	40	150/90	96	27	37.2	0.81	0.95	9.9	0.85	7.42	22	118	39	72	25	34	9	43	37	0.39
2.5	50		97	30	40.4	0.85	0.98	10.1	0.87			121			24			45	39	
3.0	60		100	33	40.2	0.90	1.03	10.3	0.87			119			25			42	36	
3.5	70		103	32	40.6	0.94	1.06	10.3	0.89			120			26			40	36	
4.0	80	162/90	102	34	46.2	0.95	1.09	10.7	0.87	7.42	22	121	39	73	25	34	9	46	40	0.42
4.5	90		111	32	58.2	1.16	1.24	11.2	0.94			119			26			48	45	
5.0	100		111	36	63.6	1.25	1.28	11.5	0.98			123			24			48	47	
5.5	110		115	35	63.7	1.30	1.35	11.7	0.96			119			27			47	45	
6.0	120	174/96	122	38	69.0	1.42	1.44	11.8	0.99	7.38	20	124	39	76	24	35	11	46	46	0.45
6.5	130		127	39	73.7	1.54	1.53	12.0	1.01			124			25			46	46	
7.0	140		136	44	90.2	1.76	1.70	12.5	1.05			126			23			49	51	
7.5	150		161	43	92.9	1.90	1.80	11.2	1.06			126			24			47	50	
8.0	160	180/90	149	41	91.5	1.93	1.84	12.3	1.05	7.36	20	121	39	76	27	36	9	46	48	0.46
8.5	170		154	53	115.0	2.23	2.03	13.2	1.10			125			24			50	54	
9.0	180	180/96	160	53	123.3	2.42	2.19	13.7	1.11	7.31	19	127	39	76	23	38	15	49	54	0.52
	Recovery		162	49	115.0	2.12	1.84	11.4	1.15			129			28			52	60	
	Recovery		140	45	106.9	1.75	1.37	9.8	1.28			132			20			59	75	
	Recovery		125	41	86.4	1.32	0.99	7.9	1.33			134			18			63	84	
	Recovery	156/84	124	41	73.7	1.15	0.88	7.1	1.31	7.30	16	134	43	79	19	34	15	61	80	0.56

Conclusion

The patient has a large right-to-left shunt at rest and during exercise because of pulmonary arteriovenous malformations. The high V_D/V_T and positive $P(a - ET)_{CO_2}$ values indicate that ventilation is relatively ineffective in removing CO_2 from the blood, consistent with a high fraction of right ventricular output bypassing the alveolar capillaries. In this patient, the wide $P(A - a)_{O_2}$, positive $P(a - ET)_{CO_2}$, and high V_D/V_T that increase with exercise, indicate a large right-to-left shunt during rest and exercise rather than the ordinary maldistribution of ventilation found in lung diseases without a right-to-left shunt.

Case 65 Poor Effort

Clinical Findings

This 37-year-old male electrician was referred for evaluation because of his 5-year exposure to asbestos while working in a shipyard. He stated that he had had a daily productive cough for a year and that he could only climb six or seven steps before he had to stop to catch his breath. He stated that he had smoked approximately half a package of cigarettes daily for the last 13 years. He denied other problems and took no medications. Physical and chest roentgenographic examinations were normal.

Exercise Findings

The patient performed exercise on a cycle ergometer. He pedaled at 60 rpm without an added load for 3 minutes. The work rate was then increased 25 W per minute to his symptom-limited maximum. Blood was sampled every second minute, and intraarterial blood pressure was recorded from a percutaneously passed brachial artery catheter. The patient was apprehensive and was unhappy about having a test performed. He breathed rapidly and shallowly on the mouthpiece despite reassurance and encouragement. He slowed his pedaling frequency after 2 minutes of incremental work and stopped pedaling at a work rate of 100 W, complaining of generalized fatigue, tingling in the hands, and lightheadedness. These symptoms resolved within 5 minutes. After an hour of rest, explanation, and encouragement to breathe at a slower rate, the test was repeated using an increment of 20 W/min. This time, the patient began to hyperventilate as soon as exercise began. He stopped cycling at a work rate of 60 W with a heart rate of 99. Complete data from the first test and selected data from the second test are presented. Resting and exercise ECGs were normal.

Interpretation

Comments

Resting respiratory function was normal (Table 10.65.1).

Analysis

Referring to flowchart 1, the peak $\dot{V}_{O_2}$ was low, and the anaerobic threshold was indeterminate (Table 10.65.2). This leads to flowchart 5. The indices of ventilation–perfusion matching at maximum work

rate are normal (branch point 5.1). The heart rate reserve is high (branch point 5.2), and $\Delta\dot{V}_{O_2}/\Delta WR$ is normal (branch point 5.5). This leads to the diagnosis of poor effort. The normal ECG, high breathing reserve, minimal decline in HCO_3^-, and R less than 1.0 at exercise cessation all signify the absence of organic cardiovascular or lung disease. We can also conclude that the patient gave a poor effort since he did not develop the metabolic acidosis that should be expected with a reasonable exercise effort. We were unable to encourage him to improve his performance when tested an hour later. The abrupt hyperventilation and respiratory alkalosis early in the two studies (Pa_{CO_2} decreased from 37 to 22 in the first study and from 34 to 21 in the second study. The data in Tables 10.65.3 and 10.65.4) are typical of patients with anxiety or voluntary hyperventilation. An irregular breathing pattern, re-

TABLE 10.65.1.   Selected Respiratory Function Data

Measurement	Predicted	Measured
Age, yr		37
Sex		Male
Height, cm		170
Weight, kg	80	87
Hematocrit, %		46
VC, L	4.52	4.20
IC, L	3.01	3.07
TLC, L	6.29	5.29
FEV_1, L	3.64	3.66
FEV_1/VC, %	81	87
MVV, L/min	152	129
$D_L CO$, ml/mm Hg/min	29.9	24.7

TABLE 10.65.2.   Selected Exercise Data

Measurement	Predicted	Measured
Peak $\dot{V}_{O_2}$, L/min	3.00	1.43
Maximum HR, beats/min	183	112
Maximum O_2 pulse, ml/beat	16.4	12.8
$\Delta\dot{V}_{O_2}/\Delta WR$, ml/min/W	10.3	10.1
AT, L/min	>1.26	Indeterminate
Blood pressure, mmHg (rest, max ex)		146/93, 174/105
Maximum $\dot{V}_E$, L/min		64
Exercise breathing reserve, L/min	>15	65 nn
Pa_{O_2}, mmHg (rest, max ex)		89, 117
$P(A - a)_{O_2}$, mmHg (rest, max ex)		6, 7
$P(a - ET)_{CO_2}$, mmHg (rest, max ex)		0, −3
V_D/V_T (rest, max ex)		0.37, 0.19
HCO_3^-, mEq/L (rest, recov)		23, 20
Carboxyhemoglobin, rest, %		6.5

TABLE 10.65.3.   Air Breathing

Time min	Work rate watts	BP mmHg	HR min⁻¹	f min⁻¹	V̇E L/min BTPS	V̇CO₂ L/min STPD	V̇O₂ L/min STPD	V̇O₂/HR ml/beat	R	pH	HCO₃⁻ meq/L	PO₂ ET	PO₂ a	PO₂ (A−a)	PCO₂ ET	PCO₂ a	PCO₂ (a−ET)	V̇E/V̇CO₂	V̇E/V̇O₂	VD/VT
	Rest	146/93								7.42	23		95			36				
	Rest		72	37	20.9	0.41	0.39	5.4	1.05			117			33			43	46	
	Rest		73	31	15.1	0.29	0.32	4.4	0.91			109			36			43	39	
	Rest		73	32	9.8	0.16	0.21	2.9	0.76			104			38			44	34	
	Rest	153/102	73	29	11.3	0.20	0.32	4.4	0.63	7.41	23	97	89	6	37	37	0	44	28	0.37
	Rest		74	26	12.8	0.27	0.40	5.4	0.68			95			38			39	26	
	Rest		77	31	15.8	0.33	0.46	6.0	0.72			96			38			40	29	
	Unloaded		82	33	30.3	0.72	0.69	8.4	1.04			115			32			38	40	
	Unloaded		88	42	33.3	0.71	0.61	6.9	1.16			122			30			42	49	
	Unloaded		90	49	45.5	0.90	0.68	7.6	1.32			127			28			46	61	
	Unloaded		85	50	45.7	0.88	0.67	7.9	1.31			127			27			47	62	
	Unloaded		85	57	39.6	0.68	0.51	6.0	1.33			129			25			51	68	
	Unloaded		85	50	33.0	0.58	0.49	5.8	1.18			126			25			50	59	
	Unloaded	168/105	85	53	38.7	0.66	0.54	6.4	1.22	7.52	21	128	122	6	24	26	2	52	63	0.32
	Unloaded		83	54	45.6	0.79	0.65	7.8	1.22			129			23			52	63	
0.5	25		88	54	47.2	0.79	0.65	7.4	1.22			128			23			54	66	
1.0	25		89	56	60.6	0.99	0.79	8.9	1.25			127			24			56	71	
1.5	50		94	59	62.8	1.06	0.92	9.8	1.15			130			21			55	63	
2.0	50	168/102	94	54	54.7	0.97	0.95	10.1	1.02	7.56	19	126	123	5	23	22	−1	52	53	0.22
2.5	75		103	51	61.9	1.13	1.09	10.6	1.04			123			25			51	53	
3.0	75		103	51	62.9	1.19	1.15	11.2	1.03			126			23			49	51	
3.5	100		110	46	53.2	1.13	1.21	11.0	0.93			114			30			44	41	
4.0	100	174/105	112	46	64.0	1.39	1.43	12.8	0.97	7.52	20	120	117	7	28	25	−3	43	42	0.19
	Recovery		96	47	52.5	1.13	1.20	12.5	0.94			119			28			43	40	
	Recovery		86	46	45.4	0.91	0.90	10.5	1.01			122			27			46	46	
	Recovery		79	52	46.6	0.77	0.61	7.7	1.26			130			22			55	69	
	Recovery	168/108	78	43	34.9	0.55	0.45	5.8	1.22	7.54	20	130	126	3	22	24	2	57	69	0.33

flected in the wild swings in gas exchange ratio shown in panel 8 of Figure 10.65.1, is more consistent with a volitional lack of cooperation.

Conclusion

This case study shows poor effort on the part of the patient. There is no evidence of abnormal gas exchange, ventilatory limitation, metabolic acidosis, or cardiovascular limitation. The symptoms and findings are typical of acute respiratory alkalosis of variable degree. Because of the high ventilatory equivalents that might suggest a gas exchange abnormality, blood gas analyses are helpful in excluding ventilation–perfusion mismatching.

TABLE 10.65.4.   Selected Measures Early in Second Study

Time (min)	Work Rate	f(/min)	V̇E (L/min)	R	pH	PaCO₂ (mmHg)	HCO₃⁻ (mEq/L)
0					7.42	34	22
0.5	Rest	32	26.6	1.08			
1	Rest	29	16.6	1.00			
1.5	Rest	22	17.7	0.97			
2	Rest	22	12.2	0.77	7.45	29	20
2.5	Rest	23	12.3	0.71			
3	Rest	25	18.3	0.80			
3.5	Unloaded	35	30.9	0.93			
4	Unloaded	39	34.9	1.07			
4.5	Unloaded	37	32.6	0.95			
5	Unloaded	46	44.5	1.08			
5.5	Unloaded	51	55.7	1.18			
6	Unloaded	49	51.0	1.14	7.57	21	19

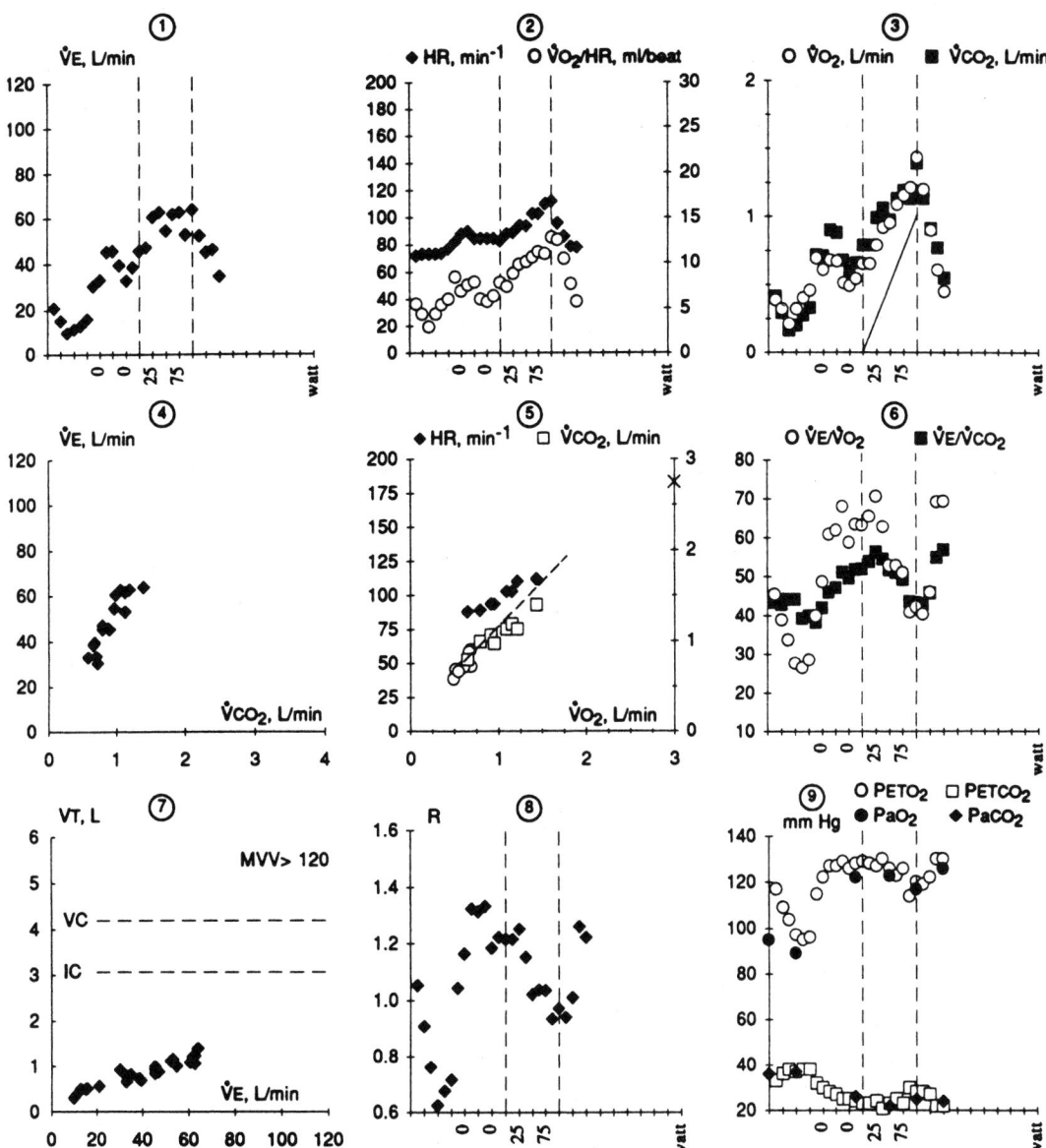

FIGURE 10.65.1.   **1:** Vertical dashed lines in panels 1 to 3 and 6, 8, and 9 indicate the beginning and the end of the increasing work period. **2:** Unloaded cycling is performed for 3 minutes before the left vertical dashed line. **3:** In panel 3, the diagonal line shows the increase of $\dot{V}O_2$ at a slope of 10 ml/min/W. **4:** In panel 5, the diagonal dashed line has a slope of 1; the x in the upper right is the predicted maximum heart rate and $\dot{V}O_2$ for the subject.

Case 66 Poor Effort

Clinical Findings

This 59-year-old shipyard worker had been made aware of an abnormality in his chest roentgenogram 1 year prior to this evaluation. Retrospectively, he felt that he had had some shortness of breath for 2 years when jogging or climbing stairs. He had smoked cigarettes for 20 years, until age 35. Results of physical, laboratory, and roentgenographic examinations were normal except for prostatic enlargement and extensive pleural calcification.

Exercise Findings

The patient performed exercise on a cycle ergometer. He pedaled at 60 rpm without added load for 3 minutes. The work rate was then increased 20 W per minute to his symptom-limited maximum. Arterial blood was sampled every second minute, and intraarterial blood pressure was recorded from a percutaneously placed brachial artery catheter. The patient pedaled irregularly during the test. He stopped pedaling, complaining of shortness of breath and leg fatigue, and stated he could go no further. Resting and exercise ECGs were normal.

Interpretation

Comments

Resting respiratory function (Table 10.66.1) is within normal limits.

Analysis

Referring to flowchart 1, the peak $\dot{V}O_2$ is significantly reduced and the anaerobic threshold is indeterminate (Table 10.66.2). See flowchart 5. The resting VD/VT is normal, but it does not decrease appropriately during exercise. Only light exercise was performed, however, and the lack of a decrease might be spurious owing to the low tidal volume, tachypnea, and low work rate performed (Table 10.66.3). Because $P(a - ET)CO_2$ and $P(A - a)O_2$ are normal (branch point 5.1), we conclude that the indices of ventilation relative to perfusion are normal. Heart rate reserve (branch point 5.2) is high, and the $\Delta\dot{V}O_2/\Delta WR$ (branch point 5.5) could not be de-

termined because the subject performed increasing work rate exercise for only 2 minutes. However, the breathing reserve and the heart rate reserve are high (Table 10.66.2). These findings place the patient in the diagnostic category of poor effort. The following findings are consistent with this diagnosis: (a) the normal exercise ECG; (b) R of only 0.82 at the peak $\dot{V}O_2$; (c) minimal decline in HCO_3^- induced by the exercise (Table 10.66.3); and the previously mentioned high heart rate reserve, high breathing reserve, normal blood gases, and normal indices of ventilation–perfusion mismatching.

Conclusion

This patient made a poor effort.

TABLE 10.66.1. Selected Respiratory Function Data

Measurement	Predicted	Measured
Age, yr		59
Sex		Male
Height, cm		173
Weight, kg	76	72
Hematocrit, %		44
VC, L	3.65	3.05
IC, L	2.44	2.44
TLC, L	5.57	4.93
FEV$_1$, L	2.87	2.49
FEV$_1$/VC, %	79	82
MVV, L/min	121	110
D$_L$CO, ml/mm Hg/min	22.6	24.6

TABLE 10.66.2. Selected Exercise Data

Measurement	Predicted	Measured
Maximum $\dot{V}O_2$, L/min	2.13	1.08
Maximum HR, beats/min	161	110
Maximum O$_2$ pulse, ml/beat	13.2	9.8
AT, L/min	>0.94	indeterminate
Blood pressure, mmHg (rest, max)		135/78, 144/78
Maximum $\dot{V}E$, L/min		30
Exercise breathing reserve, L/min	>15	80
PaO$_2$, mmHg (rest, max ex)		98, 96
P(A − a)O$_2$, mmHg (rest, max ex)		0, 10
P(a − ET)CO$_2$, mmHg (rest, max ex)		0, −3
VD/VT (rest, heavy ex)		0.35, 0.36
HCO$_3^-$, mEq/L (rest, 2-min recov)		25, 24

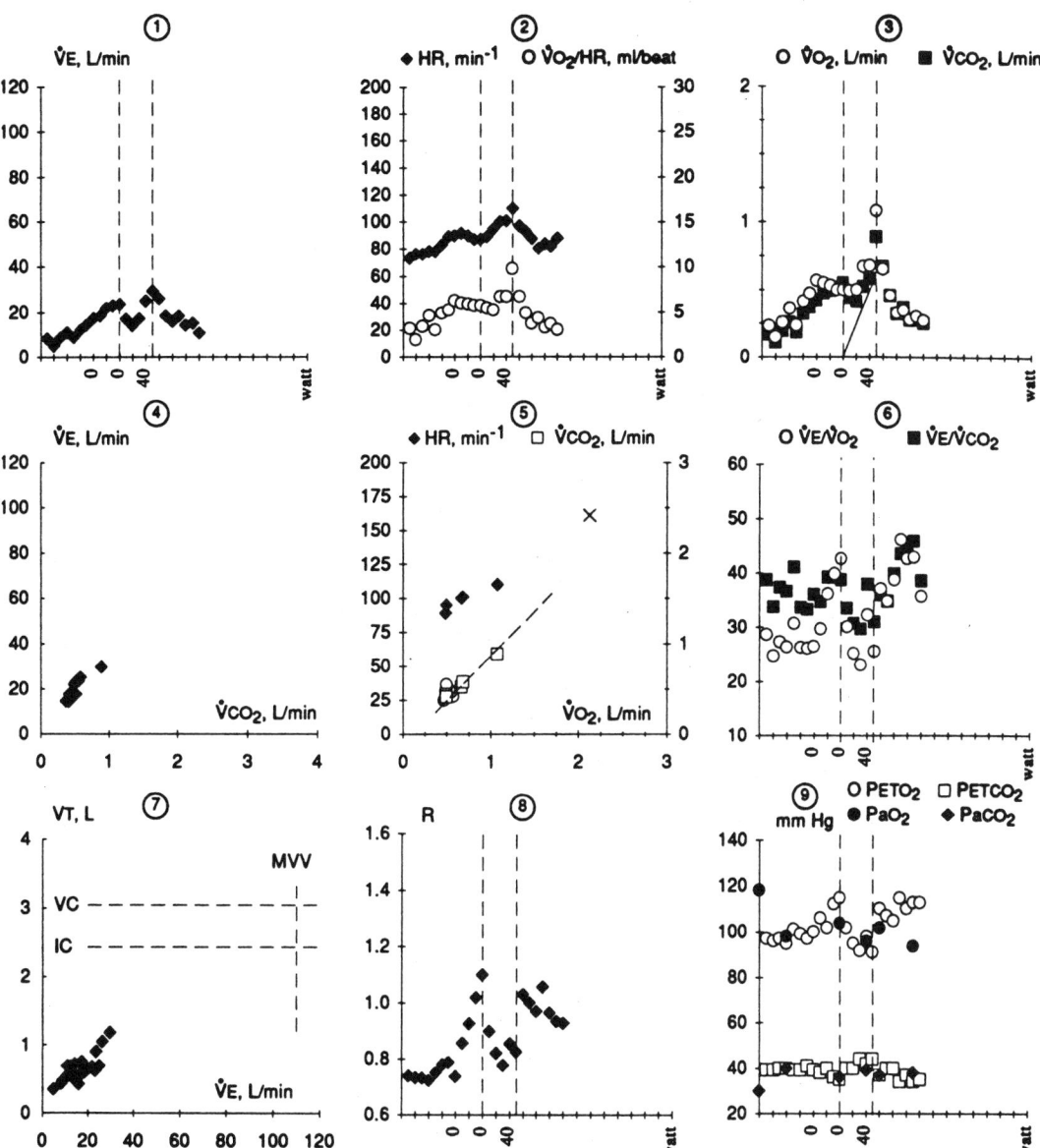

FIGURE 10.66.1. **1:** Vertical dashed lines in panels 1 to 3 and 6, 8, and 9 indicate the beginning and the end of the increasing work period. **2:** Unloaded cycling is performed for 3 minutes before the left vertical dashed line. **3:** In panel 3, the diagonal line shows the increase of $\dot{V}O_2$ at a slope of 10 ml/min/W. **4:** In panel 5, the diagonal dashed line has a slope of 1; the x in the upper right is the predicted maximum heart rate and $\dot{V}O_2$ for the subject.

TABLE 10.66.3.   Air Breathing

Time min	Work rate watts	BP mmHg	HR min⁻¹	f min⁻¹	$\dot{V}_E$ L/min BTPS	$\dot{V}_{CO_2}$ L/min STPD	$\dot{V}_{O_2}$ L/min STPD	$\dot{V}_{O_2}$/HR ml/beat	R	pH	HCO_3^- meq/L	P_{O_2}, mmHg ET	a	(A − a)	P_{CO_2}, mmHg ET	a	(a − ET)	$\dot{V}_E/\dot{V}_{CO_2}$	$\dot{V}_E/\dot{V}_{O_2}$	V_D/V_T
	Rest	135/78								7.51	24		118			30				
	Rest		73	19	8.2	0.17	0.23	3.2	0.74			97			39			39	29	
	Rest		76	14	4.9	0.11	0.15	2.0	0.73			96			39			34	25	
	Rest		76	19	8.7	0.19	0.26	3.4	0.73			97			40			37	27	
	Rest	132/78	78	20	11.2	0.26	0.36	4.6	0.72	7.41	25	95	98	0	40	40	0	37	26	0.35
	Rest		78	19	9.0	0.18	0.24	3.1	0.75			101			39			41	31	
	Rest		83	18	12.3	0.32	0.41	4.9	0.78			99			39			34	26	
	Unloaded		89	26	14.5	0.37	0.47	5.3	0.79			97			41			33	26	
	Unloaded		90	29	17.6	0.42	0.57	6.3	0.74			100			39			36	27	
	Unloaded		92	27	18.6	0.47	0.55	6.0	0.85			106			38			35	30	
	Unloaded		90	32	21.9	0.49	0.53	5.9	0.92			102			40			39	36	
	Unloaded		87	37	23.1	0.51	0.50	5.7	1.02			112			36			39	40	
	Unloaded	144/78	87	26	23.5	0.55	0.50	5.7	1.10	7.43	23	115	104	13	35	36	1	39	43	0.34
0.5	20		89	29	17.2	0.44	0.49	5.5	0.90			102			40			33	30	
1.0	20		95	20	14.3	0.41	0.50	5.3	0.82			95			40			31	25	
1.5	40		100	23	17.4	0.52	0.67	6.7	0.78			92			44			30	23	
2.0	40	144/78	101	36	25.0	0.58	0.68	6.7	0.85	7.41	24	98	96	10	42	39	−3	38	32	0.36
2.5	60		110	25	29.7	0.89	1.08	9.8	0.82			91			44			31	26	
	Recovery	150/78	97	25	26.2	0.67	0.65	6.7	1.03	7.41	23	110	102	12	37	37	0	36	37	0.32
	Recovery		93	31	18.6	0.46	0.46	4.9	1.00			107			40			35	35	
	Recovery		88	38	16.0	0.32	0.33	3.8	0.97			105			40			40	39	
	Recovery		81	28	18.5	0.37	0.35	4.3	1.06			115			34			44	46	
	Recovery		84	30	14.5	0.27	0.28	3.3	0.96			110			37			44	43	
	Recovery	132/84	82	30	15.4	0.28	0.30	3.7	0.93	7.41	24	113	94	16	34	38	4	46	43	0.42
	Recovery		88	16	11.0	0.25	0.27	3.1	0.93			113			35			39	36	

Case 67 Acute Hyperventilation and Anxiety in a Moderately Obese Man

Clinical Findings

This 56-year-old shipyard worker complained of progressive dyspnea on exertion, evident when climbing two flights of stairs. He had also noted anterior chest pain with exertion, relieved by rest, that was associated with dyspnea and diaphoresis but not with palpitations, lightheadedness, syncope, or numbness. He had stopped smoking 20 years previously after 20 pack-years. He took no medications but had been told that he had hypertension several years ago. Physical examination and resting ECG were normal. Chest roentgenogram showed mild pleural thickening bilaterally.

Exercise Findings

After percutaneous insertion of a brachial artery catheter, the patient became lightheaded and syncopal while being positioned on the cycle ergometer. The patient was placed on a gurney in the reverse Trendelenburg position. Continuous monitoring revealed a transient sinus bradycardia as low as 25 with normal blood pressure. The bradycardia lasted only a few minutes. After 15 minutes he felt well and was able to exercise. He pedaled at 60 rpm without added load for 3 minutes. The work rate was then increased 15 W every minute. Arterial blood was sampled every second minute, and intraarterial blood pressure was recorded from the brachial artery catheter. Mild chest pain began at 45 W; exercise was stopped at 90 W because of the patient's continuing and increasing chest pain, which was typical of his usual symptom. There were no ST abnormalities, nor was there arrhythmia during or after exercise.

Interpretation

Comments

Resting respiratory function studies reveal the patient to have a restrictive defect of the type generally seen with obesity (normal inspiratory capacity, but reduced expiratory reserve volume) (Table 10.67.1). The patient is, in fact, 23 kg overweight. Resting ECG is normal. As the patient was getting ready to cycle, he became lightheaded and hypotensive. His blood pressure decreased and he developed a marked bradycardia consistent with a

vasovagal reaction. When placed in a supine position, the patient's pulse and blood pressure became normal and he resumed his position on the cycle ergometer for testing; however, he acutely hyperventilated at rest, demonstrating a marked respiratory alkalosis in his arterial blood (Table 10.67.3).

Analysis

In flowchart 1, the peak $\dot{V}O_2$ is reduced and the anaerobic threshold is normal (Table 10.67.2), which directs us through branch points 1.1, 1.2, and 1.3 to flowchart 3. The breathing reserve (branch point 3.1) and ECG (branch point 3.3) are normal, directing us to "poor effort or musculoskeletal disorder." The V_D/V_T, $P(A - a)O_2$, and $P(a - ET)CO_2$ are normal, and the heart rate reserve is high. The change in bicarbonate from rest to recovery is only

TABLE 10.67.1. Selected Respiratory Function Data

Measurement	Predicted	Measured
Age, yr		56
Sex		Male
Height, cm		172
Weight, kg	75	98
Hematocrit, %		46
VC, L	4.10	3.16
IC, L	2.74	2.55
TLC, L	6.17	4.77
FEV_1, L	3.23	2.78
FEV_1/VC, %	79	88
MVV, L/min	137	98
D_LCO, ml/mm Hg/min	26.3	20.9

TABLE 10.67.2. Selected Exercise Data

Measurement	Predicted	Measured
Peak $\dot{V}O_2$, L/min	2.38	1.51
Maximum HR, beats/min	164	130
Maximum O_2 pulse, ml/beat	14.5	11.6
$\Delta\dot{V}O_2/\Delta WR$, ml/min/W	10.3	9.3
AT, L/min	>1.05	1.4
Blood pressure, mmHg (rest, max)		168/96, 228/111
Maximum $\dot{V}E$, L/min		79
Exercise breathing reserve, L/min	>15	19
PaO_2, mmHg (rest, max ex)		112, 100
$P(A - a)O_2$, mmHg (rest, max ex)		21, 25
$P(a - ET)CO_2$, mmHg (rest, max ex)		2, 0
V_D/V_T (rest, heavy ex)		0.30, 0.24
HCO_3^-, mEq/L (rest, 2-min recov)		24, 20

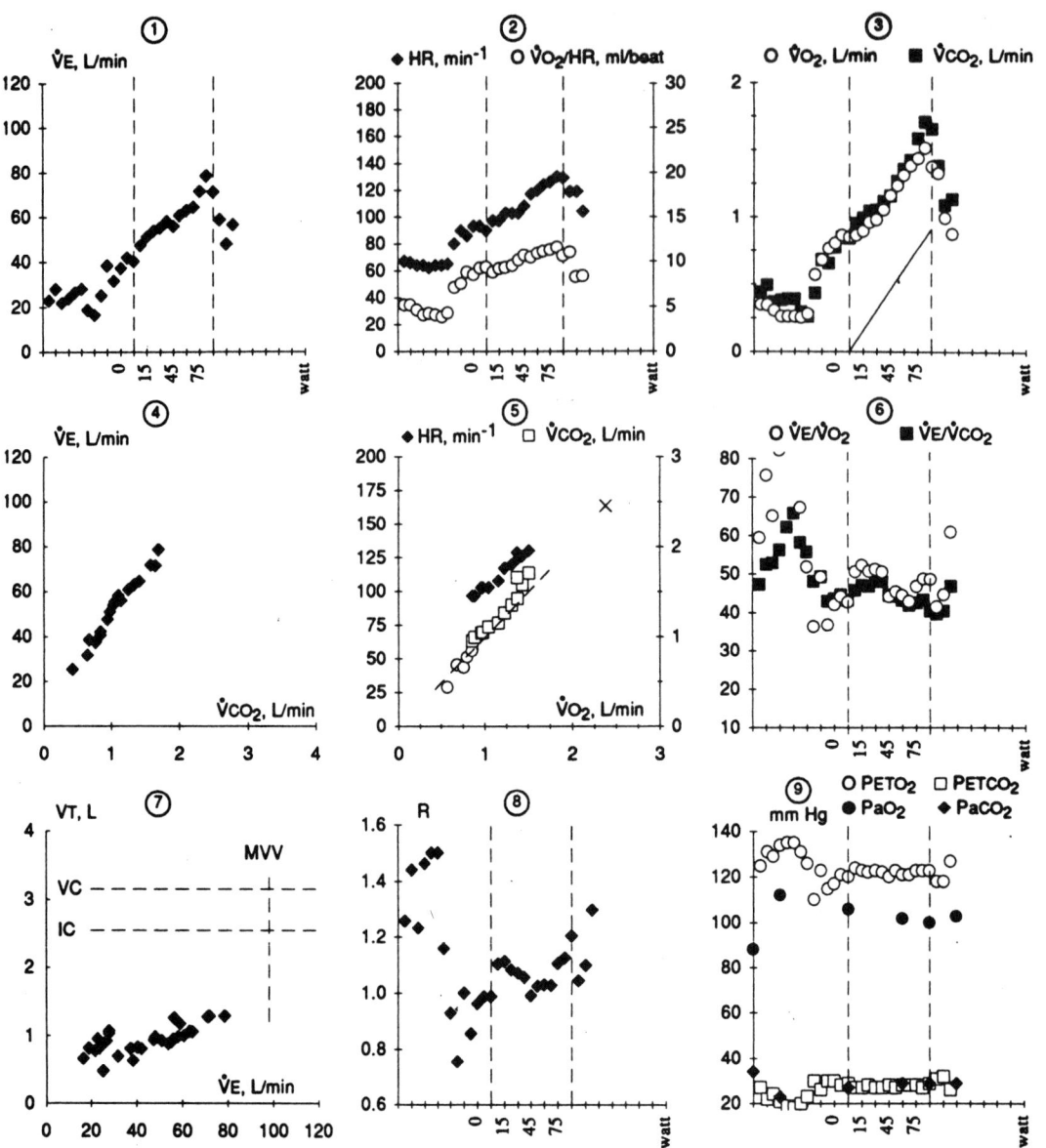

FIGURE 10.67.1. **1:** Vertical dashed lines in panels 1 to 3 and 6, 8, and 9 indicate the beginning and the end of the increasing work period. **2:** Unloaded cycling is performed for 3 minutes before the left vertical dashed line. **3:** In panel 3, the diagonal line shows the increase of $\dot{V}O_2$ at a slope of 10 ml/min/W. **4:** In panel 5, the diagonal dashed line has a slope of 1; the x in the upper right is the predicted maximum heart rate and $\dot{V}O_2$ for the subject.

4 mEq/L, which is less than expected for a normal maximal exercise effort. These findings suggest that the patient's chest pain that caused the physician to ask the patient to stop exercise was not supported by evidence of coronary artery disease, in that the ECG, $\Delta\dot{V}O_2/\Delta WR$, heart rate–$\Delta\dot{V}O_2$ relationship, and *AT* (Fig. 10.67.1, panel 5) were normal. On the other hand, the acute hyperventilation, demonstrated by the development of an abrupt alkalosis with an increase in pH from 7.47 to 7.59 and $PaCO_2$ from 34 to 23 mm Hg (Table 10.67.3), supports the

diagnosis of an anxiety state. The high and irregular respiratory exchange ratio (R) at rest (Fig 10.67.1, panel 8) also supports this diagnosis. The patient does have significant obesity and hypertension, however. Reevaluation is in order when the patient is less anxious.

Conclusion

This study shows anxiety and acute resting hyperventilation with a nonphysiologic, very irregular

TABLE 10.67.3.   Air Breathing

Time min	Work rate watts	BP mmHg	HR min⁻¹	f min⁻¹	V̇E L/min BTPS	V̇CO₂ L/min STPD	V̇O₂ L/min STPD	V̇O₂/HR ml/beat	R	pH	HCO₃⁻ meq/L	PO₂, mmHg ET	a	(A−a)	PCO₂, mmHg ET	a	(a−ET)	V̇E/V̇CO₂	V̇E/V̇O₂	VD/VT
Rest	168/96									7.47	24		88			34				
Rest		67	24	22.8	0.44	0.35	5.2	1.26			125			27			47	59	
Rest		66	26	27.9	0.49	0.34	5.2	1.44			131			22			52	76	
Rest		64	28	21.9	0.37	0.30	4.7	1.23			129			24			53	65	
Rest	156/87	64	29	23.8	0.38	0.26	4.1	1.46	7.59	22	134	112	21	21	23	2	56	82	0.30
Rest		62	29	26.7	0.39	0.26	4.2	1.50			135			19			62	93	
Rest		64	27	27.9	0.39	0.26	4.1	1.50			135			18			66	98	
Rest		64	23	18.8	0.29	0.25	3.9	1.16			131			20			58	67	
Rest		65	25	16.6	0.26	0.28	4.3	0.93			126			23			56	52	
Unloaded		80	53	25.2	0.43	0.57	7.1	0.75			110			30			48	36	
Unloaded		90	61	38.6	0.68	0.68	7.6	1.00			123			26			49	49	
Unloaded		86	45	31.7	0.65	0.76	8.8	0.86			115			30			43	37	
Unloaded		93	46	37.5	0.77	0.80	8.6	0.96			117			30			44	42	
Unloaded		93	52	42.2	0.85	0.86	9.2	0.99			121			28			44	44	
Unloaded	207/108	90	49	40.4	0.84	0.85	9.4	0.99	7.52	22	120	106	17	29	27	−2	43	43	0.23
15		97	51	47.7	0.95	0.86	8.9	1.10			124			27			46	50	
15		97	55	51.1	0.99	0.89	9.2	1.11			123			27			47	52	
30		103	61	53.9	1.04	0.96	9.3	1.08			122			28			47	51	
30		103	61	55.4	1.05	0.98	9.5	1.07			123			27			48	51	
45		103	59	58.1	1.11	1.05	10.2	1.06			122			27			48	51	
45		108	59	56.0	1.15	1.16	10.7	0.99			120			28			44	44	
60		117	61	61.0	1.26	1.23	10.5	1.02			123			27			44	45	
60	216/108	120	59	63.2	1.35	1.31	10.9	1.03	7.49	22	121	102	20	28	29	1	43	44	0.28
75		124	61	64.5	1.42	1.38	11.1	1.03			121			28			42	43	
75		126	56	71.8	1.58	1.43	11.3	1.10			123			28			42	47	
90		130	61	78.7	1.70	1.51	11.6	1.13			123			27			43	49	
90	228/111	129	56	71.3	1.65	1.37	10.6	1.20	7.46	20	123	100	25	29	29	0	40	49	024
Recovery		119	50	58.9	1.38	1.32	11.1	1.05			118			31			40	41	
Recovery		119	49	48.2	1.09	0.99	8.3	1.10			118			32			40	44	
Recovery		104	45	56.7	1.13	0.87	8.4	1.30			127			26			47	61	
										7.45	20		103			29				

breathing pattern at rest and during exercise. The combination of high heart rate reserve and normal breathing reserve without objective evidence of either myocardial, pulmonary vascular, peripheral vascular, or underlying lung disease suggests that this patient's reduced maximum oxygen uptake, and perhaps symptom of dyspnea, is psychogenic. The preexercise vasovagal reaction and the acute hyperventilation in the anticipation of exercise are consistent with this interpretation.

Case 68 Skeletal Disease Limiting Exercise

Clinical Findings

This 60-year-old former shipyard worker had enjoyed apparent good health except for arthritis of the right hip of many years' duration and hypertension, which had not been treated. He had smoked cigarettes for a short period of time 3 decades previously. Chest roentgenograms showed fibrotic changes at both bases, but no rales were heard on physical examination.

Exercise Findings

The patient felt more comfortable walking on the treadmill than pedaling the cycle ergometer. After insertion of a brachial artery catheter, he walked at 1.6 mph on the level followed by increments in grade of 2% per minute. He stopped exercise after 11 minutes because of pain in the right hip. He had no shortness of breath or palpitations. The ECG remained normal.

Interpretation

Comments

The results of the respiratory function studies are within normal limits (Table 10.68.1). The patient had significant systemic hypertension at the time of the study (Table 10.68.3). Because of arthritis of the right hip, treadmill walking was used for exercise testing. The rate of walking was slow (1.6 mph) to avoid discomfort to the patient and also so the arterial pressure could be closely monitored.

Analysis

In flowchart 1, the peak $\dot{V}O_2$ is significantly reduced but the anaerobic threshold is normal (Table 10.68.2). See flowchart 3. The breathing reserve at maximum exercise is high (branch point 3.1). The ECG is normal (branch point 3.3). The diagnosis at this point reveals either poor effort or that the patient has a musculoskeletal disorder. The normal VD/VT, borderline $P(A - a)O_2$, normal $P(a - ET)CO_2$,

high heart rate reserve, and only 1 mEq/L decrease in bicarbonate 2 minutes after the start of recovery support either of these diagnoses. However, his history, normal ventilatory pattern, and minimal acid–base changes are most consistent with a musculoskeletal disorder limiting exercise at the measured peak $\dot{V}O_2$.

Conclusion

A musculoskeletal disorder has limited this patient's exercise performance.

TABLE 10.68.1.   Selected Respiratory Function Data

Measurement	Predicted	Measured
Age, yr		60
Sex		Male
Height, cm		175
Weight, kg	78	97
Hematocrit, %		44
VC, L	3.77	4.09
IC, L	2.52	3.01
TLC, L	5.77	5.72
FEV_1, L	2.96	3.21
FEV_1/VC, %	78	78
MVV, L/min	122	94
D_LCO, ml/min Hg/min	25.0	23.9

TABLE 10.68.2.   Selected Exercise Data

Measurement	Predicted	Measured
Peak $\dot{V}O_2$, L/min	2.57	1.62
Maximum HR, beats/min	160	123
Maximum O_2 pulse, ml/beat	16.1	14.0
AT, L/min	>1.13	1.45
Blood pressure, mmHg (rest, max)		186/117, 213/123
Maximum $\dot{V}E$, L/min		52
Exercise breathing reserve, L/min	>15	42
PaO_2, mmHg (rest, max ex)		90, 80
$P(A - a)O_2$, mmHg (rest, max ex)		10, 32
$P(a - ET)CO_2$, mmHg (rest, max ex)		1, −3
VD/VT (rest, heavy ex)		0.39, 0.25
HCO_3^-, mEq/L (rest, 2-min recov)		24, 23

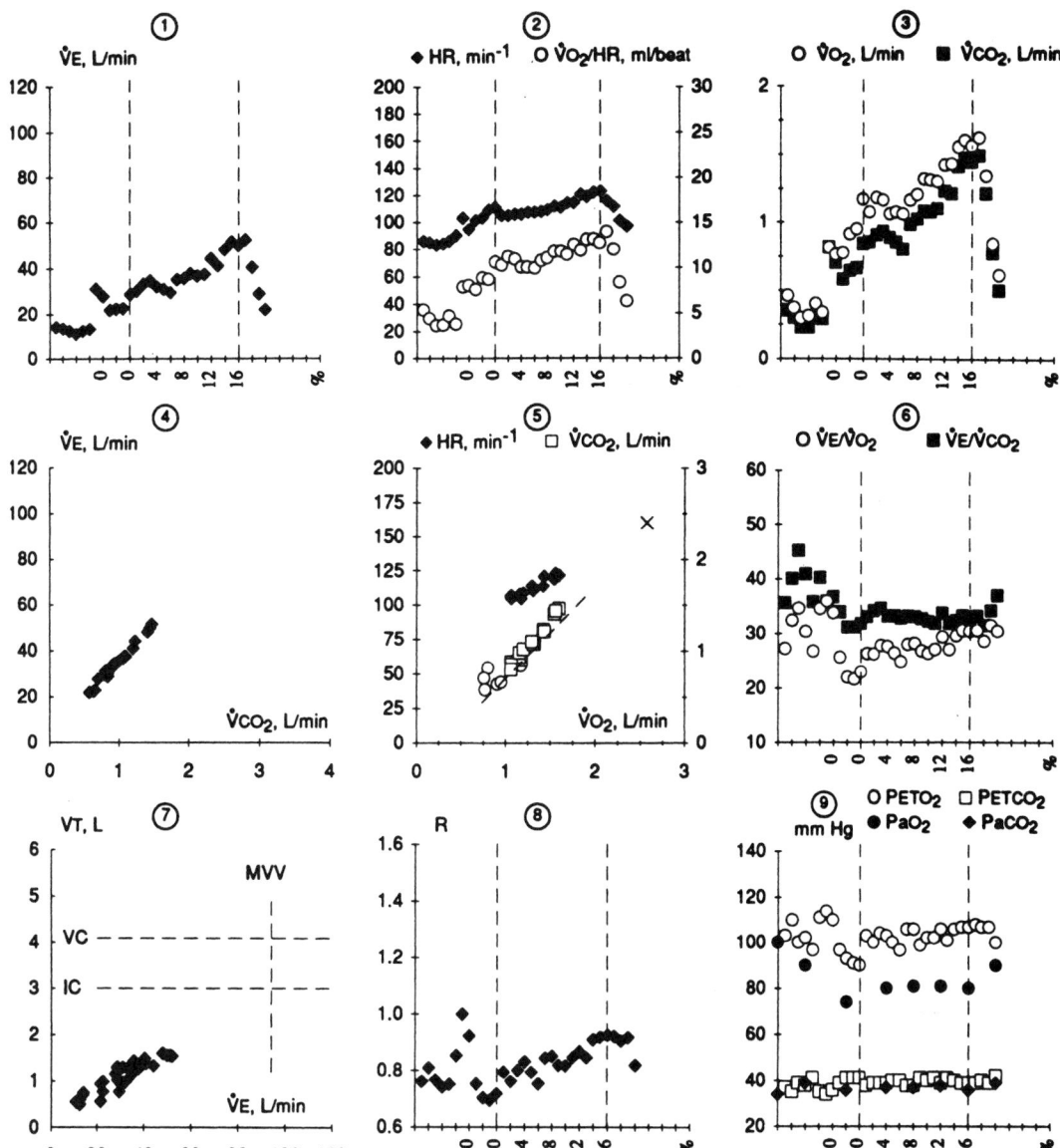

FIGURE 10.68.1.   **1:** Vertical dashed lines in panels 1 to 3 and 6, 8, and 9 indicate the beginning and the end of the increasing work period. **2:** Zero-grade walking is performed for 3 minutes before the left vertical dashed line. **3:** In panel 5, the diagonal dashed line has a slope of 1; the *x* in the upper right is the predicted maximum heart rate and $\dot{V}_{O_2}$ for the subject.

TABLE 10.68.3.   Air Breathing

Time min	Work rate watts	BP mmHg	HR min⁻¹	f min⁻¹	$\dot{V}_E$ L/min BTPS	$\dot{V}_{CO_2}$ L/min STPD	$\dot{V}_{O_2}$ L/min STPD	$\dot{V}_{O_2}$/HR ml/beat	R	pH	HCO_3^- meq/L	P_{O_2} ET	P_{O_2} a	P_{O_2} (A−a)	P_{CO_2} ET	P_{CO_2} a	P_{CO_2} (a−ET)	$\dot{V}_E/\dot{V}_{CO_2}$	$\dot{V}_E/\dot{V}_{O_2}$	V_D/V_T
	Rest	186/117								7.44	23		100			34				
	Rest		86	19	14.1	0.35	0.46	5.3	0.76			103			37			36	27	
	Rest		85	20	13.7	0.30	0.37	4.4	0.81			110			35			40	32	
	Rest		83	25	12.5	0.23	0.30	3.6	0.77			100			39			45	35	
	Rest	192/126	84	20	11.1	0.23	0.31	3.7	0.74	7.41	24	102	90	10	38	39	1	41	30	0.39
	Rest		86	21	12.5	0.30	0.40	4.7	0.75			97			41			36	27	
	Rest		90	20	13.4	0.29	0.34	3.8	0.85			111			35			40	34	
	0		103	24	31.1	0.81	0.81	7.9	1.00			114			34			36	36	
	0		95	24	27.7	0.70	0.76	8.0	0.92			110			36			37	34	
	0		101	23	21.6	0.58	0.77	7.6	0.75			97			39			34	26	
	0	216/129	103	29	22.4	0.64	0.91	8.8	0.70	7.41	22	93	74	28	41	36	−5	31	22	0.21
	0		109	23	22.5	0.66	0.95	8.7	0.69			91			41			31	22	
	0		111	22	28.6	0.84	1.17	10.5	0.72			90			41			32	23	
0.5	2		105	24	30.1	0.85	1.07	10.2	0.79			103			38			33	26	
1.0	2		105	26	33.0	0.90	1.18	11.2	0.76			100			39			34	26	
1.5	4		106	28	34.6	0.93	1.16	10.9	0.80			104			39			35	28	
2.0	4	216/126	106	33	31.9	0.88	1.06	10.0	0.83	7.41	23	103	80	27	39	37	−2	33	27	0.27
2.5	6		107	32	30.9	0.85	1.07	10.0	0.79			100			40			33	26	
3.0	6		107	38	29.4	0.80	1.06	9.9	0.75			97			40			33	25	
3.5	8		108	31	35.0	0.98	1.16	10.7	0.84			106			38			33	28	
4.0	8	210/123	109	25	35.8	1.02	1.20	11.0	0.85	7.41	23	106	81	27	38	37	−1	33	28	0.28
4.5	10		112	30	37.8	1.08	1.32	11.8	0.82			99			41			33	27	
5.0	10		111	28	36.8	1.07	1.31	11.8	0.82			102			40			32	26	
5.5	12		114	28	37.4	1.10	1.30	11.4	0.85			102			41			32	27	
6.0	12	216/123	114	33	44.3	1.23	1.42	12.5	0.87	7.40	23	106	81	26	39	38	−1	34	29	0.31
6.5	14		121	30	44.1	1.21	1.43	11.8	0.85			101			41			32	27	
7.0	14		119	30	48.3	1.41	1.55	13.0	0.91			106			40			32	30	
7.5	16		122	33	51.5	1.47	1.60	13.1	0.92			107			39			33	30	
8.0	16	213/123	123	32	49.9	1.44	1.56	12.7	0.92	7.40	22	107	80	32	39	36	−3	33	30	0.25
	Recovery		116	34	52.2	1.49	1.62	14.0	0.92			108			39			33	30	
	Recovery		112	27	40.4	1.21	1.34	12.0	0.90			107			40			31	28	
	Recovery		101	28	28.7	0.77	0.84	8.3	0.92			107			39			34	31	
	Recovery	192/126	97	38	21.7	0.50	0.61	6.3	0.82	7.39	23	100	90	14	42	39	−3	37	30	0.34

Case 69 Ankylosing Spondylitis
Clinical Findings

This 51-year-old airline employee had first developed symptoms of ankylosing spondylitis, primarily involving the neck and thoracic spine, approximately 6 years prior to evaluation. He had received some relief of pain with indomethacin. He had stopped smoking over 10 years previously. On the basis of pleural changes at the apices, he had been treated for tuberculosis several years ago, although the tuberculin skin test was negative. To maintain fitness, he had begun running approximately 3 miles a day. In recent months he had felt as if he "could not get enough air into his lungs" and found himself taking gasping breaths. Physical examination revealed reduced neck movement and thoracic expansion. Chest roentgenograms revealed apical pleural thickening. ECG was normal.

Exercise Findings

The patient performed exercise on a cycle ergometer. He pedaled at 60 rpm without added load for 3 minutes. The work rate was then increased 20 W per minute to his symptom-limited maximum. He stopped exercise because of shortness of breath. Exercise ECGs were normal except for a single interpolated ventricular premature contraction.

Interpretation
Comments

The results of spirometry and total lung capacity measurement suggest that the patient has mild restrictive disease (Table 10.69.1) consequent to his ankylosing spondylitis. This is reflected in part by a reduction in the inspiratory capacity (loss of his ability to expand his chest wall). The resting ECG is normal.

Analysis

In flowchart 1, the peak $\dot{V}O_2$ and the anaerobic threshold are normal (Table 10.69.2). See flowchart 2. The ECG and O_2 pulse at peak $\dot{V}O_2$ are normal (branch point 2.1). The subject is not obese (branch

point 2.2). The normal ventilatory equivalent for CO_2 at the anaerobic threshold suggests that ventilation–perfusion matching is normal. The observation that tidal volume reaches the inspiratory capacity (panel 7, Fig. 10.69.1) reflects the changes that would be expected from restrictive pulmonary or chest wall disease. Note that the indirect MVV is close to the maximum exercise ventilation, resulting in virtually no breathing reserve. This is further evidence of ventilatory limitation.

Conclusion

Exertional dyspnea secondary to restrictive changes in the chest wall consequent to ankylosing spondylitis.

TABLE 10.69.1.   Selected Respiratory Function Data

Measurement	Predicted	Measured
Age, yr		51
Sex		Male
Height, cm		178
Weight, kg	80	79
Hematocrit, %		39
VC, L	4.62	3.61
IC, L	3.08	2.60
FEV$_1$, L	3.67	2.76
FEV$_1$/VC, %	79	76
MVV, L/min, direct	151	132 at f = 80/min
MVV, L/min, indirect	147	110

TABLE 10.69.2.   Selected Exercise Data

Measurement	Predicted	Measured
Peak $\dot{V}O_2$, L/min	2.52	2.54
Maximum HR, beats/min	169	170
Maximum O_2 pulse, ml/beat	14.9	14.9
$\Delta\dot{V}O_2/\Delta WR$, ml/min/W	10.3	9.4
AT, L/min	>1.08	1.4
Blood pressure, mmHg (rest, max)		126/86, 206/84
Maximum $\dot{V}E$, L/min		108
Exercise breathing reserve, L/min	>15	2

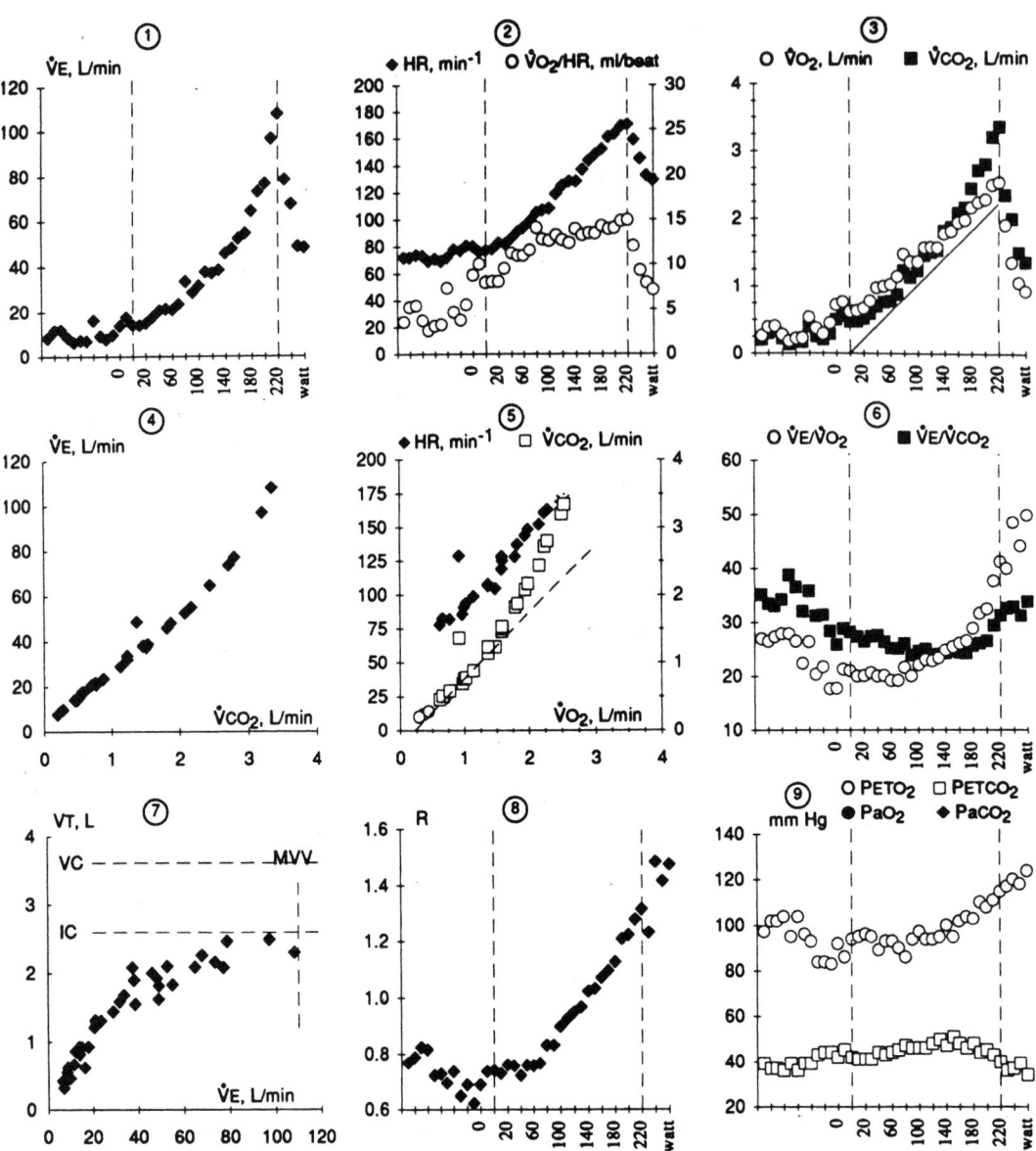

FIGURE 10.69.1.   **1:** Vertical dashed lines in panels 1 to 3 and 6, 8, and 9 indicate the beginning and the end of the increasing work period. **2:** Unloaded cycling is performed for 3 minutes before the left vertical dashed line. **3:** In panel 3, the diagonal line shows the increase of $\dot{V}O_2$ at a slope of 10 ml/min/W. **4:** In panel 5, the diagonal dashed line has a slope of 1; the x in the upper right is the predicted maximum heart rate and $\dot{V}O_2$ for the subject.

TABLE 10.69.3.   Air Breathing

Time min	Work rate watts	BP mmHg	HR min^{-1}	f min^{-1}	$\dot{V}_E$ L/min BTPS	$\dot{V}_{CO_2}$ L/min STPD	$\dot{V}_{O_2}$ L/min STPD	$\dfrac{\dot{V}_{O_2}}{HR}$ ml/beat	R	pH	HCO$_3^-$ meq/L	P_{O_2}, mmHg ET	a	(A − a)	P_{CO_2}, mmHg ET	a	(a − ET)	$\dfrac{\dot{V}_E}{\dot{V}_{CO_2}}$	$\dfrac{\dot{V}_E}{\dot{V}_{O_2}}$	$\dfrac{V_D}{V_T}$
	Rest		72	15	8.3	0.20	0.26	3.6	0.77			97			39			35	27	
	Rest		72	17	11.5	0.30	0.38	5.3	0.79			102			37			34	26	
	Rest		74	14	12.1	0.33	0.40	5.4	0.83			102			37			33	27	
	Rest		73	14	8.7	0.22	0.27	3.7	0.81			104			36			34	28	
	Rest		69	15	6.3	0.13	0.18	2.6	0.72			95			39			39	28	
	Rest	126/86	71	16	7.2	0.16	0.22	3.1	0.73			104			36			37	27	
	Rest		69	22	7.0	0.16	0.23	3.3	0.70			96			39			32	22	
	Rest		72	26	16.2	0.39	0.53	7.4	0.74			93			39			36	26	
	Unloaded		78	19	9.1	0.24	0.37	4.7	0.65			84			43			31	20	
	Unloaded		77	18	7.8	0.20	0.29	3.8	0.69			84			44			31	22	
	Unloaded		81	21	9.7	0.28	0.45	5.6	0.62			83			44			28	18	
	Unloaded		80	15	13.9	0.49	0.71	8.9	0.69			92			42			26	18	
	Unloaded		76	19	17.7	0.56	0.76	10.0	0.74			86			45			29	21	
	Unloaded		77	16	14.3	0.46	0.62	8.1	0.74			94			42			28	21	
0.5	20		78	17	14.0	0.46	0.63	8.1	0.73			95			41			27	20	
1.0	20	158/86	83	16	14.8	0.51	0.67	8.1	0.76			96			41			26	20	
1.5	40		82	19	17.7	0.59	0.78	9.5	0.76			95			41			27	21	
2.0	40	174/84	86	17	20.7	0.70	0.97	11.3	0.72			89			44			28	20	
2.5	60		91	17	21.4	0.76	1.00	11.0	0.76			93			43			26	20	
3.0	60		94	16	21.0	0.78	1.03	11.0	0.76			93			44			25	19	
3.5	80		99	18	23.5	0.88	1.15	11.6	0.77			90			45			25	19	
4.0	80	178/78	105	20	33.6	1.23	1.48	14.1	0.83			86			47			26	22	
4.5	100		107	20	28.9	1.14	1.37	12.8	0.83			94			46			24	20	
5.0	100		108	20	31.8	1.23	1.37	12.7	0.90			97			46			24	22	
5.5	120		119	20	38.0	1.46	1.58	13.3	0.92			94			46			25	23	
6.0	120	190/86	125	18	37.5	1.51	1.59	12.7	0.95			94			48			24	23	
6.5	140		128	25	38.8	1.53	1.58	12.3	0.97			95			50			24	23	
7.0	140		128	23	46.1	1.82	1.78	13.9	1.02			100			47			24	25	
7.5	160		137	25	48.3	1.88	1.82	13.3	1.03			95			51			25	25	
8.0	160	206/84	144	25	52.7	2.08	1.94	13.5	1.07			102			48			24	26	
8.5	180		148	30	55.1	2.17	1.98	13.4	1.10			104			46			24	27	
9.0	180		152	31	64.8	2.44	2.16	14.2	1.13			103			48			25	29	
9.5	200		161	34	73.6	2.71	2.24	13.9	1.21			110			44			26	32	
10.0	200		163	37	77.2	2.80	2.29	14.0	1.22			108			45			26	32	
10.5	220		169	39	97.2	3.20	2.50	14.8	1.28			111			43			29	38	
11.0	220		170	47	108.3	3.34	2.54	14.9	1.31			115			40			31	41	
	Recovery		159	32	78.9	2.35	1.91	12.0	1.23			117			36			32	40	
	Recovery		145	30	67.9	2.00	1.35	9.3	1.48			120			37			33	48	
	Recovery	160/78	133	27	49.1	1.50	1.06	8.0	1.42			118			39			31	44	
	Recovery		129	30	48.8	1.37	0.93	7.2	1.47			124			34			34	50	

Case 70 Myasthenia Gravis

Clinical Findings

This 62-year-old retired shipyard worker had been found to have myasthenia gravis 21 years earlier. He had taken 30 mg of pyridostigmine bromide with benefit for many years. He had a 20 pack-year history of smoking cigarettes but had stopped 21 years ago. He had a daily minimally productive cough. He took digoxin for an arrhythmia and reserpine for hypertension. He complained of gradually increasing shortness of breath in the last 3 years, evident when walking two to three blocks slowly or climbing a flight of stairs. There was no evidence of pulmonary or cardiovascular disease on physical examination. Chest roentgenogram was normal except for old granulomatous disease. Resting ECG showed sinus bradycardia and ST-segment depression in V_5 and V_6 consistent with digitalis effect.

Exercise Findings

The patient performed exercise on a cycle ergometer. He pedaled at 60 rpm without added load for 3 minutes. The work rate was then increased 15 W per minute to his symptom-limited maximum. Arterial blood was sampled every second minute, and intraarterial blood pressure was recorded from a percutaneously placed brachial artery catheter. He stopped exercise complaining of leg pain and generalized fatigue. A single premature ventricular contraction occurred at 60 W.

Interpretation

Comments

This patient appears to have mild restrictive lung or chest wall disease (Table 10.70.1). Because the diffusing capacity is within normal limits and the MVV is significantly reduced, the latter diagnosis is more likely. The resting ECG is normal except for the digitalis effect.

Analysis

In flowchart 1, the peak oxygen uptake is reduced but the anaerobic threshold is normal (Table 10.70.2). See flowchart 3. The breathing reserve at the maximum work rate is normal (branch point 3.1). The ECG remained normal except for the digitalis effect (branch point 3.3). This suggests that the patient either made poor effort or had a muscu-

loskeletal disorder. The indices of ventilation–perfusion mismatching are normal, supporting the concept that this patient does not have significant pulmonary disease. (V_D/V_T of 0.31 to 0.33 is considered to be normal in view of the low level of exercise performed.) The high heart rate reserve and small decrease in bicarbonate support the observation that the cardiovascular system was only minimally stressed. The reduced peak $\dot{V}_{O_2}$, with the strikingly reduced MVV, suggests that this patient is limited by a chest wall defect.

Conclusion

Exercise limitation without cardiovascular or ventilatory impairment. Limitation is most likely secondary to myasthenia gravis.

TABLE 10.70.1.   Selected Respiratory Function Data

Measurement	Predicted	Measured
Age, yr		62
Sex		Male
Height, cm		178
Weight, kg	80	80
Hematocrit, %		39
VC, L	3.87	2.96
IC, L	2.58	2.08
TLC, L	5.95	4.64
FEV_1, L	3.03	2.42
FEV_1/VC, %	78	82
MVV, L/min	123	56
D_LCO, ml/min Hg/min	24.7	25.6

TABLE 10.70.2.   Selected Exercise Data

Measurement	Predicted	Measured
Peak $\dot{V}_{O_2}$, L/min	2.21	1.09
Maximum HR, beats/min	158	102
Maximum O_2 pulse, ml/beat	14.0	10.8
$\Delta\dot{V}_{O_2}/\Delta$WR, ml/min/W	10.3	10.5
AT, L/min	>0.97	>1.1
Blood pressure, mmHg (rest, max)		158/84, 210/84
Maximum $\dot{V}_E$, L/min		37
Exercise breathing reserve, L/min	>15	19
Pa_{O_2}, mmHg (rest, max ex)		95, 86
P(A − a)$_{O_2}$, mmHg (rest, max ex)		8, 21
P(a − ET)$_{CO_2}$, mmHg (rest, max ex)		3, 1
V_D/V_T (rest, heavy ex)		0.39, 0.31
HCO_3^-, mEq/L (rest, 2-min recov)		25, 23

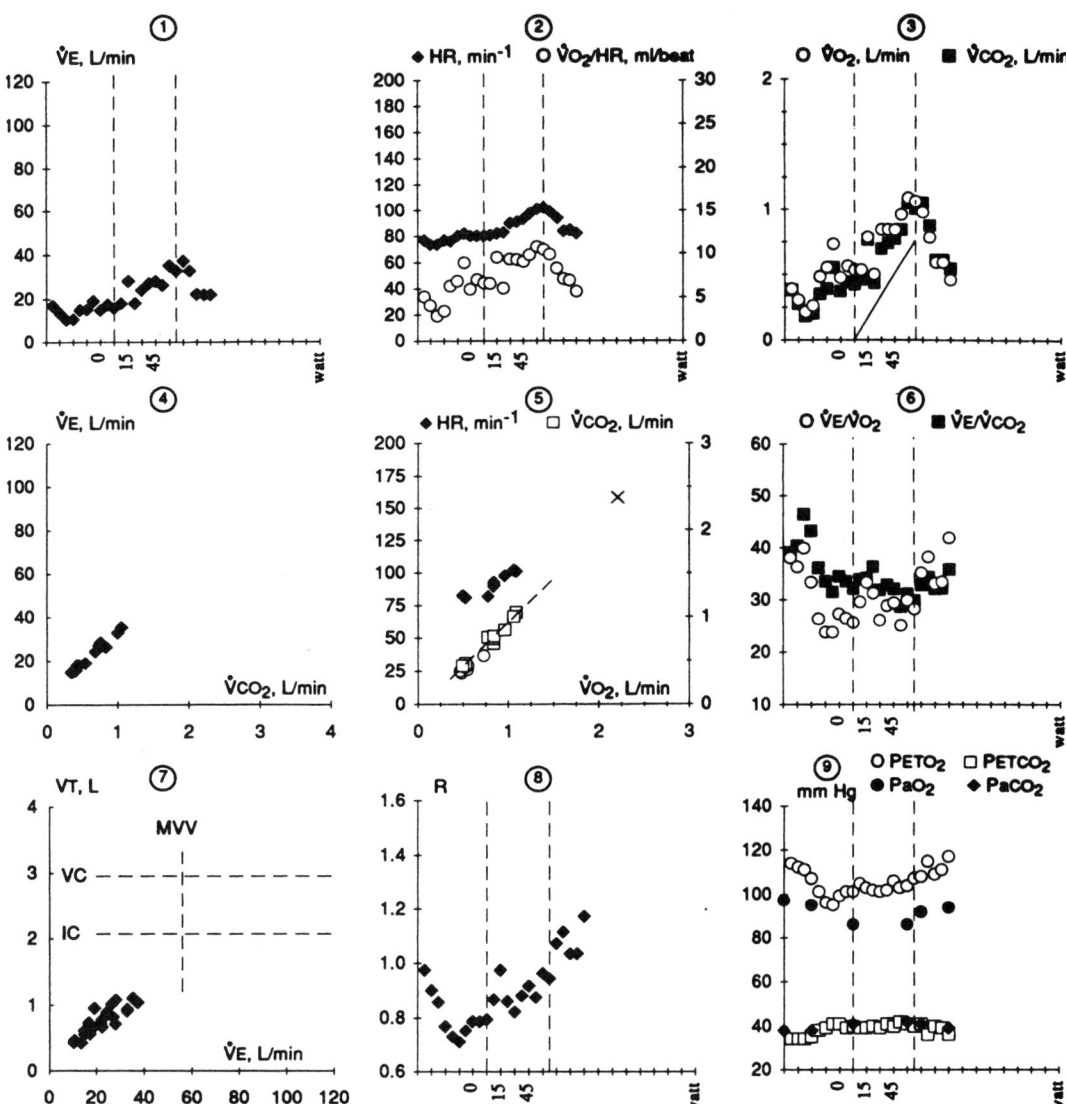

FIGURE 10.70.1.   **1:** Vertical dashed lines in panels 1 to 3 and 6, 8, and 9 indicate the beginning and the end of the increasing work period. **2:** Unloaded cycling is performed for 3 minutes before the left vertical dashed line. **3:** In panel 3, the diagonal line shows the increase of $\dot{V}O_2$ at a slope of 10 ml/min/W. **4:** In panel 5, the diagonal dashed line has a slope of 1; the x in the upper right is the predicted maximum heart rate and $\dot{V}O_2$ for the subject.

TABLE 10.70.3. **Air Breathing**

Time min	Work rate watts	BP mmHg	HR min⁻¹	f min⁻¹	$\dot{V}_E$ L/min BTPS	$\dot{V}_{CO_2}$ L/min STPD	$\dot{V}_{O_2}$ L/min STPD	$\dot{V}_{O_2}$/HR ml/beat	R	pH	HCO₃⁻ meq/L	P_{O_2}, mmHg ET	a	(A−a)	P_{CO_2}, mmHg ET	a	(a−ET)	$\dot{V}_E/\dot{V}_{CO_2}$	$\dot{V}_E/\dot{V}_{O_2}$	V_D/V_T
	Rest	153/84								7.42	24		97			38				
	Rest		77	23	16.8	0.38	0.39	5.1	0.97			114			34			39	38	
	Rest		74	32	13.6	0.27	0.30	4.1	0.90			112			34			40	36	
	Rest		74	24	10.4	0.18	0.21	2.8	0.86			111			34			46	40	
	Rest	138/78	77	23	10.6	0.20	0.26	3.4	0.77	7.43	25	107	95	8	35	38	3	43	33	0.39
	Unloaded		76	27	14.9	0.35	0.48	6.3	0.73			101			38			36	26	
	Unloaded		80	25	15.2	0.39	0.55	6.9	0.71			96			39			34	24	
	Unloaded		82	20	19.0	0.55	0.73	8.9	0.75			95			41			31	24	
	Unloaded		80	24	14.8	0.37	0.47	5.9	0.79			99			41			34	27	
	Unloaded		80	31	17.4	0.44	0.56	7.0	0.79			101			39			34	26	
	Unloaded	165/81	80	27	15.8	0.42	0.53	6.6	0.79	7.41	26	101	86	15	40	41	1	32	25	0.30
0.5	15		81	27	17.9	0.46	0.53	6.5	0.87			105			39			34	29	
1.0	15		82	26	28.1	0.76	0.78	9.5	0.97			103			39			34	33	
1.5	30		83	28	18.0	0.43	0.50	6.0	0.86			102			40			36	31	
2.0	30	162/78	90	27	24.2	0.69	0.84	9.3	0.82			101			39			32	26	
2.5	45		91	33	27.0	0.74	0.84	9.2	0.88			102			41			33	29	
3.0	45		93	39	28.0	0.77	0.84	9.0	0.92			106			40			32	29	
3.5	60		98	26	26.2	0.84	0.96	9.8	0.88			103			42			29	25	
4.0	60	192/81	101	32	35.3	1.05	1.09	10.8	0.96	7.38	24	104	86	21	41	42	1	31	30	0.31
4.5	75		102	35	32.8	1.00	1.06	10.4	0.94			107			40			30	28	
	Recovery		99	36	37.4	1.05	0.98	9.9	1.07	7.38	24	108	92	19	41	41	0	33	35	0.33
	Recovery		94	36	32.8	0.87	0.78	8.3	1.12			115			36			34	38	
	Recovery		84	33	22.3	0.61	0.59	7.0	1.03			109			40			32	33	
	Recovery		85	28	22.0	0.61	0.59	6.9	1.03			111			39			32	33	
	Recovery	174/84	82	30	21.8	0.54	0.46	5.6	1.17	7.38	23	117	94	22	36	39	3	26	42	0.33

Case 71 Aortic and Mitral Stenosis and Obstructive Airway Disease

Clinical Findings

This 43-year-old man developed dyspnea and precordial pain at rest and on exertion 3 weeks prior to study. He had a history of "passing out" with or without prior feelings of lightheadedness. He also noted cough and sputum production with exertion. He was a welder and an extremely heavy smoker, but he stated that he had reduced his smoking to several cigarettes daily. Evaluation, including cardiac catheterization, revealed severe aortic stenosis (1.4 cm^2 valvular area), normal coronary arteries, and an elevated pulmonary artery pressure of 50/25 mm Hg and wedge pressure of 16 mm Hg. Medications included an oral β-adrenergic blocker, theophylline, and an α-agonist inhaler. Physical examination was consistent with aortic stenosis and mitral valve disease, but the patient had no rales or wheezes.

Exercise Findings

The patient performed exercise on a cycle ergometer. He pedaled at 60 rpm without an added load for 3 minutes. The work rate was then increased 15 W per minute to tolerance. Blood was sampled every second minute, and intraarterial blood pressure was recorded from a percutaneously placed brachial artery catheter. The resting ECG was normal except for an intraventricular conduction defect. The patient had neither chest pain nor ectopy during exercise, but he had expiratory wheezes and frequent premature atrial and ventricular contractions early in recovery. The arterial pressure tracing showed a delayed upstroke (200 milliseconds to peak pressure).

Interpretation

Comments

Resting respiratory function tests reveal moderately severe obstructive lung disease with some response to inhaled albuterol and with a decreased $D_{L}CO$ for the subject (Table 10.71.1). Wheezing was noted during recovery from exercise. The carboxyhemoglobin level is increased. The patient has known significant valvular heart disease. The systemic blood pressure tracing showed a delayed upstroke (200 milliseconds to peak pressure), pulse pressure was low at rest, and systolic pressure did not increase normally during exercise.

Analysis

In flowchart 1, peak $\dot{V}O_2$ and the anaerobic threshold are decreased (Table 10.71.2). Proceeding to flowchart 4, the low breathing reserve (branch point 4.1) and high exercise V_D/V_T (branch point 4.2) lead us to the diagnosis of lung disease with impaired peripheral oxygenation. This is an acceptable, but incomplete, diagnosis because the impaired peripheral oxygenation was not due primarily to the increase in pulmonary vascular resistance, but rather to left-sided failure from valvular heart disease. The low anaerobic threshold, low $\Delta\dot{V}O_2/\Delta WR$, and low,

TABLE 10.71.1.   Selected Respiratory Function Data

Measurement	Predicted	Before Bronchodilator	After Bronchodilator
Age, yr		43	
Sex		Male	
Height, cm		171	
Weight, kg	74	89	
Hemoglobin, g/100 ml		15.4	
VC, L	4.47	3.03	3.14
IC, L	2.98	2.03	2.23
TLC, L	6.32	6.54	
FEV$_1$, L	3.58	1.65	1.84
FEV$_1$/VC, %	80	54	
MVV, L/min	154	62	73
D$_L$CO, ml/mm Hg/min	27.2	19.8	

TABLE 10.71.2.   Selected Exercise Data

Measurement	Predicted	Measured
Peak $\dot{V}O_2$, L/min	2.70	1.48
Maximum HR, beats/min	177	140
Maximum O$_2$ pulse, ml/beat	15.3	10.6
$\Delta\dot{V}O_2/\Delta WR$, ml/min/W	10.3	8.5
AT, L/min	>1.13	>1.0
Blood pressure, mmHg (rest, max ex)		96/69, 132/69
Maximum $\dot{V}E$, L/min		59
Exercise breathing reserve, L/min	>15	14
PaO$_2$, mmHg (rest, mod ex)		84, 95
P(A − a)O$_2$, mmHg (rest, mod ex)		16, 14
P(a − ET)CO$_2$, mmHg (rest, mod ex)		3, 3
VD/VT (rest, max ex)		0.33, 0.32
HCO$_3^-$, mEq/L (rest, 2-min recov)		25, 24
Carboxyhemoglobin, %		4.3

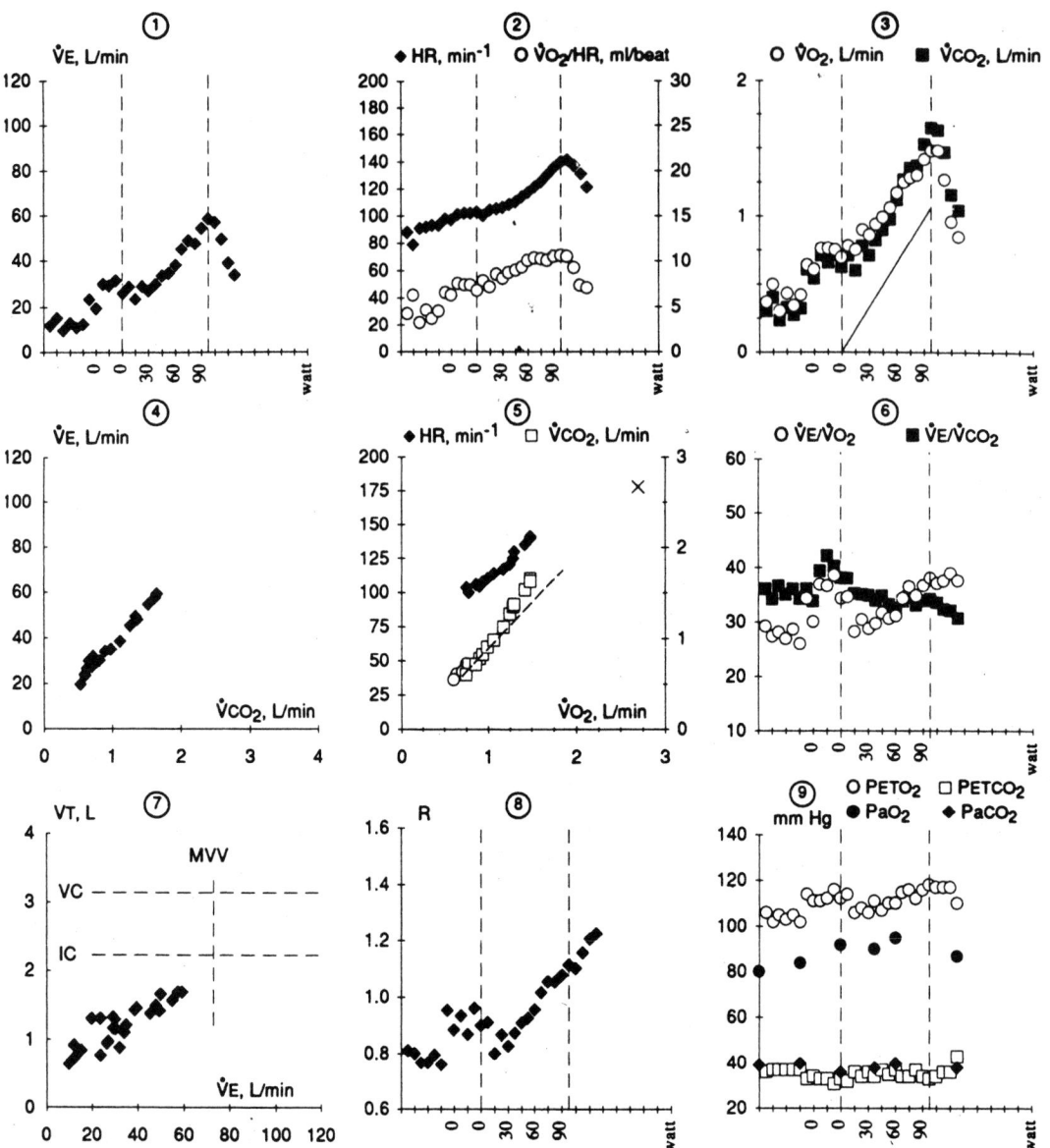

FIGURE 10.71.1.   **1:** Vertical dashed lines in panels 1 to 3 and 6, 8, and 9 indicate the beginning and the end of the increasing work period. **2:** Unloaded cycling is performed for 3 minutes before the left vertical dashed line. **3:** In panel 3, the diagonal line shows the increase of $\dot{V}O_2$ at a slope of 10 ml/min/W. **4:** In panel 5, the diagonal dashed line has a slope of 1; the x in the upper right is the predicted maximum heart rate and $\dot{V}O_2$ for the subject.

nearly flat O_2 pulse despite β-adrenergic blockade are all evidence of a low maximal cardiac output. Could the low cardiac output be exclusively due to pulmonary vascular disease secondary to heart failure or emphysema? This is possible, but it seems unlikely, considering the symptoms of recurrent lightheadedness and the findings of severe aortic valve disease confirmed by cardiac catheterization

and the slow upstroke in the arterial pressure tracing with exercise.

Conclusion

Exercise intolerance is due to the inability to increase cardiac output appropriately with exertion, primarily related to aortic valvular disease.

TABLE 10.71.3.   Air Breathing

Time min	Work rate watts	BP mmHg	HR min⁻¹	f min⁻¹	$\dot{V}_E$ L/min BTPS	$\dot{V}_{CO_2}$ L/min STPD	$\dot{V}_{O_2}$ L/min STPD	$\dot{V}_{O_2}$/HR ml/beat	R	pH	HCO₃⁻ meq/L	PO₂ ET	PO₂ a	PO₂ (A−a)	PCO₂ ET	PCO₂ a	PCO₂ (a−ET)	$\dot{V}_E$/$\dot{V}_{CO_2}$	$\dot{V}_E$/$\dot{V}_{O_2}$	VD/VT
	Rest	93/63								7.42	25		80			39				
	Rest		88	13	11.9	0.30	0.37	4.2	0.81			106			36			36	29	
	Rest		79	18	15.2	0.40	0.50	6.3	0.80			102			37			34	27	
	Rest		91	15	9.7	0.23	0.30	3.3	0.77			105			37			37	28	
	Rest		92	17	13.0	0.33	0.43	4.7	0.77			103			37			35	27	
	Rest		93	16	11.1	0.27	0.34	3.7	0.79			105			37			36	29	
	Rest	96/69	93	17	12.4	0.32	0.42	4.5	0.76	7.41	25	102	84	16	37	40	3	34	26	0.33
	Unloaded		98	18	23.5	0.61	0.64	6.5	0.95			114			33			36	34	
	Unloaded		97	15	19.6	0.54	0.61	6.3	0.89			111			34			34	30	
	Unloaded		101	26	30.2	0.71	0.76	7.5	0.93			111			33			39	37	
	Unloaded		102	23	29.8	0.66	0.76	7.5	0.87			112			33			42	37	
	Unloaded		102	36	32.0	0.72	0.75	7.4	0.96			116			31			40	39	
	Unloaded	114/75	103	28	26.4	0.63	0.70	6.8	0.90	7.46	25	112	92	19	33	36	3	38	34	0.34
0.5	15		100	25	29.1	0.71	0.78	7.8	0.91			114			32			38	35	
1.0	15		104	31	23.8	0.60	0.75	7.2	0.80			106			36			35	28	
1.5	30		105	22	29.2	0.78	0.90	8.6	0.87			106			34			35	30	
2.0	30		106	28	27.2	0.71	0.86	8.1	0.83			106			36			35	29	
2.5	45	117/78	108	26	30.1	0.82	0.94	8.7	0.87	7.43	25	111	90	18	34	38	4	34	30	0.31
3.0	45		110	31	34.0	0.90	0.99	9.0	0.91			107			37			35	32	
3.5	60		114	29	35.0	0.98	1.06	9.3	0.92			110			35			33	31	
4.0	60	114/69	117	27	38.7	1.12	1.17	10.0	0.96	7.35	22	110	95	14	37	40	3	33	31	0.32
4.5	75		121	33	45.6	1.27	1.25	10.3	1.02			115			34			34	34	
5.0	75		125	35	49.6	1.35	1.28	10.2	1.05			116			34			35	36	
5.5	90		130	32	48.0	1.37	1.30	10.0	1.05			112			37			33	35	
6.0	90	132/69	135	35	54.9	1.53	1.42	10.5	1.08			116			34			34	37	
6.5	105		140	35	59.2	1.65	1.48	10.6	1.11			118			33			34	38	
7.0			141	34	57.6	1.63	1.48	10.5	1.10			117			34			34	37	
	Recovery		137	30	50.0	1.47	1.27	9.3	1.16			117			36			32	37	
	Recovery		131	27	39.5	1.16	0.96	7.3	1.21			117			36			32	39	
	Recovery	114/72	121	29	34.3	1.04	0.85	7.0	1.22	7.42	24	110	87	30	43	38	−5	31	37	0.24

Case 72 Left Ventricular Failure and Mild Obstructive Airway Disease: Cycle and Treadmill Studies

Clinical Findings

This 64-year-old shipyard worker was referred for evaluation. He stated that he was not limited in any of his activities; he had no shortness of breath walking on the level and only mild dyspnea after climbing 25 steps. He had smoked a half a pack of cigarettes daily until 1 year prior to this evaluation. Physical examination revealed no abnormality of the cardiovascular or respiratory systems except for a resting blood pressure of 160/84. Questionable pleural thickening was noted on chest roentgenographic studies. There was a small but consistent improvement in expiratory flow rates and MVV following inhalation of aerosolized isoproterenol.

Exercise Findings

The patient performed exercise on a cycle ergometer and, 1 month later, on a treadmill. He first pedaled at 60 rpm without added load for 3 minutes. The work rate was then increased 20 W per minute to his symptom-limited maximum. Arterial blood was sampled every second minute, and intraarterial blood pressure was recorded from a percutaneously placed brachial artery catheter. The resting ECG was normal. He stopped exercising because of leg fatigue. Near the end of cycle exercise, 1-mm horizontal ST depression was noted in leads II, III, and aVF. On repeat testing 1 month later on the treadmill, the patient stopped exercising because he "could not get a good deep breath" and felt tired. There were no abnormal ECG findings on that test.

Interpretation

Comments

This case is presented to contrast cycle with treadmill incremental exercise testing. Respiratory function measurements at rest suggest that this patient has mild obstructive lung disease (Table 10.72.1). Moreover, note that the patient hyperventilated at rest ($PaCO_2$ and R values in Table 10.72.3) when first starting to breathe on the mouthpiece.

TABLE 10.72.1.   Selected Respiratory Function Data

Measurement	Predicted	Measured
Age, yr		64
Sex		Male
Height, cm		182
Weight, kg	83	80
Hematocrit, %		47
VC, L	4.49	4.25
IC, L	2.99	3.85
TLC, L	6.94	7.61
FEV_1, L	3.51	2.96
FEV_1/VC, %	78	70
MVV, L/min	140	121
D_LCO, ml/mm Hg/min	28.8	28.1

TABLE 10.72.2.   Selected Exercise Data

Measurement	Predicted Cycle	Predicted Treadmill	Measured Cycle	Measured Treadmill
Peak $\dot{V}O_2$, L/min	2.19	2.43	1.56	1.65
Maximum HR, beats/min	156	156	143	157
Maximum O_2 pulse, ml/beat	14.1	15.6	10.9	10.5
$\Delta \dot{V}O_2/\Delta WR$, ml/min/W	10.3		9.7	
AT, L/min	>0.97	>1.08	1.0	1.1
Blood pressure, mmHg (rest, max)			194/98, 230/98	
Maximum $\dot{V}E$, L/min			68	77
Exercise breathing reserve, L/min			53	44
PaO_2, mmHg (rest, max ex)			98, 104	
$P(A - a)O_2$, mmHg (rest, max ex)			22, 18	
$P(a - ET)CO_2$, mmHg (rest, max ex)			2, −3	
VD/VT (rest, heavy ex)			0.30, 0.24	
HCO_3^-, mEq/L (rest, 2-min recov)			24, 17	

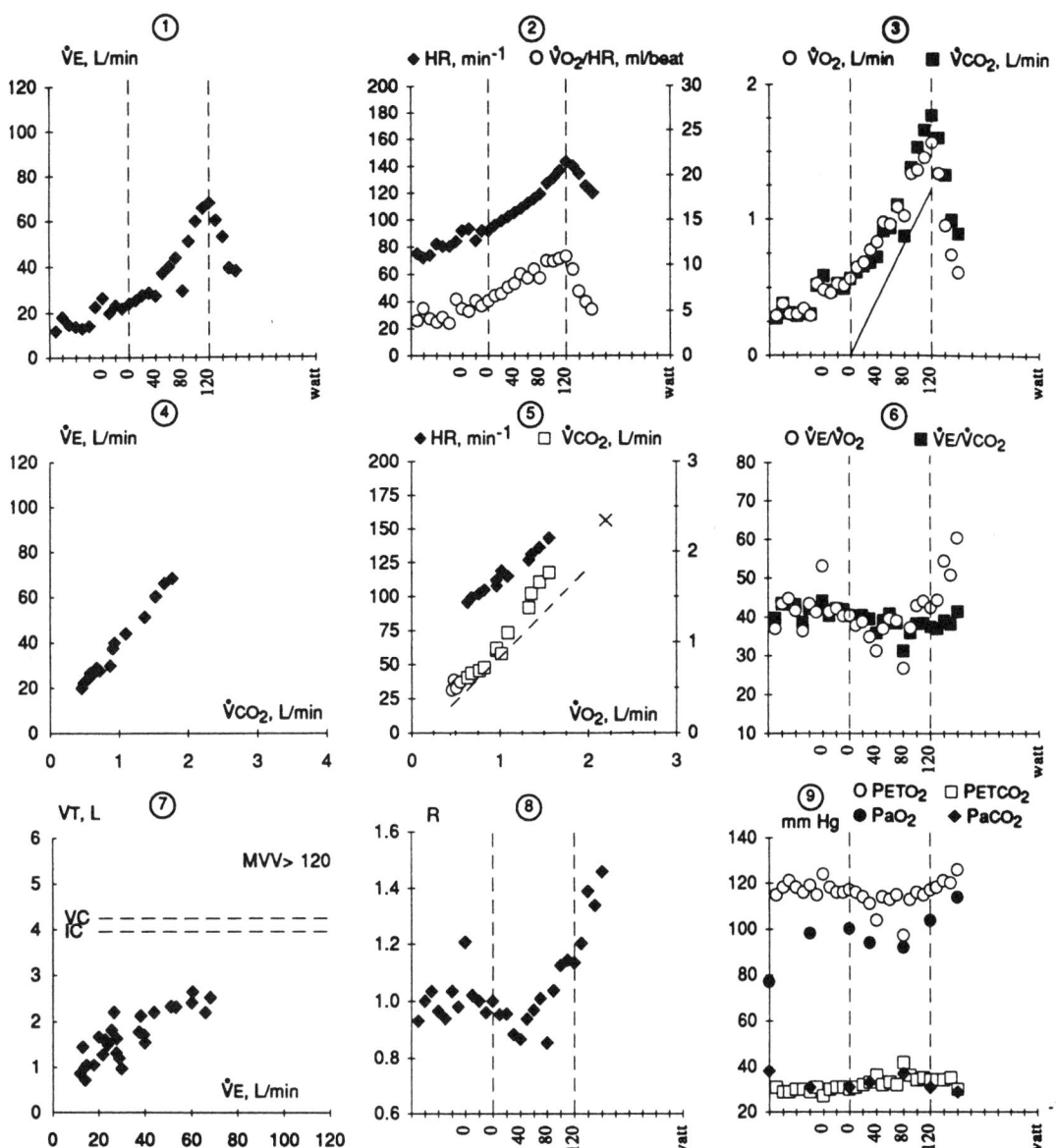

FIGURE 10.72.1.   Cycle ergometry. **1:** Vertical dashed lines in panels 1 to 3 and 6, 8, and 9 indicate the beginning and the end of the increasing work period. **2:** Unloaded cycling is performed for 3 minutes before the left vertical dashed line. **3:** In panel 3, the diagonal line shows the increase of $\dot{V}O_2$ at a slope of 10 ml/min/W. **4:** In panel 5, the diagonal dashed line has a slope of 1; the x in the upper right is the predicted maximum heart rate and $\dot{V}O_2$ for the subject.

Analysis

The peak $\dot{V}O_2$ is reduced in both the cycle and treadmill exercise studies, and the anaerobic threshold is low normal (Table 10.72.2). Using flowchart 3, the breathing reserve is high (branch point 3.1), whereas the exercise ECGs (branch point 3.3) are equivocally abnormal. The patient did not have chest pain and the $\Delta\dot{V}O_2/\Delta WR$ is normal, but the O_2 pulse is abnormally low, indicating a circulatory ab-

normality—either pulmonary vascular or cardiac. The patient hyperventilated at rest and had evidence of ventilation–perfusion mismatching or pulmonary vascular disease. The significant resting systemic hypertension did not increase inordinately during exercise, and $\Delta\dot{V}O_2/\Delta WR$ was normal, implying that peripheral arterial disease was not the primary disorder. The ECG findings, steep heart rate–$\dot{V}O_2$ relationship in both forms of ergometry (panel 5 in Figs. 10.72.1 and 10.72.2), constant and

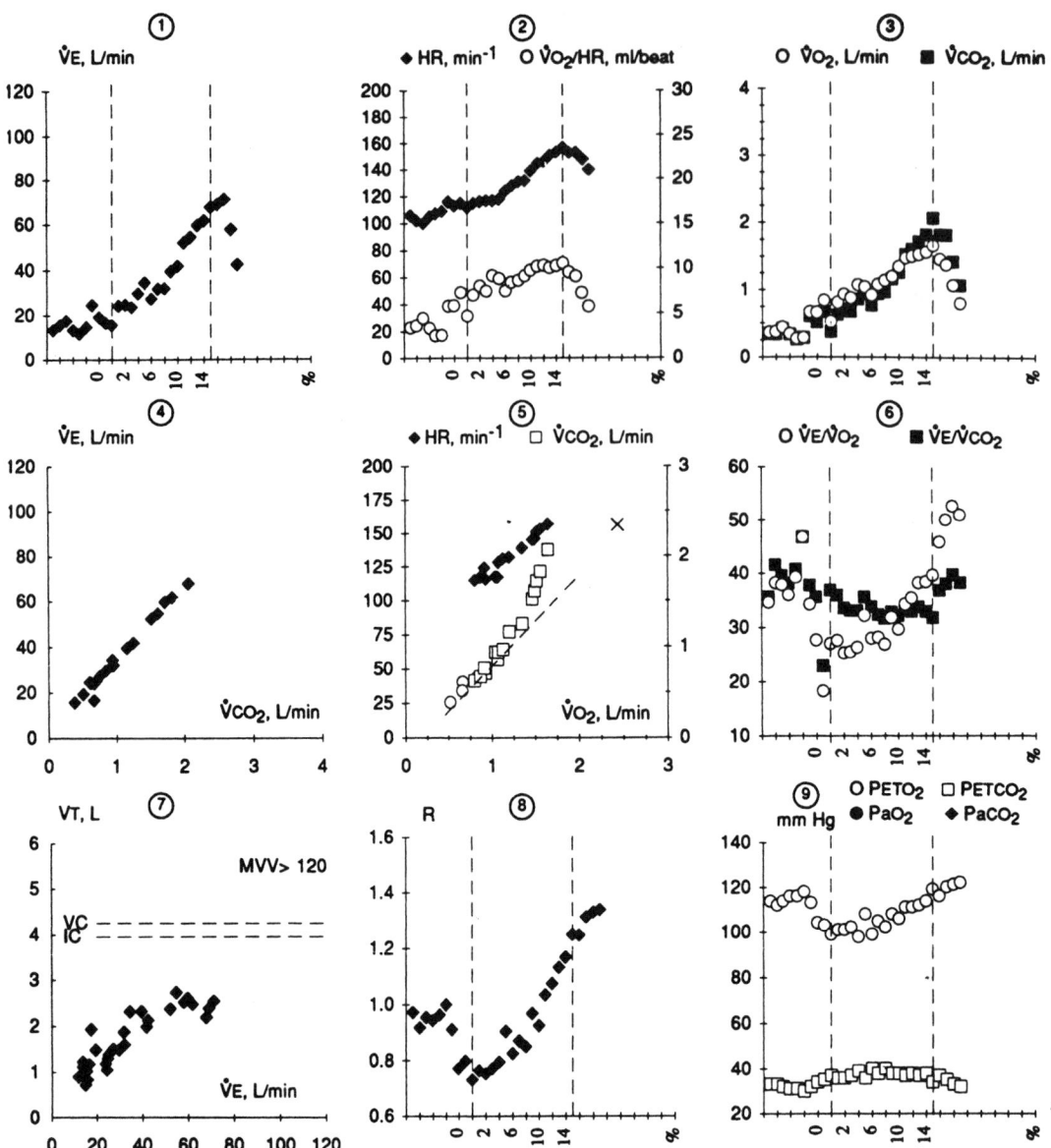

FIGURE 10.72.2.   Treadmill ergometry. **1:** Vertical dashed lines in panels 1 to 3 and 6, 8, and 9 indicate the beginning and the end of the increasing work period. **2:** Zero-grade walking is performed for 2 minutes before the left vertical dashed line. **3:** In panel 5, the diagonal dashed line has a slope of 1; the x in the upper right is the predicted maximum heart rate and $\dot{V}O_2$ for the subject.

reduced O_2 pulse, and elevated ventilatory equivalents all suggest that the primary diagnosis is left ventricular failure, presumably due to cardiac disease.

Conclusion

Left ventricular failure limiting exercise performance. This is confirmed by the absence of a cardiac reserve at the reduced maximum work rate, failure for $\dot{V}O_2$ to rise normally with increasing work rate (treadmill exercise study), and the reduced maximum O_2 pulse in both forms of ergometry.

TABLE 10.72.3. Cycle Ergometry

Time min	Work rate watts	BP mmHg	HR min⁻¹	f min⁻¹	V̇E L/min BTPS	V̇CO₂ L/min STPD	V̇O₂ L/min STPD	V̇O₂/HR ml/beat	R	pH	HCO₃⁻ meq/L	PO₂ ET	PO₂ a	PO₂ (A−a)	PCO₂ ET	PCO₂ a	PCO₂ (a−ET)	V̇E/V̇CO₂	V̇E/V̇O₂	VD/VT
	Rest	194/98								7.42	24		77			38				
	Rest		75	14	11.9	0.27	0.29	3.9	0.93			115			31			40	37	
	Rest		72	17	17.9	0.38	0.38	5.3	1.00			118			29			43	43	
	Rest		74	14	14.6	0.31	0.30	4.1	1.03			121			29			43	45	
	Rest	176/95	82	14	13.7	0.29	0.30	3.7	0.97			118			30			43	42	
	Rest		80	9	13.1	0.32	0.34	4.3	0.94			116			30			39	36	
	Rest		80	20	14.3	0.30	0.29	3.6	1.03	7.48	23	119	98	22	29	31	2	42	43	0.30
	Unloaded		84	14	22.6	0.51	0.52	6.2	0.98			115			31			42	41	
	Unloaded		92	12	26.5	0.58	0.48	5.2	1.21			124			27			44	53	
	Unloaded		93	12	20.0	0.47	0.46	4.9	1.02			118			30			40	41	
	Unloaded	194/95	85	15	23.2	0.52	0.52	6.1	1.00			116			31			42	42	
	Unloaded		92	17	21.9	0.49	0.51	5.5	0.96			116			31			42	40	
	Unloaded		92	16	24.0	0.56	0.56	6.1	1.00	7.47	22	117	100	19	30	31	1	40	40	0.29
0.5	20		96	14	25.4	0.61	0.64	6.7	0.95			116			31			40	38	
1.0	20	209/92	99	17	27.7	0.65	0.68	6.9	0.96			114			32			40	39	
1.5	40		102	24	28.8	0.68	0.77	7.5	0.88	7.44	22	111	94	20	33	33	0	39	35	0.31
2.0	40		105	21	27.6	0.72	0.83	7.9	0.87			104			36			36	31	
2.5	60		108	21	37.4	0.91	0.97	9.0	0.94			114			32			39	37	
3.0	60	212/92	112	26	40.0	0.93	0.96	8.6	0.97			113			33			41	39	
3.5	80		115	20	44.0	1.10	1.09	9.5	1.01			115			32			38	39	
4.0	80		119	31	29.8	0.87	1.02	8.6	0.85	7.40	23	97	92	16	42	37	−5	31	27	0.23
4.5	100		127	22	51.3	1.38	1.33	10.5	1.04			113			36			36	37	
5.0	100	230/98	131	25	60.3	1.53	1.36	10.4	1.13			116			34			38	43	
5.5	120		136	30	66.1	1.66	1.45	10.7	1.14			115			35			38	44	
6.0	120		143	27	68.2	1.77	1.56	10.9	1.13	7.40	19	117	104	18	34	31	−3	37	42	0.24
	Recovery		140	23	60.7	1.60	1.33	9.5	1.20			118			34			37	44	
	Recovery	221/95	134	23	53.4	1.32	0.95	7.1	1.39			121			34			39	54	
	Recovery		125	23	39.5	0.99	0.74	5.9	1.34			120			35			38	51	
	Recovery		120	18	38.2	0.89	0.61	5.1	1.46	7.38	17	126	114	14	30	29	−1	41	60	0.27

TABLE 10.72.4. Treadmill Ergometry

Time min	Work rate watts	BP mmHg	HR min⁻¹	f min⁻¹	V̇E L/min BTPS	V̇CO₂ L/min STPD	V̇O₂ L/min STPD	V̇O₂/HR ml/beat	R	pH	HCO₃⁻ meq/L	PO₂ ET	PO₂ a	PO₂ (A−a)	PCO₂ ET	PCO₂ a	PCO₂ (a−ET)	V̇E/V̇CO₂	V̇E/V̇O₂	VD/VT
	Rest		106	12	13.5	0.35	0.36	3.4	0.97			114			33			36	35	
	Rest		102	15	15.4	0.34	0.37	3.6	0.92			112			33			42	38	
	Rest		100	9	17.4	0.42	0.44	4.4	0.95			114			32			40	38	
	Rest		105	11	13.5	0.33	0.35	3.3	0.94			116			31			38	36	
	Rest		107	13	11.7	0.26	0.27	2.5	0.96			116			31			41	39	
	Rest		109	21	14.9	0.28	0.28	2.6	1.00			118			30			47	47	
	0		116	19	24.6	0.61	0.67	5.8	0.91			113			32			38	34	
	0		113	13	19.3	0.51	0.66	5.8	0.77			104			34			36	28	
	0		115	14	16.5	0.67	0.84	7.3	0.80			103			35			23	18	
	0		112	19	15.6	0.38	0.52	4.6	0.73			99			37			37	27	
0.5	2		115	23	24.2	0.62	0.81	7.0	0.77			101			36			36	27	
1.0	2		116	18	24.9	0.70	0.93	8.0	0.75			101			36			33	25	
1.5	4		117	20	23.8	0.67	0.87	7.4	0.77			102			37			33	25	
2.0	4		117	20	29.7	0.85	1.07	9.1	0.79			98			39			33	26	
2.5	6		118	15	34.6	0.94	1.04	8.8	0.90			108			36			35	32	
3.0	6		124	18	27.2	0.76	0.92	7.4	0.83			99			40			34	28	
3.5	8		128	17	31.8	0.94	1.08	8.4	0.87			105			38			32	28	
4.0	8		131	20	32.0	0.96	1.13	8.6	0.85			102			40			32	27	
4.5	10		132	17	39.5	1.16	1.20	9.1	0.97			108			38			33	32	
5.0	10		139	21	41.8	1.25	1.35	9.7	0.93			106			38			32	30	
5.5	12		145	22	52.3	1.52	1.47	10.1	1.03			111			37			33	34	
6.0	12		146	20	54.7	1.61	1.50	10.3	1.07			111			38			33	35	
6.5	14		151	23	59.9	1.72	1.52	10.1	1.13			112			37			34	38	
7.0	14		153	25	61.9	1.82	1.56	10.2	1.17			114			38			33	38	
7.5	16		157	31	67.8	2.06	1.65	10.5	1.25			119			34			32	39	
	Recovery		153	29	69.2	1.82	1.46	9.5	1.25			116			37			37	46	
	Recovery		153	28	71.2	1.81	1.38	9.0	1.31			120			35			38	50	
	Recovery		148	23	58.1	1.42	1.07	7.2	1.33			121			33			40	52	
	Recovery		140	20	42.4	1.07	0.80	5.7	1.34			122			32			38	51	

Case 73 β-Adrenergic Blockade, Systemic Hypertension, Pulmonary Vascular Disease, and Mild Chronic Bronchitis

Clinical Findings

A 55-year-old former shipyard worker had first noted exertional dyspnea and a morning cough with small amounts of sputum approximately 5 years earlier. He retired 3 years previously because of an injury to the left foot. The patient had a 60 pack-year smoking history but had stopped 1 year ago. Hypertension, diagnosed 1 year previously, was being treated with hydrochlorothiazide and propranolol. There is no history of angina or congestive heart failure. Examination revealed normal breath sounds, cardiovascular examination, and peripheral pulses. Chest roentgenograms showed minimal pleural plaques without evidence of parenchymal lung disease.

Exercise Findings

The patient performed exercise on a cycle ergometer. He pedaled at 60 rpm without added load for 3 minutes. The work rate was then increased 20 W per minute to his symptom-limited maximum. Arterial blood was sampled every second minute, and intraarterial blood pressure was recorded from a percutaneously placed brachial artery catheter. Resting and exercise ECGs were normal except for relative bradycardia. The patient stopped exercise complaining of general fatigue and shortness of breath.

Interpretation

Comments

The mechanics of breathing are normal, but the diffusing capacity is significantly reduced (Table 10.73.1). The resting ECG is normal.

Analysis

In flowchart 1, peak $\dot{V}O_2$ and the anaerobic threshold are reduced (Table 10.73.2). See flowchart 4. The breathing reserve is high (branch point 4.1). The ventilatory equivalent for CO_2 at the anaerobic threshold is high (branch point 4.3). This suggests that the patient has an abnormal pulmonary circulation. Confirmation of this is demonstrated by high VD/VT, $P(A - a)O_2$, and $P(a - ET)CO_2$ values (indices of ventilation–perfusion mismatching). Be-

cause there is no associated disturbance in respiratory mechanics, we must conclude that these findings are on the basis of primary pulmonary vascular disease. The significant reduction in diffusing capacity ($DLCO$) is compatible with this conclusion. There is no abrupt decrease in PaO_2 or O_2 saturation at the start of exercise (branch point 4.5), indicating that a right-to-left shunt does not accompany the pulmonary vascular disease. Because the patient is being treated with propranolol, the heart rate response is unusually low for this kind of abnormality. Thus, the low heart rate and the systemic hypertension likely contribute to the low peak $\dot{V}O_2$ and anaerobic threshold.

Conclusion

Exercise limitation is caused by pulmonary vascular disease, systemic hypertension, and impaired heart rate response secondary to β-adrenergic blockade.

TABLE 10.73.1.   Selected Respiratory Function Data

Measurement	Predicted	Measured
Age, yr		55
Sex		Male
Height, cm		173
Weight, kg	76	85
Hematocrit, %		48
VC, L	4.20	4.54
IC, L	2.80	3.66
TLC, L	6.26	6.88
FEV_1, L	3.32	3.16
FEV_1/VC, %	79	70
MVV, L/min	140	121
D_LCO, ml/mm Hg/min	28.1	16.6

TABLE 10.73.2.   Selected Exercise Data

Measurement	Predicted	Measured
Peak $\dot{V}O_2$, L/min	2.35	1.59
Maximum HR, beats/min	165	113
Maximum O_2 pulse, ml/beat	14.3	14.4
$\Delta\dot{V}O_2/\Delta WR$, ml/min/W	10.3	9.8
AT, L/min	>1.01	0.95
Blood pressure, mmHg (rest, max)		181/107, 206/113
Maximum $\dot{V}E$, L/min		72
Exercise breathing reserve, L/min	>15	49
PaO_2, mmHg (rest, max ex)		73, 71
$P(A - a)O_2$, mmHg (rest, max ex)		31, 46
$P(a - ET)CO_2$, mmHg (rest, max ex)		3, 4
VD/VT (rest, heavy ex)		0.33, 0.35
HCO_3^-, mEq/L (rest, 2-min recov)		24, 18

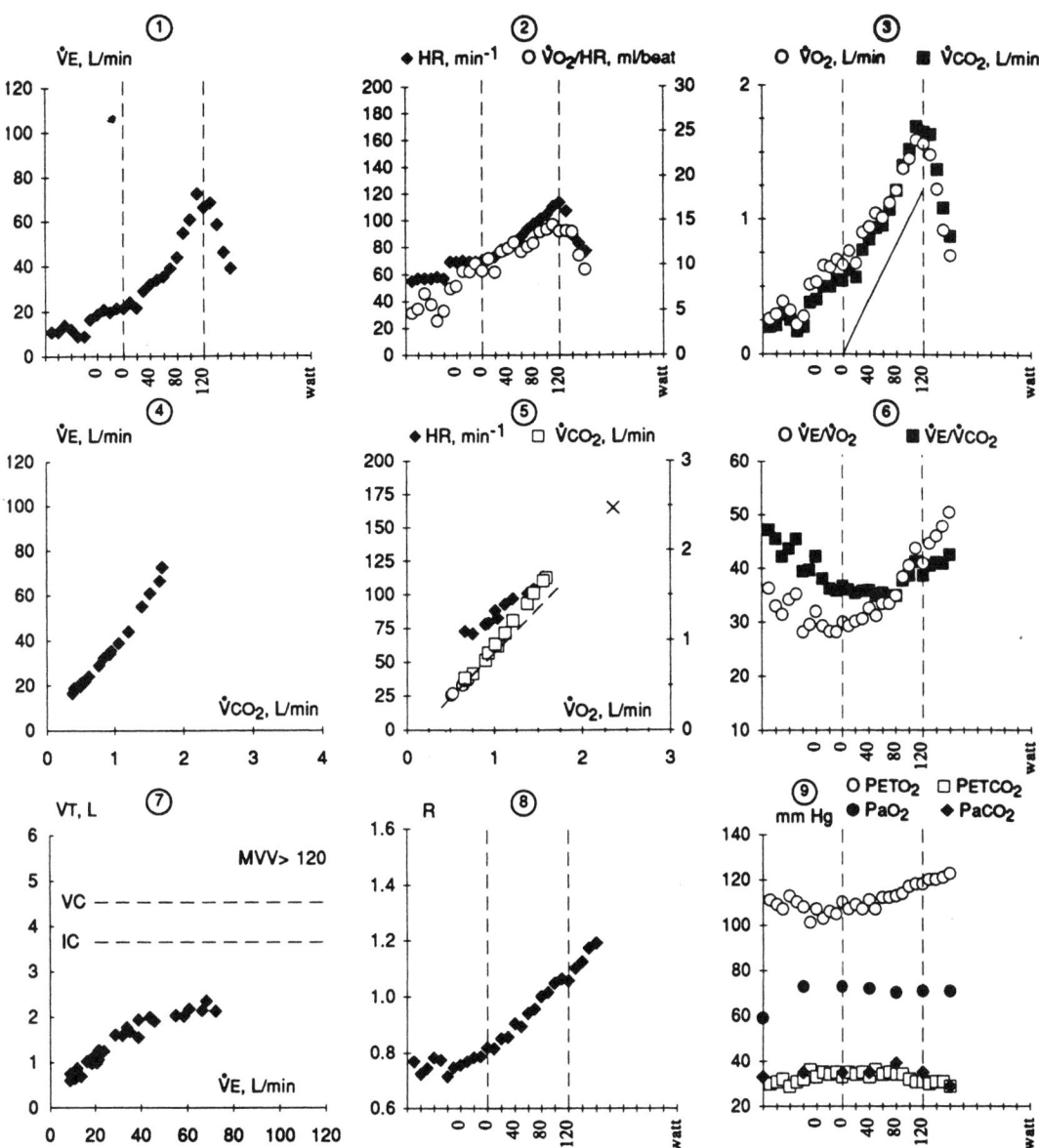

FIGURE 10.73.1.   **1:** Vertical dashed lines in panels 1 to 3 and 6, 8, and 9 indicate the beginning and the end of the increasing work period. **2:** Unloaded cycling is performed for 3 minutes before the left vertical dashed line. **3:** In panel 3, the diagonal line shows the increase of $\dot{V}O_2$ at a slope of 10 ml/min/W. **4:** In panel 5, the diagonal dashed line has a slope of 1; the x in the upper right is the predicted maximum heart rate and $\dot{V}O_2$ for the subject.

TABLE 10.73.3.   Air Breathing

Time min	Work rate watts	BP mmHg	HR min⁻¹	f min⁻¹	V̇E L/min BTPS	V̇CO₂ L/min STPD	V̇O₂ L/min STPD	V̇O₂/HR ml/beat	R	pH	HCO₃⁻ meq/L	Po₂ ET	Po₂ a	Po₂ (A−a)	Pco₂ ET	Pco₂ a	Pco₂ (a−ET)	V̇E/V̇CO₂	V̇E/V̇O₂	VD/VT
	Rest									7.47	24		59			33				
	Rest		55	15	10.7	0.20	0.26	4.7	0.77			111			30			47	36	
	Rest		57	17	11.0	0.21	0.29	5.1	0.72			109			31			46	33	
	Rest		57	20	13.9	0.29	0.39	6.8	0.74			107			32			42	31	
	Rest	182/107	57	14	12.1	0.25	0.32	5.6	0.78			113			29			44	34	
	Rest		58	15	9.0	0.17	0.22	3.8	0.77			110			31			45	35	
	Rest		57	12	8.9	0.20	0.28	4.9	0.71	7.44	23	108	73	31	32	55	2	39	28	0.33
	Unloaded		69	16	16.4	0.38	0.51	7.4	0.75			101			36			40	29	
	Unloaded	193/107	69	19	18.5	0.40	0.53	7.7	0.75			107			33			42	32	
	Unloaded		70	21	20.8	0.50	0.65	9.3	0.77			103			35			38	29	
	Unloaded		69	17	19.5	0.50	0.64	9.3	0.78			106			34			36	28	
	Unloaded		69	20	21.4	0.55	0.70	10.1	0.79			105			35			36	28	
	Unloaded		70	19	21.4	0.54	0.66	9.4	0.82	7.44	23	110	73	36	33	35	2	37	30	0.30
0.5	20		71	19	23.9	0.62	0.76	10.7	0.82			107			35			36	29	
1.0	20	194/107	73	17	21.6	0.57	0.67	9.2	0.85			109			34			35	30	
1.5	40		78	18	29.0	0.77	0.90	11.5	0.86			107			35			36	31	
2.0	40		79	20	32.2	0.85	0.94	11.9	0.90	7.44	23	111	72	40	33	35	2	36	32	0.30
2.5	60		83	19	33.9	0.93	1.04	12.5	0.89			107			36			35	31	
3.0	60	197/110	88	21	35.4	0.95	1.01	11.5	0.94			112			34			35	33	
3.5	80		93	20	39.0	1.07	1.12	12.0	0.96			112			35			35	33	
4.0	80		97	22	44.0	1.21	1.21	12.5	1.00	7.42	25	113	70	41	34	39	5	35	35	0.35
4.5	100		101	27	55.0	1.40	1.38	13.7	1.01			114			34			38	38	
5.0	100	206/113	104	28	61.0	1.52	1.45	13.9	1.05			117			32			39	40	
5.5	120		110	34	72.4	1.69	1.59	14.5	1.06			118			31			41	44	
6.0	120		113	31	66.4	1.65	1.56	13.8	1.06	7.42	22	118	71	46	31	35	4	39	41	0.35
	Recovery		107	29	68.4	1.63	1.48	13.8	1.10			120			30			40	45	
	Recovery	213/107	89	29	58.6	1.37	1.22	13.7	1.12			120			31			41	46	
	Recovery		83	24	46.0	1.08	0.92	11.1	1.17			121			31			41	48	
	Recovery		77	25	39.0	0.87	0.73	9.5	1.19	7.40	18	123	71	54	29	29	0	42	51	0.28

Case 74 β-Adrenergic Blockade, Obesity, and Asbestosis

Clinical Findings

This 61-year-old man was referred for follow-up cardiopulmonary exercise testing because of his 30-year work exposure to asbestos. He had stopped smoking 13 years before but had a 100 pack-year history of cigarette smoking. He had noted dyspnea in the past 2 years (associated with an 11-kg weight gain) but denied cough, chest pain, claudication, or ankle edema. He had hypertension; his only medications were atenolol and nifedipine. Examination revealed rare crackles at the right lung base, normal heart sounds, and peripheral pulses. Resting ECG showed a prolonged PR interval, J-point elevations in leads V_2 and V_3, and nonspecific T-wave abnormalities in the lateral chest leads. Chest roentgenograms revealed some diaphragmatic calcification, pleural thickening, and parenchymal scarring.

Exercise Findings

The patient performed exercise on a cycle ergometer. He pedaled at 60 rpm without an added load for 3 minutes. The work rate was then increased 15 W per minute to tolerance. Heart rate and rhythm were continuously monitored; 12-lead ECGs were obtained during rest, exercise, and recovery. Blood pressure was measured with a sphygmomanometer, and oxygen saturation with an ear oximeter. The patient appeared to give a good effort and stopped exercise because of general fatigue; he denied chest pain or dyspnea during or after the study. The patient had no ectopy or abnormal ECG changes during or after exercise. Ear oximetry studies were normal.

Interpretation

Comments

The reduced lung volumes are compatible with mild restrictive disease due to obesity (reduced expiratory reserve volume) and asbestosis. The nearly normal inspiratory capacity (Table 10.74.1) suggests that the restriction is primarily caused by obesity.

Analysis

In flowchart 1, peak $\dot{V}O_2$ is reduced (branch point 1.1), but the anaerobic threshold is normal (Table 10.74.2) (branch points 1.2 and 1.3), despite the patient's inability to raise his exercise heart rate above 105 beats per minute. Going next to flowchart 3, the normal breathing reserve (branch point 3.1) and probably normal ECG (branch point 3.2) lead to the diagnosis of poor effort or musculoskeletal disorder. There are no measures of VD/VT or arterial–alveolar pressure differences, but the normal ventilatory equivalents and normal ear oximetry are evidence against any major gas exchange abnormality during exercise. The high heart rate reserve might lead one to consider poor effort, but the high recovery R of 1.40 (indicating a significant metabolic acidosis) is evidence against this diagnosis. The low maximum heart rate and accompanying high maximum O_2 pulse are best explained by a high degree of β-blockade from atenolol, which gives more time than usual for filling of the ventricles. The high $\dot{V}O_2$ at unloaded pedaling (nearly 1.0 L/min) is typical of obesity.

TABLE 10.74.1.   Selected Respiratory Function Data

Measurement	Predicted	Measured
Age, yr		61
Sex		Male
Height, cm		179
Weight, kg	81	120
Hematocrit, %		42
VC, L	4.41	2.97
IC, L	2.94	2.67
TLC, L	6.75	5.04
FEV_1, L	3.46	2.34
FEV_1/VC, %	78	78
MVV, L/min	140	92
D_LCO, ml/mm Hg/min	27.2	26.6

TABLE 10.74.2.   Selected Exercise Data

Measurement	Predicted	Measured
Peak $\dot{V}O_2$, L/min	2.50	1.92
Maximum HR, beats/min	159	105
Maximum O_2 pulse, ml/beat	15.7	18.8
$\Delta\dot{V}O_2$/ΔWR, ml/min/W	10.3	9.6
AT, L/min	>1.10	1.3
Blood pressure, mmHg (rest, max)		140/90, 160/80
Maximum $\dot{V}E$, L/min		69
Exercise breathing reserve, L/min	>15	23

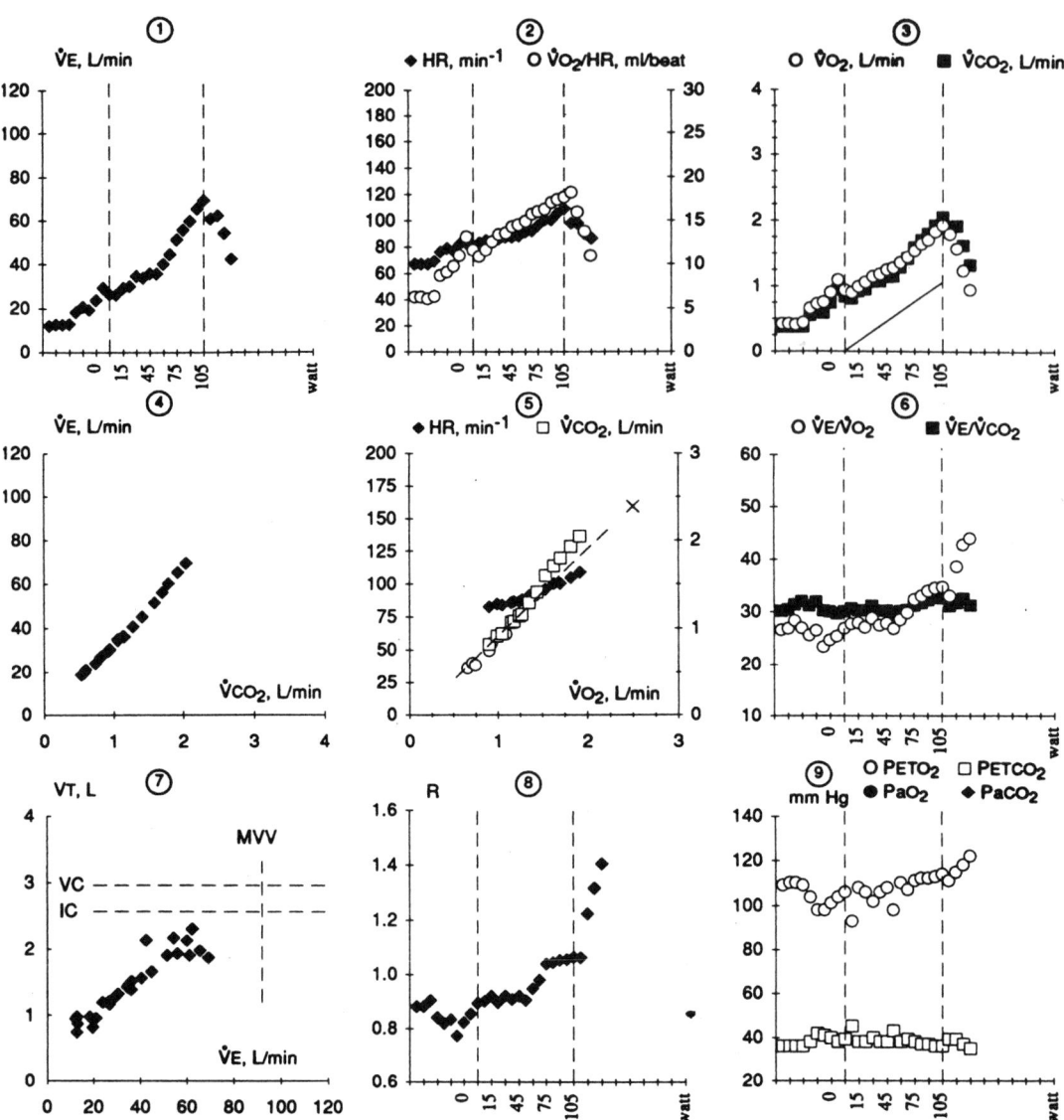

FIGURE 10.74.1.   **1:** Vertical dashed lines in panels 1 to 3 and 6, 8, and 9 indicate the beginning and the end of the increasing work period. **2:** Unloaded cycling is performed for 3 minutes before the left vertical dashed line. **3:** In panel 3, the diagonal line shows the increase of $\dot{V}O_2$ at a slope of 10 ml/min/W. **4:** In panel 5, the diagonal dashed line has a slope of 1; the x in the upper right is the predicted maximum heart rate and $\dot{V}O_2$ for the subject.

Conclusion

β-Adrenergic blockade therapy of hypertension can cause significant reduction in maximum heart rate, peak $\dot{V}O_2$, and maximum work rate. Usually, as in this patient, the increase in O_2 pulse is an important factor in overcoming the effect of reduction in maximum heart rate and minimizing the effect on maximum $\dot{V}O_2$. Obesity and the limited ability to increase heart rate can lead to the symptom of fatigue, as found in this case.

TABLE 10.74.3. Air Breathing

Time min	Work rate watts	BP mmHg	HR min⁻¹	f min⁻¹	$\dot{V}_E$ L/min BTPS	$\dot{V}_{CO_2}$ L/min STPD	$\dot{V}_{O_2}$ L/min STPD	$\dot{V}_{O_2}$/HR ml/beat	R	pH	HCO₃⁻ meq/L	P_{O_2} ET	a	(A − a)	P_{CO_2} ET	a	(a − ET)	$\dot{V}_E/\dot{V}_{CO_2}$	$\dot{V}_E/\dot{V}_{O_2}$	V_D/V_T
	Rest	140/90																		
	Rest		67	13	12.3	0.37	0.42	6.3	0.88			109			36			30	27	
	Rest		67	17	12.7	0.37	0.42	6.3	0.88			110			36			30	27	
	Rest		67	13	12.7	0.37	0.41	6.1	0.90			110			36			31	28	
	Rest	130/80	69	15	13.1	0.37	0.44	6.4	0.84			109			36			32	27	
	Unloaded		76	19	18.5	0.54	0.66	8.7	0.82			104			38			31	26	
	Unloaded		79	22	21.0	0.60	0.72	9.1	0.83			98			42			32	27	
	Unloaded		77	24	19.6	0.58	0.75	9.7	0.77			98			41			30	23	
	Unloaded	130/80	82	20	23.9	0.74	0.90	11.0	0.82			101			40			30	25	
	Unloaded		83	23	29.6	0.93	1.09	13.1	0.85			104			38			30	25	
	Unloaded		80	23	26.9	0.83	0.93	11.6	0.89			106			39			30	27	
0.5	15		83	22	26.7	0.81	0.90	10.8	0.90			93			45			31	28	
1.0	15	145/80	85	23	29.5	0.91	0.99	11.6	0.92			108			38			30	28	
1.5	30		84	23	30.4	0.94	1.05	12.5	0.90			106			38			30	27	
2.0	30		86	24	35.0	1.06	1.15	13.4	0.92			102			40			31	29	
2.5	45		87	24	34.4	1.07	1.18	13.6	0.91			106			38			30	27	
3.0	45	140/80	87	24	36.4	1.14	1.24	14.3	0.92			108			38			30	28	
3.5	60		88	26	36.1	1.15	1.27	14.4	0.91			98			43			29	27	
4.0	60		91	26	40.6	1.28	1.35	14.8	0.95			110			38			30	28	
4.5	75		92	27	45.0	1.41	1.44	15.7	0.98			107			39			30	30	
5.0	75	150/90	96	27	51.6	1.59	1.53	15.9	1.04			111			38			31	32	
5.5	90		100	29	56.1	1.70	1.63	16.3	1.04			112			37			32	33	
6.0	90		100	28	60.0	1.79	1.70	17.0	1.05			112			37			32	34	
6.5	105		105	33	65.5	1.92	1.82	17.3	1.05			113			36			33	34	
7.0	105	160/80	109	37	69.4	2.04	1.92	17.6	1.06			114			36			32	35	
	Recovery		98	32	61.2	1.89	1.78	18.2	1.06			111			39			31	33	
	Recovery		98	27	62.4	1.91	1.56	15.9	1.22			115			39			31	39	
	Recovery		90	25	54.5	1.62	1.23	13.7	1.32			118			37			32	43	
	Recovery		86	20	42.8	1.32	0.94	10.9	1.40			122			35			31	44	

Case 75 Pulmonary Vascular Disease, Chronic Bronchitis, Asbestosis, and Myocardial Ischemia

Clinical Findings

This 51-year-old shipyard worker had noted increased dyspnea on exertion for 2 years, until he was unable to finish cleaning his one-bedroom apartment. For several years he had a morning cough productive of small amounts of yellow sputum. He had over 40 pack-years of cigarette smoking and continued to smoke. He denied chest pain, tightness, or pressure. Chest roentgenographic studies showed a streaky infiltrate in the lower lung fields with nodular scarring in the upper lung zones. Physical examination of the chest was normal. There was equivocal clubbing of the digits. Peripheral pulses were normal. ECG showed left axis deviation.

Exercise Findings

The patient performed exercise on a cycle ergometer. He first pedaled at 60 rpm, without added load, for 3 minutes. The work rate was then increased 15 W per minute to his symptom-limited maximum. Arterial blood was sampled every second minute, and intraarterial blood pressure was recorded from a percutaneously placed brachial artery catheter. The patient stopped exercising because of severe knee cramps. During incremental exercise, he developed premature atrial and ventricular contractions and 3- to 4-mm ST-segment depression in leads V_4 and V_5. He denied any chest pain or discomfort, dizziness, or lightheadedness. The ST segments returned to normal within 1 minute of recovery.

Interpretation

Comments

Resting respiratory function tests are compatible with mild airflow obstruction (Table 10.75.1). The diffusing capacity is at the lower limits of normal. The resting ECG is essentially normal.

Analysis

In flowchart 1, the peak $\dot{V}O_2$ and the anaerobic threshold are normal (Table 10.75.2). See flowchart 2. The ECG at maximum exercise is abnormal, suggesting ischemic changes. The arterial blood gases are also significantly abnormal during exercise (branch point 2.1). The indices of ventilation–perfusion matching [VD/VT, $P(a - ET)CO_2$, and $P(A - a)O_2$] (branch point 2.3) are clearly abnormal, suggesting that this patient has lung disease and/or pulmonary vascular disease. Because the results of the resting respiratory function tests are not consistent with a diagnosis of restrictive lung disease and suggest that the patient's airflow obstruction is only mild, it is likely that the major abnormalities in ventilation–perfusion mismatching observed in this patient are attributable to pulmonary vascular disease. The ECG abnormalities that this patient developed as he approached his maximum work rate, despite the absence of chest pain, suggest that the patient also develops myocardial ischemia under exercise stress.

TABLE 10.75.1.   Selected Respiratory Function Data

Measurement	Predicted	Measured
Age, yr		51
Sex		Male
Height, cm		166
Weight, kg	70	55
Hematocrit, %		49
VC, L	3.88	3.83
IC, L	2.59	2.37
TLC, L	5.71	6.81
FEV_1, L	3.07	2.41
FEV_1/VC, %	79	63
MVV, L/min, direct	136	120
MVV, L/min, indirect	123	96
D_LCO, ml/mm Hg/min	26.9	21.5

TABLE 10.75.2.   Selected Exercise Data

Measurement	Predicted	Measured
Peak $\dot{V}O_2$, L/min	1.99	1.77
Maximum HR, beats/min	169	150
Maximum O_2 pulse, ml/beat	11.8	11.8
$\Delta\dot{V}O_2/\Delta WR$, ml/min/W	10.3	9.7
AT, L/min	>0.86	1.2
Blood pressure, mmHg (rest, max)		132/72, 189/99
Maximum $\dot{V}E$, L/min		79
Exercise breathing reserve, L/min	>15	17
PaO_2, mmHg (rest, max ex)		69, 63
$P(A - a)O_2$, mmHg (rest, max ex)		30, 44
$P(a - ET)CO_2$, mmHg (rest, max ex)		10, 6
VD/VT (rest, heavy ex)		0.53, 0.47
HCO_3^-, mEq/L (rest, 2-min recov)		25, 17

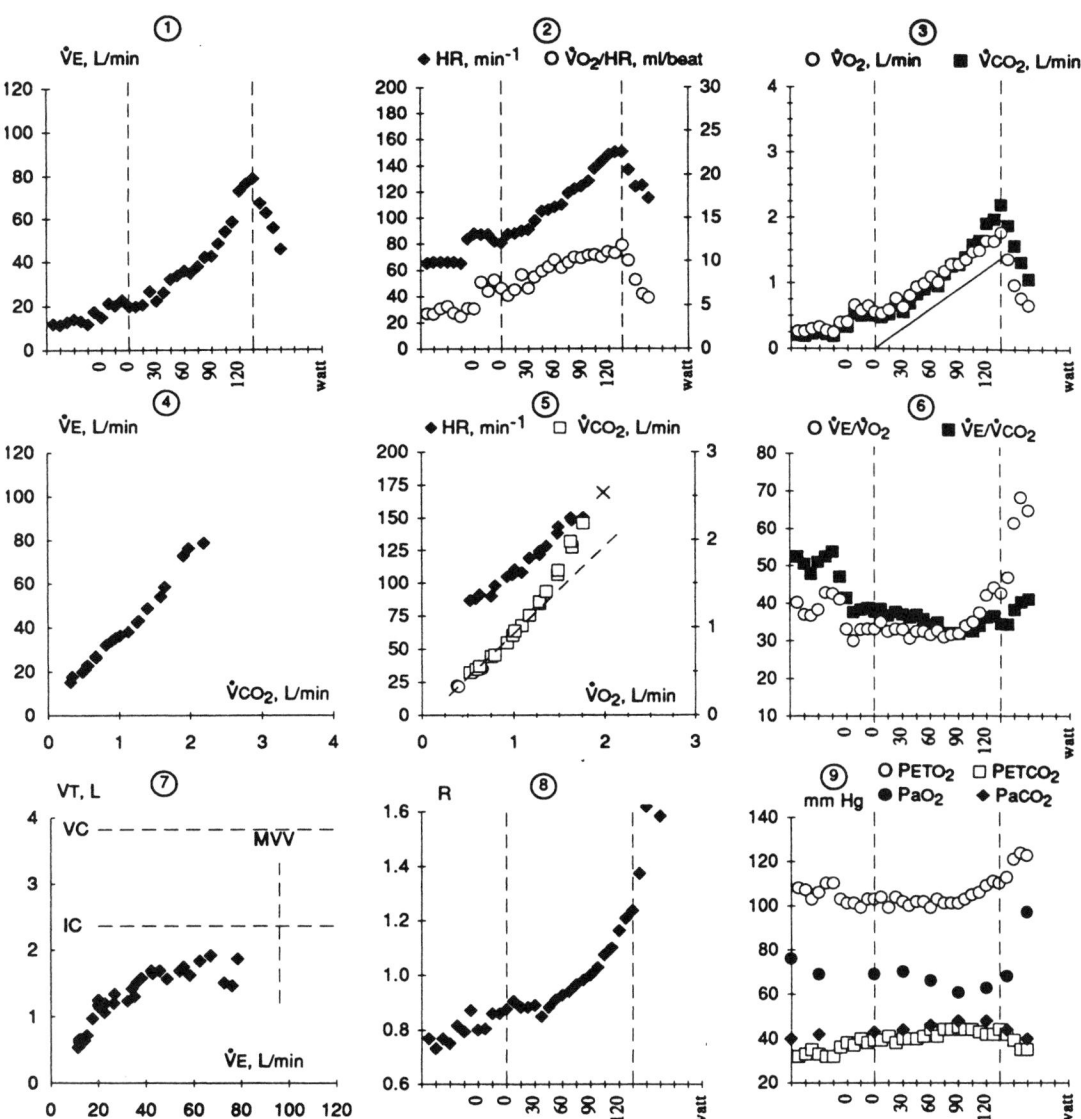

FIGURE 10.75.1.   **1:** Vertical dashed lines in panels 1 to 3 and 6, 8, and 9 indicate the beginning and the end of the increasing work period. **2:** Unloaded cycling is performed for 3 minutes before the left vertical dashed line. **3:** In panel 3, the diagonal line shows the increase of $\dot{V}O_2$ at a slope of 10 ml/min/W. **4:** In panel 5, the diagonal dashed line has a slope of 1; the x in the upper right is the predicted maximum heart rate and $\dot{V}O_2$ for the subject.

Conclusion

This study shows normal maximum exercise capacity in a patient with pulmonary vascular disease and myocardial ischemia. There is clear evidence of significant ventilation–perfusion mismatching of the type seen with pulmonary vascular disease; however, his pulmonary mechanics are only mildly abnormal. Presumably, this is an instance of changes in the pulmonary circulation disproportionate to airway or parenchymal disease. Additionally, the exercise-induced ST-segment depression and arrhythmia, typical of myocardial ischemia, suggest coronary artery disease. The pulmonary vascular disease and exercise hypoxemia possibly contribute to this cardiac abnormality.

TABLE 10.75.3.   Air Breathing

Time min	Work rate watts	BP mmHg	HR min⁻¹	f min⁻¹	V̇E L/min BTPS	V̇CO₂ L/min STPD	V̇O₂ L/min STPD	V̇O₂/HR ml/beat	R	pH	HCO₃⁻ meq/L	PO₂, mmHg ET	PO₂, mmHg a	PO₂, mmHg (A−a)	PCO₂, mmHg ET	PCO₂, mmHg a	PCO₂, mmHg (a−ET)	V̇E/V̇CO₂	V̇E/V̇O₂	VD/VT
	Rest	132/72								7.42	25		76			40				
	Rest		65	18	12.0	0.20	0.26	4.0	0.77			108			32			52	40	
	Rest		66	21	11.4	0.19	0.26	3.9	0.73			107			33			51	37	
	Rest		66	19	12.6	0.23	0.30	4.5	0.77			103			35			48	37	
	Rest	159/81	66	22	14.1	0.24	0.32	4.8	0.75	7.39	25	106	69	28	33	42	9	51	38	0.52
	Rest		66	21	13.3	0.22	0.27	4.1	0.81			110			32			52	43	
	Rest		65	19	11.8	0.19	0.24	3.7	0.79			110			32			54	42	
	Unloaded		84	18	17.5	0.34	0.39	4.6	0.87			103			36			47	41	
	Unloaded		88	21	15.0	0.32	0.40	4.5	0.80			101			38			41	33	
	Unloaded		87	18	21.4	0.53	0.66	7.6	0.80			101			37			37	30	
	Unloaded	165/90	87	16	20.1	0.49	0.57	6.6	0.86			99			40			38	33	
	Unloaded		82	19	22.8	0.55	0.64	7.8	0.86			103			38			39	33	
	Unloaded		81	16	19.9	0.49	0.56	6.9	0.88	7.38	25	103	69	33	39	43	4	38	33	0.44
0.5	15		87	17	19.9	0.48	0.53	6.1	0.91			104			39			38	35	
1.0	15	180/93	88	18	20.6	0.52	0.59	6.7	0.88			99			41			37	32	
1.5	30		90	20	26.9	0.67	0.76	8.4	0.88			104			38			38	33	
2.0	30		91	21	22.5	0.56	0.63	6.9	0.89	7.37	25	102	70	32	40	44	4	37	33	0.43
2.5	45		98	22	26.4	0.68	0.80	8.2	0.85			100			40			36	31	
3.0	45	186/93	105	26	32.3	0.82	0.93	8.9	0.88			102			40			37	32	
3.5	60		106	24	34.2	0.90	0.99	9.3	0.91			102			41			36	32	
4.0	60		108	24	36.4	1.01	1.09	10.1	0.93	7.35	25	99	66	35	44	46	2	34	32	0.42
4.5	75		110	27	35.3	0.95	1.01	9.2	0.94			103			41			35	33	
5.0	75	189/93	119	24	38.1	1.13	1.17	9.8	0.97			101			44			32	31	
5.5	90		122	25	42.4	1.26	1.28	10.5	0.98			101			44			32	31	
6.0	90		124	26	43.0	1.28	1.28	10.3	1.00	7.31	24	101	61	41	45	48	3	32	32	0.41
6.5	105		128	31	48.8	1.40	1.36	10.6	1.03			103			44			33	34	
7.0	105	191/99	138	32	54.2	1.59	1.48	10.7	1.07			105			44			32	35	
7.5	120		143	36	58.6	1.64	1.49	10.4	1.10			106			43			34	37	
8.0	120		148	48	72.8	1.91	1.64	11.1	1.16	7.28	22	109	63	44	42	48	6	36	42	0.47
8.5	135		150	52	76.2	1.97	1.63	10.9	1.21			111			42			36	44	
9.0	135	189/99	150	42	78.7	2.19	1.77	11.8	1.24			110			44			34	42	
	Recovery		137	35	67.2	1.88	1.37	10.0	1.37	7.25	19	113	68	47	42	44	2	34	47	0.41
	Recovery	184/84	124	34	62.6	1.57	0.97	7.8	1.62			121			39			38	62	
	Recovery		125	32	55.9	1.32	0.78	6.2	1.69			124			35			40	68	
	Recovery		115	27	45.8	1.06	0.67	5.8	1.58	7.24	17	123	97	25	35	40	5	41	65	0.45

Case 76 "CHF," "COPD," Obesity, and Anemia

Clinical Findings

This 50-year-old meatcutter and former smoker had severe exertional dyspnea and had been hospitalized on several occasions for what had been considered to be congestive heart failure with wheezing, leg edema, and orthopnea. He was referred for exercise testing to aid in distinguishing between cardiac and respiratory disease. He was anemic from unknown cause. Breath sounds were distant.

Exercise Findings

The patient performed exercise on a cycle ergometer. He pedaled at 60 rpm without an added load for 3 minutes. The work rate was then increased 15 W per minute to tolerance. Arterial blood was sampled every second minute, and intraarterial pressure was recorded from a percutaneously placed brachial artery catheter. Heart rate and rhythm were continuously monitored; 12-lead ECGs were obtained during rest, exercise, and recovery. The patient appeared to give an excellent effort and stopped exercise because of severe dyspnea and exhaustion. He denied chest pain during or after the study. No arrhythmias or ischemic changes were noted on the ECGs.

Interpretation

Comments

Resting respiratory function studies showed severe obstructive lung disease with hyperinflation, no improvement in flow rates following inhaled albuterol, and an above-predicted $D_{L}CO$ (Table 10.76.1). The predicted value for $D_{L}CO$ was adjusted for the patient's anemia. The patient was also overweight, with arterial blood gases and pH suggesting a chronic compensated respiratory acidosis and an acute respiratory alkalosis. The respiratory acidosis increases with exercise.

Analysis

Referring to flowchart 1, the peak $\dot{V}O_2$ and anaerobic threshold were both decreased (Table 10.76.2). Most striking is the ventilatory limitation accompanied by increasing respiratory acidosis and a low O_2 pulse. We are directed through branch points 1.1, 1.2, and 1.3 to flowchart 4. The low breathing re-

serve (branch point 4.1) and the high V_D/V_T (branch point 4.2) lead to the diagnosis labeled "lung disease with impaired peripheral oxygenation." The patient's data do not fit the conditions listed under this diagnosis perfectly, but he does have a low arterial O_2 content (anemia and slightly decreased arterial O_2 saturation) and many of the factors listed in the pulmonary vascular disease category. If we had used flowchart 5, we might have arrived through branch points 5.1, 5.3, and 5.7 at the diagnosis of "obstructive lung disease." This is satisfactory, especially because of the severe respiratory acidosis that developed during exercise, but it accounts poorly for his low $\Delta\dot{V}O_2/\Delta WR$ and flat O_2 pulse, which indicate an O_2 flow problem. These latter abnormalities, with normal $P(A - a)O_2$, can be accounted for by anemia and left ventricular failure.

TABLE 10.76.1.   Selected Respiratory Function Data

Measurement	Predicted	Measured
Age, yr		50
Sex		Male
Height, cm		174
Weight, kg	77	91
Hemoglobin, g/100 ml		10.3
VC, L	4.40	3.11
IC, L	2.94	2.15
TLC, L	6.44	9.78
FEV_1, L	3.49	1.14
FEV_1/VC, %	79	37
MVV, L/min	147	45
$D_{L}CO$, ml/mm Hg/min	24.4	28.8

TABLE 10.76.2.   Selected Exercise Data

Measurement	Predicted	Measured
Peak $\dot{V}O_2$, L/min	2.55	1.20
Maximum HR, beats/min	170	147
Maximum O_2 pulse, ml/beat	14.3	8.4
$\Delta\dot{V}O_2/\Delta WR$, ml/min/W	10.3	7.6
AT, L/min	>1.10	0.95
Blood pressure, mmHg (rest, max)		135/90, 180/84
Maximum $\dot{V}E$, L/min		41
Exercise breathing reserve, L/min	>15	4
PaO_2, mmHg (rest, max ex)		84, 76
$P(A - a)O_2$, mmHg (rest, max ex)		19, 21
$P(a - ET)CO_2$, mmHg (rest, max ex)		5, 5
V_D/V_T (rest, heavy ex)		0.43, 0.46
HCO_3^-, mEq/L (rest, 2-min recov)		31, 29

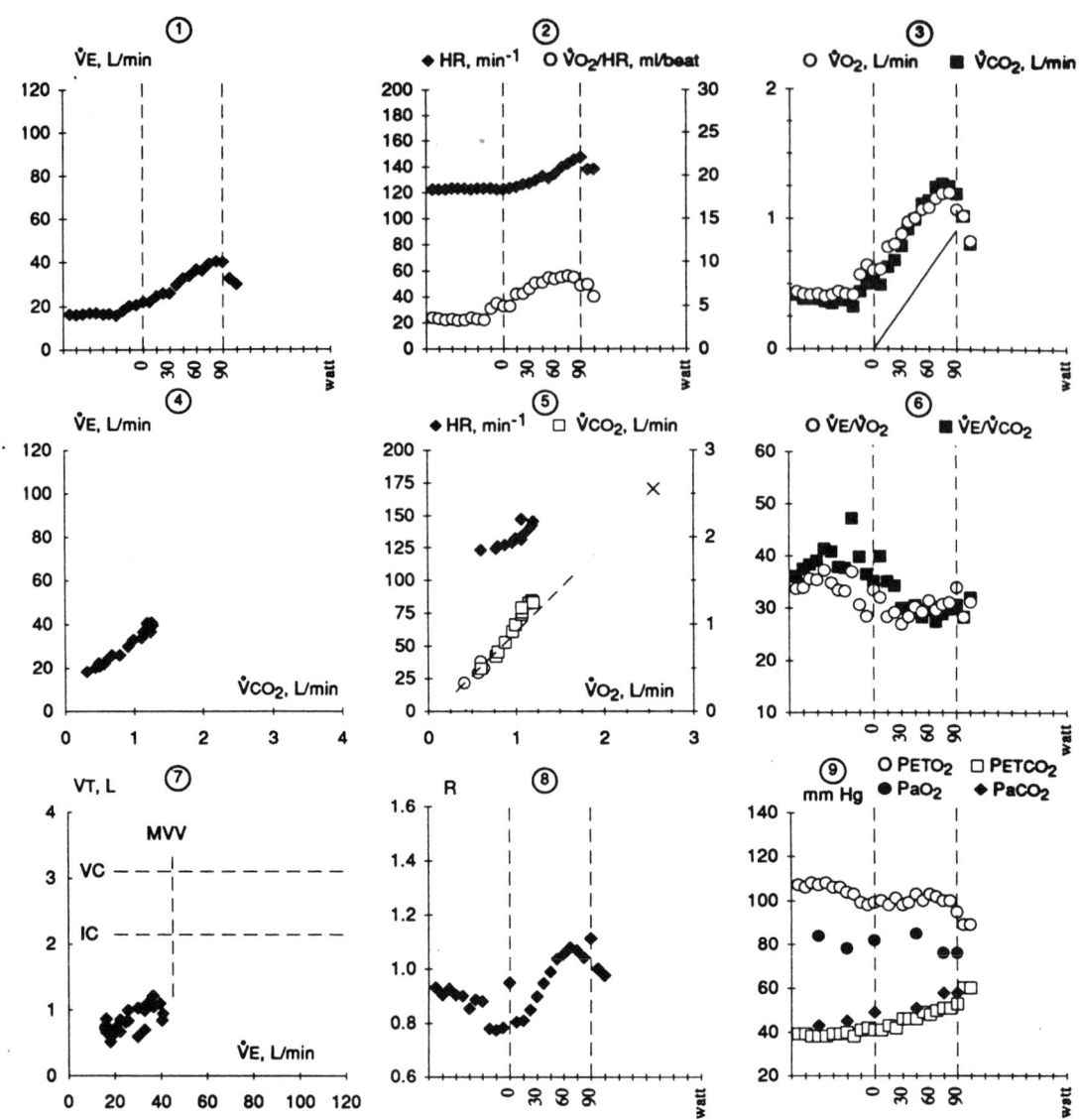

FIGURE 10.76.1. **1:** Vertical dashed lines in panels 1 to 3 and 6, 8, and 9 indicate the beginning and the end of the increasing work period. **2:** Unloaded cycling is performed for 2 minutes before the left vertical dashed line. **3:** In panel 3, the diagonal line shows the increase of $\dot{V}O_2$ at a slope of 10 ml/min/W. **4:** In panel 5, the diagonal dashed line has a slope of 1; the x in the upper right is the predicted maximum heart rate and $\dot{V}O_2$ for the subject.

Conclusion

As noted in Chapter 8, the flowcharts cannot, and should not, always come to a single diagnosis. This is because the patient may have pathophysi-ologic features involving more than one organ system. In this patient, the primary problem appears to be severe obstructive lung disease. Pulmonary vascular disease is secondary, complicated by anemia.

TABLE 10.76.3. Air Breathing

Time min	Work rate watts	BP mmHg	HR min⁻¹	f min⁻¹	V̇E L/min BTPS	V̇CO₂ L/min STPD	V̇O₂ L/min STPD	V̇O₂/HR ml/beat	R	pH	HCO₃⁻ meq/L	PO₂, mmHg ET	a	(A−a)	PCO₂, mmHg ET	a	(a−ET)	V̇E/V̇CO₂	V̇E/V̇O₂	VD/VT
	Rest		122	19	16.4	0.41	0.44	3.6	0.93			107			39			36	34	
	Rest		122	21	16.0	0.38	0.42	3.4	0.90			106			39			37	34	
	Rest		122	22	16.4	0.38	0.41	3.4	0.93			108			38			38	35	
	Rest	135/90	123	23	16.8	0.38	0.42	3.4	0.90	7.48	31	107	84	19	38	43	5	39	35	0.43
	Rest		123	25	17.0	0.36	0.40	3.3	0.90			108			38			41	37	
	Rest		123	25	16.4	0.35	0.41	3.3	0.85			106			39			41	35	
	Rest		122	22	16.6	0.39	0.44	3.6	0.89			106			39			38	33	
	Rest	126/84	123	22	15.8	0.37	0.42	3.4	0.88	7.46	31	104	78	22	40	45	5	38	33	0.43
	Unloaded		123	35	18.1	0.32	0.41	3.3	0.78			103			38			47	37	
	Unloaded		123	31	20.1	0.44	0.57	4.6	0.77			99			41			40	31	
	Unloaded		122	28	20.6	0.50	0.64	5.2	0.78			98			42			36	28	
	Unloaded	138/90	122	26	22.2	0.57	0.60	4.9	0.95	7.42	31	99	82	17	41	49	8	35	33	0.45
0.5	15		123	33	22.3	0.49	0.61	5.0	0.80			100			41			40	32	
1.0	15		124	30	24.6	0.63	0.78	6.3	0.81			98			43			35	28	
1.5	30		126	31	25.9	0.68	0.80	6.3	0.85			101			42			34	29	
2.0	30		127	26	25.9	0.79	0.88	6.9	0.90			98			46			30	27	
2.5	45		129	29	30.0	0.92	0.97	7.5	0.95			99			46			30	28	
3.0	45	140/78	132	33	32.9	0.99	1.00	7.6	0.99	7.38	30	103	85	14	46	51	5	30	30	0.41
3.5	60		131	31	33.9	1.11	1.07	8.2	1.04			100			49			28	29	
4.0	60		134	35	36.8	1.14	1.08	8.1	1.06			103			48			30	31	
4.5	75		139	30	36.6	1.24	1.15	8.3	1.08			102			50			27	30	
5.0	75	132/84	142	36	39.6	1.27	1.19	8.4	1.07	7.32	29	100	76	19	51	58	7	29	31	0.45
5.5	90		145	43	40.8	1.25	1.20	8.3	1.04			100			51			30	31	
6.0	90	180/84	147	48	40.4	1.19	1.07	7.3	1.11	7.32	29	95	76	21	53	58	5	31	34	0.46
	Recovery		138	47	32.8	1.02	1.02	7.4	1.00			89			60			28	28	
	Recovery		138	50	30.1	0.81	0.83	6.0	0.98			89			60			32	31	

Case 77 Mild Obstructive Airway Disease Complicated by Systemic Hypertension and Pulmonary Vascular Disease

Clinical Findings

This 64-year-old retired shipyard worker was evaluated because of increasing shortness of breath that had begun 7 years previously and had increased to become evident with walking two blocks or climbing a flight of stairs. He had smoked half a pack of cigarettes daily from age 40 to 60. He had been treated with isoniazid and ethambutol for pulmonary tuberculosis for 4 years, 2 decades ago. Prostatic carcinoma had been diagnosed 8 months previously while he was having a transurethral prostatectomy. He took triamterene, hydrochlorothiazide, and methyldopa for the treatment of hypertension. Pulse was irregular without other evidence of cardiovascular disease. The chest roentgenographic studies revealed a single small pleural plaque on the left, evidence of old granulomatous disease in the right apex, and a flat diaphragm. Respiratory function tests done several days prior to exercise showed airway obstruction.

Exercise Findings

The patient performed exercise on a cycle ergometer. He pedaled at 60 rpm without added load for 3 minutes. The work rate was then increased 15 W per minute to his symptom-limited maximum. Arterial blood was sampled every second minute, and intraarterial blood pressure was recorded from a percutaneously placed brachial artery catheter. Resting ECG showed some premature atrial and ventricular contractions, poor R-wave progression from leads V_1 through V_3, and left atrial enlargement. At 90 W there were occasional pairs of premature ventricular contractions and two episodes of ventricular bigeminy. The patient stopped exercising because of shortness of breath. Under questioning, he also conceded that he had felt some substernal tightness at the highest work rate.

Interpretation

Comments

This case is presented to illustrate the considerable amount of gas exchange abnormality that can occur during exercise, even with only mild abnormalities in spirometry, if there is considerable pulmonary vascular disease.

The results of the resting respiratory function studies indicate that this patient has mild airflow obstruction, hyperinflation, and a moderately severe abnormality in diffusing capacity (Table 10. 77.1). The resting ECG is abnormal, as evidenced by premature atrial and ventricular contractions and poor R-wave progression from V_1 to V_3. The arterial blood pressure is elevated. In such instances, one might have considered deferring the exercise test until blood pressure was under better control. The cuff-measured blood pressure is on the average 10 mm Hg lower than the

TABLE 10.77.1.   Selected Respiratory Function Data

Measurement	Predicted	Measured	
Age, yr		64	
Sex		Male	
Height, cm		178	
Weight, kg	80	82	
Hematocrit, %		47	

	Predicted	Before Bronchodilator	After Bronchodilator
VC, L	3.82	4.52	4.75
IC, L	2.55	3.25	
TLC, L	5.93	8.66	
FEV_1, L	2.98	2.69	2.78
FEV_1/VC, %	78	60	58
MVV, L/min	121	90	112
$D_L CO$, ml/mm Hg/min	24.8	14.0	

TABLE 10.77.2.   Selected Exercise Data

Measurement	Predicted	Measured
Peak $\dot{V}O_2$, L/min	2.16	1.42
Maximum HR, beats/min	156	159
Maximum O_2 pulse, ml/beat	13.9	8.9
$\Delta \dot{V}O_2/\Delta WR$, ml/min/W	10.3	8.1
AT, L/min	>0.95	0.7
Blood pressure, mmHg (rest, max)		186/116, 263/128
Maximum $\dot{V}E$, L/min		91
Exercise breathing reserve, L/min	>15	91
PaO_2, mmHg (rest, max ex)		79, 57
$P(A-a)O_2$, mmHg (rest, max ex)		38, 65
$P(a-ET)CO_2$, mmHg (rest, max ex)		4, 9
VD/VT (rest, heavy ex)		0.38, 0.47
HCO_3^-, mEq/L (rest, 2-min recov)		24, 17

TABLE 10.77.3.   Air Breathing

Time min	Work rate watts	BP mmHg	HR min⁻¹	f min⁻¹	$\dot{V}_E$ L/min BTPS	$\dot{V}_{CO_2}$ L/min STPD	$\dot{V}_{O_2}$ L/min STPD	$\dfrac{\dot{V}_{O_2}}{HR}$ ml/beat	R	pH	HCO_3^- meq/L	P_{O_2}, mmHg ET	a	(A − a)	P_{CO_2}, mmHg ET	a	(a − ET)	$\dfrac{\dot{V}_E}{\dot{V}_{CO_2}}$	$\dfrac{\dot{V}_E}{\dot{V}_{O_2}}$	$\dfrac{V_D}{V_T}$
	Rest	185/116								7.42	24		67			38				
	Rest		103	16	13.6	0.27	0.30	2.9	0.90			116			30			45	41	
	Rest		102	16	16.3	0.33	0.36	3.5	0.92			117			29			45	42	
	Rest		102	22	18.3	0.33	0.35	3.4	0.94			121			26			50	47	
	Rest		103	12	8.6	0.15	0.15	1.5	1.00			118			29			51	51	
	Rest		105	15	14.2	0.26	0.28	2.7	0.93			119			27			50	46	
	Rest	185/116	108	23	13.2	0.23	0.24	2.2	0.96	7.46	22	120	79	38	28	32	4	49	47	0.38
	Unloaded		114	12	17.9	0.37	0.37	3.2	1.00			115			31			46	46	
	Unloaded		115	21	22.9	0.50	0.55	4.8	0.91			116			30			42	38	
	Unloaded		116	17	28.4	0.64	0.67	5.8	0.96			112			33			42	40	
	Unloaded		117	19	28.5	0.64	0.65	5.6	0.98			117			30			42	41	
	Unloaded		117	27	35.8	0.72	0.69	5.9	1.04			120			28			47	49	
	Unloaded	236/126	119	27	35.6	0.74	0.71	6.0	1.04	7.43	22	122	72	46	28	33	5	45	47	0.39
0.5	15		121	23	38.1	0.78	0.73	6.0	1.07			118			30			46	50	
1.0	15		123	28	43.1	0.85	0.80	6.5	1.06			123			26			48	51	
1.5	30		128	29	44.5	0.85	0.79	6.2	1.08			125			25			49	53	
2.0	30	236/128	128	30	50.9	0.95	0.89	7.0	1.07	7.44	21	123	68	52	26	32	6	51	54	0.45
2.5	45		129	33	49.9	0.93	0.89	6.9	1.04			124			25			51	53	
3.0	45		133	38	49.8	0.91	0.92	6.9	0.99			121			27			51	51	
3.5	60		139	44	62.7	1.07	1.04	7.5	1.03			125			24			55	57	
4.0	60		143	39	63.2	1.12	1.08	7.6	1.04	7.44	21	126	61	59	24	31	7	53	55	0.45
4.5	75		146	40	62.7	1.15	1.13	7.7	1.02			123			26			52	52	
5.0	75		148	44	71.3	1.26	1.21	8.2	1.04			123			26			54	56	
5.5	90		153	50	86.6	1.46	1.35	8.8	1.08			127			23			56	61	
6.0	90		157	52	88.2	1.49	1.34	8.5	1.11	7.42	20	128	60	61	22	31	9	56	63	0.48
6.5	105	263/128	159	47	90.8	1.59	1.42	8.9	1.12	7.41	19	128	57	65	22	31	9	55	61	0.47
	Recovery		161	43	84.4	1.54	1.25	7.8	1.23			128			23			52	65	
	Recovery		160	41	78.6	1.39	1.22	7.6	1.14			127			23			54	62	
	Recovery		161	44	75.2	1.31	1.14	7.1	1.15			122			29			55	63	
	Recovery	233/139	138	35	60.3	1.12	0.95	6.9	1.18	7.39	17	127	73	51	24	29	5	51	60	0.40

directly recorded blood pressure, as described in Chapter 7. Because of the blood pressure elevation, the patient was exercised especially cautiously. The objective was to determine if this patient was primarily limited by his heart or lung disorder.

Analysis

Referring to flowchart 1, the peak $\dot{V}_{O_2}$ and AT are reduced (Table 10.77.2), which directs us through branch points 1.1, 1.2, and 1.3 to flowchart 4. The breathing reserve is low (branch point 4.1). The V_D/V_T is high (branch point 4.2), leading us to lung disease with impaired peripheral oxygenation. However, the V_T/IC ratio is not high as in restrictive lung disease. Nor does a respiratory acidosis develop as in obstructive lung disease. The breathing reserve is zero despite the presence of only mild obstructive lung disease. The reason for the absence of a breathing reserve is the increasing ventilatory drive with exercise due to an increasing V_D/V_T and decreasing Pa_{O_2} (Table 10.77.3) as work rate is increased.

The diagnosis box for lung disease with impaired peripheral oxygenation asks that we confirm with abnormalities in the pulmonary circulation box. The presence of O_2 flow limitation due to pulmonary vascular disease is confirmed by an increasing V_D/V_T with work rate, a systematic increase in P(A − a)O_2 with work rate, an increase in P(a − ET)CO_2 with work rate, steep heart rate–$\Delta\dot{V}_{O_2}$ relationship with no heart rate reserve, low O_2 pulse, and low and decreasing $\Delta\dot{V}_{O_2}/\Delta WR$ with increasing work rate. These findings implicate the pulmonary circulation as the organ of major dysfunction. This abnormality may be complicated by changes in gas exchange accounted for by a right-to-left shunt due to the opening of a foramen ovale during exercise (see the last item in the pulmonary vascular disease box). One hundred percent O_2 breathing during exercise might have confirmed the development of a right-to-left shunt.

Other gas exchange characteristics of a right-to-left shunt developing during exercise are an increasing rather than a decreasing $\dot{V}_E/\dot{V}_{CO_2}$ ratio dur-

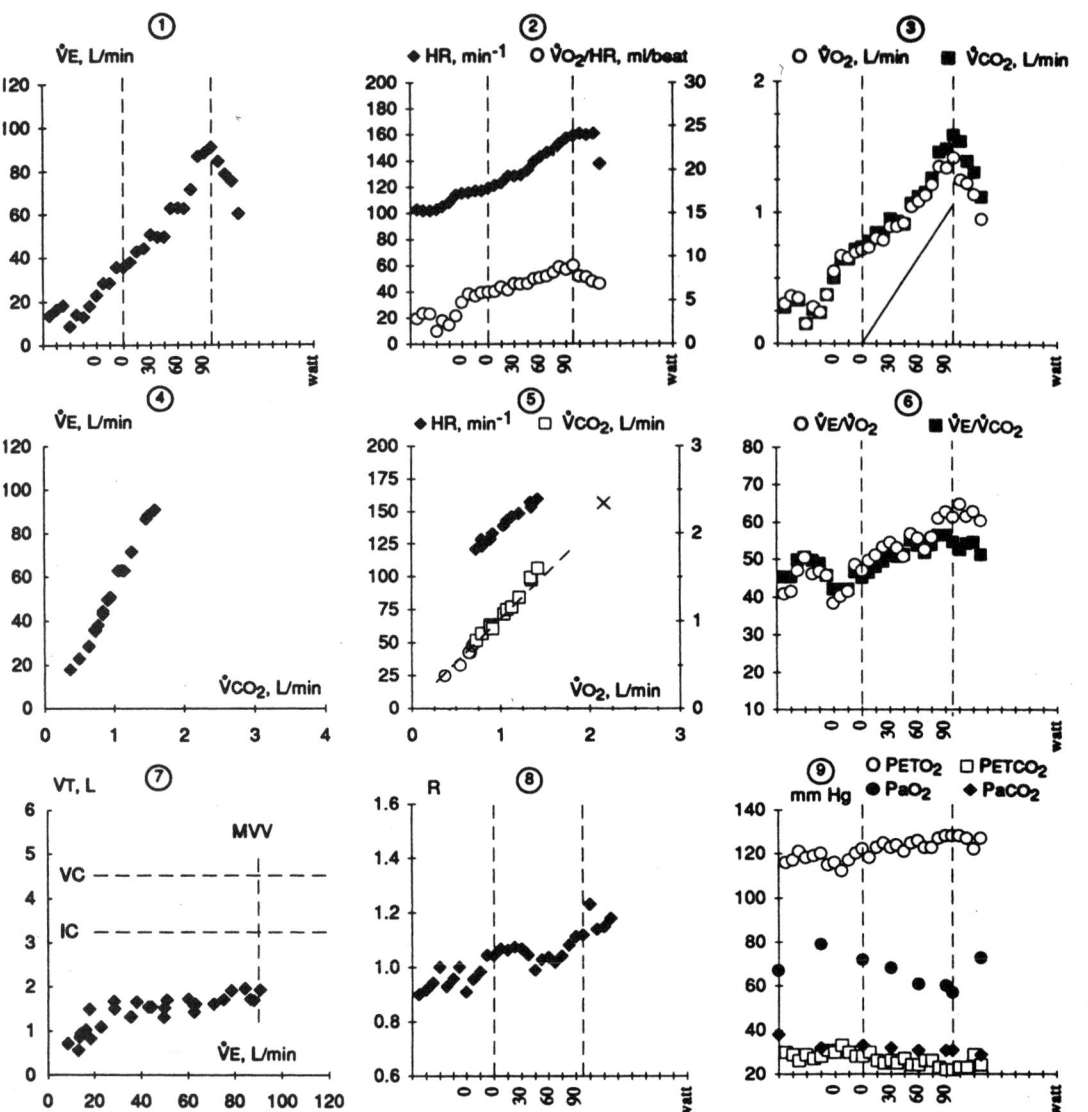

FIGURE 10.77.1.   **1:** Vertical dashed lines in panels 1 to 3 and 6, 8, and 9 indicate the beginning and the end of the increasing work period. **2:** Unloaded cycling is performed for 3 minutes before the left vertical dashed line. **3:** In panel 3, the diagonal line shows the increase of $\dot{V}O_2$ at a slope of 10 ml/min/W. **4:** In panel 5, the diagonal dashed line has a slope of 1; the x in the upper right is the predicted maximum heart rate and $\dot{V}O_2$ for the subject.

ing exercise below the *AT* (indicating the lung getting less efficient as a gas exchanger), R becoming greater than 1 throughout exercise (panel 8, Fig. 10.77.1), P_{ETCO_2} decreasing with increasing work rate (panel 9, Fig. 10.77.1), and the calculated V_D/V_T and $P(a - ET)CO_2$ not only remaining abnormal but becoming more abnormal as work rate increases (Table 10.77.3). These changes are explained by venous blood bypassing the lungs and mixing with arterial blood during exercise.

Conclusion

This patient has mild airflow obstruction but considerable pulmonary vascular disease, possibly secondary to emphysema. The probable opening of a foramen ovale during exercise can account for this patient's increasing V_D/V_T, exercise-induced hypoxemia, and high ventilatory drive reflected in an increasing rather than a decreasing $\dot{V}E/\dot{V}CO_2$ from the onset of exercise.

Case 78 Pulmonary Vascular Disease, Obstructive Airway Disease, and Talc Pneumoconiosis

Clinical Findings

This 63-year-old man had complained of progressive dyspnea for 10 years, but denied cough, sputum, wheezing, chest pain, or ankle edema. He had hypertension of 5 years' duration and was being treated with clonidine and Dyazide (hydrochlorothiazide and triamterene). For several months he had noted epigastric burning pain, occasionally relieved by meals. He had been exposed to talc for over 40 years in his work and was an ex-smoker with a 40 pack-year history of cigarette smoking. He had no heart murmurs. The chest roentgenogram showed pulmonary fibrosis. Resting ECG showed left anterior hemiblock and T-wave abnormalities in the anteroseptal region suggestive of ischemia. The patient was tested to evaluate the pathophysiology of his exertional dyspnea.

Exercise Findings

The patient performed exercise on a cycle ergometer. He pedaled at 60 rpm without an added load for 3 minutes. The work rate was then increased 20 W per minute to tolerance. Arterial blood was sampled every second minute, and intraarterial pressure was recorded from a percutaneously placed brachial artery catheter. The patient stopped exercise because of shortness of breath. He had no chest pain and no further ECG abnormalities.

Interpretations

Comments

Resting studies showed a mild obstructive ventilatory defect with a severely reduced D_LCO (Table 10.78.1). The patient had systemic hypertension at rest with a mildly abnormal ECG.

Analysis

Referring to flowchart 1, peak $\dot{V}O_2$ is decreased and the anaerobic threshold is borderline abnormal (Table 10.78.2). If one goes next to flowchart 3, the

high breathing reserve and mildly abnormal ECG lead to the diagnosis of myocardial ischemia, but this is unsatisfactory because it does not take into account the severe gas exchange disturbances elicited. Flowcharts 4 or 5 are preferable. Referring to flowchart 5, at branch point 5.1 we note abnormal VD/VT, $P(a - ET)CO_2$, and $P(A - a)O_2$. The breathing reserve is normal (branch point 5.3), and the PaO_2 progressively decreases (branch point 5.6), leading to the diagnosis of pulmonary vascular disease, with all the confirmatory findings described in the diagnostic box. The patient does have mild obstructive lung disease, but this is physiologically less important than the pulmonary vascular dis-

TABLE 10.78.1.   Selected Respiratory Function Data

Measurement	Predicted	Measured
Age, yr		63
Sex		Male
Height, cm		163
Weight, kg	68	67
Hematocrit, %		53
VC, L	3.28	3.56
IC, L	2.19	2.28
TLC, L	5.17	6.00
FEV$_1$, L	2.55	2.20
FEV$_1$/VC, %	78	62
MVV, L/min	115	96
D$_L$CO, ml/mm Hg/min	23.9	10.7

TABLE 10.78.2.   Selected Exercise Data

Measurement	Predicted	Measured
Peak $\dot{V}O_2$, L/min	1.84	1.02
Maximum HR, beats/min	157	161
Maximum O$_2$ pulse, ml/beat	11.7	6.7
$\Delta\dot{V}O_2/\Delta WR$, ml/min/W	10.3	5.2
AT, L/min	>0.81	0.8
Blood pressure, mmHg (rest, max)		162/84, 249/145
Maximum $\dot{V}E$, L/min		66
Exercise breathing reserve, L/min	>15	30
PaO$_2$, mmHg (rest, max ex)		79, 57
P(A − a)O$_2$, mmHg (rest, max ex)		33, 64
P(a − ET)CO$_2$, mmHg (rest, max ex)		4, 6
VD/VT (rest, max ex)		0.42, 0.44
HCO$_3^-$, mEq/L (rest, 2-min recov)		22, 17

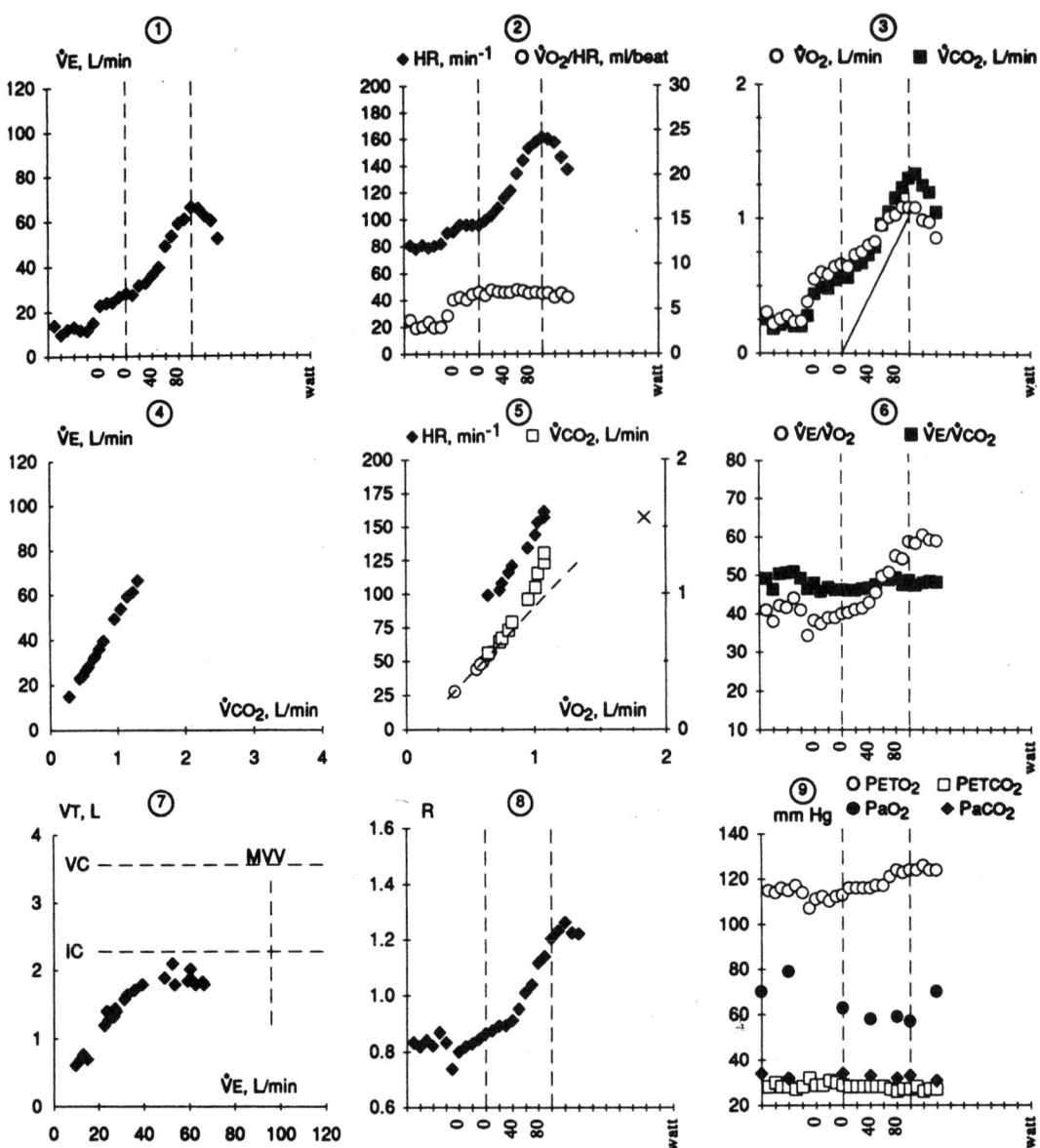

FIGURE 10.78.1. **1:** Vertical dashed lines in panels 1 to 3 and 6, 8, and 9 indicate the beginning and the end of the increasing work period. **2:** Unloaded cycling is performed for 3 minutes before the left vertical dashed line. **3:** In panel 3, the diagonal line shows the increase of $\dot{V}O_2$ at a slope of 10 ml/min/W. **4:** In panel 5, the diagonal dashed line has a slope of 1; the x in the upper right is the predicted maximum heart rate and $\dot{V}O_2$ for the subject.

ease, as evidenced by the low and decreasing $\Delta\dot{V}O_2/\Delta WR$ (panel 3, Fig. 10.78.1), very steep heart rate–$\dot{V}O_2$ relationship (panel 5, Fig. 10.78.1), high VD/VT, increased $P(A - a)O_2$, positive $P(a - ET)CO_2$, high ventilatory equivalents, and low and unchanging O_2 pulse despite polycythemia. The systemic hypertension could also be contributing to a high afterload and low cardiac output state.

Conclusion

This patient has pulmonary vascular disease that is more severe than can be explained by uncomplicated obstructive lung disease, as well as coexistent exercise arterial hypertension. A subsequent lung biopsy demonstrated talc pneumoconiosis.

TABLE 10.78.3.   Air Breathing

Time min	Work rate watts	BP mmHg	HR min⁻¹	f min⁻¹	$\dot{V}_E$ L/min BTPS	$\dot{V}_{CO_2}$ L/min STPD	$\dot{V}_{O_2}$ L/min STPD	$\dfrac{\dot{V}_{O_2}}{HR}$ ml/beat	R	pH	HCO_3^- meq/L	P_{O_2}, mmHg ET	a	(A − a)	P_{CO_2}, mmHg ET	a	(a − ET)	$\dfrac{\dot{V}_E}{\dot{V}_{CO_2}}$	$\dfrac{\dot{V}_E}{\dot{V}_{O_2}}$	$\dfrac{V_D}{V_T}$
	Rest	162/84								7.43	22		70			34				
	Rest		81	19	13.9	0.25	0.30	3.7	0.83			115			28			49	41	
	Rest		78	16	9.7	0.18	0.22	2.8	0.82			114			30			46	38	
	Rest		81	17	12.0	0.21	0.25	3.1	0.84			116			28			50	42	
	Rest		79	17	13.1	0.23	0.28	3.5	0.82	7.46	22	115	79	33	28	32	4	51	42	0.42
	Rest		80	17	11.6	0.20	0.23	2.9	0.87			117			27			51	44	
	Rest	192/96	82	17	11.3	0.20	0.24	2.9	0.83			114			28			49	41	
	Unloaded	240/117	90	21	14.8	0.28	0.38	4.2	0.74			107			32			46	34	
	Unloaded		91	19	22.7	0.44	0.55	6.0	0.80			111			29			48	38	
	Unloaded		96	17	23.8	0.49	0.60	6.3	0.82			112			29			46	37	
	Unloaded		96	19	24.1	0.48	0.58	6.0	0.83			110			31			47	39	
	Unloaded		96	20	26.6	0.54	0.64	6.7	0.84			112			30			46	39	
	Unloaded	237/111	96	20	28.0	0.57	0.66	6.9	0.86	7.44	23	113	63	49	29	34	5	46	40	0.42
0.5	20		99	19	27.4	0.56	0.64	6.5	0.88			116			28			46	40	
1.0	20		103	20	31.6	0.65	0.73	7.1	0.89			116			28			46	41	
1.5	40		108	20	32.7	0.67	0.75	6.9	0.89			116			28			46	41	
2.0	40	240/114	116	21	35.9	0.73	0.80	6.9	0.91	7.45	23	116	58	56	28	33	5	47	43	0.42
2.5	60		121	22	39.4	0.79	0.83	6.9	0.95			117			28			48	45	
3.0	60		134	26	49.3	0.96	0.95	7.1	1.01			117			28			49	50	
3.5	80		144	30	53.7	1.05	1.01	7.0	1.04			121			27			49	51	
4.0	80	246/123	153	32	59.2	1.15	1.03	6.7	1.12	7.44	21	124	59	62	26	32	6	49	55	0.43
4.5	100		157	33	61.2	1.23	1.08	6.9	1.14			123			27			47	54	
5.0	100	249/145	161	37	66.4	1.30	1.08	6.7	1.20	7.40	20	124	57	64	27	33	6	49	59	0.44
	Recovery		160	36	65.8	1.33	1.08	6.8	1.23			124			28			47	58	
	Recovery		157	35	62.8	1.25	0.99	6.3	1.26			126			26			48	60	
	Recovery		146	30	60.5	1.20	0.98	6.7	1.22			124			27			48	59	
	Recovery	234/108	137	25	52.6	1.05	0.86	6.3	1.22	7.35	17	124	70	53	27	31	4	48	59	0.40

Case 79 Systemic Sclerosis and Primary Lung Cancer: Preoperative Evaluation

Clinical Findings

This 59-year-old woman with progressive systemic sclerosis was found to have a potentially operable squamous cell carcinoma of the lung by fiberoptic bronchoscopy. She had a 26 pack-year history of cigarette smoking, complained of dyspnea after walking one block, and denied having a productive cough or hemoptysis. She had no history or overt signs or symptoms of heart disease. Her only medications were thyroid supplements and estrogens. A cardiopulmonary exercise test was done to evaluate cardiac and lung function reserves in response to stress.

Exercise Findings

The patient performed exercise on a cycle ergometer. She pedaled at 60 rpm without an added load for 3 minutes. The work rate was then increased 5 W per minute to her symptom-limited maximum. Arterial blood was sampled every second minute, and intraarterial blood pressure was recorded from a percutaneously passed brachial artery catheter. Resting and exercise ECGs were normal. The patient stopped exercise complaining of tired thighs.

Interpretation

Comments

The resting respiratory function studies show mild restriction and mild obstruction, severe loss of available pulmonary capillary bed, and mild hypoxemia (Table 10.79.1). She had no known cardiac disease.

Analysis

Referring to flowchart 1, the patient had a low peak $\dot{V}O_2$ and borderline anaerobic threshold (Table 10.79.2). If we use flowchart 3, we proceed through branch point 3.1 (normal breathing reserve) and branch point 3.3 (normal ECG) to poor effort or musculoskeletal disorder. This impression does not fit our patient well because she has unequivocal evidence of gas exchange abnormalities. If her anaerobic threshold were low, we would work through flowchart 4.

Because her breathing reserve is normal (branch point 4.1), we are directed to the right branch. Because the $\dot{V}E/\dot{V}CO_2$ is high at the AT (branch point 4.3), we arrive at the diagnosis of abnormal pulmonary circulation. The patient has all the physiologic abnormalities that define this disorder. While the VC is reduced (probably from systemic sclerosis), the increasing $P(A - a)O_2$ with increasing work rate suggests that the abnormal pulmonary circulation is due to pulmonary vascular disease rather than left ventricular failure (branch point 4.5).

Conclusion

This patient has mild restrictive and obstructive lung disease but does not have ventilatory limitation during exercise. Rather, she demonstrates significant gas exchange abnormalities characteristic of pulmonary vascular disease. This may be part of her systemic sclerosis and associated interstitial lung disease. Her peak $\dot{V}O_2$ of 11.5 ml/min/kg places her in a high-risk category for pulmonary resection.

TABLE 10.79.1.   Selected Respiratory Function Data

Measurement	Predicted	Measured
Age, yr		59
Sex		Female
Height, cm		165
Weight, kg	62	75
Hematocrit, %		43
VC, L	2.73	2.26
IC, L	1.82	1.36
TLC, L	4.57	3.34
FEV$_1$, L	2.18	1.58
FEV$_1$/VC, %	80	70
MVV, L/min	82	73
D$_L$CO, ml/mm Hg/min	18.0	8.4

TABLE 10.79.2.   Selected Exercise Data

Measurement	Predicted	Measured
Peak $\dot{V}O_2$, L/min	1.43	0.86
Maximum HR, beats/min	161	135
Maximum O$_2$ pulse, ml/beat	8.9	6.4
$\Delta\dot{V}O_2/\Delta WR$, ml/min/W	10.3	9.1
AT, L/min	>0.7	0.7
Blood pressure, mmHg (rest, max ex)		135/69, 180/81
Maximum $\dot{V}E$, L/min		38
Exercise breathing reserve, L/min	>15	35
PaO$_2$, mmHg (rest, max ex)		66, 55
P(A − a)O$_2$, mmHg (rest, max ex)		24, 51
P(a − ET)CO$_2$, mmHg (rest, max ex)		7, 13
VD/VT (rest, max ex)		0.40, 0.47
HCO$_3^-$, mEq/L (rest, recov)		25, 23

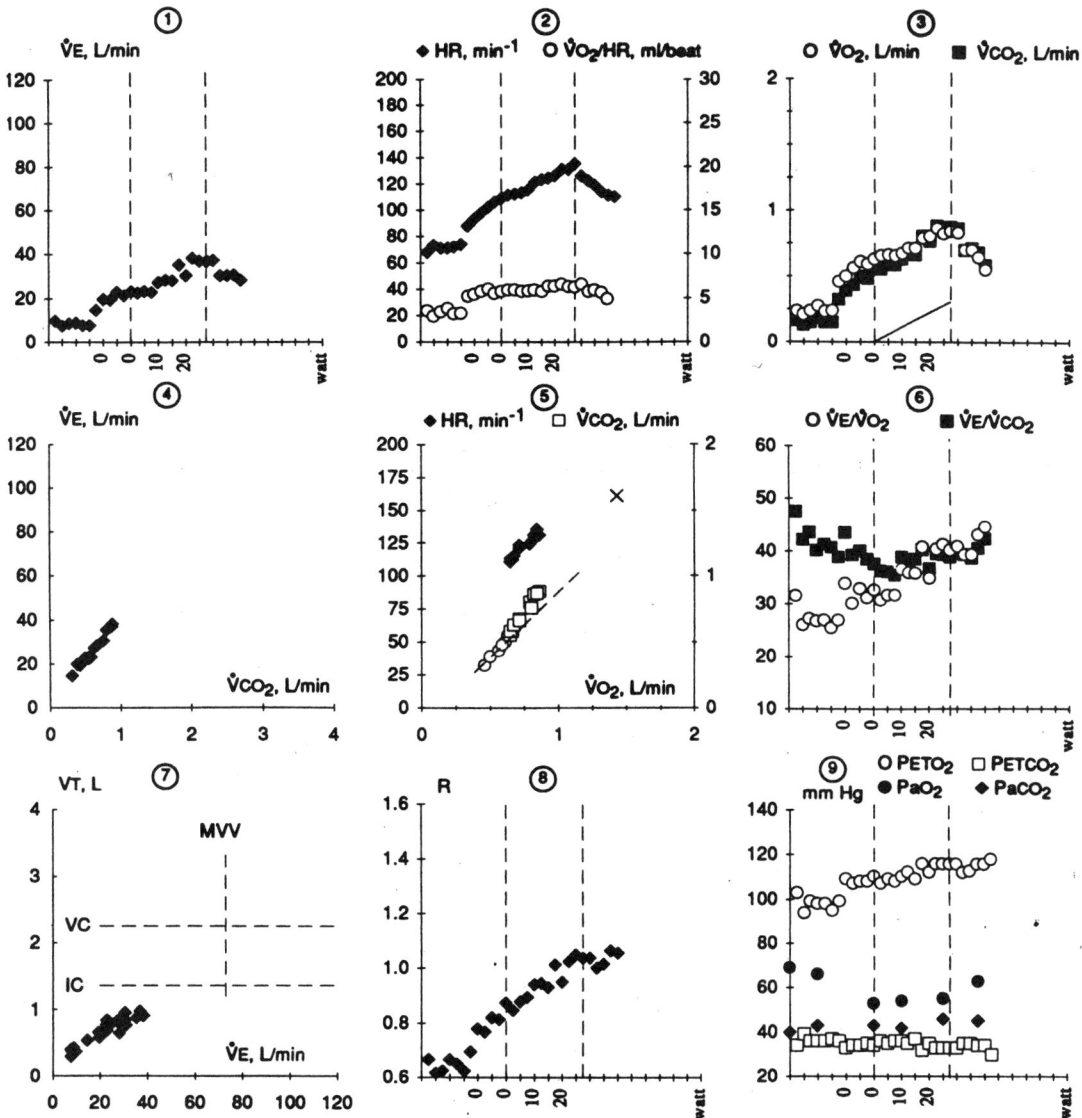

FIGURE 10.79.1.   **1:** Vertical dashed lines in panels 1 to 3 and 6, 8, and 9 indicate the beginning and the end of the increasing work period. **2:** Unloaded cycling is performed for 3 minutes before the left vertical dashed line. **3:** In panel 3, the diagonal line shows the increase of $\dot{V}O_2$ at a slope of 10 ml/min/W. **4:** In panel 5, the diagonal dashed line has a slope of 1; the x in the upper right is the predicted maximum heart rate and $\dot{V}O_2$ for the subject.

TABLE 10.79.3. Air Breathing

Time min	Work rate watts	BP mmHg	HR min⁻¹	f min⁻¹	$\dot{V}_E$ L/min BTPS	$\dot{V}_{CO_2}$ L/min STPD	$\dot{V}_{O_2}$ L/min STPD	$\dfrac{\dot{V}_{O_2}}{HR}$ ml/beat	R	pH	HCO₃⁻ meq/L	PO₂, mmHg ET	a	(A − a)	PCO₂, mmHg ET	a	(a − ET)	$\dfrac{\dot{V}_E}{\dot{V}_{CO_2}}$	$\dfrac{\dot{V}_E}{\dot{V}_{O_2}}$	$\dfrac{V_D}{V_T}$
	Rest	132/69								7.40	24		69			40				
	Rest		68	26	9.8	0.16	0.24	3.5	0.67			103			34			47	32	
	Rest		73	25	7.6	0.13	0.21	2.9	0.62			94			39			42	26	
	Rest		71	22	8.4	0.15	0.24	3.4	0.63			99			36			44	27	
	Rest	135/69	71	21	9.0	0.18	0.27	3.8	0.67	7.38	25	98	66	24	36	43	7	40	27	0.40
	Rest		72	19	7.8	0.15	0.23	3.2	0.65			98			36			41	27	
	Rest		74	20	7.8	0.15	0.24	3.2	0.63			95			37			41	25	
	Unloaded		88	27	14.7	0.32	0.46	5.2	0.70			99			36			39	27	
	Unloaded		93	34	19.8	0.39	0.50	5.4	0.78			109			33			43	34	
	Unloaded		98	29	19.3	0.43	0.56	5.7	0.77			107			34			39	30	
	Unloaded		102	33	22.8	0.50	0.61	6.0	0.82			108			34			40	33	
	Unloaded		106	33	21.2	0.48	0.59	5.6	0.81			108			35			38	31	
	Unloaded	171/81	109	31	23.2	0.55	0.63	5.8	0.87	7.37	24	110	53	49	34	43	9	37	33	0.41
0.5	5		111	29	22.4	0.55	0.65	5.9	0.85			107			36			36	31	
1.0	5		112	28	23.2	0.58	0.66	5.9	0.88			109			35			36	32	
1.5	10		113	27	22.8	0.58	0.65	5.8	0.89			108			36			35	32	
2.0	10	174/78	115	33	27.2	0.63	0.67	5.8	0.94	7.35	23	110	54	52	36	42	6	39	36	0.42
2.5	15		121	34	28.3	0.67	0.71	5.9	0.94			112			35			38	36	
3.0	15		123	33	28.1	0.66	0.71	5.8	0.93			109			37			38	36	
3.5	20		124	40	35.5	0.80	0.79	6.4	1.01			116			32			40	41	
4.0	20		126	32	30.5	0.76	0.80	6.3	0.95			112			35			37	35	
4.5	25		131	42	38.3	0.88	0.86	6.6	1.02			116			33			39	40	
5.0	25	180/81	131	39	37.0	0.86	0.82	6.3	1.05	7.35	25	116	55	51	33	46	13	39	41	0.47
5.5	30		135	38	36.9	0.87	0.84	6.2	1.04			116			33			39	40	
	Recovery		126	39	37.2	0.86	0.83	6.6	1.04			116			33			39	41	
	Recovery		122	36	30.5	0.70	0.70	5.7	1.00			112			35			39	39	
	Recovery		119	36	30.5	0.71	0.70	5.9	1.01			113			35			39	39	
	Recovery	162/69	114	40	30.9	0.68	0.64	5.6	1.06	7.32	23	116	63	44	34	45	11	40	43	0.47
	Recovery		111	43	28.1	0.58	0.55	5.0	1.05			116			34			42	44	
	Recovery		110									118			30					

Case 80 Primary Pulmonary Hypertension Before and After Treatment

Clinical Findings

This 51-year-old woman was referred for cardiopulmonary exercise testing to evaluate the severity of her pulmonary hypertension. She experienced progressive exertional dyspnea for 2 to 3 years, leading to marked exertional dyspnea, the cause of which remained undiagnosed until a right heart catheterization demonstrated pulmonary hypertension. After ruling out other causes of pulmonary hypertension, the diagnosis of primary pulmonary hypertension (PPH) was made, possibly secondary to having been on a phentermine and fenfluramine (Phen-Fen) regimen for 7 months for weight reduction 5 years previously. She also had systemic hypertension and was being treated with verapamil, benazepril (Lotensin), atorvastatin (Lipitor), and baby aspirin.

Two cardiopulmonary exercise tests are presented on this patient: The first was performed soon after diagnosis was made (Fig. 10.80.1), and the second 6 weeks after being on an oral endothelin-1 receptor antagonist (Fig. 10.80.2). The first cardiopulmonary exercise test was done to obtain objective information on the severity of her disease. The second was done to obtain objective information on the effect of the endothelin-1 receptor antagonist on her functional state and exercise tolerance; the patient reported clinical improvement.

Exercise Findings

On both occasions of testing, the patient performed exercise on a cycle ergometer while breathing through a mouthpiece with a nose clip in place for breath-by-breath measurements of gas exchange. Heart rate and rhythm were continuously monitored. Arterial pressure was monitored and measured every 2 minutes with an automated cuff device. The protocol consisted of 3 minutes of rest and 3 minutes of unloaded cycling at 60 rpm, followed by a progressive increase in work rate of 10 W per minute until she became too short of breath to continue. Twelve-lead ECG recordings were obtained during rest, every minute of exercise, and recovery. Arterial oxyhemoglobin saturation was continuously monitored with a pulse oximeter on her index finger. The patient performed the exercise test with good effort.

TABLE 10.80.1.   Selected Respiratory Function Data

Measurement	Predicted	Measured
Age, yr		51
Sex		Female
Height, cm		164
Weight, kg		99
Hematocrit, %		41
VC, L	3.20	3.01
IC, L	2.13	2.25
ERV, L	1.07	0.76
FEV_1, L	2.63	2.53
FEV_1/VC, %	82	84
MVV, L/min	97	112
D_LCO, ml/mm Hg/min	22.7	25.7

TABLE 10.80.2.   Selected Exercise Data

Measurement	Predicted	Baseline	After treatment
Peak $\dot{V}O_2$, L/min	1.70	0.86	0.93
Maximum HR, beats/min	168	134	136
Maximum O_2 pulse, ml/beat	10.0	6.4	6.8
$\Delta\dot{V}O_2$/ΔWR, ml/min/W	10.3	7.3	8.7
AT, L/min	>0.83	0.57	0.57
Blood pressure, mmHg (rest, max)		131/89, 201/79	125/73, 165/96
Maximum $\dot{V}E$, L/min		51	45
Exercise breathing reserve, L/min	>15	61	67
$\dot{V}E/\dot{V}CO_2$@AT	<32	52	39
$P_{ET}CO_2$@AT	≥40	24	30
$\dot{V}E$ vs $\dot{V}CO_2$	<32	48	34
SaO_2 rest, ex − pulse oximeter (%)	>95	96, 81	96, 93

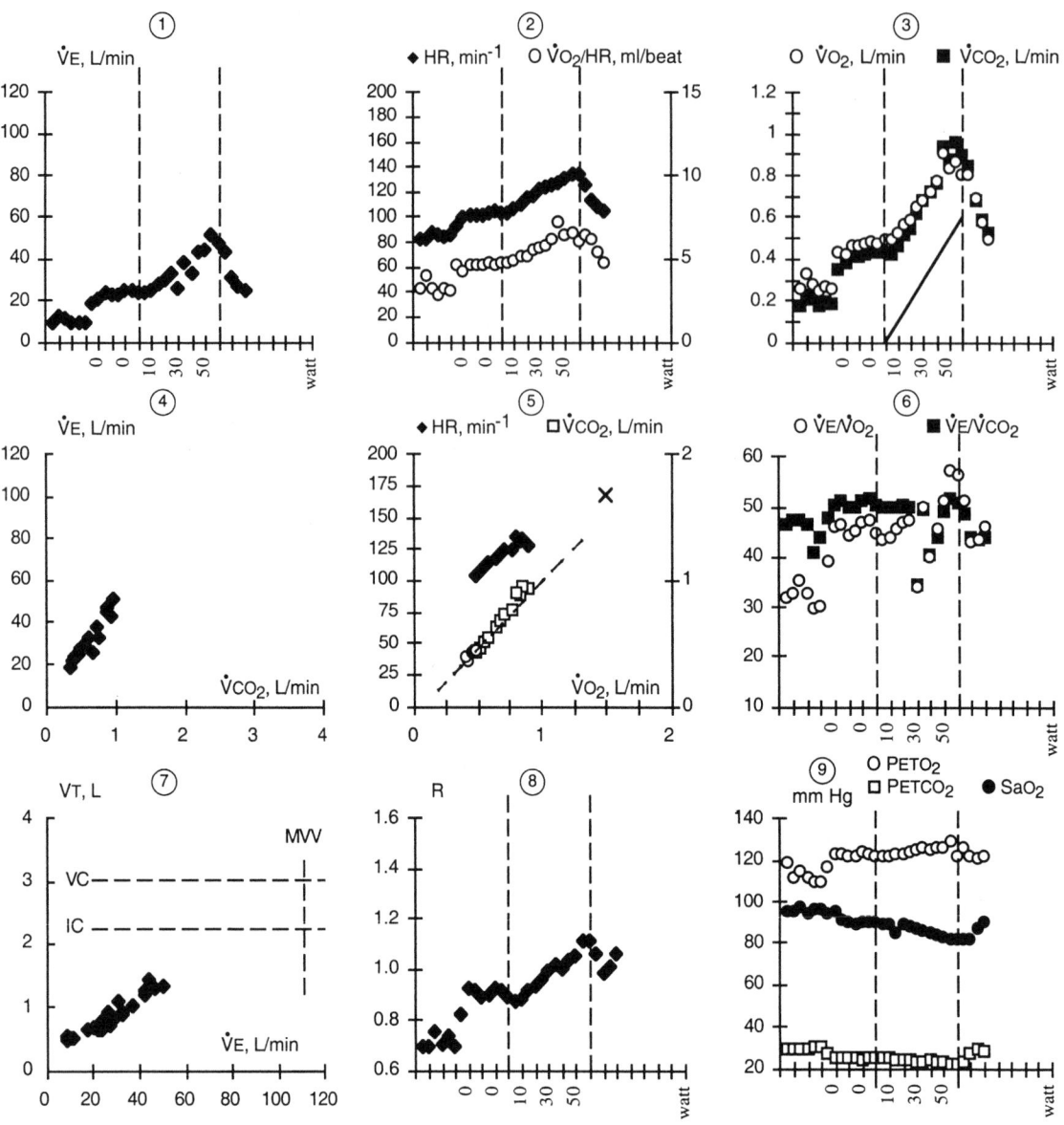

FIGURE 10.80.1. **1:** Vertical dashed lines in panels 1 to 3 and 6, 8, and 9 indicate the beginning and the end of the increasing work period. **2:** Unloaded cycling is performed for 3 minutes before the left vertical dashed line. **3:** In panel 3, the diagonal line shows the increase of $\dot{V}O_2$ at a slope of 10 ml/min/W. **4:** In panel 5, the diagonal dashed line has a slope of 1; the x in the upper right is the predicted maximum heart rate and $\dot{V}O_2$ for the subject.

Interpretation

Comments

Resting pulmonary function was normal (Table 10.80.1). Her ECG showed right ventricular hypertrophy and strain pattern. Her exercise ECGs were unchanged from rest except for rate.

Analysis

Referring to the baseline study (prior to endothelin-1 receptor antagonist treatment) in Tables 10.80.1 and 10.80.2, the accompanying nine-panel graphical array (Fig. 10.80.1), and the flowcharts, we are led to the diagnosis of pulmonary vascular disease. The analysis starts with flowchart 1. Her peak $\dot{V}O_2$ and *AT* are low, bringing us through branch points 1.1, 1.2, and 1.3 to flowchart 4. The breathing reserve is normal (branch point 4.1), and the ventilatory equivalent for $\dot{V}CO_2$ at the *AT* (branch point 4.3) is high, bringing us to abnormal pulmonary circulation. The exercise oxyhemoglobin saturation is low (branch point 4.5), bringing us to the diagnosis of pulmonary vascular disease in con-

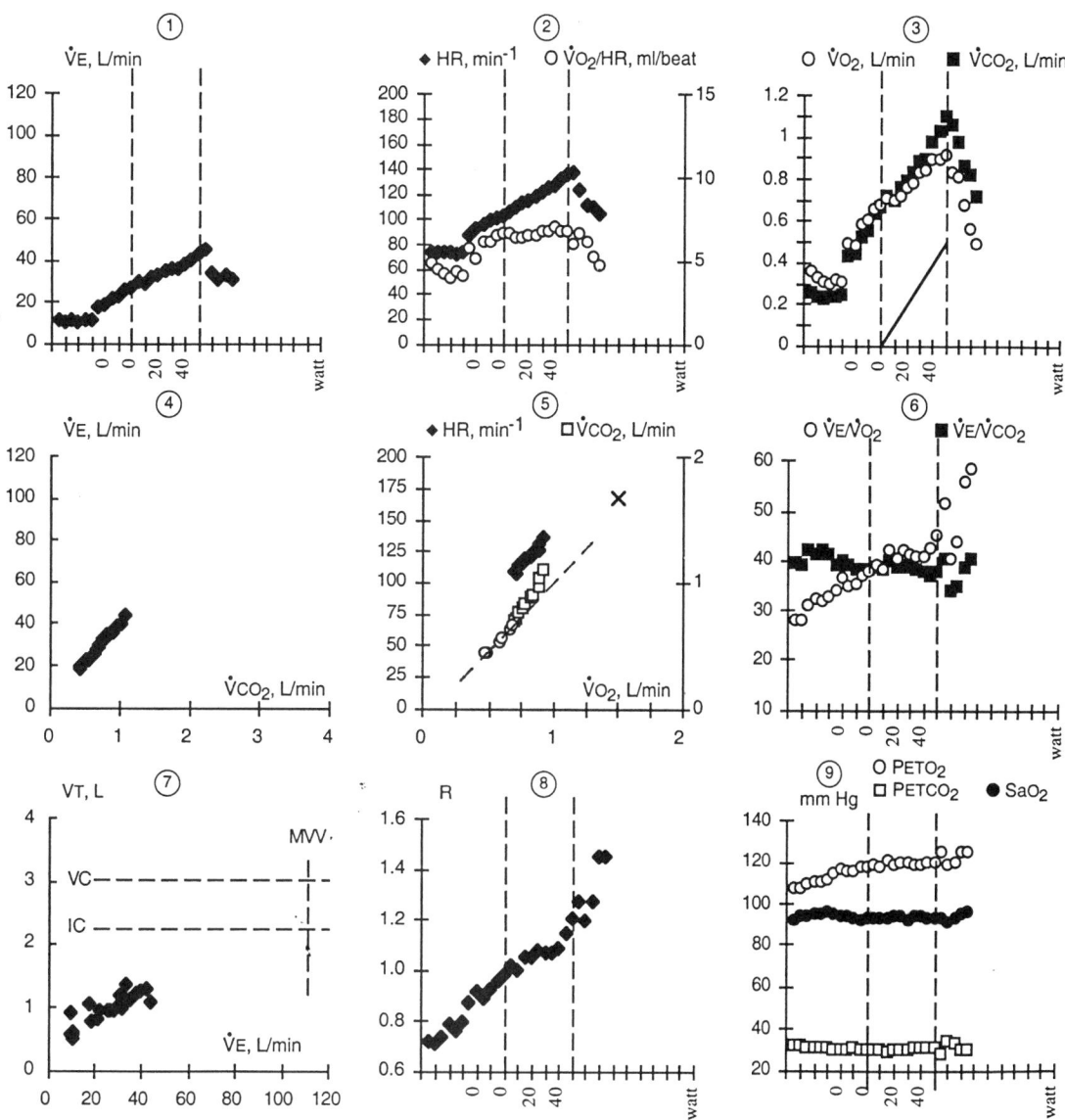

FIGURE 10.80.2.   **1:** Vertical dashed lines in panels 1 to 3 and 6, 8, and 9 indicate the beginning and the end of the increasing work period. **2:** Unloaded cycling is performed for 3 minutes before the left vertical dashed line. **3:** In panel 3, the diagonal line shows the increase of $\dot{V}O_2$ at a slope of 10 ml/min/W. **4:** In panel 5, the diagonal dashed line has a slope of 1; the x in the upper right is the predicted maximum heart rate and $\dot{V}O_2$ for the subject.

trast to the alternate diagnosis of left ventricular failure. She did not have direct arterial blood gas measurements. Therefore, we cannot use items 2 through 4 in the confirmatory box to support the diagnosis. However, other noninvasive measurements support the diagnosis.

Beside having low peak $\dot{V}O_2$ and *AT* values, which are often the only measurements examined by investigators treating these patients, the independent physiologic markers of impaired perfusion of ventilated lung characteristic of the pulmonary vasculopathy leading to pulmonary hypertension, are evidenced by the abnormally steep slope of $\dot{V}E$ versus

$\dot{V}CO_2$ and high $\dot{V}E/\dot{V}CO_2$ at the anaerobic threshold. The latter is 51 in this patient, with a normal value predicted between 25 and 32. This reflects the failure to perfuse ventilated lung, thereby requiring an approximate twice-normal ventilation to perform a given level of exercise such as walking.

An additional important abnormality is evident in the study shown in Figure 10.80.1. At the start of exercise (3 minutes), $PETCO_2$ abruptly decreases and $PETO_2$ abruptly increases, with a decrease in SaO_2 and increase in R, $\dot{V}E/\dot{V}O_2$, and $\dot{V}E/\dot{V}CO_2$. These directional changes are the opposite of normal and are almost always due to an opening of a right-to-left

TABLE 10.80.3. Baseline

Time min	Work rate watts	BP mmHg	HR min⁻¹	f min⁻¹	$\dot{V}_E$ L/min BTPS	$\dot{V}_{CO_2}$ L/min STPD	$\dot{V}_{O_2}$ L/min STPD	$\dot{V}_{O_2}$/HR ml/beat	R	pH	HCO₃⁻ meq/L	PO₂, mmHg ET	a	(A−a)	PCO₂, mmHg ET	a	(a−ET)	$\dot{V}_E$/$\dot{V}_{CO_2}$	$\dot{V}_E$/$\dot{V}_{O_2}$	VD/VT
	Rest		82	19	9.1	0.18	0.26	3.1	0.69			119			29			46	32	
	Rest		82	23	11.7	0.22	0.32	3.9	0.69			111			39			47	33	
	Rest		87	21	10.8	0.21	0.28	3.2	0.75			115			29			47	35	
	Rest	132/91	86	19	8.9	0.17	0.25	2.8	0.70			111			29			46	32	
	Rest		84	17	8.8	0.20	0.27	3.2	0.73			109			30			41	30	
	Rest		86	18	8.7	0.18	0.26	3.0	0.69			109			30			44	30	
	Unloaded		92	29	18.2	0.35	0.43	4.7	0.82			117			27			48	39	
	Unloaded		99	31	20.7	0.38	0.42	4.2	0.92			123			25			50	46	
	Unloaded		100	35	22.9	0.42	0.46	4.6	0.91			123			25			51	46	
	Unloaded		101	34	22.1	0.41	0.46	4.6	0.89			122			25			50	44	
	Unloaded		101	36	22.8	0.42	0.47	4.6	0.90			122			25			50	45	
	Unloaded		102	37	24.3	0.44	0.48	4.7	0.92			124			24			51	47	
	Unloaded		104	39	24.3	0.43	0.48	4.6	0.91			123			25			52	47	
	Unloaded		103	36	23.6	0.43	0.49	4.7	0.89			122			25			50	45	
0.5	5		103	36	23.0	0.42	0.49	4.7	0.87			122			25			50	44	
1.0	10		106	37	24.6	0.46	0.52	4.9	0.88			122			25			50	44	
1.5	15		110	39	27.3	0.51	0.56	5.1	0.91			123			24			50	45	
2.0	20		114	37	29.2	0.55	0.59	5.1	0.93			123			24			50	47	
2.5	25		117	38	32.7	0.62	0.65	5.6	0.95			124			24			50	47	
3.0	30		121	36	24.9	0.67	0.68	5.6	0.99			125			23			34	34	
3.5	35		123	37	37.5	0.72	0.71	5.8	1.01			126			23			49	50	
4.0	40		124	36	32.6	0.76	0.77	6.2	0.99			125			24			40	40	
4.5	45		127	36	43.0	0.94	0.91	7.1	1.03			126			23			44	45	
5.0	50		130	31	44.3	0.88	0.83	6.4	1.05			126			23			49	51	
5.5	55		133	39	51.0	0.96	0.86	6.5	1.11			129			22			51	57	
6.0	60	214/106	134	37	46.9	0.89	0.80	6.0	1.11			122			22			51	56	
	Recovery		125	34	42.5	0.84	0.80	6.4	1.06			126			23			49	51	
	Recovery		113	29	31.0	0.68	0.69	6.1	0.98			122			27			44	43	
	Recovery		108	29	26.6	0.58	0.58	5.4	1.01			121			29			43	44	
	Recovery	169/96	105	31	24.3	0.52	0.49	4.7	1.06			122			28			44	46	

shunt through a foramen ovale at the start of exercise, as described by Sun and associates (1). The mechanism can be attributed to the sudden increase in right atrial filling causing the right atrial pressure to increase above the left atrial pressure at the start of exercise, thereby diverting some of the venous return through the foramen ovale. This causes entry of humoral ventilatory stimuli (decreased Pa_{O_2} and increased Pa_{CO_2} and H⁺), ordinarily corrected in the lungs, to reach arterial chemoreceptors, thereby driving ventilation higher than would be predicted from the ventilation–perfusion mismatching caused by the underlying pulmonary vasculopathy. When this is observed during a cardiopulmonary exercise testing (CPET) study, the diagnostic possibilities are few. In patients without other disease evident, such as this patient, the diagnosis of PPH is almost a certainty.

This woman was restudied 6 weeks after treatment. At the time, she reported considerable symptomatic improvement. The posttreatment study is compared with the pretreatment study in Table 10.80.2 and Figures 10.80.1 and 10.80.2. The peak $\dot{V}_{O_2}$ is modestly improved, and the AT is unchanged. The major improvement is evident in the reduction in the arterial desaturation at end of exercise in the posttreatment study as compared with the pretreatment study (Sa_{O_2} of 93% as compared with 81%). This must be due to less right atrial pressure increase at the start of exercise. Improved matching of perfusion to ventilation is also reflected in the reduction in $\dot{V}_E$/$\dot{V}_{CO_2}$ at the AT after treatment as compared with before treatment (39 as compared to 52) and in the improved efficiency in ventilatory gas exchange evidenced by the increase in P_{ETCO_2} at the AT after treatment (30 compared with 24) (Table 10.80.4).

Conclusion

This 51-year-old woman, although symptomatic for several years, was recently diagnosed as having PPH after a right heart catheterization. Her exercise gas exchange was characteristic of PPH with an exercise-induced right-to-left shunt. She had a reduced peak $\dot{V}_{O_2}$ and AT, a marked increase in venti-

TABLE 10.80.4.   After Treatment

Time min	Work rate watts	BP mmHg	HR min⁻¹	f min⁻¹	V̇E L/min BTPS	V̇CO₂ L/min STPD	V̇O₂ L/min STPD	V̇O₂/HR ml/beat	R	pH	HCO₃⁻ meq/L	PO₂, mmHg ET	a	(A−a)	PCO₂, mmHg ET	a	(a−ET)	V̇E/V̇CO₂	V̇E/V̇O₂	VD/VT
	Rest		74	18	11.0	0.26	0.36	4.9	0.71			107			32			39	28	
	Rest		73	17	9.9	0.23	0.33	4.5	0.71			107			32			39	28	
	Rest		74	21	10.6	0.23	0.31	4.2	0.74			109			31			42	31	
	Rest	125/73	73	11	10.0	0.23	0.29	4.0	0.78			110			31			41	32	
	Rest		72	22	11.1	0.24	0.31	4.3	0.76			110			31			42	32	
	Rest		74	20	11.0	0.24	0.31	4.1	0.79			111			31			41	33	
	Unloaded		87	17	17.6	0.43	0.50	5.7	0.87			115			30			39	34	
	Unloaded		93	24	18.6	0.44	0.48	5.1	0.91			117			30			40	36	
	Unloaded		96	27	21.7	0.52	0.59	6.1	0.89			116			30			39	35	
	Unloaded		99	24	22.5	0.56	0.60	6.1	0.92			116			31			38	35	
	Unloaded		101	27	25.5	0.63	0.66	6.5	0.96			118			30			38	37	
	Unloaded	125/58	102	28	26.8	0.66	0.68	6.6	0.98			118			30			38	38	
0.5	10		106	30	29.2	0.71	0.71	6.7	1.01			119			30			39	39	
1.0	10		109	30	28.1	0.69	0.70	6.4	1.00			118			30			38	38	
1.5	20		113	33	31.9	0.76	0.72	6.4	1.05			121			29			40	42	
2.0	20	155/90	115	31	32.2	0.79	0.76	6.6	1.05			119			30			39	41	
2.5	30		118	32	34.2	0.84	0.78	6.6	1.07			120			30			39	42	
3.0	30		121	32	35.8	0.89	0.83	6.8	1.07			120			30			39	41	
3.5	40		124	32	35.7	0.90	0.84	6.8	1.07			119			31			38	41	
4.0	40		126	31	38.1	0.97	0.89	7.1	1.09			119			31			38	41	
4.5	50		131	32	39.6	1.03	0.89	6.8	1.15			120			31			37	43	
5.0	50		135	34	43.1	1.10	0.92	6.8	1.20			120			31			38	45	
	Recovery		137	41	44.7	1.06	0.83	6.1	1.27			125			28			40	51	
	Recovery		123	25	34.1	0.97	0.82	6.6	1.19			119			34			34	40	
	Recovery		111	26	31.0	0.86	0.68	6.1	1.27			120			33			35	44	
	Recovery		109	29	33.1	0.82	0.57	5.2	1.45			125			30			39	56	
	Recovery	171/82	104	30	30.5	0.72	0.50	4.8	1.45			125			30			40	58	

latory requirement because of ventilation–perfusion mismatch and exercise-induced hypoxemia secondary to the development of an exercise-induced right-to-left shunt, and hyperventilation of pulmonary blood flow. Aerobic function improved modestly during treatment with an endothelin-1 receptor antagonist, but the greatest gain in reducing her symptom of exertional dyspnea was due to the decrease in right-to-left shunt. Consequently, her ventilatory requirement during exercise was greatly reduced. The reduction in right-to-left shunt is attributed to a lowering of right atrial pressure accompanying a reduction in pulmonary vascular resistance. Without CPET, physicians man-

aging this patient would be blind to the pathophysiology of the patient's impairment. They would be unaware that she developed a right-to-left shunt during exercise before treatment, and that pulmonary vascular resistance decreased after treatment, sufficient to greatly reduce the size of her right-to-left shunt and ventilatory requirement.

Reference

1. Sun XG, Hansen JE, Oudiz RJ, Wasserman K. Gas exchange detection of exercise-induced right-to-left shunt in patients with primary pulmonary hypertension. *Circulation* 2002;105:54–60.

Case 81 Cardiomyopathy Due to Diastolic Dysfunction

Clinical Findings

This 29-year-old male executive has had exercise intolerance due to fatigue and dyspnea for about a year. He had been evaluated by a pulmonologist, allergist, and cardiologist, none of whom felt that they had an understanding of the cause of his symptoms. He had a history of asthma, but his physical signs and pulmonary function tests were not compatible with his symptoms. He was referred for cardiopulmonary exercise testing in order to get some help in understanding his symptoms and pathophysiology.

He had three exercise tests, the one presented here being the third. The first two were very similar to the one presented here and showed that the peak $\dot{V}O_2$ and *AT* were significantly reduced with high CO_2 output, reflecting a low work rate metabolic acidosis that was confirmed by arterial blood gases and lactate measurements on tests 2 and 3. Also, the O_2 pulse was significantly reduced and did not increase normally. The arterial blood gases and VD/VT were normal. Therefore, we knew that the low peak $\dot{V}O_2$ and *AT* were not due to lung or primary pulmonary vascular disease. Also, they were not due to peripheral arterial disease because the pattern of increase in $\dot{V}O_2$ and $\dot{V}CO_2$ was not compatible with this diagnosis (see Chapter 8). In the absence of a murmur, ECG changes suggestive of myocardial ischemia, or history of congenital heart disease, he was diagnosed as either having a cardiomyopathy with diastolic dysfunction, or, less likely, a skeletal muscle myopathy in which the patient's muscles could not consume O_2 normally. Assuming that he did not have a skeletal muscle myopathy, the low O_2 pulse at peak $\dot{V}O_2$ indicates that his maximal stroke volume was about 65 mL.

To distinguish between cardiac and muscle bioenergetic dysfunction, the cardiopulmonary exercise test was repeated for a third time with systemic and pulmonary arterial and femoral venous catheters with blood gas and pH measurements and direct arterial blood pressure tracings in search of a possible diagnosis of hypertrophic cardiomyopathy, other cardiomyopathy with diastolic dysfunction, or peripheral skeletal muscle myopathy.

Exercise Findings

Catheters were placed in the patient's right femoral vein, pulmonary artery, and brachial artery for the purpose of measuring blood gases, lactate, and arterial pressures and wave form. The patient performed exercise on a cycle ergometer while breathing through a mouthpiece with a nose clip in place for breath-by-breath measurements of gas exchange. Heart rate and rhythm were continuously monitored. The protocol consisted of 3 minutes of rest and 3 minutes of unloaded pedaling at 60 rpm, followed by a progressive increase in work rate of 20 W per minute until the patient became too symptomatic to continue. Blood was sampled for

TABLE 10.81.1.   Selected Respiratory Function Data

Measurement	Predicted	Measured
Age, yr		20
Sex		Male
Height, cm		180
Weight, kg	81	86
Hematocrit, %		47
VC, L	4.95	4.29
IC, L	3.30	2.94
FEV$_1$, L	4.13	2.74
FEV$_1$/VC, %	83	64
MVV, L/min	163	110

TABLE 10.81.2.   Selected Exercise Data

Measurement	Predicted	Measured
Peak $\dot{V}O_2$, L/min	3.28	1.69
Maximum HR, beats/min	192	176
Maximum O_2 pulse, ml/beat	17.2	9.8
$\Delta\dot{V}O_2/\Delta WR$, ml/min/W	10.3	7.9
AT, L/min	>1.41	0.90
Blood pressure, mmHg (rest, max ex)		155/85, 160/90
Maximum $\dot{V}E$, L/min		90
Exercise breathing reserve, L/min	>15	20
PaO$_2$, mmHg (rest, max ex)		86, 105
P(A − a)O$_2$, mmHg (rest, max ex)		11, 17
P(a − ET)CO$_2$, mmHg (rest, max ex)		4, 7
VD/VT (rest, max ex)		0.47, 0.41
HCO$_3^-$, mEq/L (rest, recov)		26, 17
Lactate, mEq/L (recovery)		13.7

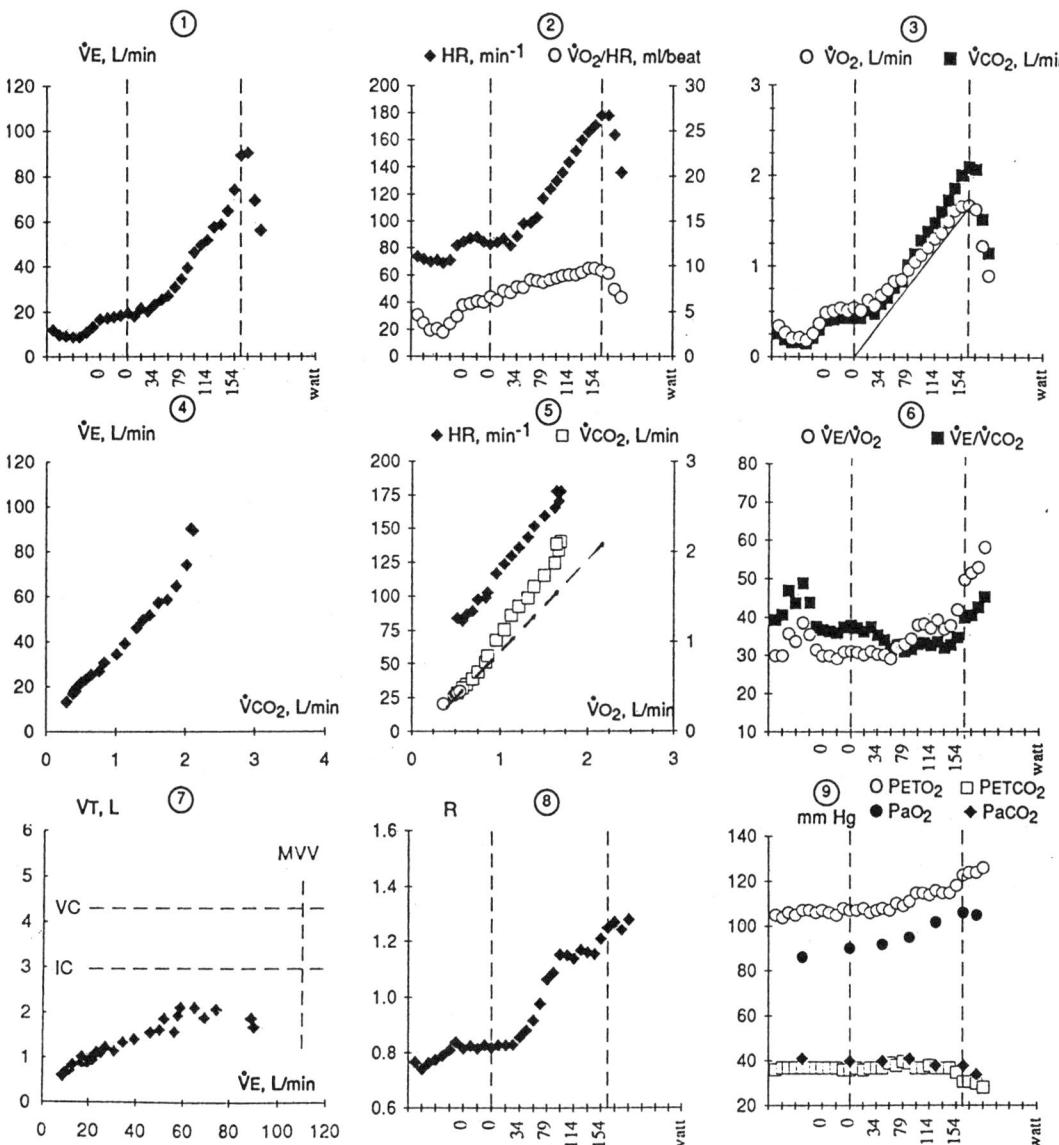

FIGURE 10.81.1.   **1:** Vertical dashed lines in panels 1 to 3 and 6, 8, and 9 indicate the beginning and the end of the increasing work period. **2:** Unloaded cycling is performed for 3 minutes before the left vertical dashed line. **3:** In panel 3, the diagonal line shows the increase of $\dot{V}O_2$ at a slope of 10 ml/min/W. **4:** In panel 5, the diagonal dashed line has a slope of 1; the x in the upper right is the predicted maximum heart rate and $\dot{V}O_2$ for the subject.

blood gases, pH, and lactate at rest, at the end of 3 minutes of unloaded cycling, every minute during the incremental exercise period, and at 6 minutes of recovery from the three sites. Twelve-lead ECG recordings were obtained during rest, every minute of exercise, and recovery. The patient performed the exercise test with good effort. His resting and exercise electrocardiograms were normal. No ectopic beats were noted.

The patient had a near syncopal event during the immediate recovery period as well as during spirometry. During these events he complained of dizziness and was diaphoretic. He admitted to these symptoms having occurred previously after exercise. His blood pressure was noted to drop to 82/64, while his pulse remained in the 90 range. Lying flat with his legs raised helped him recover from these two episodes. The typical cardiac slowing of a vasovagal event was not observed.

Interpretation

Comments

Respiratory function tests showed mild airflow obstruction (Table 10.81.1).

TABLE 10.81.3.   Air Breathing

Time min	Work rate watts	BP mmHg	HR min⁻¹	f min⁻¹	$\dot{V}_E$ L/min BTPS	$\dot{V}_{CO_2}$ L/min STPD	$\dot{V}_{O_2}$ L/min STPD	$\dot{V}_{O_2}$/HR ml/beat	R	pH	HCO_3^- meq/L	P_{O_2}, mmHg ET	a	(A−a)	P_{CO_2}, mmHg ET	a	(a−ET)	$\dot{V}_E/\dot{V}_{CO_2}$	$\dot{V}_E/\dot{V}_{O_2}$	V_D/V_T
	Rest																		30	
	Rest		74	17	12.0	0.26	0.34	4.6	0.76			105			36			39	30	
	Rest		72	15	9.7	0.20	0.27	3.8	0.74			104			37			41	36	
	Rest		70	16	9.2	0.16	0.21	3.0	0.76			106			37			47	34	
	Rest		71	15	9.0	0.17	0.22	3.1	0.77			105			37			44	39	
	Rest	155/85	69	15	8.9	0.15	0.19	2.8	0.79	7.40	25	107	86	14	37	41	4	49	35	0.47
	Rest		71	16	10.9	0.21	0.26	3.7	0.81			107			37			44		
	Unloaded		82	16	13.3	0.31	0.37	4.5	0.84			106			37			37	31	
	Unloaded		85	19	16.7	0.40	0.49	5.8	0.82			107			37			37	30	
	Unloaded		87	17	17.1	0.42	0.51	5.9	0.82			106			37			36	30	
	Unloaded		88	19	17.8	0.44	0.54	6.1	0.81			105			37			36	29	
	Unloaded		85	20	18.2	0.43	0.52	6.1	0.83			108			36			37	31	
	Unloaded	145/85	83	22	19.4	0.45	0.55	6.6	0.82	7.41	25	107	90	13	36	40	4	38	31	0.38
0.5	4		84	20	18.1	0.43	0.52	6.2	0.83			107			37			37	31	
1.0	14		87	23	21.4	0.52	0.63	7.2	0.83			108			36			37	30	
1.5	24		82	21	20.3	0.48	0.58	7.1	0.83			106			37			38	31	
2.0	34		89	21	23.1	0.59	0.69	7.8	0.86			107			37			35	30	
2.5	44	155/85	98	23	25.0	0.66	0.75	7.7	0.88	7.40	24	108	92	14	37	40	3	34	30	0.33
3.0	54		99	22	26.8	0.77	0.84	8.5	0.92			107			39			32	29	
3.5	64		103	27	30.5	0.84	0.86	8.3	0.98			110			38			33	32	
4.0	79		117	26	34.4	1.02	0.96	8.2	1.06			109			40			31	33	
4.5	85	175/90	124	28	39.2	1.14	1.05	8.5	1.09	7.38	24	111	95	17	39	41	2	32	35	0.31
5.0	94		130	30	46.2	1.30	1.13	8.7	1.15			115			37			33	38	
5.5	104		136	31	49.7	1.39	1.21	8.9	1.15			115			37			33	38	
6.0	114		144	28	51.7	1.49	1.31	9.1	1.14			114			38			33	37	
6.5	124	160/90	152	30	57.5	1.61	1.38	9.1	1.17	7.39	23	116	102	14	37	38	1	34	39	0.31
7.0	134		160	28	58.7	1.74	1.50	9.4	1.16			115			37			32	37	
7.5	144		166	31	64.7	1.87	1.62	9.8	1.15			115			37			33	38	
8.0	154		171	36	74.1	2.02	1.67	9.8	1.21			118			35			35	42	
8.5	164		178	48	89.3	2.11	1.69	9.5	1.25	7.35	21	123	106	12	31	38	7	40	50	0.41
9.0	152		178	54	90.2	2.08	1.64	9.2	1.27			124			31			41	52	
	Recovery		164	37	69.2	1.53	1.23	7.5	1.24	7.32	17	124	105	16	30	34	4	43	53	0.38
	Recovery		136	36	56.1	1.15	0.90	6.6	1.28			126			28			45	58	

TABLE 10.81.4.   Hemodynamic Responses to Exercise

Status	VO_2 (ml/min)	Heart rate (beats/min)	Systemic artery O_2 cont (ml/100 ml)	PO_2 (mmHg)	O_2 sat (%)	Pulmonary artery O_2 cont (ml/100 ml)	PO_2 (mmHg)	O_2 sat. (%)	Femoral vein O_2 cont (ml/100 ml)	PO_2 (mmHg)	O_2 sat (%)	$C(a-\bar{v})_{O_2}$ (ml/100 ml)	S.V. (ml)	C.O. (L/min)
Rest	250	71	20.0	86	97	12.1	33	60	6.0	20	32	7.9	44	3.1
O load	520	83	21.0	90	97	8.7	26	47	5.0	18	25	12.3	51	4.2
44 watts	720	98	21.0	92	97	8.6	26	44	4.9	18	25	12.4	59	5.8
85 watts	1000	124	21.0	95	97	8.2	25	39	5.8	21	29	12.8	63	7.8
124 watts	1340	152	21.5	102	97	7.9	25	37	7.4	26	35	13.6	65	9.8
164 watts	1680	176	22.0	106	97	6.1	23	29	6.7	25	31	15.9	60	10
(Max ex)	1640	164	22.0	105	97	4.8	20	22	5.1	23	24	17.2	58	9.5
6 min rec			21.0	99	97	14.5	45	69	17.0	55	80	6.5		

Analysis

Referring to Table 10.81.2 and flowchart 1, his peak $\dot{V}_{O_2}$ and anaerobic threshold are low, bringing us through branch points 1.1, 1.2, and 1.3 to flowchart 4. The breathing reserve is normal (branch point 4.1) and the ventilatory equivalent for $\dot{V}_{CO_2}$ at the anaerobic threshold (branch point 4.3) is borderline normal, bringing us to the diagnosis of O_2 flow problem of nonpulmonary origin. The hematocrit is normal (branch point 4.4), and he has a low O_2 pulse that is nonchanging as peak $\dot{V}_{O_2}$ is approached. This brings us to heart disease. Although his electrocardiogram is normal, he has an abnormally steep heart rate increase relative to $\dot{V}_{O_2}$ increase, and a reduced $\Delta\dot{V}_{O_2}/\Delta WR$, supporting the diagnosis of heart disease.

For the hemodynamic measurements, see Table 10.81.4. The stroke volume calculated by the direct Fick method was abnormally low at about 65 mL per beat on repeated measurements, which explained the low peak $\dot{V}_{O_2}$ and steep heart rate–$\dot{V}_{O_2}$ relationship. The O_2 extraction across the leg is normal, indicating that the patient does not have a skeletal muscle myopathy that prevents normal O_2 extraction. Note that his femoral vein P_{O_2} increased as work rate continued past the subject's anaerobic threshold. This paradoxical phenomenon has been previously observed in heart failure patients by Koike and associates (1). O_2 extraction across the central circulation was normal, although the maximum O_2 extraction (75% to 80%) is reached at a lower $\dot{V}_{O_2}$ than expected.

Conclusion

This 29-year-old man had a low stroke volume and cardiac output state judged to be due to diastolic cardiomyopathy. Pulmonary vascular disease, lung disease, peripheral arterial disease, skeletal muscle disease, and other forms of heart disease were excluded.

Reference

1. Koike A, Wasserman F, Taniguchi K, et al. Critical capillary oxygen partial pressure and lactate threshold in patients with cardiovascular disease. *J Am Coll Cardiol* 1994;23:1644–1650.

Case 82 Transition from Normal to Left Ventricular Failure

Clinical Findings

This 71-year-old white-collar worker was evaluated by cardiopulmonary exercise testing 4.5 years earlier (at age 66) and again at this time because of a recent worsening in exercise tolerance. The earlier studies showed that he had mild underlying lung or pulmonary vascular disease evidenced by a reduced diffusing capacity and slightly elevated ventilatory equivalent for CO_2 at the anaerobic threshold but normal lung mechanics. He tried to maintain a personalized exercise training program. He was doing well until about 9 months earlier, when he developed painless hematuria. Workup for this was complicated by a respiratory arrest. It was eventually revealed that the hematuria was due to a renal calculus. He now experiences dyspnea with exercise. His medications consist of a cholesterol-lowering drug and an inhaled bronchodilator.

Exercise Findings

For both evaluations, the patient performed exercise on a cycle ergometer while breathing through a mouthpiece with a nose clip in place for breath-by-breath measurements of gas exchange. Heart rate and rhythm were continuously monitored. The protocol consisted of 3 minutes of rest and 3 minutes of unloaded pedaling at 60 rpm, followed by a progressive increase in work rate of 15 W per minute until he became too symptomatic to continue. He stopped exercise because of leg fatigue on both occasions; 12-lead ECG recordings were obtained during rest, every minute of exercise, and recovery. For the first test at age 66, he had a normal ECG.

For the test at age 71, he had a prolonged PR interval (0.21 sec) and some premature atrial contractions at rest, which disappeared during exercise. There was no ectopy during exercise. The patient performed the exercise test with good effort.

TABLE 10.82.1.   Selected Respiratory Function Data

Measurement	Predicted	Measured
Age, yr		66
Sex		Male
Height, cm		164
Weight, kg	69	72
Hematocrit, %		43
VC, L	3.05	2.90
IC, L	2.03	2.00
FEV_1, L	2.48	2.30
FEV_1/VC, %	81	79
MVV, L/min	105	118
$D_L CO$, ml/mm Hg/min	23	19

TABLE 10.82.2.   Selected Respiratory Function Data

Measurement	Predicted	Measured
Age, yr		71
Sex		Male
Height, cm		164
Weight, kg	69	74
Hematocrit, %		43
VC, L	2.96	3.01
IC, L	1.98	2.22
FEV_1, L	2.30	2.64
FEV_1/VC, %	78	88
MVV, L/min	93	110
$D_L CO$, ml/mm Hg/min	23	12.3

TABLE 10.82.3.   Selected Exercise Data

Measurement	Predicted Age 66	Predicted Age 71	Measured Age 66	Measured Age 71
Peak $\dot{V}O_2$, L/min	1.80	1.67	1.88	1.24
Maximum HR, beats/min	154	149	125	116
Maximum O_2 pulse, ml/beat	11.7	11.2	15.9	10.7
$\Delta\dot{V}O_2/\Delta WR$, ml/min/W	10.3	10.3	14	7.2
AT, L/min	>0.85	>0.78	1.0	0.65
Maximum $\dot{V}E$, L/min			90	63
Exercise breathing reserve, L/min	>15	>15	28	47

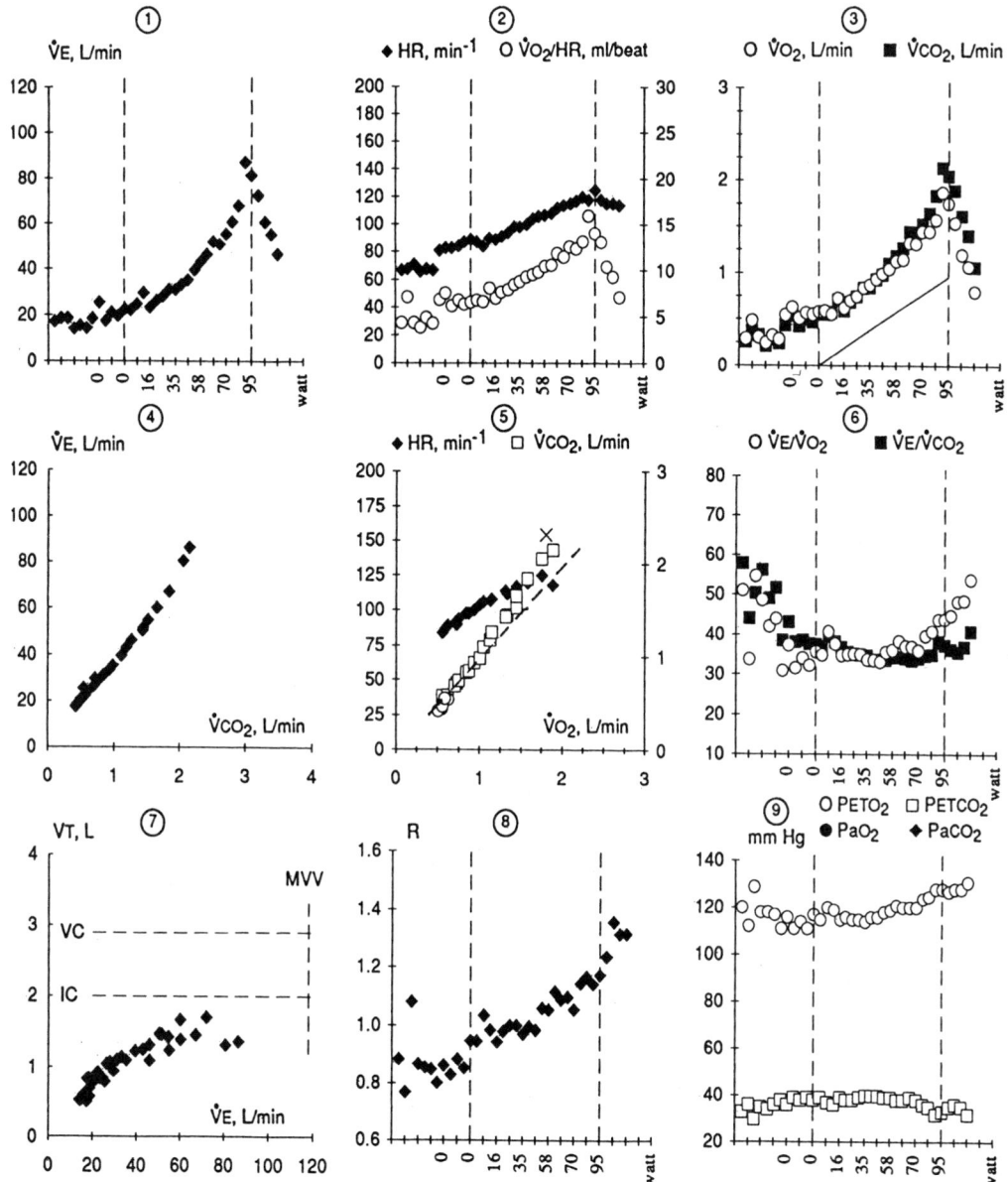

FIGURE 10.82.1. Age 66. **1:** Vertical dashed lines in panels 1 to 3 and 6, 8, and 9 indicate the beginning and the end of the increasing work period. **2:** Unloaded cycling is performed for 3 minutes before the left vertical dashed line. **3:** In panel 3, the diagonal line shows the increase of $\dot{V}O_2$ at a slope of 10 ml/min/W. **4:** In panel 5, the diagonal dashed line has a slope of 1; the x in the upper right is the predicted maximum heart rate and $\dot{V}O_2$ for the subject.

Interpretation

Comments

Resting pulmonary function tests were normal at age 66 (Table 10.82.1). DLCO was reduced at age 71.

Analysis

Age 66. Referring to Table 10.82.3 and flowchart 1, his peak $\dot{V}O_2$ and *AT* are normal, bringing us through branch point 1.1 to flowchart 2. At branch point 2.2

we find that he is not obese and would conclude that he would benefit from reassurance of his ability to continue his exercise program. However, the somewhat elevated $\dot{V}E/\dot{V}CO_2$ (Fig. 10.82.1) suggested some uneven ventilation–perfusion relationships, accompanied by a good breathing reserve.

Age 71. Referring to Table 10.82.3 and flowchart 1, his peak $\dot{V}O_2$ and *AT* are now reduced. We are directed through branch points 1.2 and 1.3 to flowchart 4. The breathing reserve is normal (branch

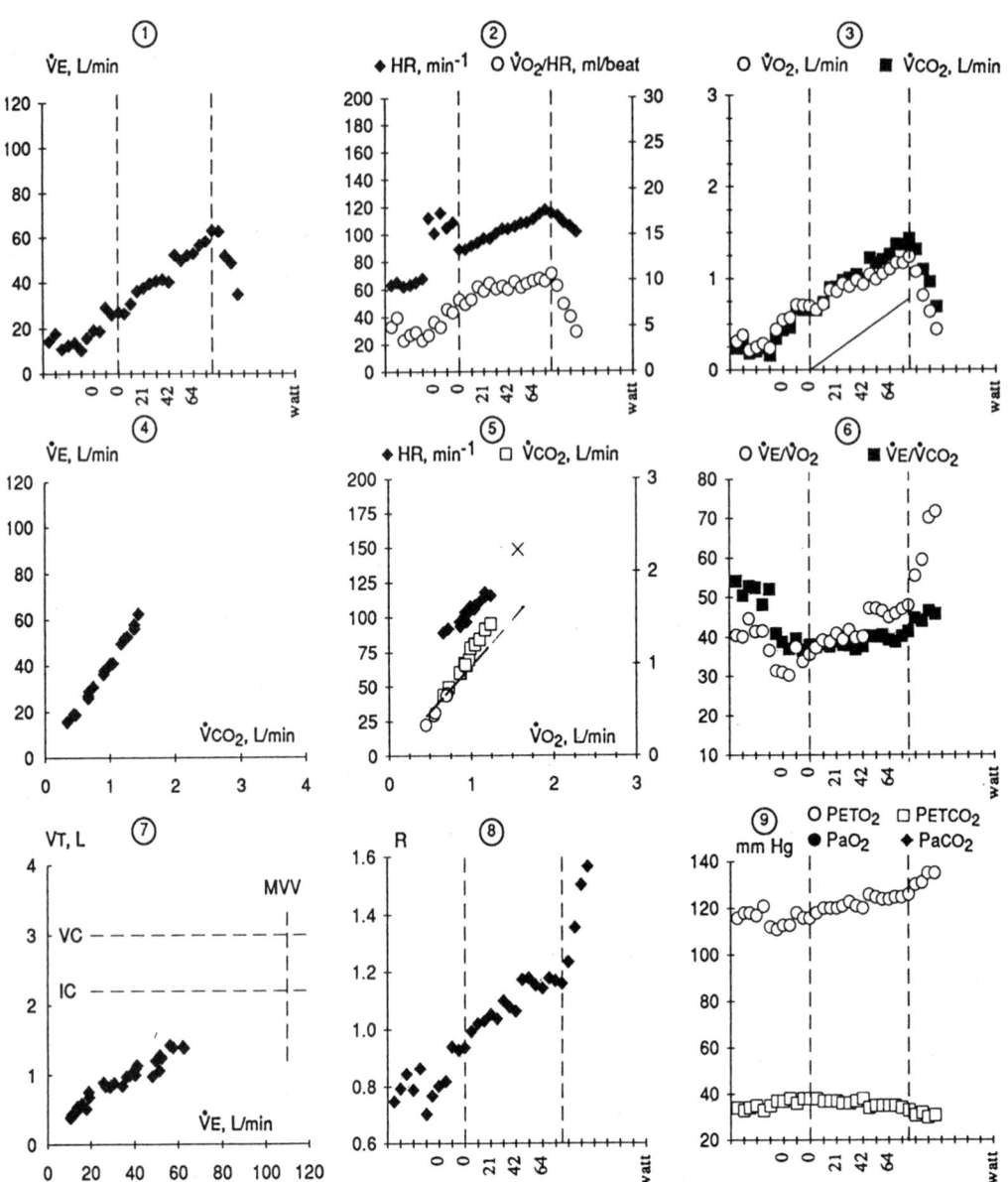

FIGURE 10.82.2.   Age 71. **1:** Vertical dashed lines in panels 1 to 3 and 6, 8, and 9 indicate the beginning and the end of the increasing work period. **2:** Unloaded cycling is performed for 3 minutes before the left vertical dashed line. **3:** In panel 3, the diagonal line shows the increase of $\dot{V}O_2$ at a slope of 10 ml/min/W. **4:** In panel 5, the diagonal dashed line has a slope of 1; the *x* in the upper right is the predicted maximum heart rate and $\dot{V}O_2$ for the subject.

point 4.1), and the ventilatory equivalent for $\dot{V}CO_2$ at the *AT* (branch point 4.3) is high, bringing us to abnormal pulmonary circulation. The vital capacity is normal (branch point 4.5), suggesting a diagnosis of pulmonary vascular disease rather than left ventricular failure. He did not have arterial blood gas measurements; therefore, we cannot use items 2 through 4 in the confirmatory box to support the diagnosis. Referring to items 5 through 6 (noninvasive measurements), he does not have a steep heart rate response to exercise. In fact, he has a low maximum heart rate. His oxygen saturation by pulse

oximetry was normal. Thus, we conclude that a better choice of diagnosis would have been heart disease with left ventricular failure. This is an example in which the flowcharts get you close to the diagnosis. However, when the confirming data do not fit, another selection with similar pathophysiology should be considered.

This case was selected because of the sequential measurements at a 4.5-year interval and a telephonic follow-up to the second study. The predicted peak $\dot{V}O_2$ decreased 0.13 L/min, but his actual peak $\dot{V}O_2$ decreased 0.64 L/min over the 4.5-year

TABLE 10.82.4. Age 66

Time min	Work rate watts	BP mmHg	HR min⁻¹	f min⁻¹	V̇E L/min BTPS	V̇CO₂ L/min STPD	V̇O₂ L/min STPD	V̇O₂/HR ml/beat	R	pH	HCO₃⁻ meq/L	PO₂ ET	PO₂ a	PO₂ (A−a)	PCO₂ ET	PCO₂ a	PCO₂ (a−ET)	V̇E/V̇CO₂	V̇E/V̇O₂	VD/VT
	Rest																			
	Rest		67	34	17.2	0.26	0.29	4.4	0.88			120			33			58	51	
	Rest		68	32	18.6	0.37	0.49	7.2	0.77			112			36			44	34	
	Rest		71	27	18.7	0.34	0.31	4.4	1.08			129			30			51	55	
	Rest		66	27	14.2	0.22	0.26	3.9	0.87			118			35			56	49	
	Rest		68	26	15.6	0.28	0.33	4.9	0.85			118			34			49	42	
	Rest		67	27	14.4	0.24	0.29	4.3	0.85			117			36			52	44	
	Unloaded		81	22	18.5	0.44	0.55	6.8	0.80			111			38			39	31	
	Unloaded		83	32	25.4	0.54	0.63	7.5	0.86			116			36			43	37	
	Unloaded		83	21	17.5	0.42	0.51	6.1	0.83			111			39			38	32	
	Unloaded		84	26	21.0	0.50	0.57	6.8	0.88			114			38			39	34	
	Unloaded		87	25	19.5	0.47	0.56	6.4	0.85			111			39			38	32	
	Unloaded		89	24	22.4	0.56	0.59	6.6	0.95			117			38			38	36	
0.5	2		87	24	22.1	0.56	0.59	6.8	0.95			115			39			37	35	
1.0	7		84	29	24.6	0.58	0.56	6.6	1.03			120			37			39	41	
1.5	11		90	31	29.4	0.72	0.73	8.1	0.98			119			36			38	38	
2.0	16		89	28	23.4	0.59	0.62	7.0	0.94			115			39			37	35	
2.5	23		91	25	26.2	0.69	0.70	7.7	0.98			116			38			36	35	
3.0	26		94	26	28.0	0.75	0.75	7.9	1.00			115			38			35	35	
3.5	32		98	28	31.0	0.84	0.84	8.5	1.00			115			39			35	35	
4.0	35		98	28	31.1	0.85	0.87	8.9	0.97			114			40			35	34	
4.5	42		100	29	33.3	0.93	0.94	9.4	1.00			116			40			34	34	
5.0	44		104	32	35.3	0.98	1.00	9.6	0.99			116			40			34	33	
5.5	50		106	32	39.5	1.11	1.05	9.9	1.06			118			39			34	36	
6.0	58		107	34	43.0	1.19	1.13	10.5	1.05			119			39			34	36	
6.5	59		108	35	46.1	1.27	1.14	10.6	1.11			121			38			34	38	
7.0	70		112	35	51.6	1.45	1.33	11.9	1.09			120			38			34	37	
7.5	72		114	34	50.5	1.44	1.31	11.5	1.10			120			39			34	37	
8.0	70		115	44	54.9	1.53	1.45	12.6	1.06			120			38			34	36	
8.5	82		117	43	60.2	1.65	1.45	12.4	1.14			124			36			35	40	
9.0	87		120	46	67.2	1.84	1.58	13.1	1.17			125			35			35	41	
9.5	94		118	63	86.4	2.15	1.88	15.9	1.14			128			32			38	44	
10.0	95		125	61	80.5	2.06	1.75	14.0	1.17			128			33			37	44	
	Recovery		118	42	71.8	1.90	1.54	13.1	1.24			127			35			36	45	
	Recovery		115	36	60.1	1.62	1.20	10.4	1.35			128			36			36	48	
	Recovery		115	38	54.7	1.41	1.07	9.3	1.31			128			35			37	49	
	Recovery		114	42	46.2	1.06	0.81	7.1	1.32			131			32			41	54	

interval. Further, his maximum O₂ pulse decreased from 15.9 to 10.7 at similar maximum heart rates. The patient, in a telephone follow-up that he initiated, stated that his cardiologist, seeing the results of cardiopulmonary exercise testing, decided to do a coronary angiogram despite the absence of ECG changes to support myocardial ischemia. Several major coronary vessels had high-grade stenoses, which were treated with angioplasty. The patient called back to inform us that since angioplasty, he had improved exercise tolerance, felt better, and would return for follow-up study at a later date.

Conclusion

This 71-year-old man developed chronic heart failure over a 4.5-year interval, probably due to myocardial ischemia.

TABLE 10.82.5. Age 71

Time min	Work rate watts	BP mmHg	HR min⁻¹	f min⁻¹	$\dot{V}_E$ L/min BTPS	$\dot{V}_{CO_2}$ L/min STPD	$\dot{V}_{O_2}$ L/min STPD	$\dfrac{\dot{V}_{O_2}}{HR}$ ml/beat	R	pH	HCO₃⁻ meq/L	P_{O_2}, mmHg ET	a	(A − a)	P_{CO_2}, mmHg ET	a	(a − ET)	$\dfrac{\dot{V}_E}{\dot{V}_{CO_2}}$	$\dfrac{\dot{V}_E}{\dot{V}_{O_2}}$	$\dfrac{V_D}{V_T}$
	Rest																			
	Rest		63	28	14.5	0.23	0.31	5.0	0.75			116			34			54	41	
	Rest		65	35	17.8	0.31	0.39	5.9	0.79			118			33			51	40	
	Rest		62	26	11.2	0.18	0.21	3.4	0.85			118			34			53	45	
	Rest		63	28	12.4	0.20	0.26	4.0	0.79			117			35			53	41	
	Rest		65	25	13.5	0.25	0.29	4.4	0.86			121			33			48	42	
	Rest		68	27	10.4	0.17	0.24	3.5	0.70			112			35			52	37	
	Unloaded		112	27	15.8	0.34	0.45	4.0	0.77			111			37			41	31	
	Unloaded		101	28	19.0	0.44	0.55	5.5	0.80			113			37			39	31	
	Unloaded		116	25	18.9	0.47	0.57	4.9	0.82			113			38			37	30	
	Unloaded		105	35	29.0	0.67	0.72	6.8	0.94			118			36			40	37	
	Unloaded		109	29	25.9	0.66	0.71	6.5	0.93			116			38			37	34	
	Unloaded		89	32	27.0	0.66	0.70	7.9	0.94			116			38			38	36	
0.5	8		89	32	26.7	0.66	0.66	7.4	0.99			118			38			37	37	
1.0	11		92	35	30.7	0.74	0.72	7.9	1.02			120			37			38	39	
1.5	16		94	37	36.2	0.90	0.87	9.2	1.03			120			37			38	39	
2.0	21		97	38	37.7	0.90	0.86	8.8	1.05			120			37			39	41	
2.5	25		97	38	39.6	0.98	0.94	9.7	1.04			121			36			38	39	
3.0	32		101	37	40.6	1.01	0.91	9.0	1.10			123			36			38	42	
3.5	35		104	36	41.1	1.05	0.97	9.4	1.08			121			37			37	40	
4.0	42		104	40	40.2	0.99	0.93	9.0	1.06			120			38			38	40	
4.5	45		106	41	52.0	1.22	1.04	9.8	1.17			126			34			40	47	
5.0	52		108	41	49.6	1.17	0.99	9.2	1.18			125			35			40	47	
5.5	57		109	40	51.7	1.21	1.05	9.7	1.15			124			35			40	47	
6.0	64		111	42	52.5	1.26	1.11	10.0	1.14			124			35			39	45	
6.5	67		115	39	56.2	1.38	1.17	10.2	1.18			125			35			39	46	
7.0	70		118	41	57.8	1.37	1.17	9.9	1.17			125			34			40	47	
7.5	77		116	45	62.6	1.44	1.24	10.7	1.16			126			33			42	48	
	Recovery		114	44	62.2	1.32	1.07	9.4	1.24			130			31			45	55	
	Recovery		109	48	51.3	1.10	0.81	7.4	1.36			131			32			44	60	
	Recovery		106	49	48.2	0.96	0.64	6.0	1.50			135			30			47	70	
	Recovery		102	41	34.5	0.70	0.44	4.4	1.57			135			31			46	72	

Case 83 Psychogenic Dyspnea

Clinical Findings

This 73-year-old woman was referred for cardio-pulmonary exercise testing because of exertional dyspnea that has been a progressive problem over the past year and had been worked up by internal medicine, cardiology, and pulmonary specialists without reaching a diagnosis. A number of therapeutic options were tried without relief of symptoms. She had no problem at rest and had experienced no orthopnea or nocturnal dyspnea. She admitted to mild ankle edema toward evening. She did not experience typical angina-type pain but did report pressure in the xiphoid area at times that was not related to breathing and which might also take place at rest. She had no history of gastroesophageal reflux. She had no breathing noises, although her daughter does say that she can hear her inhale at times (possibly a sigh, not stridor). She had no difficulty in getting air out of her chest. She had right heart catheterization and left heart catheterization and selective right and left coronary angiography. The only abnormality reported was a somewhat elevated pulmonary artery pressure. She had an ejection fraction of 0.76. Her chest roentgenogram and CT scans of her chest and abdomen were normal. Ventilation and perfusion scans and echocardiogram were reported to be normal. Her medications are metaproterenol, nifedipine (Procardia), conjugated estrogens (Premarin), sertraline (Zoloft), levothyroxine (Synthroid), and magnesium.

Exercise Findings

An arterial catheter was inserted percutaneously in the left brachial artery under lidocaine anesthesia. The patient performed exercise on a cycle ergometer while breathing through a mouthpiece with a nose clip in place for breath-by-breath measurements of gas exchange. Heart rate and rhythm were continuously monitored. The protocol consisted of 3 minutes of rest and 3 minutes of unload pedaling at 60 rpm, followed by a progressive increase in work rate of 10 W per minute until she became too symptomatic to continue. Twelve-lead ECG recordings were obtained during rest, every minute of exercise, and recovery. Blood pressure was monitored from the arterial catheter and recorded on a strip chart recorder. Arterial blood samples were taken at rest, at the end of 3 minutes of unloaded cycling, and at 1-minute intervals (every 10 W) to maximum exercise and at 2 minutes of recovery. A pulse oximeter was used for monitoring arterial O_2 saturation during the test.

The patient made good effort. She started hyperventilating at rest and increased her breathing rate to 50 breaths per minute as soon as she started to exercise. She started pedaling very rapidly, so that unloaded cycling was equivalent to 10 W. She stated that she stopped exercise because she found it difficult to continue to pedal and because of shortness of breath. There were no ectopic beats or evidence of myocardial ischemia on the electrocardiogram.

TABLE 10.83.1.   Selected Respiratory Function Data

Measurement	Predicted	Measured
Age, yr		73
Sex		Female
Height, cm		163
Weight, kg	63	76
Hematocrit, %		45
VC, L	2.79	2.35
IC, L	1.86	2.23
FEV_1, L	2.19	1.80
FEV_1/VC, %	78	77
MVV, L/min	84	67
D_LCO, ml/mm Hg/min	20.1	17.1

TABLE 10.83.2.   Selected Exercise Data

Measurement	Predicted	Measured
Peak $\dot{V}O_2$, L/min	1.18	1.00
Maximum HR, beats/min	147	104
Maximum O_2 pulse, ml/beat	8.0	9.6
$\Delta\dot{V}O_2/\Delta$WR, ml/min/W	10.3	7.0
AT, L/min	>0.64	0.8
Blood pressure, mmHg (rest, max ex)		150/75, 175/95
Maximum $\dot{V}E$, L/min		53
Exercise breathing reserve, L/min	>15	14
PaO_2, mmHg (rest, max ex)		105, 122
P(A − a)O_2, mmHg (rest, max ex)		21, 6
P(a − ET)CO_2, mmHg (rest, max ex)		0, −1.4
VD/VT (rest, max ex)		0.28, 0.17
HCO_3^-, mEq/L (rest, recov)		19, 14
Lactate, mEq/L (rest, recov)		1.7, 9.7

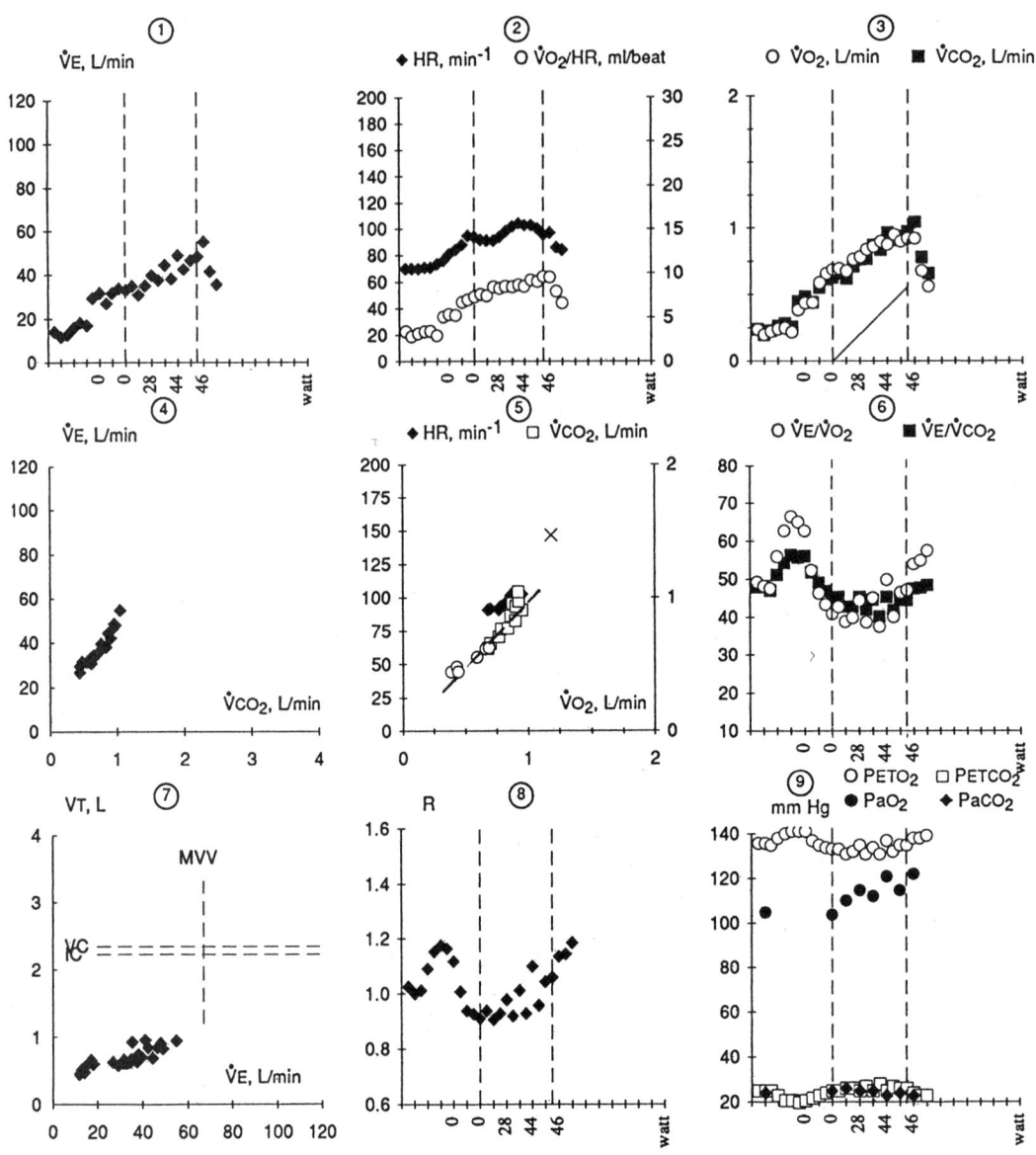

FIGURE 10.83.1.   **1:** Vertical dashed lines in panels 1 to 3 and 6, 8, and 9 indicate the beginning and the end of the increasing work period. **2:** Unloaded cycling is performed for 3 minutes before the left vertical dashed line. **3:** In panel 3, the diagonal line shows the increase of $\dot{V}O_2$ at a slope of 10 ml/min/W. **4:** In panel 5, the diagonal dashed line has a slope of 1; the *x* in the upper right is the predicted maximum heart rate and $\dot{V}O_2$ for the subject.

Interpretation

Comments

Resting spirometry was normal (Table 10.83.1).

Analysis

Referring to Table 10.83.2 and flowchart 1, her peak $\dot{V}O_2$ is low normal, and the *AT* is normal, bringing us through branch point 1.1 to flowchart 2. Her ECG, arterial blood gases, and O_2 pulse at peak $\dot{V}O_2$ are normal (branch point 2.1), and she is overweight (branch point 2.2), but not excessively so.

Her major problems with respect to her symptoms are twofold. First and foremost is that she starts to hyperventilate with a very small tidal volume (almost panting), as evident from panel 7 and the nonphysiological changes in the gas exchange ratio and the arterial blood gas measurements (panels 8 and 9) showing acute hyperventilation. The pattern of breathing is also abnormal in that she maintains a breathing rate of 50 to 60 breaths per minute from shortly after the start of unloaded cycling, with a low tidal volume relative to her inspiratory capacity. Second, her heart rate response to exercise is impaired (low and very shallow slope of heart rate

TABLE 10.83.3. Air Breathing

Time min	Work rate watts	BP mmHg	HR min^{-1}	f min^{-1}	$\dot{V}_E$ L/min BTPS	$\dot{V}_{CO_2}$ L/min STPD	$\dot{V}_{O_2}$ L/min STPD	$\dot{V}_{O_2}$/HR ml/beat	R	pH	HCO$_3^-$ meq/L	P_{O_2}, mmHg ET	a	(A−a)	P_{CO_2}, mmHg ET	a	(a−ET)	$\dfrac{\dot{V}_E}{\dot{V}_{CO_2}}$	$\dfrac{\dot{V}_E}{\dot{V}_{O_2}}$	$\dfrac{V_D}{V_T}$
	Rest																			
	Rest		70	30	14.2	0.24	0.24	3.4	1.03			136		21	25			48	49	
	Rest	150/75	70	26	11.8	0.20	0.20	2.8	1.00	7.50	18	136	105		25	24	−1	48	48	0.21
	Rest		70	25	12.8	0.23	0.22	3.2	1.01			135			25			47	48	
	Rest		71	26	15.7	0.26	0.24	3.4	1.09			138			23			51	56	
	Rest		71	30	18.0	0.28	0.25	3.5	1.15			140			21			54	63	
	Rest		74	26	16.9	0.26	0.22	3.0	1.18			141			21			57	66	
	Unloaded		76	51	29.3	0.45	0.38	5.1	1.16			141			20			56	65	
	Unloaded		81	52	31.5	0.48	0.43	5.3	1.12			141			21			56	63	
	Unloaded		84	43	26.8	0.45	0.44	5.3	1.01			137			22			52	52	
	Unloaded		88	48	31.5	0.56	0.59	6.7	0.94			135			23			49	46	
	Unloaded		95	54	33.4	0.61	0.66	7.0	0.93			134			24			47	44	
	Unloaded	155/85	94	54	32.8	0.63	0.69	7.3	0.91	7.50	19	133	104	19	25	25	0	45	41	0.20
0.5	10		92	55	34.5	0.66	0.70	7.6	0.94			133			25			45	43	
1.0	7	165/90	91	50	30.8	0.62	0.68	7.5	0.91	7.47	19	131	110	12	26	26	0	43	39	0.20
1.5	16		91	52	34.9	0.71	0.76	8.4	0.93			132			26			43	40	
2.0	28	175/100	94	56	39.6	0.77	0.78	8.3	0.98	7.48	18	135	115	10	25	25	0	46	45	0.21
2.5	25		98	59	37.4	0.77	0.84	8.5	0.92			131			27			42	39	
3.0	31	190/100	102	64	44.3	0.87	0.86	8.4	1.01	7.47	18	134	112	13	25	25	0	45	45	0.20
3.5	31		104	51	38.0	0.83	0.90	8.6	0.93			131			28			40	38	
4.0	44	185/95	103	59	48.8	0.96	0.87	8.5	1.10	7.47	16	137	121	8	25	23	−2	46	50	0.16
4.5	47		103	50	42.3	0.91	0.95	9.2	0.96			132			27			42	40	
5.0	50	175/95	100	55	46.6	0.94	0.90	9.0	1.04	7.45	16	135	115	12	26	24	−2	45	47	0.17
5.5	55		96	53	48.1	0.98	0.92	9.6	1.06			135			26			45	47	
6.0	46	150/65	97	58	54.8	1.05	0.92	9.5	1.14	7.43	15	138	122	7	24	23	−1	48	54	0.19
	Recovery		86	43	41.1	0.78	0.68	7.9	1.15			138			23			48	55	
	Recovery		84	38	35.4	0.66	0.56	6.7	1.18			139			23			49	58	

versus $\dot{V}_{O_2}$), presumably due to being on a β-adrenergic blocking drug in a dose that limits ability of heart rate, and therefore cardiac output, to increase normally (heart rate at maximum exercise = 104). Thus, there are psychogenic and iatrogenic causes for this patient's symptoms.

Conclusion

Psychogenic dyspnea in a 73-year-old woman, complicated by heavy β-adrenergic blockade.

Case 84 Hypertension Treated with β-Adrenergic Blockade

Clinical Findings

This 60-year-old woman was evaluated because of chronic cough and moderate exertional dyspnea. She was a nonsmoker and never smoked. She had systemic arterial hypertension, for which she was treated with a β-adrenergic blocking drug and diuretic. An angiotensin-converting enzyme inhibitor was not used because of the chronic cough. In her exercise evaluation, it was noted that she had a reduced exercise tolerance, with a reduced heart rate response and poor control of her hypertension. To determine if the limited heart rate response accounted for her reduced exercise capacity, she was asked to not take her β-adrenergic blocking drug for 2 days and then have her blood pressure during exercise and her exercise tolerance reevaluated. Two cardiopulmonary exercise tests were done. The first (Fig. 10.84.1) was done during her first visit, and the second (Fig. 10.84.2) was done 2 days later after the β-adrenergic blocking drug had been withheld.

Exercise Findings

On both tests, the patient performed exercise on a cycle ergometer while breathing through a mouthpiece with a nose clip in place for breath-by-breath gas exchange measurements. Heart rate and rhythm were continuously monitored. Arterial pressure was monitored and measured every 2 minutes with cuff and stethoscope. The protocol consisted of 3 minutes of rest and 3 minutes of unloaded cycling at 60 rpm, followed by a progressive increase

in work rate of 10 W per minute until she could not continue. Twelve-lead ECG recordings were obtained during rest, every minute of exercise, and recovery. Arterial oxyhemoglobin saturation was continuously monitored with a pulse oximeter on her index finger. The patient performed the exercise test with good effort.

Interpretation

Comments

Resting pulmonary function showed moderate airway obstruction with significant reduction in her diffusing capacity (Table 10.84.1). Her exercise electrocardiogram was thought to be normal. Her maximum heart rate was 113 with and 156 without β-adrenergic blockade (Table 10.84.2). Her blood

TABLE 10.84.1.   Selected Respiratory Function Data

Measurement	Predicted	Measured
Age, yr		60
Sex		Female
Height, cm		165
Weight, kg		59
Hematocrit, %		41
VC, L	3.22	2.74
IC, L	2.15	1.75
ERV, L	1.07	1.00
FEV_1, L	2.53	1.76
FEV_1/VC, %	78	64
MVV, L/min	104	70
D_LCO, ml/mm Hg/min	25.2	11.1

TABLE 10.84.2.   Selected Exercise Data

Measurement	Predicted	With β blockade	Without β blockade
Peak $\dot{V}O_2$, L/min	1.31	1.07	1.22
Maximum HR, beats/min	160	113	156
Maximum O_2 pulse, ml/beat	8.2	9.5	7.8
$\Delta\dot{V}O_2$/ΔWR, ml/min/W	10.3	6.8	8.7
AT, L/min	>0.68	0.50	0.80
Blood pressure, mmHg (rest, max)		180/85, 200/100	170/90, 220/100
Maximum $\dot{V}E$, L/min		54	55
Exercise breathing reserve, L/min	>15	16	15
$\dot{V}E/\dot{V}CO_2$ @AT	<33	31	30
$P_{ET}CO_2$ @AT	≥40	38	40
$\dot{V}E$ vs $\dot{V}CO_2$	<32	29	27
SaO_2 rest, ex — pulse oximeter (%)	>95	97, 97	95, 95

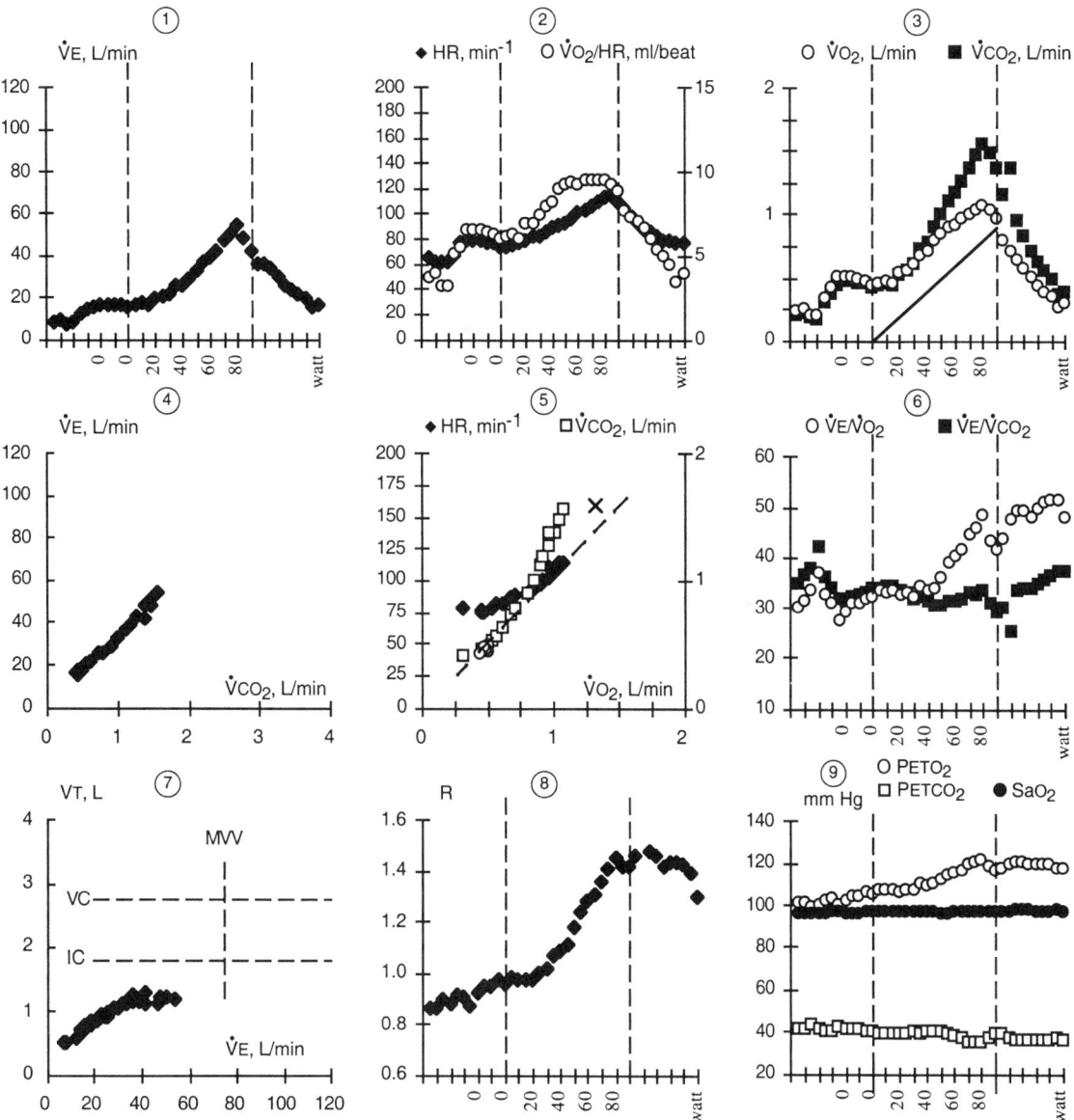

FIGURE 10.84.1.   **1:** Vertical dashed lines in panels 1 to 3 and 6, 8, and 9 indicate the beginning and the end of the increasing work period. **2:** Unloaded cycling is performed for 3 minutes before the left vertical dashed line. **3:** In panel 3, the diagonal line shows the increase of $\dot{V}O_2$ at a slope of 10 ml/min/W. **4:** In panel 5, the diagonal dashed line has a slope of 1; the x in the upper right is the predicted maximum heart rate and $\dot{V}O_2$ for the subject.

pressure response was similar on both days of testing. Her SaO_2 during exercise was normal for both tests. She stopped both tests because of leg fatigue.

Analysis

Referring to this woman's first test (Table 10.84.2 and Fig. 10.84.1) and using the flowcharts shown in Chapter 8, her peak $\dot{V}O_2$ and AT are low, bringing us through branch points 1.1, 1.2, and 1.3 to flowchart 4. The breathing reserve is borderline normal (branch point 4.1), and the ventilatory equivalent for $\dot{V}CO_2$ at

the AT (branch point 4.3) is normal, bringing us to a diagnosis of O_2 flow problem of nonpulmonary origin (anemia, heart disease, or peripheral arterial disease). She was not anemic (Table 10.84.1). Her ECG was normal during this test. She had no symptoms of claudication, and the increase in $\dot{V}O_2$ as related to work rate started out normal at low work rates but became more shallow as peak $\dot{V}O_2$ was approached, making the calculated $\Delta\dot{V}O_2/\Delta W\dot{R}$ slope low (panel 3, Fig. 10.84.1; Table 10.84.2).

Two days later, the patient repeated the exercise test after withholding her β-adrenergic blocking

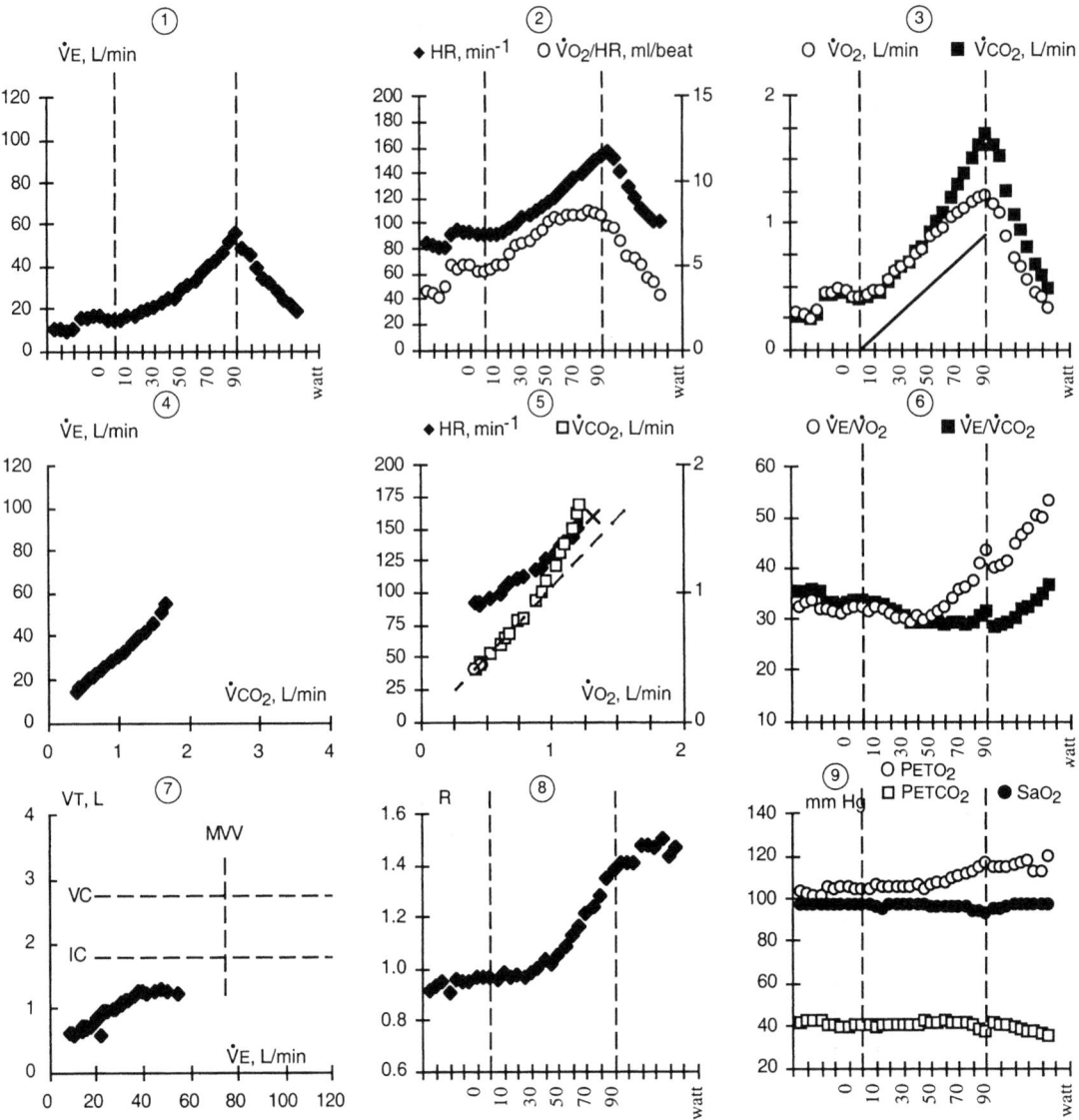

FIGURE 10.84.2.   **1:** Vertical dashed lines in panels 1 to 3 and 6, 8, and 9 indicate the beginning and the end of the increasing work period. **2:** Unloaded cycling is performed for 3 minutes before the left vertical dashed line. **3:** In panel 3, the diagonal line shows the increase of $\dot{V}O_2$ at a slope of 10 ml/min/W. **4:** In panel 5, the diagonal dashed line has a slope of 1; the x in the upper right is the predicted maximum heart rate and $\dot{V}O_2$ for the subject.

drug. On this occasion, her peak $\dot{V}O_2$ and anaerobic threshold were normal. Her $\Delta\dot{V}O_2/\Delta WR$ was also now normal. With the peak $\dot{V}O_2$, $A\tilde{T}$, $\Delta\dot{V}O_2/\Delta WR$, O_2 pulse, $\dot{V}E/\dot{V}CO_2$ and $PETCO_2$ at the anaerobic threshold, and ECG being normal, we have no evidence of cardiac or pulmonary vascular disease. She has hypertension that does not seem to limit exercise tolerance as much as the drug that she was taking to treat it. The etiology of her lung disease remained to be determined.

Conclusion

The patient had reduced exercise tolerance on the drug regimen that she was taking for treating her systemic hypertension. Unfortunately, it had reduced her exercise tolerance without effectively treating her hypertension. This case illustrates that cardiopulmonary exercise testing may help in the proper selection and dosing of medication.

TABLE 10.84.3.   On β-Adrenergic Blockade Medication

Time min	Work rate watts	BP mmHg	HR min⁻¹	f min⁻¹	$\dot{V}_E$ L/min BTPS	$\dot{V}_{CO_2}$ L/min STPD	$\dot{V}_{O_2}$ L/min STPD	$\dfrac{\dot{V}_{O_2}}{HR}$ ml/beat	R	pH	HCO₃⁻ meq/L	P_{O_2} ET	a	(A − a)	P_{CO_2} ET	a	(a − ET)	$\dfrac{\dot{V}_E}{\dot{V}_{CO_2}}$	$\dfrac{\dot{V}_E}{\dot{V}_{O_2}}$	$\dfrac{V_D}{V_T}$
	Rest		64	16	8.0	0.21	0.24	3.7	0.86			101			41			35	30	
	Rest		62	17	8.5	0.21	0.24	3.9	0.86			101			41			36	31	
	Rest		62	15	7.3	0.17	0.20	3.1	0.89			99			43			38	34	
	Rest		61	16	8.1	0.17	0.20	3.2	0.88			100			41			42	37	
	Rest	180/85	66	21	12.1	0.31	0.34	5.1	0.91			102			40			36	33	
	Rest		76	22	14.0	0.38	0.42	5.5	0.90			103			40			34	31	
	Unloaded		78	21	15.1	0.44	0.51	6.5	0.87			100			42			32	28	
	Unloaded		78	21	15.8	0.47	0.51	6.5	0.92			102			41			32	29	
	Unloaded		78	21	16.6	0.48	0.51	6.5	0.95			104			41			32	31	
	Unloaded		77	21	16.1	0.46	0.49	6.3	0.95			104			41			33	31	
	Unloaded		76	22	16.4	0.47	0.48	6.3	0.97			106			40			33	32	
	Unloaded		74	22	15.3	0.42	0.44	6.0	0.95			105			40			34	32	
0.5	5		74	23	16.4	0.45	0.46	6.2	0.98			107			39			34	33	
1.0	10		75	23	16.8	0.46	0.47	6.3	0.97			107			39			34	33	
1.5	15		76	23	16.6	0.45	0.46	6.1	0.97			107			39			34	34	
2.0	20	190/90	78	24	18.7	0.52	0.54	6.9	0.97			106			39			34	32	
2.5	25		81	25	19.8	0.56	0.56	6.9	1.00			107			39			33	33	
3.0	30		82	25	21.0	0.62	0.61	7.4	1.02			107			40			32	32	
3.5	35		86	28	24.9	0.73	0.69	8.0	1.07			110			39			32	34	
4.0	40		88	28	25.6	0.78	0.72	8.2	1.08			109			40			31	34	
4.5	45	200/96	90	28	28.6	0.90	0.81	9.0	1.11			110			40			30	34	
5.0	50		93	29	32.2	1.00	0.86	9.2	1.17			112			40			31	36	
5.5	55		96	32	36.5	1.11	0.90	9.4	1.24			114			39			31	39	
6.0	60		100	34	38.9	1.18	0.92	9.2	1.28			116			38			31	40	
6.5	65		102	38	42.2	1.26	0.97	9.5	1.30			117			37			32	42	
7.0	70		106	42	47.4	1.37	1.01	9.6	1.36			120			35			33	45	
7.5	75		110	42	50.3	1.47	1.05	9.5	1.41			121			35			33	46	
8.0	80	200/100	113	47	54.2	1.56	1.07	9.5	1.45			122			35			33	48	
8.5	85		114	39	47.6	1.48	1.05	9.2	1.41			119			37			31	44	
9.0	90		110	33	42.0	1.38	0.97	8.8	1.41			117			39			29	41	
	Recovery		104	29	36.2	1.16	0.80	7.7	1.46			118			39			30	44	
	Recovery		98	30	35.7	1.36	0.72	7.3	1.90			120			37			25	48	
	Recovery	196/90	92	30	33.5	0.95	0.65	7.0	1.47			121			36			34	49	
	Recovery		87	29	29.9	0.84	0.57	6.6	1.46			121			36			34	50	
	Recovery		85	27	25.8	0.72	0.51	6.0	1.42			120			36			34	48	
	Recovery		82	25	23.0	0.63	0.44	5.3	1.43			120			36			35	50	
	Recovery		79	24	21.2	0.56	0.39	5.0	1.44			120			36			35	51	
	Recovery		78	23	19.1	0.50	0.35	4.5	1.42			120			36			36	52	
	Recovery		77	21	14.6	0.37	0.26	3.4	1.39			118			37			37	52	
	Recovery		77	21	15.8	0.40	0.31	4.0	1.29			118			36			37	48	

TABLE 10.84.4. Off β-Adrenergic Blockade Medication

Time min	Work rate watts	BP mmHg	HR min⁻¹	f min⁻¹	$\dot{V}_E$ L/min BTPS	$\dot{V}_{CO_2}$ L/min STPD	$\dot{V}_{O_2}$ L/min STPD	$\dot{V}_{O_2}$/HR ml/beat	R	pH	HCO₃⁻ meq/L	P_{O_2}, mmHg ET	a	(A − a)	P_{CO_2}, mmHg ET	a	(a − ET)	$\dot{V}_E$/$\dot{V}_{CO_2}$	$\dot{V}_E$/$\dot{V}_{O_2}$	V_D/V_T
	Rest		84	17	10.0	0.26	0.28	3.4	0.92			103			41			35	32	
	Rest	160/80	82	16	9.7	0.25	0.27	3.3	0.93			102			42			35	33	
	Rest		80	15	8.8	0.23	0.24	3.0	0.95			101			42			35	34	
	Rest		80	18	10.4	0.27	0.30	3.8	0.90			101			42			35	32	
	Unloaded		90	22	15.2	0.42	0.44	4.9	0.96			105			40			33	32	
	Unloaded	170/90	94	22	15.0	0.42	0.44	4.7	0.95			104			40			33	31	
	Unloaded		93	23	15.6	0.44	0.47	5.0	0.95			105			39			33	31	
	Unloaded		92	22	15.7	0.44	0.46	5.0	0.97			105			39			33	32	
	Unloaded		91	21	14.4	0.40	0.41	4.5	0.97			104			40			33	32	
	Unloaded		90	23	14.3	0.40	0.41	4.6	0.96			104			40			33	32	
0.5	5		91	22	14.4	0.41	0.42	4.7	0.96			104			40			33	31	
1.0	10		90	24	15.7	0.44	0.45	5.0	0.98			106			39			33	32	
1.5	15		92	24	15.8	0.45	0.46	5.0	0.97			105			40			33	32	
2.0	20	190/90	95	25	17.8	0.52	0.54	5.7	0.97			105			40			32	31	
2.5	25		99	25	19.6	0.59	0.61	6.1	0.97			105			40			31	30	
3.0	30		104	25	20.7	0.64	0.65	6.3	0.98			105			40			30	30	
3.5	35		106	39	21.9	0.68	0.68	6.4	1.00			105			40			29	29	
4.0	40		110	26	24.2	0.77	0.75	6.8	1.03			106			40			30	31	
4.5	45		112	26	24.7	0.80	0.79	7.1	1.02			104			42			29	30	
5.0	50	200/100	117	29	28.4	0.92	0.88	7.5	1.05			106			41			29	31	
5.5	55		119	29	30.7	1.00	0.93	7.8	1.08			107			41			29	32	
6.0	60		125	29	32.6	1.08	0.96	7.7	1.12			107			42			29	32	
6.5	65		130	31	36.8	1.21	1.04	8.0	1.16			109			41			29	34	
7.0	70		135	32	39.9	1.31	1.08	8.0	1.21			110			41			29	35	
7.5	75		139	34	41.6	1.38	1.11	8.0	1.24			111			41			29	36	
8.0	80		143	37	45.6	1.50	1.17	8.2	1.28			112			40			29	37	
8.5	85	220/100	149	41	51.0	1.62	1.20	8.1	1.35			115			38			30	41	
9.0	90		153	45	55.0	1.69	1.22	8.0	1.39			117			37			31	43	
	Recovery		156	37	47.7	1.61	1.15	7.3	1.41			114			41			28	40	
	Recovery	220/100	150	36	45.5	1.52	1.08	7.2	1.41			115			40			29	40	
	Recovery		140	31	38.3	1.26	0.89	6.4	1.41			115			40			29	41	
	Recovery		129	30	33.4	1.06	0.72	5.6	1.47			116			39			30	44	
	Recovery	220/100	119	29	31.3	0.95	0.64	5.4	1.47			117			38			32	46	
	Recovery		111	28	27.5	0.81	0.55	4.9	1.47			118			37			32	48	
	Recovery		106	25	23.5	0.66	0.44	4.2	1.50			112			37			34	50	
	Recovery	198/90	101	25	21.1	0.57	0.40	4.0	1.43			112			36			35	50	
	Recovery		100	25	18.5	0.47	0.32	3.2	1.46			120			35			36	53	

Case 85 Ischemic Cardiomyopathy, Restrictive Lung Disease, and β-Adrenergic Blockade

Clinical Findings

This patient is a 72-year-old man, a former contractor, who was referred for cardiopulmonary exercise testing to clarify the mechanism for his exercise intolerance. He complains of decreasing energy and shortness of breath with activity starting 2 years previous to this evaluation. He had a "heart attack" 10 years previously, following which he had a coronary artery bypass graft. With the onset of his current symptoms, his bypass graft and coronary blood vessels were reevaluated by coronary angiography. It was concluded by his cardiologist that his symptoms were unlikely to be due to his heart. He then had pulmonary function tests, which showed a restrictive pattern. High-resolution scans did not show pulmonary fibrosis, but the right leaf of the diaphragm moved poorly and there was atelectasis of the right middle lobe. Ventilation and perfusion scans were thought to be normal. He was a nonsmoker. He had no orthopnea or paroxysmal nocturnal dyspnea. Medications included ipratropium (Atrovent), atenolol, simvastatin (Zocor), and aspirin.

Except for the scar over the sternum, his physical exam was normal for his age. His diaphragm appeared to move well. He had no peripheral edema. His electrocardiogram showed sinus rhythm with a rate of 57 per minute and abnormal Q waves in leads III, aVF, and V_1 through V_5.

Exercise Findings

The patient performed exercise on a cycle ergometer while breathing through a mouthpiece with a nose clip in place for breath-by-breath gas exchange measurements. Heart rate and rhythm were continuously monitored. Arterial pressure was monitored and measured every 2 minutes with cuff and stethoscope. The protocol consisted of 3 minutes of rest and 3 minutes of unloaded cycling at 60 rpm, followed by a progressive increase in work rate of 15 W per minute until the patient was too symptomatic to continue. Twelve-lead ECG recordings were obtained during rest, every minute of exercise, and recovery. Arterial oxyhemoglobin saturation was continuously monitored with a pulse oximeter on his index finger. The patient performed the exercise test with good effort.

TABLE 10.85.1.   Selected Respiratory Function Data

Measurement	Predicted	Measured
Age, yr		72
Sex		Male
Height, cm		185
Weight, kg		105
Hematocrit, %		43
VC, L	4.72	2.60
IC, L	3.15	2.35
ERV, L	1.57	0.25
FEV_1, L	3.71	1.83
FEV_1/VC, %	79	71
MVV, L/min	135	78
D_LCO, ml/mm Hg/min	26.9	17.0

TABLE 10.85.2.   Selected Exercise Data

Measurement	Predicted	Measured
Peak $\dot{V}O_2$, L/min	2.05	1.38
Maximum HR, beats/min	148	90
Maximum O_2 pulse, ml/beat	13.9	15.3
$\Delta\dot{V}O_2/\Delta WR$, ml/min/W	10.3	8.9
AT, L/min	>0.97	0.85
Blood pressure, mmHg (rest, max)		147/92, 176/70
Maximum $\dot{V}E$, L/min		47
Exercise breathing reserve, L/min	>15	31
$\dot{V}E/\dot{V}CO_2$ @AT	<34	30
$PETCO_2$ @AT	≥40	40
$\dot{V}E$ vs $\dot{V}CO_2$	<33	27
SaO_2 rest, ex − pulse oximeter (%)	>95	96, 94

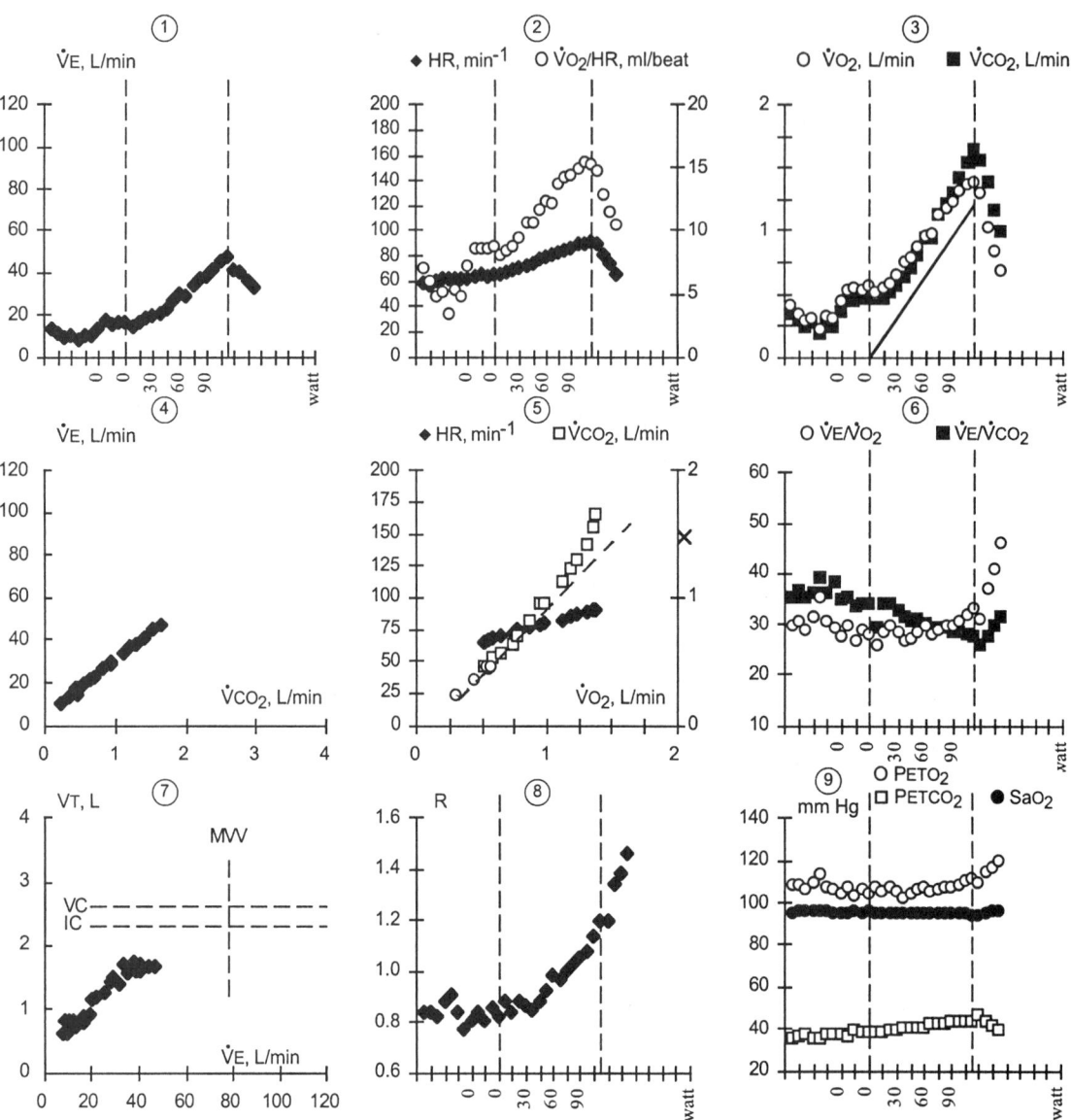

FIGURE 10.85.1. **1:** Vertical dashed lines in panels 1 to 3 and 6, 8, and 9 indicate the beginning and the end of the increasing work period. **2:** Unloaded cycling is performed for 3 minutes before the left vertical dashed line. **3:** In panel 3, the diagonal line shows the increase of $\dot{V}O_2$ at a slope of 10 ml/min/W. **4:** In panel 5, the diagonal dashed line has a slope of 1; the x in the upper right is the predicted maximum heart rate and $\dot{V}O_2$ for the subject.

Interpretation

Comments

The patient stopped cycling at 120 W because he was "running out of air." He had no chest pain during exercise. There were no changes in his ECG complexes or cardiac ectopy during exercise. His SaO_2 during exercise was normal. He had no physical signs of airflow limitation. He had a very adequate breathing reserve.

Analysis

Referring to the flowcharts, his peak $\dot{V}O_2$ and *AT* are low, bringing us through branch points 1.1, 1.2, and 1.3 to flowchart 4. The breathing reserve is normal (branch point 4.1), and the ventilatory equivalent for $\dot{V}CO_2$ at the *AT* (branch point 4.3) is normal, bringing us to a diagnosis of O_2 flow problem of nonpulmonary origin (anemia, heart disease, or peripheral arterial disease). He was not anemic (Table 10.85.1). Also, his normal $\Delta\dot{V}O_2/\Delta$WR argues against

TABLE 10.85.3.   Air Breathing

Time min	Work rate watts	BP mmHg	HR min⁻¹	f min⁻¹	V̇E L/min BTPS	V̇CO₂ L/min STPD	V̇O₂ L/min STPD	V̇O₂/HR ml/beat	R	pH	HCO₃⁻ meq/L	PO₂, mmHg			PCO₂, mmHg			V̇E/V̇CO₂	V̇E/V̇O₂	VD/VT
												ET	a	(A − a)	ET	a	(a − ET)			
	Rest		58	16	12.7	0.34	0.40	6.9	0.84			108			35			35	30	
	Rest	147/92	56	14	10.9	0.28	0.33	6.0	0.84			108			36			37	31	
	Rest		60	11	8.7	0.23	0.28	4.7	0.82			106			37			35	29	
	Rest		62	13	10.4	0.27	0.31	5.0	0.87			109			35			36	31	
	Rest		61	13	8.0	0.19	0.21	3.4	0.90			113			35			39	35	
	Rest		61	14	10.4	0.27	0.32	5.2	0.84			107			37			36	30	
	Unloaded		62	16	9.5	0.23	0.30	4.8	0.77			106			37			38	29	
	Unloaded		62	19	13.3	0.36	0.45	7.2	0.80			104			37			35	28	
	Unloaded		63	22	16.8	0.45	0.53	8.5	0.84			107			36			35	29	
	Unloaded		64	19	15.4	0.43	0.54	8.5	0.80			103			39			33	27	
	Unloaded	141/77	63	20	16.4	0.46	0.53	8.5	0.85			106			38			34	29	
	Unloaded		64	19	16.5	0.46	0.56	8.8	0.82			104			38			34	28	
0.5	15		64	19	14.1	0.45	0.51	8.0	0.88			107			38			29	26	
1.0	15		66	21	16.6	0.46	0.55	8.3	0.84			105			38			34	28	
1.5	30		68	21	18.5	0.52	0.59	8.6	0.88			107			39			34	30	
2.0	30	191/70	69	21	19.3	0.56	0.65	9.4	0.86			105			39			33	28	
2.5	45		71	18	20.7	0.63	0.75	10.5	0.84			102			40			31	26	
3.0	45		74	19	22.1	0.69	0.78	10.6	0.88			104			40			31	27	
3.5	60	184/70	76	21	25.9	0.81	0.88	11.5	0.92			106			40			31	28	
4.0	60		78	20	29.4	0.94	0.96	12.3	0.98			107			40			30	30	
4.5	75		80	20	28.3	0.94	0.98	12.2	0.97			105			42			29	28	
5.0	75		82	20	33.6	1.12	1.13	13.7	0.99			106			42			29	29	
5.5	90	215/67	84	22	36.3	1.22	1.19	14.1	1.02			107			42			29	30	
6.0	90		86	22	37.8	1.30	1.24	14.4	1.05			107			43			28	30	
6.5	105		88	24	40.9	1.41	1.31	14.9	1.08			108			43			28	30	
7.0	105		89	27	44.5	1.55	1.37	1.54	1.13			110			43			28	32	
7.5	120	176/70	90	28	46.7	1.65	1.38	15.3	1.20			111			43			27	33	
	Recovery		88	26	41.3	1.55	1.30	14.8	1.19			109			46			26	31	
	Recovery		80	25	39.5	1.39	1.03	12.9	1.34			114			43			28	37	
	Recovery		73	23	35.5	1.16	0.84	1.15	1.38			117			41			30	41	
	Recovery		65	23	32.1	0.99	0.68	10.4	1.46			120			39			31	46	

peripheral arterial disease as being the cause of his symptoms of shortness of breath. This leaves heart disease as the cause of his exercise intolerance. However, his O₂ pulse is above predicted; further, applying the concepts developed for calculating stroke volume from V̇O₂ and O₂ pulse described in Chapters 4 and 9, the patient's stroke volume must be at least 100 ml. Thus, his heart problem is not due to poor contractility. Rather, the study shows that he has a chronotropic problem, probably pharmacologically induced by a high level of β-adrenergic blockade. His heart rate response to exercise is poor, the peak heart rate being 90.

Conclusion

This patient is limited during exercise due to inadequate heart rate response to exercise. β-Adrenergic blockade therapy is now standard for treating patients with coronary artery disease. However, dosing is critical: A high-enough dose is needed to be cardioprotective, but not so high as to incapacitate the patient by restricting too heavily the sympathetic changes in cardiovascular function needed to exercise.

Symbols and Abbreviations

A bar ($^{-}$) above any symbol indicates a mean value.
A dot ($^{\cdot}$) above any symbol indicates a time derivative.

GASES

	PRIMARY SYMBOLS		EXAMPLES
V	Gas volume	V_A	Volume of alveolar gas
$\dot{V}$	Gas volume per unit time	$\dot{V}_{O_2}$	Oxygen uptake per minute
P	Gas pressure	P_{AO_2}	Alveolar O_2 pressure
$\bar{P}$	Mean gas pressure	$\bar{P}_{CO_2}$	Mean capillary O_2 pressure
F	Fractional concentration of a gas	F_{IO_2}	Fractional concentration of O_2 in inspired gas
f	Respiratory frequency		
D	Diffusing capacity	D_{LCO}	Diffusing capacity of lung for carbon monoxide
R	Respiratory exchange ratio		
RQ	Respiratory quotient		
Q	Gas quantity		
$\dot{Q}$	Gas quantity per unit time (gas flow)	$\dot{Q}_{O_2}$	Oxygen consumed per minute
STPD	standard temperature and pressure (0°C, 760 mm Hg), dry		
BTPS	body temperature and pressure, saturated with water vapor		

	SECONDARY SYMBOLS		EXAMPLES
I	Inspired gas	F_{IO_2}	Fractional concentration of O_2 in inspired gas
E	Expired gas	V_E	Volume of expired gas
A	Alveolar gas	$\dot{V}_A$	Alveolar ventilation per minute
ET	End tidal	P_{ETCO_2}	End-tidal CO_2 tension
T	Tidal gas	V_T	Tidal volume
D	Dead space gas	V_D	Physiological dead space volume
B	Barometric	P_B	Barometric pressure

BLOOD

PRIMARY SYMBOLS			EXAMPLES
$\dot{Q}$	Volume flow of blood per unit time	$\dot{Q}c$	Blood flow through pulmonary capillaries per minute
C	Concentration of gas in blood phase	Ca_{O_2}	Content of O_2 in arterial blood
S	Percent saturation of Hb with O_2	$S\bar{v}_{O_2}$	Saturation of Hb with O_2 in mixed venous blood

SECONDARY SYMBOLS			EXAMPLES
a	Arterial blood	Pa_{CO_2}	Partial pressure of CO_2 in arterial blood
v	Venous blood	$P\bar{v}_{O_2}$	Partial pressure of O_2 in mixed venous blood
c	Capillary blood	Pcc_{O_2}	Partial pressure of CO_2 in pulmonary capillary blood

LUNG VOLUMES AND FLOWS

V_T	Tidal volume = Volume of air inhaled or exhaled with each breath
VC	Vital capacity = Maximal volume that can be expired after maximal inspiration
IC	Inspiratory capacity = Maximal volume that can be inspired from the resting end-expiratory level
ERV	Expiratory reserve volume = Maximal volume that can be expired from the resting end-expiratory level
FRC	Functional residual capacity = Volume of gas in lungs at end-expiration
RV	Residual volume = Volume of gas in lungs after maximal expiration
TLC	Total lung capacity = Volume of gas in lungs after maximal inspiration
FEV_x	Forced expired volume in x seconds (e.g., FEV_1 = forced expiratory volume in 1 second)
MVV	Maximal voluntary ventilation

VARIABLES AND PARAMETERS

$\dot{V}_{O_2}$	Oxygen uptake
$\dot{V}_{O_2}max$	Maximal aerobic power
$\dot{V}_{CO_2}$	Carbon dioxide output
$\dot{Q}_{O_2}$	Oxygen consumption
$\dot{Q}_{CO_2}$	CO_2 production
AT	Anaerobic threshold
LT	Lactate threshold
LAT	Lactic acidosis threshold
R	Gas exchange ratio
RQ	Respiratory quotient
$\dot{V}_E/\dot{V}_{O_2}$	Ventilatory equivalent for O_2
$\dot{V}_E/\dot{V}_{CO_2}$	Ventilatory equivalent for CO_2
V_D/V_T	Physiological dead space–tidal volume ratio
V_D	Physiological dead space
BR	Breathing reserve
HR	Heart rate
HRR	Heart rate reserve
WR	Work rate
$\Delta\dot{V}_{O_2}/\Delta WR$	Change in $\dot{V}_{O_2}$/change in WR

Glossary

Aerobic: Having molecular oxygen present; describes a metabolic process utilizing oxygen.

Alveolar to arterial P_{O_2} difference [$P(A - a)_{O_2}$]: The difference between the ideal alveolar P_{O_2} (estimated) and the arterial P_{O_2}. A larger difference reflects an increase in the lungs' inefficiency with respect to oxygen exchange.

Alveolar ventilation ($\dot{V}_A$): The theoretic alveolar ventilation necessary to eliminate the metabolic CO_2 at the current arterial CO_2 tension. It assumes that $\dot{V}_A/\dot{Q}$ is uniform in all the acini so that their mean P_{CO_2} is equal to the arterial P_{CO_2}.

Anaerobic: Lacking or inadequate molecular oxygen; describes any metabolic process that does not use molecular oxygen.

Anaerobic threshold (AT): The exercise $\dot{V}_{O_2}$ above which anaerobic high-energy P_{O_4} production supplements aerobic high-energy P_{O_4} production, with the consequent lower redox state, increase in lactate-to-pyruvate (L/P) ratio, and net increase in lactate production at the site of anaerobiosis. Exercise above the AT is reflected by an increase in lactate concentration and L/P ratio in the muscle effluent and central blood, and a metabolic acidosis. Gas exchange is also affected by an increase in CO_2 output over that produced from aerobic metabolism, resulting from HCO_3^- buffering of lactic acid.

Analog-to-digital converter: A device for transforming continuously changing information into discrete units over some small time frame within which the value is considered to be relatively constant. This transforms continuous signals to a form that can be analyzed by a digital computer.

Arterial to end-tidal P_{CO_2} difference [$P(a - ET)_{CO_2}$]: The difference between the mean arterial P_{CO_2} and the end-tidal P_{CO_2}. This is positive when the arterial P_{CO_2} is higher than the end-tidal P_{CO_2}. An increased positive difference generally reflects increased inefficiency of lung CO_2 exchange.

Arterial–mixed venous O_2 content difference [$C(a - \bar{v})_{O_2}$]: The difference in the O_2 content of the arterial and venous blood, usually expressed in milliliters of O_2 per deciliter or liter of blood.

ATPS: A convention for expressing gas volume conditioned to the ambient (e.g., room) temperature and pressure, and saturated with water vapor at ambient temperature.

Breath-by-breath: The expression of a particular physiological value averaged over one entire respiratory cycle, usually expressed as the value that variable would have if maintained over an entire minute (e.g., ventilation expressed as L/min). Breath-by-breath is also used to describe a method for measurement of respiratory gas exchange in a breath during which respired gas volume and simultaneously measured expired gas concentration are integrated and reported.

Breathing reserve (BR): The difference between the maximum voluntary ventilation (measured at rest) and the maximum exercise minute ventilation. Hence, this represents the body's potential for further increasing ventilation at maximum exercise.

BTPS: A convention for expressing gas volume conditioned to body temperature and the ambient atmospheric pressure and fully saturated with water vapor at the subject's body temperature.

Carbon dioxide output ($\dot{V}CO_2$): The amount of CO_2 exhaled from the body into the atmosphere per unit time, expressed in milliliters or liters per minute, STPD. This differs from CO_2 production rate under conditions in which additional CO_2 may be evolved from the body's stores ($\dot{V}CO_2$ is higher than production rate) or CO_2 is added to the body's stores ($\dot{V}CO_2$ is lower than production rate). In the steady state, CO_2 output equals CO_2 production rate. In rare circumstances, appreciable quantities of CO_2 can be eliminated from the body as bicarbonate via the gastrointestinal tract or by hemodialysis.

Carbon dioxide production ($\dot{Q}CO_2$): The amount of carbon dioxide produced by the body's metabolic processes and, in some circumstances, released by buffering reactions within the body, expressed in milliliters or liters per minute, STPD.

Cardiac output ($\dot{Q}$): The flow of blood from the heart in a particular period of time, usually expressed as liters per minute. It is the product of the average stroke volume per beat and the heart rate (i.e., number of beats per minute).

Constant work rate test: An exercise test in which a constant power output is required of the subject.

Dead space or physiological dead space (VD): The theoretic volume of gas taken into the lung that is not involved in gas exchange, assuming that the remaining volume (i.e., the alveolar volume) consists of acini having uniform $\dot{V}A/\dot{Q}$ so that their mean PCO_2 equals the mean PCO_2 of the pulmonary capillary blood. The physiological dead space is made up of the anatomic dead space (the volume of the upper airways, trachea, and bronchi) and the alveolar dead space (the theoretical volume of alveoli that are ventilated but are unperfused).

Dead space–tidal volume ratio (VD/VT): The proportion of the tidal volume that is made up of the physiological dead space. This is an index of the relative inefficiency of pulmonary gas exchange to eliminate CO_2.

Diffusing capacity: A measure of the rate of uptake of a particular gas across the alveolar–capillary bed for a specified driving pressure for that gas. It is measured, therefore, as the volume of gas per unit time per pressure difference (e.g., mL/min/mm Hg). It is also referred to as the pulmonary gas transfer index (a term that more properly reflects the measurement). It is most practical to use carbon monoxide as the test gas for measurement of diffusing capacity of the lungs, in which case it is referred to as D_{LCO}.

Diffusion defect: A defect in the lungs' capacity for gas diffusion. This is typically caused either by an abnormally increased diffusion path length or by conditions in which the transit time of the red cell through the pulmonary capillary bed is so fast that insufficient time is available for complete diffusion equilibrium.

Disability: A legal term that considers the effect of a functional impairment on the patient's ability to perform a specific work task, along with other factors such as age, sex, education, social environment, job availability, and the energy requirements of the occupation.

End-tidal PCO_2 ($PETCO_2$): The PCO_2 of the respired gas determined at the end of a spontaneous exhalation. This is commonly the highest PCO_2 measured during the alveolar phase of the exhalation.

End-tidal PO_2 ($PETO_2$): The PO_2 determined in the respired gas at the end of a spontaneous exhalation. This is typically the lowest PO_2 determined during the alveolar portion of the exhalation.

Exponential: A process in which the instantaneous rate of change of a variable is proportional to the "distance" from a steady-state or required level; hence, the rate of change of the function under consideration is rapid when it is far from its steady-state value and slows progressively as the function approaches its steady state. If the process is known to be, or may be reasonably estimated to be, exponential, the time to reach 63% of the final value (i.e., to approach within 37% of the final value) is termed the time constant (τ) of the response. If the process is exponential, this time constant is related to the half time (the time to reach 50% of the final value) by the equation $t_{1/2} = 0.693 \times \tau$.

Fick method for cardiac output: A means of estimating cardiac output from the uptake of O_2 by the lungs and the arterial–mixed venous O_2 content difference. $\dot{Q} = \dot{V}O_2/C(a - \bar{v})O_2$. When the same principle is used to measure cardiac output with CO_2 as the test gas, the CO_2 output is divided by the $C(\bar{v} - a)CO_2$.

Frequency response: This reflects the fidelity with which a measuring device can track rapidly changing physiologic information. The frequency response of the device is determined by applying rapidly changing signals of a particular amplitude, spanning a range of frequencies, and then establishing the frequency range over which the device tracks the signal at a predetermined level of accuracy.

Gas exchange ratio (R): The ratio of the carbon dioxide output to the oxygen uptake per unit time. This ratio reflects not only tissue metabolic exchange of the gases but also the influence of transient change in gas storage of O_2, and especially of CO_2. For example, the gas exchange ratio exceeds the respiratory quotient during hyperventilation as additional CO_2 is evolved from the body's stores, whereas the gas exchange ratio is less than the respiratory quotient during transient hypoventilation when CO_2 is retained in the body's stores.

Half time ($t_{1/2}$): Unlike the time constant, which requires evidence of exponentiality for its determination, the half time of a response is a simple description of the time to reach half of the change to the final value, regardless of the function. It is, therefore, generally representative of the speed of approaching the steady state.

Heart rate reserve (HRR): The difference between the predicted highest heart rate attainable during maximum exercise and the actual highest heart rate, usually during exercise testing involving large muscle masses, such as during cycle or treadmill ergometry.

Ideal alveolar PO_2: The hypothetical alveolar PO_2 that would be obtained if the lung were an ideal gas exchanger, that is, with ventilation uniformly matched to perfusion.

Impairment: A medical term reflecting a physiological abnormality. For exercise, it could represent any defect in the ventilatory-circulatory-metabolic coupling of external to internal respiration.

Incremental exercise test: An exercise test designed to provide a graded stress to the subject. The work rate required by the subject is usually increased over uniform periods of time; for example, every 4 minutes, every minute, every 15 seconds, or even continuously (e.g., ramp pattern increment).

Lactate: The anion of lactic acid.

Lactate threshold (LT): The exercise $\dot{V}O_2$ above which a net increase in lactate production results in a sustained increase in central blood lactate concentration.

Lactic acid: A three-carbon carboxylic acid ($CH_3CHOHCOOH$) that is one of the potential end products of glucose oxidation. Another major product is pyruvic acid ($CH_3COCOOH$), which can undergo conversion to acetyl coenzyme A and can thereby be further oxidized. The relative amounts of lactic acid and pyruvic acid are determined by the cytosolic redox state; a low redox state, reflected by a high ratio of NADH to NAD^+, favors the generation of lactic acid, which in turn maintains the supply of NAD^+ necessary for glycolysis to continue. The presence of lactic acid is a marker of anaerobic metabolism.

Lactic acidosis threshold (LAT): The exercise $\dot{V}O_2$ above which arterial standard HCO_3^- decreases because of a net increase in lactate production. This can be detected by an increase in CO_2 output (from dissociation of H_2CO_3 as HCO_3^- buffers lactic acid) above that which would be predicted from aerobic metabolism alone during a progressively increasing work rate exercise test.

Laminar flow: A condition in which the flow of a fluid (gas or liquid) through a conduit is characterized by the uniform direction of flow of any plane sheet of the fluid, each of which flows parallel to any other in the direction of flow. Under conditions of laminar flow, the pressure difference between two fixed points upstream and downstream is directly proportional to flow and with the proportionality constant the resistance of the conduit.

Mass spectrometer: A device that separates and measures molecules of gas of a particular type in a mixed gas stream on the basis of their mass.

Maximum exercise heart rate: The highest obtainable heart rate during a maximum-effort test.

Maximum exercise ventilation: The highest minute ventilation achieved during a maximum–work rate test. This is usually determined by tests that tax large muscle masses, such as cycle or treadmill ergometry.

Maximum voluntary ventilation (MVV): The upper limit of the body's ability to ventilate the lungs. This is conventionally measured from maximal volitional effort for short periods of time (e.g., 12 seconds) and expressed in units of liters per minute, BTPS.

Mets: Mets, or metabolic equivalents, are the multiple of the resting metabolic rate expressed as O_2 uptake per minute per kilogram. The resting metabolic rate used in this calculation is usually 3.5 ml/min/kg, which is the average for a 40-year-old, 70-kg man. The weakness in applying this concept is that the exercise $\dot{V}O_2$ is usually not measured but assumed for a given treadmill grade and speed or cycle work rate. A further weakness is the assumption that the resting $\dot{V}O_2$ is 3.5 mL/min/kg for everyone.

Minute ventilation ($\dot{V}I$ or $\dot{V}E$): The volume of air taken into or exhaled from the body in 1 minute. This is conventionally expressed at body temperature, saturated with water at atmospheric pressure (BTPS).

Mixed venous blood: A sample of blood representative of the flow-weighted venous blood returning from all the organs of the body. Usually, blood obtained from the pulmonary artery is considered to be mixed venous blood.

Mixed venous O_2 or CO_2: The average partial pressure or gas content of the blood returning from all the tissues of the body and, having been fully mixed in the right heart, normally represented by the concentration or partial pressure of that substance in the pulmonary arterial blood.

Mixing chamber: A device that mixes the dead space and alveolar gas to produce a gas that is representative of the mixed expired gas. This is typically achieved by exhaling into a baffled chamber that mixes several breaths. The mixed expired concentration of a gas can be measured downstream from the chamber.

Oximeter: A device that uses light transmission or reflectance techniques to estimate the saturation of hemoglobin with oxygen. Direct oximetry is done on blood samples. For indirect oximetry, a site for measurement, such as the earlobe or finger, is selected because blood comes close to the skin and traverses the capillary bed with little loss of oxygen; hence, the mean capillary value will reflect arterial values. See *pulse oximeter*.

Oxygen consumption ($\dot{Q}O_2$): The amount of oxygen utilized by the body's metabolic processes in a given time, expressed in milliliters or liters per minute, STPD.

Oxygen content (CO_2): The volume of O_2 (STPD) in a given volume (L, dl, or ml) of blood. This includes the major component that is bound to hemoglobin and the amount physically dissolved in the blood.

Oxygen debt: The additional oxygen utilized in excess of the baseline needs of the body following a bout of exercise.

Oxygen deficit: The oxygen equivalent of the total energy utilized to perform the work that did not derive from reactions utilizing atmospheric oxygen taken into the body after the start of the exercise. Consequently, for moderate-intensity exercise, this O_2 deficit represents the energy equivalent of the depletion of the high-energy phosphate stores and oxygen stored in the body at the start of the work. For heavy or severe exercise, the oxygen deficit also includes the energy equivalent of the anaerobic processes.

Oxygen delivery: The amount of oxygen delivered to a tissue per unit time. It is, therefore, the product of the oxygen content of arterial blood and the blood flow to that tissue.

Oxygen pulse: The oxygen uptake divided by the heart rate. Hence, it is the amount of oxygen extracted by the tissues of the body from the O_2 carried in each stroke volume.

Oxygen uptake ($\dot{V}O_2$): The amount of oxygen extracted from the inspired gas in a given period of time, expressed in milliliters or liters per minute, STPD. This can differ from oxygen consumption under conditions in which oxygen is flowing into or being utilized from the body's stores. In the steady state, oxygen uptake equals oxygen consumption.

Phase I: The period of time following the onset of exercise that is required for the products of exercise metabolism to reach the lungs. During phase I, the mixed venous blood entering the pulmonary capillary bed has not changed its composition. Phase I is a result of the transit delay from the site of increased metabolism. Normally, this period is about 15 seconds.

Phase II: The period of time following the onset of exercise when the mixed venous blood gas concentrations continue to change because of changes in the effluent from the exercising muscles. Phase II reflects the "kinetic phase" of the gas exchange that begins at the end of phase I and continues until a steady state is obtained.

Phase III: The steady-state phase of gas exchange during exercise. For moderate exercise, it reflects the period in which the mixed venous gas concentrations have become constant. For heavy exercise, $\dot{V}O_2$ is observed to increase slowly during this phase, likely related to lactate metabolism.

Physiological dead space: See *dead space*.

Pneumotachograph: A device used to measure gas flow. It is typically composed of a screen across which the pressure drop stemming from the flow of gas may be measured. Flow may be integrated over time to yield the volume of air respired.

Power: See *work rate*.

Pulse oximeter: A noninvasive device for estimating arterial blood oxygen saturation using a combination of spectrophotometry and pulse plethysmography. The pulse oximeter probe is designed to be placed on the earlobe, finger tip, or forehead.

Pulse pressure: The difference between the systolic and the diastolic blood pressure.

Pump calibrator: A device that simulates the airflow and gas concentration waveforms encountered during respiration. Because the "metabolic rate" of such a device can be precisely calculated, it is useful for calibration of an exercise gas exchange measurement system.

R: See *gas exchange ratio*.

Ramp exercise test: An exercise testing protocol in which the work rate is continuously increased at a constant rate, (e.g., 10 W/min). See *incremental exercise test*.

Response time: A means of characterizing the rate at which a device or system responds to a given signal. For example, in response to a sudden application of a constant level of input, how long does the output take to become constant? This can be characterized by the time constant, half time, or the time to reach 90% of the final value.

RQ (respiratory quotient): The ratio of the rate of carbon dioxide production to oxygen consumption. This ratio reflects the metabolic exchange of the gases in the body's tissues and is dictated by the percentage of substrate species (carbohydrates, fatty acids, and amino acids) used in energy production by the cells.

Set point: A term used in control system theory that reflects the particular value of a variable that the output of the system regulates. For example, a CO_2 set point is considered to be the operating level of arterial P_{CO_2}, which is maintained at its relatively constant (i.e., set-point) value by changes in ventilation at a given level of CO_2 output.

Steady state: A characteristic of a physiologic system in which its functional demands are being met such that its output per unit time becomes constant. The time to achieve a steady state commonly differs for different physiologic systems. For example, following the onset of constant-load exercise, oxygen uptake rises to reach its steady state appreciably faster than CO_2 output or ventilation. A constant value attained by the system is not sufficient, however, to determine that the system is in a steady state. If the system reaches the limit of its output, and, as a result, its output becomes constant (as in the case of oxygen uptake reaching its maximum value), a steady state does not prevail. The system in this instance is in a limited state, not a steady state.

STPD: A convention for expressing gas volume at standard conditions of temperature and pressure, free of water vapor. The standard conditions are 0°C, 760 mm Hg, and dry gas.

Stroke volume: The volume of blood ejected from either ventricle of the heart in a single beat.

Sustainable work rate: A relative term that reflects the extent to which a particular work rate may be sustained for sufficient time for the successful completion of a particular occupational, recreational, or laboratory-induced work rate. Therefore, at a sustainable work rate, the subject does not fatigue within the time constraints of the requirements of the test.

Thermodilution blood flow measurement: A technique in which a measured bolus of physiologic fluid of known temperature, usually at 0°C, is injected into a vascular stream, such as in the right atrium, and the temperature of the blood is measured at a mixed downstream point, such as in the pulmonary artery. The addition of the cold bolus of fluid decreases the blood temperature at the downstream point; the amount of cooling is a function of the blood flow. Thermodilution cardiac output measurements are usually performed using a thermistor-tipped pulmonary artery catheter (Swan-Ganz type).

Tidal volume to inspiratory capacity ratio (V_T/IC): The ratio of the volume of air exhaled during a breath (V_T) to the volume potentially available for that breath, the latter measured from the end-expiratory lung volume to the maximum inspiratory volume (IC). Hence, it reflects the proportion of the potential inspiratory volume excursion that is actually utilized for a particular breath.

Transcutaneous gas tension: A technique for estimating the partial pressure of the gas in the capillary blood perfusing a region of skin with high flow and low metabolic rate. When the intent of this measurement is to estimate arterial blood gases, it must be interpreted with caution, especially with rapid changes in arterial blood gases.

Transducer: A device that transforms energy from one form to another. Consequently, a pressure transducer is a device that changes fluid pressure into an electrical signal that can be analyzed and used for display or recording.

Turbulent flow: A condition in which the fluid (gas or liquid) flow has characteristic eddies, whorls, and diverse directional currents, such that additional energy needs to be applied to create a given fluid flow. Under conditions of turbulent flow, the relation between flow and pressure is nonlinear.

V-slope method: A method for determining the anaerobic or lactic acidosis threshold by plotting the volume of CO_2 output against the O_2 uptake on equal scales. The onset of lactic acidosis during an incremental exercise test is detected when CO_2 output increases relative to O_2 uptake, reflecting the increased CO_2 generated from bicarbonate as it buffers lactic acid.

$\Delta\dot{V}O_2$ (6 − 3): The difference in oxygen uptake between the sixth and the third minute of a constant-load exercise test. Normal subjects typically attain a steady state for constant-load exercise within 3 minutes during moderate exercise; hence, the $\Delta\dot{V}O_2$ (6 − 3) is zero. A positive value for this index reflects a degree of continuing non–steady state for the work and usually signals fatiguing exercise.

$\dot{V}O_2$max: The highest oxygen uptake obtainable for a given form of ergometry despite further work rate increases and effort by the subject. This is characterized by a plateau of oxygen uptake despite further increases in work rate.

$\Delta\dot{V}O_2/\Delta WR$: The increase in oxygen uptake in response to a simultaneous increase in work rate. Under appropriate conditions (e.g., steady-state aerobic work), this may be used to estimate the efficiency for muscular work.

Wasted ventilation ($\dot{V}D$): The difference between the computed alveolar ventilation and the measured minute ventilation. Also known as the physiological dead space ventilation, this term is meant to reflect the volume of the respired air that did not participate in alveolar capillary gas exchange; it is equal to $V_D \times f$.

Work: A physical quantification of the force operating on a mass that causes it to change its location. Under conditions in which force is applied and no movement results (e.g., during an isometric contraction), no work is performed, despite increased metabolic energy expenditure. The unit of work is the joule (kg m^2/sec^2).

Work rate or power: This reflects the rate at which work is performed (i.e., work per unit time). Work rate is usually measured in watts (kg m^2/sec^3 or joule/sec) or in kilopond meters per minute (kp-m/min); 1 W is equivalent to 6.12 kp-m/min.

APPENDIX C

Calculations, Formulas, and Examples

T HIS APPENDIX PRESENTS the most essential formulas for calculating gas exchange and other related variables during exercise. An example accompanies the formula for each variable, using typical data acquired during exercise testing. Calculation of these variables uses well-defined and tested formulas, but several areas deserve particularly close attention. We address the specific problems of water vapor in the calculation of $\dot{V}O_2$, of making corrections for the dead space of the breathing valve, and of collecting data for breath-by-breath gas exchange analysis.

With computerized systems for collecting expired gas, measuring gas concentrations and ventilation, and calculating and displaying the relevant variables, some might be curious why one would need to understand how these calculations are made. It is important to understand how and how much variables can be affected by changes in the environment or by dysfunction of measurement devices. This understanding can be helpful in troubleshooting or deciding on the need to recalibrate the systems or obtain service for the equipment.

FORMULAS AND EXAMPLES OF GAS EXCHANGE CALCULATION

The formula for calculating each variable takes into account the condition under which each measurement is made and certain conventions. For the example calculations, we assume that expired gas is collected for exactly 2 minutes into a sealed meteorological balloon or Douglas bag. Assume that the gas volume is measured in a large spirometer or other suitable device, that fractional concentrations of O_2 and CO_2 are measured to within 0.04% using gas analyzers or a mass spectrometer, and that these are fractions of total gas volume excluding water vapor. An arterial blood sample is obtained during the collection of expired gas.

The measurements used for the example calculations are given in Table C.1.

TABLE C.1. Measurements Used for Example of Calculation of Gas Exchange

Measured volume: 54.2 (ATPS)
Collection time: 2 min
Number of breaths: 41 in 2 min
Heart rate (HR) = 120/min
Body temperature = 37°C
F_{IO_2} = 0.2093 (20.93%)
F_{ICO_2} = 0.0004 (0.04%)
F_{EO_2} = 0.162 (16.2%)
F_{ECO_2} = 0.041 (4.1%)
(Fractions of dry gas volume)

Hemoglobin − 15 g/100mL
Valve dead space = 63 ml
Ambient temperature (T) = 22°C
Barometric pressure (P_B) = 760 mmHg
Partial pressure of water, saturated gas at 22°C (P_{H_2O}) = 19 mmHg
Pa_{O_2} = 91 mmHg
Pa_{CO_2} = 36 mmHg
pH = 7.44
Sa_{O_2} = 95%
P_{ETCO_2} = 38 mmHg
$P\bar{v}_{O_2}$ = 27 mmHg
$S\bar{v}_{O_2}$ = 50%

Minute Ventilation ($\dot{V}_E$)

The volume of gas exhaled divided by the time of collection in minutes is minute ventilation ($\dot{V}_E$). By convention, $\dot{V}_E$ is reported at body temperature saturated with water vapor at ambient pressure (BTPS), as in Eq. 1. It may be necessary during calculation to obtain $\dot{V}_E$ at standard temperature and pressure (STPD) using Eq. 2 or the appropriate tables (see Appendix E).

Most commonly, ventilation is measured at ambient temperature and the gas is fully saturated with water vapor at ambient temperature (ATPS). Equation 1 is used to adjust volume from ATPS to BTPS. The temperature and water vapor correction factors can also be found in Appendix E.

$$\dot{V}_E \text{ (L/min, BTPS)} = \dot{V}_E \text{ (L/min, ATPS)} \times \frac{(273 + 37)}{273 + T}$$
$$\times \frac{P_B - P_{H_2O} \text{ (at } T)}{P_B - 47} \quad (1)$$

where T is ambient temperature (°C), body temperature is 37°C, P_{H_2O} at 37°C is 47 mm Hg (fully saturated), and P_B is barometric pressure.

Alternatively, ventilation can be measured at STPD. From $\dot{V}_E$ (BTPS), $\dot{V}_E$ (STPD) can be obtained using Eq. 2, which converts BTPS to STPD (at 273°

K, barometric pressure = 760 mm Hg, and no water vapor present) for $\dot{V}_{CO_2}$ and $\dot{V}_{CO_2}$ calculations.

$\dot{V}_E$ (L/min, STPD)
$$= \dot{V}_E \text{ (L/min, BTPS)} \times \frac{273}{(273 + 37)} \times \frac{(P_B - 47)}{760}$$

which becomes

$$\dot{V}_E \text{ (L/min, STPD)} = \dot{V}_E \text{ (L/min, BTPS)} \times 0.826 \quad (2)$$

if P_B = 760 mm Hg.

Example

$$\dot{V}_E \text{ (L/min, ATPS)} = \frac{\text{Total volume (ATPS)}}{\text{Total collection time}}$$

$$= \frac{54.2}{2 \text{ min}} = 27.1$$

Then, from Eq. 1,

$$\dot{V}_E \text{ (L/min, BTPS)} = 27.1 \times \frac{310}{(273 + 22)} \times \frac{(760 - 19)}{(760 - 47)}$$

$$= 29.6$$

and, from Eq. 2,

$$\dot{V}_E \text{ (L/min, STPD)} = 29.6 \times 0.826 = 24.3$$

Respiratory Frequency (f)

$$f \text{ (min}^{-1}) = \frac{\text{Number of complete breaths}}{\text{Total time for complete breaths}} \quad (3)$$

Example

$$f \text{ (min}^{-1}) = \frac{41 \text{ breaths}}{2 \text{ min}} = 20.5$$

Tidal Volume (V_T)

$$V_T \text{ (L, BTPS)} = \frac{\dot{V}_E \text{ (L/min, BTPS)}}{f} \quad (4)$$

Example

$$V_T \text{ (L, BTPS)} = \frac{29.6}{20.5} = 1.44$$

Carbon Dioxide Output ($\dot{V}_{CO_2}$)

The CO_2 output and O_2 uptake are reported, by convention, under STPD conditions. If $\dot{V}_E$ and $\dot{V}_I$ are measured at or converted to STPD conditions, F_{ECO_2} is the fraction of dry gas volume, and F_{ICO_2} is zero or negligible, then

$$\dot{V}_{CO_2} \text{ (L/min, STPD)} = \dot{V}_E \text{ (L/min, STPD)} \times F_{ECO_2} \quad (5)$$

or, for $P_B = 760$ mm Hg,

$$\dot{V}_{CO_2} \text{ (L/min, STPD)} = \dot{V}_E \text{ (L/min, BTPS)}$$
$$\times\, 0.826 \times F_{ECO_2} \quad (6)$$

Example

Substituting $\dot{V}_E$ and F_{ECO_2} (Table C.1) into Eq. 5,

$$\dot{V}_{CO_2} \text{ (L/min, STPD)} = 24.3 \times 0.041 = 0.997$$

Oxygen Uptake ($\dot{V}_{O_2}$)

For the derivation of the formula for $\dot{V}_{O_2}$ and consideration of water vapor, see "Special Considerations for Calculation of Gas Exchange Variables," later in this appendix. Equation 7 should be used only for expired gas containing no water vapor (or measured as such).

If $\dot{V}_E$ is measured at or converted to STPD, F_{IO_2} is 0.2093 (dry room air), F_{ECO_2} and F_{EO_2} are fractions of CO_2 and O_2 in dry gas, respectively, and F_{ICO_2} is 0, then

$$\dot{V}_{O_2} \text{ (L/min, STPD)} = \dot{V}_E \text{ (L/min, STPD)}$$
$$\times\, (\Delta F_{O_2}) \text{ true, dry} \quad (7)$$

where (ΔF_{O_2}) true, dry $= 0.265 - 1.265 \times F_{EO_2} - 0.265 \times F_{ECO_2}$ for a person breathing room air. The (ΔF_{O_2}) true, dry can also be obtained from the nomogram in Appendix E.

Example

Substituting from Table C.1 into Eq. 7:

$$(\Delta F_{O_2}) \text{ true, dry} = 0.265 - 0.205 - 0.0108 = 0.049$$
$$\dot{V}_{O_2} \text{ (L/min, STPD)} = 24.3 \times 0.049 = 1.19$$

Gas Exchange Ratio (R)

$$R = \frac{\dot{V}_{CO_2} \text{ (L, min STPD)}}{\dot{V}_{O_2} \text{ (L, min STPD)}} \quad (8)$$

Example

$$R = \frac{0.997}{1.19} = 0.84$$

Ventilatory Equivalents for Carbon Dioxide and Oxygen ($\dot{V}_E/\dot{V}_{CO_2}$, $\dot{V}_E/\dot{V}_{O_2}$)

The ventilatory equivalents for CO_2 and O_2 are measurements of the ventilatory requirement for that metabolic rate. By convention, they are expressed as $\dot{V}_E$ (L/min, BTPS) divided by $\dot{V}_{CO_2}$ or $\dot{V}_{O_2}$ (L/min, STPD). Because the portion of the ventilation wasted in clearing the breathing valve dead space is disregarded in determining the ventilatory requirement, the product of valve dead space (V_{D_m}) and respiratory frequency (f) is subtracted from the total $\dot{V}_E$:

$$\dot{V}_E/\dot{V}_{CO_2} = \frac{\dot{V}_E \text{ (L/min, BTPS)} - [f\,\text{min}^{-1} \times V_{D_m} \text{(L)}]}{\dot{V}_{CO_2} \text{ (L/min, STPD)}} \quad (9)$$

$$\dot{V}_E/\dot{V}_{O_2} = \frac{\dot{V}_E \text{ (L/min, BTPS)} - [f\,\text{min}^{-1} \times V_{D_m} \text{(L)}]}{\dot{V}_{O_2} \text{ (L/min, STPD)}} \quad (10)$$

Example

$$\dot{V}_E/\dot{V}_{CO_2} = \frac{29.6 - [20.5 \times 0.064]}{0.997} = 28.4$$

$$\dot{V}_E/\dot{V}_{O_2} = \frac{29.6 - [20.5 \times 0.064]}{1.19} = 23.8$$

Oxygen Pulse ($\dot{V}_{O_2}$/HR)

$\dot{V}_{O_2}$/HR (mL, STPD/beat)

$$= \frac{\dot{V}_{O_2} \text{ (L/min, STPD)} \times 1000 \text{ ml/L}}{\text{HR (beats/min)}} \quad (11)$$

Example

$$\dot{V}_{O_2}\text{/HR (ml, STPD/beat)} = \frac{1.19 \times 1000}{120} = 9.9$$

Alveolar P_{O_2} ($P_{A O_2}$)

$P_{A O_2}$ (mm Hg)

$$= F_{IO_2} \times (P_B - 47) - \frac{P_{A CO_2}}{R} [1 - F_{IO_2} (1 - R)] \quad (12)$$

where barometric pressure is in mm Hg, $P_{A CO_2}$ is ideal alveolar P_{CO_2} in mm Hg, R is the gas exchange ratio, and F_{IO_2} is the fraction of inspired O_2, dry. Usually, the assumption that $P_{ACO_2} = P_{aCO_2}$ is used, and the term $F_{IO_2} \times (1 - R)$ may be dropped because it is so small that it has an insignificant effect on the calculated P_{AO_2}, especially during air breathing. This simplifies the formula to the following:

$$P_{AO_2} \text{ (mm Hg)} = F_{IO_2} \times (P_B - 47) - \frac{P_{aCO_2}}{R} \quad (13)$$

Whereas R in the fasting state is often assumed to be 0.8 at rest, R should always be calculated during exercise because it may range from 0.7 to 1.4 or more, which will have an appreciable effect on alveolar P_{O_2} calculation.

Example

Substituting into Eq. 13,

$$P_{AO_2} \text{ (mm Hg)} = (0.2093 \times 713) - \frac{36}{0.84} = 106$$

Alveolar–Arterial P_{O_2} Difference [$P(A - a)O_2$]

$$P(A - a)O_2 \text{ (mm Hg)} = P_{AO_2} - P_{aO_2} \quad (14)$$

where P_{AO_2} is determined as above and P_{aO_2} is arterial P_{O_2}.

Example

$$P(A - a)O_2 \text{ (mm Hg)} = 106 - 91 = 15$$

Arterial End-Tidal P_{CO_2} Difference [$P(a - ET)CO_2$]

$$P(a - ET)CO_2 = P_{aCO_2} - P_{ETCO_2} \quad (15)$$

where P_{aCO_2} is arterial P_{CO_2} and P_{ETCO_2} is end-tidal P_{CO_2}.

Example

$$P(a - ET)CO_2 = 36 - 38 = -2 \text{ mm Hg}$$

Physiological Dead Space (V_D)

$$V_D \text{ (L)} = V_T \text{ (L)} \times \frac{(P_{aCO_2} - P_{\bar{E}CO_2})}{P_{aCO_2}} - V_{D_m} \text{ (L)} \quad (16)$$

where V_T is tidal volume, P_{aCO_2} is arterial P_{CO_2}, $P_{\bar{E}CO_2}$ is mixed expired P_{CO_2}, and V_{D_m} is breathing valve dead space. Mixed expired P_{CO_2} can be calculated as follows:

$$P_{\bar{E}CO_2} = \frac{\dot{V}_{CO_2} \text{ (L/min, STPD)}}{\dot{V}_E \text{ (L/min, STPD)}} \times (P_B - 47 \text{ mm Hg})$$

Example

$$P_{\bar{E}CO_2} = \frac{0.997}{24.3} \times 713 = 29$$

$$V_D \text{ (L)} = 1.44 \times \frac{36 - 29}{36} - 0.064 = 0.22$$

Physiological Dead Space–Tidal Volume Ratio (V_D/V_T)

$$\frac{V_D}{V_T} = \frac{(P_{aCO_2} - P_{\bar{E}CO_2})}{P_{aCO_2}} - \frac{V_{D_m} \text{ (L)}}{[V_T \text{ (L)} - V_{D_m} \text{ (L)}]} \quad (17)$$

Example

$$\frac{V_D}{V_T} = \frac{39 - 29}{36} - \frac{0.064}{1.44} = 0.15$$

V_D/V_T must be calculated using the arterial P_{CO_2}. There has been an unfortunate trend of calculating V_D/V_T "noninvasively" during exercise by substituting P_{ETCO_2} for P_{aCO_2} in the foregoing formulas, or by estimating P_{aCO_2} from P_{ETCO_2} using a regression formula derived from normal subjects. As shown in Chapters 3 and 4, P_{ETCO_2} and P_{aCO_2} are nearly equal only in normal subjects at rest. During exercise, the $P(a - ET)CO_2$ becomes negative in normal subjects, whereas it becomes larger and more positive in patients with lung disease who have increased V_D/V_T. Therefore, the relation between P_{aCO_2} and P_{ETCO_2} during exercise ranges widely and unpredictably [1]. Furthermore, even small errors in P_{aCO_2} may result in clinically important differences in the calculated V_D/V_T.

Cardiac Output

The cardiac output ($\dot{Q}$) can be determined by thermal indicator dilution or by the Fick method using $\dot{V}_{O_2}$ and arterial–mixed venous O_2 content difference:

$$\dot{Q} \text{ (L/min)} = \frac{\dot{V}_{O_2} \text{ (ml/min, STPD)}}{(C_{aO_2} - C_{\bar{v}O_2}) \text{ (ml } O_2/\text{L blood)}} \quad (18)$$

where Ca_{O_2} is O_2 content in arterial blood and $C\bar{v}_{O_2}$ is O_2 content in mixed venous blood. These can be calculated as follows:

$$C_{O_2} \text{ (ml } O_2/100 \text{ ml)}$$
$$= (S_{O_2} \times 0.01 \times 1.34 \text{ ml } O_2/g \text{ Hb} \times [\text{Hb}]) \quad (19)$$
$$+ (0.003 \text{ ml } O_2/mm \text{ Hg}/100 \text{ ml} \times P_{O_2})$$

where [Hb] is hemoglobin concentration in g/100 ml blood and S_{O_2} is the percentage of oxyhemoglobin saturation. Note that this calculation gives O_2 content in ml $O_2/100$ ml of blood and is converted to ml O_2/L blood by multiplying by 10.

Example

$$Ca_{O_2}\text{(ml } O_2/100 \text{ ml)}$$
$$= (95\% \times 0.01 \times 1.34 \times 15) + (0.003 \times 91) = 19.4$$
$$C\bar{v}_{O_2} \text{ (ml } O_2/100 \text{ ml)}$$
$$= (50\% \times 0.01 \times 1.34 \times 15) + (0.003 \times 27) = 10.1$$
$$(Ca_{O_2} - C\bar{v}_{O_2})$$
$$= 19.4 - 10.1 = 9.3 \text{ ml } O_2/100 \text{ ml} = 93 \text{ ml } O_2/L$$

$$\dot{Q} \text{ (L/min)} = \frac{1190 \text{ (ml/min, STPD)}}{93 \text{ ml } O_2/L \text{ blood}} = 12.8$$

A noninvasive determination of cardiac output has been described using an analogous formula for CO_2 and an estimate of mixed venous CO_2 content (indirect Fick method) from a single-exhalation (2) or a rebreathing (3) method. With the rebreathing method, as a mixture of CO_2 and high inspired O_2 is rebreathed, the P_{CO_2} of the rebreathed gas rapidly approaches that of mixed venous blood. This value is then referred to a CO_2 dissociation curve to determine CO_2 content. However, as shown in Chapter 3, estimating mixed venous CO_2 content ($C\bar{v}_{CO_2}$) has great pitfalls during exercise.

Sun et al. (4,5), using direct measurements of blood gases and pH, addressed the problem of indirectly determining CO_2 contents in arterial and mixed venous blood. pH profoundly affects the CO_2 dissociation curve, making it impossible to get a reasonably reliable estimate of C_{CO_2}, particularly for $C\bar{v}_{CO_2}$. This study showed that $C\bar{v}_{CO_2}$ did not increase in proportion to $P\bar{v}_{CO_2}$ during exercise. In fact, $C\bar{v}_{CO_2}$ actually decreased as $P\bar{v}_{CO_2}$ increased above the anaerobic threshold because of the shift downward of the CO_2 dissociation curve as pH decreased. Also, as discussed in reference to calculating V_D/V_T, it is invalid to derive Pa_{CO_2} and Ca_{CO_2} from P_{ETCO_2} because the difference between these

two measures of P_{CO_2} is variable, particularly in patients, and is too large to obtain reliable estimates of CO_2 content with the precision required for valid measurements.

Using direct measures of arterial and mixed venous O_2 and CO_2 gas tensions, pH, and hemoglobin concentrations, Sun et al. (4,5) compared the O_2 and CO_2 values determined by direct Fick cardiac output measurements during exercise from rest to peak $\dot{V}_{O_2}$. They found that the two test gases gave the same results, but the variability was greater with CO_2. The reader is referred to the two papers by Sun et al. (4,5) on this topic, where the problems of measuring cardiac output by the indirect Fick method are thoroughly discussed.

CALCULATIONS AT MAXIMUM EXERCISE
Breathing Reserve (BR)

$$BR \text{ (L/min)} = MVV \text{ (L/min)}$$
$$- \dot{V}_E \text{ (L/min) at maximum exercise} \quad (20)$$

$$BR \text{ (\%)}$$
$$= \frac{MVV \text{ (L/min)} - \dot{V}_E \text{ (L/min) at maximum exercise}}{MVV \text{ (L/min)}}$$
$$\times 100 \quad (21)$$

where MVV is maximum voluntary ventilation at rest.

Example

If MVV is 82 L/min and $\dot{V}_E$ at maximum exercise is 65 L/min, then

$$BR \text{ (L/min)} = 82 - 65 = 17 \text{ L/min}$$
$$BR \text{ (\%)} = \frac{82 - 65}{82} \times 100 = 21\%$$

Heart Rate Reserve (HRR)

$$HRR \text{ (beats/min)} = \text{Predicted maximum HR}$$
$$- \text{HR at maximum exercise} \quad (22)$$
$$HRR \text{ (\%)} =$$
$$\frac{\text{Predicted maximum HR} - \text{HR at maximum exercise}}{\text{Predicted maximum HR}}$$
$$\times 100 \quad (23)$$

where predicted maximum HR (adults) = 220 − age (years).

Example

For a 60-year-old man, predicted maximum HR = $220 - 60 = 160$ beats/min. If HR at maximum exercise is 145 beats/min, then

$$HRR \ (beats/min) = 160 - 145 = 15$$

$$HRR \ (\%) = \frac{160 - 145}{160} \times 100 = 9\%$$

SPECIAL CONSIDERATIONS FOR CALCULATION OF GAS EXCHANGE VARIABLES
Water Vapor and Oxygen Uptake

Oxygen uptake ($\dot{V}_{O_2}$) is determined most often by collection and analysis of expired gas. The usual calculation method determines $\dot{V}_{O_2}$ from expired ventilation, expired CO_2 fraction, and expired O_2 fraction, and is based on the assumption that the inspired and expired volumes of nitrogen (and other inert gases) do not differ during the collection period. During rest and exercise, this method has been found to be satisfactory (6,7). Nevertheless, errors may be introduced if careful attention is not paid to methods and calculations. This is especially true of how water vapor is handled because this variable can greatly affect the calculation of $\dot{V}_{O_2}$.

If the Scholander or Haldane method of gas analysis or a mass spectrometer is used, or water vapor is removed by drying the gas prior to measurement, then measured gas concentration is relative to total gas minus the volume of water vapor. Thus, the dilution of the concentration of each gas caused by water vapor can be ignored and calculations are relatively simple:

$$\dot{V}_{O_2} \ (L/min, \ STPD) = [F_{IO_2} \times \dot{V}_I \ (L/min, \ STPD)]$$
$$- [F_{EO_2} \times \dot{V}_E \ (L/min, \ STPD)]$$

where F_{IO_2} and F_{EO_2} are the O_2 fractions of dry gas volumes. If, over the period of collection, the volumes of inspired and expired nitrogen (and other inert gases) are equal during breathing, then

$$\dot{V}_I \times F_{IN_2} = \dot{V}_E \times F_{EN_2}$$

and

$$\dot{V}_I = (F_{EN_2}/F_{IN_2}) \times \dot{V}_E$$

where F_{IN_2} and F_{EN_2} are the fractional concentrations of nitrogen and other inert gases.

Because $(F_{IN_2} + F_{IO_2} + F_{ICO_2}) = 1$ and $(F_{EN_2} + F_{EO_2} + F_{ECO_2}) = 1$, then

$$\dot{V}_I = \frac{(1 - F_{EO_2} - F_{ECO_2})}{(1 - F_{IO_2} - F_{ICO_2})} \times \dot{V}_E$$

and

$$\dot{V}_{O_2} \ (L/min, \ STPD) = \left[\frac{F_{IO_2} \times (1 - F_{EO_2} - F_{ECO_2})}{(1 - F_{IO_2} - F_{ICO_2})} \right]$$
$$\times \dot{V}_E \ (L/min, \ STPD) \qquad (24)$$

The quantity in brackets is called the true O_2 difference, (ΔF_{O_2})true.

If we assume that $F_{ICO_2} = 0$, or is negligible, then

$$(\Delta F_{O_2}) \ true = \frac{(F_{IO_2} - F_{EO_2} - F_{IO_2} \times F_{ECO_2})}{(1 - F_{IO_2})}$$

and

$$\dot{V}_{O_2} \ (L/min, \ STPD) = \dot{V}_E \ (L/min, \ STPD) \times (\Delta F_{O_2}) true$$

For room-air inspired gas, F_{IO_2} (dry) = 0.2093, and

$$\dot{V}_{O_2} \ (L/min, \ STPD) = \dot{V}_E \ (L/min, \ STPD)$$
$$\times (0.265 - 1.265 \times F_{EO_2} - 0.265 \times F_{ECO_2}) \quad (25)$$

If water vapor is not removed from the gas and the method of gas analysis measures gas fraction of the total gas volume including water vapor, as is the case for most discrete O_2 analyzers, then the water vapor will reduce each dry gas fraction by the following factor:

$$\frac{(P_B - P_{H_2O})}{P_B} \ or \ (1 - F_{H_2O})$$

In this case, the determination of $\dot{V}_{O_2}$ is affected by water vapor as follows. First, $\dot{V}_{O_2}$ can be expressed using $\dot{V}_I$ and $\dot{V}_E$ determined under the conditions of measurement (i.e., at temperature T and containing some water vapor):

$$\dot{V}_{O_2} \ (L/min, \ STPD) = \frac{273}{273 + T} \times \frac{P_B}{760}$$
$$\times (\dot{V}_I \times F_{IO_2} - \dot{V}_E \times F_{EO_2}) \quad (26)$$

where $\dot{V}I$ and $\dot{V}E$ are L/min at temperature T, and F_{IO_2} and F_{EO_2} are fractions of $\dot{V}I$ and $\dot{V}E$, respectively, including the volume of water vapor.

Because $\dot{V}I = (F_{EN_2}/F_{IN_2}) \times \dot{V}E$, and $(F_{EN_2} + F_{EO_2} + F_{ECO_2} + F_{EH_2O}) = 1$ and $(F_{IN_2} + F_{IO_2} + F_{ICO_2} + F_{IH_2O}) = 1$, then substituting into Eq. 26 gives

$$\dot{V}O_2 \text{ (L/min, STPD)} = \dot{V}E \text{ (L/min at } T)$$
$$\times k(T, P_{H_2O}) \times (\Delta F_{O_2})\text{true} \quad (27)$$

where

$$k(T, P_{H_2O}) = \frac{273}{273 + T} \times \frac{P_B}{760}$$

and

$$(\Delta F_{O_2})\text{true} =$$
$$\frac{F_{IO_2} \times (1 - F_{ECO_2} - F_{EH_2O}) - F_{EO_2} \times (1 - F_{IH_2O})}{(1 - F_{IO_2} - F_{IH_2O})}$$

The calculation of $\dot{V}O_2$ is simpler if the expired gas is dried prior to analysis for O_2 and CO_2. However, Beaver (8) provides a nomogram for calculation of oxygen uptake in the presence of water vapor that can be used to determine $\dot{V}O_2$ and R from a sample of mixed expired gas assumed to be fully saturated with water vapor at a known temperature (see Appendix E). The subject is assumed to be breathing room air, and the O_2 and CO_2 analyzers display the fractions of total expired gas including water vapor. Substantial errors would result if water vapor were not taken into account. Again, the correction is not needed when gas fractions are measured as fractions of dry gas.

Breath-by-breath measurement systems must deal with the effect of water vapor on calculation of $\dot{V}O_2$. Rapidly responding gas analyzers or a respiratory mass spectrometer are used. A mass spectrometer may be adjusted to "ignore" water vapor if the sum of ion voltages is made up of only those measuring N_2, O_2, CO_2, and argon, with water vapor ignored in both inspired and expired gases. If this method is used, then the volume to be multiplied by true O_2 fraction should be adjusted to the dry volume.

Rapidly responding O_2 analyzers and infrared CO_2 analyzers used without drying the analyzed gas read fractions of total gas volume and therefore read lower concentrations than if the same gas were measured after being dried. As shown in Eq. 27, the values can be used in a breath-by-breath system if F_{EH_2O} and F_{IH_2O} are known (9). The as-

sumption that expired gas is fully saturated at some known temperature is the starting point for several approaches to dealing with this in breath-by-breath systems.

First, the expired gas sample can be kept warm to prevent condensation. If gas is fully saturated at a known temperature, F_{EH_2O} can be estimated. A heated sampling tube is necessary, and the temperature must be accurately known. For example, assuming a value of 37°C when actual expired gas temperature is 32°C can result in a 7% to 8% error in $\dot{V}O_2$. During exercise, expired gas rapidly cools in the mouthpiece and breathing valve to as low as 32°C. Because gas for analysis is most often sampled at this location in breath-by-breath systems, then even if the gas is rewarmed, there will have been some unknown loss of water vapor to condensation. A second approach is to allow the sampled gas to cool to a known temperature. This avoids the problem of indeterminate loss of water vapor from cooling followed by rewarming.

Another approach used by many exercise systems employs conducting tubing that allows water vapor to pass out of the gas being conveyed to the gas analyzer until water vapor equilibrium is reached with the atmosphere. Thus, water vapor partial pressure in the gas analyzers is equal to the ambient P_{H_2O} rather than saturated at some imprecisely known temperature. This method avoids the need to know the precise temperature of the respired gas and does not adversely affect the response time.

Oxygen Uptake and Oxygen Breathing

The foregoing calculation of $\dot{V}O_2$ is intended for measurement during room-air breathing. The use of the same equations during breathing of oxygen-enriched inspired gas mixtures has several potential problems. The relation of $\dot{V}I$ to $\dot{V}E$ is sensitive to small measurement errors when F_{IO_2} and F_{EO_2} are high and F_{IN_2} and F_{EN_2} are low. In addition, the assumption that $\dot{V}I \times F_{IN_2} = \dot{V}E \times F_{EN_2}$ is not valid during the transient wash-out period during which hyperoxic gas is inspired and more nitrogen is removed during expiration than is added during inspiration. Finally, if the subject is breathing 100% oxygen, the equations given previously cannot be used at all because there is no inspired or expired nitrogen.

Although calculation of $\dot{V}O_2$ during enriched oxygen breathing is theoretically possible, the accuracy of $\dot{V}O_2$ using conventional equations and measurements is almost certainly less than when the subject is breathing room air. $\dot{V}O_2$ calculated with FIO_2 greater than 0.21 should be interpreted with caution. Some investigators have demonstrated that accurate determination of $\dot{V}O_2$ can be achieved with FIO_2 up to 0.30 to 0.50.

An alternative approach to testing subjects during oxygen breathing is to ignore or not make measurements of $\dot{V}O_2$. Often, a reason for exercise testing is to determine the need for supplemental oxygen in a particular patient. This question can usually be answered by comparison of maximum work rate, heart rate, respiratory frequency, minute ventilation, $\dot{V}E/\dot{V}CO_2$, and exercise endurance between a maximum exercise test on room air with a similar test during oxygen breathing. An objective improvement in exercise capacity and decreased $\dot{V}E$ and $\dot{V}E/\dot{V}CO_2$ are encouraging signs of a beneficial effect of supplemental O_2.

Valve Dead Space and Physiological Dead Space

The physiological dead space consists of the anatomic dead space and the alveolar dead space. During measurement, the volumes of the breathing valve and mouthpiece apparatus are considered to be in series with the anatomic dead space. This apparatus dead space is usually subtracted from the VD calculated by the Engoff modification of the Bohr equation:

$$VD = VT\ (L) \times \frac{PaCO_2 - P\overline{E}CO_2}{PaCO_2} - VD_m\ (L)$$

where VD is subject dead space, VT is tidal volume, and VD_m is the volume of the apparatus (or valve dead space).

Bradley and Younes (10), Suwa and Bendixen (11), and Singleton et al. (12) reported that the effective dead space of the valve (the correction term VD_m) may be different from the measured mechanical dead space. The reader is referred to their thorough analyses of the proper correction value under various conditions.

In practice, most reports of VD during exercise have corrected for apparatus dead space by subtracting the entire mechanical dead space. Any potential error can be minimized if the valve dead space is small and the subject's tidal volume is relatively large compared with VD_m. Valves with large dead spaces may be necessary, however, because they usually offer smaller breathing resistances at high inspiratory and expiratory flows. These high flows would be encountered when studying healthy normal subjects with large tidal volumes during exercise. On the other hand, patients with small tidal volumes will usually not generate high flows during exercise, and the valves with small dead spaces are recommended.

Calculations for Breath-by-Breath Analysis

Breath-by-breath methods use the same formulas as for mixed expired gas collection. Conceptually, the expired volume is divided into small sequential samples. The volume of each is determined and, when multiplied by the gas concentrations appropriate for that sample (adjusted for the time difference between the flow and gas concentration signals), gives the volume of CO_2 eliminated or O_2 taken up for that sample. The results are summed and then reported either per breath or per unit time. Thus, the phrase "breath-by-breath" applies to the method of expired gas analysis and data reduction and does not necessarily mean that each breath is individually reported.

If VE is the sum of all volume exhaled between time 0 and time T, then

$$VE = \sum_{t=0}^{T} Vexp(t + \Delta t)$$

where $Vexp(t + \Delta t)$ is the volume expired between time t and $(t + \Delta t)$, Δt is a time interval, and T is the total time of expiration for single or multiple breaths.

This is satisfactory if volume is directly measured over small time intervals. If expired flow rather than volume is measured, then

$$VE = \int_0^T \dot{V}exp(t)\ dt$$

where $\dot{V}exp(t)$ is the expired flow over the infinitesimally small time interval dt at time t. The volume exhaled over that time is the product $\dot{V}exp(t) \times dt$. In practice, a small constant Δt is substituted for dt, and the mean flow during the time interval $(t + \Delta t)$ is used as $\dot{V}exp(t)$:

$$VE = \sum_{t=0}^{T} \dot{V}exp(t + \Delta t) \times \Delta t$$

where $\dot{V}exp(t + \Delta t)$ is the mean flow rate during the time interval $t + \Delta t$. The minute ventilation ($\dot{V}E$) is the volume per unit time.

In a breath-by-breath system, the $\dot{V}CO_2$ is calculated by multiplying the nearly instantaneous $FECO_2$ for each small time interval by the simultaneous expired volume during that interval. These products are then integrated:

$$VCO_2 = \int_{t=0}^{T} \dot{V}exp(t)dt \times FECO_2(t)$$

where $\dot{V}exp(t)dt$ is the instantaneous expired volume, and $FECO_2(t)$ is the instantaneous expired CO_2 concentration at time t, adjusted for the delay between when the gas is sampled and when the analyzer reads the appropriate concentration. In practice, the small time interval Δt is substituted for dt:

$$VCO_2 = \sum_{t=0}^{T} \dot{V}exp(t + \Delta t) \times \Delta t \times FECO_2(t)$$

where $\dot{V}exp(t + \Delta t)$ is the mean flow for the time period t to $(t + \Delta t)$, $FECO_2(t)$ is the mean expired CO_2 during this time period, and Δt is a small time interval. For the volume of O_2 taken up, the true O_2 difference [(ΔFO_2) true] is substituted for $FECO_2$ in this equation. The $\dot{V}CO_2$ and $\dot{V}O_2$ are equal to the volume of CO_2 or O_2 divided by the time during exhalation, whether expressed per breath or per minute or other time unit.

An analog-to-digital converter and digital computer perform the necessary multiplications and summations. The respired gas is not, strictly speaking, measured and analyzed continuously, but instead data are rapidly sampled (e.g., every 20 milliseconds). The resultant expired flow versus time curve is, therefore, made up of sequential points sampled at intervals of Δt or at a frequency $f = 1/\Delta t$. The rate of sampling is important because rapid and large changes in expired flow (or gas concentration) may occur during exercise and could be missed if the data are sampled at too slow a rate. Bernard (13), using generalized simulated curves of expired flow and expired CO_2, found that a sample rate of 30 Hz was adequate during exercise, and that rates of 40, 50, and 100 Hz achieved little improvement in fidelity. Beaver et al. (14), in their analysis, suggested that a sampling frequency equal to twice the highest frequency occurring in the signal to be measured should be used. They suggested

that for human exercise testing, a frequency of 50 Hz is satisfactory to record flow and mass spectrometer signals.

A serious potential problem deals with time alignment of the appropriate expired flow (or volume) and expired gas concentration because of the appreciable time required for gas transport and measurement by most gas analyzers. For breath-by-breath analysis, it is essential that the appropriate instantaneous flow rate be multiplied by the proper time-matched expired gas concentration. Flow rates can be determined accurately and nearly instantaneously, because flow at the mouth will reach the measuring transducer with a delay determined by the speed of sound (approximately 100 ft/sec) and the distance to the transducer. However, gas analyzer measurements cannot with current technology be made without some delay and distortion inherent to the transport of gas to the analyzer and the intrinsic characteristics of the analyzer. The accuracy of a breath-by-breath system is dependent on the ability of the system to match flow rate and appropriate gas concentration prior to integration. Thus, each flow sampled must be stored until the appropriate expired gas concentration value has been determined. This matching process is performed as part of the computer program for online exercise systems.

Bernard (13) used simulated curves of expired CO_2 and expired flow to estimate potential error caused by the time delay between measurements of these two variables. Using perfectly time-matched hypothetical curves, less than a 5% difference in calculated $\dot{V}CO_2$ was found if the time misalignment was less than or equal to 25 milliseconds. Of importance is that the theoretic sampling rate was 100 Hz, the signals were given random noise, and the product of flow and CO_2 was integrated using the trapezoid rule.

Two factors contribute to the time-alignment problem. Most systems use a capillary tube to draw a continuous expired gas sample into the analyzer. The gas transport time depends on the dimensions of the tube and the flow rate; transport time is on the order of 200 milliseconds. Second, the gas analyzer output itself has an intrinsic response time that further adds to the delay. For infrared CO_2 analyzers, electrochemical O_2 analyzers, and respiratory mass spectrometers, the time constants for response are approximately 50 milliseconds. The result is a delay in the measurement of any instantaneous change in gas concentration at the sampling end of the tubing.

To account for the gas analyzer delay and response time, the transport time plus an additional correction factor are usually used. This function is derived from analysis of the total response of the gas analyzer system. Beaver et al. (14) indicated that the most significant wave shape distortion is removed by a total delay correction equal to transport delay plus one time constant, and analyzed the magnitude of potential errors. We (15) found that an equal-area method for analyzer delay time adds a one-time-constant delay if the analyzer response curve is exponential, and an empirically determined longer delay time if the curve is sigmoid.

The importance of matching flow rate and appropriate gas concentration cannot be overly stressed for a breath-by-breath system. Although not all investigators agree on the optimal way of dealing with gas analyzer response time, a satisfactory balance among degree of accuracy, speed, and reproducibility can be reached.

References

1. Lewis D, Sietsema KE, Casaburi R, et al. Inaccuracy of noninvasive estimates of VD/VT in clinical exercise testing. *Chest* 1994;106:1476–1480.
2. Kim TS, Rahn H, Farhi LE. Estimation of the true venous and arterial P_{CO_2} by gas analysis of a single breath. *J Appl Physiol* 1996;21:1338–1344.
3. Jones NL, Campbell EJM, McHardy GJR, et al. The estimation of carbon dioxide pressure of mixed venous blood during exercise. *Clin Sci* 1967;32:311–327.
4. Sun XG, Hansen JE, Ting H, et al. Comparison of exercise cardiac output by the Fick principle using oxygen and carbon dioxide. *Chest* 2000;118:631–640.
5. Sun XG, Hansen JE, Stringer WW, et al. Carbon dioxide pressure-concentration relationship in arterial and mixed venous blood during exercise. *J Appl Physiol* 2001;90:1798–1810.
6. Wagner JA, Horvath SM, Dahms TE, et al. Validation of open-circuit for the determination of oxygen consumption. *J Appl Physiol* 1973;34:859–863.
7. Wilmore JH, Costill DL. Adequacy of the Haldane transformation in the computation of exercise $\dot{V}_{O_2}$ in man. *J Appl Physiol* 1973;35:85–89.
8. Beaver WL. Water vapor corrections in oxygen consumption calculations. *J Appl Physiol* 1973;35:928–931.
9. Beaver WL, Wasserman K, Whipp BJ. On-line computer analysis and breath-by-breath graphical display of exercise function tests. *J Appl Physiol* 1973;34:128–132.
10. Bradley PW, Younes M. Relation between respiratory valve dead space and tidal volume. *J Appl Physiol* 1980;49:528–532.
11. Suwa K, Bendixen HH. Change in $PaCO_2$ with mechanical dead space during artificial ventilation. *J Appl Physiol* 1968;24:556–563.
12. Singleton GJ, Olsen CR, Smith RL. Correction for mechanical dead space in the calculation of physiological dead space. *J Clin Invest* 1972;51:2768–2772.
13. Bernard TE. Aspects of on-line digital integration of pulmonary gas transfer. *J Appl Physiol* 1977;43:375–378.
14. Beaver WL, Lamarra N, Wasserman K. Breath-by-breath measurement of true alveolar gas exchange. *J Appl Physiol* 1981;51:1662–1675.
15. Sue DY, Hansen JE, Blais M, et al. Measurement and analysis of gas exchange during exercise using a programmable calculator. *J Appl Physiol* 1980;49:456–461.

Placement of a Brachial Artery Catheter

EQUIPMENT

Appropriate catheter
Cournand-type needle with sharp, hollow stylus
A 2-ml syringe with a 26-gauge needle for local anesthesia
Sterile saline suitable for intravascular injection
Heparinized saline, 50 ml, for catheter flushing

SELECTION OF CATHETER

Because we most often insert the catheter into a brachial artery, we use a polyethylene catheter that is 25 cm long and has a diameter of 1.37 mm. The tip is tapered to fit a guidewire (50.0 cm × 0.63 mm) that fits through a 19-gauge thin-walled Cournand-style needle. The catheter is long enough so that the end used for collection can be brought around the back of the arm and sampling can be done without the subject altering the position of his or her arm or being aware of when blood is sampled.

For radial artery catheterization, any number of small, short polyethylene catheters designed for insertion into the radial artery can be used.

ARTERY SELECTION

The brachial or radial artery is generally used. Complications such as thrombosis are exceedingly rare when appropriate precautions are taken. We find the brachial artery to be preferable, however, because it is larger and the catheter has less effect on compromising its lumen. Moreover, the patient's arm need not be secured to a board, and sliding of the catheter in and out of the artery when the patient moves is not a problem. The radial pulse should be palpated to check for continued patency. If the radial artery is used for the arterial catheterization, do an Allen test to verify that there is blood flow through the ulnar artery to the hand.

POSITIONING THE ARM FOR BRACHIAL ARTERY CATHETERIZATION

Positioning the arm is extremely important.

1. Extend the arm; place a rolled towel or cushion under the elbow for maximum extension.
2. Pronate the hand.
3. Palpate the brachial artery on the medial side of the antecubital fossa.

LOCAL ANESTHESIA

If the patient is not allergic to the local anesthetic agent, anesthetize the skin and area around the artery. If time allows (approximately 1 hour before placing the catheter), a topical local anesthetic ointment (e.g., lidocaine plus prilocaine) can be used to anesthetize the skin surface. For injection, we use 1% or 2% lidocaine without epinephrine. After positioning the arm, inject the local anesthetic (a) intradermally above the artery, (b) subcutaneously just above the artery, and (c) subcutaneously on either side of the artery. The total amount should be about 1 to 2 ml, because excessive amounts of anesthetic can make palpation of the brachial pulse more difficult.

ARTERIAL PUNCTURE AND CATHETER INSERTION

1. Locate the artery between the fingers in the area of anesthesia.
2. Use a 19-gauge Cournand-style needle with the sharp, hollow stylus inserted.
3. Holding the needle by its shield while keeping the stylus in the needle with one's thumb (be sure not to cover the hole in the stylus), penetrate the skin over the artery. Position the tip of the needle above the artery. Then abruptly insert the stylus and the needle tip into the artery.
4. When the tip of the stylus enters the artery, blood will flow out of the proximal hole in the stylus.
5. Advance the needle 1 mm to be sure that the tip of the needle is in the artery (the stylus protrudes a little beyond the tip of the needle).
6. Remove the stylus. At this point, blood should shoot out of the needle with arterial pressure, indicating that the needle tip is well within the lumen of the artery. If blood does not flow readily, withdraw the needle slightly (it might have gone into the posterior wall of the artery). Once a strong stream of arterial blood is evident, it is safe to advance the needle further into the lumen of the artery using the continu-

ous stream of blood to document the needle's position. The needle advance may be facilitated by depressing the hub slightly to reduce the possibility of impaling the posterior wall of the artery with the needle tip. Do not advance the needle without the stylus in place if there is no flow of blood. It may damage the artery.

7. If there is no blood flow, slowly withdraw the needle without the stylus because the needle tip may have passed through the inner wall of the artery. If there is still no blood flow, withdraw the tip of the needle to the skin. Clear the needle and stylus of any blood or clot, and then try again.
8. With the needle tip in the lumen of the artery (documented by freely flowing blood), thread the guidewire for the catheter through the needle and slide it about 3 inches into the lumen of the artery. If the guidewire does not slip easily past the needle tip, the needle lumen is not centered in the lumen of the artery, and the needle must be repositioned. Do not try to advance the guidewire if any resistance is encountered.
9. Remove the needle, leaving the guidewire in place. To avoid a hematoma at the site, compress over the site at which the needle was inserted because the guidewire is narrow relative to the withdrawn needle.
10. Now slide the smoothly tapered end of the catheter over the wire. When the catheter reaches the skin, slide it through the skin and arterial wall using a gently rotating motion while holding the skin back so that it does not move with the catheter.
11. When the catheter is well established several inches into the artery, remove the guidewire. Blood should readily flow out of the end of the catheter.
12. Attach a Luer-lock stopcock to the end of the catheter and flush the system immediately with heparinized saline.
13. Cover the site of insertion with sterile gauze and fix the catheter with tape.

DIFFICULT PUNCTURES

Limit yourself to 15 minutes of effort. If you are not successful by then, stop trying and ask someone with more experience to help or rely only on noninvasive measurements. The latter will provide a considerable amount of information.

Tables and Nomogram

TABLE E.1. Partial Pressure of Water of Saturated Gas at Centigrade Temperature T

T	P_{H_2O}	T	P_{H_2O}	T	P_{H_2O}
10	9.20	20	17.53	30	31.83
11	9.84	21	18.65	31	33.70
12	10.51	22	19.82	32	35.67
13	11.23	23	21.07	33	37.73
14	11.98	24	22.38	34	39.90
15	12.78	25	23.76	35	42.18
16	13.63	26	25.21	36	44.57
17	14.53	27	26.74	37	47.08
18	15.47	28	28.35	38	49.70
19	16.47	29	30.04	39	52.45
20	17.53	30	31.83	40	55.34

TABLE E.2. Factors for Conversion from ATPS to BTPS (37°C)

$T°C$ P_B	16	17	18	19	20	21	22	23	24	25	26	27	28	29	30
600	1.138	1.132	1.126	1.120	1.115	1.109	1.103	1.097	1.090	1.084	1.078	1.071	1.065	1.058	1.051
610	1.136	1.131	1.125	1.119	1.114	1.108	1.102	1.096	1.090	1.083	1.077	1.071	1.064	1.058	1.051
620	1.135	1.130	1.124	1.118	1.113	1.107	1.101	1.095	1.089	1.083	1.076	1.070	1.064	1.057	1.050
630	1.134	1.129	1.123	1.117	1.112	1.106	1.100	1.094	1.088	1.082	1.076	1.069	1.063	1.056	1.050
640	1.133	1.128	1.122	1.116	1.111	1.105	1.099	1.093	1.087	1.081	1.075	1.069	1.062	1.056	1.049
650	1.132	1.127	1.121	1.116	1.110	1.104	1.098	1.092	1.087	1.081	1.074	1.068	1.062	1.056	1.049
660	1.131	1.126	1.120	1.115	1.109	1.103	1.098	1.092	1.086	1.080	1.074	1.068	1.061	1.055	1.049
670	1.130	1.125	1.119	1.114	1.108	1.103	1.097	1.091	1.085	1.079	1.073	1.067	1.061	1.055	1.048
680	1.129	1.124	1.118	1.113	1.107	1.102	1.096	1.090	1.085	1.079	1.073	1.067	1.060	1.054	1.048
690	1.128	1.123	1.118	1.112	1.107	1.101	1.095	1.090	1.084	1.078	1.072	1.066	1.060	1.054	1.047
700	1.128	1.122	1.117	1.111	1.106	1.100	1.095	1.089	1.083	1.077	1.072	1.066	1.059	1.053	1.047
710	1.127	1.121	1.116	1.111	1.105	1.100	1.094	1.088	1.083	1.077	1.071	1.065	1.059	1.053	1.047
720	1.126	1.121	1.115	1.110	1.104	1.099	1.093	1.088	1.082	1.076	1.070	1.065	1.059	1.052	1.046
730	1.125	1.120	1.115	1.109	1.104	1.098	1.093	1.087	1.082	1.076	1.070	1.064	1.058	1.052	1.046
740	1.124	1.119	1.114	1.109	1.103	1.098	1.092	1.087	1.081	1.075	1.070	1.064	1.058	1.052	1.046
750	1.124	1.118	1.113	1.108	1.102	1.097	1.092	1.086	1.080	1.075	1.069	1.063	1.057	1.051	1.045
760	1.123	1.118	1.113	1.107	1.102	1.096	1.091	1.086	1.080	1.074	1.069	1.063	1.057	1.051	1.045
770	1.122	1.117	1.112	1.107	1.101	1.096	1.090	1.085	1.079	1.074	1.068	1.062	1.057	1.051	1.045
780	1.122	1.116	1.111	1.106	1.101	1.095	1.090	1.084	1.079	1.073	1.068	1.062	1.056	1.050	1.044

$T°C$, ambient temperature in degrees centigrade; P_B, barometric pressure.

TABLE E.3. Factors for Conversion from ATPS to STPD

T°C PB	16	17	18	19	20	21	22	23	24	25	26	27	28	29	30
600	0.729	0.725	0.722	0.718	0.714	0.710	0.706	0.703	0.699	0.695	0.691	0.686	0.682	0.678	0.674
610	0.741	0.738	0.734	0.730	0.726	0.723	0.719	0.715	0.711	0.707	0.703	0.698	0.694	0.690	0.685
620	0.754	0.750	0.746	0.742	0.739	0.735	0.731	0.727	0.723	0.719	0.715	0.710	0.706	0.702	0.697
630	0.766	0.762	0.759	0.755	0.751	0.747	0.743	0.739	0.735	0.731	0.727	0.722	0.718	0.714	0.709
640	0.779	0.775	0.771	0.767	0.763	0.759	0.755	0.751	0.747	0.743	0.739	0.734	0.730	0.726	0.721
650	0.791	0.787	0.783	0.779	0.775	0.771	0.767	0.763	0.759	0.755	0.751	0.746	0.742	0.737	0.733
660	0.803	0.800	0.796	0.792	0.788	0.784	0.780	0.775	0.771	0.767	0.763	0.758	0.754	0.749	0.745
670	0.816	0.812	0.808	0.804	0.800	0.796	0.792	0.788	0.783	0.779	0.775	0.770	0.766	0.761	0.757
680	0.828	0.824	0.820	0.816	0.812	0.808	0.804	0.800	0.795	0.791	0.787	0.782	0.778	0.773	0.768
690	0.841	0.837	0.833	0.829	0.824	0.820	0.816	0.812	0.807	0.803	0.799	0.794	0.790	0.785	0.780
700	0.853	0.849	0.845	0.841	0.837	0.832	0.828	0.824	0.820	0.815	0.811	0.806	0.802	0.797	0.792
710	0.866	0.861	0.857	0.853	0.849	0.845	0.840	0.836	0.832	0.827	0.823	0.818	0.813	0.809	0.804
720	0.878	0.874	0.870	0.865	0.861	0.857	0.853	0.848	0.844	0.839	0.835	0.830	0.825	0.821	0.816
730	0.890	0.886	0.882	0.878	0.873	0.869	0.865	0.860	0.856	0.851	0.847	0.842	0.837	0.833	0.828
740	0.903	0.899	0.894	0.890	0.886	0.881	0.877	0.872	0.868	0.863	0.859	0.854	0.849	0.844	0.840
750	0.915	0.911	0.907	0.902	0.898	0.894	0.889	0.885	0.880	0.875	0.871	0.866	0.861	0.856	0.851
760	0.928	0.923	0.919	0.915	0.910	0.906	0.901	0.897	0.892	0.887	0.883	0.878	0.873	0.868	0.863
770	0.940	0.936	0.931	0.927	0.923	0.918	0.913	0.909	0.904	0.900	0.895	0.890	0.885	0.880	0.875
780	0.953	0.948	0.944	0.939	0.935	0.930	0.926	0.921	0.916	0.912	0.907	0.902	0.897	0.892	0.887

T°C, ambient temperature in degrees centigrade; PB, barometric pressure.

TABLE E.4. Estimated Oxygen Uptake ($\dot{V}_{O_2}$) for Various Activities

Activity	Estimated $\dot{V}_{O_2}$ (ml/kg/min)	Activity	Estimated $\dot{V}_{O_2}$ (ml/kg/min)
Basic postures		Hitching trailers, operating jacks or heavy levers	12.25
Sitting only (desk work, writing, calculating)	4.25	Masonry, painting, paperhanging	14.0
Standing only (bartending)	8.75		
Walking 3.0 mph	10.5	**Walking: Moderate work**	
Walking 3.5 mph	14.0	Carrying trays, dishes	14.70
		Gas station mechanical work (changing tires, etc.)	15.75
Sitting: Light or moderate work			
Driving a car	4.25	**Heavy arm work**	
Driving a truck	5.30	Lifting and carrying	
Hand tools, light assembly	5.30	20–44 lb	15.75
Working heavy levers	7.0	45–64 lb	21.0
Riding a mower	8.75	65–84 lb	26.25
Crane operator	8.75	85–100 lb	29.75
Driving heavy truck (including frequent on and off with some arm work)	10.5	**Heavy tools**	
		Jackhammers, pneumatic drills	21.0
Standing: Moderate work		Shovel, pick	28.0
Light assembly at slow pace	8.75		
Gas station operator	9.45	**Carpentry**	
Scrubbing, waxing, polishing (floors, walls)	9.45	Light interior repair (tile laying)	14.0
Heavy assembly (farm machinery, plumbing)	10.5	Building and finishing interior	15.75
Light welding	10.5	Putting in sidewalk	17.5
Stocking shelves (light objects)	10.5	Exterior remodeling (hammering, sawing)	21.0
Janitorial work	10.5		
Assembly line with light or medium parts at moderate pace	12.25	**Miscellaneous**	
		Pushing objects of 75 lb or more (desks, file cabinets)	28.0
Assembly line with brief lifting every 5 minutes (45 lb or less)	12.25	Laying railroad track	24.5
		Cutting trees or chopping wood	
Same as above (parts > 45 lb)	14.0	Hand saw	19.25
		Automatic	10.5

From Tennessee Heart Association. *Physician's handbook for evaluation of cardiovascular and physical fitness.* Nashville: Tennessee Heart Association, 1972, with permission.

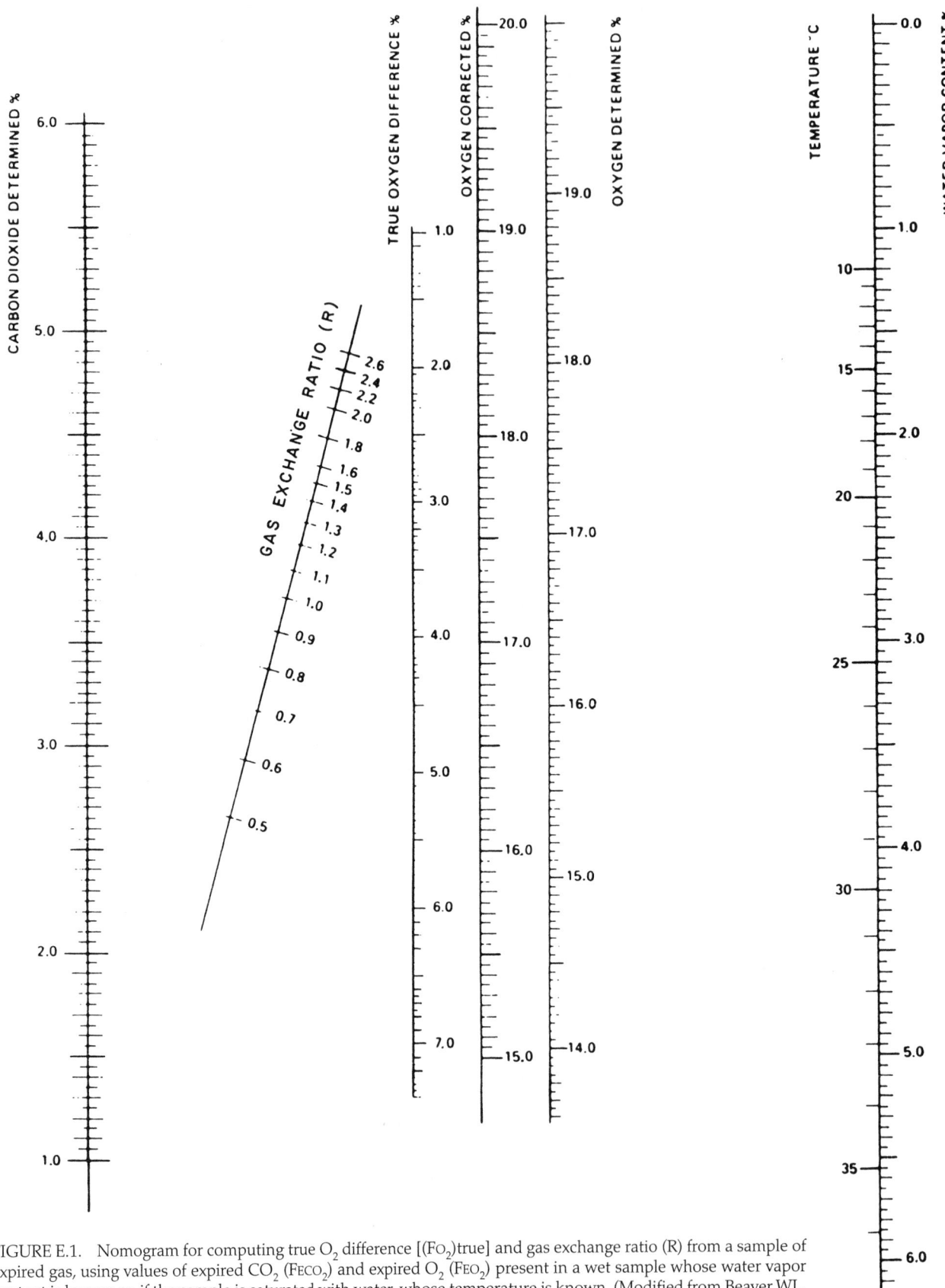

FIGURE E.1.   Nomogram for computing true O_2 difference [(FO_2)true] and gas exchange ratio (R) from a sample of expired gas, using values of expired CO_2 ($FECO_2$) and expired O_2 (FEO_2) present in a wet sample whose water vapor content is known or, if the sample is saturated with water, whose temperature is known. (Modified from Beaver WL. Water vapor corrections in oxygen consumption calculations. *J Appl Physiol* 1973;35:928–931.)

Index

Page numbers followed by the letter *f* refer to figures; those followed by the letter *t* refer to tabular material.